Comparative Spermatology

Comparative Spermatology

Proceedings of the International Symposium, held in Rome and Siena, 1–5 July 1969

EDITED BY

BACCIO BACCETTI

Institute of Zoology – University of Siena

1970

ACCADEMIA NAZIONALE DEI LINCEI – ROME
ACADEMIC PRESS – NEW YORK – LONDON

Distributed throughout the world by
ACADEMIC PRESS, INC.
111 Fifth Avenue, New York, New York 10003

and

ACADEMIC PRESS, INC. (LONDON) LTD.
Berkeley Square House, London W1X 6BA

LIBRARY OF CONGRESS CATALOG CARD NUMBER: 74-107938

Printed in Italy by Dott. G. Bardi, Tipografo dell'Accademia Nazionale dei Lincei

TABLE OF CONTENTS

PARTICIPANTS

H. ADAM, Universität Salzburg, Zoologisches Institut, SALZBURG (Austria).

B. AFZELIUS, University of Stockholm, Wenner-Gren Institute, STOCKHOLM (Sweden).

W. ANDERSON, Department of Anatomy, Harvard Medical School, BOSTON (U.S.A.).

J. ANDRÉ, Laboratoire de Biologie Cellulaire, Faculté des Sciences, ORSAY (France).

B. BACCETTI, Istituto di Zoologia dell'Università, SIENA (Italy).

A. BAIRATI Jr., Istituto Anatomico dell'Università, MILANO (Italy).

K. R. BARKER, Department of Zoology, University, JOHANNESBURG (South Africa).

S. R. BAWA, Department of Biophysics, Panjab University, CHANDIGARH (India).

C. BEDINI, Istituto di Biologia generale dell'Università, PISA (Italy).

E. BIGLIARDI, Istituto di Zoologia dell'Università, SIENA (Italy).

R. BILLARD, Institut National des Recherches Agronomiques, JOUY EN JOSAS (France).

L. BOISSIN, Laboratoire de Zoologie, Faculté des Sciences, MONTPELLIER (France).

G. BOUIX, Laboratoire de Zoologie, Faculté des Sciences, MONTPELLIER (France).

C. J. BROKAW, Division of Biology, Institute of Technology, PASADENA (U.S.A.).

G. G. BROWN, Duke University Marine Laboratory, BEAUFORT, NORTH CAROLINA (U.S.A.).

J. BRUSLÉ, Biologie Cellulaire, Faculté des Sciences, ORLÉANS LA SOURCE (France).

A. G. BURRINI, Istituto di Zoologia dell'Università, SIENA (Italy).

A. M. CANTACUZÈNE, Laboratoire de Biologie Animale, Faculté des Sciences, PARIS (France).

PH. CHEVAILLIER, Groupe de Recherches de Biologie Cellulaire, Faculté des Sciences, RENNES (France).

R. DALLAI, Istituto di Zoologia dell'Università, SIENA (Italy).

J. DAN, Department of Biology, Ochanumizu University, BENKYO-KU, TOKYO (Japan).

C. D. EDDLEMAN, Department of Biology, Union College, LINCOLN, NEBRASKA (U.S.A.).

M. FAIN MAUREL, Laboratoire d'Évolution des Êtres Organisés, PARIS (France).

P. FAVARD, Laboratoire de Biologie Cellulaire, Faculté des Sciences, PARIS (France).

D. FAWCETT, Department of Anatomy, Harvard Medical School, BOSTON (U.S.A.).

R. FOLLIOT, Groupe de Recherches de Biologie Cellulaire, Faculté des Siences, RENNES (France).

Å. FRANZÉN, Institute of Zoology, University, UPPSALA (Sweden).

P. FURIERI, Istituto di Anatomia Comparata dell'Università, FIRENZE (Italy).

V. GALANGAU, Laboratoire de Zoologie, Faculté des Sciences, MONTPELLIER (France).

L. GENEVES, Laboratoire de Botanique, École Normale Supérieure, PARIS (France).

F. GIUSTI, Istituto di Zoologia dell'Università, SIENA (Italy).

I. GRAEBNER, Zoologisches Institut der Universität, SALZBURG (Austria).

B. L. GUPTA, Department of Zoology, University of CAMBRIDGE (England).

J. HENDELBERG, Institute of Zoology, University, UPPSALA (Sweden).

E. HORSTMANN, Anatomisches Institut, Universität, HAMBURG (Germany).

R. G. KESSEL, Department of Zoology, University of Iowa, IOWA-CITY, IOWA (U.S.A.).

J. K. KOEHLER, Department of Biological Structure, University of Washington, SEATTLE, WASHINGTON (U.S.A.).

I. MANTON, Department of Botany, University of LEEDS (England).

X. MATTEI, Laboratoire de Zoologie, Faculté des Sciences, DAKAR–FANN (Sénégal).

G. MEYER, Max–Planck Institut für Biologie, TUBINGEN (Germany).

G. MONTALENTI, Istituto di Genetica, Università, ROMA (Italy).

L. NELSON, Department of Physiology, Medical College, TOLEDO, OHIO (U.S.A.).

L. NICANDER, Department of Anatomy, Veterinary College, STOCKHOLM (Sweden).

V. PALLINI, Istituto di Chimica Biologica dell'Università, SIENA (Italy).

F. PAPI, Istituto di Biologia Generale dell'Università, PISA (Italy).

H. PEDERSEN, Division of Electron Microscopy, Institute of Anatomy, University of ÅRHUS (Denmark).

M. E. PEROTTI, Istituto Anatomico dell'Università, MILANO (Italy).

P. PERSONNE, Laboratoire de Biologie Animale, Faculté des Sciences, AMIENS (France).

D. PHILLIPS, Department of Biology, Washington University, St. LOUIS, MISSOURI (U.S.A.).

J. POCHON MASSON, Laboratoire d'Evolution des Etres Organisés, PARIS (France).

S. PRATT, Department of Anatomy, School of Medicine, ALBUQUERQUE, NEW MEXICO (U.S.A.).

J. F. REGER, Department of Anatomy, University of Tennessee, Medical University, MEMPHIS TENNESSEE (U.S.A.).

J. G. RIEMANN, Metabolism and Radiation Research Laboratory, State University Station, FARGO, NORTH DAKOTA (U.S.A.).

W. G. ROBISON Jr., Department of Biology, University of Virginia, CHARLOTTESVILLE, VIRGINIA (U.S.A.).

F. ROSATI, Istituto di Zoologia dell'Università, SIENA (Italy).

D. SANDOZ, Centre de Recherches d'Ivry–sur–Seine (France).

M. H. WALKER, Department of Zoology, University, ST. ANDREWS (Scotland).

G. WERNER, Institut für Zytologie und Elektronenmikroskopie, Universität des Saarlandes, HOMBURG, SAAR (Germany).

G. YASUZUMI, Electron Microscope Research Laboratory, Department of Anatomy, Nara Medical University, KASHIHARA CITY, NARA (Japan).

INTRODUCTION

Since the general occurrence of the 9 + 2 pattern in cilia and flagella was discovered by MANTON (1952) and by FAWCETT and PORTER (1954), researchers have made numerous attempts to understand the significance of this pattern and to determine its possible role in flagellar motility, which is typical of most spermatozoa. In the past few years, submicroscopic histochemistry has led to a more precise functional interpretation, and a large number of works on the comparative ultrastructure of spermatozoa have shown the great variety of morphological solutions in the spermatozoa of living animals.

Scientists interested in the problems of sperm function have previously convened in symposia (New York, 1960; Oxford, 1967), devoted to fertility, or sperm motility and the morphologists in this field have also met at the various electron microscopy congresses. There was need, however, of a broader discussion, in which results obtained by morphologists, histochemists and physiologists could be considered together in order, on the one hand, to correlate better the structure and function of the sperm cell, which is the ultimate achievement of the most specialized cell line, and, on the other, to give to the comparative spermatology its due place in systematic and phylogenetic studies.

Thus the idea of an International Symposium of Comparative Spermatology was born and sponsored by the Accademia Nazionale dei Lincei, which offered its hospitality and substantial financial aid, assisted by the Consiglio Nazionale delle Ricerche and the Università di Siena.

BACCIO BACCETTI

PRESENTAZIONE

Da quando fu scoperto il valore generale del dispositivo 9 + 2 in ciglia e flagelli per merito di MANTON (1952) e di FAWCETT e PORTER (1954) sono stati fatti molti tentativi per meglio definire il significato di questa formula, e collegare con essa la possibilità di movimento flagellare, che è tipico della generalità degli spermi. In tempi più recenti, l'istochimica submicroscopica ha fornito ulteriori suggerimenti per più precise interpretazioni funzionali, mentre un grande numero di lavori di ultrastrutturistica comparata hanno mostrato una vasta possibilità di soluzioni morfologiche nella costituzione dello spermatozoo dei vari esseri viventi.

Già più volte studiosi interessati al problema della funzionalità dello spermatozoo si sono riuniti in simposio (New York, 1960; Oxford, 1967, quest'ultima volta nell'ambito dello studio della motilità cellulare in genere) ed ugualmente si sono incontrati, nei vari congressi di Microscopia Elettronica, i morfologi della spermatologia. Sinora è però mancato del tutto un colloquio di più ampio raggio, in cui le talora ampie casistiche oramai a disposizione dei morfologi, degli istochimici e degli studiosi del movimento venissero messe direttamente a confronto, con lo scopo sia di ottenere più precise correlazioni fra struttura e funzione dello spermio in sè come peculiare tipo di cellula variamente evoluto nel mondo vivente, sia di inserire le attuali cognizioni di spermatologia comparata in quell'inquadramento filogenetico che la sistematica botanica e zoologica oggi prospettano, e che sinora ha dovuto forzatamente prescindere dalle conoscenze sullo spermatozoo.

È nata così l'idea di un Simposio Internazionale di Spermatologia Comparata, che l'Accademia Nazionale dei Lincei ha accolto sotto la propria ègida accordando la propria ospitalità ed un aiuto finanziario determinante, e che il Consiglio Nazionale delle Ricerche e l'Università di Siena hanno pure sensibilmente facilitato.

BACCIO BACCETTI

DON W. FAWCETT (*) and D. M. PHILLIPS (*)

RECENT OBSERVATIONS ON THE ULTRASTRUCTURE AND DEVELOPMENT OF THE MAMMALIAN SPERMATOZOON (**)

SUMMARY. — The current concept of the ultrastructure of the mammalian spermatozoon is reviewed and new observations reported on interspecific differences in size and shape of the acrosome; on the role of the centrioles in formation of the connecting piece; on the origin of the outer dense fibers of the flagellum as lateral outgrowths of the axonemal doublets; and on the development of the satellite fibrils from the cortex of the outer coarse fibers and their possible role as accessory motor elements. The formation of the fibrous sheath is described and its local attachments to the axoneme and to outer fibers 3 and 8 are considered in relation to the restraints it may impose upon tail movements.

RIASSUNTO. — Viene riveduto il concetto corrente dell'ultrastruttura degli spermatozoi dei mammiferi e vengono riportate nuove osservazioni su differenze interspecifiche in grandezza e forma dell'acrosoma; sul ruolo dei centrioli nella formazione della regione di connessione; sull'origine delle fibre esterne del flagello come emissioni laterali dei doppietti dell'assonema; sullo sviluppo delle fibrille satelliti dalla corteccia delle fibre esterne accessorie e sul loro possibile ruolo come elementi motori accessori. Viene descritta la formazione della guaina fibrosa; il suo aggancio con l'assonema e con le fibre esterne 3 e 8 viene considerato in relazione alle limitazioni che esso può imporre sui movimenti della coda.

The ultrastructure of the mammalian spermatozoon was first reviewed a few years after methods were developed for ultrathin sectioning of tissues for electron microscopy (FAWCETT, 1958). It was possible then to correct a number of misinterpretations of structures that were previously poorly resolved and to define relationships just beyond the reach of the light microscope. The greatly accelerated pace of cytological investigation in the ensuing ten years has yielded a rich harvest of new discoveries about the structure of mammalian spermatozoa. Much of this is included in the recent review by HANCOCK (1966). In a symposium of specialists, familiarity with this literature is assumed. This presentation will therefore describe additional findings which have resulted from work of the past few years by members of our own laboratories and will direct attention to some of the intriguing problems of structure and function which still await solution.

(*) Department of Anatomy and Laboratories of Human Reproduction and Reproductive Biology, Harvard Medical School, Boston, Massachusetts, U.S.A.

(**) Supported by grant HD-02344 from the Research Grants Division of the Institute of Child Health and Human Development and Contract NIH-69-2107 from the Center for Population Studies, National Institutes of Health, United States Public Health Service.

Acrosome.

Increasing interest in the changes in spermatozoa immediately prior to fertilization has focused investigative attention upon the acrosome. With the light microscope the full extent of the acrosome and its relations to the cell membrane, to the so-called galea capitis, and to the nucleus could not be resolved. The electron microscope has shown that the mammalian acrosome is not simply a crescentic body at the apex of the nucleus but is a membrane-limited, cap-like structure covering the anterior two thirds of the nucleus and extending for variable distances beyond its anterior margin. It has become useful for purposes of description to distinguish a thickened, *apical segment* projecting anteriorly beyond the edge of the nucleus, a *main segment* extending back over the anterior portion of the nucleus and a thinner *equatorial segment* of varying length comprising the caudal portion of the acrosomal cap.

As sperm were usually examined in smears, the flattened heads presented only their broad face to the viewer and the light microscopist could neither appreciate the depth of the acrosome in the plane perpendicular to the slide nor gain an accurate impression of the three dimensional configuration of the apical portion of the acrosome. The opportunity to examine sperm in thin sagittal and transverse sections with the electron microscope has revealed in some species entirely unexpected complexities in the form of sperm heads and particularly in the shapes of the apical portion of the acrosome (FAWCETT and PHILLIPS, 1969 a). Striking differences have been shown from species to species in the volume and shape of the acrosome (Fig. 1). In a number of species there is also a marked deviation of the acrosome from the long axis of the nucleus. The head, as a whole, is often at an angle to the axis of the flagellum. These features of head shape and orientation passed unnoticed until recently because of the single orientation imposed upon sperm in smears. It has also been found that the specific configuration of the apical portion of the acrosome in hystricomorph rodents, and the angulation of the head develop late in spermiogenesis, usually during passage through the epididymis (FAWCETT and HOLLENBERG, 1963; FAWCETT and PHILLIPS, 1969 a).

In monkey, man, bull, boar, rabbit and bat the apical segment of the acrosome is relatively small, simple in form, and extends but little beyond the tip of the nucleus, but in chinchilla, guinea pig, and ground squirrel it is very much larger and quite elaborate in its form (Fig. 1). These remarkable differences from species to species in the volume and shape of the apical segment of the acrosome raise a number of puzzling questions. If the function of the acrosome is simply to release lytic enzymes that facilitate access of the sperm to the ovum, any shape would seem to be as good as any other. Do the specific shapes of the acrosome have any significance or are they meaningless accidents of evolution? Are the variations in acrosome volume correlated with variations in the difficulty of penetrating the cumulus and the zona pellucida in the respective species? Do the various shapes of the head and their deviations from the axis of the flagellum have important hydrodynamic consequences for the pattern of swimming?

Little is known about the intracellular forces responsible for early events in shaping the sperm head. Although there is good circumstantial evidence in birds and reptiles implicating microtubules in the cytoplasm of the spermatids (McIntosh and Porter, 1967; Clark 1967) this explanation does not seem to be applicable to mammals. The only ordered arrays of microtubules found in spermatids are those of the manchette. While these might

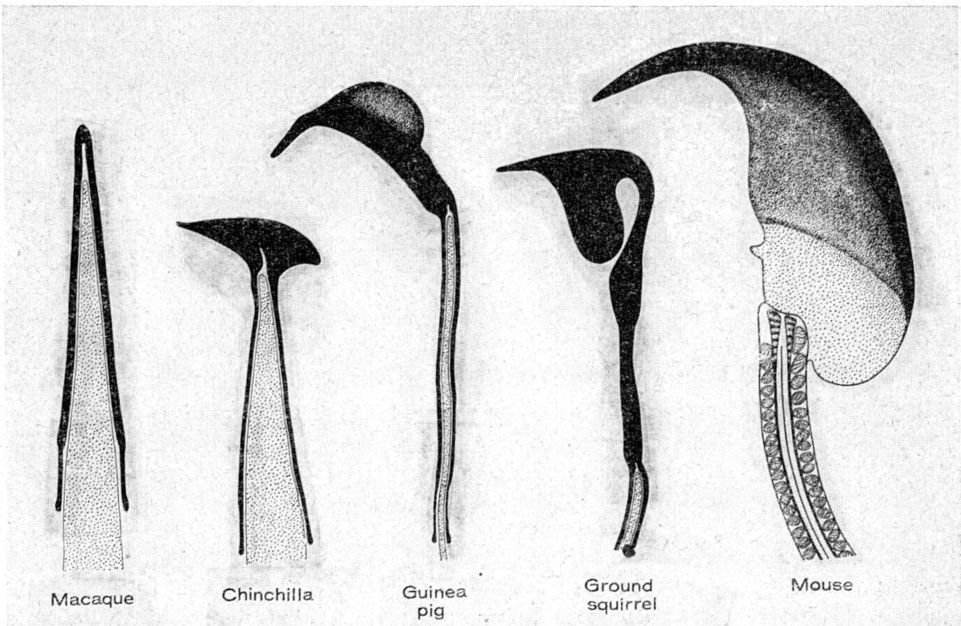

Fig. 1. – Drawing illustrating some variations in the size and shape of the apical portion of the acrosomal cap. All are mid-sagittal sections except the mouse sperm which is sectioned in the transverse axis of the flat, scimitar-shaped head.

possibly play a role in modelling the most caudal portion of the nucleus, the manchette is never associated with the acrosome or the anterior two thirds of the head where the most extensive and characteristic shape changes occur. The late changes in form of the acrosome which take place in the epididymis pose even more difficult questions as to the mechanism of morphogenesis, for they occur when the sperm heads have no surrounding cytoplasm and while they are freely floating in the epididymal fluid (Fawcett and Hollenberg, 1963).

The origin and nature of the striated connecting piece.

The neck of the spermatozoon has been one of its least understood regions. The nature of the cross-striated connecting piece; the role of the centrioles in its development; and its relation to the outer coarse fibers of the flagellum are problems which have proven difficult to solve and the morphological observations on this region have been subject to widely differing interpretations.

In the development of this region the first elements of the connecting piece appear around the centrioles shortly after the spermatid first develops a simple flagellum, and before the pair of centrioles has become fixed to the nucleus. A thin, curved plate deposited parallel to the rostral surface of the proximal centriole is destined to form the articular surface of the future connecting piece (Fig. 2 a). A series of ill-defined densities aligned parallel to the wall of the distal centriole are the precursors of the striated columns

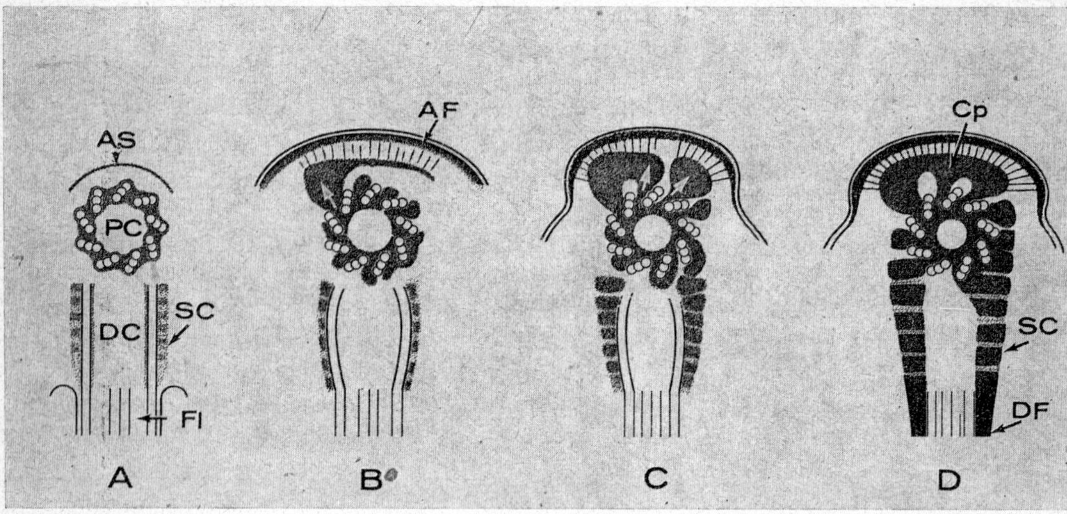

Fig. 2. – Diagrammatic representation of four successive stages in the differentiation of the connecting piece.

A. At the periphery of an early spermatid, the distal centriole (DC) gives rise to a simple flagellum (Fl). A series of periodic densities (SC) appear arrayed parallel to the wall of the centriole. These represent the beginnings of the striated columns. Arching over the proximal centriole (PC) is a thin lamina representing the anlage of the articular surface (AS) of the future connecting-piece; B and C. After the centrioles have become associated with the implantation fossa (IF) of the nucleus, dense strands of matrix emerge from the interspaces between triplets on the juxtanuclear side of the proximal centriole and extend toward the anlage of the articular surface. They fuse with it in clockwise sequence to form the capitulum. Similar extensions of matrix from between triplets on the lateral and caudal aspects of the proximal centriole, polymerize to form the anterior ends of the striated columns and their connections to the capitulum; D. As the development of the distal ends of the striated columns (SC) progresses and they become attached to the outer dense fibers of the flagellum (DF), the distal centriole gradually disappears.

(Fig. 2 a). In sections transverse to the centrioles at this stage it is evident that the precursor material of the connecting piece is first deposited between the triplets in the wall of the centrioles and extends radially from these interspaces to accumulate around the centrioles (Fig. 2 b). As a consequence of this mode of origin, the nine-part radial symmetry of the distal centriole is expressed in the formation of the nine columns of the connecting piece. Although we had earlier thought that the proximal centriole was passive in the process of formation of the striated neck piece and remained unmodified (FAWCETT, 1958; FAWCETT and ITO, 1965), more detailed examination of developmental stages has shown that it is as actively involved as the distal centriole. Dense precursor material emerges from the interspaces between its uppermost triplets in a precise clockwise sequence in several species studied. These contributions fuse with the anlage of the articular surface and with each other to form the capitulum (Fig. 2 c and d). Contributions from the interspaces between triplets on the lateral aspects of the proximal centriole become aligned in register with the columns developing around the distal centriole and form the rostral ends of the columns and their connections with the capitulum.

Other workers have frequently referred to the broader dense bands in the striated neck-piece as " laminae " and have interpreted the narrower light bands as clefts or incisures between them (NICANDER and BANE, 1962; SAACKE and ALMQUIST, 1964). In our own recent studies (FAWCETT and PHILLIPS, 1969 b) we have found that the cross-banded elements that arise from pericentriolar polymerization of a dense precursor material, are composed of a cross-striated fibrous protein with a 665 Å major period and a 9 or 10 banded symmetrical intraperiod structure. The connecting piece thus appears to be homologous with satellites, rhizoplasts, ciliary rootlets and similar appendages of centrioles and basal bodies (AUSTIN, 1965; FAWCETT and PHILLIPS, 1969 b). Although these observations clarify the nature and mode of origin of the connecting piece, they leave unanswered the question as to whether the centrioles are a site of synthesis, or simply attract and organize the assembly of molecular subunits synthesized elsewhere in the cell.

These studies have helped to correct the prevalent misconception that the nine, striated columns of the neck–piece are simply local specializations of the outer dense fibers with which they are continuous in the mature spermatozoon. It is now clear that they are fundamentally different in their fine structure. They have different times and modes of origin, and only secondarily become joined end-to-end with the outer fibers late in spermiogenesis.

The origin of the outer dense fibers of the flagellum.

Formation of the doublets of the axonemal complex of cilia and flagella appears to be initiated by accumulation and polymerization of microtubule protein at the ends of subfibrils A and B of the triplets in the wall of the distal centriole. The microtubules then elongate by accretion to their distal ends until the flagellum has reached its definitive length. The origin of the outer dense fibers of the tail seems not to have been carefully studied in the mammal.

In earlier work, the connecting piece of the sperm neck was interpreted as a modified or transformed distal centriole (FAWCETT, 1958; FAWCETT and ITO, 1965). At that time it was considered probable that the outer dense fibers which appear continuous with the nine, segmented columns of the connecting piece arose at its distal end and elongated from base toward tip by accretion of material to the ends of the fibers. More careful study has made this interpretation untenable. The outer fibers do not take origin from the connecting piece and grow distally, but instead, each arises as a lateral outgrowth from the wall of the corresponding doublet (FAWCETT and PHILLIPS, 1969 b). The first indication of their beginning to form is the appearance of a small dense ridge which, in cross sections, projects radially from the groove between subfibrils *a* and *b* of the doublet (Figs. 3 a and 4). However, the projection clearly arises from the wall of subfiber *a* (Fig. 17 inset). The subsequent formation of the fibers involves accretion of material to the free edge and sides of this initial ridge-like outgrowth (Figs. 3 b, c, d). The initiation of the development of these fibers seems to take place at about the same time along their entire length. The taper of the fibers in the mature sperm must be a result of a proximo-distal gradient in the rate of their subsequent thickening. There must also be characteristic differences among the individual fibers in the rate or duration of accretion to account for the distinctive shapes which they assume (Figs. 7 and 8) and the consistently greater cross-sectional area of outer fibers 1, 5, and 6, or 1, 9, 5 and 6.

Soon after the initiation of outer fiber formation in mammalian spermatids, the fibers detach from the walls of the doublets but they nevertheless continue to thicken after their separation. Their detachment from the axonemal complex seems to start near the base of the flagellum and to progress along the tail. The process never goes to completion in the distal part of the principal piece, for the ends of the outer fibers there remain continuous with the wall of the corresponding doublet even in mature spermatozoa (FAWCETT and ITO, 1965; FAWCETT and PHILLIPS, 1969).

The progressive thickening of the developing outer fibers has been illustrated in a previous publication (FAWCETT and PHILLIPS, 1969). The process is similar in most particulars in the development of avian spermatozoa, illustrated in cross section in Figs. 3 A to 3 D, but here, the nine outer fibers are identical in cross-sectional area, and they remain in contact with the walls of the doublets. In insects, the outer or accessory elements of the flagellum are not solid, dense fibers but are tubular. They too form as lateral outgrowths from the axonemal doublets, appearing first as a C-shaped projection from subfiber b (Fig. 5). This incomplete tubule is then cast off from the wall of the doublet and the hiatus in its wall is filled in to form a cylindrical microtubule with a typical circular profile (Fig. 6). The process has been described in greater detail by PHILLIPS (1970).

These observations have interesting implications for the unresolved question as to the nature of the outer fibers in mammals and birds and of the accessory fibers or tubules in insects. In has been widely assumed that these represent additional motor elements developed in relation to the acquisition of internal fertilization with its attendant requirement for progression in a more viscous fluid environment. Immunocytochemical evidence suggests that the outer fibers are composed of proteins with actin and myosin-like antigenic properties (PLOWMAN and NELSON, 1962; NELSON, 1967), but there is as yet, no more compelling evidence for their contractility. That the doublets of the axoneme are the active agents of sperm motility seems generally accepted although their contractile mechanism is not well understood. The finding that the outer fibers arise as outgrowths from the wall of the axonemal doublets provides additional circumstantial evidence that they are of similar composition and therefore are probably also composed of contractile protein.

The origin and possible significance of the satellite fibrils.

A number of investigators have noticed small punctate or angular profiles along the sides of the outer dense fibers in cross sections of the middle piece (Fig. 7). Some have referred to these as granules but in studies on bat sperm, it was shown (FAWCETT and ITO, 1965) that in longitudinal sections they appeared as linear profiles, coarsing parallel to the axoneme and to the outer fibers. They were therefore given the name *satellite fibrils* to describe their topographical relation to the dense fibers from which they appeared to be derived. The outer fibers have a clearly defined cortical layer 200–300 A thick which has staining affinities differing somewhat from those of the interior of the fiber (Fig. 1, 7 and 9). This thin cortex is most obvious on the convex outer aspect of the fibers, and is often lacking on their sides, along which the satellite fibrils are deployed. The cortex of the outer fibers often ends abruptly and the satellite fibrils seem to arise by exfoliation from this free edge (Fig. 9).

Since these fibrils were first described in bat sperm, additional evidence for their derivation from the outer coarse fibers has been accumulated from the study of sperm in other species, particularly *Citellus lateralis*, the golden-mantled ground squirrel. The thickness of the middle piece in this rodent species is quite exceptional, having a diameter at least three times that of sperm in many ruminant species. The outer dense fibers are very large, oddly shaped and widely separated from each other and from the axonemal complex (Fig. 8). In transverse sections, the space between all of these elements is occupied by an elaborate filigree pattern (Figs. 10, 11), which can be resolved at higher magnification into meandering rows of closely associated punctate profiles like those of the satellite fibrils of other species. Examination of longitudinal sections leaves no doubt that the pattern seen in cross sections is made up of laterally associated fibrils of appreciable length running parallel to the long axis of the mid-piece (Fig. 13). The claim for identity of the substance of the satellite fibrils and the cortex of the outer fibers is further supported by their similar staining properties. When sperm are fixed in glutaraldehyde and post-fixed with 2 % phosphotungstic acid in the fixatives and dehydrating solutions, the cortex of the outer fibers of sperm tails is deeply stained and the medulla unstained (GORDON and BENSCH, 1968). Upon application of this procedure to sperm of the golden-mantle ground squirrel, the extensive pattern of interstitial satellite fibrils is deeply stained as is the cortex of the outer fibers (Fig. 12). Although the chemical nature of the cortex and its functional significance remain unknown, it seems evident that the satellite fibrils are derived from it and are of similar composition.

In describing the sperm of the bandicoot, *Parameles nasuta*, CLELAND and ROTHSCHILD (1959) observed that the outer fibers were displaced radially and that all save those which would now be designated as numbers 3 and 8 were quite a long distance from the axis of bending. Between each peripheral dense fiber and the corresponding doublet there was a pair of linear densities which they called the *connecting laminae*. In longitudinal sections, it was apparent that the two halves of each lamina consisted of long fibrils 200–250 A in diameter separated from one another by about 250 Å. The fibrils were oriented obliquely and seemed to run from the outer coarse fiber to the corresponding member of the axonemal complex. The outer fibers were considered by CLELAND and ROTHSCHILD to be contractile and it was suggested that the very considerable distance between them and the axoneme represented an adaptation in which moved the fibers were moved away from the hinge point thus enhancing their effectiveness as motor elements in bending this unusually thick sperm tail. A similar, but less extreme, radial displacement of the outer fibers is seen in the opossum, *Didelphys virginiana*. It seems likely that the " satellite fibrils " described here are homogous with the " laminar filaments " of CLELAND and ROTHSCHILD.

In considering the possible function of the satellite fibrils it is probably significant that they are most extensively developed in spermatozoa that are uncommonly thick. The principal piece of the bandicoot sperm is 155 mμ in diameter compared to 30 mμ for the rat sperm. In the ground squirrel illustrated here we have again a remarkably thick spermatozoon. By extension of the same reasoning that led us to suggest that the outer coarse fibers developed from the doublets of the axoneme as an adaptation to internal fertilization and progression in a viscous medium, it is tempting to speculate that when the thickness and resistance of sperm to bending increases beyond a certain value, satellite fibrils arise from the outer fibers as accessory tensile elements. Although this is highly conjectural, the occurrence of an elaborate system of satellite fibrils in the exceptionally thick sperm of two quite unrelated species, the bandicoot and the ground squirrel, strongly suggests that this unusual feature has evolved independently in relation to large sperm diameter.

The origin of the fibrous sheath.

Because of its proximity to the beginning of the fibrous sheath, the annulus was formerly suspected of taking part in formation of this sheath. Indeed it seemed possible that the fibrous sheath was formed ring by ring, conceivably by delamination from the annulus, as the tail elongated. Further study of the sequence of developmental events makes it clear that this interpretation is erroneous.

The fibrous sheath is already well-advanced in its development before the caudal migration of the annulus has occurred (Figs. 14 and 15). Thus it now seems unlikely that this organelle plays any significant role in initiating fibrous sheath formation.

The beginnings of the sheath are first detectable in the free portion of flagellum that projects beyond the sleeve of spermatid cytoplasm into the lumen of the seminiferous tubule. Examination of cross sections, suggests that deposition of the dorsal and ventral longitudinal columns between the flagellar membrane and doublets 3 and 8 precedes, by a short time, the development of the circumferential elements of the sheath (Fig. 16). The latter first appear as very slender circumferential rings deposited inmmediately beneath the plasma membrane of the flagellum (Fig. 17). Seen in longitudinal sections, these are of uniform thickness and very regularly spaced (Fig. 23). There is some indication that these circumferential elements may be complete rings, and not simply semicircular ribs, for in sagittal sections coinciding with the plane of the longitudinal columns, the cross sectional profiles of the rings can be identified within the substance of the columns (Fig. 22).

In subsequent development, the slender rings deposited first, appear to thicken, and become dissociated from the plasma membrane. They also seem to aggregate in groups of 2, 3 or 4, fusing with one another to form the much coarser and less regularly spaced ribs of the definitive fibrous sheath (Fig. 24). The multipartite nature of the ribs of the fully formed fibrous sheath is evident in their frequent bicuspid or tricuspid cross sectional appearance in sagittal sections of the tail (Fig. 24). Although the original circumferential elements of the sheath develop very close to the membrane, the sheath in the mature sperm is some distance within the flagellar membrane and is no longer fixed to it (Figs. 21 and 24). Indeed, the membrane appears to be rather loose fitting over the anterior part of the principal piece, but farther caudal is smoother and more closely associated with the fibrous sheath. It is possible that this looseness of the flagellar membrane provides the necessary slack to accommodate the bending movements of the principal piece.

In the anterior half of the principal piece during development of the sheath, the cross-sectional outline of the flagellum for a time becomes markedly elliptical with the long transverse axis of the ellipse perpendicular to the axis of the central pair (Figs. 18, 19). As the longitudinal columns and ribs of the sheath thicken later in development, the cross-sectional shape changes so that the longer axis is the one passing through the dorsal and ventral columns and doublets 3 and 8 (Figs. 20 and 21). This change in cross-sectional shape of the tail has been observed in guinea pig, chinchilla and chinese hamster. Its significance is not immediately apparent.

Attachments of the fibrous sheath.

In the middle-piece and beginning of the principal piece there are nine outer dense fibers in the sperm tail. A short distance beyond the annulus, in most mammalian species, outer fibers 3 and 8 terminate rather abruptly.

A feature that does not seem to have been fully appreciated heretofore, is the fact that just proximal to the termination of these two fibers, inward projections from the dorsal and ventral longitudinal columns come into contact with fibers 3 and 8 and seem to be attached to them. This is shown in chinese hamster (Fig. 25) and guinea pig (Fig. 21). In the ground squirrel, dorsal and ventral columns are not obvious at this level but there is, nevertheless, a small site of apparent continuity between the fibrous sheath and the convex outer surface of fibers 3 and 8 which are unusually large in this species (Fig. 26). From this sampling of three mammalian species, we suggest that an attachment of the columns of the fibrous sheath to outer fibers 3 and 8 may prove to be a feature common to all mammalian spermatozoa.

Distal to the termination of fibers 3 and 8, the two longitudinal columns of the sheath have a wedge-shaped cross section and their tapering inner edges extend into the spaces between fibers 2 and 4 and 7 and 9 to attach to short radial projections from the wall of doublets 3 and 8 respectively (Fig. 25 C). Some authors have suggested that the triangular cross section of these columns result from incorporation of fibers 3 and 8 into them (See Fig. 2, Nelson 1967). This interpretation does not seem to be correct. With staining methods currently in use, the density and texture of the outer fibers in cross sections is very different from that of the fibrous sheath. Other authors have indicated that the bulbous tip of the minute stud-like radial projection from doublets 3 and 8 (Fig. 17 inset) represents a continuation of the outer fibers very greatly reduced in diameter. Though this view is more difficult to exclude, we feel that these two outer fibers terminate and that the small stud-like structure on the corresponding doublets simply provides attachment for the tapering inner edge of the dorsal and ventral columns of the sheath.

The precise significance of these attachments of the fibrous sheath to outer fibers 3 and 8 near their termination and to the corresponding doublets distal to this point, is not clear but it seems likely that if the sheath were attached neither to the flagellar membrane nor to the axoneme, it might well be displaced caudally by the propagated wave of contraction passing along the tail. Considering that the movement of mammalian sperm tails is believed to be a resultant of a major wave in the plane perpendicular to the central pair and a minor wave at right angles to it (Rikmenspoel, 1964) one can speculate further, that if an attachment of the sheath to the axoneme is necessary to maintain the relative positions of these components it would interfere least with the bending movements in the major plane, if the attachment were on or near the 3–8 axis.

References

AUSTIN C. R., (1965) – *Fine structure of the snake sperm tail.* « J. Ultrastructure Res. », 12, 452–462.

CLARK A. W., (1967) – *Some aspects of spermiogenesis in a lizard.* « Am. J. Anat. » 121, 369–400.

CLELAND K. W. and ROTHSCHILD Lord, (1959) – *The bandicoot spermatozoon: An electron microscopic study of the tail.* « Proc. Roy. Soc. » (London), B150, 24–42.

FAWCETT D. W., (1958) – *The structure of the mammalian spermatozoon.* « Int. Rev. Cytol. », 7, 195–235.

FAWCETT D. W. and HOLLENBERG R. D., (1963) – *Changes in the acrosome of guinea-pig spermatozoa during passage through the epididymis.* « Z. Zellforsch. », 60, 276–292.

FAWCETT D. W. and ITO S., (1965) – *The fine structure of bat spermatozoa.* « Am. J. Anat. », 116, 567–610.

FAWCETT D. W. and PHILLIPS D. M., (1969 a) – *Observations on the release of spermatozoa and on changes in the head during passage through the epididymis.* « J. Reprod. Fert. », Suppl. 6, 405–418.

FAWCETT D. W. and PHILLIPS D. M., (1969 b) – *The fine structure and development of the neck region of the mammalian spermatozoon.* « Anat. Rec. », 165, 153.

GORDON M. and BENESCH K. G., (1968) – *Cytochemical differentiation of the guinea pig sperm flagellum with phosphotungstic acid.* « J. Ultrastructure Res. », 24, 33–50.

HANCOCK J. L., (1966) – *The ultrastructure of mammalian spermatozoa.* « Recent Advances in Reproduction and Fertility », 1, 125.

MCINTOSH J. R. and PORTER K. R., (1967) – *Microtubules in the spermatids of the domestic fowl.* « J. Cell. Biol. », 36, 153–173.

NELSON L., (1967) – *Sperm motility,* in « Fertilization », Vol. I, pp. 27–97 (C. B. Metz and A. Monroy, eds.) Academic Press, New York.

NICANDER L. and BANE A., (1962) – *Fine structure of boar spermatozoa.* « Zeitschr. f. Zellforsch. », 57, 390–405.

PHILLIPS D. W., (1970) – *The insect spermatozoan.* « J. Cell Biol. », 44, 243.

PLOWMAN K. M. and NELSON L. (1962) – *An actin-like protein isolated from starfish spermatozoa.* « Biol. Bull. », 123, 478.

RIKMENSPOEL R., (1965) – *The tail movements of bull spermatozoa. Observations and model calculations.* « Biophys. J. », 5, 365–391.

SAACKE R. G. and ALMQUIST J. O., (1964) – *The ultrastructure of bovine spermatozoa II The neck and tail of normal ejaculated sperm.* « Am. J. Anat. », 115, 163–184.

Explanation of figures 3–26.

Fig. 3. – Electron micrographs showing four successive stages in the formation of the outer dense fibers of the sperm flagellum in a bird. In *A* a small ridge originates in the sulcus between subfiber a and b of each doublet and extends radially (arrows). These small lateral outgrowths from the doublets represent very early stages in formation of the outer fibers. In *B* there has been further accretion of material to the end and sides of the radial projection from the doublets. In *C* and *D* continued deposition has resulted in further thickening of the fibers. In birds, the outer fibers remain very intimately related to the wall of the corresponding doublets throughout their development.

Fig. 4. – A cross section through the base of the flagellum on a mammalian spermatid at a stage soon after initiation of outer fiber formation. Thin radial projections from the walls of the doublets are visible at the arrows. The process is initiated earlier or proceeds more rapidly on doublets 1, 5, and 6 for, even at this early stage, these outer fibers are thicker than the others. Soon after this stage the outer fibers separate from the wall of the doublets.

Figs. 5, 6. – Two stages in the formation of the accessory fibers in insect sperm. These arise as shown in Fig. 5 at the arrow, as C-shaped outgrowths from subfiber b of the doublets. They subsequently separate from the doublets and close the gap in their wall to form 9 outer microtubules as in Fig. 6. In some species the lumen of the microtubule is occupied by dense material, in others it remains clear.

Fig. 7. – Electron micrograph of a cross section through the middle-piece of a chinese hamster spermatozoan, showing the typical 9+2 axonemal complex surrounded by 9 outer dense fibers. A cortex and medulla are discernible in the outer fibers. Between them are small punctate profiles that are transverse sections of the so-called satellite fibrils.

Fig. 8. – Cross section through the middle piece of ground-squirrel sperm. The sperm of this species are extraordinarily thick. If shown at the same magnification, this cross section would have twice the diameter of the hamster sperm above. The outer fibers are very large and far removed from the axonemal complex. The spaces between them are filled with a filigree pattern composed of thin satellite fibrils laterally associated to produce meandering linear profiles.

Fig. 9. – A sector of chinese hamster midpiece at higher magnification, illustrating the differentiation of the outer fibers into cortex and medulla. The cortex is often lacking on the medial surface of the fibers and may present a free edge (at arrows). The satellite fibers are most often found adjacent to those surfaces of the outer fibers which lack a cortical layer. It is suggested that the satellites arise from disintegration of the cortex or by delamination from its free edge.

Fig. 10. – A sector from the principal piece of a ground squirrel sperm. The satellite fibrils appear either as punctate profiles or as discontinuous sheets or laminae. Continuity between the cortex of the outer fibers and these satellite fibrils or laminae is often observed, as at the arrow on the left side of the figure.

Figs. 11 and 12. – Cross section of the mid-piece of a sperm of *Citellus lateralis* shown here for purposes of orientation of other figures. With routine staining the outer fibers may appear dense and homogeneous, but the presence of a thin cortex can be demonstrated by special stains as in Fig. 12. The interrupted line represents the approximate orientation of the longitudinal section presented in Fig. 13. (Fig. 12 courtesy of Dr. W. ANDERSON).

Fig. 13. – A longitudinal section of the mid-piece of Citellus sperm illustrating that the filigree pattern seen in Figs. 11 and 12 is in fact composed of long, predominantly fibrillar, elements. The close lateral association of these fibrils results in their appearing in cross-sections as if they were laminae. The interrupted line of Fig. 11 suggests the approximate orientation of the section shown here which intersects the inner end of only one of the outer fibers.

Fig. 14. – Longitudinal section of the flagellum of a chinchilla spermatid showing the anterior margin of the fibrous sheath which is well advanced in its development before the annulus has migrated caudally. This makes it unlikely that the annulus plays any significant role in formation of the fibrous sheath.

Fig. 15. – Longitudinal section of the differentiating flagellum in a chinchilla spermatid slightly more advanced than that shown in Fig. 14. The annulus has now taken up its definitive position at the anterior end of the fibrous sheath and the mitochondria are gathering around the flagellum to complete the formation of the middle piece. (From FAWCETT and PHILLIPS, *Biology of Reproduction*, 1969).

Fig. 16. – Cross sections of differentiating flagella of guinea pig spermatids. Condensations of material (at arrows) between the flagellar membrane and doublets 3 and 8 represent the developing longitudinal columns of the fibrous sheath. These appear to differentiate before the circumferential elements. They also extend a short distance into the end piece beyond the termination of the sheath.

Fig. 17. – The circumferential elements of the sheath first appear as ring-like concentrations of amorphous material close to the flagellar membrane (see at arrows). The inset shows that the stud-like projection from fibers 3 and 8 along which the longitudinal columns develop, arises from subfiber A of the doublet.

Fig. 18. – In the sections shown here both the longitudinal columns and the ribs of the fibrous sheath have thickened and become more dense. The cross-section is beginning to assume an elliptical shape with the long axis perpendicular to the plane of the central pair.

Fig. 19. – Another example of the transient deformation of the cross sectional outline of the tail, seemingly due to elongation of the ribs at a more rapid rate than the elongation of the inward projections of the longitudinal columns of the sheath which bind the sheath to doublets 3 and 8.

Fig. 20. – At this later stage of sheath development, the outer fibers of the flagellum and ribs of the sheath have both thickened noticeably. The tapering inward-projecting portions of the dorsal and ventral longitudinal columns have elongated and the long axis of the cross section is now parallel to the plane of the central pair.

Fig. 21. – In the mature guinea pig sperm tail the fibrous sheath is no longer closely associated with the flagellar membrane. Indeed the membrane in the anterior half of the tail usually appears loose fitting and irregular in outline. Notice here the apparent attachment of the sheath to outer fibers 3 and 8 near their termination.

Fig. 22. – Longitudinal section of the flagellum of a guinea-pig spermatid, coinciding with the developing dorsal and ventral columns of the fibrous sheath. These are composed of longitudinally oriented fine filaments. The end-on sections of the circumferential elements of the sheath can be made out in the dense substance of the columns (at arrows).

Fig. 23. – Longitudinal section of a flagellum not in the plane of the longitudinal columns, illustrating the regularly spaced slender circumferential fibers deposited very near the flagellar membrane.

Fig. 24. – Longitudinal section of a fully differentiated fibrous sheath. The ribs of the fibrous sheath are very much thicker than the circumferential fibers first deposited, and often appear bipartite or tripartite (see at arrows) suggesting that they may develop by aggregation and fusion of the more slender elements deposited early in the development of the sheath. Notice also that the flagellar membrane is no longer close to the sheath but appears to be loose and free of attachment to the underlying structures of the tail.

Fig. 25. – Transverse sections at three closely-spaced successive levels in the first part of the principal piece. In *A*, just distal to the annulus, inward extensions of the fibrous sheath appear to attach to fibers 3 and 8 (at arrows). In *B*, fibers 3 and 8 are smaller but still seem to be in contact with the thin edges of ridges projecting inward from the dorsal and ventral longitudinal columns of the sheath (at arrows). In *C*, fibers 3 and 8 have terminated and their places are now occupied by the tapering inner edges of the longitudinal columns which attach to doublets

3 and 8. This is the condition which prevails throughout the greater part of the length of the principal piece. (The flagellar membrane was opaqued out of the negative and hence is not seen here).

Fig. 26. – Transverse sections of the initial portion of the principal piece of ground squirrel sperm. At the levels shown here, just caudal to the annulus, the dorsal and ventral longitudinal columns are not easily identified but the sheath nevertheless appears (at the arrows) to be attached to or continuous with the surface of outer fibers 3 and 8 which are uncommonly thick in this species.

Discussion

AFZELIUS. – When describing the material close to the proximal centriole you have numbered the nine triplet tubules 1, 2,... 9. What convention do you use? One made specifically to describe the situation in the proximal centriole or one which agrees with the situation in the sperm tail?

FAWCETT. – The system of numbering follows no convention and is not related to the numbering of the doublets in the axoneme. The number of the triplets of the proximal centriole in this work has been done arbitrarily, simply to facilitate description of the observations.

HORSTMANN. – Is there any connection between the material around the proximal centriole and the nucleus? Especially have you found material or structures in the gaps of the nuclear membrane?

FAWCETT. – The light zone usually observed between the articular surface of the connecting piece and the implantation fossa of the nucleus is traversed by exceedingly fine filaments. In addition, the two layers of the nuclear envelope are very closely approximated in this region and the narrow interspace between them is bridged by very regularly spaced periodic densities. These structures, I presume, are local specializations of the nuclear envelope and of the basal plate to assure a firm union of head to tail.

BACCETTI. – Could you give us some details on the chemical nature of the material constituting the centriolar adjunct of vertebrates? It seems to be very different from that of insects.

FAWCETT. – The " centriolar adjunct " of vertebrate sperm is entirely different from the structure bearing that name in invertebrate sperm. I may have been unwise to use a term already preempted for a different component of the sperm in invertebrates. I considered " centriolar extension " but abandoned this because it carried the implication that the added segment was identical in its structure to the original centriole, and I wished to emphasize that its structure was somewhat different. The word *adjunct* seemed appropriate because it is defined as « something added or joined to another thing, but not essentially a part of it ". I hope this terminology will not prove to be too confusing.

ANDRÉ. – As usual, Dr. FAWCETT gave us today a magnificient masterpiece, demonstrating elegantly a number of new important data. But masterpieces make us more eager to learn still more. What I would like to ask Dr. FAWCETT is what is the evidence for the property of contractility for the coarse fibers, and how the solid appearance of the coarse fibers can be paralleled with the fibrous structure of the other contractile organelles such as myofibrils.

FAWCETT. – The evidence for contractility of the outer fibers is at present largely suggestive and circumstantial. (1) Their appearance in the phylogenetic scale, concurrently with acquisition of internal fertilization and the requirement for locomotion in a more viscous medium. (2) The concurrent development of a long mitochondrial sheath presumed to be an energy source in close apposition to the outer dense fibers. (There is little to indicate that the axoneme requires close proximity of mitochondria for vigorous motility). (3) The finding in some very thick sperm, that the outer fibers are so massive that it seems inconceivable that the axoneme alone could bend the midpiece if the outer fibers were passive stiffening structures. The only other evidence of which I am aware is immunohistochemical evidence suggesting that the outer fibers have antigenic properties that relate them to actin and myosin. I believe Dr. Leonard Nelson could comment more authoritatively on this point.

NELSON. – Evidence for the contractile nature of the outer coarse longitudinal fibers of sperm flagella comes from immunocytochemical electron microscopic studies on rat sperm. We used actin, myosin and actomyosin antibodies (rabbit muscle proteins injected into chickens) and rat muscle protein injected into rabbits). In frozen dried sperm the actin antibodies reacted with the cortical region of the coarse fibers, while the myosin antibodies combined with the medullar region of the coarse longitudinal fibers in the mid piece and principal piece of the flagellum. When the spermatozoa were previously extracted with 0.6M KI or 0.6M KCl and then treated with the antibodies, there was no longer any immunocytochemical reaction. 0.6M KCl and 0.6M KI are used for the extraction of the contractile proteins from muscle, myosin and actomyosin, and also for the preparation of actin from the extracts. These studies support previous cytochemical evidence we obtained showing the localization of ATP ase in the same regions of the coarse fibers in rat sperm. The work is reported in the AAAS Symposium on Spermatozoan Motility in my Chapter on Cytochemical Aspects of Sperm Motility, published in 1962.

BROKAW to ANDRÉ. – I believe that consideration of my own work on the energetics of movement of simple spermatozoa such as sea urchin spermatozoa, and Dr. RIKMENSPOEL'S work on the energetics of bull spermatozoa shows us that bull spermatozoa do work at rates about five times greater than the maximum work of sea urchin spermatozoa. I believe that mammalian spermatozoa therefore must have some work–generating mechanism in addition to the central axoneme which is also found in sea urchin spermatozoa.

Brokaw. – Do mammalian spermatozoa have " arms " on the outer doublet microtubules of the central axoneme?

Fawcett. – The doublets of the axoneme in mammalian sperm flagella do have " arms " projecting toward the next doublet. They are assymetrical. The outermost arm has an appendage which gives it a hatchet-like or flag-like appearance in cross sections. This appendage is not seen on the inward directed arm.

Don W. Fawcett and D. M. Phillips – *Recent observations on the ultrastructure and development of the mammalian spermatozoon.*

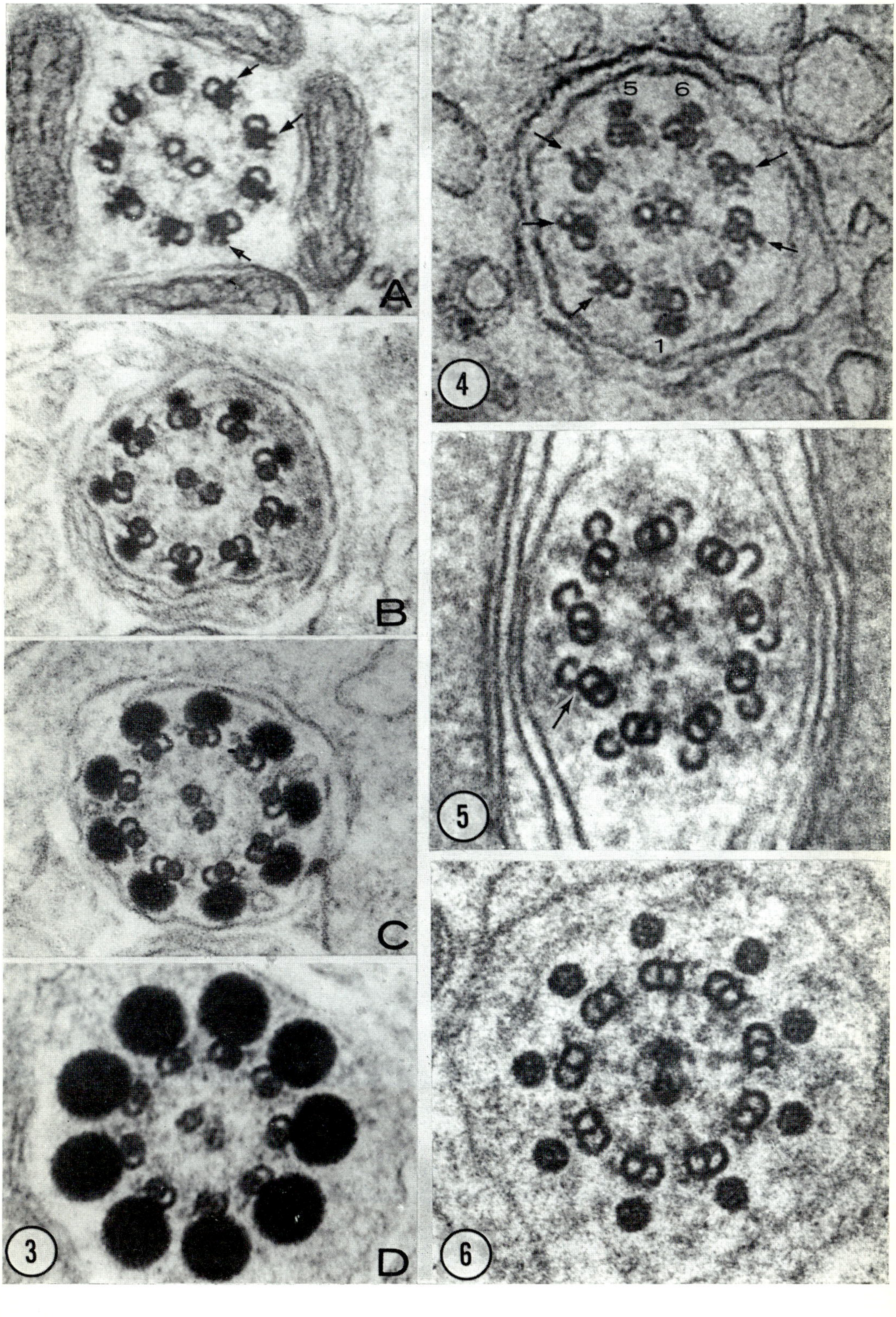

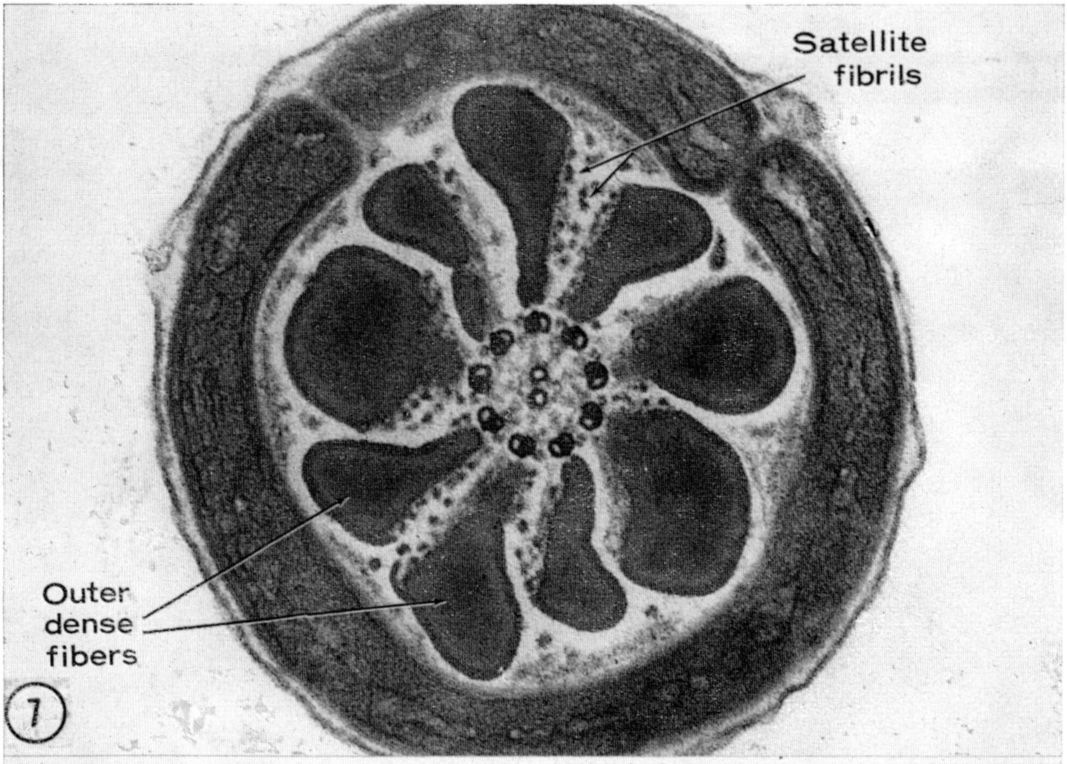
Satellite
fibrils
Outer
dense
fibers
7

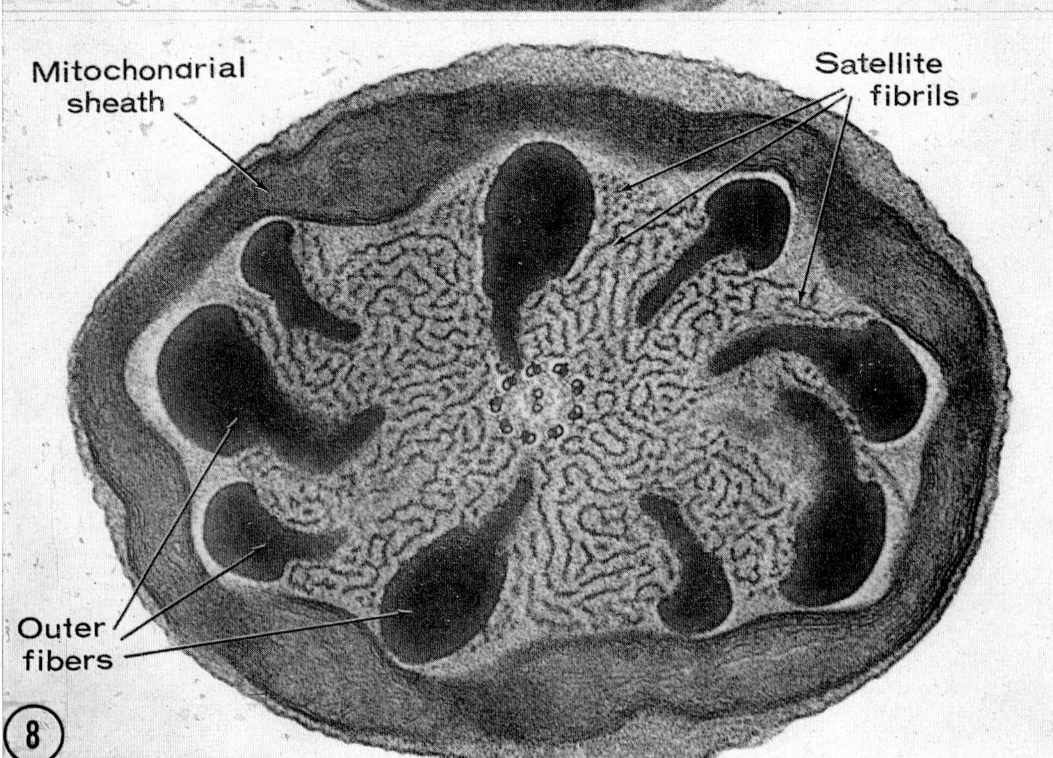
Mitochondrial
sheath
Satellite
fibrils
Outer
fibers
8

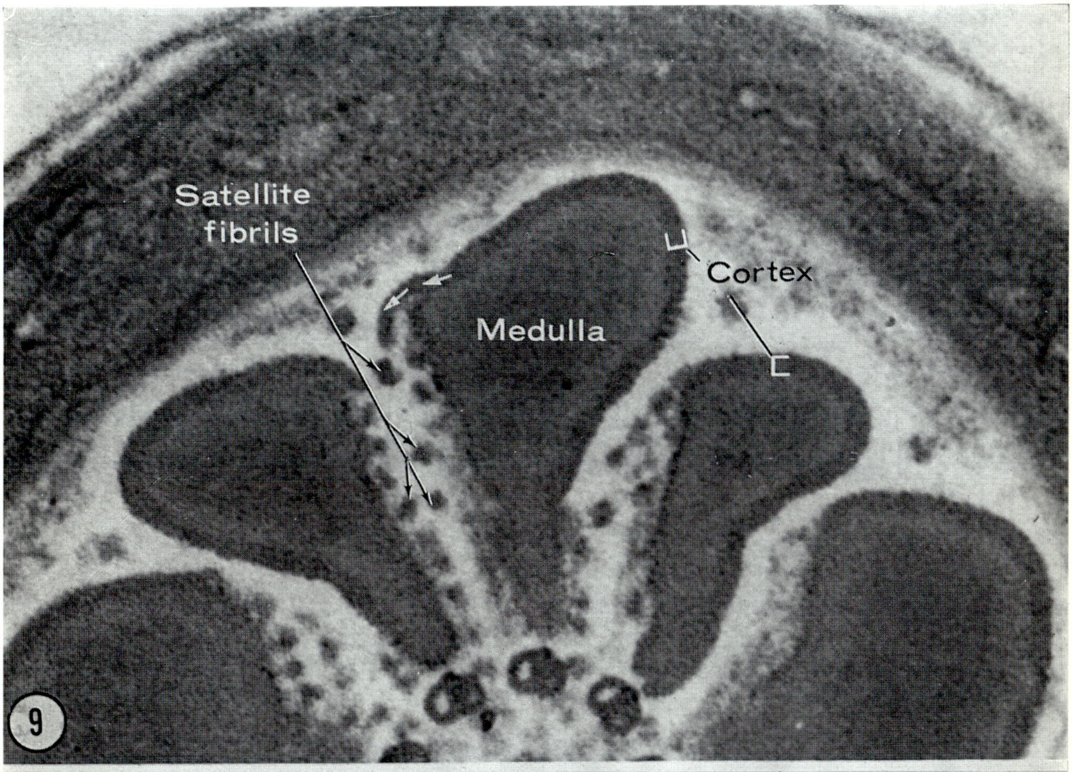
Satellite
fibrils
Cortex
Medulla
9

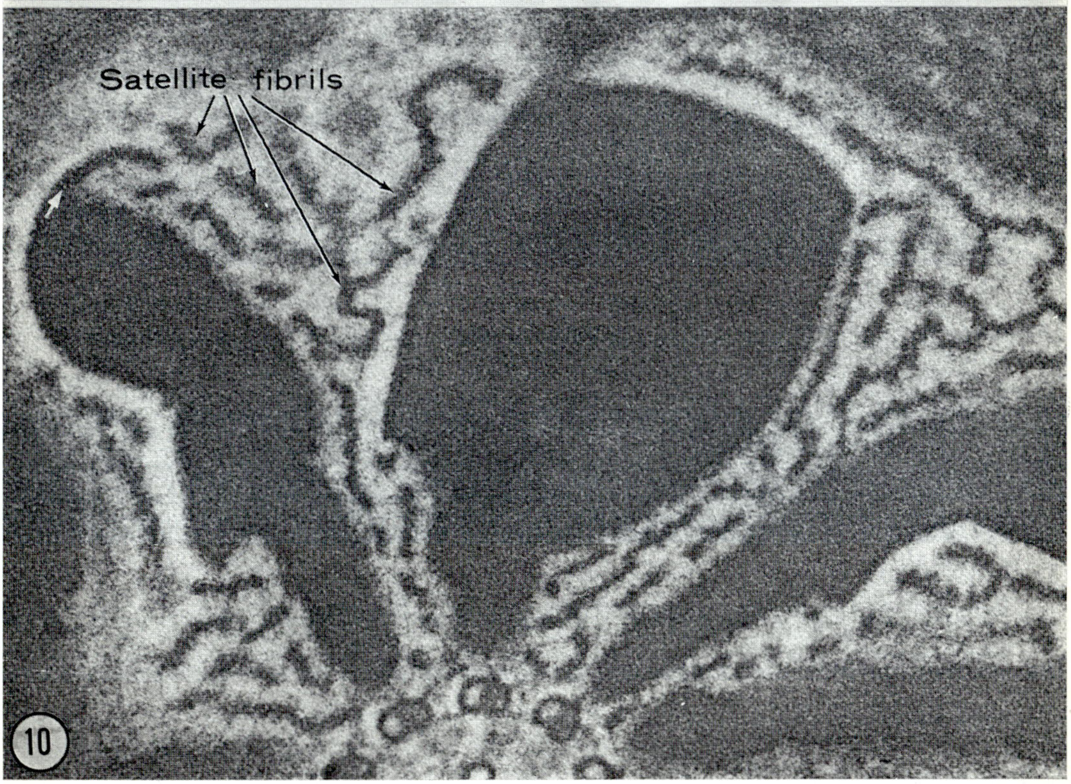
Satellite fibrils
10

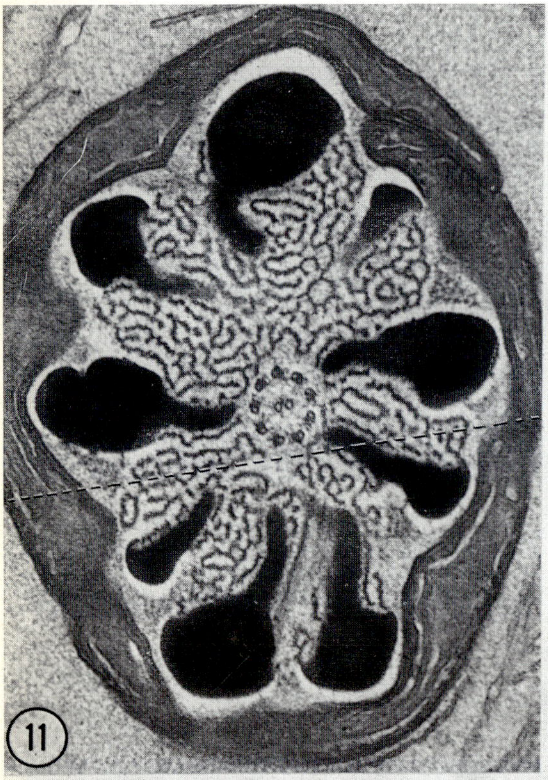

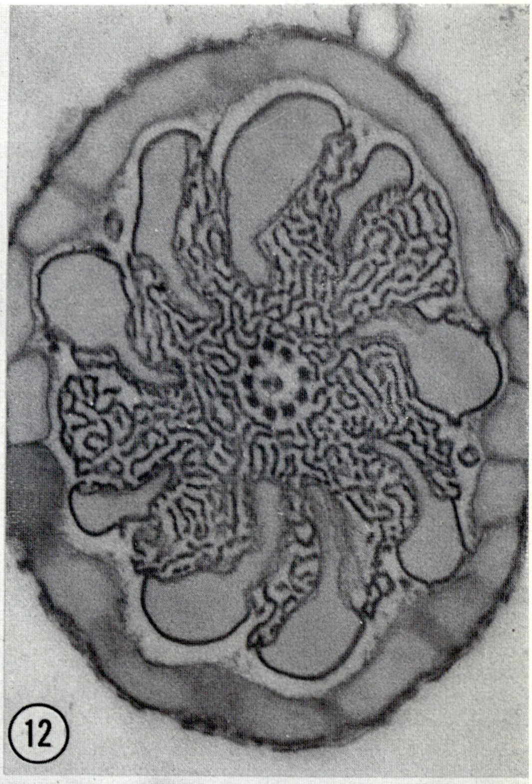

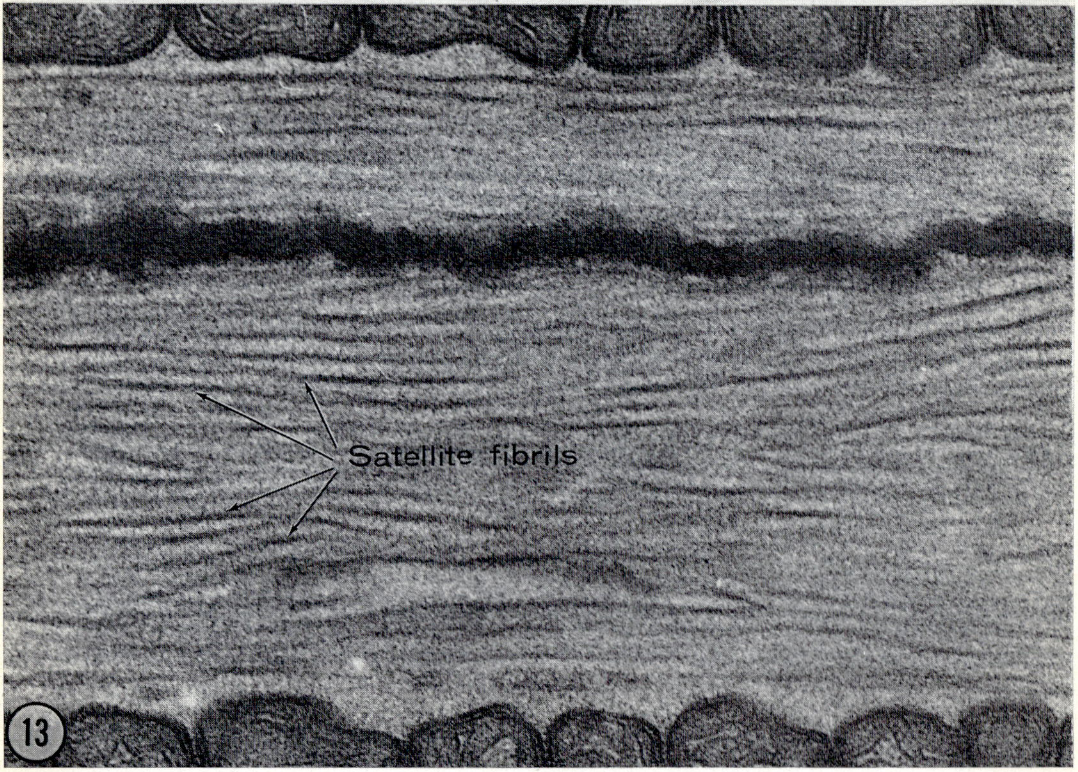
Satellite fibrils

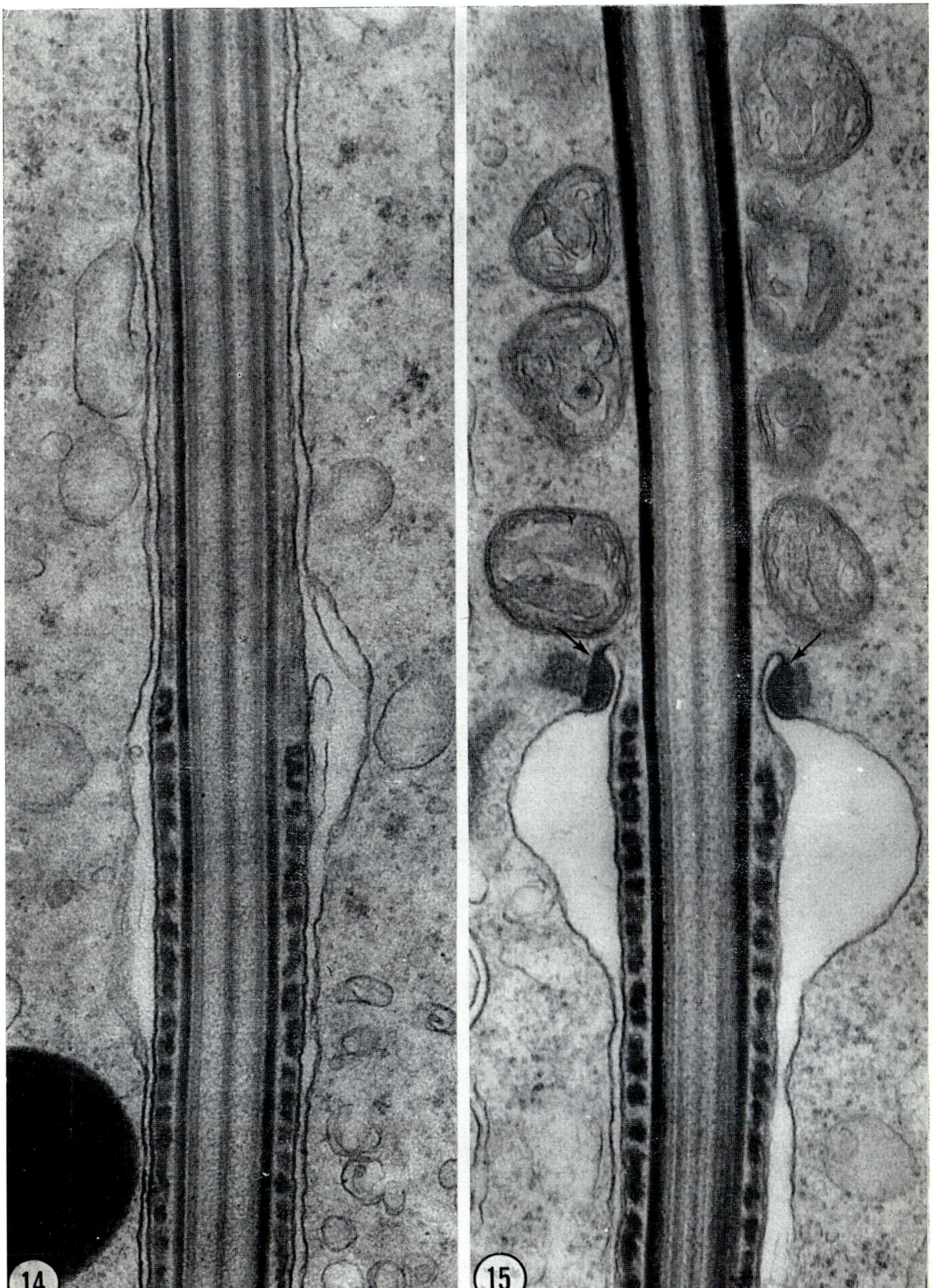
14
15

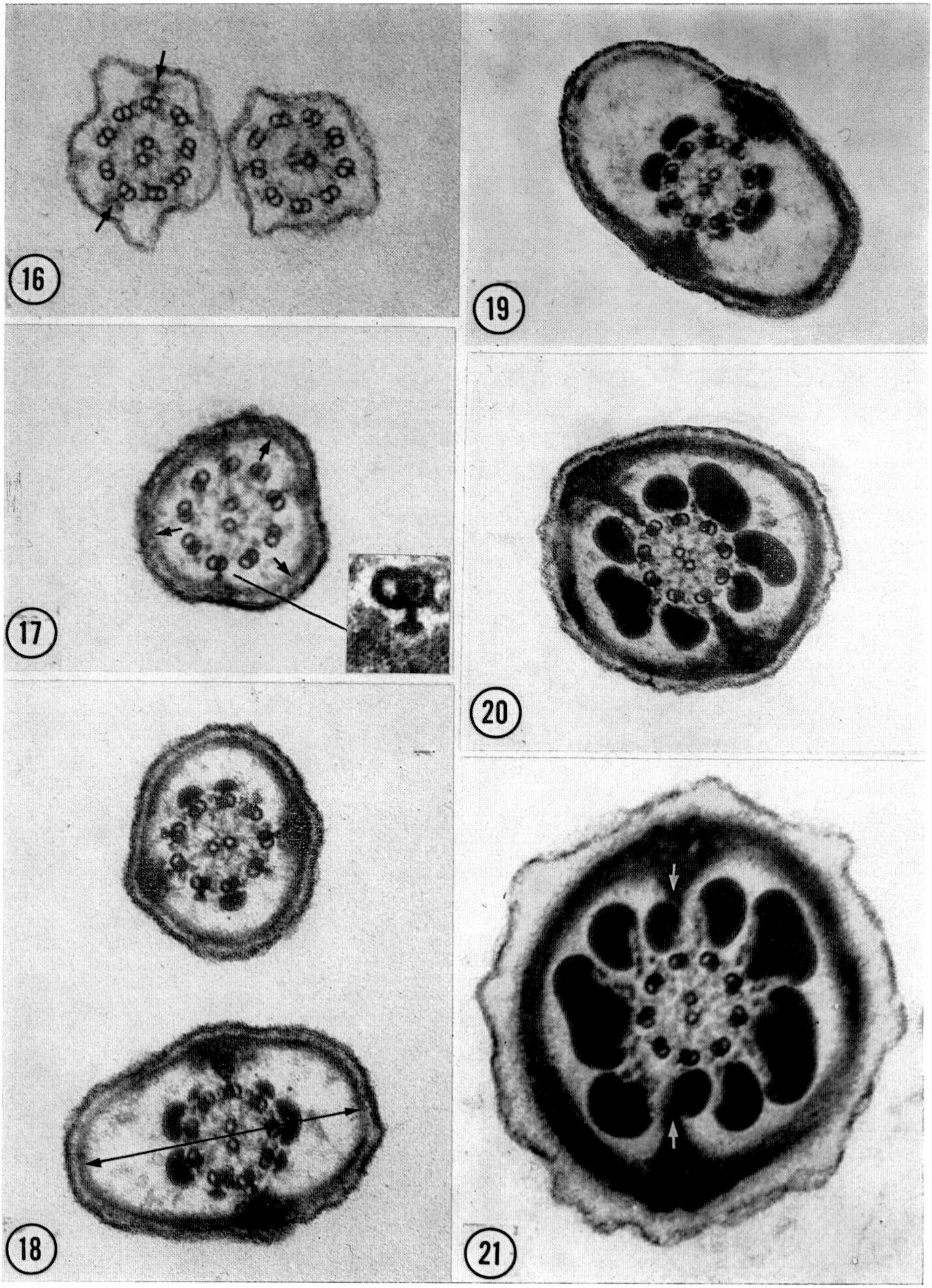
16
17
18
19
20
21

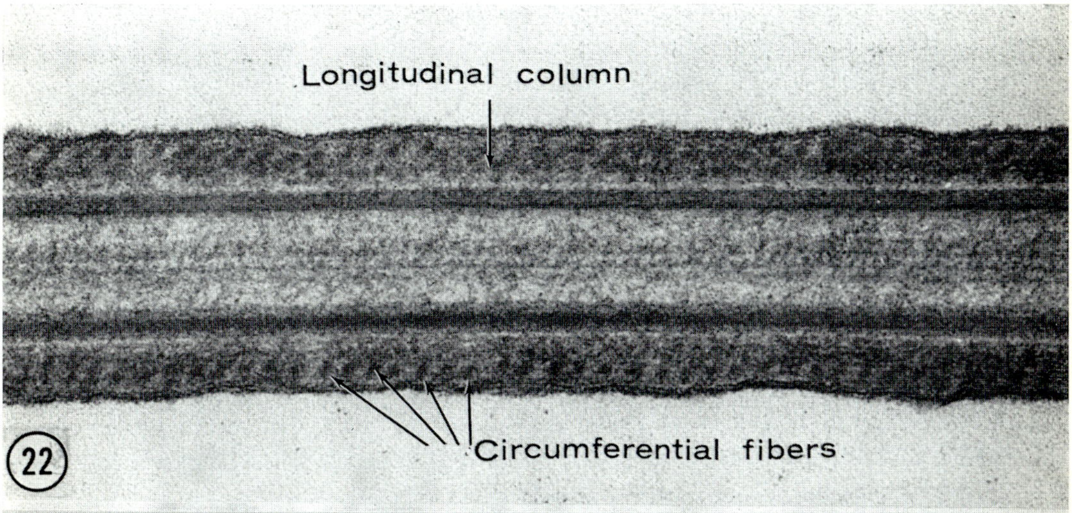

22

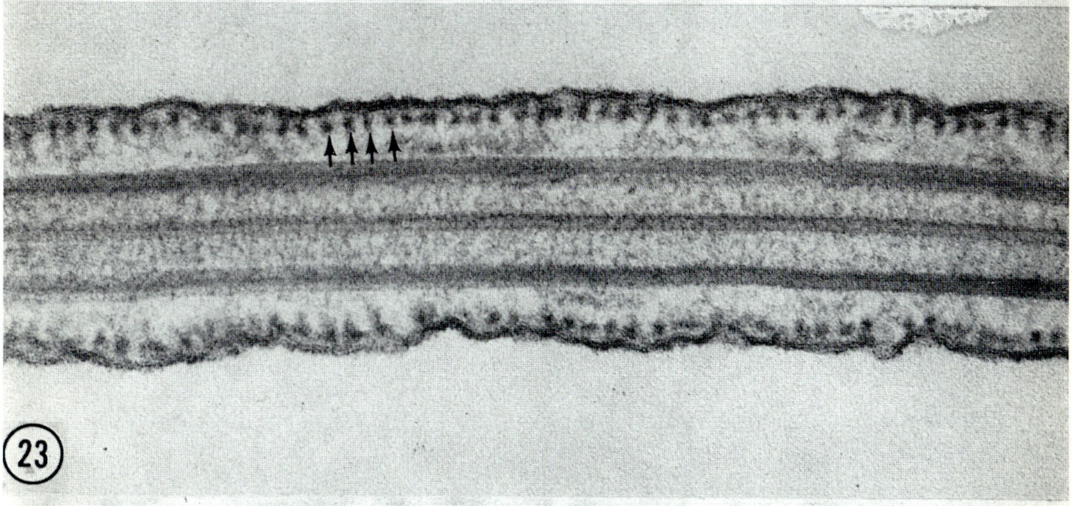

23

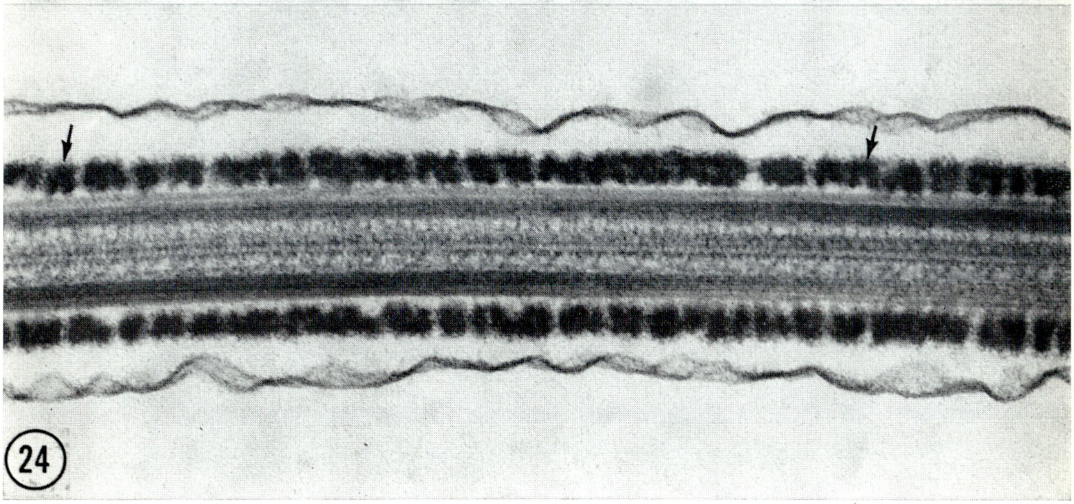

24

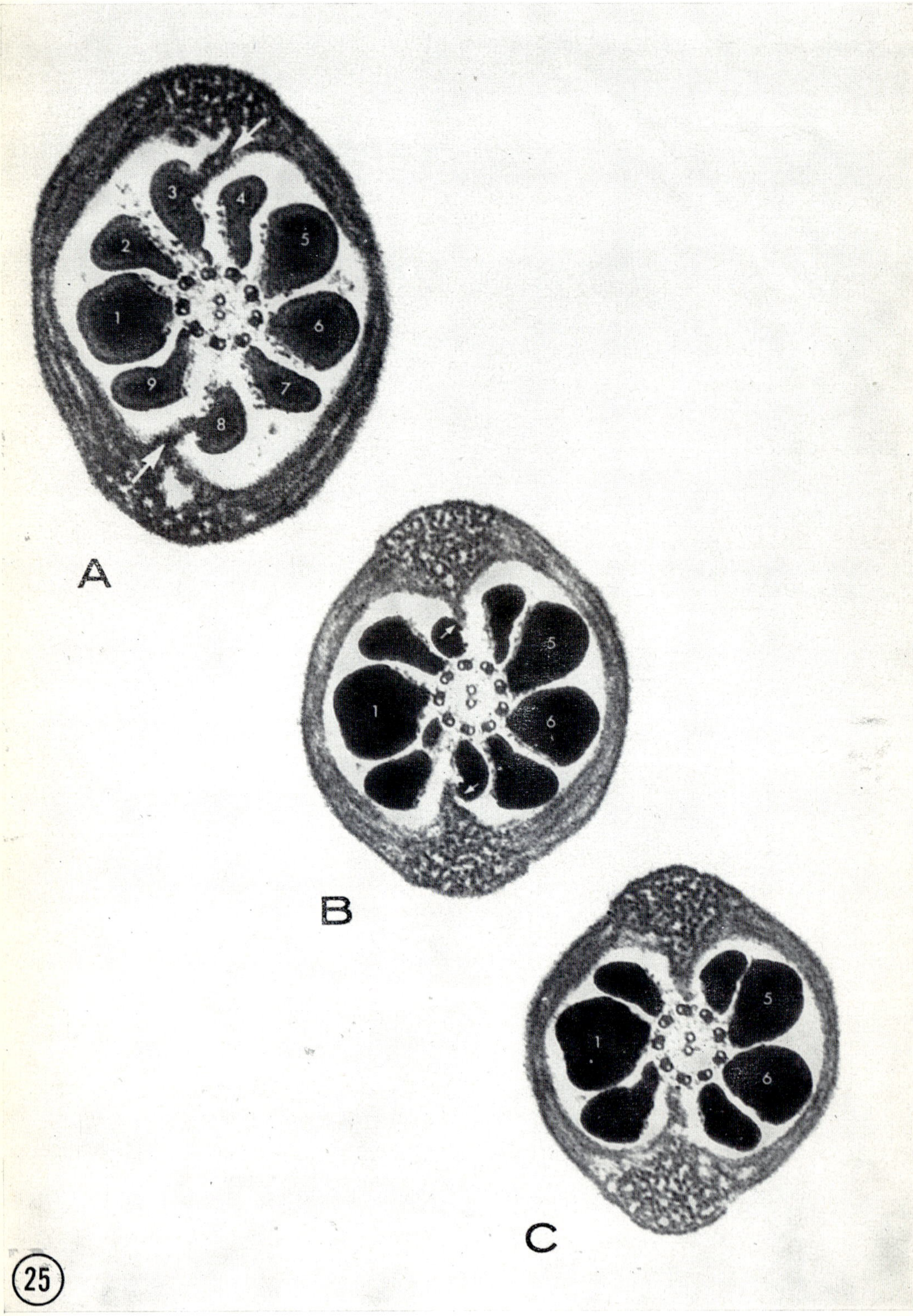
1
2
3
4
5
6
7
8
9
A
1
5
6
B
1
5
6
C
25

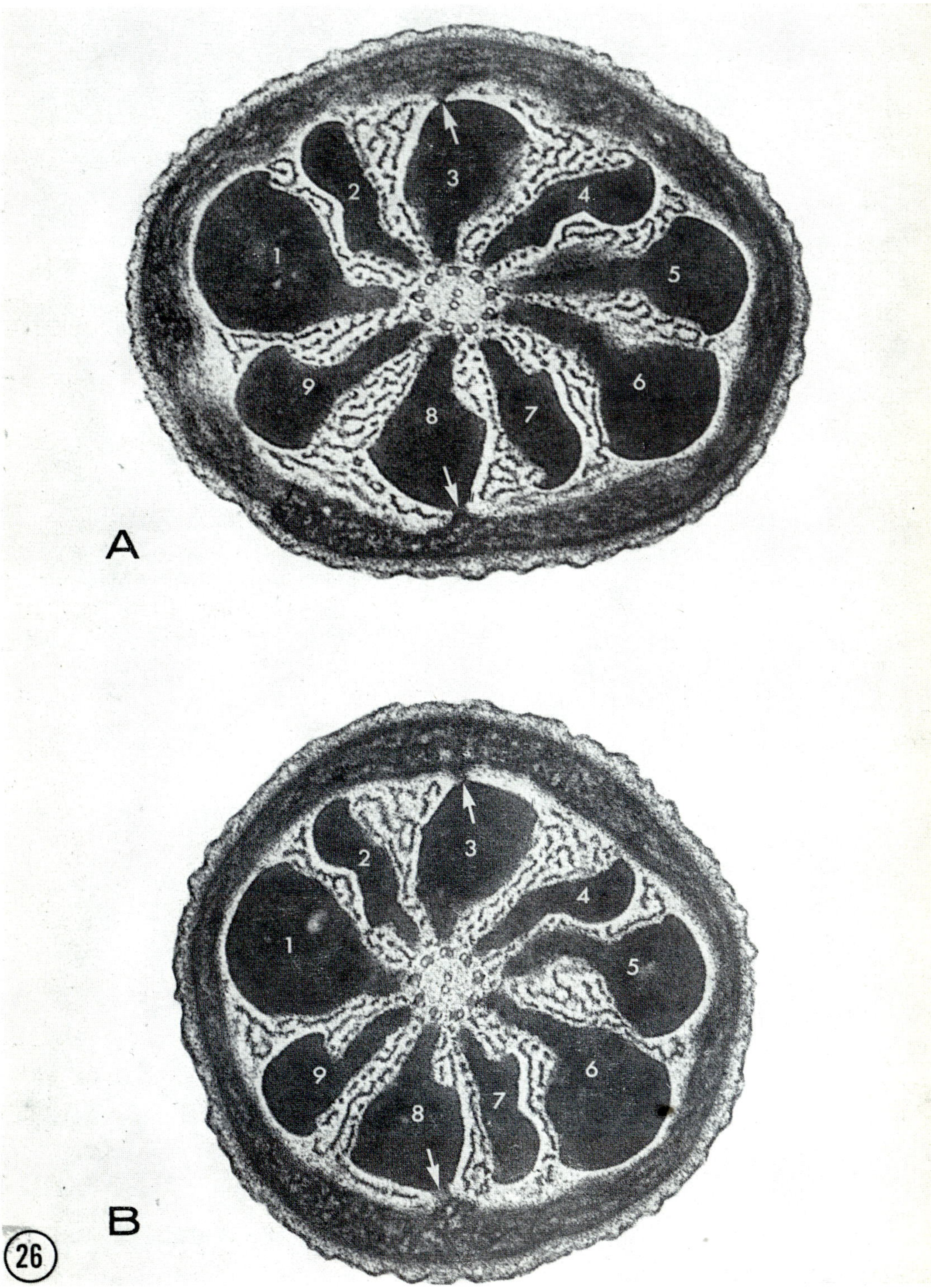
1
2
3
4
5
6
7
8
9
A
1
2
3
4
5
6
7
8
9
B

Å. FRANZÉN (*)

PHYLOGENETIC ASPECTS OF THE MORPHOLOGY OF SPERMATOZOA AND SPERMIOGENESIS

SUMMARY. — To sum up one can say that in the Metazoa the morphology of the spermatozoon is in some way related to the mode of fertilization. Forms releasing their spermatozoa freely into the water retain the primitive type of spermatozoon. When on the other hand internal fertilization takes place or the spermatozoa are released in the immediate proximity of the female genital opening, the morphology of the spermatozoa diverges to varying degrees from the primitive type. During the cytogenesis of the spermatozoon in Nemertini, Annelida, and Mollusca it is possible to follow the changes in the cell as it differentiates from a spermatid with primitive features into a modified type of spermatozoon. Differences from the primitive condition are mainly confined to the head and the middle piece. Of special importance to my argument is the characteristic redistribution of the mitochondrial material.

These main types of spermatozoan constructions especially with respect to the location of the energy—providing mitochondria, might be related to the locomotory demands of the forms. In external fertilization more swimming is needed and so the mitochondria are functionally related to the organelle of motility, the flagellum. With respect to internal fertilization the distance needed to be covered by the spermatozoon is negligible.

Particularly strongly aberrant types of spermatozoa occur within Platyhelminthes, Aschelminthes, Myzostomida and Arthropoda. The modified types of spermatozoa in these phyla are related to a strongly modified and specialized biology of fertilization.

RIASSUNTO. — Nei Metazoi la morfologia dello spermatozoo è in relazione col modo di fecondazione. Le forme che liberano gli spermatozoi nell'acqua mantengono un tipo primitivo di spermatozoo. Quando invece la fecondazione è interna o gli spermatozoi vengono liberati nelle immediate vicinanze della apertura genitale femminile, la morfologia differisce in vari gradi dal tipo primitivo. Durante la citogenesi dello spermatozoo nei Nemertini, Anellidi e Molluschi è possibile seguire i cambiamenti nella cellula non appena essa si differenzia da uno spermatidio con costituzione primitiva in un tipo modificato di spermatozoo. Differenze dalla costituzione primitiva sono limitate alla testa e alla regione intermedia. Di particolare importanza è la caratteristica ridistribuzione del materiale mitocondriale.

Questi particolari modelli di spermatozoi, specialmente rispetto alla posizione dei mitocondri che provvedono l'energia, può essere relativa alle esigenze di locomozione. Nella fecondazione esterna è necessario un maggior movimento e così i mitocondri sono funzionalmente in relazione con l'organulo della motilità, il flagello. Nella fecondazione interna, la distanza che lo spermatozoo deve coprire è insignificante.

Tipi di spermatozoi particolarmente aberranti si trovano nei Platelminti, Aschelminti e Artropodi. I tipi modificati di spermatozoi in questi phyla sono relativi ad una biologia di fecondazione fortemente modificata e specializzata.

(*) Institute of Zoology, University, Uppsala, Sweden.

I. – The primitive type of spermatozoon in the Metazoa

My conception of the morphology of the primitive type of spermatozoon is based on a comparative study of spermiogenesis and the biology of fertilization in some different phyla in the Metazoa.

Gametes with two flagella have long been known from several unicellular organisms and " lower " plants. In the Metazoa turbellarian spermatozoa with two flagella or " nebengeisseln " have been described in several species. The similarity of many turbellarian spermatozoa to the gametes in unicellular organisms has given rise to the theory that the occurrence of two flagella in the turbellarian spermatozoa is a primitive feature surviving from the stage before the evolution of the metazoan organization. In this theory the Turbellaria are interpreted as a very primitive group; however, the reproductive system of the Turbellaria is one of the most complicated in the animal kingdom. According to Ax (1963) the turbellarian archetype had internal fertilization. In my opinion the spermatozoa in Turbellaria are highly specialized, and this specialization can be explained as depending on a strongly changed biology of propagation.

The primitive type of spermatozoon in the Metazoa is made up of a short roundish or conical head, a middle piece (mp) containing usually 4–5 spherical mitochondrial aggregates, and a tail (t) consisting of a long flagellum. The head is mainly composed of the nucleus (n), but the tip usually contains an acrosome (a) of variable morphology. The flagellum or tail filament begins at the centriolar apparatus (c) at the posterior part of the head, penetrates the middle piece, extends for about 50 μ, and terminates with a tiny end – piece (e). The middle piece contains the mitochondria, collected in usually 4–5 spherical or egg–shaped aggregates, the proximal part of the flagellum, and the centriolar apparatus.

The centriolar apparatus lies at the basal end of the nucleus and consists of two short cylindrical components, often called the proximal and distal centrioles.

The ultrastructure of the spermatozoon's flagellum is similar to the structure found in cilia and flagella! Thus two microtubules are found in the centre of the flagellum.

The acrosome consists of an acrosomal vesicle, which is bounded by a membrane. The ultrastructure of the acrosome is often very complex, and the term acrosome may be used to refer to the acrosomal membrane and all elements encosed therein.

The strongest argument for my opinion that this spermatozoon represents the primitive metazoon type is provided by its occurrence in so numerous and so widely separated phyla as the Cnidaria, Ctenophora, Porifera, Tentaculata (only Brachiopoda), Aschelminthes (only Priapuloidea) Nemertini, Sipunculoidea, Mollusca, Annelida, Echinodermata, Enteropneusta, Tunicata (only few species) and Acrania.

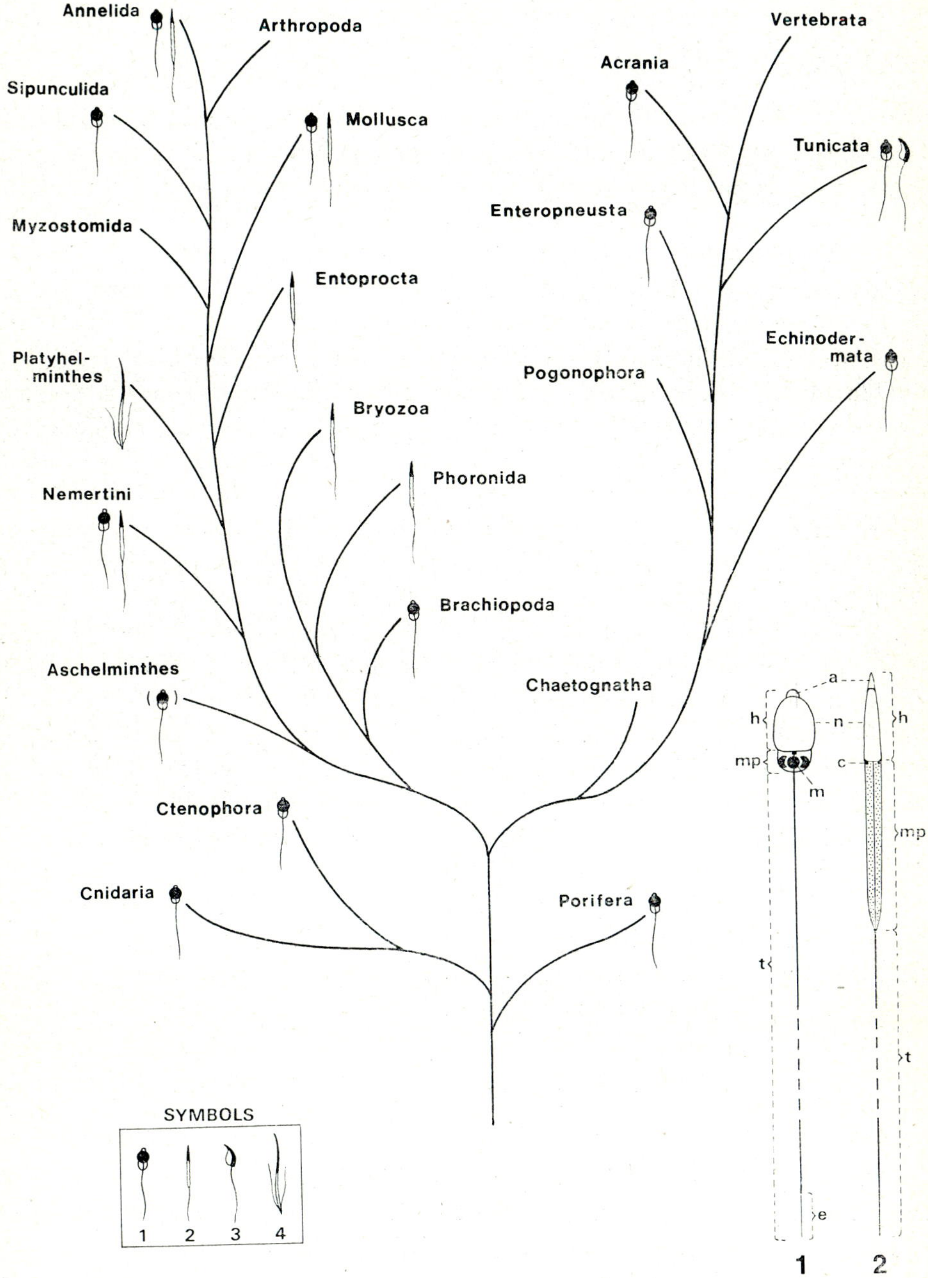

Fig. 1. – The occurrence of the primitive type of spermatozoon (1) as found in the metazoon phylogenetic tree. Symbols: 1. The primitive type of spermatozoon. 2. Modified spermatozoon, evolved from the primitive type. The head and the middle piece are more or less elongated. Primitive characters are often retained during the spermiogenesis. The occurrence of this type of modified spermatozoon is associated with a changed biology of fertilization. 3. Modified spermatozoon, usually characterized by the presence of a lateral structure containing mitochondria (phylum Tunicata). 4. Biflagellate spermatozoa in the phylum Platyhelminthes.

a, acrosome; c, centriole; e, end piece; f, flagellum; h, head; m, mitochondria; mp, middle piece; n, nucleus; rc, residual cytoplasm; Sc, stereocilia; t, tail.

A definite relationship has been demonstrated to exist between spermiogenesis and the biology of fertilization. The primitive type of spermatozoon is retained in groups and species which have retained the primitive metazoan way for the discharge of spermatozoa, viz. freely into the water. If the spermatozoa are not discharged freely into the water for the fertilization of the eggs but are transferred directly to the receiving female animal by spermatophores or by organs of copulation, the morphology of the spermatozoon is altered in some way or other.

This connexion between the morphology of the spermatozoon and the method of sperm transmission is particularly evident in the phyla Nemertini, Annelida and Mollusca. These groups contain several species where it is possible during spermiogenesis to follow the earliest and most conspicuous steps in the spermatozoon's modification, viz. the transformation of the middle piece and the elongation of the head. Here we have examples of phylogenetically early modifications of the spermatozoon. Thus it is possible to derive other types of spermatozoa from the type I consider to be the primitive one.

Types of spermatozoa evolved from the primitive one are indicated in Fig. 1 symbol 2. These types consist of a rod-shaped, more or less elongated middle piece, and a tail formed by a long flagellum. Primitive characters are often retained during the spermiogenesis. The mitochondria assemble into four spherical accumulations at the base of the nucleus. Later the cytogenesis is complicated by a phase in which the mitochondrial mass is evenly distributed in an elongated middle piece of variable length. The modification and final disappearance of the four mitochondrial spheres is often marked by their temporary fusion into two spheres. A stage of this kind has been observed by me (FRANZÉN, 1956) in several species within the following groups: Entoprocta, Polychaeta, Bryozoa, and Nemertini. After this stage the mitochondrial mass extends. The most modified type of spermatozoon of this type is thread-shaped.

II. – TENTACULATA

Bryozoa.

On comparing the different species within the Stelmatopoda most species examined during their cytogenesis exhibit certain primitive features and on the whole the cytogenesis seems to follow a similar course. The most interesting detail from the comparative point of view is that of an ephemeral stage characterized by four spheres of mitochondria more or less regularly arranged around the flagellum. A stage with two large mitochondrial spheres often dominates the picture of the preparations. These mitochondrial spheres give rise to two dark ribbons of mitochondrial material.

In some species, e.g. *Flustra foliacea* (L) (Fig. 2 d) the middle piece of the mature spermatozoon consists (in addition to these mitochondrial portions) of a central layer of lighter cytoplasm near the central flagellum. In

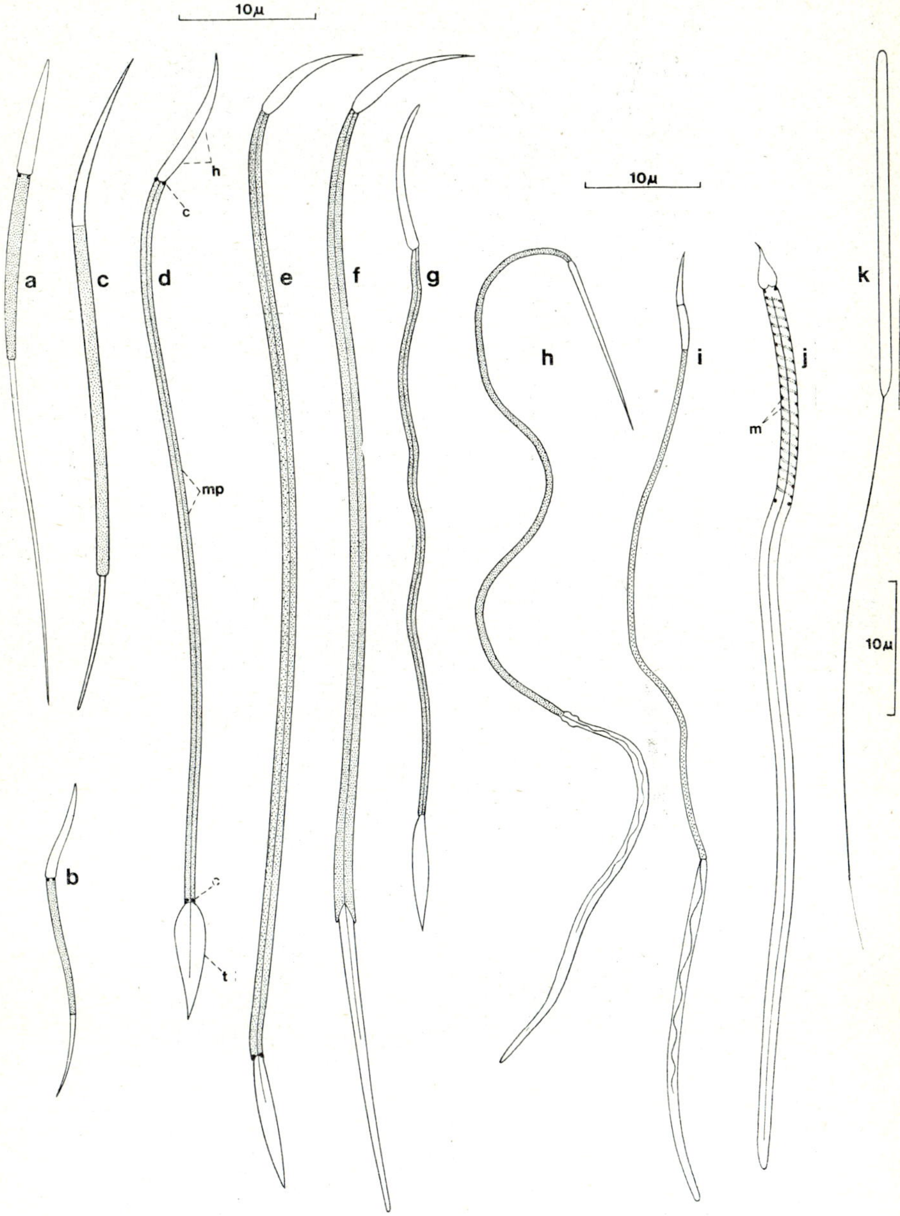

Fig. 2. – Diagrams of spermatozoa within the Bryozoa and the Phoronidea.

a – b, Bryozoa, Cyclostomata. c – g, Bryozoa, Cheilostomata. h – i, Bryozoa, Ctenostomata. j, Bryozoa, Lophopoda. k, Phoronidea.

a, *Diplosolen obelia* (JOHNSTON); b, *Berenicea patina* (LAMARCK); c, *Bicellariella ciliata* (L.); d, *Flustra foliacea* (L.); e, *Caberea ellisii* (FLEMMING); f, *Cryptosula pallasiana* (MOLL); g, *Scrupocellaria scruposa* (L.); h, *Triticella korenii* G. O. SARS; i, *Monobryozoon limicola* FRANZÉN; j, *Plumatella fungosa* (PALL.); k, *Phoronis ovalis* Str. WRIGHT.

a – h, after FRANZÉN (1956). i, after FRANZÉN (1960). c, j, and k original.

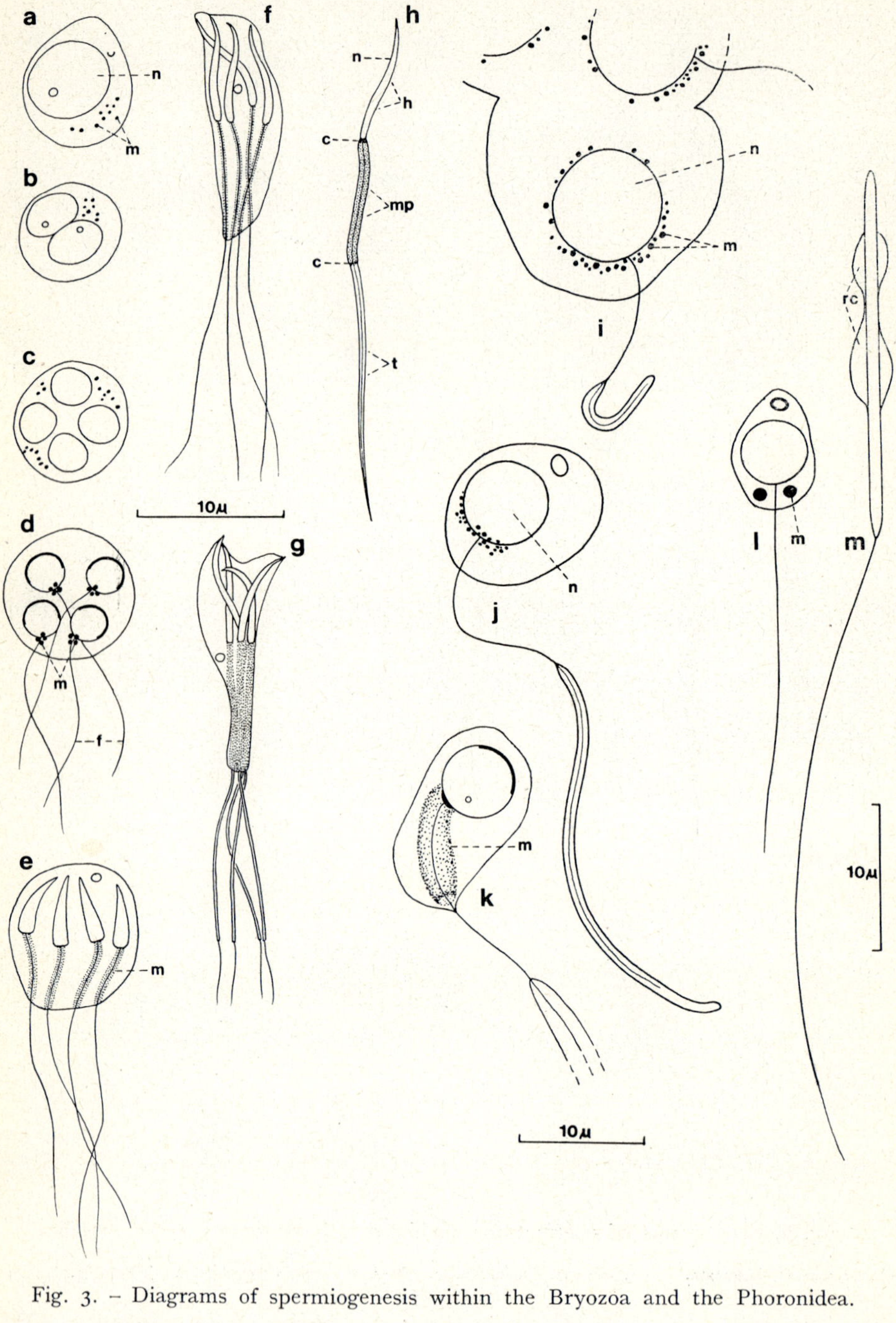

Fig. 3. – Diagrams of spermiogenesis within the Bryozoa and the Phoronidea.

a – g, consecutive stages in spermatid development of the bryozoan *Tubulipora liliacea* (Pallas) (Bryozoa Cyclostomata). h, mature spermatozoon of *T. liliacea*. i – k, consecutive stages in the development of the spermatid in *Plumatella fungosa* (Bryozoa, Lophopoda). l – m, *Phoronis ovalis* (Phoronidae): l, spermatid with mitochondrial material collected in two spheres at the base of the flagellum. m, late spermatid.

a – h after FRANZÉN (1956). i – m original.

other species (Fig. 2 a-c) the mitochondria either form a more homogeneous layer in the cytoplasm of the middle piece or the boundaries of the two strands remain in all cases more diffuse. (Indicated by stippling in the figures).

Fig. 3 i-k show some stages in the development of the spermatozoon in the Lophopoda. Fig. 3 i shows a young spermatid in a cluster of several spermatids. The flagellum has grown out from the future base of the nucleus and mitochondria are collected round the nucleus. A characteristic feature already seen at this stage is a large lump of cytoplasm surrounding the distal end of the flagellum. The mitochondria are collected in a ring near the base of the nucleus, and later in the cytogenesis the mitochondrial material extends backwards along the flagellum. Finally, in the spermatozoon, the mitochondria form a helix in the middle piece (Fig. 2 j).

The two main groups of the Bryozoa, the Stelmatopoda and the Lophopoda, each has its own type of spermatozoon. The most aberrant type is found in the Lophopoda, which are commonly considered as the more primitive group.

Phoronidea.

The spermiogenesis in *Phoronis pallida* Schneider has been described in an earlier paper, FRANZÉN (1956) and I want to add only a few words on an other phoronid, *Phoronis ovalis* Str Wright. When the flagellum of this spermatid has grown out, the mitochondria have collected into two large spheres on either side of the flagellum. The appearance at first of a few then later of two larger mitochondrial spheres is an interesting similarity to the conditions in the bryozoon sub-group Stelmatopoda.

The nucleus undergoes a longitudinal stretching. Initially the cytoplasm is collected around the middle of the nucleus of the late spermatid. In the spermatozoon the mitochondrial-containing middle piece is directly connected with the head (Fig. 2 i) and the tail consists of the long flagellum. The spermatozoon is of a thread-shaped, modified type.

ZIMMER (1967) has studied the morphology and function of accessory reproductive glands in two phoronids. In both species spermatozoa are accumulated within the nephridia later to pass into spermatophoral organs where each sperm mass is molded into a characteristic shape and encased with membranes. The structure of the spermatophore is characteristic for each species. These observations on spermatophore formation provide an explanation why the spermatozoon in the Phoronides is not primitive. This modified type of spermatozoon is related to spermatophore formation.

III. – ANNELIDA

Polychaeta and Archiannelida.

The spermatozoa of Polychaetes have been described already by RETZIUS (1904) who deals with altogether twelve different forms and gives good drawings of the mature spermatozoon. All these spermatozoa are of the pri-

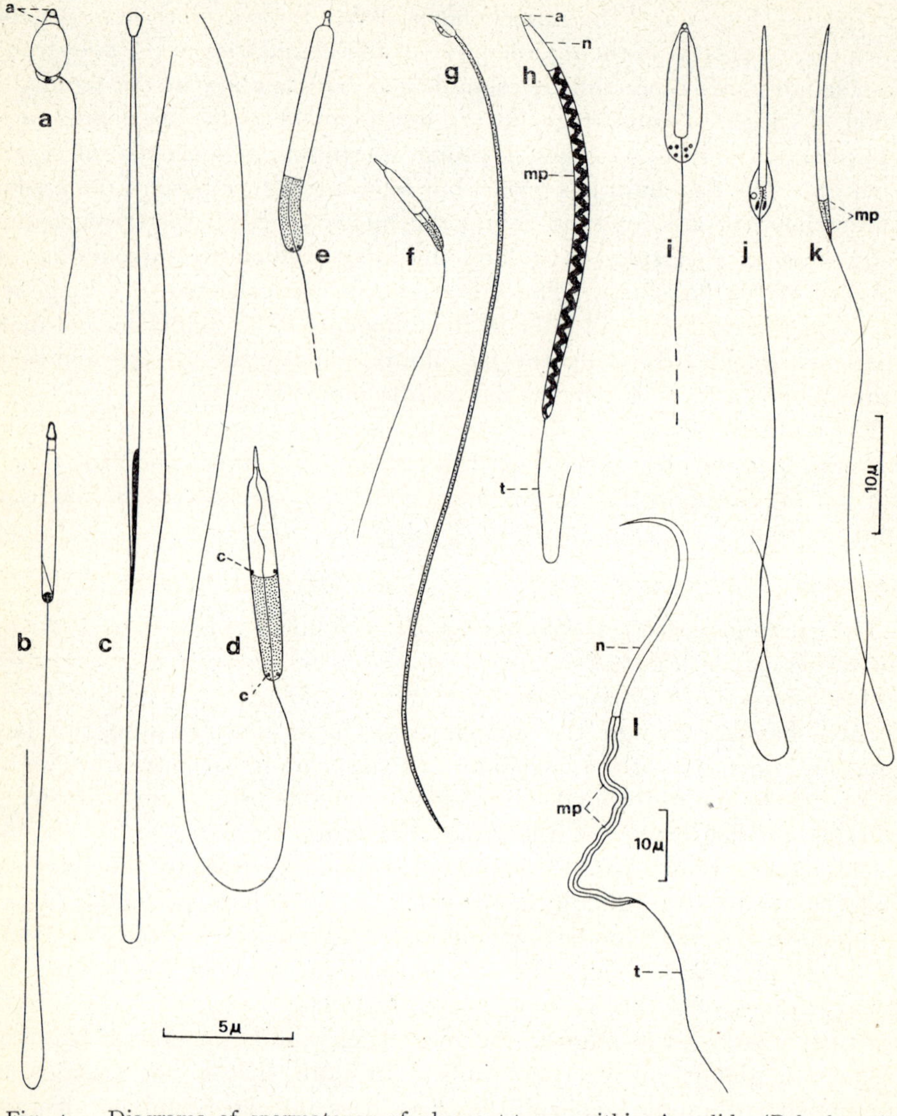

Fig. 4. – Diagrams of spermatozoa of aberrant types within Annelida (Polychaeta).

All figures except i, and j, represent spermatozoa: a, b, and c, family Syllidae: a, *Exogone gemmifera* (Pagenstecher). b, *Grubea clavata* (Clavata). c, *Sphaerosyllis hystrix* Claparede. d, and e, family Spionidae: d, *Polydora ciliata* (Johnston). e, *Pygospio elegans* Claparede. f, family Capitellidae: *Capitella capitata* Fabricius. g, and h, family Sabellidae: g, *Fabricia sabella* (Ehrenberg), h, *Manayunkia aestuarina* Bourne. i – k, family Serpulidae: *Salmacina dysteri* (Huxley). i, and j, spermatids in successive stages of development. k, spermatozoon. l, family Hesionidae: *Hesionides arenaria* Friedrich.

a – h, after Franzén (1956). i – k, after Franzén (1958), 1 after Westheide (1967).

mitive type and it is obvious that this type is retained in most Polychaetes. By a comparative study of the spermiogenesis in several families of Polychaetes I have, however, observed the occurence of aberrant morphology of the spermatozoon in many species (Fig. 4-6). In a number of cases the changes have led to very similar results, and also the spermiogenesis is very similar e.g. in the Spionids (Fig. 4 d, e), the Serpulids (Fig. 4 i - k) and the

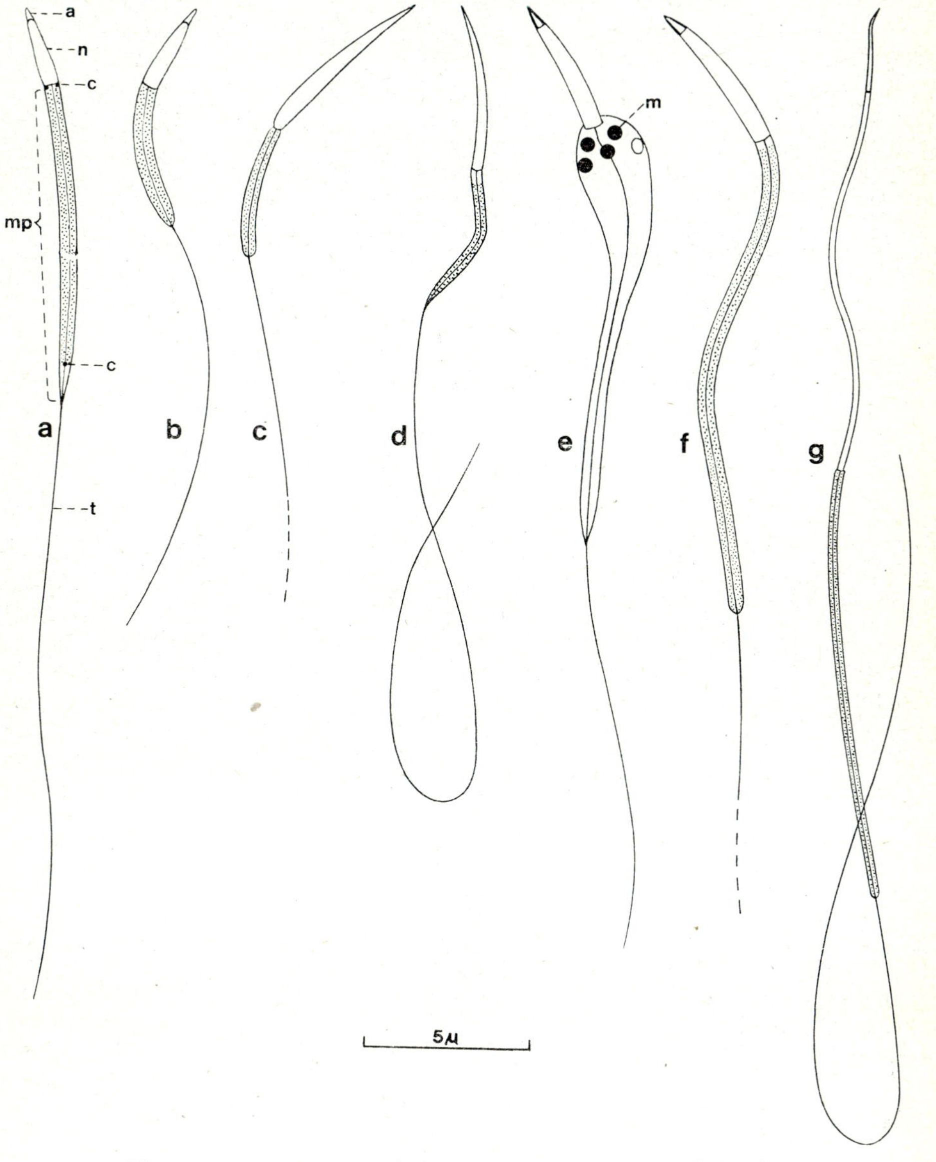

Fig. 5. – Spermatozoa within the polychete genus *Spirorbis*.

a, *S. borealis* Daudin. b, *S. granulatus* (L.). c, *S. spirillum* (L). d, *S. vitreus* (FABRICIUS). e, and f, *S. militaris* Claparede: e, spermatid. f, spermatozoon. g, *S. pagenstecheri* Quatrefages. a – d, after FRANZÉN (1956). e – g, after FRANZÉN (1958).

Capitellid (Fig. 4 f). In other species and families the changes have led in partly other directions, as within the families Syllidae (Fig. 4 a - c), Sabellidae (Fig. 4 g and h) and Hesionidae (Fig. 4 l). The divergences are furthermore greater in the Sabellidae, and this applies to a still higher degree to *Dinophilus*, *Protodrilus* and *Diurodrilus* among the Archiannelida. In some of the Archiannelids, e.g. *Protodrilus* (Fig. 6 c) no primitive characters can

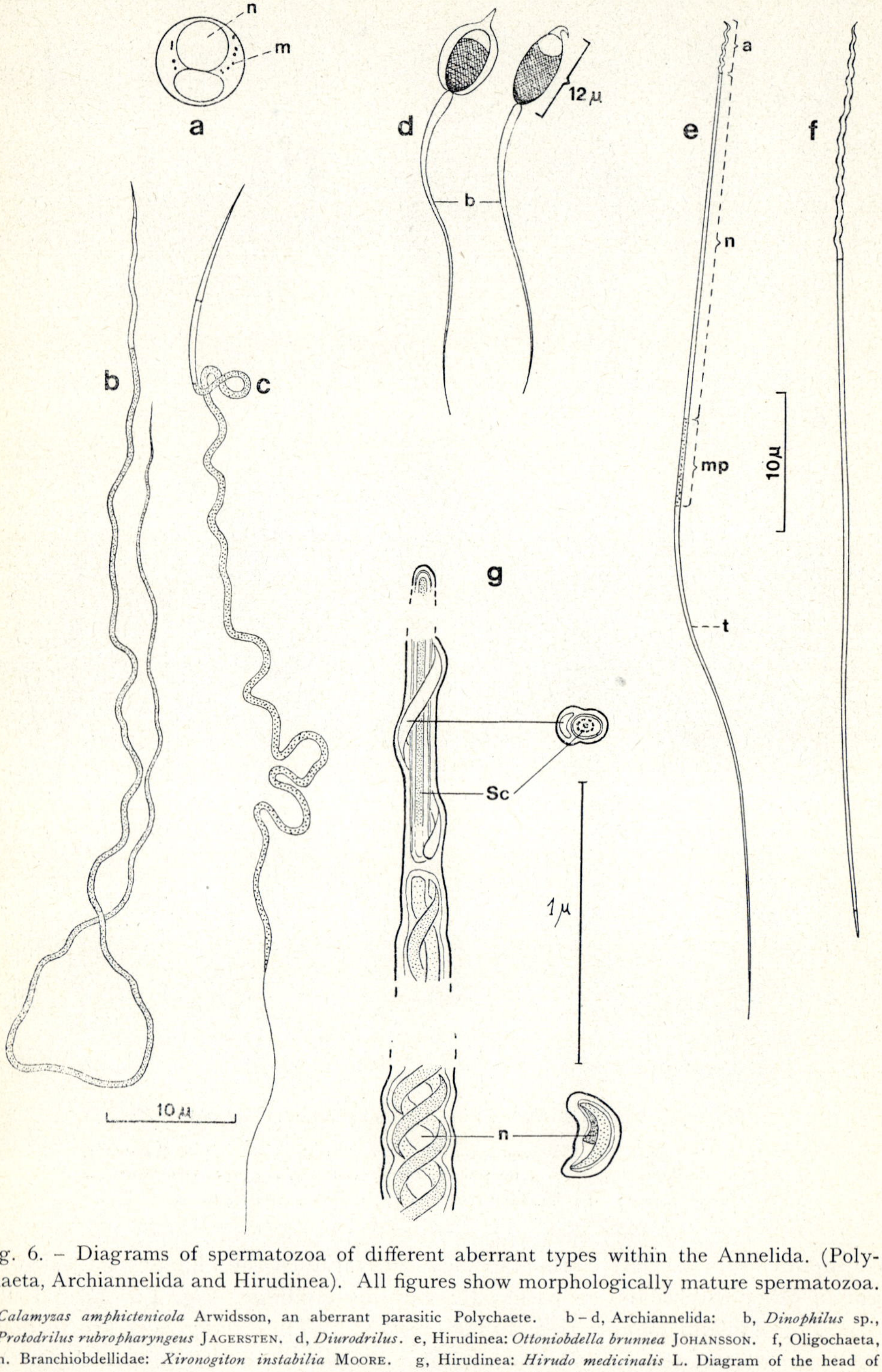

Fig. 6. – Diagrams of spermatozoa of different aberrant types within the Annelida. (Polychaeta, Archiannelida and Hirudinea). All figures show morphologically mature spermatozoa.

a, *Calamyzas amphictenicola* Arwidsson, an aberrant parasitic Polychaete. b – d, Archiannelida: b, *Dinophilus* sp., c, *Protodrilus rubropharyngeus* JAGERSTEN. d, *Diurodrilus*. e, Hirudinea: *Ottoniobdella brunnea* JOHANSSON. f, Oligochaeta, fam. Branchiobdellidae: *Xironogiton instabilia* MOORE. g, Hirudinea: *Hirudo medicinalis* L. Diagram of the head of the spermatozoon. Sc = stereocilia.

a, original. b, and c, after FRANZÉN (1956). e, and f, after FRANZÉN (1962). d, after AX (1967). g, after PASTISSON (1966), somewhat simplified.

be traced during the cytogenesis. In the aberrant Polychaete *Calamyzas* (Fig. 6 a) the spermatozoon agrees superficially with ordinary cells. Neither in the spermatids, nor in the spermatozoa of *Calamyzas amphictenicola*, studied by phase contrast microscopy only, have I found any flagella. The absence of flagellum in the spermatozoon of this species is obviously the result of reduction. The genus *Spirorbis* shows a variation of the morphology of the spermatozoon within one genus (Fig. 5). The spermatozoa are here of three morphological types. So far as is known all species of *Spirorbis* are hermaphrodite, and the embryos are incubated in the tube or in the operculum.

In all species of Polychaeta and Archiannelida with modified types of spermatozoa it is possible to link up the changes in sperm morphology with an altered biology of propagation.

Oligochaeta and Hirudinea.

In these two groups of Annelids the spermatozoa are of modified types in all species studied. The nucleus generally is very elongated (Fig. 6 e, f and g). PASTISSON (1966) has described a complicated helicoidal structure in the head. The total lack in the spermiogenesis of stages with four mitochondrial aggregates, so characteristic in the Polychaeta indicates that in these groups the spermatozoon is more modified than in the polychaetes.

In Oligochaeta and Hirudinea also the biology of fertilization is more modified from the primitive conditions than in most polychaetes.

IV. – MOLLUSCA

Gastropoda.

The spermatozoon in Diotocardia (with the exception of the fam. Neritidae) is the original type of spermatozoon in Metazoa. Both head and middlepiece are short, the most remarkable characteristic of the middle piece being the presence of distinct mitochondrial spheres. In Monotocardia this is a transient stage in the spermiogenesis. The mitochondrial spheres dissolve and the mitochondrial material is distributed evenly over a more or less elongated cytoplasm cylinder behind the nucleus. The length of the head varies greatly but compared with Diotocardia one may say that the nucleus tends to be elongated. Since the middle piece is elongated as well, the whole spermatozoon looks like a thread of even width, and the thin tail flagellum is often relatively short.

A good example of the visible changes during spermiogenesis may be seen in development of the sperm of the gastropod *Partulida* (fam. Pyramidellidae). During spermiogenesis the cytoplasm glides down along the filament at the same time as the cell assumes an oval shape. The nucleus moves to the pole of the cell opposite the filament. Gradually the latter develops a

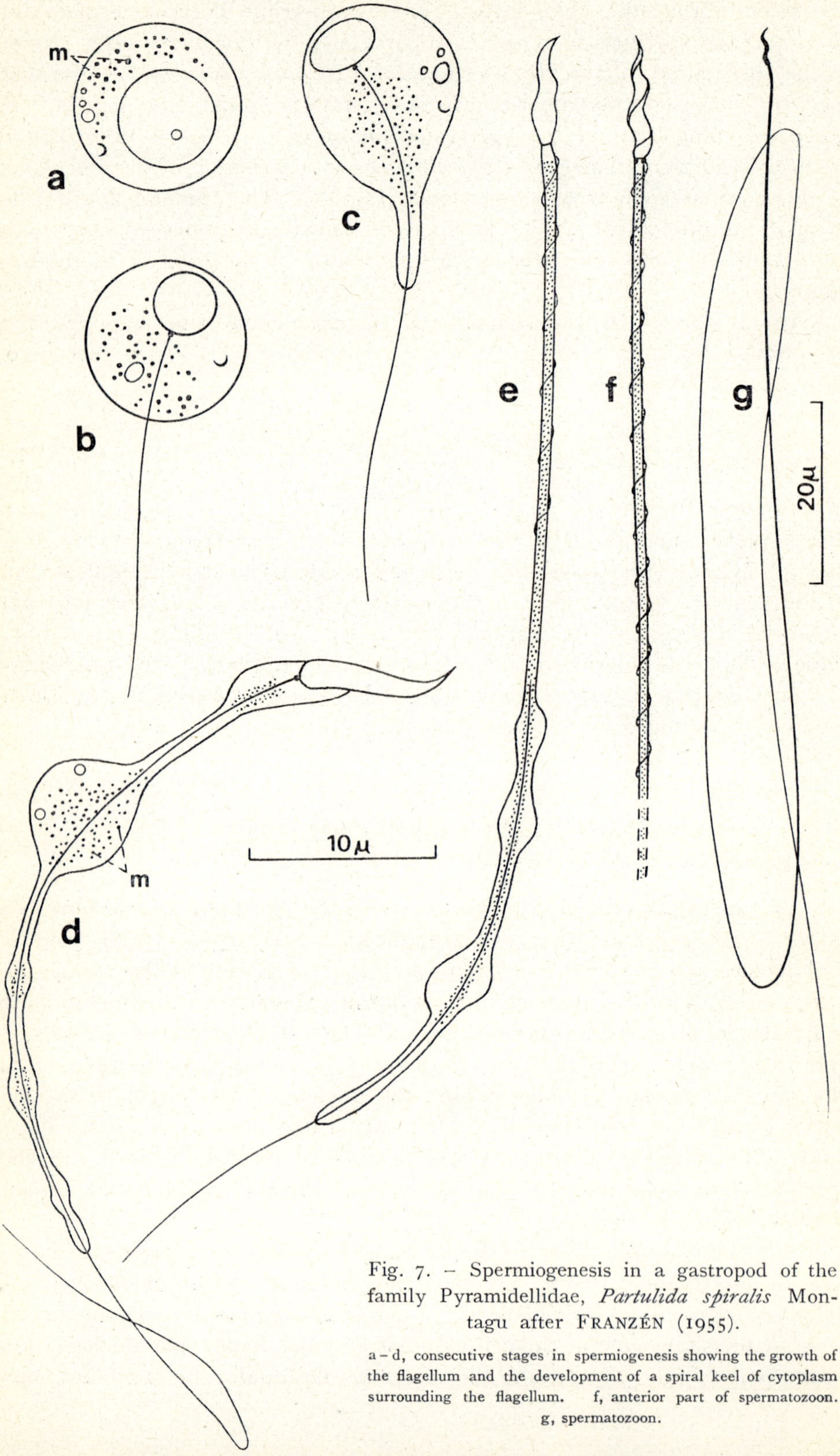

Fig. 7. – Spermiogenesis in a gastropod of the family Pyramidellidae, *Partulida spiralis* Montagu after FRANZÉN (1955).

a–d, consecutive stages in spermiogenesis showing the growth of the flagellum and the development of a spiral keel of cytoplasm surrounding the flagellum. f, anterior part of spermatozoon. g, spermatozoon.

cytoplasmic sheath. The mitochondria, which to begin with are more or less irregularly distributed in the cell gather along the flagellum in an elliptical mass. However, they do not form big spheres, but the mitochondrial mass divides into several parts at the same time the cytoplasm continues to move down the flagellum, forming drop-like swellings. At the centre of these cytoplasm drops or lumps the thin flagellum can be seen, and scattered around this in the cytoplasm are numerous still small mitochondria. Gradually these mitochondria form an apparently homogeneous cylindrical sheath around the filament. This sheath of cytoplasm and mitochondria gets so dense that in a mature sperm it is impossible to detect the flagellum it envelops.

As the development proceeds the outer surface of cytoplasm around the filament forms a spiral-formed, light elevation or keel. In mature spermatozoa this looks more or less like a spiral thread wound around the central axis, which consists of the flagellum and its adjacent covering of cytoplasm and mitochondrial sheath. The spiral thread as well as the central rod taper off towards the tip. Of the morphologically mature spermatozoon, which is 300 μ long, the head forms a very small part. Most of the threadlike spermatozoon consists of a middle piece, which without any sharp demarcation merges into the tail filament. By middle piece I mean that part of the flagellum where the cytoplasmic sheath with its mitochondrial material is thickest. Since the structures in the posterior part get extremely fine it is impossible to determine where the mitochondrial sheath stops and the actual sperm tail begins. The cytoplasm not used in the formation of the plasma sheath is shed as so-called residual cytoplasm, and some of it flows into the cytophore that forms the centre of the radial " aster " of spermatids during one phase of histogenesis. It is impossible ot see any special nutrient cells in the mass of cytoplasm around which the spermatids are arranged.

The investigation into the cytogenesis shows that in *Partulida* the central strand of the spermatozoon tail at least in its anterior part directly corresponds to the mitochondrial sheath around the axial filament in the sperms of the primitive type, but there are great differences as to the details of the part played by the cytoplasm and the components of the cytoplasm during histogenesis. I shall return to this subject below.

At the same time as the flagellum grows out and the cytoplasm glides down it the nucleus elongates and assumes a conical shape. At the same time it twists into a spiral and decreases in size. The spiral effect is enhanced by the presence of a surrounding spiral seam or keel. This keel appears to be composed of differentiated cytoplasm. The spiral twist and tapering towards the tip gives the head of the mature sperm the appearance of a corkscrew. The tip is capped by an insignificant acrosome.

When comparing the spermiogenesis and the morphology of the sperm of different members of Gastropoda it is impossible to ignore the rather close similarities between Opistobranchia and Pulmonata.

TUZET (1940) does indeed point out certain differences, such as that in Opistobranchia. The head of the sperm is surrounded by a perinuclear, spiral filament while in Pulmonata it has an intranuclear, straight filament. Other authors show, however, that in many pulmonates the filament does not traverse the whole nucleus, but stops short off the centre counting from the base of the nucleus. Conditions are thus the same as those I have described for *Actaeon tornalis* (L.), *Philine aperta* (L.) and other species. The length of the head of the spermatozoon is no distinguishing mark either. It is true that in *Acera*, *Cylidina* and *Aplysia* the head of the sperm is relatively longer than in the pulmonates, but other opistobranchids, such as *Actaeon*, *Philine*, *Tritonia*, *Onchidoris* and others, agree with the pulmonates in this respect. The spiral twist of the head in opistobranchid sperms may possibly be a trait peculiar to this group, but *Philine aperta* forms an exception, and so does one pyramidellid, *Brachystomia* where I have not been able to find a true spiral filament.

To sum up, the argument may be stated as follows. The spermiogenesis and morphology of the spermatozoon are essentially similar in Opistobranchia and Pulmonata. The similarities are especially marked in comparison with Prosobranchia, where the type of sperm and spermiohistogenesis are quite different. These facts support the hypothesis that Opistobranchia and Pulmonata are closely related, a belief that has led to the inclusion of these two groups in Eutyneura as distinct from Prosobranchia or Streptoneura.

Polyplacophora, Bivalvia and Scaphopoda.

In these groups nearly all the species investigated are found to retain the primitive type of spermatozoon. A common feature regarding the reproduction of all these groups is that there are no copulative organs and that both ovum and sperm are usually simply shed into the water, where the egg is fertilized. This is undoubtedly the original mode of fertilization in Metazoa. It is true that in Bivalvia there has been a change in the reproductive process of several species, especially fresh water forms. Here the eggs are not released into the water but remain inside the mother animal, where they are fertilized and undergo part of their embryonic development. However, though fertilization is internal there are no male copulative organs and the sperms are released in the usual manner directly into the water. They are then sucked with the breathing water into the mantle cavity of the female, where fertilization apparently takes place.

However, deviations from the primitive type of spermatozoon occur in some groups of bivalves too. According to OCKELMAN (1964) the typical Veneracean spermatozoon shows a slightly bent conical head with a distinct acrosome and four mitochondrial spheres in the middle piece. In *Turtonia minuta* (Fabricius) the head of the spermatozoon is elongated and spirally coiled. Its acrosome also differs somewhat from the Veneracean type. *Turtonia* shows certain specializations with respect to reproduction. Fertilization seems to take place in the mantle cavity prior to the formation of the egg– capsule.

Cephalopoda.

As is well known, it is a common feature of the differentiation of most types of flagellated spermatozoa that the mitochondria are located adjacent to the proximal part of the axial filament in the region posterior to the nucleus. The concentrations, in the decapodan cephalopods, of the mitochondria in a single large mass separated from the issuing point of the tail filament is a surprising exception from this rule. It is also surprising that the two main groups of recent cephalopods differ so much concerning the morphology of their male genital cells. In the octopodan cephalopods the sperm is atypical in having a head and tail but no distinct middlepiece. Most spermatozoa, even of highly aberrant types, have an obvious middle piece.

A study of the spermiogenesis in the two octopodan genera *Eledone* and *Octopus* shows that the spermatozoon in *Eledone* has arisen from the type found in *Octopus*.

To me it appears natural to interpret the difference in size of eggs and in appearance and biology of the juvenile stage in *Octopus* and *Eledone* as expressing an evolution from the *Octopus*-type towards the *Eledone*-type. The difference in the morphology of the sperm and in spermiogenesis is another expression of this evolution, and is connected with the difference in size of egg and ontogeny. The evolution has proceeded towards eggs of larger size containing more yolk and towards a more complicated sperm provided with spiral structure. The spermogenesis has been lengthened by a phase that has given rise to an extremely strongly altered spermatozoon. The whole biology of propagation has undergone a major alteration.

V. – Tunicata.

The spermatozoa of many ascidians are characterized by a moderately elongated head followed immediately by a tail-flagellum. A middle piece of the usual construction and position is lacking; however, the lateral body visible at the side of the nucleus, (Fig. 8 b, c and in Fig. 1, symbol 3) contains the cell's mitochondria.

In my earlier study on ascidian spermatozoa Franzén (1956) I did not find mature spermatozoa of *Trididemnum tenerum*. All specimens studied contained only spermatids which still possessed a considerable remnant of cytoplasm. In such late spermatids (Fig. 8 d) the nucleus is bent in a characteristic zigzag way. During the later phases in spermiogenesis the nucleus becomes very elongated and blends in with the mitochondria of the lateral body.

In order to discuss the ascidian spermatozoa I shall describe cytology of the spermatozoa of *Doliolum* (Fig. 8 f). Head and middle piece with mitochondria not clearly visible merge into one another without marked external boundary. In an earlier paper (1958) I gave a short description of the spermatozoa in *Pyrosoma* and *Salpa*.

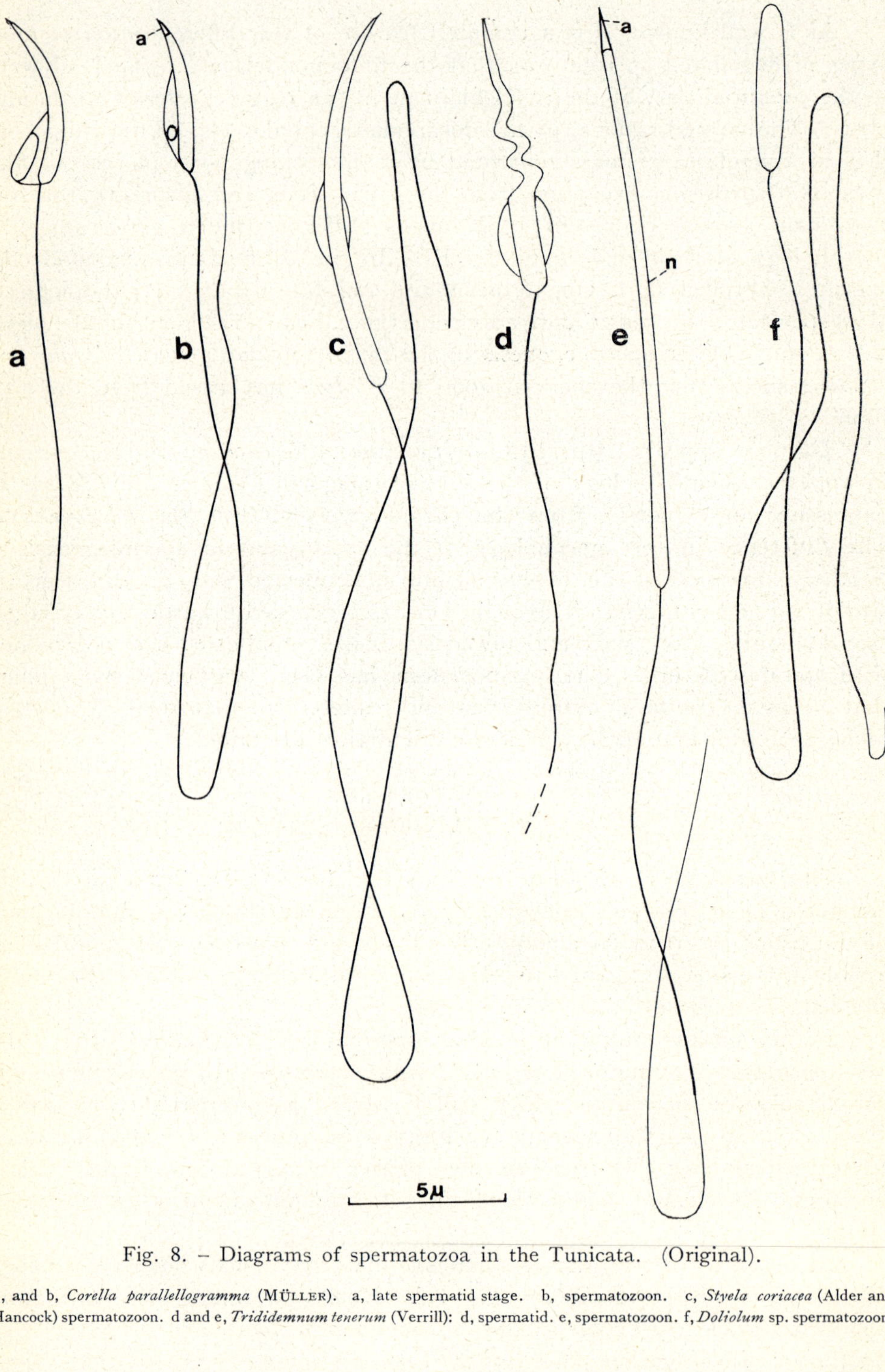

Fig. 8. – Diagrams of spermatozoa in the Tunicata. (Original).

a, and b, *Corella parallellogramma* (MÜLLER). a, late spermatid stage. b, spermatozoon. c, *Styela coriacea* (Alder and Hancock) spermatozoon. d and e, *Trididemnum tenerum* (Verrill): d, spermatid. e, spermatozoon. f, *Doliolum* sp. spermatozoon.

It is important to note that in all species from the two tunicate subgroups studied by me, Ascidiacea and Thaliacea, the spermatozoa have a wide range of head lengths and have a tail consisting of a long flagellum often terminating in an end piece. A middle piece with mitochondrial spheres as in the primitive type of spermatozoon is lacking. The mitochondria in the spermatozoon of ascidians are generally collected in a lateral body. It should be mentioned, however, that TUZET and HARANT have described ascidian spermatozoa which correspond to the primitive type.

REFERENCES

AX P. (1963) – *Relationships and phylogeny of the Turbellaria,* in E. C. Dougherty (edit.), The lower Metazoa, Berkeley and Los Angeles, Univ. California Press, 191–224.

AX P. (1967) – Diurodrilus ankeli *nov. spec.* (*Archiannelida*) *von der nordamerikanischen Pazifikküste.* « Z. Morph. Ökol. Tiere », 60, 5–16.

DAMAS D. (1968) – *Les cellules germinales mâles de* Glossiphonia complanata (*L.*), (Hirudinee, Rhynchobdelle). *Origine, évolution et structure.* « Bull. Soc. Zool. Fr. », 93, 375–385.

EZELL S. D. (1963) – *The lateral body of* Ciona intestinalis *spermatozoa.* « Exp. Cell Res. », 30, 615–617.

FRANZÉN Å. (1955) – *Comparative morphological investigations into the spermiogenesis among Mollusca.* « Zool. Bidr. », Uppsala, 30, 399–456.

FRANZÉN Å. (1956) – *On spermiogenesis, morphology of the spermatozoon, and biology of fertilization among invertebrates.* Ibid., 31, 355–482.

FRANZÉN Å. (1958) – *On sperm morphology and acrosome filament formation in some Annelida, Echiuroidea and Tunicata.* Ibid., 33, 1–28.

FRANZÉN Å. (1960) – Monobryozoon limicola *n. sp., a ctenostomatous bryozoan from the detritus layer on soft sediment.* Ibid., 33, 135–148.

FRANZÉN Å. (1962). – *Notes on the morphology and histology of* Xironogiton instabilia (*Moore 1893*) (*Fam. Branchiobdellidae*) *with special references to the muscle cells.* Ibid., 35, 369–383.

FRANZÉN Å. (1967 a) – *Spermiogenesis and spermatozoa of the Cephalopoda.* « Ark. Zool. », ser. 2, 19, 323–334.

FRANZÉN Å. (1967 b) – *Remarks on spermiogenesis and morphology of the spermatozoon among the lower Metazoa.* Ibid., 19, 335–342.

OCKELMANN K. W. (1964) – Turtonia minuta (*Fabricius*), *a neotenous veneracean bivalve.* « Ophelia », 1, 121–146.

PASTISSON C. (1966) – *Anatomie ultrastructurale du spermatozoide de la sangsue* Hirudo medicinalis *L.* « Ann. Université et A.R.E.R.S. », 4, 67–75.

RETZIUS G. (1904) – *Zur Kenntnis des Spermien der Evertebraten.* « Biol. Untersuch. N. F. », 11, N : o 1, 1–32.

TUZET O. and HARANT H. (1930) – *Sur la spermatogenèse d'une Ascidie* Stylea partita (Stimpson). « C. R. Soc. Biol. Paris », 105, 299–301.

TUZET O. (1940) – *Sur la spermatogenèse de l'*Oncidiella celtica *Cuv.* « Arch. Zool. exp. gén. », 81, 371–394.

WESTHEIDE W. (1967) – *Monographie der Gattungen* Hesionides *Friedrich und* Microphthalmus *Mecznikow* (Polychaeta, Hesionidae). « Z. Morph. Tiere », 61, 1–159.

ZIMMER R. L. (1967) – *The morphology and function of accessory reproductive glands in the Lophophores of* Phoronis vancouverensis *and* Phoronopsis harmeri. « J. Morph. », 121, 159–178.

Discussion

MEYER. – A short question about the length of sperm. Is there any relation with the evolutionary pattern you have demonstrated so beautifully?

FRANZÉN. – No! There is a marked difference in the length of the primitive type of sperm in the primitive gastropod group Archaeogastropoda and the modified type of sperm in the gastropod group Opistobranchia, but there is no simple answer to the question of the length of the sperm. It can be noted that the spermatozoon of the polychaete *Tomopteris* has two flagella. Each flagellum is about half as long as would be expected in a spermatozoon with so big a head (FRANZÉN 1958).

REGER. – Dr. FRANZÉN, you commented on spermatophore in *Phoronidae,* either on the basis of your own work or that of Dr. ZIMMER. Could you clarify and detail this? We have also studied *Phoronid* sperm and have not seen spermatophore formation. Perhaps this is a species difference because some species self-fertilize.

FRANZÉN. – My comment on spermatophore in Phoronida was based on the study by ZIMMER. In the simultaneous hermaphroditic *Phoronis vancouverensis*, both accessory spermatophoral organs and nidamental glands are found. The accessory spermatophoral organs are paired glands placed to either side of the midline in the floor of the lophophoral cavity. Being accessory male reproductive organs, accessory spermatophoral organs are limited to males of the dioecious *Phoronopsis harmeri.* They undergo cyclic changes related to the breeding season.

The spermatophore of *Phoronopsis harmeri* consists of two portions, a spherical part containing the packed spermatozoa and a long spiral membrane. The spermatophora of *Phoronis vancouverensis* consists only of a capsule of spermatozoa.

ZIMMER mention that the unique role of the enclosed lophophoral organs in spermatophore formation and the presence of such organs in all but one species of Phoronida indicates that spermatophore production is practiced by all phoronids with enclosed lophophoral glands.

ANDRÉ. – In view of what you just said about the acrosome, how would you propose to apply your theory to Teleosts, which have no acrosome?

FRANZÉN. – What I said about the acrosome is not intended to be a theory. I only wanted to emphasize the fact that there are some types of spermatozoa where an acrosomal structure in front of the nucleus is not observed. On the other hand, observations on Teleost spermatozoa comfirm my theory that the morphology of the spermatozoon is related to the mode of fertilization. The direct dependence of the morphology of the spermatozoon on the biology of fertilization limits of course greatly the possibility of utilizing the spermatozoa for systematic purposes.

L. Nicander (*)

COMPARATIVE STUDIES ON THE FINE STRUCTURE OF VERTEBRATE SPERMATOZOA

SUMMARY. — A survey is given of the fine structure of spermatozoa in vertebrates, especially the acrosome region, the centriolar region, and accessory tail structures. A true acrosome is present except in teleost fishes. It is most often cap-shaped, but lateral in frogs and an apical body in passerine birds and lampreys. Some subacrosomal material is generally present, except in frogs, passerine birds and possibly some mammals. It forms a rod that penetrates into the nucleus in some birds and urodele amphibians, and runs through the nucleus into the tail in lampreys, where it plays an important role in fertilization. Nothing is known about its function in the other sperm types.

The centriolar region generally shows two centrioles, except in passerine birds. Pericentriolar material often forms complicated structures in the neck region. The centrioles are often modified. The distal one may show a structure similar to the region of transfer from the basal body to the shaft in cilia. The mitochondrial sheath seen in some groups with external fertilization may have importance for the penetration of the thick egg coatings in these groups. A helical structure of the whole cell is seen in eslasmobranchs and passerine birds, where the spermatozoa rotate around their longitudinal axis. Accessory tail structures are often present in a plane through the two central filaments of the flagellum.

RIASSUNTO. — Viene esposto un esame sulla fine struttura degli spermatozoi dei Vertebrati, specialmente della regione acrosomale, della regione centriolare, e delle strutture accessorie della coda. Un vero acrosoma è presente in tutti tranne che nei pesci Teleostei. Generalmente è a forma di cappuccio, si presenta lateralmente nella Rana e come un corpo apicale nel Passero e nella Lampreda. Materiale subacrosomale è quasi sempre presente tranne che nella Rana nel Passero e in alcuni mammiferi. Esso forma un bastone che penetra nel nucleo in alcuni uccelli e anfibi urodeli, e corre attraverso il nucleo fino alla coda nelle lamprede, dove gioca un importante ruolo nella fertilizzazione. Non si conoscono le sue funzioni negli altri tipi di spermi.

La regione centriolare presenta generalmente due centrioli salvo che nel Passero. Il materiale pericentriolare spesso forma complicate strutture nella regione del collo. I centrioli sono spesso modificati. Quello distale può mostrare una struttura simile alla regione prossima al corpuscolo basale delle ciglia. La guaina mitocondriale vista in alcuni gruppi a fecondazione esterna può avere importanza per la penetrazione nelle uova dal guscio robusto di questi gruppi. Una struttura elicata dell'intera cellula si nota negli Elasmobranchi e nel Passero, in cui gli spermatozoi ruotano intorno al loro asse longitudinale. Strutture accessorie della coda sono spesso presenti in un piano passante per i due filamenti centrali del flagello.

(*) Department of Anatomy and Histology and Laboratory of Electron Microscopy, Royal Veterinary College, Stockholm, Sweden.

No survey of the fine structure of vertebrate sperm has been found in the literature. The present paper gives such a survey, based on my own observations and available literature. The paper will discuss the acrosomal region, characteristics of the tail, and some features of the centrioles and the pericentriolar structures. A short report of some of the original observations has been published (NICANDER, 1968).

MATERIAL AND METHODS

Material was collected from cyclostomes (*Lampetra fluviatilis*, *Myxine glutinosa*), an elasmobranch (*Raja clavata*), teleosts (*Salmo solar*, *Esox lucius*, *Xiphophorus helleri*), urodele (*Triturus cristatus*) and anuran (*Rana temporaria*, *Bufo vulgaris*) amphibians, birds (*Gallus domesticus*, *Taeniopyga castanotis*), and the common domestic and laboratory mammals. Pieces of testis and excurrent ducts were fixed in osmium tetroxide, or in glutaraldehyde followed by osmium tetroxide, and embedded in Epon. Sections were cut with glass knives, stained with lead acetate and uranyl acetate, and studied in a Siemens Elmiskop I electron microscope.

OBSERVATION AND DISCUSSION

The acrosomal region generally comprises an *acrosome*, derived from the Golgi apparatus, and some *subacrosomal material*. The most common type of acrosome is cap-shaped. It is found in *Myxine* (Fig. 2), a lungfish, *Protopterus annectens* (BOISSON, MATTEI and MATTEI, 1967), skates, salamanders (Fig. 5; BARKER and BIESELE, 1967, PICHERAL, 1967), toads (Fig. 1; BURGOS and FAWCETT, 1956), reptiles (BOISSON and MATTEI, 1966, FURIERI, 1962–63, 1965, YASUZUMI and YASUDA, 1968), the domestic fowl (Fig. 4; NAGANO, 1962, LAKE, SMITH and YOUNG, 1968), and mammals (cfr. NICANDER and BANE, 1966). Frogs have a lateral cap (Fig. 3). An apical vesicle is seen in lampreys (Fig. 8; cfr. STANLEY, 1967), and an apical, solid body in passerine birds (Fig. 27; FURIERI, 1961, 1962–63). The absence of any acrosomal structure in teleost fishes (Fig. 9; FURIERI, 1962) has been repeatedly confirmed by others. No differentiation of the acrosomal cap reminiscent of the equatorial segment in mammals has been observed in the sperm of submammalian groups. *Subacrosomal material* is scanty or absent in frogs (Fig. 3), passerine birds, and some mammals. In sperm types with a cap-shaped acrosome it may be a thin, amorphous layer, as in the hagfish (Fig. 2) and most reptiles (BOISSON and MATTEI, 1966, FURIERI, 1965) and mammals, or form small rods above and along the tip of the nucleus, as in toads (Fig. 1; BURGOS and FAWCETT, 1956). In salamanders (Figs. 5, 6; PICHÉRAL, 1967) and the domestic fowl (Fig. 4; NAGANO, 1962) there is a long, dense subacrosomal rod that penetrates deep into the nucleus and is surrounded by some substance of different opacity. In *Triturus* a honey-comb structure is suggested in cross sections of the rod (Fig. 6). The subacrosomal material in lampreys is still more complicated, with a dense, subacrosomal ring and a long, helical fibre running through the nucleus and far back in the tail, surrounded by the membranes of the nuclear envelope (Figs. 8, 14, 15; *cf.* STANLEY, 1967). This structure plays a prominent rôle during fertilization in lampreys. It is extruded to form the core of a true acrosomal tubule during the acrosome reaction (NICANDER and SJÖDÉN, 1968). This seems to be the only known example in a vertebrate of an acrosome reaction with the formation of a true acrosomal tubule, which makes the first contact with the egg surface as in many invertebrates (cfr. COLWIN and COLWIN, 1967). The mammalian sperm also shows a typical acrosome reaction, but the first contact with the plasma membrane of the egg is made by the postacrosomal region of the sperm head (cfr. BEDFORD, 1968). The function, if any, of the subacrosomal material in other vertebrates than lampreys thus remains obscure, though recent cytochemical studies (BUONGIORNO and BERTOLINI, 1967) suggest the presence of lysosomal enzymes in this material in *Triturus*.

The absence of an acrosome in teleost fishes corresponds to the presence of micropyles in the egg envelopes.

Structures similar to the postacrosomal dense lamina ("postnuclear cap") of mammalian spermatozoa have not been observed in other vertebrate sperm types. A material with a fine structure reminiscent of this dense lamina is present in salamander sperm heads (Fig. 6; PICHERAL, 1967), but it is located inside the nuclear envelope and probably constitutes non-chromatin nuclear material. This also applies to a band with similar location in skate sperm heads (Fig. 7), known from light microscopy (BALLOWITZ, 1890) to form a helix.

The spermatozoa of vertebrates generally show two centrioles instead of the single basal body of cilia. Structural modifications of one or both centrioles and the formation of some pericentriolar material are common features (cfr. SOTELO and TRUJILLO-CENÓZ, 1958). Vertebrate sperm tails also have at least some accessory structures around the flagellum proper with its 9 + 2 pattern of microtubules. A mitochondrial collar or sheath is the best known structure. Other common features are extra structures in a plane through the two central microtubules which is perpendicular to the plane of the beat in cilia.

Teleost fishes have a low mitochondrial collar (Fig. 9; BOISSON, MATTEI and MATTEI, 1968, FURIERI, 1962, STANLEY, 1969) if fertilization is external but a high collar with many mitochondria in viviparous species (DADONE and NARBAITZ, 1967, PORTE and FOLLENIUS, 1960). Folds of the tail plasma membrane form ridges in a plane through the two central microtubules in many species (Fig. 10; BOISSON, MATTEI and MATTEI, 1968, SOTELO and TRUJILLO-CENÓZ, 1958, STANLEY, 1969). Only one high ridge is seen in *Esox lucius* (Fig. 11). These ridges probably increase the efficiency of the tail beat. The proximal centriole is small and sometimes modified (BOISSON, MATTEI and MATTEI, 1969, DADONE and NARBAITZ, 1967, STANLEY, 1969). Dense material forms around this centriole (Fig. 12), especially between it and the distal one. This material may show cross-striation or "segmentation" reminiscent of that in the neck region of spermatozoa in mammals and passerine birds and in ciliary rootlets. Part of the distal centriole shows tubular doublets instead of triplets (BOISSON, MATTEI and MATTEI, 1968, 1969, STANLEY, 1969). This arrangement is similar to that seen in the "neck" of common cilia, between the basal body proper and the ciliary shaft. Fish spermatozoa with two tails have been observed in a lungfish (BOISSON, MATTEI and MATTEI, 1967) and a teleost (STANLEY, 1965 b), and aflagellar spermatozoa with two centrioles have also been reported in a fish (MATTEI, BOISSON, MATTEI, and REIZER, 1967).

Cyclostome spermatozoa have a mitochondrial sheath (Figs. 15, 16), which is long and irregular in lampreys (Fig. 15; STANLEY, 1967) and supported by longitudinal microtubules. Lamprey spermatozoa also have nine peripheral dense fibres along the peripheral doublets. Their typical centrioles lie side by side in a deep pit in the base of the nucleus (Fig. 14).

Sharks (STANLEY, 1965 a) and skates (Fig. 25) have a mitochondrial sheath around a pile of dense plates probably formed from pericentriolar material. The rather simple distal centriole is situated at the end of this middle piece. The tail comprises two dense, coarse longitudinal columns, always situated in a plane through the two central doublets of the flagellum (Fig. 26). As the columns obviously run a helical course (Fig. 25), this means that the flagellum proper is twisted in these spermatozoa, which seem to rotate around their longitudinal axis (STANLEY, 1965 a).

Sperm tails in amphibians show a variety of accessory structures. Frogs have a simple flagellum with a long mitochondrial sheath (Fig. 13). The presence of a true mitochondrial sheath in frogs and lampreys, which have external fertilization, seems surprising. FRANZÉN (1956) has published a theory, based on extensive comparative studies on sperm types in invertebrates, according to which primitive sperm types, discharged into water, have a low mitochondrial collar. A modified middle piece would be associated with discharge in more viscous media than water. However, in lampreys and frogs the spermatozoa have to swim through thick egg coatings. Similar conditions are present in toads, where the sperm tail has a high mitochondrial collar as well as an undulating membrane in the plane of the central microtubules (Figs. 17, 18; BURGOS and FAWCETT, 1956, FURIERI, 1961). FRANZÉN's (1956) theory may thus be valid for vertebrate sperm types, too.

Urodele amphibians have sperm tails with an undulating membrane (BARKER and BIESELE, 1967, PICHERAL, 1967) attached to a coarse rod originating from pericentriolar material in the base of the head (Fig. 19). The mitochondria form a sheath around the rod (Figs. 19, 20) and the flagellum runs in the free margin of the undulating membrane, with a dense, flattened column in the plane of the two central flagellar microtubules (Fig. 20).

Reptile spermatozoa (AUSTIN, 1965, FURIERI, 1965, HAMILTON and FAWCETT, 1968) have a complicated neck piece, a mitochondrial sheath, and a fibrous sheath that continues under the mitochondrial sheath up to the neck, in snakes (AUSTIN, 1965, HAMILTON and FAWCETT, 1968). Nine coarse peripheral fibres are also seen, as in mammals (cfr. FAWCETT, 1965) but those two in a plane through the central flagellar fibres are largest and are attached to the fibrous sheath.

Bird sperm tails have been studied in the domestic fowl and in passerine species only. Fowl spermatozoa have short tails with the mitochondrial sheath surrounding the very long distal centriole and the proximal part of the flagellum proper (Figs. 21–24; LAKE, SMITH and YOUNG, 1968). Thin, dense peripheral fibres are present in the proximal part of the tail (Fig. 24), and an amorphous substance (Fig. 22) surrounds the flagellum proper in most of the principal piece. The report by LAKE, SMITH and YOUNG (1968) that the two central microtubules run through the distal centriole in this species could not be confirmed in any single spermatozoon (Figs. 21, 23), not even after glutaraldehyde fixation.

Passerine birds have very different sperm tails (Figs. 27–30; FURIERI, 1961, 1962–63). One modified centriole only is present, and both segmented pericentriolar material and the nine identical coarse peripheral tail fibres anchor the neck to the base of the head (Fig. 28). The mitochondria form one long helix along the helical tail (Figs. 27, 30). No other sheath is seen. The development of the helical character of this sperm type involves a helical bundle of twisted microtubules formed in early elongated spermatids. This microtubular complex is shed during the passage of the spermatozoa through the ductus deferens, in a similar way to the cytoplasmic droplet in mammals. The movement of these spermatozoa is known to involve rapid rotation around their longitudinal axis.

REFERENCES

AUSTIN C. R., (1965) – *Fine structure of the snake sperm tail.* « J. Ultrastruct. Res. », 12, 452–462.

BALLOWITZ E., (1890) – *Untersuchungen über die Struktur der Spermatozoen.* « Arch. mikr. Anat. », 36, 225–290.

BARKER K. R. and BIESELE J. J., (1967) – *Spermateleosis of a salamander Amphiuma tridactylum Cuvier. A correlated light and electron microscope study.* « La Cellule », 67, 91–118.

BEDFORD J. M., (1968) – *Ultrastructural changes in the sperm head during fertilization in the rabbit.* « Amer. J. Anat. », 123, 329–358.

BOISSON C. and MATTEI X., (1966) – *La spermiogenèse de Python sebae Gmelin observée au microscope electronique.* « Ann. Sci. Naturelles. Zool. », 12, Série 8, 363–390.

BOISSON C., MATTEI C. and MATTEI X., (1967) – *Troisième note sur la spermiogenèse de Protopterus annectens (Dipneuste) du Sénégal.* « Bulletin de l'institut fondamental d'Afrique noire », Série A, 29, 1079–1121.

BOISSON C., MATTEI X. and MATTEI C., (1968) – *Le spermatozoide de Dactylopterus volitans, Linné (Poisson Cephalacanthidae), étudié au microscope electronique.* « C. R. Soc. Biol. », 162, 820–823.

BOISSON C., MATTEI X. and MATTEI C., (1969) – *Mise en place et évolution du complexe centriolaire au cours de la spermiogenèse d'Upeneus prayensis C. V. (Poisson Mullidae).* « J. Microscopie », 8, 103–112.

BUONGIORNO-NARDELLI M. and BERTOLINI B., (1967) – *Subcellular localization of some acid hydrolases in Triturus cristatus spermatozoa.* « Histochemie », 8, 34–44.

BURGOS M. H. and FAWCETT D. W., (1956) – *An electron microscope study of spermatid differentiation in the toad, Bufo arenarium Hensel.* « J. Biophys. Biochem. Cytol. », 2, 223–240.

COLWIN A. L. and COLWIN L. H., (1967) – *Behavior of the spermatozoon during sperm-blastomere fusion and its significance for fertilization (Saccoglossus kowalevskii: Hemichordata).* « Z. Zellforsch. », 78, 208–220.

DADONE L. and NARBAITZ R., (1967) – *Submicroscopic structure of spermatozoa of a cyprinodontiform teleost, Jenynsia lineata.* « Z. Zellforsch », 80, 214–219.

FAWCETT D. W., (1965) – *The anatomy of the mammalian spermatozoon with particular reference to the guinea pig.* « Z. Zellforsch. », 67, 279–296.

FRANZÉN Å., (1956) – *Investigations into spermiogenesis and sperm morphology among invertebrates.* Thesis. Almqvist och Wiksells Boktryckeri AB, Uppsala 1–13.

FURIERI P., (1961) – *Caratteri ultrastrutturali di spermi flagellati di Anfibi e Uccelli. Studio al microscopio elettronico.* « Arch. Zool. Ital. », 46, 123–147.

FURIERI P., (1962) – *Prime osservazioni al microscopio elettronico sullo spermatozoo di Salmo trutta L.*, « Boll. Soc. Ital. Biol. Sper. », 38, 1030–1032.

FURIERI P., (1962–63) – *La morfologia degli spermi di Fringilla coelebs L. e di Tarentola mauritanica* L. *studiata al microscopio elettronico.* « Mon. Zool. Ital. », 70–71, 159–174.

FURIERI P., (1965) – *Osservazioni ultrastrutturali sullo spermio di Testudo Hermanni Gmelin.* « Boll. Soc. Ital. Biol. Sper. », 41, 144–145.

GRÖNBERG R. and TELKKÄ A., (1968) – *Juxtanuclear changes during the early spermatogenesis in Lebistes reticulatus (Guppy).* « Z. Zellforsch. », 84, 342–349.

HAMILTON D. W. and FAWCETT D. W., (1968) – *Unusual features of the neck and middle-piece of snake spermatozoa.* « J. Ultrastruct. Res. », 23, 81–97.

LAKE P. E., SMITH W. and YOUNG D., (1968) – *The ultrastructure of the ejaculated fowl spermatozoon.* « Quart. J. Exp. Physiol. », 53, 356–366.

MATTEI X. and BOISSON C., (1966) – *Le complexe centriolaire du spermatozoïde de Lebistes reticulates.* « C. R. Acad. Sc. Paris. », Série D, 262, 2620–2622.

MATTEI X., BOISSON C., MATTEI C. and REIZER C., (1967) – *Spermatozoïdes aflagellés chez un Poisson: Gymnarchus niloticus (Téléostéen, Gymnarchidae).* « C. R. Acad. Sc. Paris », Série D, 265, 2010–2012.

NAGANO T., (1962) – *Observations on the fine structure of the developing spermatid in the domestic chicken.* « J. Cell Biol. », 14, 193–205.

NICANDER L., (1967) – *Microtubules in spermatids of mammals and birds.* « J. Ultrastruct. Res. », 18, 230.

NICANDER L., (1968) – *Gametogenesis and the ultrastructure of germ cells in vertebrates.* VIe Cong. Intern. Reprod. Anim. Insem. Artif., Paris, 1, 89–107.

NICANDER L. and BANE A., (1966) – *Fine structure of the sperm head in some mammals, with particular reference to the acrosome and the subacrosomal substance.* « Z. Zellforsch. », 72, 496–515.

NICANDER L. and SJÖDÉN I., (1968) – *The acrosomal complex and the acrosomal reaction in spermatozoa of the river lamprey.* « J. Ultrastruct. Res. », 25, 167–168.

PICHÉRAL B., (1967) – *Structure et organisation du spermatozoïde de Pleurodeles waltlii Michah. (Amphibien Urodèle).* « Arch. Biol. », 78, 193–221.

PORTE A. and FOLLENIUS E., (1960) – *La spermiogénèse chez Lebistes reticulatus, étude au microscope électronique.* « Bull. Soc. Zool. France », 85, 82–88.

SOTELO J. R. and TRUJILLO-CENÓZ O., (1958) – *Electron microscope study of the kinetic apparatus in animal sperm cells.* « Z. Zellforsch. », 48, 565–601.

STANLEY H. P., (1965 a) – *Fine structure of the tail flagella in the spermatozoa of two chondrichthyan fishes, Squalus suckleyi and Hydrolagus colliei.* « Anat. Rec. », 151, 419.

STANLEY H. P., (1965 b) – *Electron microscopic observations on the biflagellate spermatids of the teleost fish Porichthys notatus.* « Anat. Rec. », 151, 477.

STANLEY H. P., (1967) – *The fine structure of spermatozoa in the Lamprey Lampetra planeri.* « J. Ultrastruct Res. », 19, 84–99.

STANLEY H. P., (1969) – *An electron microscope study of spermiogenesis in the teleost fish Oligocottus maculosus.* « J. Ultrastruct. Res. », 27, 230–243.

YASUZUMI G. and YASUDA M., (1968) – *Spermatogenesis in animals as revealed by electron microscopy.* XVIII. *Fine structure of developing spermatids of the Japanese freshwater turtle fixed with potassium permanganate.* « Z. Zellforsch. », 85, 18–33.

EXPLANATION OF FIGURES.

Fig. 1. – Cap-shaped acrosome (A) of toad (*Bufo vulgaris*), with dense subacrosomal material (S) above and around apex of nucleus (N). Osmium fixation. × 37.000.

Fig. 2. – Apical region of sperm head in hag-fish (*Myxine glutinosa*), with small, cap-shaped acrosome (A) and subacrosomal substance (S) at tip of nucleus (N). Osmium fixation. × 40.000.

Fig. 3. – Cross-section of frog (*Rana temporaria*) sperm head, with acrosome (A) along one side of nucleus (N). Osmium fixation. × 65.000.

Fig. 4. – Apex of spermatid of domestic fowl, with acrosome (A) and subacrosomal rod (S) penetrating into tip of nucleus (N). Glutaraldehyde fixation. ×55.000.

Fig. 5. – Cross-sections of acrosome (A) and subacrosomal (S) rod in late spermatids of newt (*Triturus cristatus*). Glutaraldehyde fixation. ×55.000.

Fig. 6. – Cross-section of sperm head in *Triturus cristatus*. Subacrosomal rod (S) and nuclear mantle (NM) both show honey-comb structure. Osmium fixation. ×120.000.

Fig. 7. – Cross-section of nucleus with « mantle » (NM) in *Raja clavata*. Osmium fixation. ×35.000.

Fig. 8. – Tip of sperm head in *Lampetra fluviatilis*, with acrosome (A), subacrosomal ring (SR), and part of the subacrosomal fibre (SF). Osmium fixation. ×55.000.

Fig. 9. – Survey of sperm head and tail in *Salmo salar*. Two centrioles in a nuclear pit, a low mitochondrial collar (m), and a simple tail (t). Glutaraldehyde fixation. ×25.000.

Fig. 10. – Cross-section of sperm tails in *Salmo salar*, to show ridges (arrows) of the cell surface. Glutaraldehyde fixation. ×65.000.

Fig. 11. – Cross section of sperm tails in *Esox lucius*, to show high ridge (R) in the plane of the central microtubules. Glutaraldehyde fixation. ×50.000.

Fig. 12. – Neck region in a viviparous teleost, *Xiphophorus helleri*, with small modified proximal centriole (arrow), and long distal centriole (C). Part of the high mitochondrial collar (m) around the simple tail (t) is seen. Glutaraldehyde fixation. ×40.000.

Fig. 13. – Part of spermatozoon in a frog (*Rana temporaria*), with base of nucleus (N), distal centriole (C), and proximal part of mitochondrial sheath around the simple tail (t). Osmium fixation. ×35.000.

Fig. 14. – Cross section of nucleare base in a lamprey (*Lampetra fluviatilis*), with two typical centrioles and the subacrosomal fibre (arrow). Glutaraldehyde fixation. ×55.000.

Fig. 15. – Cross section of sperm tail in *Lampetra fluviatilis*, to show dense fibres along the doublets, dense mitochondria (m), microtubules (arrows), and the subacrosomal filament (Sf) surrounded by four membranes. Glutaraldehyde fixation. ×95.000.

Fig. 16. – Cross section of immature sperm tail in *Myxine glutinosa*, to show mitochondrial sheath. Glutaraldehyde fixation. ×50.000.

Fig. 17. – Neck region of immature sperm in a toad (*Bufo vulgaris*), with proximal centriole (PC), distal centriole (DC) anchored to the nucleus, and a forming mitochondrial collar. Osmium fixation. ×35.000.

Fig. 18. – Cross section of three sperm tails in *Bufo vulgaris*, to show undulating membrane (UM). Osmium fixation. ×35.000.

Fig. 19. – Neck region, *Triturus cristatus*. The proximal (PC) and distal (DC) centrioles are embedded in pericentriolar material in the base of the nucleus, surrounded by a shell of chromatin (N). Mitochondria (m) line up along the proximal part of the rod (R). Glutaraldehyde fixation. ×35.000.

Fig. 20. – Cross section of sperm tail, *Triturus cristatus*, to show flagellum (f) with satellite material in free margin of undulating membrane (UM). Mitochondria (M) lie along the stiff rod (R). Glutaraldehyde fixation. ×35.000.

Fig. 21. – Centriolar region, domestic fowl. Short proximal (PC) and very long distal (DC) centriole, surrounded by dense mitochondria (m). Osmium fixation. ×40.000

Fig. 22. – End of middle piece, same spermatozoon as in Fig. 21, to show amorphous sheath (AS) in the principle piece. Osmium fixation. ×40.000.

Fig. 23. – Cross section of atypical distal centriole in domestic fowl. Glutaraldehyde fixation. ×90.000.

Fig. 24. – Cross section of anterior end of flagellum, domestic fowl, to show peripheral dense fibres. Glutaraldehyde fixation. ×85.000.

Fig. 25. – Immature centriolar region in *Raja clavata*, to show mitochondria around pile of dense plates (arrow), distal centriole (DC) behind the mitochondrial sheath, and dense columns (HC) winding around the flagellum (f). Glutaraldehyde fixation. ×25.000.

Fig. 26. – Cross section of sperm tail in *Raja clavata*, to show dense helical columns (HC) in a plane though the central fibrils of the flagellum (f). Osmium fixation. ×55.000.

Fig. 27. – Survey picture of spermatozoa in the ductus deferens of a passerine bird (*Taeniopyga castanata*). Both solid acrosome (A), nucleus (N) and tail have a helical shape, and the mitochondria (M) also form a helix. Glutaraldehyde fixation. ×10.000.

Fig. 28. – Neck region, same species, to show a modified single centriole (C) surrounded by dense, partly segmented material anchored to the nucleus (N). Glutaraldehyde fixation. ×55.000.

Fig. 29. – Cross section of immature neck region, same species, to show dense material within the centriole and the transitory, helical sheath of microtubules (arrow). Glutaraldehyde fixation. ×45.000.

Fig. 30. – Cross section of mature sperm tail, same species, to show mitochondrial spiral (m) and nine identical, peripheral dense fibers. Glutaraldehyde fixation. ×45.000.

Discussion

ANDRÉ. – I would simply add here a simple piece of information about the acrosomal reaction. There is another example of acrosomal reaction very similar to the one you have just shown. It is in the horse–shoe crab *Limulus*. Here, a very long rod is preformed in the mature sperm. It goes through the whole nucleus in an intranuclear canal, is wound in a 6–10 turn helix at the base of the nucleus and points its fore end just beneath the acrosomal membrane, on the nuclear side. At the time of fertilization, this preformed acrosomal filament unwinds, slides abruptly into the nuclear canal, pointing stiffly a long distance ahead of the nucleus. Here also it is this acrosomal filament which first makes contact with the egg surface.

MEYER. – You showed intranuclear, honey-comb like structure. Could it be partially transformed chromosomal material as observed in spermatids of grasshoppers.

NICANDER. – This is possible, but the stainability of the structure suggests the absence of nucleic acids.

BACCETTI. – Why do lampreys have 9 + 9 + 2 sperms, as shown by Follenius?

AFZELIUS. – I think I have an answer to your question, although I must confess that I do not think that there is a necessary correlation between internal fertilization and the presence of coarse fibers. It is true however that the spermatozoon of the lamprey is much more complicated than could be expected for a fairly primitive animal having a fairly primitive type of fertilization. At least they have external fertilization. One may compare the complicated lamprey sperm with that of the herring, carp or trout.

The explanation may be like this: the lamprey has external fertilization, but it is believed that its ancestors did have internal fertilization. The lamprey has a penis but it has come out of the habit of using the penis at copulation, for reasons I have difficulties to understand. Possibly, the lamprey retains features in its sperm morphology as well as its gross morphology reflecting the conditions of its ancestors.

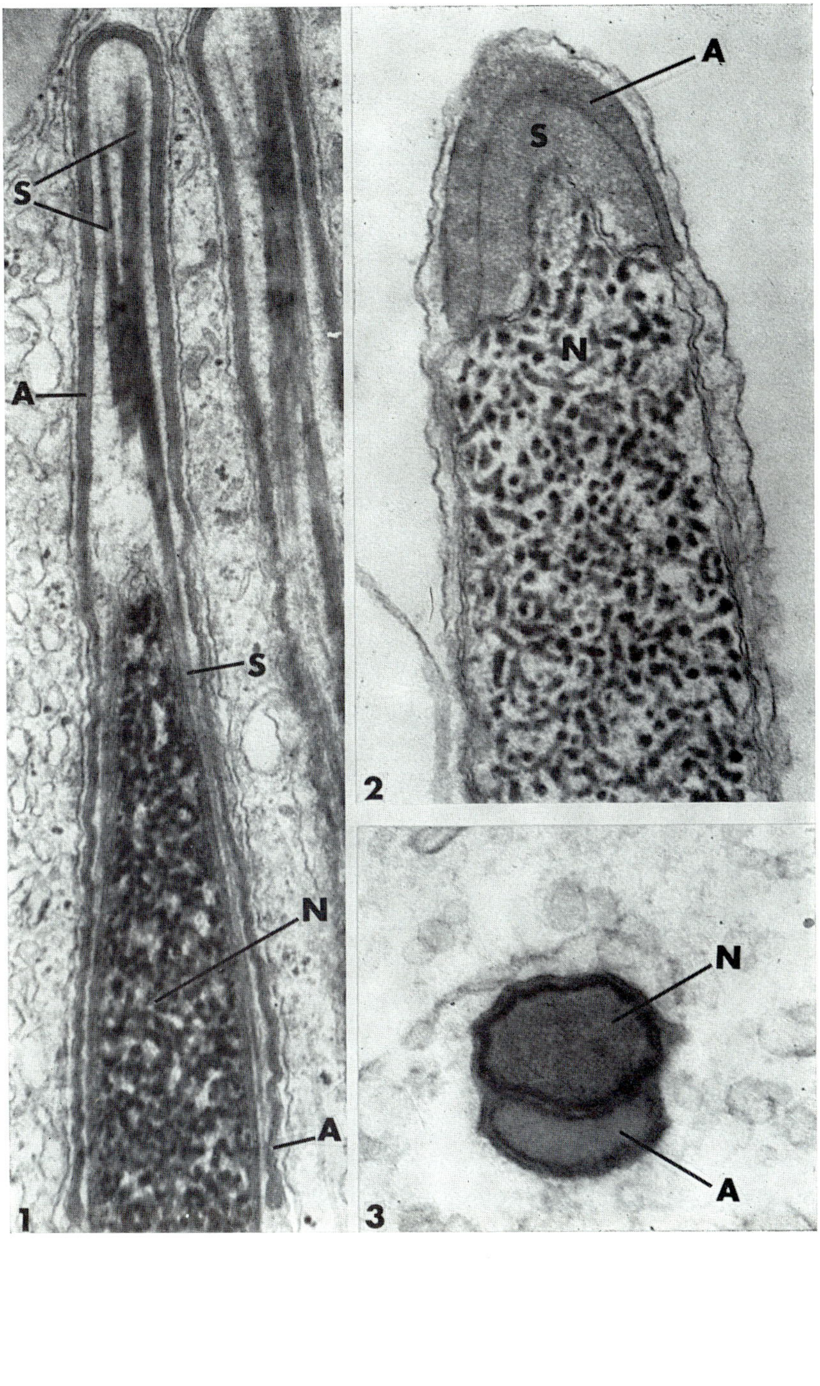
S
A
S
N
A
1
A
S
N
2
N
A
3

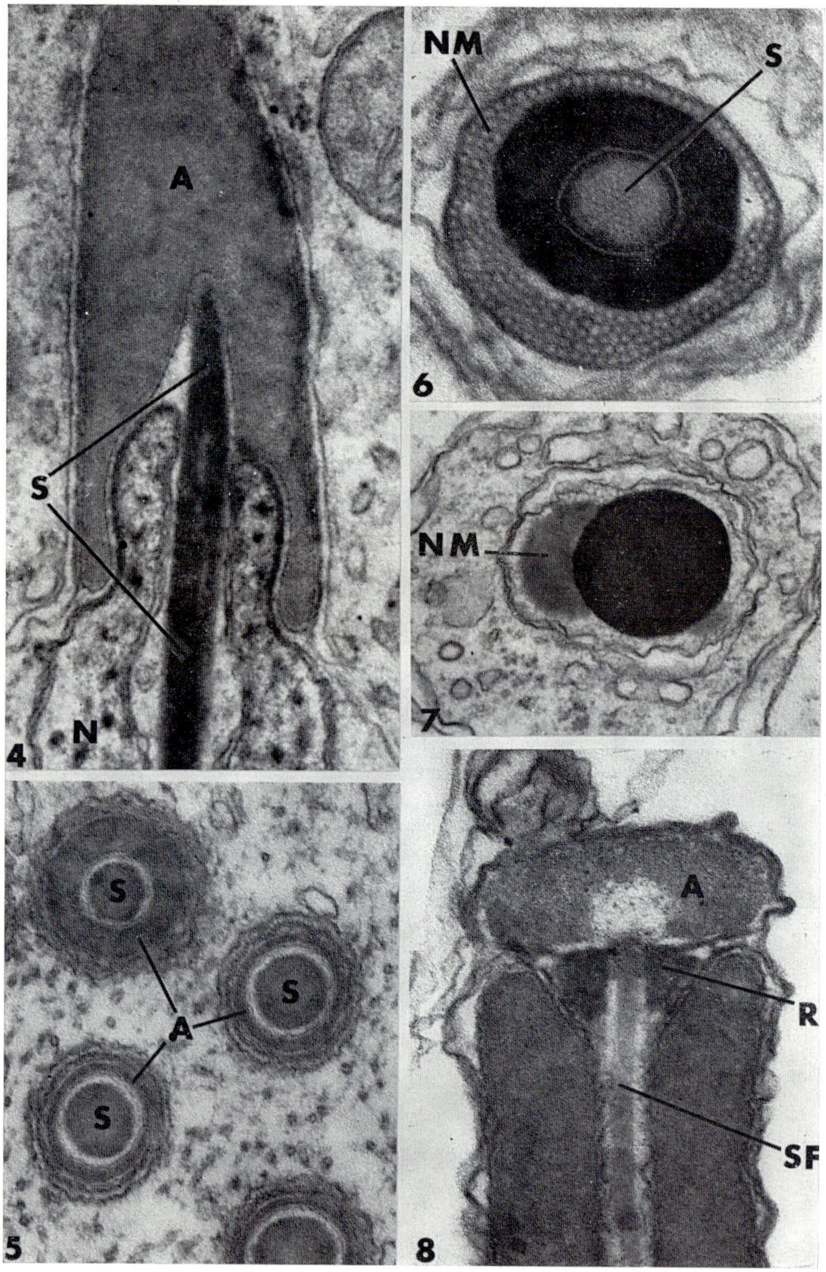
A
S
N
4
NM
S
6
NM
7
S
S
A
S
5
A
R
SF
8

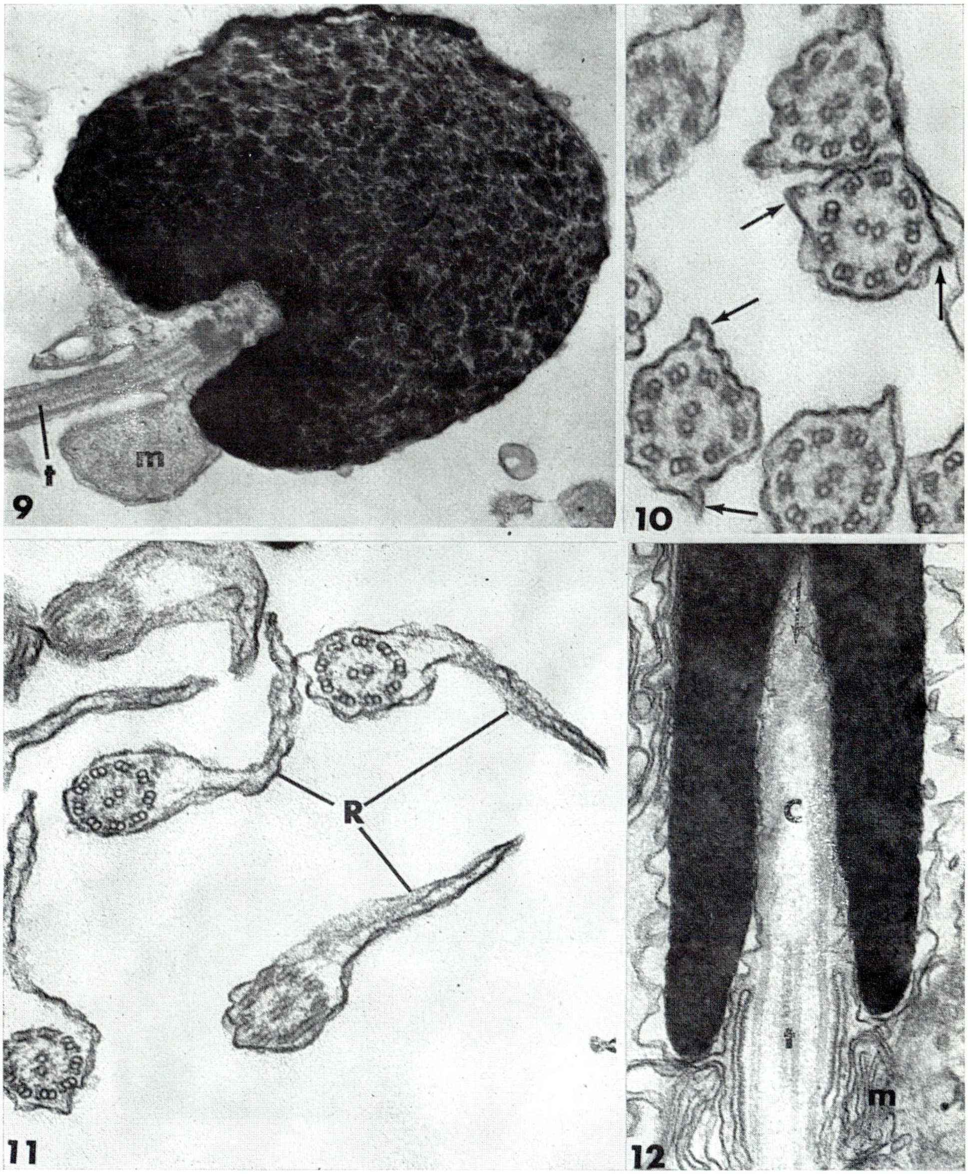
t
m
9
10
R
11
c
i
m
12

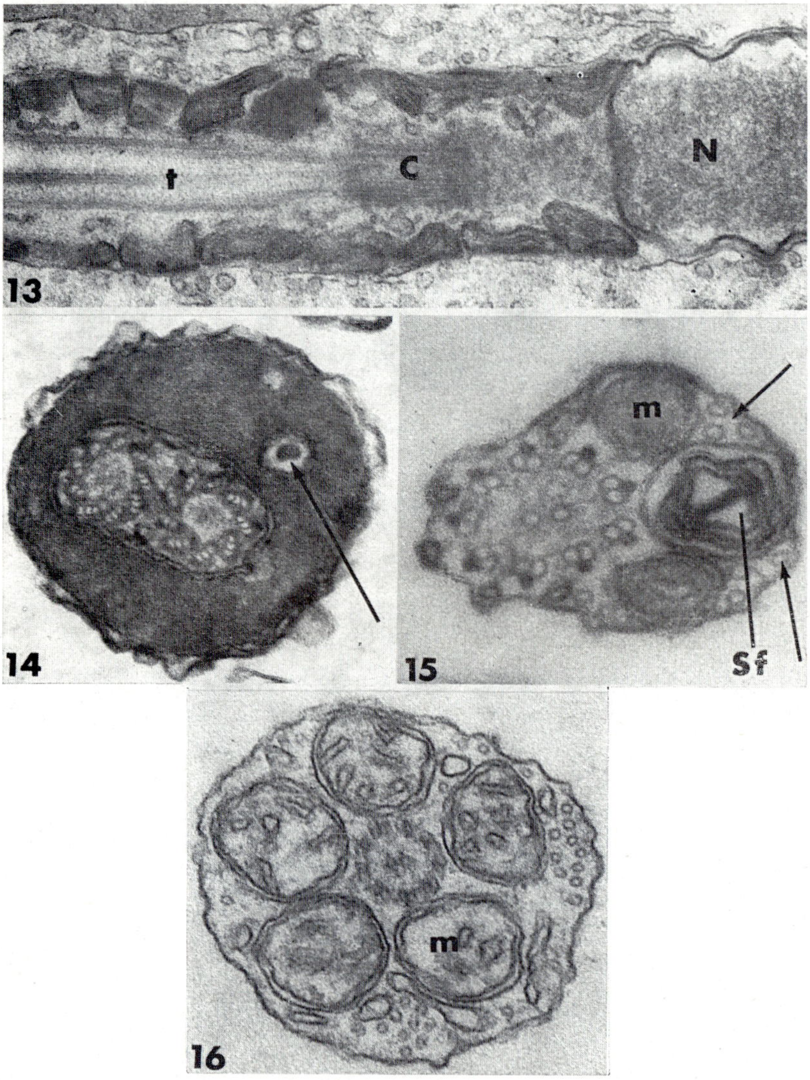
13
t
C
N
14
15
m
Sf
16
mf

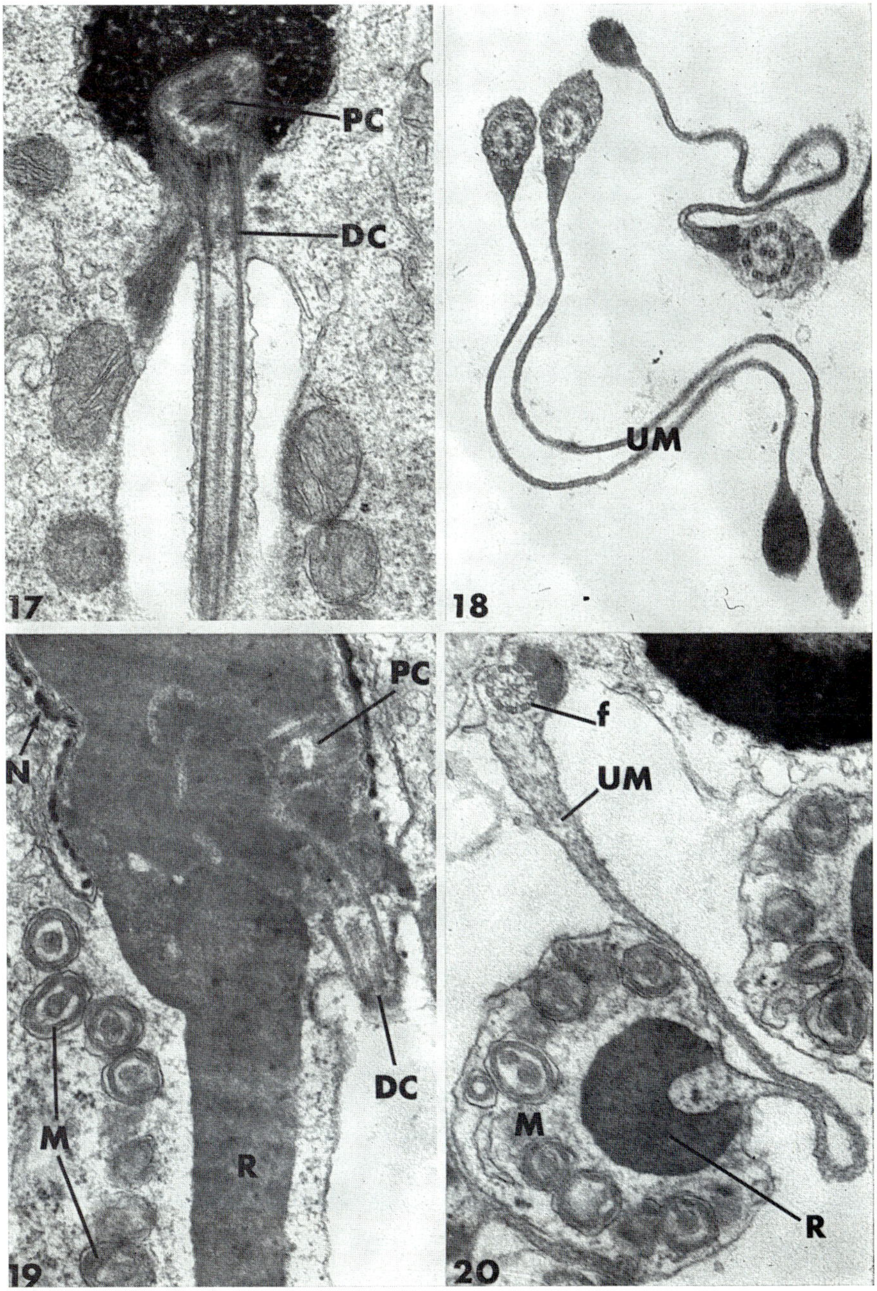
PC
DC
17
UM
18
PC
N
M
R
DC
19
f
UM
M
R
20

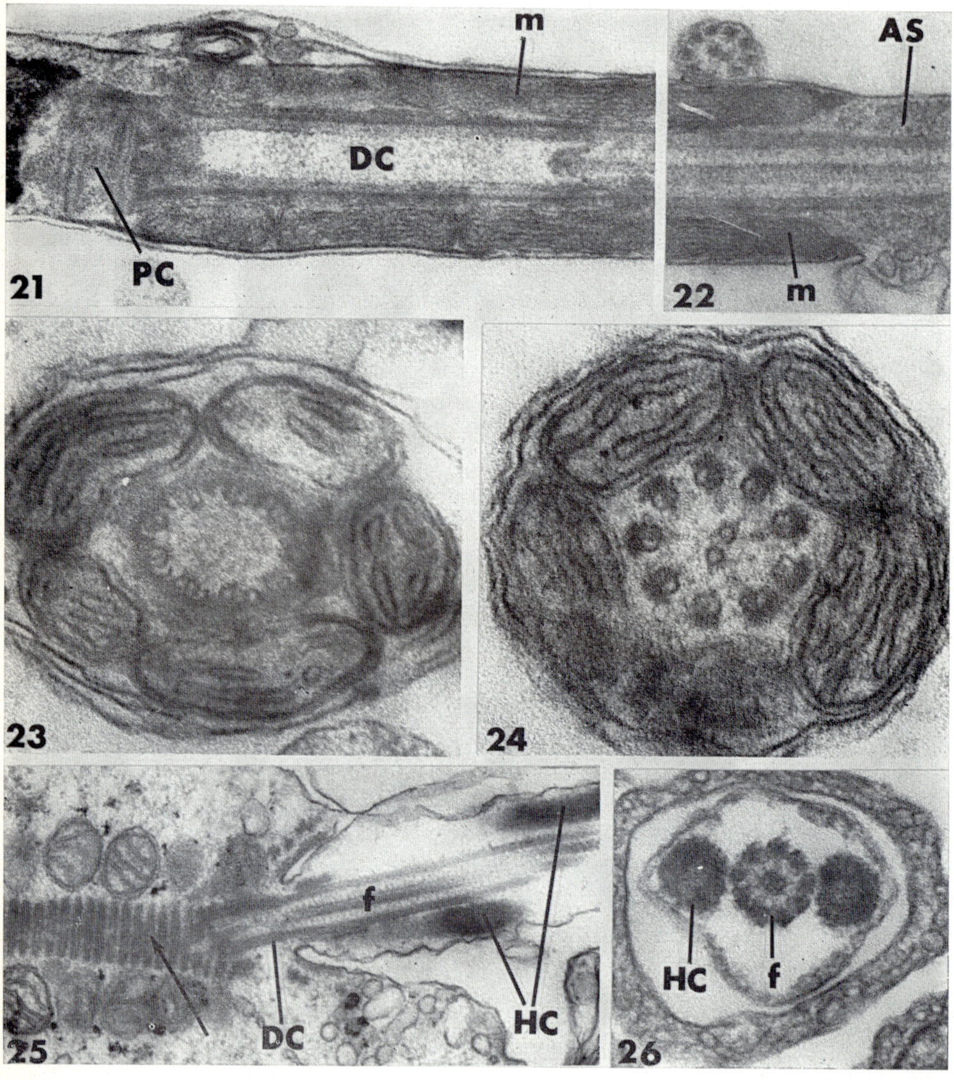
m
DC
PC
21
AS
22
m
23
24
f
DC
HC
25
HC
f
26

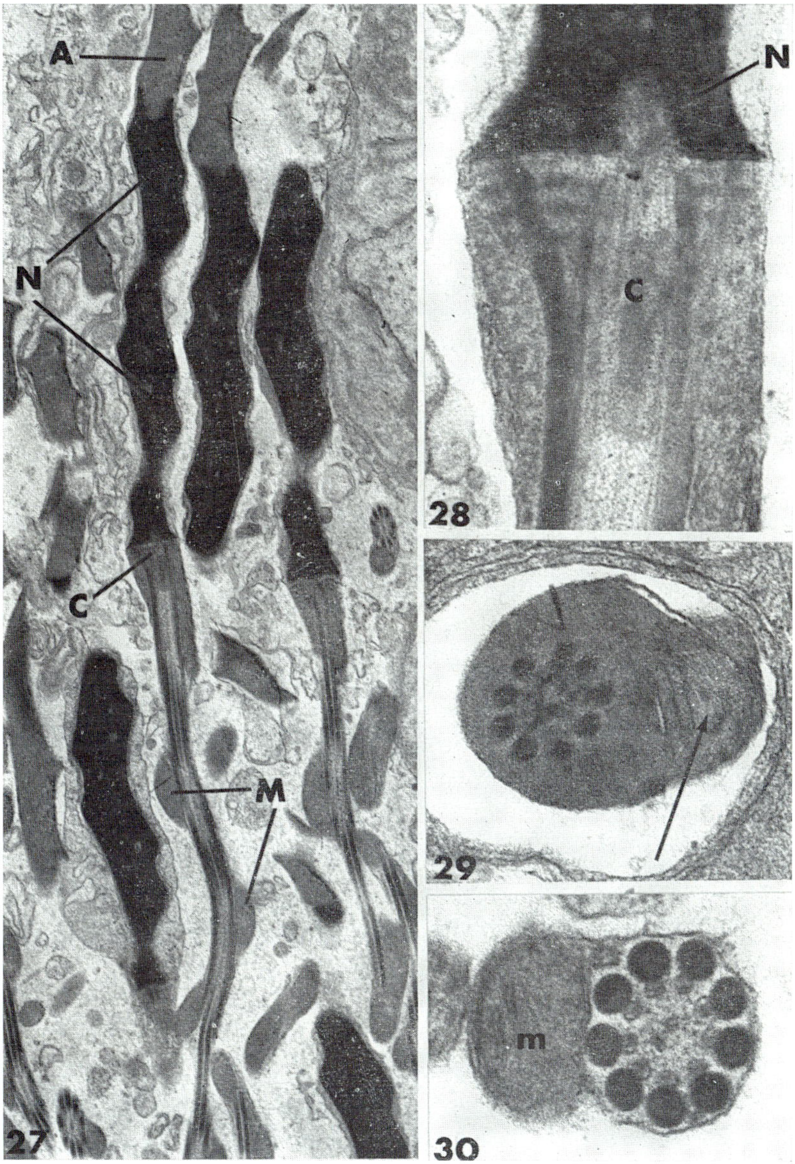
A
N
C
M
27
N
C
28
29
m
30

X. MATTEI (*)

SPERMIOGENÈSE COMPARÉE DES POISSONS

SUMMARY. — Les spermatozoïdes de Poissons présentent une grande diversité de forme et de structure. Il est impossible d'établir un type de gamète Poisson ni même un type de gamète Téléostéen.

RIASSUNTO. — Gli spermatozoi dei Pesci presentano una grande diversità di forma e di struttura. È impossibile stabilire un tipo di gamete Pesce e tanto meno un tipo di gamete Teleosteo.

Notre étude a porté sur 82 espèces de Poissons: 1 Dipneuste, 1 Brachioptérigien, 4 Sélaciens et 76 Téléostéens.

Les Sélaciens

La jeune spermatide du Sélacien que nous avons plus particulièrement étudié, *Rhinobatos cemiculus*, est une cellule sphérique d'environ 9 μ de diamètre; elle contient un noyau volumineux, un diplosome proche de la membrane cellulaire, un dictyosome au voisinage des centrioles, une baguette fibreuse et des mitochondries éparses dans le cytoplasme (Fig. 1 a).

Au cours de la spermiogenèse cette cellule subit de grandes modifications. Tout d'abord, le dictyosome se porte au pôle antérieur du noyau et sécrète une vésicule acrosomienne qui s'appuie fortement sur le noyau. Au pôle opposé de la spermatide, les centrioles demeurent proches de la membrane cellulaire. Habituellement dans les spermatides en évolution, le diplosome se déplace vers le noyau et se loge dans une fossette creusée à la base de celui–ci; chez les Sélaciens, deux formations naissent à partir des centrioles, se développent en direction du noyau et insèrent leur extrémité antérieure dans la fossette nucléaire (Fig. 1 b). Nous avons donné les noms de rhizoplaste amorphe et rhizoplaste structuré à ces formations paracentriolaires (BOISSON, MATTEI et MATTEI, 1968).

Le noyau s'allonge de même que les rhizoplastes et la baguette fibreuse; l'acrosome coiffe l'extrémité antérieure du noyau tandis que des filaments de chromatine s'individualisent. Les mitochondries se rassemblent dans la région antérieure de la spermatide (Fig. 1 c et d). A la fin de l'allongement nucléaire le contenu du noyau devient compct; la baguette fibreuse a un développement maximum (Fig. 1 e).

(*) Laboratoire de Zoologie et de Microscopie Electronique, Faculté des Sciences, Dakar, Sénégal.

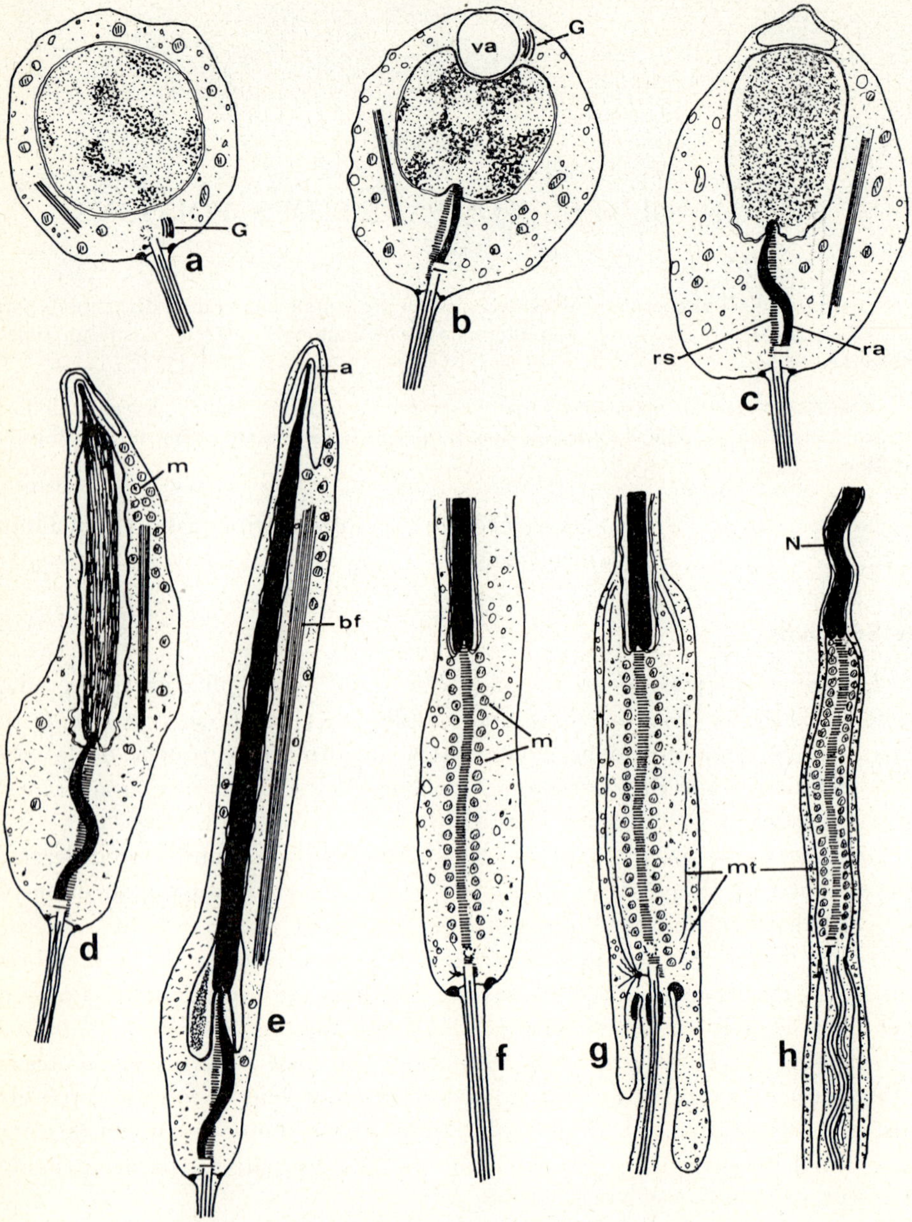

Fig. 1. – La spermiogenèse de *Rhinobatos cemiculus.*

a) La jeune spermatide. *b*) Sécrétion de la vésicule acrosomienne et développement des rhizoplastes. *c*, *d* et *e*) Allongement du noyau, des rhizoplastes et de la baguette fibreuse. Dans les schémas f, g et h, seule la région distale de la spermatide est représentée. *f*) Migration des mitochondries. *g*) Mise en place de la manchette. *h*) Le spermatozoïde. *a*, acrosome; *bf*, baguette fibreuse; G, appareil de Golgi; *m*, mitochondries; *mt*, microtubules de la manchette; N, noyau; *ra*, rhizoplaste amorphe; *rs*, rhizoplaste structuré; *va*, vésicule acrosomienne.

La baguette fibreuse et le rhizoplaste amorphe disparaissent ensuite; les mitochondries migrent vers la région distale de la cellule et se disposent autour du rhizoplaste structuré (Fig. 1 f).

Des microtubule cytoplasmisques associés à un satellite du centriole distal se développent en direction du noyau et constituent la manchette qui se dispose autour de la gaine mitochondriale (Fig. 1 g).

Le spermatozoïde des Sélaciens (Fig. 1 h) comprend trois parties bien distinctes: le noyau, le segment intermédiaire et le flagelle.

Deux particularités essentielles se dégagent de cette spermiogenèse: d'une part, comme le remarquait STANLEY en 1964, l'axe du segment intermédiaire n'est pas constitué par la portion antérieure du flagelle mais par un dérivé centriolaire; d'autre part, la manchette se singularise par son origine, sa structure, son emplacement et sa persistance dans le spermatozoïde. Le rôle de protection passagère qui lui est habituellement attribué est mis en défaut dans ce cas.

Le Dipneuste *Protopterus annectens.*

La jeune spermatide de Protoptère mesure 12 à 15 μ de diamètre. Le noyau est sphérique; le cytoplasme est différencié en deux régions: une zone ectoplasmique vésiculeuse qui est probablement le lieu d'accumulation des réserves nutritives et une zone endoplasmique homogène où sont rassemblés les divers organites cellulaires (BOISSON, 1963) (Fig. 2 a).

Deux particularités sont à signaler chez ce Poisson, au niveau de l'acrosome et du segment intermédiaire.

1) La mise en place de l'acrosome.

L'appareil de Golgi qui est bien développé dans les spermatocytes (BOISSON, MATTEI et MATTEI, 1967) fait une apparition fugace dans la spermatide. Dans la très jeune spermatide, les saccules golgiens sont mal différenciés et s'émiettent rapidement en petites vésicules qui se dispersent dans le cytoplasme sans réaliser de vésicule acrosomienne.

Pendant cette désagrégation de l'appareil de Golgi, une lamelle dense se dépose à la surface du noyau; elle est toujours indépendante de l'enveloppe nucléaire et sa structure rappelle celle d'un saccule golgien dont les parois seraient plus rapprochées que la normale. Par la suite, cette lamelle s'allonge et se plie en angle au sommet du noyau pour constituer l'acrosome (Fig. 2 b à f).

Ainsi la formation de l'acrosome de *Protopterus annectens* ne semble pas résulter d'une sécrétion golgienne comme nous l'avons vu chez les Sélaciens, mais de la transformation d'un seul saccule du Golgi.

2) Le segment intermédiaire.

Le segment intermédiaire est constitué du diplosome, du chondriome et d'un amas dense aux électrons que nous avons appelé « corps rétronucléaire ».

Les deux centrioles sont identiques et ne se différencient pas en centriole proximal et centriole distal; chacun d'eux élabore son propre flagelle.

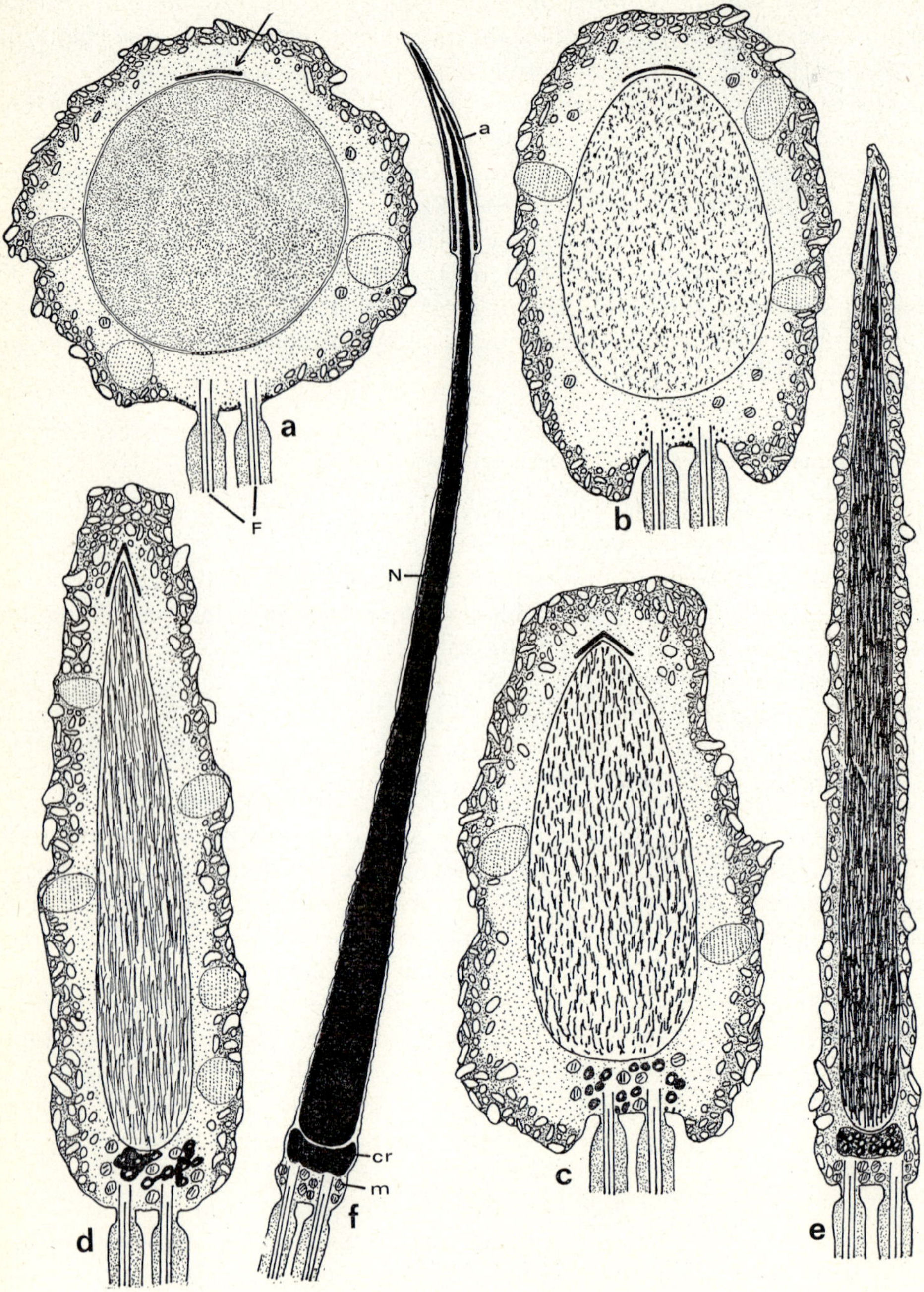

Fig. 2. – La spermiogenèse de *Protopterus annectens*.

a) La jeune spermatide après le dépôt du saccule acrosomien (Flèche) et le développement des deux flagelles. *b*) Allongement du noyau et apparition de granules denses autour des centrioles. *c* et *d*) Des filaments de chromatine s'individualisent dans le noyau qui continue son allongement. Le saccule acrosomien se plie en angle au sommet du noyau. Dans la région distale de la spermatide, les granules denses se rassemblent en amas mêlés aux mitochondries. *e*) Séparation nette du chondriome et du « corps rétronucléaire ». *f*) Le spermatozoïde.

a, acrosome; *cr*, « corps rétronucléaire »; *F*, flagelles; *m*, mitochondries; *N*, noyau.

Le « corps rétronucléaire » est une formation énigmatique dont nous avons pu suivre le mode de formation. Dans la région distale de la jeune spermatide, des granules denses sont élaborés au niveau de la membrane cellulaire; ils se réunissent en grains plus volumineux (Fig. 2 c) puis en amas qui sont toujours plus ou moins mélés aux mitochondries (Fig. 2 d). Il se produit ensuite une séparation nette entre le chondriome et le « corps rétronucléaire » (Fig. 2 e); ce dernier s'applique à la base du noyau et constitue un bloc compact dans le spermatozoïde (Fig. 2 f).

Le Brachioptérygien *Polypterus senegalus.*

La jeune spermatide est une cellule volumineuse de forme très variable, pouvant atteindre 30 µ dans sa plus grande dimension. La membrane cellulaire est ornée à sa périphérie de microvillosités.

Le noyau peut également présenter des formes très diverses; son contenu est homogène avec cependant, une concentration chromatinienne contre la membrane nucléaire. Le noyau occupe toujours une position excentrique dans la cellule, il est placé contre la membrane cellulaire (Fig. 3 a). Les centrioles sont situés non loin de la zone de tangence; ils sont proches de la membrane cellulaire, ce qui est un caractère commun pour une jeune spermatide et également proches du noyau qui présente à leur niveau un petit mamelon.

L'appareil de Golgi, bien individualisé, est situé dans le voisinage du diplosome. Chez ce Poisson, l'appareil de Golgi et les centrioles ne sont pas disposés à deux pôles opposés du noyau comme nous l'avons vu précédemment chez les Sélaciens et le Dipneuste.

Le cytoplasme est abondant, il renferme des gouttes lipidiques volumineuses, mesurant 3 à 4 µ de diamètre. Les mitochondries, de petite taille, sont disséminées dans le cytoplasme à l'exception de certaines, associées aux centrioles. En effet, chaque fois que nous avons obtenu le coupe d'un centriole, nous avons observé une mitochondrie comprimée entre ce centriole et le mamelon nucléaire qui lui fait face.

Chacun des centrioles donne naissance à un flagelle. L'appareil de Golgi sécréte une vésicule acrosomienne qui se dépose à la surface du noyau (Fig. 3 d).

Dans le noyau, une concentration chromatinienne apparaît sous la vésicule acrosomienne et se prolonge sur les 2/3 de la superficie du noyau; le reste du noyau est homogène et achromatique. L'amas chromatinien est percé d'une sorte de cheminée sous la vésicule acrosomienne; il semble également que la membrane nucléaire soit perforée à cet endroit. Il se constitue un canal endonucléaire qui contient un réseau de fibres parallèles.

Le noyau se déplace ensuite et vient buter par son pôle antérieur contre la membrane cellulaire, la vésicule acrosomienne faisant saillie à sa surface (Fig. 3 c).

Le noyau s'allonge tandis que le nucléoplasme achromatique se résorbe progressivement (Fig. 3 d) jusqu'à disparaître à la fin de la rétraction nucléaire.

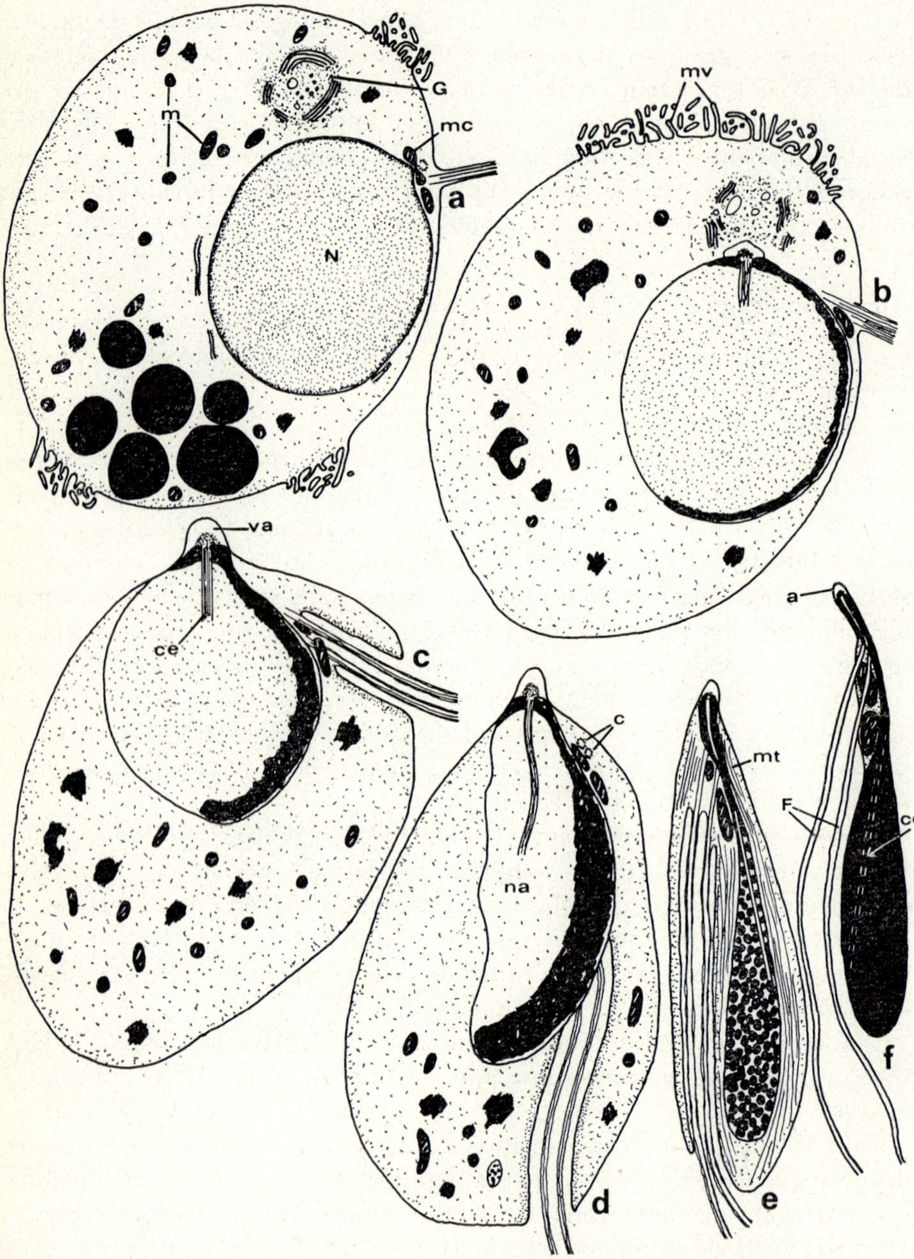

Fig. 3. – La spermiogenèse de *Polypterus senegalus*.

a) La très jeune spermatide. *b*) Sécrétion de la vésicule acrosomienne, ébauche du canal endonucléaire et condensation chromatinienne dans le noyau. *c*) Déplacement du noyau et invagination des flagelles dans la spermatide. *d*) Allongement et rétraction nucléaire. *e*) Dans la spermatide âgée, des grains de chromatine s'individualisent dans le noyau; des microtubules cytoplasmiques réalisent la manchette. *f*) Le spermatozoïde.

a, acrosome; *c*, centriole; *ce*, canal endonucléaire; *F*, flagelle; *G*, appareil de Golgi; *m*, mitochondries; *mc*, mitochondries associées aux centrioles; *mt*, microtubules de la manchette; *mv*, microvillosités; *N*, noyau; *na*, nucléoplasme achromatique; *va*, vésicule acrosomienne.

Dans la spermatide âgée (Fig. 3 e), les grains de chromatine s'organisent dans le noyau; des microtubules cytoplasmiques réalisent une manchette classique. Dans le spermatozoïde (Fig. 3 f), le noyau est compact, tout le cytoplasme spermatique a été éliminé de même que la manchette et les mitochondries non associées aux centrioles. La région nucléaire antérieure est étroite, c'est à ce niveau que s'insèrent les centrioles; à cette région fait suite une portion de noyau amincie, creusée d'une concavité où se logent les mitochondries; la région distale du noyau est renflée.

Le canal endonucléaire occupe une position axiale dans la région antérieure; vers l'arrière, il traverse obliquement le noyau et se termine contre la membrane nucléaire, près de l'extrémité distale du noyau.

Nous ferons quelques remarques pour conclure l'étude de ce Brachioptérygien:

– Les spermatides sont de grande taille et biflagellées comme chez le Dipneuste, mais ce sont là les seules ressemblance entre les gamètes de ces deux Poissons. Des spermatozoïdes biflagellés ont également été décrits dans une famille de Téléostéens, les BATRACHOIDIDAE (HOFFMAN, 1963 et STANLEY, 1965 b).

– La manchette a une structure et un emplacement classiques; sa présence est fugace, ce sont autant de caractères qui l'éloignent de la manchette des Sélaciens.

– Nous avons observé un canal endonucléaire uniquement chez le Polyptère. Une formation semblable a cependant été décrite dans les deux classes voisines des Poissons; chez un Agnathe, *Lampetra planeri* par FOLLENIUS (1965) et STANLEY (1967) et chez un Batracien, *Pleurodeles waltlii* par PICHERAL (1967).

– Parmi les mitochondries, certaines apparaissent associées très tôt aux centrioles. La migration des mitochondries vers les centrioles qui est généralement un phénomène tardif dans la spermiogenèse semble se produire ici avant que les centrioles aient élaboré leurs flagelles.

Les Téléostéens.

La spermiogenèse des Téléostéens nous a révélé une grande diversité de forme et de structure des spermatozoïdes; la Fig. 4 donne une idée de cette diversité. Tous ces gamètes possèdent cependant un caractère commun qui est l'absence d'acrosome.

L'existence d'un acrosome a été longtemps discuté par les spermiologistes qui travaillaient en microscopie photonique, mais depuis l'utilisation du microscope électronique, aucun auteur n'a mentionné d'acrosome dans ce groupe de Poissons.

Dans les 76 espèces de Téléostéens que nous avons étudiées, les spermatozoïdes sont dépourvus d'élément golgien ou de toute autre formation susceptible d'évoquer un acrosome. Cette absence d'acrosome est peut-être

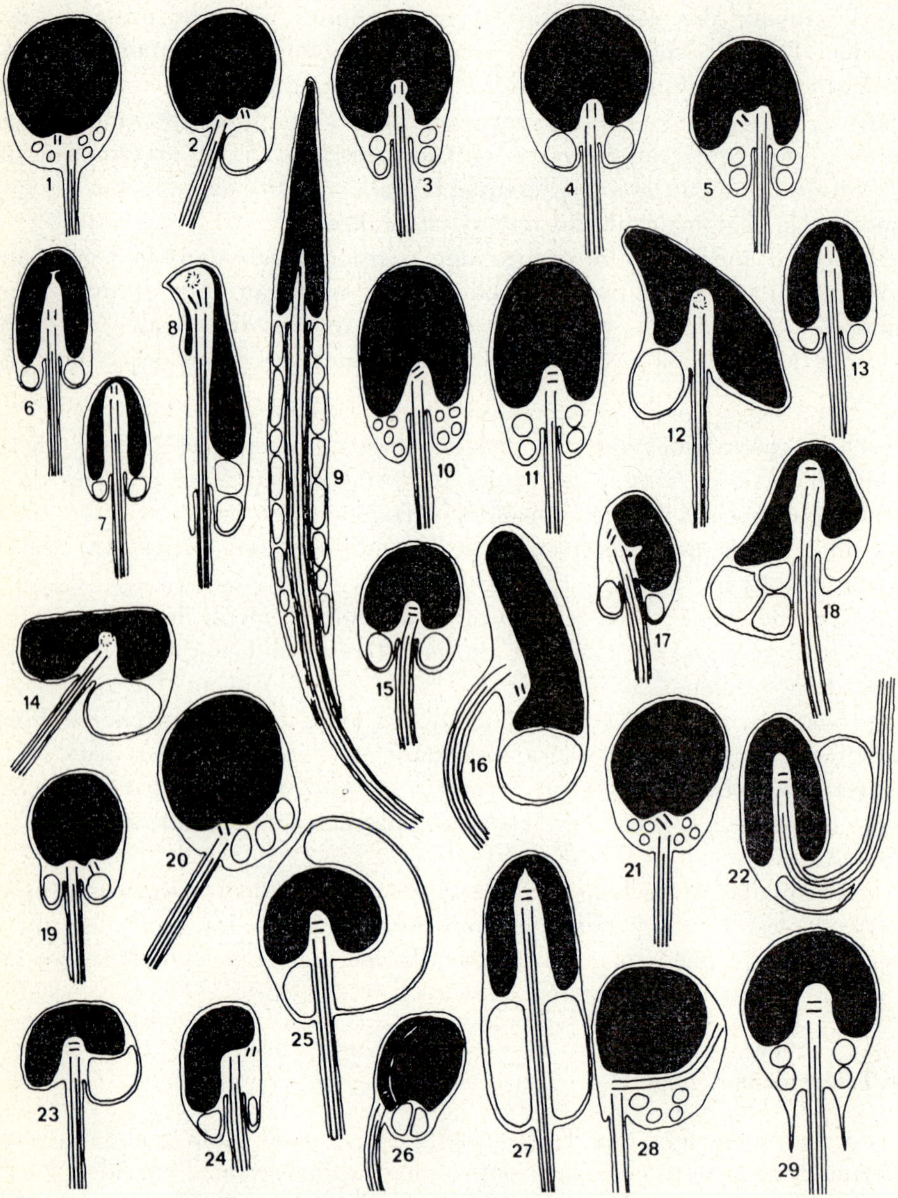

Fig. 4. – Représentation schématique de quelques spermatozoïdes de Téléostéens.

1) *Epiplatys senegalensis.* 2) *Clinus nuchipinnis.* 3) *Scorpaena angolensis.* 4) *Chilomycterurus antennatus.* 5) *Fistularia tabacaria.* 6) *Balistes forcipatus.* 7) *Upeneus prayensis.* 8) *Cephalacanthus volitans.* 9) *Lebistes reticulatus.* 10) *Clarias senegalensis.* 11) *Hemichromis fasciatus.* 12) *Trachinocephalus myops.* 13) *Pegusa triophthalmus.* 14) *Boops boops.* 15) *Antennarius senegalensis.* 16) *Ophioblennius atlanticus.* 17) *Parapristipoma octolineatum.* 18) *Zeus faber.* 19) *Fodiator acutus.* 20) *Blennius cristatus.* 21) *Papyrocranus afer.* 22) *Sardinella aurita.* 23) *Periophthalmus papilio.* 24) *Galeoides decadactylus.* 25) *Ethmalosa fimbriata.* 26) *Blennius vandervekeni.* 27) *Engraulis guineensis.* 28) *Lycodontis afer.* 29) *Tilapia nilotica.*

en corrélation avec la présence d'un micropyle dans l'oeuf des Téléostéens (PASTEELS, 1965 a et b; GINSBURG, 1968).

Devant cette diversité de forme des spermatozoïdes, nous avons essayé d'établir une classification en nous basant sur les variations de la spermiogenèse. En tenant compte principalement des déplacements des organites

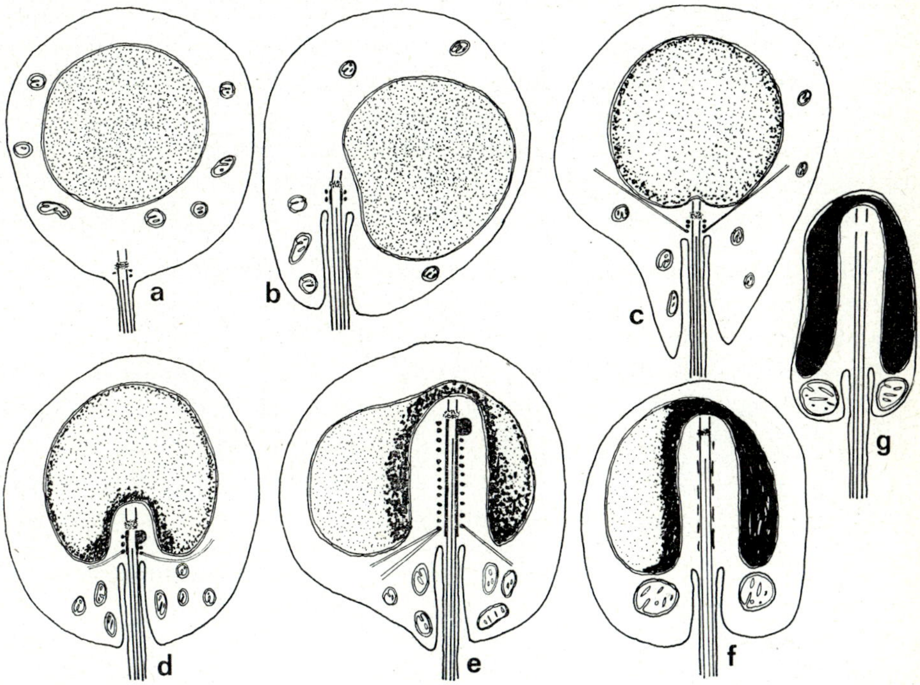

Fig. 5. – La spermiogenèse d'*Upeneus prayensis.*

a) La jeune spermatide. *b*) Migration des centrioles. *c*) Rotation amenant les centrioles dans la fossette nucléaire. *d*, *e* et *f*) Migration des mitochondries; mise en place et évolution du complexe centriolaire. *g*) Le spermatozoïde.

cellulaires qui se produisent pendant l'évolution de la spermatide, nous distinguons 4 temps dans le déroulement de la spermiogenèse:

1) La jeune spermatide.
2) La migration des centrioles.
3) La rotation du noyau.
4) La migration des mitochondries.

En fonction de ceci, les Téléostéens que nous avons examinés se répartissent en deux types principaux:

– Le type I, dans lequel la spermiogenèse comporte les 4 temps que nous venons d'indiquer.

– Le type II, dans lequel le troisième temps, c'est-à-dire la rotation du noyau ne se produit pas.

Spermiogenèse d'un Téléostéen de type I: *Upeneus prayensis* (MULLIDAE).

1) La jeune spermatide (Fig. 5 a) possède une noyau central, un diplosome proche de la membrane cellulaire et des mitochondries éparses dans le cytoplasme.

2) Les centrioles se déplacent en direction du noyau entrainant le flagelle et la membrane cellulaire, de sorte que le flagelle présente une portion invaginée dans la spermatide. En général, l'axe flagellaire se dispose tangentiellement par rapport au noyau (Fig. 5 b).

3) Une rotation de 90° amène le diplosome dans la fossette creusée à la base du noyau (Fig. 5 c).

4) Les mitochondries migrent à la base du noyau (Fig. 5 d).

Après ces quatre temps principaux, des transformations très variées peuvent affecter le noyau, le chondriome ou le complexe centriolaire d'où la grande diversité de forme des spermatozoïdes (MATTEI, 1969).

La spermiogenèse d'*Upeneus prayensis* constitue un exemple bien particulier. (BOISSON, MATTEI et MATTEI, 1969).

Spermiogenèse d'un Téléostéen de type II: *Parapristipoma octolineatum* (POMADASYIDAE).

1) La jeune spermatide est semblable à celle décrite dans le type I, (Fig. 6 a).

2) La migration des centrioles amène, de la même manière, l'axe flagellaire à se disposer tangentiellement par rapport au noyau (Fig. 6 b).

3) Il se produit ensuite le creusement de la fossette nucléaire et la migration des mitochondries autour des centrioles (Fig. 6 c).

La rotation du noyau n'a pas lieu; des transformations nucléaires (Fig. 6 d et e) réalisent le spermatozoïde (Fig. 6 f). Dans ce dernier, l'axe flagellaire demeure tangent au noyau; les centrioles sont placés en dehors de la fossette nucléaire.

Cas particuliers: *Galeoides decadactylus* (POLYNEMIDAE) et *Gymnarchus niloticus* (GYMNARCHIDAE).

1) Dans la jeune spermatide de *Galeoides decadactylus*, après la migration des centrioles, la rotation du noyau se fait partiellement. Les centrioles sont placés sensiblement dans la fossette nucléaire et l'axe flagellaire est disposé obliquement dans cette fossette.

Nous considérons ce Poisson comme un intermédiaire entre les types I et II.

2) *Gymnarchus niloticus* représente le seul Téléostéen et également le seul Vertébré connu à ce jour, possèdant un spermatozoïde aflagellé.

Une coupe de testicule observée en microscopie photonique (Fig. 7) montre des tubes séminifères contenant à leur périphérie des cystes où sont rassemblées des cellules sexuelles en évolution. La lumière du tube est emplie de spermatozoïdes aflagellés, pourvus d'un noyau plus ou moins dense, en position centrale dans un cytoplasme abondant, peu coloré que limite une membrane cellulaire très nette.

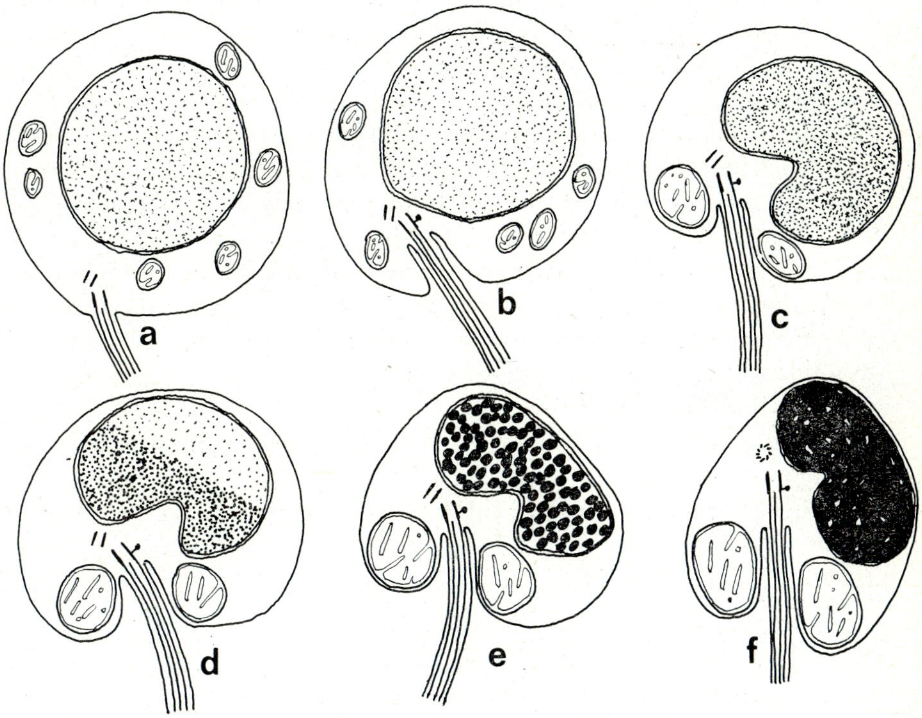

Fig. 6. – La spermiogenèse de *Parapristipoma octolineatum.*

a) La jeune spermatide. *b*) Migration des centrioles. *c*) Creusement de la fossette nucléaire et migration des mitochondries. *d* et *e*) Modifications nucléaires. *f*) Le spermatozoïde.

En microscopie électronique (Fig. 8), le noyau du spermatozoïde est quiescent, le cytoplasme est constitué de tubules ou de vésicules, les centrioles sont proches du noyau et la membrane cellulaire apparait doublée intérieurement d'un réseau de microtubules (Mattei, Boisson, Mattei et Reizer, 1967).

Les spermatozoïdes de ce Poisson ont conservé des caractères juvéniles et semblent figés au premier temps de leur évolution.

Conclusion

Si nous ajoutons à ces observations les études ultrastructurales réalisées par Stanley (1965 a) chez un Bradyodonte et Ginsburg (1968) chez des Chondrostéens, en tenant compte également des travaux effectués en microscopie photonique par TUZET et MILLOT (1959) sur le Coelacanthe et RETZIUS (1905) sur un Holostéen, l'idée principale qui ressort de cette étude de la spermiogenèse des Poissons est la grande diversité que présentent les spermatozoïdes du point de vue morphologique. Il est impossible d'établir un type de gamète Poisson comme on peut le faire pour les Reptiles et les Mammifères par exemple.

Si nous considérons les Téléostéens, leurs spermatozoïdes rappellent davantage ceux des Mollusques Bivalves, des Annélides et des Echinodermes que les spermatozoïdes des autres Poissons.

Les Poissons de la Classe des Chondrichthyens qui sont groupés par leur parenté morphologique, le sont également par leur « parenté spermatique ». Les représentants de la Classe des Ostéichthyens ne présentent pas cette « parenté spermatique » et constituent un ensemble au sperme hétérogène.

En tenant compt seulement de la « parenté spermatique », on pourrait imaginer plusieurs phylums dérivant comme suit: à l'origine, le type Chondrichthyen duquel se sépareraient très tôt les types Brachioptérygien, Dipneuste et Crossoptérygien; ces derniers ayant conservé jusqu'à nos jours avec le Coelacanthe, une structure spermatique ancestrale qui serait proche de celle des Vertébrés terrestres.

L'évolution se serait poursuivie par ailleurs vers le type Actinoptérygien avec une simplification progressive réalisant les Téléostéens qui présentent actuellement une sorte d'explosion en plusieurs types spermatiques simplifiés.

BIBLIOGRAPHIE

BOISSON C. (1963) – *La spermiogenèse de* Protopterus annectens (*Dipneuste*) *du Sénégal étudiée au microscope optique et quelques détails au microscope électronique.* « Ann. Fac. Sc. Dakar », 10, 43–72.

BOISSON C., MATTEI C. et MATTEI X. (1967) – *Troisième note sur la spermiogenèse de* Protopterus annectens (*Dipneuste*) *du Sénégal.* « Bull. IFAN », série A, 29, 1097–1121.

BOISSON C., MATTEI X. et MATTEI C. (1968) – *La spermiogenèse de* Rhinobatus cemiculus *Geof. St. Hilaire* (*Sélacien, Rhinobatidae*). *Etude au microscope électronique.* « Bull. IFAN » série A, 30, 659–673.

BOISSON C., MATTEI X. et MATTEI C. (1969) – *Mise en place et évolution du complexe centriolaire au cours de la spermiogenèse* d'Upeneus prayensis *C. V.* (*Poisson Mullidae*). « J. Microscopie », 8, 103–112.

FOLLENIUS E. (1965) – *Particularités de structure des spermatozoïdes de* Lampetra planeri, *étude au microscope électronique.* « J. Ultrastructure Res. », 13, 459–468.

GINSBURG A. S. (1968) – *Fertilization in fishes and the problem of polyspermy.* Publishing House « Nauka », 1–358.

HOFFMAN R. A. (1963) – *Gonads, spermatic ducts, and spermatogenesis in the reproductive system of male toadfish,* Opsanus tau, « Chesapeake Sc. », 4, 21–29.

MATTEI X. (1969) – *Contribution à l'étude de la spermiogenèse et des spermatozoïdes de Poissons par les méthodes de la microscopie électronique. Thèse de Doctorat enrégistrée au C.N.R.S.*: N° A. O. 3263.

MATTEI X., BOISSON C., MATTEI C. et REIZER C. (1967) – *Spermatozoïdes aflagellés chez un Poisson:* Gymnarchus niloticus (*Téléostéen, Gymnarchidae*). « C. R. Acad. Sc. », 265, 2010–2012.

PASTEELS J. J. (1965 a) – *La fécondation étudiée au microscope électronique. Etude comparative.* « Bull. Soc. Zool. France », 90, 195–224.

PASTEELS J. J. (1965 b) – *Aspects structuraux de la fécondation vus au microscope électronique.* « Arch. Biol. Belg. », 76, 463–509.

PICHERAL B. (1967) – *Structure et organisation du spermatozoïde de* Pleurodeles waltlii *Michah.* (*Amphibien Urodèle*). « Arch. Biol. Belg. », 78, 193–221.

RETZIUS G. (1905) – *Die Spermien der Leptokardier, Teleostier und Ganoidien.* « Biol. Untersuch. », 12, 103–115.

STANLEY H. P. (1964) – *Fine structure and development of the spermatozoan midpiece in the elasmobranch fish* Squalus suckleyi. « J. Cell. Biol. », 23, 88 A.

STANLEY H. P. (1965 a) – *Fine structure of the tail flagella in the spermatozoa of two chondrichthyan fishes,* Squalus suckleyi *and* Hydrolagus colliei. « Anat. Rec. », 151, 419.

STANLEY H. P. (1965 b) – *Electron microscopic observations on the biflagellate spermatids of the teleost fish* Porichtys notatus. « Anat. Rec. », 151, 477.

STANLEY H. P. (1967) – *The fine structure of spermatozoa in the Lamprey* Lampetra planeri. « J. Ultrastructure Res. », 19, 84–99.

TUZET O. et MILLOT J. (1959) – *La spermatogenèse de* Latimeria chalumnae *Smith* (*Crossopterygien Coelacanthidae*). « Ann. Sc. Nat. Zool. », 1, 61–69.

LÉGENDES DES FIGURES 7–8.

Fig. 7. – Coupe d'un tube séminifère de *Gymnarchus niloticus.* Les cellules sexuelles en évolution sont groupées par cystes. La lumière du tube est emplie de spermatozoïdes.

Fig. 8. – Spermatozoïdes de *Gymnarchus niloticus.*

Discussion

AFZELIUS. – Is anything known about the fertilization of *Gymnarchus nilotus*?

MATTEI. – La fécondation n'a pas été étudiée chez *Gymnarchus niloticus.* L'absence de tout organe copulateur laisse supposer que le mâle arrose les oeufs que la femelle dépose dans son nid. L'ultrastructure des spermatozoïdes et la présence du réseau de tubules sous–membranaires sont en faveur d'un déplacement amiboïde. Il n'est pas impossible que des modifications accélérées du gamète se produisent au moment de la fécondation.

Ce matériel est difficile à se procurer et nous n'avons pu jusqu'ici mettre en évidence le processus de la fécondation.

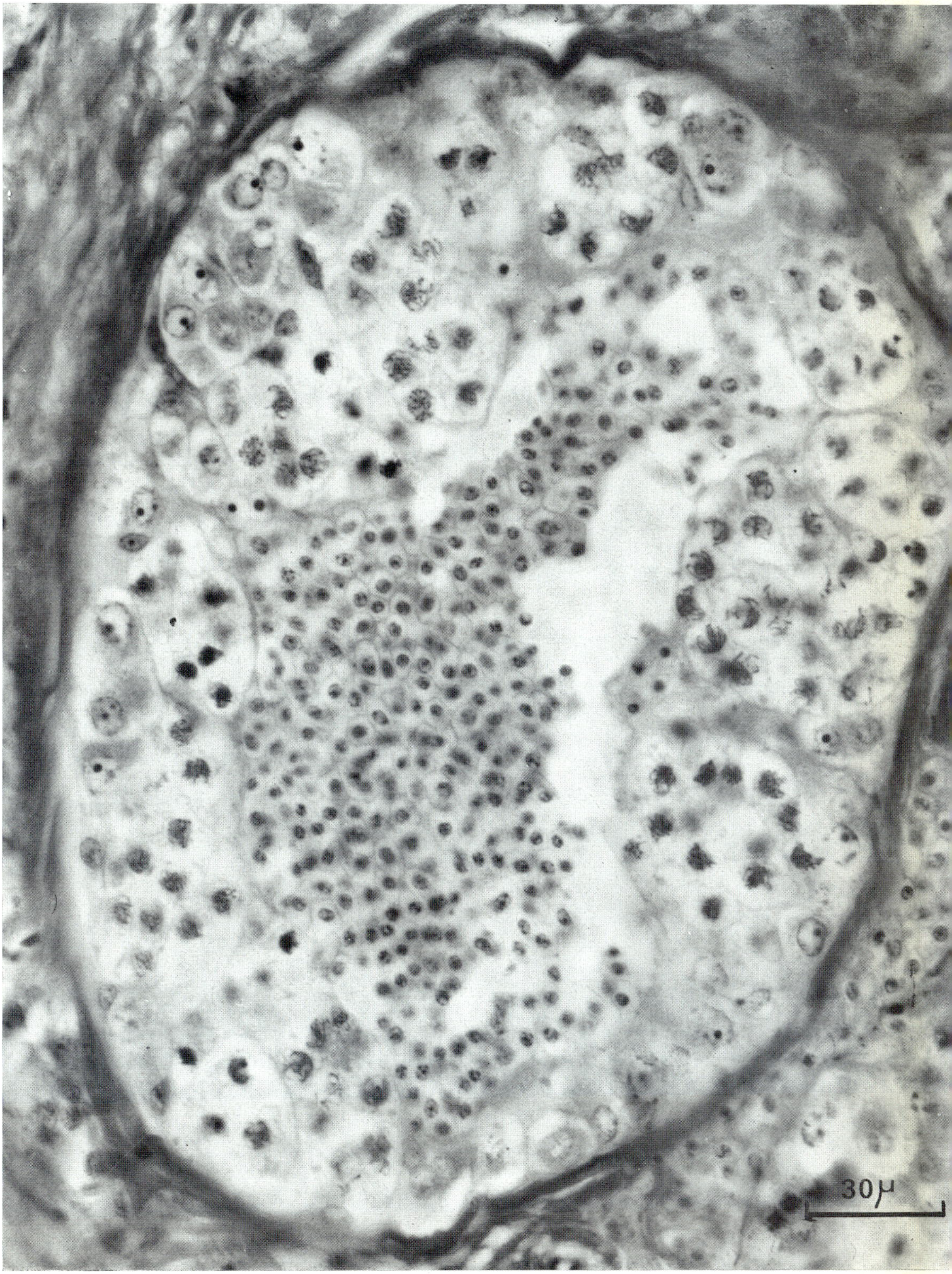

Fig. 7.

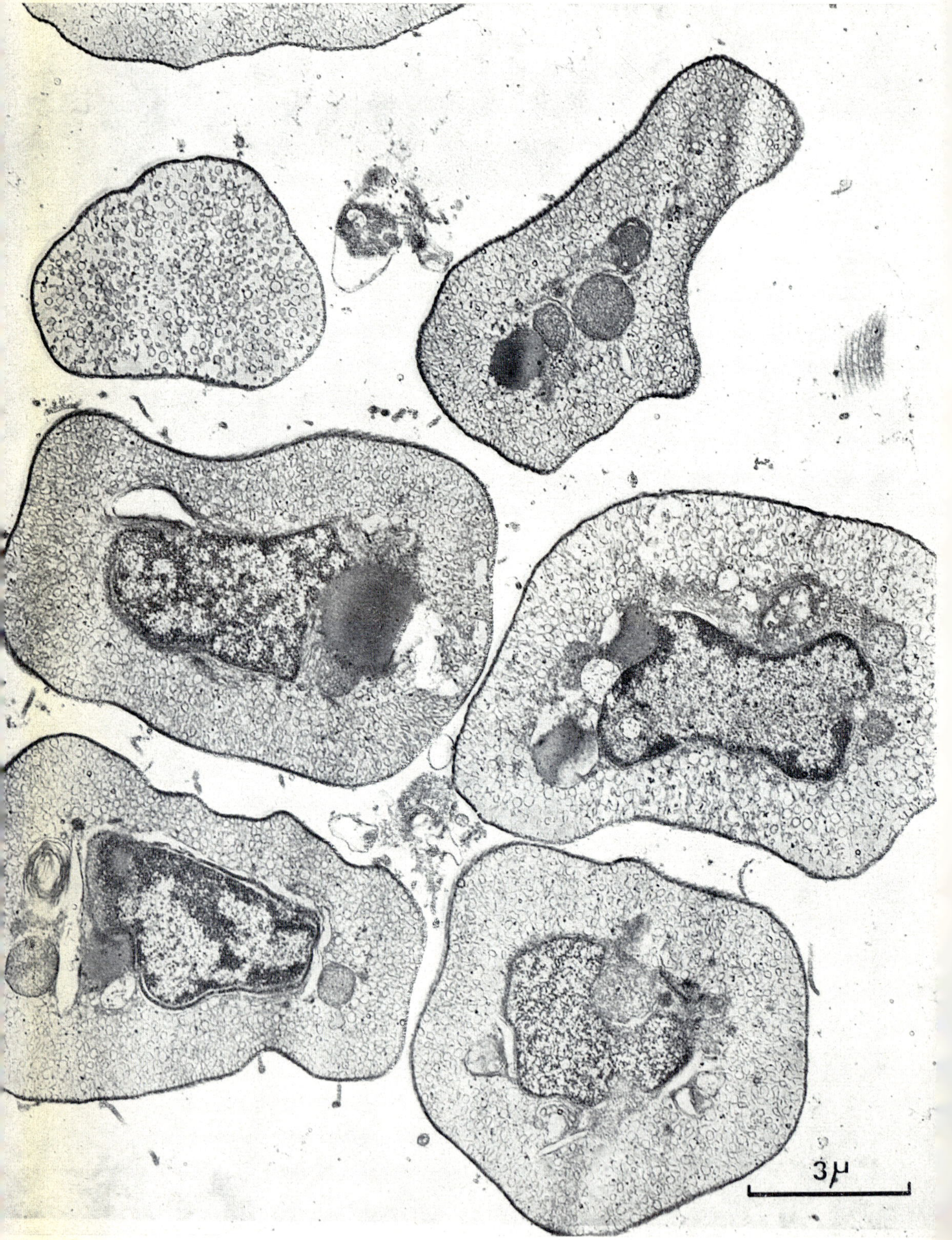

Fig. 8.

R. Billard (*)

ULTRASTRUCTURE COMPARÉE DE SPERMATOZOÏDES DE QUELQUES POISSONS TÉLÉOSTÉENS

Résumé. — L'étude comparée de la morphologie des spermatozoïdes de quelques espèces de poissons Téléostéens permet de distinguer 3 catégories de spermatozoïdes d'après leur degré d'évolution.

Groupe 1 (Carpe et Brochet): spermatozoïdes peu elaborés, tête ovoïde, mitochondries et cytoplasme simplement rejetés dans la partie postérieure de la tête spermatique et ne constituant pas une véritable pièce intermédiaire, flagelle inseré sur un coté de la tête spermatique.

Groupe 2 (Truite): la tête spermatique subit un allongement et acquiert une symétrie de révolution. Les mitochondries peuvent fusionner et forment une collerette autour du flagelle dans la partie postérieure de la tête.

Groupe 3 (Guppy). La tête spermatique est très allongée et présente une symétrie bilatérale. Les mitochondries s'organisent sous la forme d'un long manchon dans la partie postérieure de la tête mais restent séparées du flagelle par le canal cytoplasmique comme dans les 2 groupes précedents.

La morphologie du spermatozoïde parait donc susceptible de rendre compte du degré d'évolution phylogénétique des processus de reproduction dans les différents groupes de poissons Téléostéens.

Riassunto. — Lo studio comparato della morfologia degli spermatozoi di alcune specie di pesci Teleostei permette di distinguere tre categorie di spermatozoi a seconda del loro grado di evoluzione.

Gruppo I (Carpa e Luccio): spermatozoi poco elaborati, testa ovoidale, mitocondri e citoplasma confinati semplicemente nella parte posteriore della testa e non costituenti un vero pezzo intermedio, flagello inserito sul lato della testa spermatica.

Gruppo II (Trota): La testa spermatica subisce un allungamento ed acquista una simmetria di rivoluzione. I mitocondri possono fondersi e formano un collaretto intorno al flagello nella parte posteriore della testa.

Gruppo III (Guppy): La testa spermatica è molto allungata e presenta una simmetria bilaterale. I mitocondri si organizzano sotto forma di un lungo manicotto nella parte posteriore della testa ma restano separati dal flagello dal canale citoplasmatico come nei due gruppi precedenti.

La morfologia dello spermatozoo sembra dunque suscettibile di rendere conto del grado di evoluzione filogenetica dei processi di riproduzione nei differenti gruppi di pesci Teleostei.

(*) Institut National de la Recherche Agronomique, 78 Jouy en Josas – France.

Introduction

Les informations ultrastructurales concernant la morphologie des spermatozoïdes de Poissons étudiés ici sont dues principalement à des études par métallisation (Rotheli *et al.*, 1950; Fischer *et al.*, 1952; Hug *et al.*, 1953; Lowman, 1953, chez la Truite et Fujimura *et al.*, 1956, chez la Carpe). Quelques études plus récentes faites à partir de coupes ont été réalisées par Porte et Follenius (1960) et Mattei *et al.*, (1967) chez le Guppy et par Furieri (1962), chez la Truite.

Les descriptions complémentaires apportées par ce travail permettent une comparaison des spermatozoïdes de Carpe (*Cyprinus carpio*), de Brochet (*Esox lucius*), de Truite (*Salmo gairdneri* et *Salmo trutta fario*) et du Guppy (*Poecilia reticulata* = *Lebistes reticulatus*).

Matériel et méthodes

Les observations ont porté sur des spermatozoïdes émis pendant la période de reproduction. Les conditions de fixation et d'inclusion pour la Truite et le Gyppy ont déjà été décrites (Billard et Fléchon, 1969 a). Les spermatozoïdes de Carpe et de Brochet ont été fixés dans une solution d'acide osmique à 2% pendant 1 heure. La terminologie d'Afzelius (1959) et de Gibbons et Grimstone (1960) est utilisée pour la description des flagelles et celle de André (1962), pour la pièce intermédiaire.

Resultats

La tête spermatique.

Les têtes des spermatozoïdes de Carpe et de Brochet ont une forme à peu près identique (Fig. 2 et 4), mais une taille différente (Tableau 1). La tête est ovoïde, légèrement aplatie, parallèlement au plus grand axe antero–postérieur, ce qui définit une symétrie bilatérale avec 2 faces latérales, une face dorsale et une face ventrale – qui est la face sur laquelle s'insère le flagelle. Cette morphologie se retrouve dans le spermatozoïde de Tilapia. L'allongement présenté par la tête du spermatozoïde de Truite (Figs. 6 et 7) est encore plus marqué chez le Guppy (Fig. 12).

Tableau 1.

Taille de la tête spermatique de quelques poissons téléostéens (en μ).

(Après fixation glutaraldéhyde – O_sO_4).

	Carpe	Brochet	Truite	Guppy
Longueur antéro–postérieure . .	3,3	2	2,5	4
Diamètre maximum	2,5	1,8	1,5–2	1
Diamètre orthogonal correspondant	2	1,5	1,5–2	0,7

La chromatine qui apparait sous la forme de gros amas chez le Brochet et la Truite (Figs. 4, 6 et 7) est finement granulaire chez la Carpe (Fig. 2) et presque homogène chez le Guppy (Fig. 12). Dans tous les cas, la membrane nucléaire est fortement ondulée, de même que la membrane plasmique qui entoure le noyau et qui peut quelquefois emprisonner du cytoplasme (Fig. 7). Il n'y a pas d'acrosome.

Le complexe centriolaire.

Le complexe centriolaire est caractérisé par:

– L'absence de centriole proximal (qui disparait au cours de la spermiogénèse) et une modification du centriole distal chez le Guppy (Figs. 13 et 14).

– L'existence, chez la Truite, de relations complexes entre les 2 centrioles (Fig. 1), qui sont totalement engagés dans une profonde encoche nucléaire (Figs. 10 et 11).

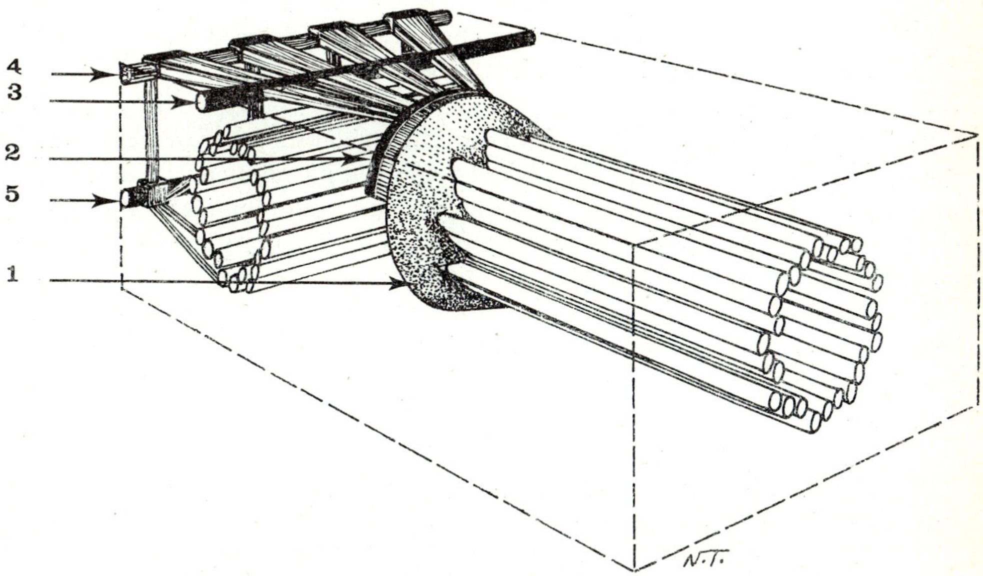

Fig. 1. – Schéma du complexe centriolaire du spermatozoïde de Carpe.

1. anneau osmiophile; 2. croissant osmiophile; 3. barre latérale; 4. barre antérieure latérale; 5. barre antérieure médiane.

– Une insertion latérale chez la Carpe et le Brochet ou une extrémité du centriole proximal est engagée dans une encoche nucléaire située sur la face ventrale de la tête spermatique et l'autre extrémité vient s'appuyer contre le centriole distal (Figs. 2, 3 et 4).

La piece intermediaire.

Les originalités de la pièce intermédiaire sont les suivantes:

– Elle est peu développée; elle est dissymétrique chez la Carpe et le Brochet (Fig. 2 et 4) et se présente chez la Truite sous la forme d'une collerette dans la partie postérieure de la tête spermatique (Figs. 6 et 7). Seule la pièce intermédiaire du spermatozoïde de Guppy a l'aspect d'un véritable manchon mitochondrial (Fig. 18).

– Elle est constituée par une association inorganisée de mitochondries et de cytoplasme avec des vésicules. Cependant, chez le Guppy, les vésicules n'existent pas et le cytoplasme est organisé sous la forme d'un manchon qui double les mitochondries du côté interne (Fig. 18).

– Dans tous les cas, les mitochondries sont séparées du flagelle par une invagination de la membrane plasmique qui est l'équivalent du canal cytoplasmique des spermatides de mammifères.

– Les transformations morphologiques des mitochondries sont peu marquées. Il n'y a pas de modification chez la Carpe (Figs. 2 et 19). Par contre, la dilatation de l'espace intermembranaire au niveau des crêtes et la fusion des mitochondries qui sont esquissées chez le Brochet (Figs. 4 et 20), sont beaucoup plus affirmées chez la Truite (Fig. 21). Chez le Guppy, il n'y a pas fusion des mitochondries qui sont aplaties et dont les crêtes qui ne présentent pas de gonflement tendent à devenir concentriques à la membrane mitochondriale exterme (Figs. 16, 18 et 22). Dans tous les cas, la matrice des mitochondries est opaque aux électrons.

– Sur toute la longueur de la pièce intermédiaire, la membrane plasmique qui limite le canal cytoplasmique est doublée par une couche de matériel dense. Cette dernière est très marquée chez la Truite (Fig. 21), discontinue chez la Carpe (Fig. 2) et à l'état d'ébauche chez le Guppy au sein du manchon cytoplasmique (Fig. 22), mais n'entre jamais en contact avec une autre accumulation de matériel osmiophile qui se trouve associée à la membrane plasmique au fond du canal cytoplasmique (Figs. 10 et 11).

Le flagelle.

L'axonème du flagelle est de structure classique; les 9 doublets périphériques portent une paire de bras sur les sous fibres A, lesquelles sont reliées par 9 rayons à une gaine qui entoure la paire de fibres centrales. Les 2 fibres de cette paire sont reliées entre elles par un filament rectiligne. Chez le Guppy, la sous–fibre A est généralement comblée par du matériel dense. Dans la partie antérieure du flagelle, chez la Truite et le Brochet, les 9 doublets périphériques sont reliés entre eux, du côté interne, par un manchon de matériel dense (Figs. 8 et 9) et une autre particularité consiste en l'existence de bras externes (Fig. 9). Chez la Truite, à l'extrémité distale du flagelle, les sous–fibres B disparaissent les premières, en même temps que les sous fibres A correspondantes perdent leurs bras (Fig. 25).

Les structures annexées à l'axonème varient d'une espèce à l'autre; chez la Carpe, dans la partie antérieure du flagelle, une gaine cytoplasmique riche en vésicules, entoure l'axonème sur une longueur d'environ 4 μ (Figs. 2 et 19). Dans les spermatozoïdes des autres espèces, des expansions cytoplasmiques sont identifiables d'un seul côté (Brochet) ou opposées de chaque côté (Truite, Figs. 22, 23 et 24; Guppy, fig. 22). Chez la Truite, des comptages réalisés sur 200 coupes transversales de flagelles, montrent que ces expansions sont au nombre de 2 et opposées (92,4 % des cas), plus rarement disposées à 90° (6,4 % des cas). Elles sont parfois au nombre de 3 (12 % des cas). Le plan des expansions cytoplasmiques passe en général dans le plan de la paire de fibres centrales, mais seulement dans 38 % des cas chez la Truite.

Conclusion

La morphologie de spermatozoïdes des poissons Téléostéens apparait donc variable. Il nous semble possible de les grouper en 3 catégories, compte tenu de leur degré d'évolution et de la complexité de la spermiogénèse:

Groupe 1.

Les spermatozoïdes sont peu évolués (Carpe et Brochet); la tête reste ovoïde et ne subit pas de transformation au cours de la spermiogénèse. Le flagelle s'insère sur un côté de la tête spermatique. Les mitochondries non modifiées, associées à du cytoplasme, sont rassemblées à la partie postérieure de la tête et ne réalisent pas une véritable pièce intermédiaire. A ce groupe se rattache le spermatozoïde de Tilapia.

Groupe 2.

Ce groupe est représenté par le spermatozoïde de Truite où la tête spermatique subit un léger allongement, mais reste cylindrique, ce qui lui confère une symétrie de révolution. Les mitochondries qui fusionnent le plus souvent, forment une colerette dans la partie postérieure de la tête. Des spermatozoïdes tel celui d'Hemichronis peuvent s'integrer à ce groupe (MATTEI, 1969).

Groupe 3.

Le type le plus évolué correspond au spermatozoïde de Guppy, dont l'allongement s'opère au cours d'une spermiogénèse complexe (BILLARD, à paraître). Le spermatozoïde d'*Oligocotus maculosus* (STANLEY, 1969), se rattache à ce groupe.

La pièce intermédiaire reste toujours sommaire chez les Poissons Téléostéens (BILLARD et FLÉCHON, 1969 b). Elle n'atteint jamais le degré d'élaboration acquis chez les vertébrés plus évolués et reste toujours séparée du flagelle par le canal cytoplasmique (NICANDER, 1968).

Il apparait donc que la morphologie des spermatozoïdes puisse rendre compte du degré d'évolution phyllogénétique des différents groupes de Téléostéens.

BIBLIOGRAPHIE.

AFZELIUS B. A. (1959) – *Electron microscopy of the sperm tail.* « J. Biophys. Biochem. Cytol. », 5, 269–279.

ANDRÉ J. (1962) – *Contribution à la connaissance du chondriome.* « J. Ultrast. Res. », suppl. 3, 1–185.

BILLARD R. et FLÉCHON J. E. (1969 a) – *Spermatogonies et spermatocytes flagellés chez* Poecilia reticulata (*Téléostéen cypronodontiforme*). « Ann. Biol. Anim. Bioch. Biophys. », 9, 281–286.

BILLARD R. et FLÉCHON J. E. (1969 b) – *Particularités de la pièce intermédiaire des spermatozoides de quelques Poissons Téléostéens.* « J. Microscopie », 8, 36 a.

FISHER H., HUG O. et LIPPERT W. (1952) – *Electronenmikroscopische studien an Florellen spermatozoen und ihrer zellkernen.* « Chromosoma », 5, 69–80.

FUJIMURA W. (1956) – *Electron microscope study of sections of carp sperms.* « J. Nara. Med. Ass. », 7, 122 (cité par PORTE et FOLLENIUS 1960).

FURIERI P. (1962) – *Prime osservazioni al microscopio electronico sullo spermatozoo de* Salmo trutta *L.* « Bull. Soc. Ital. Biol. sperm. », 38, 1030–1032.

GIBBONS I. R. et GRIMSTONE A. V. (1960) – *On flagellar structure in certain flagellates.* « J. Biophys. Biochem. cytol. », 7, 697–716.

HUG O., LIPPERT W. et FISCHER H. (1953) – *Das elektronenoptische Bild der Salmonidenspermatozoen.* « Protoplasma », 42, 95–99.

LOWMAN F. G. (1953) – *Electron microscope studies of silver salmon spermatozoa* (Oncorhynchus kisutch *Walbaum*). « Exp. Cell. Res. », 5, 335–360.

MATTEI X., MATTEI C. et BOISSONS C. (1967) – *L'extrémité flagellaire du spermatozoïde de* Lebistes reticulatus (*Poecilidae*), « C. R. Soc. Biol. », 161, 884–887.

MATTEI X., (1969) – *Contribution a l'étude de la spermiogenese et des spermatozoïdes de poissons par les méthodes de la mesoscopie éléctronique.*

NICANDER L. (1968) – *Gametogenesis and the ultrastruture of germ cells in vertebrates.* VI^{éme} Cong. Intern. Reprod. Anim. Insem. Artif., Paris, 1, 89–107.

PORTE A. et FOLLENIUS E. (1960) – *La spermiogénèse chez* Lebistes reticulatus. *Etude au microscope électronique.* « Bull. Soc. Zool. France », 85, 82–88.

ROTHELI A., ROTH H. et MEDEM F. (1950) – *Elektronenoptische untersuchungen der strukturveränderung agglutinierter fishpermien.* « Exp. Cell. Res. », 1, 115–126.

STANLEY H. P. (1969) – *A electron microscope study of spermiogenesis in the teleost fish* Oligocottus maculosus. « J. Ultrastruct. Res. », 27, 230–243.

LÉGENDES DES FIGURES 2–25.

Abreviations utilisées dans les figures.

am.o.	=	amas osmiophile
a.o.	=	anneau osmiophile
b.a.m.	=	barre antérieure médiane
bal	=	barre antérieure latérale
bl	=	barre latérale
c.o.	=	croissant osmiophile
c.cyt.	=	canal cytoplasmique
c.d.	=	centriole distal
c.p.	=	centriole proximal

ch = chromatine
cyt. = résidus cytoplasmiques
f. = flagelle
f.d. = face dorsale de la spermatide ou du spermatozoïde
f.v. = face ventrale de la spermatide ou du spermatozoïde
g.f. = gaine du flagelle (chez la Carpe)
m.cyt. = manchon cytoplasmique
m.m. = manchon mitochondrial
m.o. = manchon osmiophile (condensation de la formation intercentriolaire)
m.n. = membrane nucléaire
r.a. = renflement antérieur du flagelle
v. = vésicules.

Fig. 2–3. – *Spermatozoïdes de carpe.* La tête, légèrement ovoïde, contient une chromatine finement granulaire. Autour de la tête, les membranes plasmiques et nucléaires présentent de fortes ondulations.
Les 2 centrioles insérés sur la face ventrale (f.v.) se disposent à 90° (Fig. 2). A la base de la tête spermatique, quelques mitochondries non modifiées à matrice sombre sont groupées avec du cytoplasme et des vésicules. La couche de matériel dense qui double la membrane plasmique du côté du canal cytoplasmique (c.cyt.) présente quelques interruptions (flêche).
La partie antérieure du flagelle est entourée par une gaine riche en vésicules (g. f.), mais cette gaine ne subsiste pas sur toute la longueur du flagelle; la coupe transversale du flagelle (f.) en est dépourvue. ×30.000.

Fig. 4–5. – *Spermatozoïdes de Brochet.* Comme chez la Carpe, la tête est ovoïde, mais plus petite et la chromatine se présente sous la forme de gros amas. Le centriole proximal engagé dans une encoche nucléaire (coupe transversale, Fig. 5) est entouré d'amas de matériel osmiophile. Les mitochondries, dont les espaces intermembranaires au niveau des crêtes peuvent être dilatés, sont, comme chez la Carpe, disposées de façon dissymétrique dans la partie postérieure de la tête. (fig. 4 – ×30.000); (Fig. 5 – ×60.000).

Fig. 6–7. – *Spermatozoïdes de truite coupés perpendiculairement au centriole proximal* (*c.p.*), (*Fig.* 6) *et parallelement* (*Fig.* 7). La chromatine se présente sous la forme d'amas denses dont la répartition n'est pas homogène. Les centrioles sont disposés à 90° dans une profonde encoche nucléaire. La membrane plasmique qui entoure la tête spermatique peut emprisonner des résidus cytoplasmiques (cyt.). Les mitochondries peuvent ne pas être totalement fusionnées, (Fig. 7). ×40.000.

Fig. 8–9. – *Ces figures correspondent aux emplacements 8 et 9 figures sur la Fig 7.* Les doublets périphériques du flagelle qui fait suite au centriole distal, sont reliés entre eux du côté interne (Figs. 8–9). Au niveau du repli antérieur de la membrane plasmique délimitant le canal cytoplasmique, des rayons externes prennent naissance entre les 2 microtubules de chaque doublet et semblent entrer en contact avec les amas de matériel osmiophile (a.m.o.) de la Fig. 10. ×60.000.

Fig. 10–11. – *Détails montrant les relations entre les 2 centrioles* (se reporter à la Fig. 1 dans le texte). La condensation du matériel, sous la forme d'une couche dense, entre la membrane plasmique et le feuillet externe de la mitochondrie, s'interromp au niveau des flêches (Fig. 10). ×61.000.

Fig. 12. – *Coupe longitudinale sub-sagittale d'un spermatozoïde de Guppy.* Les membranes nucléaires et plasmiques sont étroitement appliquées contre la tête spermatique dans la partie antérieure, mais présentent des ondulations dans la partie postérieure. × 30.000.

Fig. 13. – *Detail de la parrie posterieure d'une tete spermatique de Guppy.* Le centriole proximal n'est plus visible et le centriole distal modifié demeure visible (c.d.), mais il est modifié et doublé par la paire de fibres centrale, qui sont à ce niveau, plus écartées que dans le flagelle. ×41.000.

Fig. 14–15. – *Coupes transversales de la tete spermatique de Guppy* passant au niveau du centriole distal (Fig. 14) et au-dessous de ce dernier (Fig. 15). Fig. 14 : ×50.000 Fig. 15 : ×40.000.

Fig. 16. – *Coupe longitudinale et tangentielle du manchon mitochondrial* montrant la forme rectangulaire des mitochondries. ×45.000.

Fig. 17. – *Coupes transversales de flagelles* passant au niveau et au delà de l'extrêmité du manchon cytoplasmique qui double intérieurement et prolonge le manchon mitochondrial. Les expansions cytoplasmiques opposées sont toutes orientées dans le même sens et passent par le plan de la paire de fibres centrales. La flêche indique un flagelle supposé en dégénérescence. (GUPPY). ×34.000.

Fig. 18. – *Coupe longitudinale de l'ensemble de la piece intermediaire* du GUPPY. ×24.000.

Figs. 19 à 22. – *Coupe transversale des « Pieces intermediaires » des spermatozoïdes,* respectivement de CARPE, BROCHET, TRUITE et GUPPY. Les flêches simples signalent la couche de matériel dense (cf. fig. 10) et la double flêche de la fig. 22 représente l'ébauche d'une condensation analogue chez le GUPPY.
Fig. 19 : ×48.000. – Fig. 20 : ×45.000. – Fig. 21 : ×58.000. – Fig. 22 : ×60.000.

Fig. 23–25. – *Coupe transversale de flagelles de spermatozoïdes de truites dans les parties anterieure (fig. 23), mediane (fig. 24) et posterieure (fig. 25).* ×60.000. Les expansions cytoplasmiques sont le plus souvent opposées et symétriques. Fig. 23 mais peuvent ne pas avoir la même longueur Fig. 24.

Discussion

MATTEI. – FURIERI (1962) décrit une mitochondrie annulaire dans le spermatozoïde de *Salmo trutta*; nous avons nous-même décrit des mitochondries à tendance annulaire dans les spermatozoïdes de Clupeidae et Engraulidae; est-ce qu'un véritable anneau mitochondrial est réalisé dans les espèces de truite que vous avez étudié.

BILLARD. – Chez *S. trutta* et *S. gairdneri* les mitochondries tendent à se condenser sous une forme annulaire mais c'est seulement sur un petit nombre de spermatozoïdes qu'il est possible d'observer un anneau mitochondrial complet.

MATTEI. – L'ensemble des microtubules que vous assimilez à une manchette nous semble provenir d'une prolifération des triplets du centriole proximal. Proposez-vous une autre origine à cette formation?

BILLARD. – L'ensemble des microtubules divergent a partir de la région du complexe centriolaire mais je n'ai jamais pu observer ces microtubules en continuité avec les triplets des centrioles.

NELSON. – The variable remoteness of mitochondria from flagellar fibers seen in electron micrographs of spermatozoa of many species indicates that while ATP is necessary for sperm motility the distances involved may make reliance on mitochondrial synthesis during ATP utilization inadequate. Many ATP regenerating enzymes occur in closer proximity to the contractile, ATP–utilizing fibers of the flagellum, e.g., creatine–phosphokinase, adenylate–kinase and the enzymes of oxidative phosphorylation, succinic–dehydrogenase and cytochrome oxidase. If ATP diffusion from the mitochondria is important, one may assume that during the quiescent period before ejaculation and mixing with seminal plasma or sea water, ATP was produced in sufficient amount to diffuse expeditionaly throughout the flagellum. After ejaculation or spawning, the other ATP–regenerating enzyme systems could sufficiently rapidly restore the ATP concentration locally to high enough levels to maintain flagellar movement, and so the flagellum would not necessarily have to depend on ATP diffusion over long distances.

ROBISON. – Upon consideration of the following facts:

1) that the mitochondria in the sperm are isolated from the motile apparatus (axial filament complex) and therefore present problems of energy transfer;

2) that there are no mitochondria in the sperm of coccid insects in spite of the the fact these sperms are motile;

3) that DNA is present in mitochondria, one is lead to the idea that perhaps we should reconsider the role of mitochondria in sperm.

It is entirely possible that mitochondria are involved in the trasmission of hereditary information in addition to or in lieu of a role in supplying energy for motility.

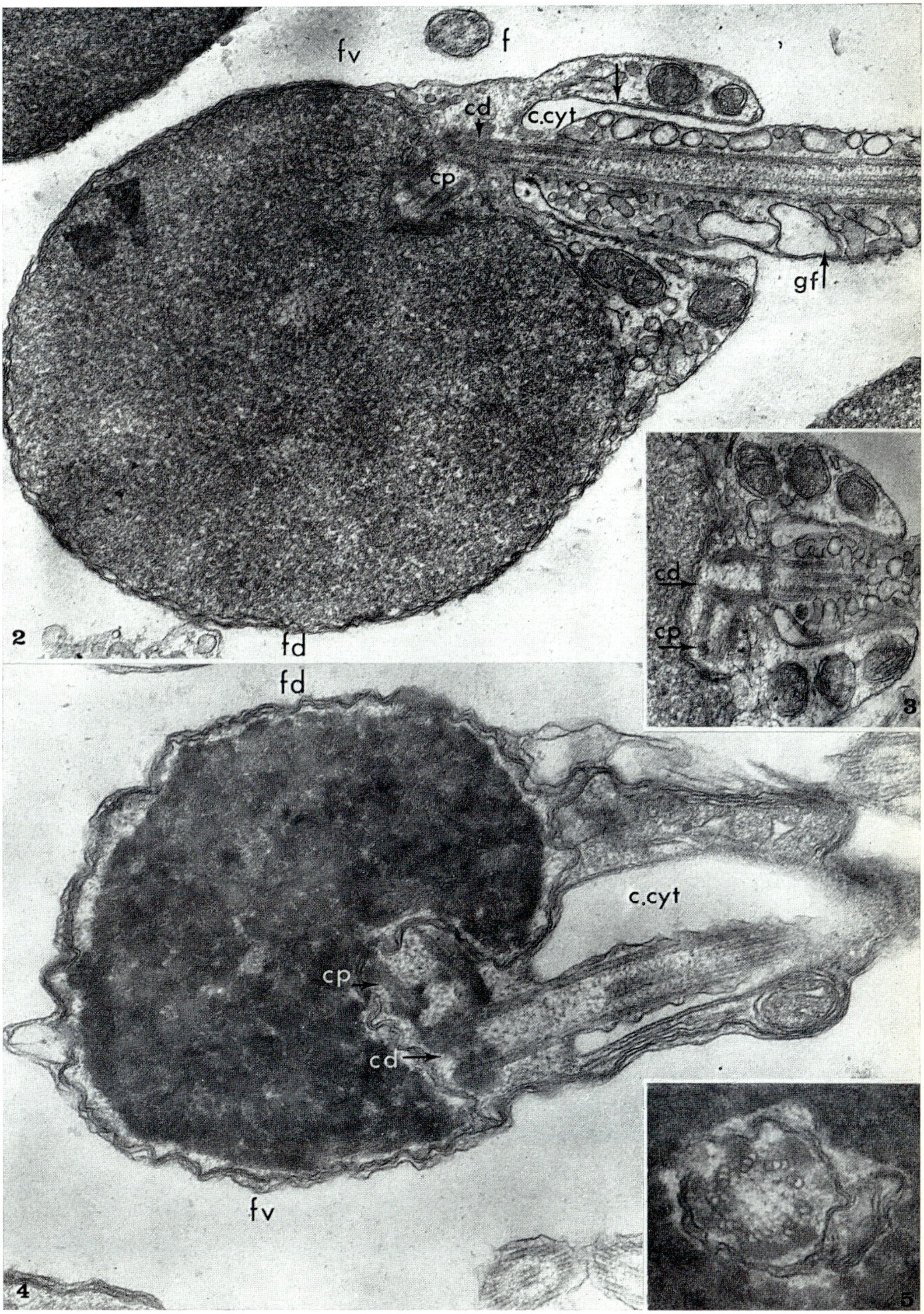
fv
f
cd
c.cyt
cp
gf
2
fd
cd
cp
3
fd
c.cyt
cp
cd
fv
4
5

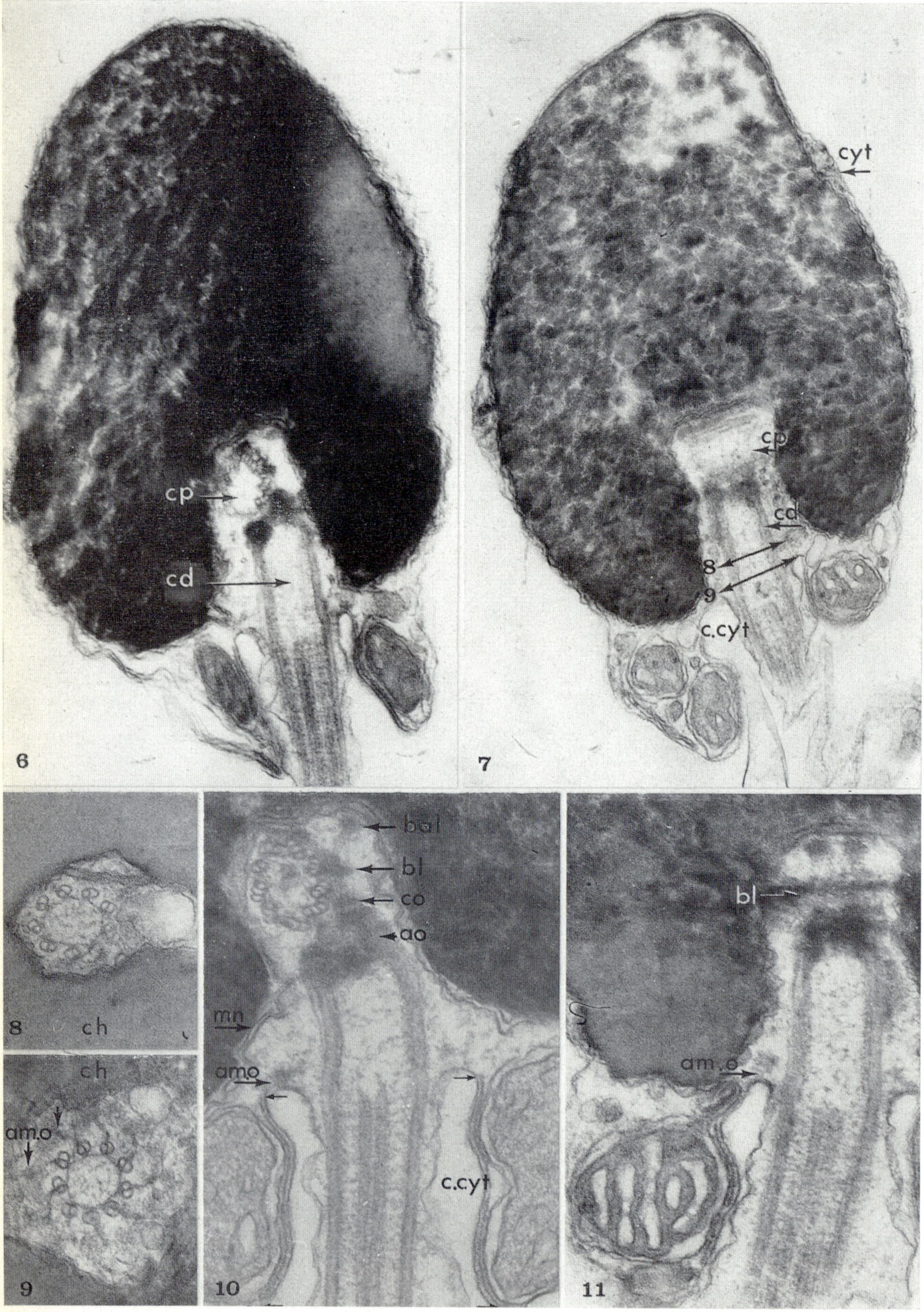
cp
cd
6
cyt
cp
cd
8
9
c.cyt
7
ch
8
ch
am.o
9
bal
bl
co
ao
mn
am.o
c.cyt
10
bl
am.o
11

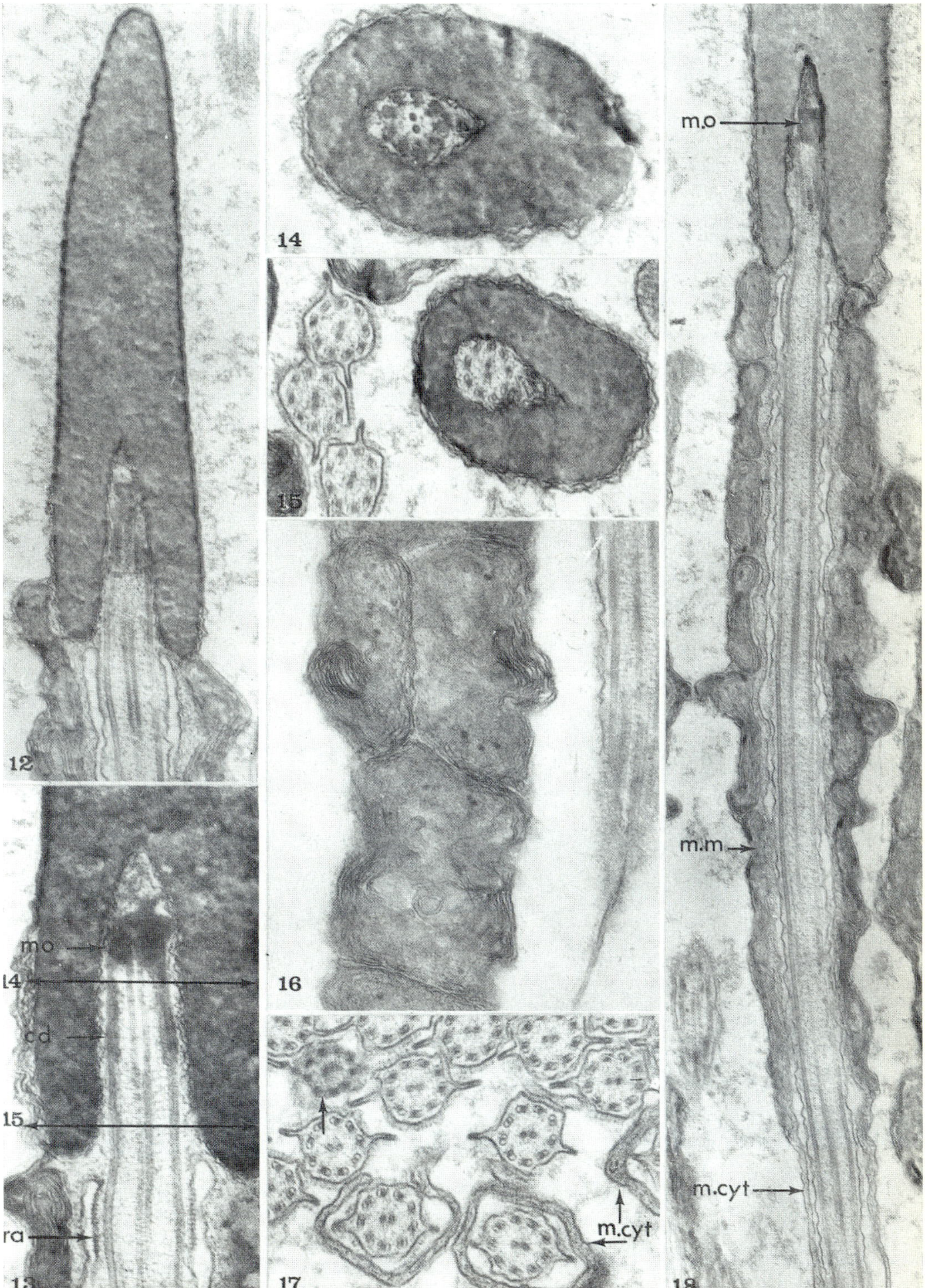
12
13
mo
14
cd
15
ra
14
15
16
17
m.cyt
m.o
m.m
m.cyt
18

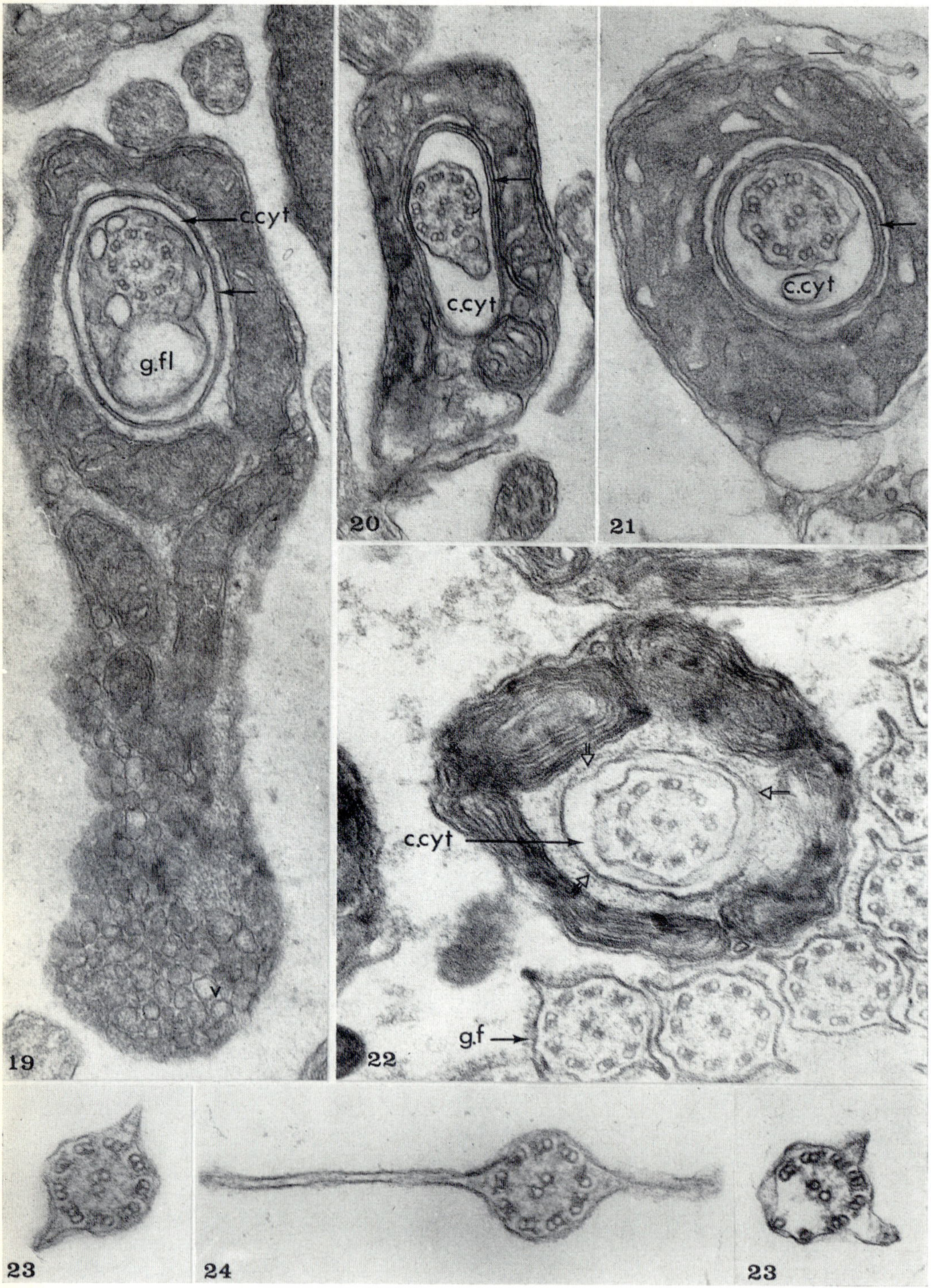
c.cyt
g.fl
v
19
c.cyt
20
c.cyt
21
c.cyt
g.f
22
23
24
23

K. R. BARKER [1] (*) and C. L. BAKER [2] (*)

URODELE SPERMATELEOSIS: A COMPARATIVE ELECTRON MICROSCOPE STUDY

SUMMARY. — The axial rod of urodele sperm varies in shape. A " ring " is typically observed in urodele spermatids, but the size of the ring depends on the species. Elongation of this ring is observed in some species, but not all. Other diagnostic features for a genus include length of middle–piece and of neck–piece.

RIASSUNTO. — Il bastoncello assiale degli spermi degli Urodeli varia per la forma. Un « anello » è tipicamente osservato negli spermatidi degli Urodeli ma la grandezza dell'anello dipende dalla specie. L'allungamento di questo anello è osservato in alcune specie e non in altre. Altre caratteristiche diagnostiche per un genere includono la lunghezza del pezzo intermedio e del collo.

There are six or seven families of American urodeles depending on the classification system to which one adheres. Many of these families are represented by only a few species and consequently it is possible to examine representatives of all families within a reasonable length of time. Light and electron microscope studies have been made by us over the past few years on specimens from the various families and this is a report of some of these findings. We give here a picture of some of the variations found in the urodele sperm and its formation. The theme is one that is well-known in biology— that of variation around a basic pattern. The basic pattern is described below.

It is important to remember that the sperm of urodeles differs from many vertebrate sperm in that the flagellum is lateral to the main axis which is occupied by a dense rod, which we shall term the axial rod, a term suggested by FAWCETT. The flagellum, which is drawn up in sine waves around the tail of the helically shaped sperm, as demonstrated by the work of BAKER (1962; 1966) and BARKER and BIESELE (1967) is held to the convex side of the curved axial rod by a thin cytoplasmic membrane which is generally called the undulating membrane.

There is no evidence from our studies of urodele sperm that this sheath has any powers of contractility or motility. It moves only when the flagellum moves. However, in other amphibian sperm, such as those of *Bufo arenarum*, this membrane may have power of independent movement, as is suggested by the work of Burgos and FAWCETT (1956).

(*) Dept. of Biology, Canisius College, New York.

(1) Current address: Canisius College, Buffalo, New York. Much of this work was completed at the University of the Witwatersrand, Johannesburg, South Africa.

(2) Current address: Southwestern at Memphis, Memphis, Tennessee.

The variation in this basic pattern occurs in the shape of the axial rod, especially as seen in cross-section, in the size of the flagellar rod along side the " nine plus two " structure of the flagellum itself, in the amount of material round the flagellum, and in the number of flagella present. The first part of this report deals with this variation, which is described in detail below.

The following families and species are represented here: Family, Amphiumidae: *Amphiuma tridactylum;* Family, Cryptobranchidae: *Cryptobranchus alleganiensis bishopi*; Family, Plethodontidae: *Desmognathus quadrimaculatus quadrimaculatus*, *D. fuscus fuscus*, *D. monticola*, and *Plethodon dorsalis*; Family, Salamandridae: *Diemictylus* (*Triturus*) *viridescens viridescens*; Family, Ambystomidae: *Ambystoma maculatum*; Family, Proteidae: *Necturus maculosus*; and Family, Sirenidae: *Pseudobranchus striatus axanthus*. All sections shown of the tail of these sperm are taken at the level of the principal-piece, with the exception of *Necturus* which has no principal-piece, and are all cross-sections.

The sperm of three species of *Desmognathus* are represented here, representing the family Plethodontidae. In each case a single flagellum is attached to the axial rod by a cytoplasmic sheath. The shape of the axial rod varies from almost spherical in *Desmognathus fuscus fuscus* (Fig. 1), bi-partite on one side in *D. monticola* (Fig. 2), and halfmoon shaped in *D. quadrimaculatus quadrimaculatus* (Fig. 5). The flagellar rod is quite large in *D. fuscus fuscus* (Fig. 1) and deserves special attention. This rod in *D monticola* (Fig. 2) is medium size and has the size relationship to the flagellum that is typical of the urodele sperm that we have studied. This rod is very reduced in size in *D. quadrimaculatus quadrimaculatus* (Fig. 5). The shape of the rod of *Ambystoma maculatum* (Fig. 3) resembles an anchor. The axial rod of *Crytobranchus* is almost cylindrical (Fig. 4) while in *Necturus maculosus* it is relatively small. Mitochondria are present the entire length of the tail of the *Necturus* sperm, so there is no area we can define as a principal-piece (BAKER; 1963). The axial rod of *Diemictylus viridescens* is tri-foliate in shape (FAWCETT; 1961; BAKER, 1966) (Fig. 9). The sperm of *Pseudobranchus* is bi-flagellate and the axial rod is very reduced in size (Fig. 6).

In all of the above cases the typical pattern is a flagellum attached to an axial rod by a cytoplasmic sheath. The flagellum, which is always a " nine plus two " without additional tubules, is on the periphery of the sperm axis. Other sperms have such a morphology, such as the insect, *Ceutophilis* (SHAY, 1968) and other amphibians, such as *Bufo arenarum* (BURGOS and FAWCETT, 1956; BARKER and RIESS, unpublished data). In the case of *Bufo arenarum* it is the axial rod that is on the outside of the sperm tail, while the flagellum is centrally placed, providing another kind of variation.

The sperm formation of certain urodeles, *Amphiuma tridactylum*, *Diemictylus viridescens*, *Necturus maculosus*, and *Cryptobranchus alleganiensis bishopi*, have been described in detail (BAKER, 1962, 1963; BARKER, and BIESELE 1967). Here we wish only to compare certain specific aspects of sperm formation, namely the size of the ring, whether or not it elongates, and the size of the neck-piece.

The ring is a typical feature of urodele spermateleosis and was often called the " distal centriole " by the early light microscopists. It has not been demonstrated to be a centriole and does not have centriolar structure. Therefore, we refer to it as the ring. It is present in all the urodele spermatids that we have investigated. In a majority of cases it elongates down the length of the middle-piece, but in *Cryptobranchus* and *Necturus* there is no evidence of any ring elongation (BAKER, 1963). Shown here are sections through the ring in *Desmognathus* (Fig. 8), *Amphiuma* (Fig. 11), and *Cryptobranchus* (Fig. 12). The ring is quite large in *Desmognathus*, medium sized in *Diemictylus* and *Amphiuma*, and very reduced in *Cryptobranchus*.

A diagnostic feature for a family of urodeles is the size of the neck-piece. In the Salamandridae the neck-piece is long, in Amphiumidae quite small, and in *Cryptobranchus* so small as to be not visible with the light microscope. MCGREGOR (1899) suggested that there might be some correlation between the size and length of the neck-piece and the length of time that the sperm is retained in the female cloaca. Our observations support his idea. In *Cryptobranchus* where sperm are utilized soon after formation and external fertilization is the rule in this family, the neckpiece is very small. In *Diemictylus* where the sperm is retained by the male or female for several months before use the neck-piece is long.

REFERENCES

BAKER C. L. (1962) – *Spermatozoa of Amphiuma: spermateleosis, helical motility and reversibility*. « J. Tenn. Acad. Sci. », 37, 23–37.

BAKER C. L. (1963) – *Spermatozoa and spermateleosis in Cryptobranchus and Necturus*. « J. Tenn. Acad. Sci. », 38, 1–11.

BAKER C. L. (1966) – *Spermatozoa and Spermateleosis in the Salamandridae with electron microscopy of Diemictylus*. « J. Tenn. Acad. Sci. », 41, 2–25.

BARKER K. R. and BIESELE J. J. (1967) – *Spermateleosis of a salamander*, Amphiuma tridactylum (*Cuvier*): *a correlated light and electron microscope study*. « La Cellule », 67, 91–118.

BURGOS MARIO H. and FAWCETT DON W. (1956) – *An electron microscope study of spermatid differentiation in the toad*, Bufo arenarum (*Hensel*). « J. Biophys. Biochem. Cytol. », 2, 223–240.

FAWCETT DON W. (1961) – *Cilia and Flagella*. In « The Cell », Vol. II. Academic Press, NYC, 217–267.

MCGREGOR J. H. (1899) – *The spermatogenesis of Amphiuma*. « J. of Morph. », 15, (Supplement), 57–104.

SHAY J. and BIESELE J. – *Ultrastructural Observations on Spermiogenesis in the Cave Cricket*, Ceutophilos Secretis, (*Seutter*). « La Cellule », 67, 269–282.

Explanation of figures.

Fig. 1. – Cross-section through principal-piece of *Desmognathus fuscus fuscus*. Note large flagellar rod. (32,000×).

Fig. 2. – Cross-section through principal-piece of *Desmognathus monticola*. (40,000×).

Fig. 3. – Cross-section through principal-piece of *Ambystoma maculatum*. (50,000×).

Fig. 4. – Cross-section through principal-piece of *Cryptobranchus alleganesis bishopi*. (37,500×).

Fig. 5. – Cross-section through principal-piece of *Desmognathus quadrimaculatus quadrimaculatus*. (44,000×).

Fig. 6. – Cross-section through bi-flagellate sperm of *Pseudobranchus striatus axanthus*. Note small axial rod at the end of arrow. (6,000×).

Fig. 7. – Cross-section through middle-piece of *Necturus maculosus*. (40,000×).

Fig. 8. – Cross-section of ring of *Desmognathus quadrimaculatus quadrimaculatus*. (12,000×).

Fig. 9. – Cross-section through principal-piece of *Diemictylus viridescens viridescens* (20,000×).

Fig. 10. – Cross-section through principal-piece of *Plethodon dorsalis dorsalis* (38,000×).

Fig. 11. – Section through neck-piece, ring, and tail complex of spermatid of *Amphiuma tridactylum*. (20,000×).

Fig. 12. – Section through spermatid of *Cryptobranchus*. The neck-piece, below centriole, is quite small. Ring is at end of arrow. (32,000×).

K. R. Barker and C. L. Baker – *Urodele spermateleosis: a comparative electron microscope study.*

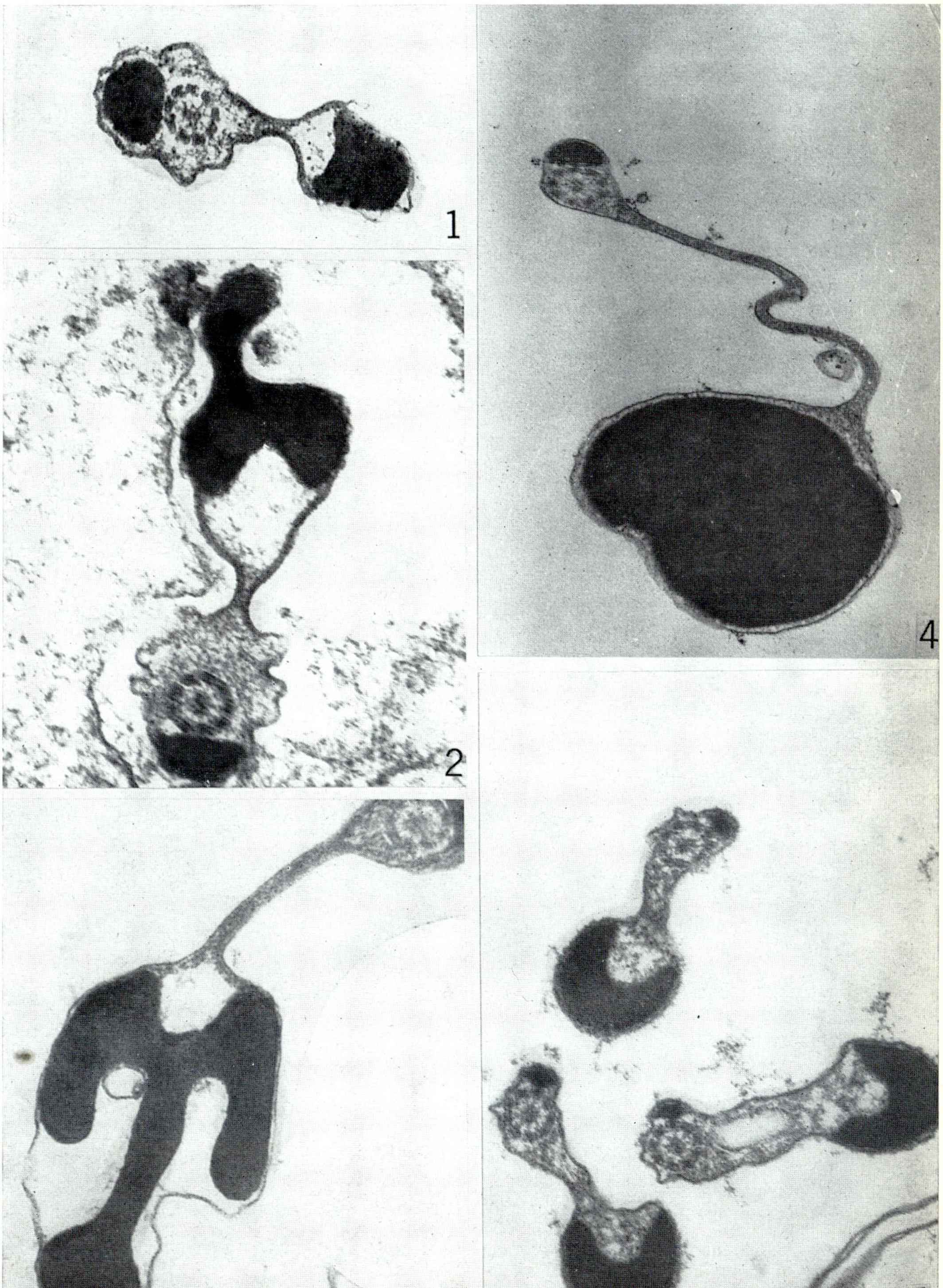

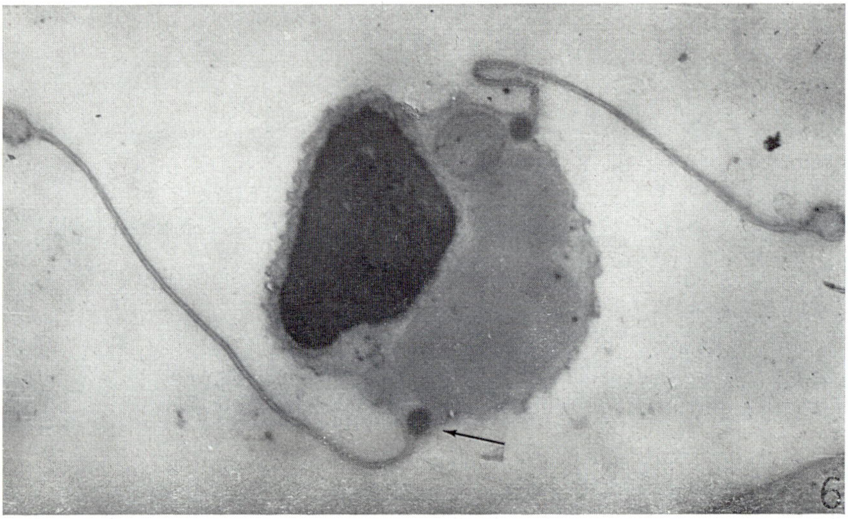
6

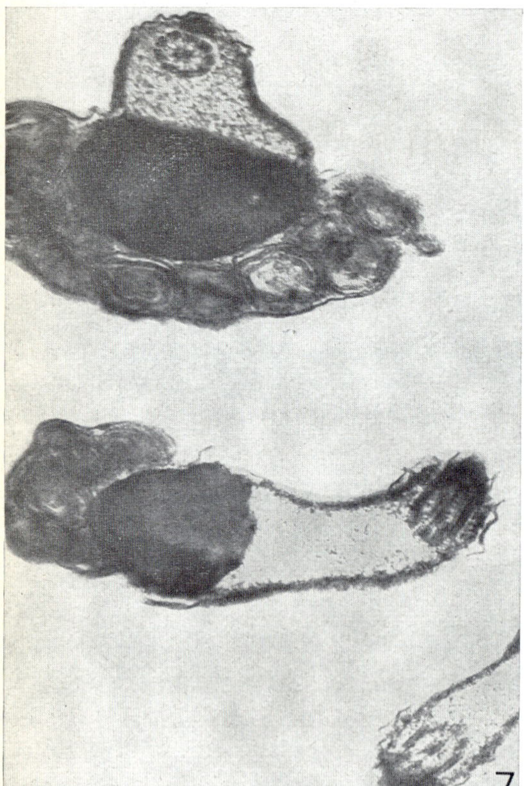
7

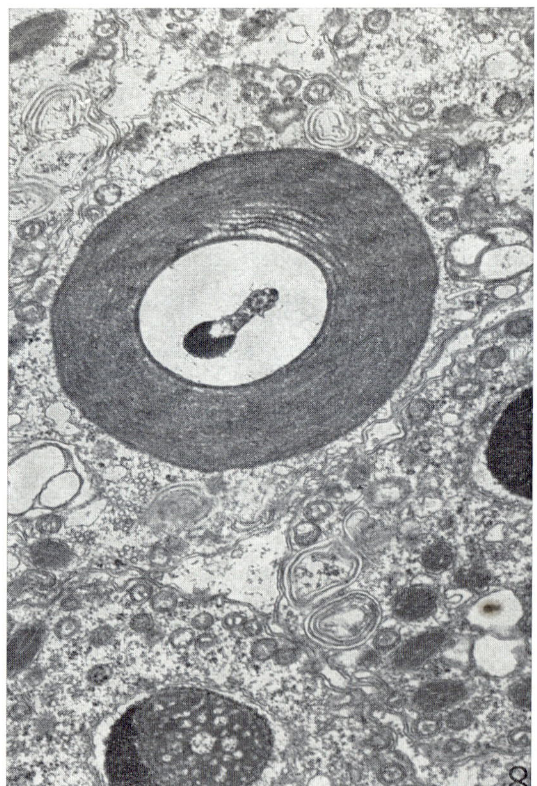
8

K. R. Barker and C. L. Baker – *Urodele spermateleosis: a comparative electron microscope study.*

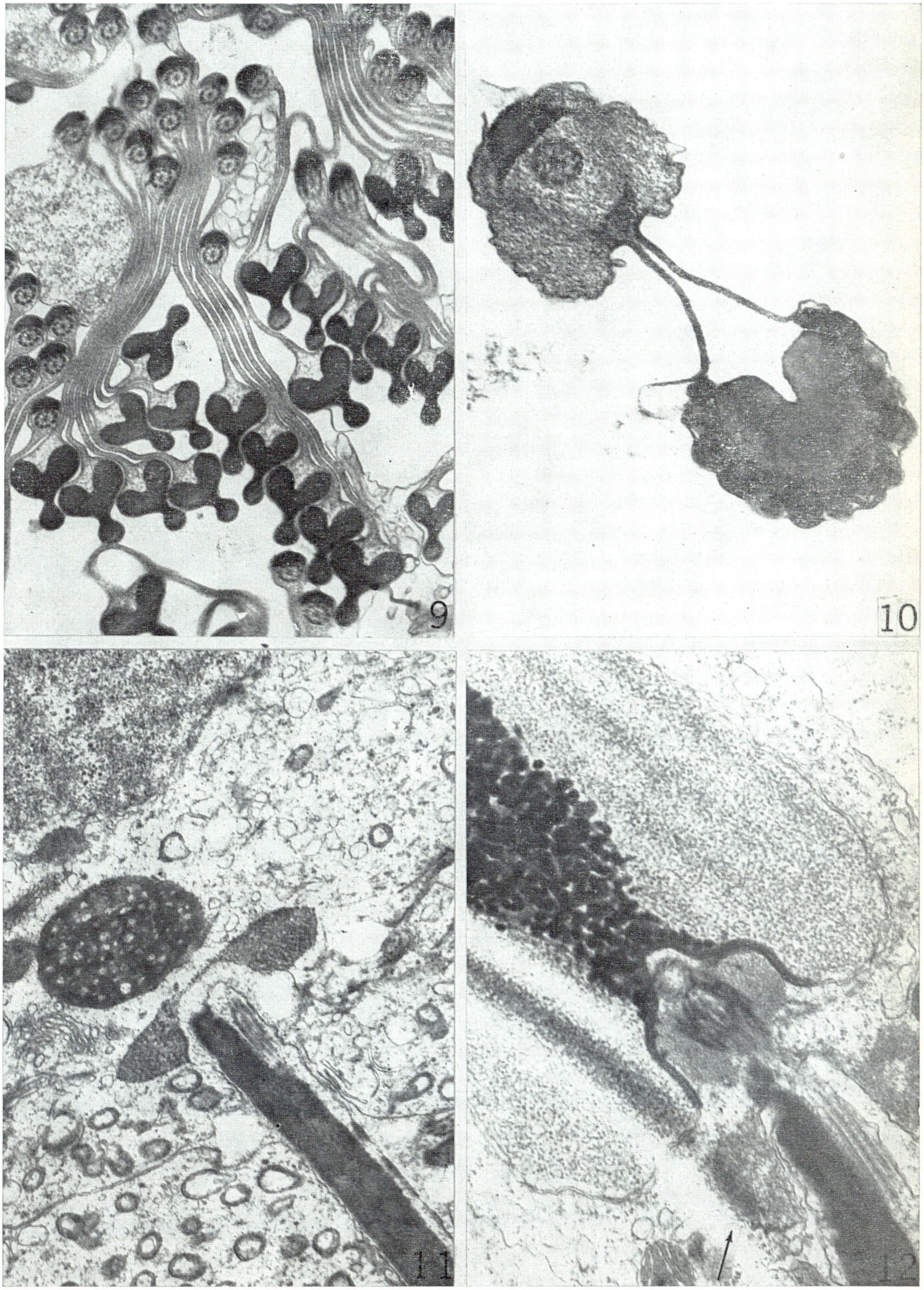

G. WERNER (*)

ON THE DEVELOPMENT AND STRUCTURE OF THE NECK IN URODELE SPERM (**)

SUMMARY. — The development and structure of the neck region has been studied in spermatids and spermatozoa of *Salamandra salamandra* and *Triturus alpestris*. Consistent in both cases a double ring is formed at the anterior end of the flagellar sheath. Apparently it is not derived from the distal centriole. A flocculant pericentriolar material and some different appearing substance at the anterior end of the developing axial rod on one side of the distal centriole are formed, before the centrioles have reached the nucleus. While the larger part of the Golgi-apparatus is involved in the formation of the acrosome, a single dictyosome remains during the formation of these structures in a constant spacial relationship to the centriolar complex, suggesting, that different parts of the same organelle may perform different functions at the same time. After the centrioles have reached the nucleus, this special dictyosome soon disappears. At this time the anlage of the neck piece will become visible, situated in an invagination of the nuclear wall above the centrioles. Simultaneously, the nuclear wall develops a multiporous area around the later caudal pole, where some granular material seems to accumulate. The temporal correspondence of these events allows to conclude, that the neck piece is derived from the nucleus and is thus the homologous structure in the vertebrates to the so called centriole adjunct or juxtanuclear body in the insects. Further conclusions are discussed.

RIASSUNTO. — Lo sviluppo e la struttura della regione del collo sono stati studiati negli spermatidi e negli spermatozoi di *Salamandra salamandra* e di *Triturus alpestris*. In entrambi i casi si nota al polo anteriore della guaina flagellare un doppio anello, che apparentemente non è derivato dal centriolo distale. Prima che i centrioli raggiungano il nucleo, materiale pericentriolare si forma al polo anteriore da un lato del centriolo distale. Mentre la maggior parte dell'apparato di Golgi forma l'acrosoma, un solo dictiosoma rimane durante la formazione di questa struttura in costante relazione spaziale con il complesso centriolare, suggerendo che diverse parti dello stesso organello possono svolgere differenti funzioni nello stesso tempo. Dopo che i centrioli hanno raggiunto il nucleo, questo dittiosoma scompare. Contemporaneamente, la membrana nucleare forma un'area multiporosa intorno al polo caudale, dove si accumula materiale granulare. La corrispondenza temporale di questi eventi permette di concludere che la regione del collo deriva dal nucleo ad è, nei vertebrati, la struttura omologa all'aggiunto centriolare degli insetti. Vengono discusse ulteriori conclusioni.

INTRODUCTION

During the classic period of light microscopy the development and structure of the spermatozoa of the tailed amphibia were the subject of numerous studies. The rings, being well visible in the light microscope, and a conspi-

(*) Institut für Zytologie und Elektronenmikroskopie der Universität des Saarlandes, 665 Homburg/Saar, Bundesrepublik Deutschland.

(**) Supported by Deutsche Forschungsgemeinschaft.

cuous enlargement in the area of the proximal centriole caused a special interest in that they were interpreted as transformations of the centrioles. Since spermatogenesis of the urodeles has been studied relatively infrequently by means of electron microscopy, it seemed promising to re-explore this problem by new methods at this time.

The development and structure of the neck were studied in *Salamandra salamandra* and *Triturus alpestris*. Preliminary results of *Triturus helveticus* which will be published elsewhere confirm the results presented here. RETZIUS (1906) and CHAMPY (1913), among others, have emphasized, that the spermatozoa of these species appear very similar in shape, differing only in the proportions of their separate parts. When examined under the electron microscope, it became evident that they differ in fine structural details as well. Under such circumstances, the individual species can be clearly differentiated from each other. On the whole, however, there are many uniform features also on this level.

The study of such a closely related group while demanding some effort does not allow to expect wide range of variation. But certain details are so inconspicuous that they become evident only by virtue of their regular appearance. In the cases presently explored, it was impressive to note that from the beginning, the development of the neck region follows a uniform chronological order and spacial relationship.

The neck always consists of the same parts clearly separated from each other: A solid cylindrical rod extending into a deep nuclear invagination is commonly called the neck in urodele sperm. For the sake of simplicity, this term is adopted, though, strictly speaking, it is not correct. By definition the neck constitutes the connection between the head and the middle piece. So we have to include the two centrioles with their pericentriolar granular material, the remnants of the former rings which seem to have a function related to the formation of the middle piece, and also the axial rod to the extent that it takes its origin by the side of the distal centriole.

RESULTS

In the very young spermatids of *Salamandra salamandra* (Fig. 1), the two centrioles form an angle of about 130° and are located in the cytoplasm. The flagellum begins to grow into a vesicle. At some distance from the distal centriole, the first sign of ring formation becomes evident in the form of a dark appearing substance. It is remarkable that one part of the Golgi-apparatus is related to the centrioles, while its greater mass is gathered around the proacrosomal vesicle.

The next stage of differentiation is illustrated in Fig. 2. Here the ring, in reality now a double ring, is located at the anterior end of the developing flagellum. It consists of an outer distal dark somewhat layered material and an inner proximal granular substance. Both centrioles are surrounded by a denser flocculant material. A single dictyosome can be seen in the adjacent area again.

Fig. 3 illustrates a similar situation, except here a new material can now be distinguished next to the flagellar centriole. If a section occurs at a particular plane, the single dictyosome always occurs in the angle formed by the two centrioles with the dark material being located at the opposite side.

When the centriolar complex approximates the nuclear membrane (Figs. 4 and 5), the accompanying dictyosome soon disappears. The nuclear wall forms an indentation at this point of contact. When the axial rod differentiates, it will appear between the flocculant pericentriolar material and the laterally displaced substance adjoining the distal centriole. It's possible that the axial rod is formed in this position, before the centrioles have reached the nucleus, as is the case in *Triturus*. Another structural entity, the anlage of the so-called neck, initially consisting of a spongy structure within a lighter flocculant area above the proximal centriole, appears only after invagination of the nucleus has occured.

As nuclear elongation commences (Fig. 6), the niche deepens and is essentially filled by the rapidly enlarging neck. Posteriorly it is deliniated by the first centriole. Granular material appears along the nuclear wall but at some distance away. At this initial stage of nuclear elongation, its contents are composed of fine fibrils. Simultaneously, in the posterior area the first appearance of pores occurs some distance from the indentation.

The Golgi-apparatus has already become displaced from the centriolar complex. Fig. 7 illustrates the spacial relationship between the two centrioles and the neck piece. By this time the two rings have become fully developed. In Fig. 8 the anterior end of the axial rod can be seen. It is bent and shows a constriction at its point of juncture to the tail, a condition which persists in the mature stage (Fig. 10). This structure is much more electron dense at first than it is in the mature spermatozoon.

As elongation of the nucleus proceeds (Fig. 9), the neck grows and the light holes become progressively smaller and finally disappear. The condensation of the contents of the nucleus initiates in front of the neck where a thin layer of chromatin is attached to the indentation of the nuclear wall. This part does not show any interruptions in contrast to those laterally displaced which display many pores in the posterior region. Before the axial rod has reached its final thickness the rings open at its dorsal side. Not until now does the formation of the middle piece occur: the mitochondria which were previously distributed around the nucleus gather in a semicircle around the axial rod. The axial rod remains oriented along the same axis as the head while the flagellum, connected to the former by the undulating membrane, is laterally displaced.

In the mature spermatozoon (Figs. 10, 11, 12) the so called neck piece is essentially homogenous except occasional few light spots. The remnants of the rings, which is mainly the proximal one, are still situated in their original place. It is not known if the two dark spots on each side of the undulating membrane represent the former distal ring as is the case in *Triturus*. The axial rod consists of a homogenous wall and a denser granular core. A short distance behind the second centriole a flagellar rod has formed. Apparently, it has no connection to any of the structures in the neck region.

In young spermatids of *Triturus alpestris* (Fig. 13) a single dictyosome is again present near the centrioles, which has become separated from the main mass of the Golgi-apparatus. The first still uniform anlage of the rings is visible. A little later a dark outer and a light inner part can be discerned (Fig. 14).

Next, denser material appears around the centrioles (Fig. 15). This figure again demonstrates the simultaneous relationship of the Golgi-apparatus to the centrioles and the developing acrosome. As in *Salamandra*, some material is added on the side opposing the Golgi-apparatus (Fig. 16), and again it is along the side of the axial rod. The separation of the two rings however is more evident than in *Salamandra*. The dark outer ring displays distinct layers.

The attachment of the centriolar complex to the nucleus takes place in the same manner as it does in *Salamandra* (Fig. 17). The proximal centriole is directed obliquely towards the nuclear wall and forms an angle of about 130° with the distal one. The axial rod has its anterior end next to the distal centriole. The neck piece begins to develop within a light substance above the centrioles. From the initial stage it consists primarily of a denser material than was found in *Salamandra*. At the place of contact, the nuclear wall is always distinctly separated into two membranes. Pores are seen only some distance away. Indeed, one has the impression here likewise, that darker material is distributed along the pores.

When nuclear elongation commences (Fig. 18) the neck piece enlarges into the deepening invagination. It contains irregularly shaped lighter areas. Apparently, the neck piece grows at the caudal end by accretion of a condensing substance. The axial rod is situated next to the distal centriole and its pericentriolar material.

In this stage the rings are fully developed (Fig. 19). The neck piece becomes longer and the lighter areas are replaced by the dense substance. At the caudal end, where it is not contiguous with the centrioles, some tortuous folds appear. The chromatin has contracted, so that a broad cleft appears. The nuclear membrane is tight except at the lateral aspect of the posterior region, where the pores are concentrated. One has the impression that surplus membrane is cast off at the end. The mitochondria are still disposed around the nucleus.

Later (Fig. 20) the nuclear wall is again loosely attached to the chromatin. The neck piece has now reached its definitive length. The folds at the base are very prominent.

In ripe spermatozoa (Figs. 21–24), the neck piece appears uniformly dense. In favourable sections the outer region displays a very regular lattice structure which is superimposed by a second wider lattice in the outermost layer (Figs. 25, 26). The neck piece is distinctly separated from the other components of this region, the centriolar complex and the anterior end of the axial rod. The axial rod has a faint periodic substructure at the lateral edges. Its anterior end now envelopes the distal centriole which is situated in a short channel as is also the case in *Salamandra*. The rings have opened, their remnants are found in the original position. The distal one has extended to a slim band along the axial rod. The structure of this rod is essentially the same as in *Salamandra*.

Conclusion

If one compares the results with each other, the close relationship of one part of the Golgi-apparatus to the centrioles is particularly striking. From the initial stage to the moment, when the centrioles reach the nucleus, a special dictyosome is found within their immediate proximity. Assuming a constant plane of section one recognizes that the spacial relationship is fixed at the initial stage of development. This means that the dictyosome is always found in the angle between the two centrioles and opposite to the later appearing material. This constant relationship suggests that there exists some functional dependence between these structures.

Besides its well known role in the formation of the acrosome we find here another activity of the Golgi-apparatus in the development of structures of the neck region. This means that different parts of the same organelle may perform different functions at the same time. A further consequence of these results seems to be very remarkable: As is the case with the acrosome, the products of the Golgi-apparatus are generally seen within an enveloping membrane originating from the cisternae. It seems possible however, that the Golgi-apparatus is also involved in the synthesis of substances not enclosed by a membrane in some manner. A similar mode of action was assumed to exist in *Lepisma* (Werner, 1964). Barker and Biesele (1967) have supposed that the Golgi-apparatus in addition to the nucleus, participates in the formation of the neck piece in *Amphiuma tridactylum*. The present results seem to allow a clearer distribution of the roles played by the Golgi-apparatus and the nucleus. In both instances the Golgi-apparatus is present only during the formation of the pericentriolar material and the substance around the origin of the axial rod. The dictyosome quickly disappears after the centrioles have reached the nucleus. On the other hand the anlage of the neck piece is visible only after this stage. The multiporous area develops while the greater parts of the nuclear wall become tight. Since the heterogenous character of the nuclear wall has now been mentioned so often, one has to regard it a general phenomenon in the course of spermatogenesis. It can not merely be explained as a preservation of the original situation, because the pores are more numerous than at any former stage. This multiporous area is particularly evident in certain coleoptera (WERNER, 1965, 1966), such as *Carabus* and *Cicindela*. In the latter species, one can observe how granular material fades out of the porous nuclear vesicle with a concomitant appearance of similar material outside around the centriole, the so called centriole adjunct or juxtanuclear body which becomes an integral part of the mature sperm. It is evident that the same mechanism functions in the development of the neck piece in urodele sperm. Therefore, the centriole adjunct of insect spermatozoa and the so called neck piece in urodele spermatatozoa are homologous structures, as has been supposed already some years ago (WERNER, 1966, p. 598). In view of the widespread occurence of a multiporous area in the nuclear wall during spermiogenesis, which has become apparent in the meantime, a further supposition made in the forementioned paper seems to prove now, i.e. that the dislocation of one part of the nuclear contents into the cytoplasm seems to be a common phenomenon.

REFERENCES

BARKER K. R. and BIESELE J. J. (1967) – *Spermateleosis of a salamander* Amphiuma tridactylum *Cuvier. A correlated light and electron microscope study.* « La Cellule », 67, 89–118.

CHAMPY C. (1913) – *Recherches sur la spermatogénèse des batraciens et les éléments accessoires du testicule.* « Arch. Zool. exptl. gén. », 52, 13–304.

RETZIUS G. (1906) – *Die Spermien der Amphibien.* « Biologische Untersuchungen », 13, 49–70.

WERNER G. (1964) – *Untersuchungen über die Spermiogenese beim Silberfischchen,* Lepisma saccharina *L.* « Z. Zellforsch. », 63, 880–912.

WERNER G. (1965) – *Untersuchungen über die Spermiogenese beim Sandläufer,* Cicindela campestris *L.* « Z. Zellforsch. », 66, 255–275.

WERNER G., (1966) – *Untersuchungen über die Spermiogenese bei einem Laufkäfer,* Carabus catenulatus *Scop., und der Skorpionwasserwanze,* Nepa rubra *L.* « Z. Zellforsch. », 73, 576–599.

EXPLANATION OF FIGURES

List of abbreviations.

AR = axial rod
D = dictyosome
DR = dense ring
FR = flagellar rod
GA = Golgi–apparatus
LR = light ring
N = neck piece
NU = nucleus
PA = proacrosome

Figs. 1–4. – Early stages in the development of the neck in spermatids of *Salamandra salamandra.* In Fig. 1 the proacrosomal vesicle (PA) is seen approaching the nucleus. In Fig. 4 the anterior end of the axial rod (AR) and the anlage of the neck piece (N) are visible. Further details are described in the text. Magnification 27.000 : 1.

Figs. 5–8. – Spermatids of *Salamandra salamandra,* different stages of nuclear elongation. Fig. 5 is cut in a plane perpendicular to the following. AR is the anterior end of the axial rod, N the anlage of the neck piece. Magnification 27.000 : 1.

Fig. 9. – Neck of a spermatid of *Salamandra salamandra,* stage of beginning nuclear condensation. Multiporous areas are seen in the posterior region of the nuclear wall. Figs 10–12 represent mature spermatozoa of *Salamandra salamandra.* The remnants of the rings are indicated. Magnification 27.000 : 1.

Figs. 13 – 16. – Early stages in the development of the neck in spermatids of *Triturus alpestris.* Details are described in the text. Magnification 16.500 : 1.

Figs. 17–20. – Different stages of elongating spermatids of *Triturus alpestris.* Magnifications: Fig. 17 16.500 : 1, Fig. 18 27.000 : 1, Figs 19 and 20 5 500 : 1.

Figs. 21–24. – The neck region of mature spermatozoa of *Triturus alpestris* in longitudinal and cross sections. The arrows indicate the remnants of the dense ring. In Figs. 22 and 24 the remnant of the light ring is also seen. Fig. 23 displays the regular pattern in the outer zone of the neck piece. Magnification 47.000 : 1.

Figs. 25, 26. – Longitudinal sections through different levels of the neck piece of *Triturus alpestris.* The crystalline structure of the outer zone is clearly visible. Magnification 47.000 : 1.

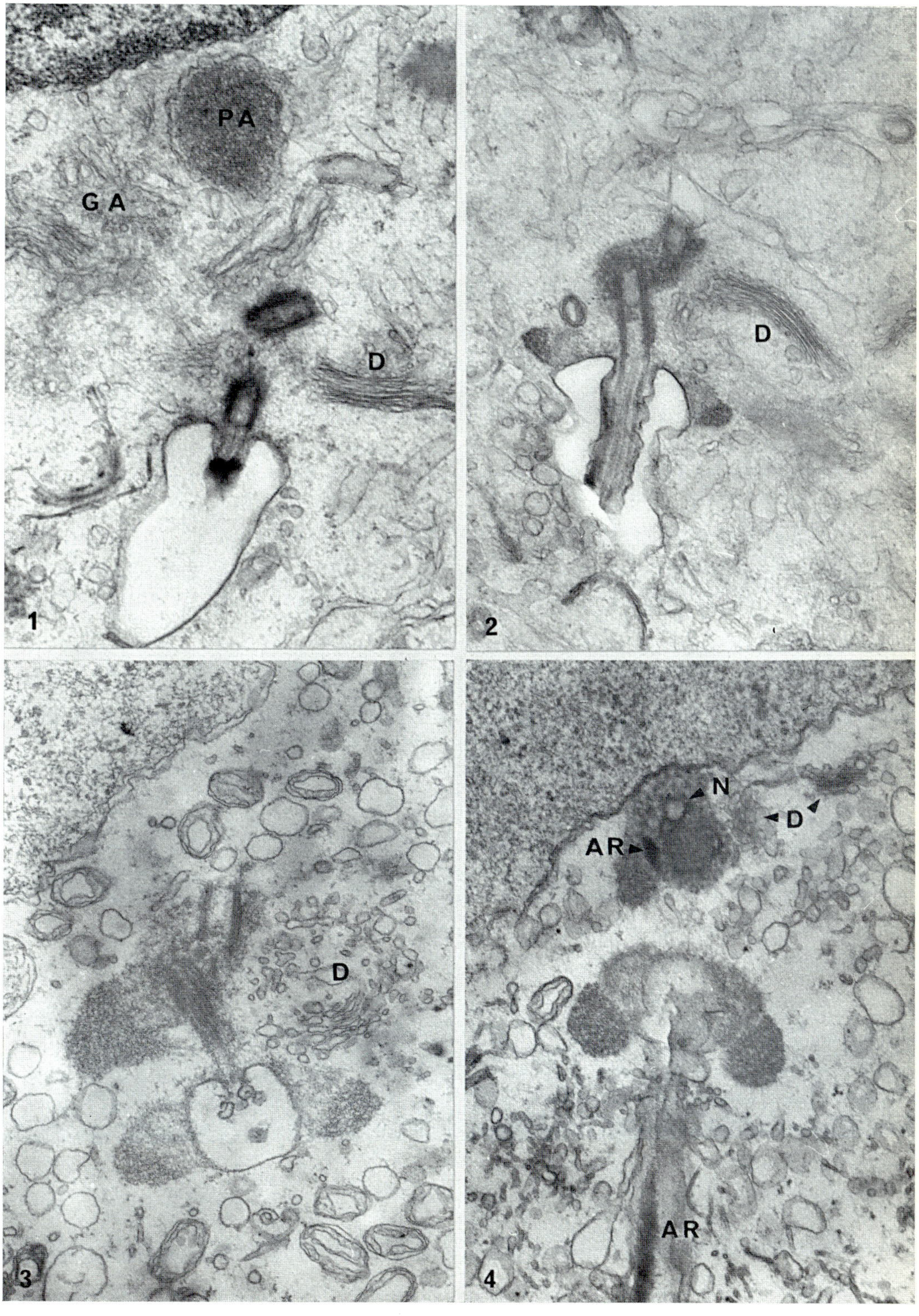
PA
GA
D
1
D
2
D
3
N
D
AR
AR
4

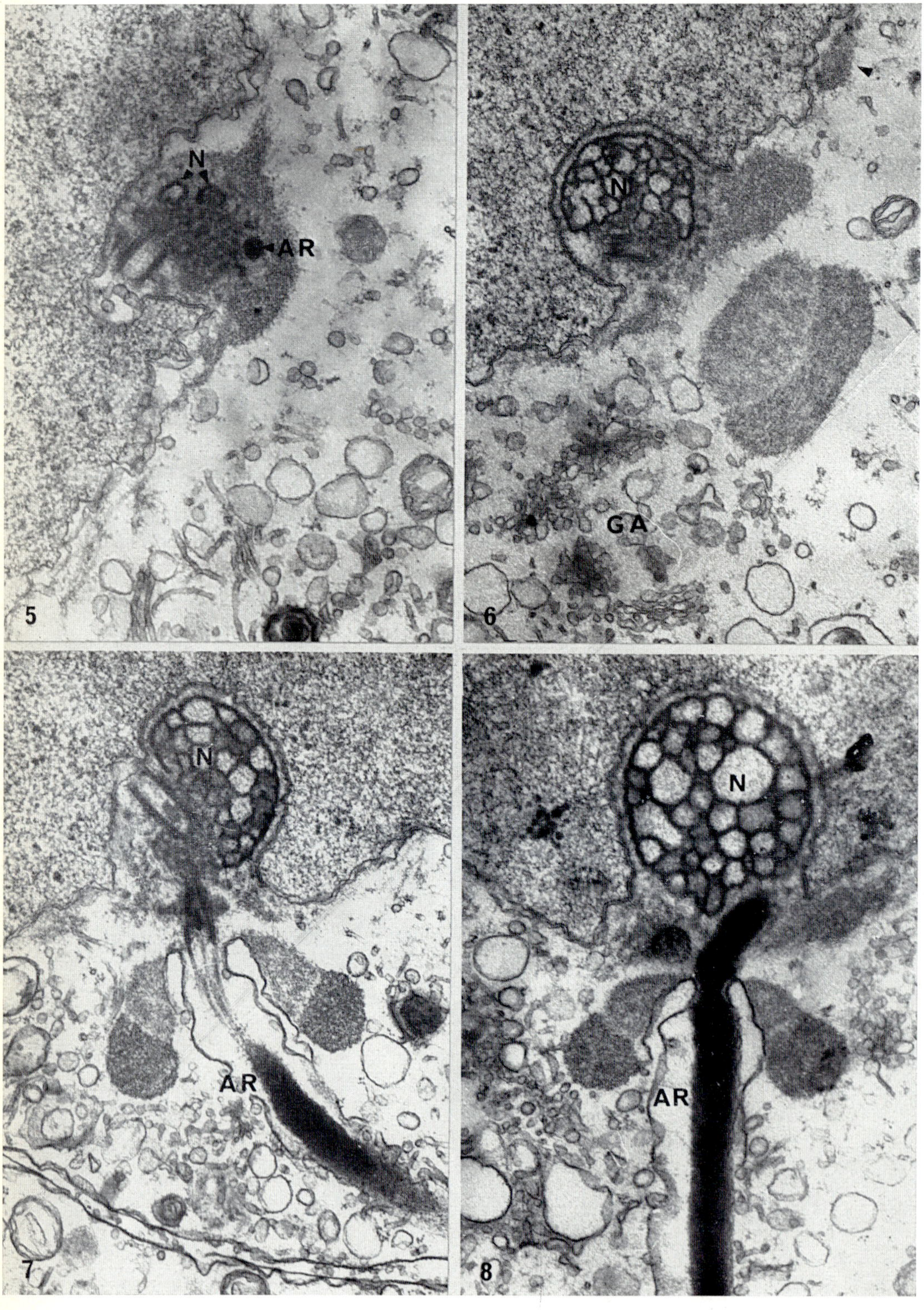
N
AR
5
N
GA
6
N
AR
7
N
AR
8

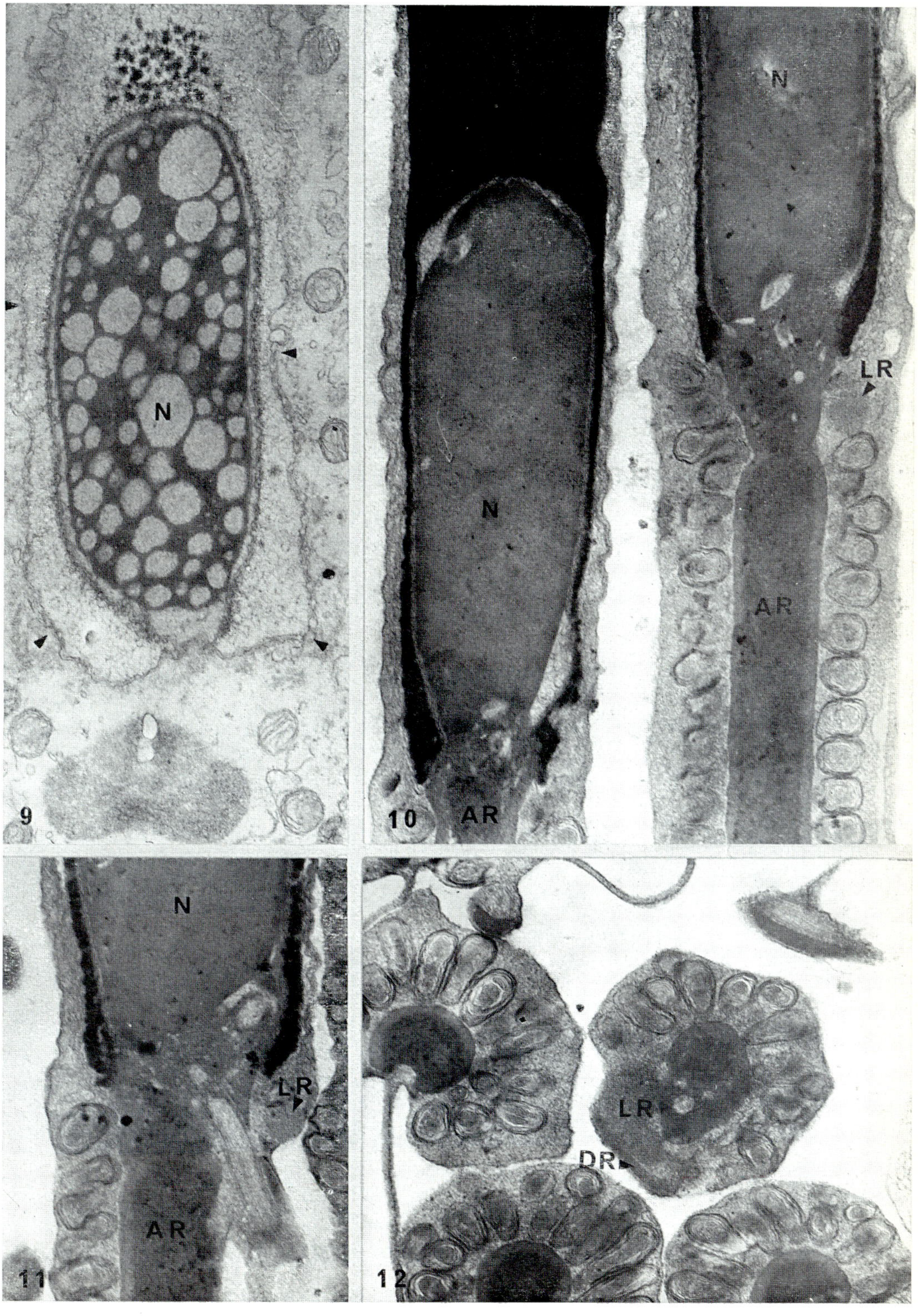
N
9
N
10
AR
N
LR
AR
N
LR
AR
11
LR
DR
12

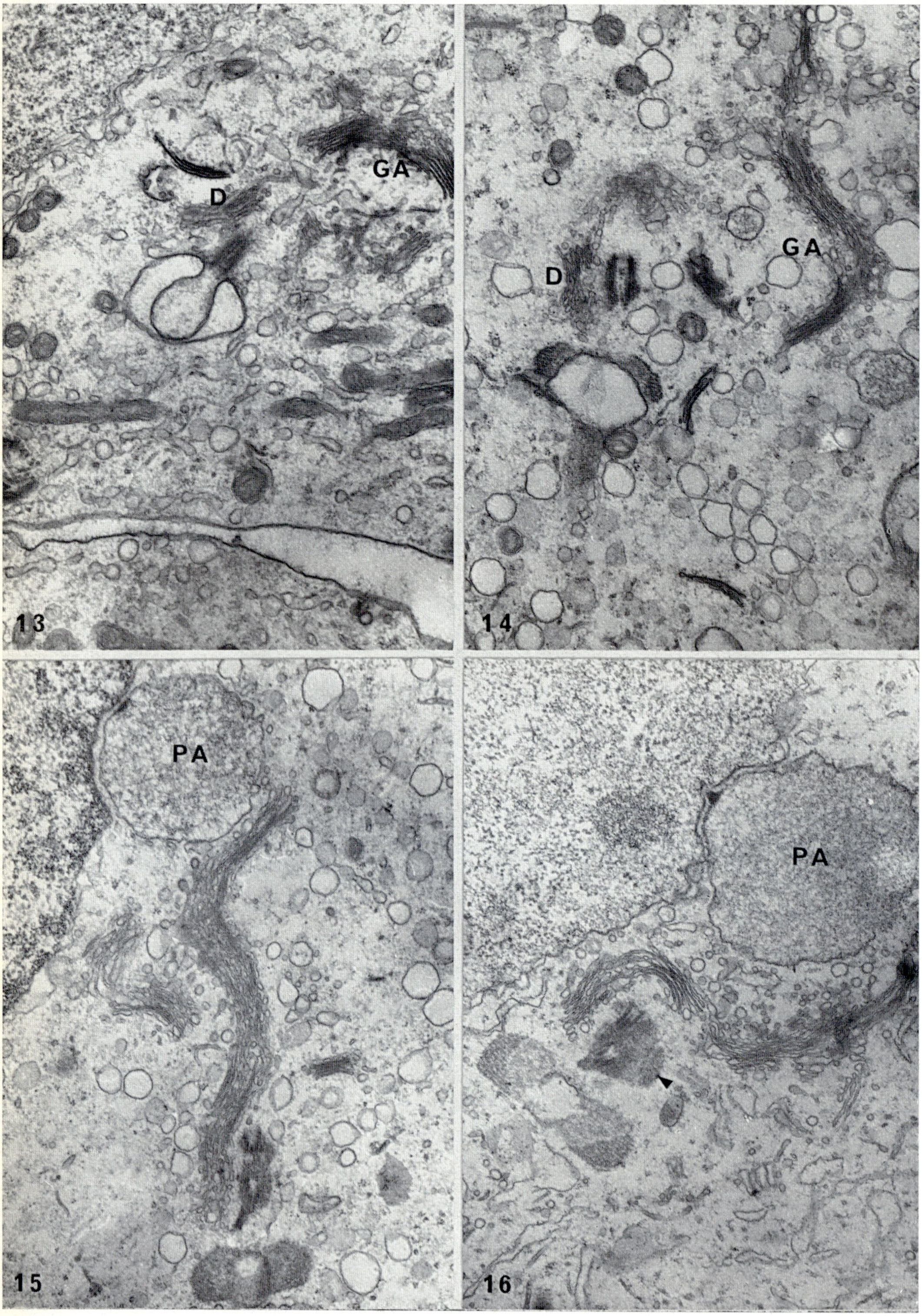
GA
D
13
GA
D
14
PA
15
PA
16

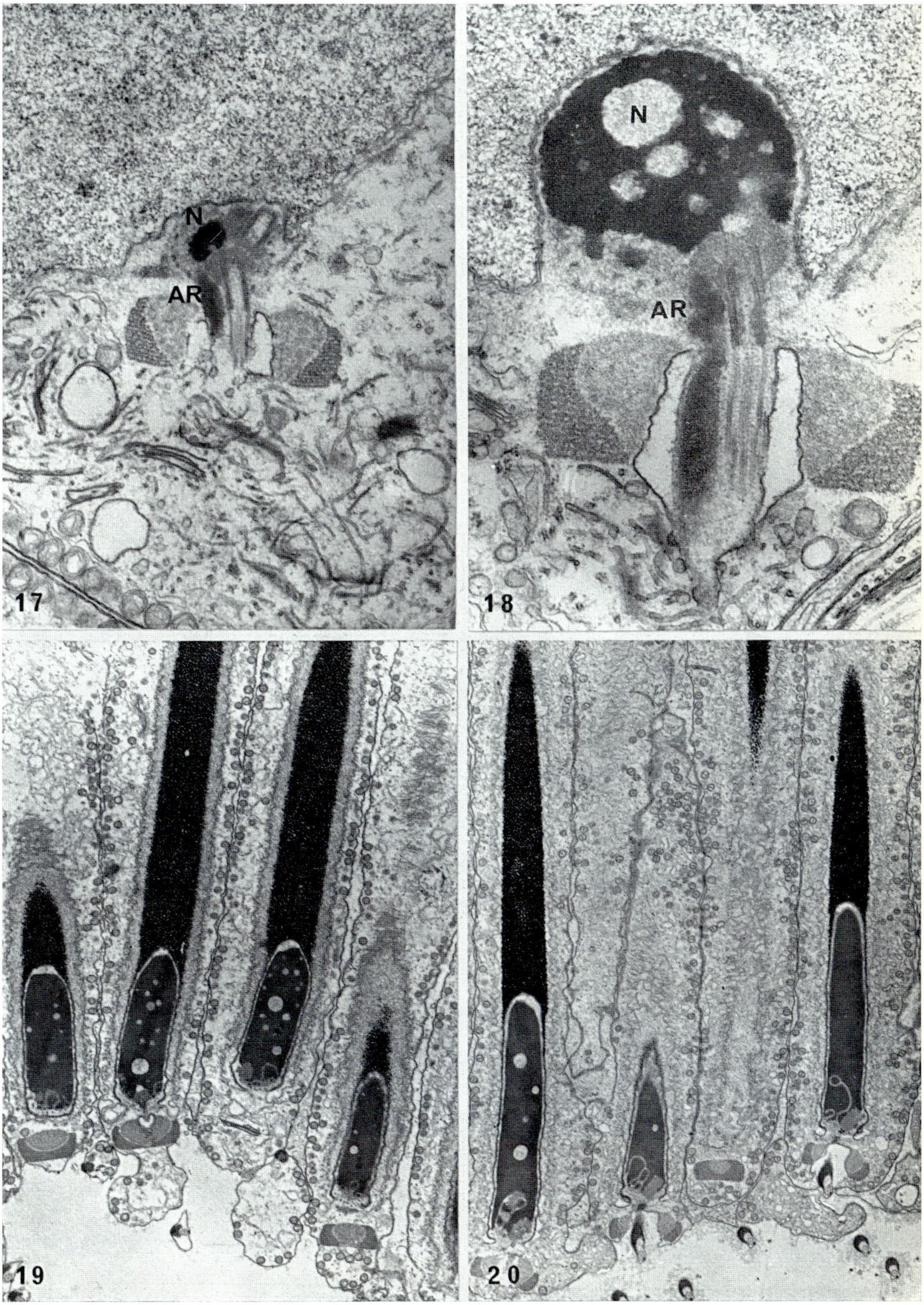
N
AR
17
N
AR
18
19
20

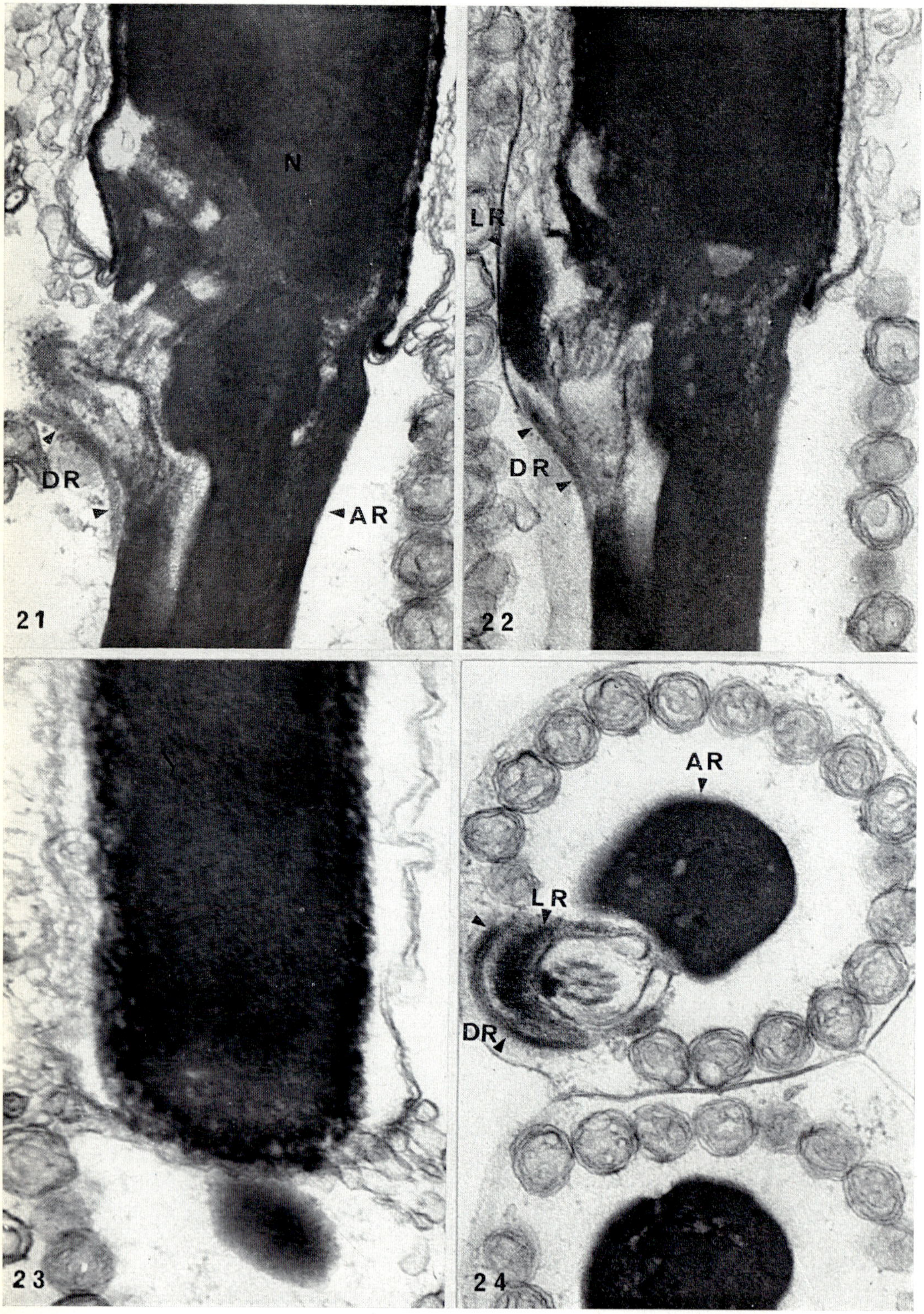
N
LR
DR
AR
21
22
23
24

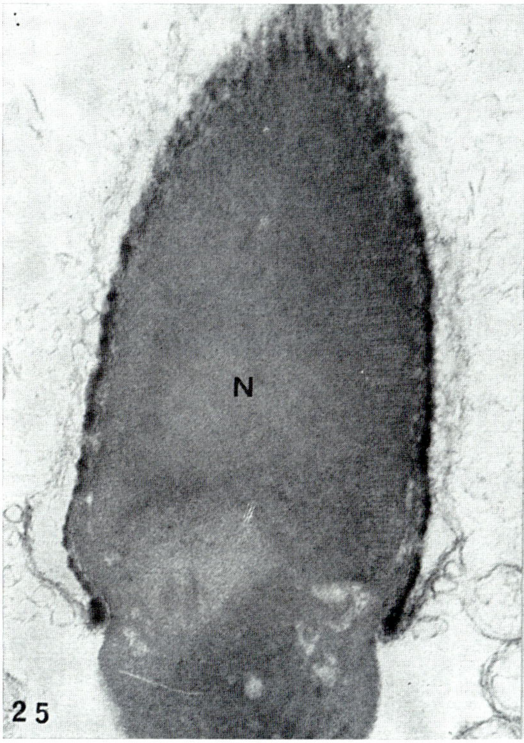
N
25

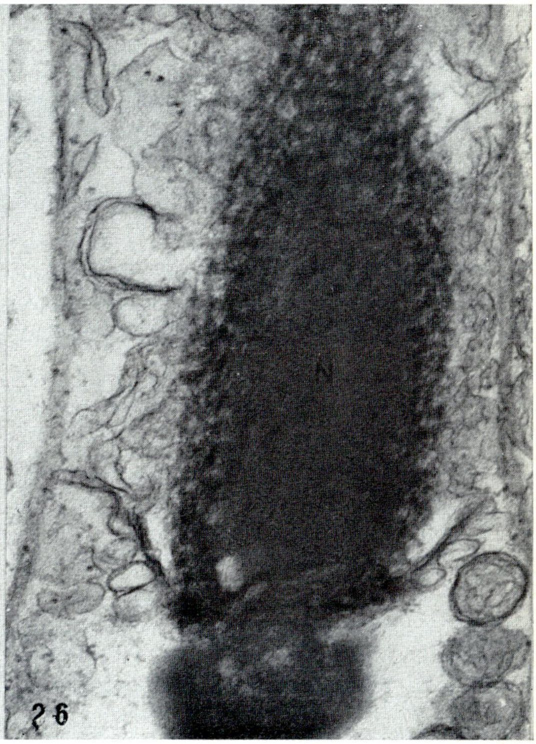
N
26

Fig. 18. – Coupe longitudinale de la tête d'une spermatide âgée; ×29.000.

Acide periodique – TCH – protéinate d'Argent.
Sur cette coupe on distingue successivement la membrane plasmique (*mp*), l'acrosome (*A*) avec une partie externe dense et une partie interne riche en polysaccharides, l'espace sous-acrosomien (*sa*), l'enveloppe nucléaire (*an*), le nucléoplasme (*N*), l'enveloppe nucléaire qui s'est invaginée (flèche), en formant le canal endonucléaire dans lequel se trouve la baguette (*b*).

Discussion

BACCETTI. – Le matériel de polysaccharides que vous avez montré est-il present d'abord au niveau des dictyosomes ou bien des faisceaux membranaires?

SANDOZ. – Mis à part une convergence morphologique, les faisceaux membranaires semblent être totalement différents des dictyosomes. On observe souvent des rapports topographiques entre ces deux formations, mais rien ne prouve que ces rapports aient une signification physiologique.

Le matériel polysaccharidique que l'on observe dans les saccules golgiens peut difficilement être comparé à celui que l'on observe uniquement à la surface des membranes constituant les faisceaux et rien n'indique que ces derniers participent à la formation du matériel acrosomien.

D. Sandoz – *Étude ultrastructurale et cytochimique de la formation de l'acrosome du Discoglosse (Amphibien Anoure).*

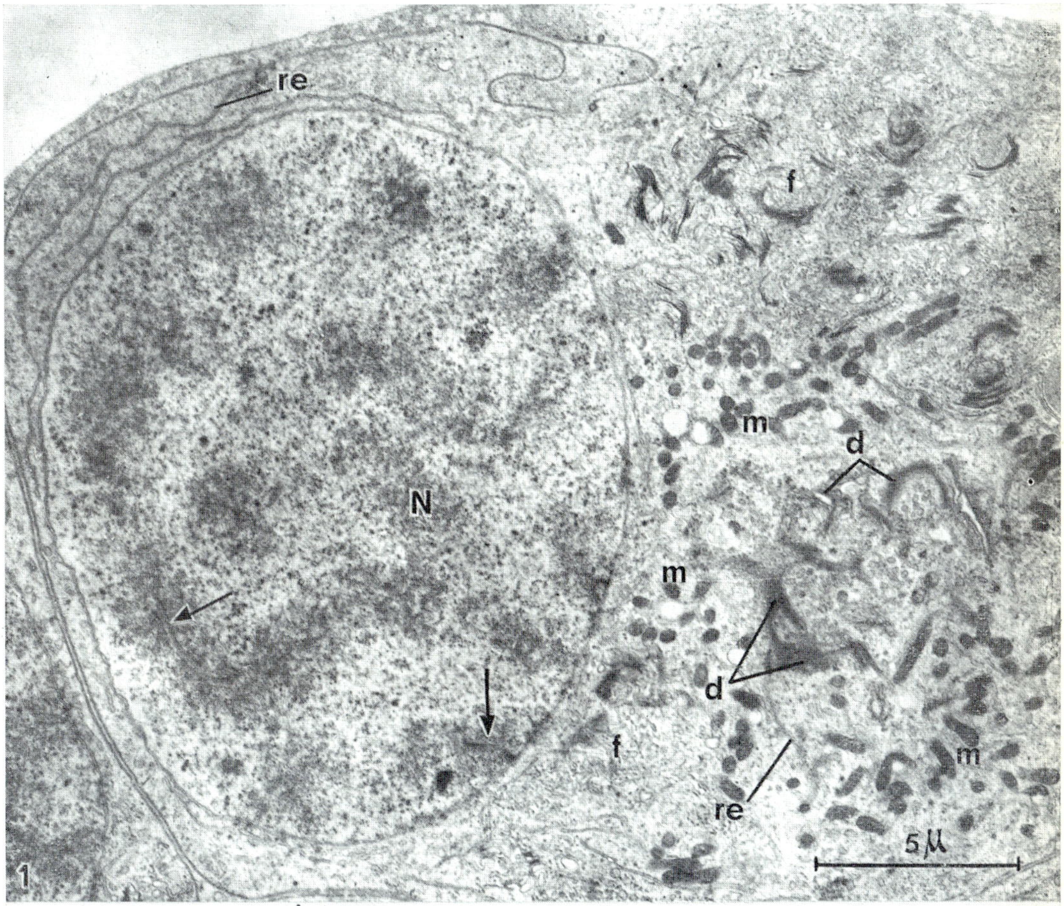

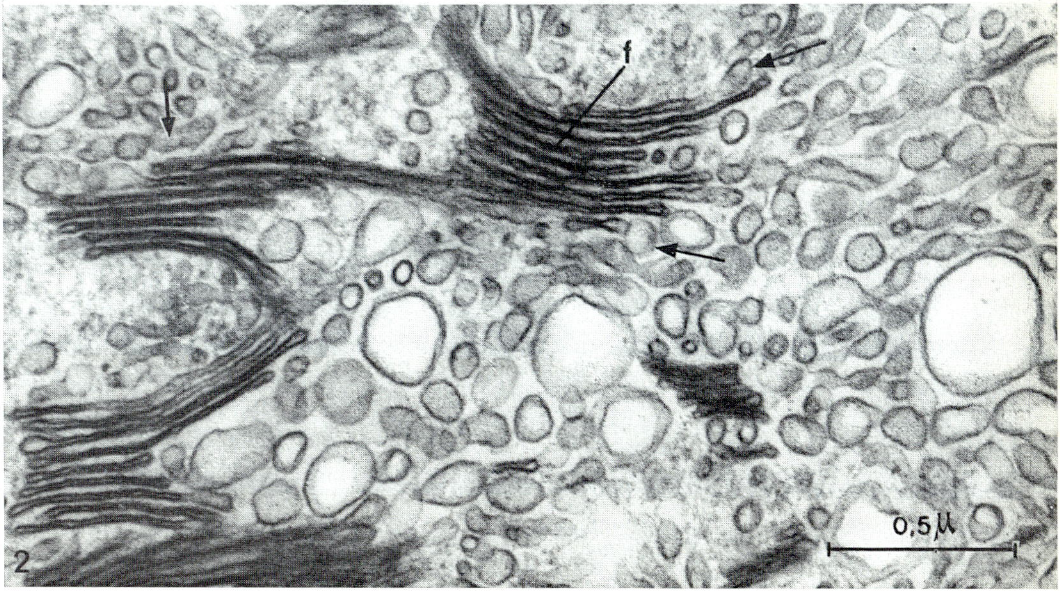

D. SANDOZ – *Étude ultrastructurale et cytochimique de la formation de l'acrosome du Discoglosse (Amphibien Anoure).*

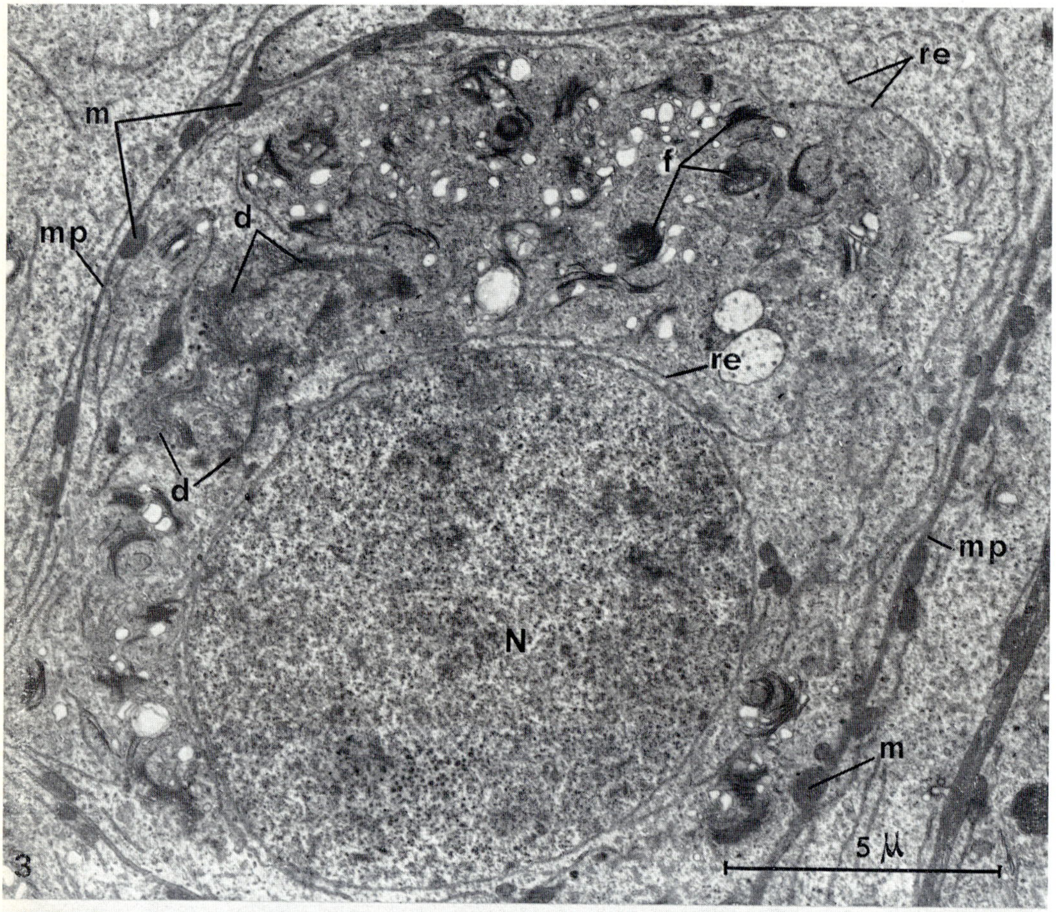

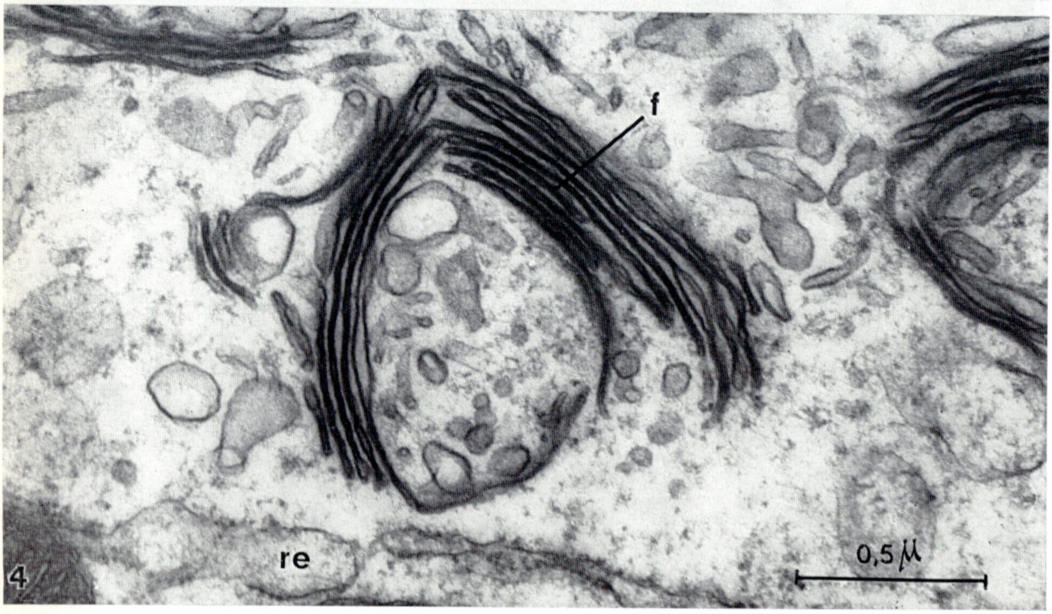

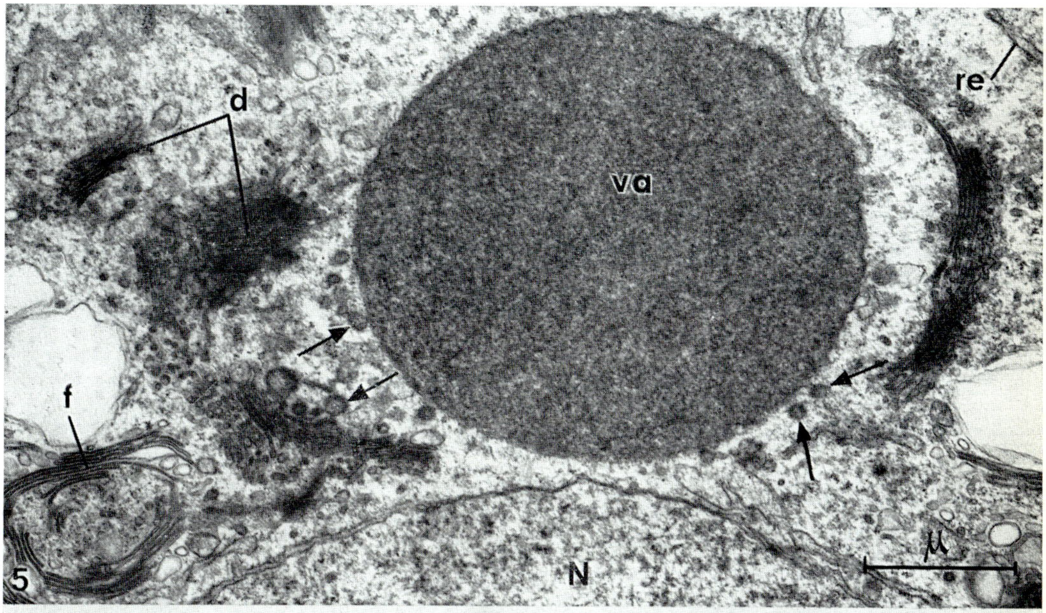
d
re
va
f
5
N
μ

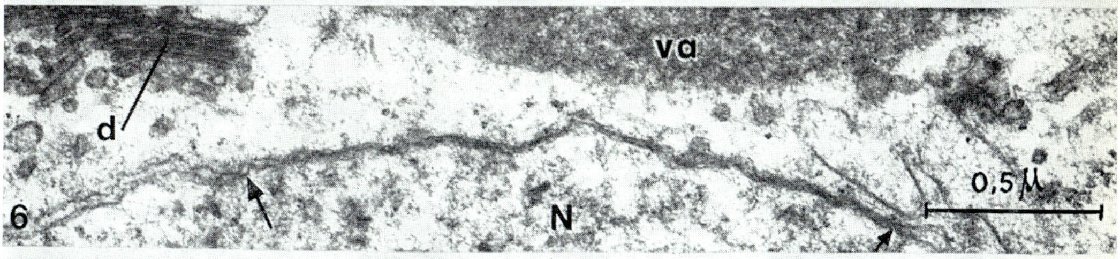
va
d
0,5 μ
6
N

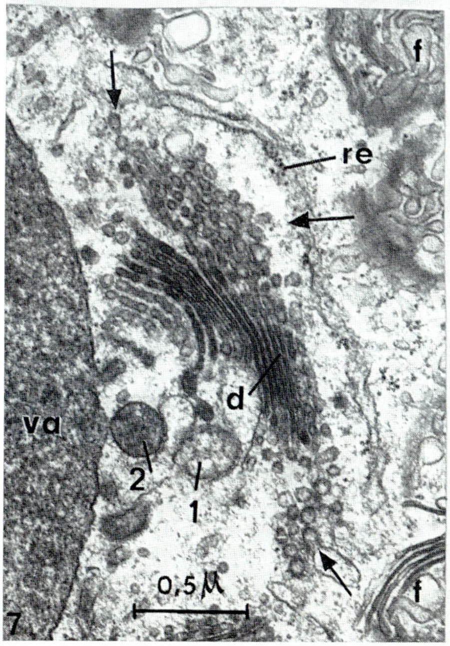
f
re
d
va
2
1
0,5 μ
f
7

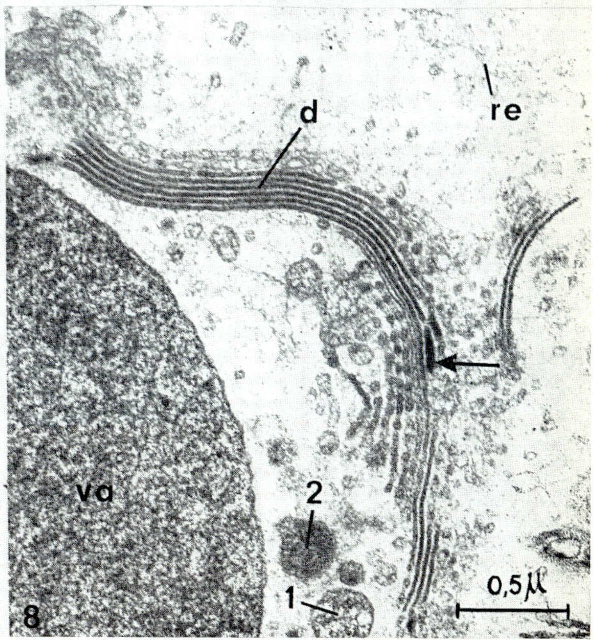
re
d
va
2
1
0,5 μ
8

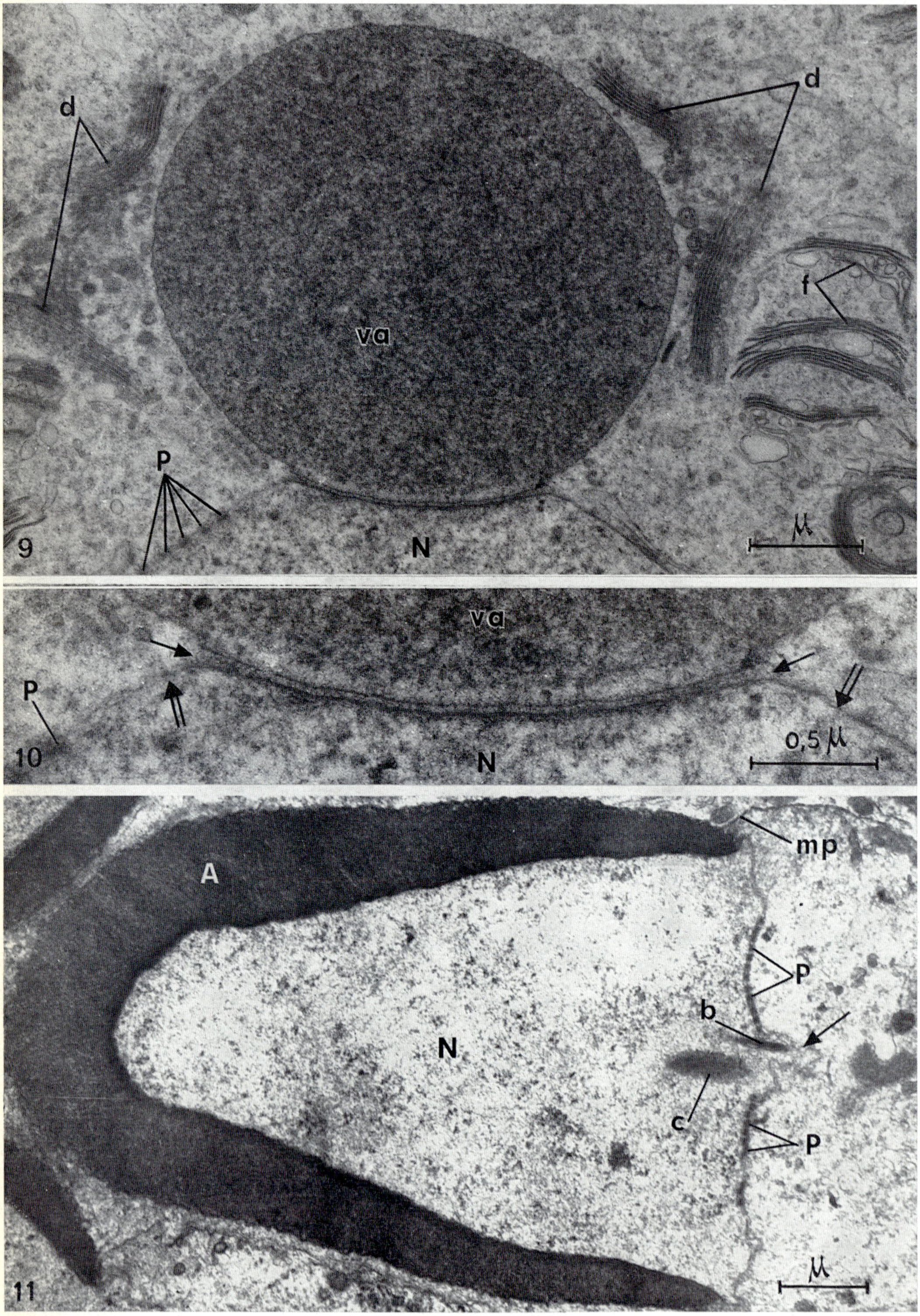
d
d
f
va
P
9
N
μ
va
P
10
N
0,5 μ
mp
A
P
b
N
c
P
11
μ

D. SANDOZ – *Étude ultrastructurele et cytochimique de la formation de l'acrosome du Discoglosse (Amphibien Anoure).*

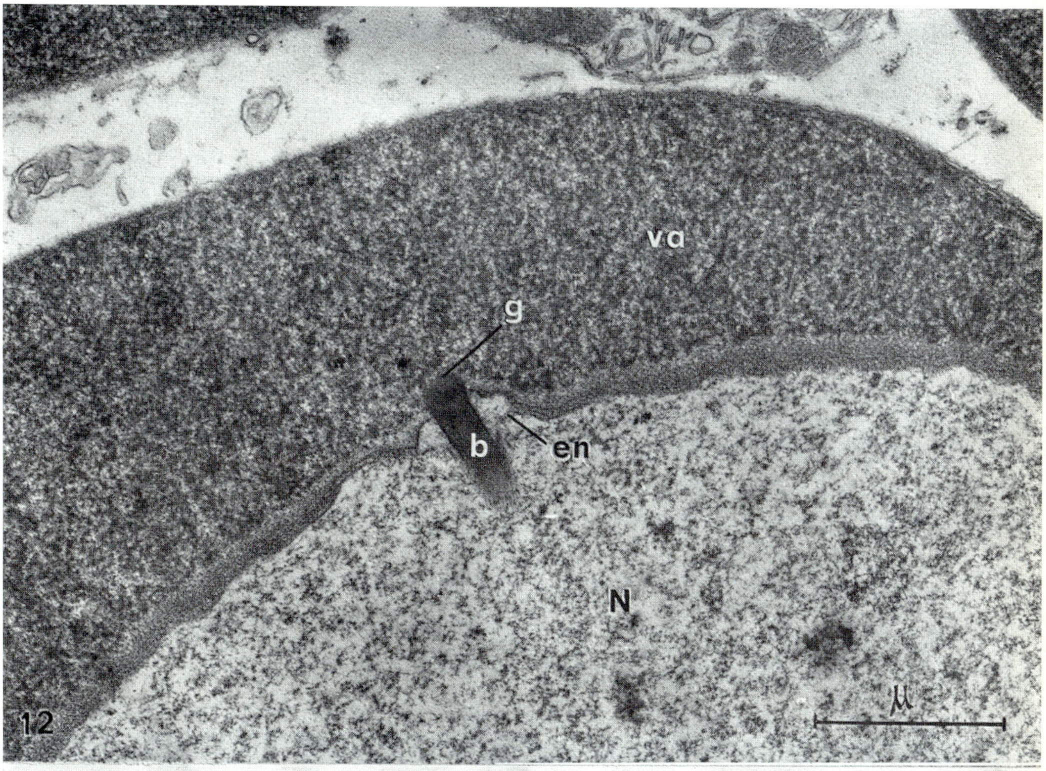

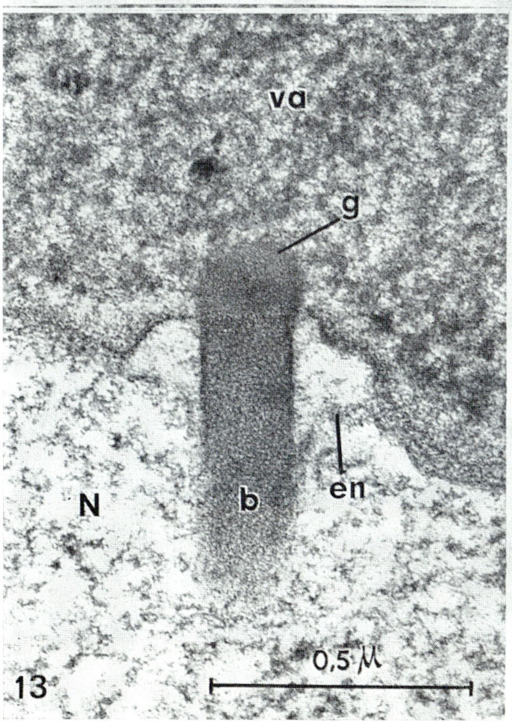

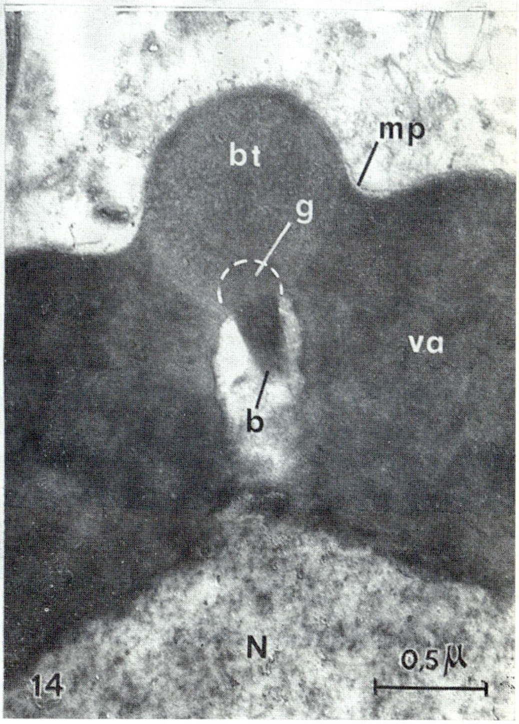

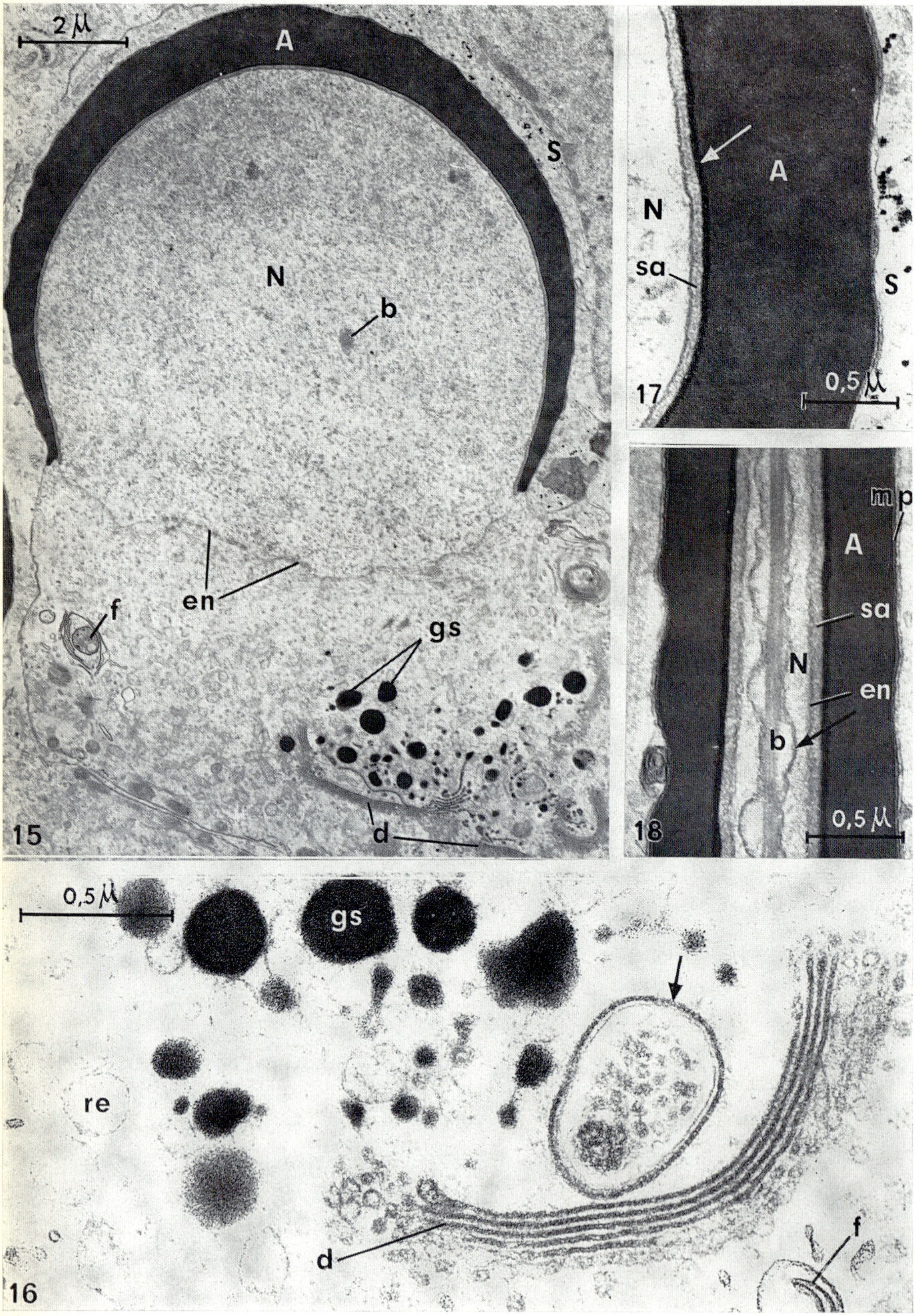
2 μ
A
S
N
b
en
f
gs
d
15
A
N
sa
S
17
0,5 μ
mp
A
sa
N
en
b
18
0,5 μ
0,5 μ
gs
re
d
f
16

PIETRO FURIERI (*)

SPERM MORPHOLOGY IN SOME REPTILES: SQUAMATA AND CHELONIA (**)

SUMMARY. — The ultrastructure of mature sperms was studied in 22 species of Reptiles belonging to the orders of Chelonia and Squamata, in order to find the relationships between sperm morphology and systematic position. Orders can be clearly distinguished; in the order of Squamata it is possible to split it further into suborders of Lacertilia and Serpentes; distinctive characters at family level were only observed in the suborder of Lacertilia; and in the family Gekkonidae, distinctive characters were observed for three genera.

RIASSUNTO. — L'A. studia la morfologia degli spermi maturi di 22 specie di Rettili appartenenti agli ordini dei Cheloni e degli Squamati per metterne in evidenza le differenze di struttura tra gruppi sistematici: sono chiaramente differenziabili gli Ordini; solo nell'ordine degli Squamata sono ulteriormente separabili i sottordini Lacertilia e Serpentes; e solo tra i Lacertilia sono riconoscibili le Famiglie dei Gekkonidae, Scincidae e Lacertidae; infine, tra i Gekkonidae si trovano differenze sufficienti a caratterizzare tre generi.

It has been well established that the sperm of animals that are taxonomically distant show great morphological differences, and that the differences diminish in groups that are more closely related. In this work I have taken a rather homogeneous group in order to see up to what point of systematic affinity these differences can still be observed.

The classification used here is that accepted by most authors, who divide living reptiles into four orders, Testudines or Chelonia, Squamata, Ryncocephala and Loricata. I have examined Testudines and Squamata in particular. Chelonia form a very homogenous order, and this homogeniety is also encountered in the morphology of the sperm, whereas notable structural differences are found in the sperm of Squamata, which is subdivided into two suborders, Lacertilia and Serpentes. Certain authors (TATARINOV, 1964) would prefer to raise these suborders to the rank of true orders, but on the basis of the differences between their sperm, I do not consider this as justified, and conforted by ROMER'S (1967) authority, shall continue to consider them as suborders.

(*) Institute of Comparative Anatomy, University of Florence, Italy.
(**) This research was supported by a grant from the C.N.R.

Materials and methods

Twenty-two species of reptiles belonging to two orders and six families (as specified in Table I) were examined.

The sperm were observed either in the ductus epididymis or in the ductus deferens. Thus they can be considered mature or almost mature even though the middle–piece of some of them is still accompanied by a droplet of cytoplasm, which is already separated from the sperm by a membrane.

Table I

Order	Suborder	Family	Species
Chelonia or Testudines		Emydidae	Emys orbicularis
			Clemmys guttata
			Clemmys insculpta
			Terrapene carolina
			Chrysemys picta picta
			Chrysemys picta belli
		Testudinidae	Testudo hermanni
Squamata	Lacertilia	Gekkonidae	Hemidactylus frenatus
			Hemidactylus mabouia
			Lygodactylus picturatus
			Tarentola mauritanica m.
		Lacertidae	Algyroides alleni
			Lacerta sicula campestris
			Lacerta lepida lepida
			Lacerta laevis
			Lacerta viridis
		Scincidae	Chalcides ocellatus tiligugu
	Serpentes	Colubridae	Coluber viridiflavus v.
			Natrix tessellata tessellata
			Natrix natrix
			Coronella austriaca
		Viperidae	Vipera aspis

The material was fixed in 1 % OsO_4, buffered in Millonig and embedded in Araldite. Sections were cut on an L.K.B. Ultrotome and collected on copper grids coated with Formvar. They were stained with warm uranyle acetate and lead citrate. The material was examined in a Hitachi H.S. 6 electron microscope and the best micrographs were obtained with a M. E. Hitachi H. U. 11. E. S. and M. E. Siemens Elmiskop 1.

For each homogenous group of sperm a diagramatic drawing has been made of the longitudinal section and of significant points of the transverse section. The scale of the latter is twice that of the longitudinal drawings and certain particulars have been reproduced on a still larger scale to show the details.

Results

Chelonia.

The anatomy of many organs of these anapsidian reptiles shows a lower level of evolution than that of Squamata.

In a previous work (FURIERI, 1964) I have already briefly described the sperm of *Testudo hermanni*. Since then I have examined those of the other species listed in Table I. Although these species belong to different genera and families, the differences between their sperm are insignificant; they are all like those of *Pseudemys scripta elegans*, recently described by KAPLAN and coll. (1966).

The drawing in Schema 1 fits the different species well: a very long curved, lanceshaped head with an opaque and homogeneous nucleus, which is anteriorly tapered and firmly engaged with the acrosome. The tapered portion of the nucleus is longitudinally indented by two or three slender tubules filled with acrosomal material, probably fluid (Figs. 1, 2, 3, 4).

The acrosome consist of two coaxial caps. The external one is more opaque and is homogeneous in structure, while the less opaque internal one, which is in direct contact with the nucleus, is composed of a finely granulated substance. However, the granules are not clearly arranged in a paracrystalline pattern as in Squamata (Figs. 2, 3, 4).

In the neck region, a connecting piece of opaque material embraces the basal portion of the nucleus with its concave anterior portion, and axially, contains the transverse or proximal centriole. In particularly successful longitudinal sections of the neck region, numerous transversely sectioned microtubules can be seen. These are lined up side by side and surround the anterior scooped-out portion of the connecting piece. The ring that is thus formed seems to lie outside the sperm membrane. It might be a residue of the " manchette ", but, whereas the microtubules of this structure are usually parallel to the sperm axis, here they are at right angles to it.

The transverse centriole is followed by the distal centriole at an angle of about 80° to it, and then the flagellum begins. The centrioles and first portion of the flagellum are wrapped by the mitochondrial sheath, which characterizes the middle piece.

In turtles, the portion of the flagellum surrounded by the mitochondrial sheath is peculiar. Its most anterior portion is wrapped by a thick electron opaque cylinder, the internal surface of which gives off nine large fibers formed of similarly opaque material. These lie in the space between the peripheral doublets of the axial filament and merge with an axial structure of opaque material that envelops the central fibrils. (Figs. 6, 7). This complicated structure resembles a centriole with its characteristic peripheral triplets, but a closer look reveals only pairs of fibrils, since the third element is only the space between the opaque reinforcing fiber and the doublet. The presence of fibers that reinforce the external doublets of the axial filament complex is certainly no novelty. In fact it has been found in distantly related groups, in birds and mammals and in many orders of insects, but with the substantial difference that in these groups the supporting fibers are peripheral to the doublets whereas in chelonians they run between the fibrils in an intrafibrillar arrangement. It is also noteworthy that at the very beginning of the flagellum, three central fibrils can be seen. However, this

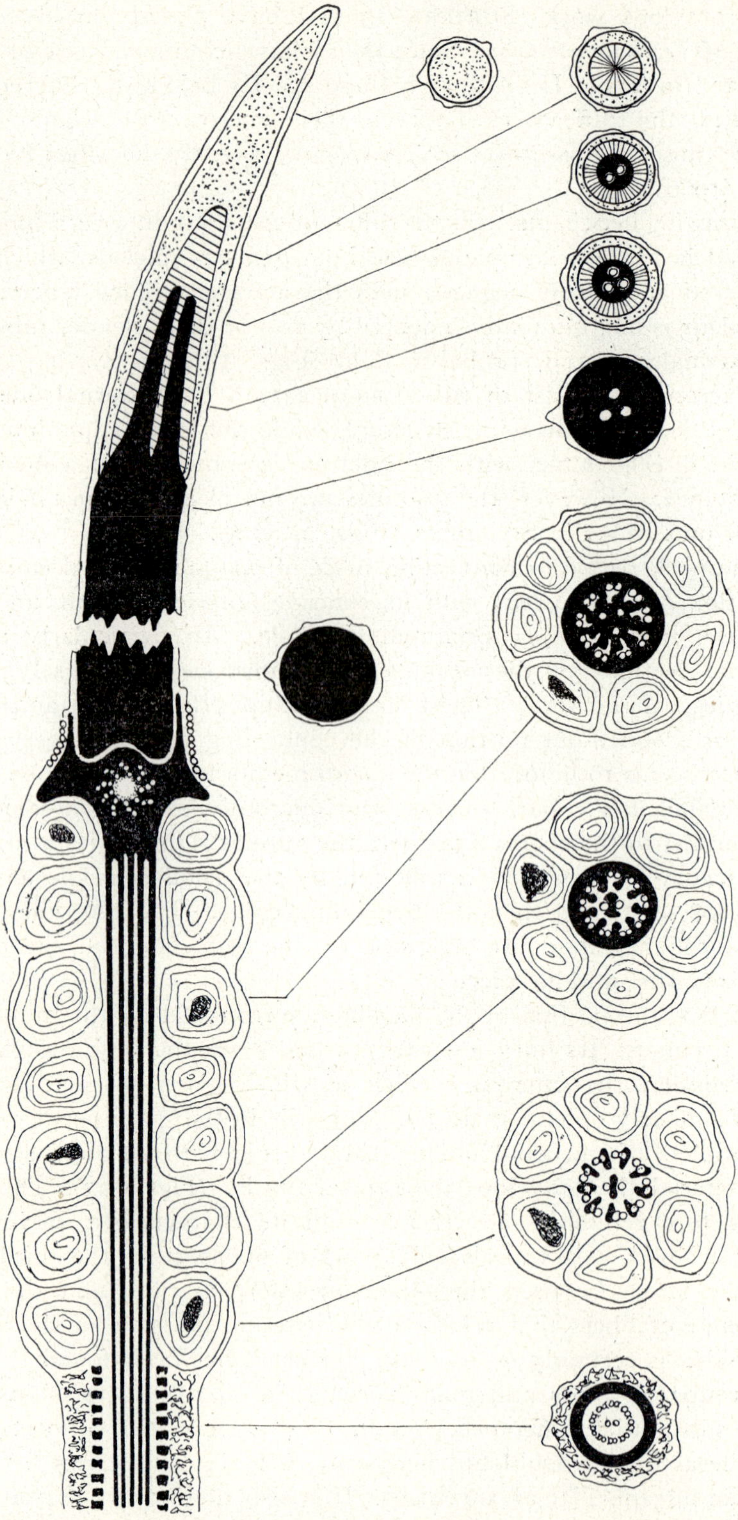

Schema 1. – Schematic drawing of sperm of Chelonia.

may be an illusion, caused, for example, by a very arched bridge joining the opaque sheath of the two usual fibrils (like a pince-nez) (Fig. 6).

Moving towards the caudal portion of the middle piece, cross sections show that the intrafibrillar fibers no longer connect with the sheath of the central fibrils, (at this point it is clear that the central fibrils form only a doublet, giving the flagellum the typical 9 + 9 + 2 pattern) and that the external cylinder, intrafibrillar fibers and the sheaths of the central fibrils gradually decrease in size until, at the distal end of the middle–piece, the peripheral and central doublets remain bare (Figs. 7, 8, 9).

The mitochondrial sheath consists of very large globular elements, distinctive because of their concentric cristae with, at times, a large mass of electron dense material at the center (Figs. 6, 7, 8, 9). The mitochondria (about fifty of them) are arranged irregularly in about ten rings piled on top of each other, with five, or occasionally six, elements per ring.

Immediately after the last ring of mitochondria, the flagellum is encircled by a complicated fibrous helix that begins like the capital of a column and extends almost to the tip of the tail. It can be subdivided into an inner and outer layer, the former made up of a few rather large, regular fibers that have an orderly arrangement, and the latter composed of many irregular slender fibers in no particular order (Fig. 10).

Regarding the middle-piece, the fact that the mitochondrial sheath ensures it a good degree of rigidity, suggests that the abundance of opaque material around and between the flagellar fibrils is not a simple reinforcement. Perhaps this material contains reserves of energy. Preliminary tests with Thiéry's method and alpha-amylase digestion, indicate that this area is rich in glycogen.

Squamata.

Comparing the sperm of Squamata and Chelonia, very clear differences in the structure and arrangement of the various parts can be observed. The sperm of Squamata appear long and slender because the middle–piece is wrapped by a sheath of slender, elongated mitochondria with quite usual cristae. The acrosome of Squamata is composed of two coaxial caps as in the chelonians, but the internal cap has a clearly paracrystalline pattern. Lesser but easily recognizable differences are also found between the spermatozoa of the suborders Serpentes and Lacertilia.

I studied ten species of Lacertilia of three families (Gekkonidae, Lacertidae, and Scincidae) belonging to the infraorder Discoglossa, superamily Anguidea. The sperm of these families are easily distinguishable by their acrosomes and the amount and arrangement of the electron opaque material between the mitochondria. I have made a schematic drawing of these differences for each family.

I shall begin with a description of the Gekkonidae sperm derived from micrographs of *Lygodactylus* (FURIERI, 1968) because this genus well exemplifies the characteristics of the family (Schema 2). The nucleus is elongated and slightly curved and ends in a sharp point, on which the acrosome is impaled. Of the two coaxial caps of the acrosome, the internal one is more-electron transparent and has a paracrystalline structure, probably hexagonal, the external cap is more opaque and is further subdivided into an inner and outer zone, with the former more electron dense than the latter (Fig. 13, 15).

The cavity of the internal cap is not completely filled by the prolongation of the nucleus; apically there remains a small chamber, which is closed anteriorly by an opaque, homogeneous stopper (Fig. 14). From this stopper a more or less cylindrical process extends forwards. It is structured and opaque and lies in an axial furrow in the denser inner zone of the external cap. (Fig. 15).

Posterior to the head are the two centrioles, embedded in an opaque, rougly cylindrical structure, the neck cylinder, according to the terminology used by AUSTIN (1965), HAMILTON & FAWCETT (1968). Distally, the neck cylinder is surrounded by the first twists of a fibrous helix that envelops the flagellum almost down to its end. The helix consists of several thick fibers that spiral very tightly and are held firm by two large fibers that run longitudinally and internal to the helix and are aligned with the central doublet of the axial filament, that is, they lie beside peripheral doublets 3 and 8. Outer dense fibers are also attached to the other doublets of the axial filament in the middle-piece and gradually become thinner and disappear at different levels in the different species (Figs. 11, 12, 13, 16, 17, 18).

A mitochondrial sheath envelops the middle-piece as is normal, but in this family the mitochondria are not in direct contact with each other but are separated by greater or smaller amounts of opaque material in the various genera. In *Lygodactylus* the opaque intermitochondrial material is so abundant that it forms a cylinder around the axial structures (filament complex and the fibrous helix). At certain points, its wall is as thick as the " chondrioma " but at other points it is deeply indented to hold the mitochondria (Figs. 11, 12). This material is less abundant in *Tarentola* (Figs. 16, 17), and even less so in *Hemidactylus* (Fig. 18).

Scincidae.

I examined (FURIERI, 1967) only one species of this family, *Chalcides ocellatus tiligugu*. The general appearance of the longitudinal section of this sperm does not differ much from that of the *Gekkonidae* (Schema 3; Fig. 19), but, upon careful examination, the differences are clear cut. In the acrosome, the apical groove in the external cap, which is perfectly axial in the Gekkonidae, is on a slant of about 120°, and begins nearly half way down the acrosome cap rather than at its apex (Fig. 2).

A second difference is the deep funnel-shaped indentation of the basal surface of the nucleus (Fig. 20), within which an extension of the connecting piece is contained. The connecting piece, in turn, encloses the two centrioles.

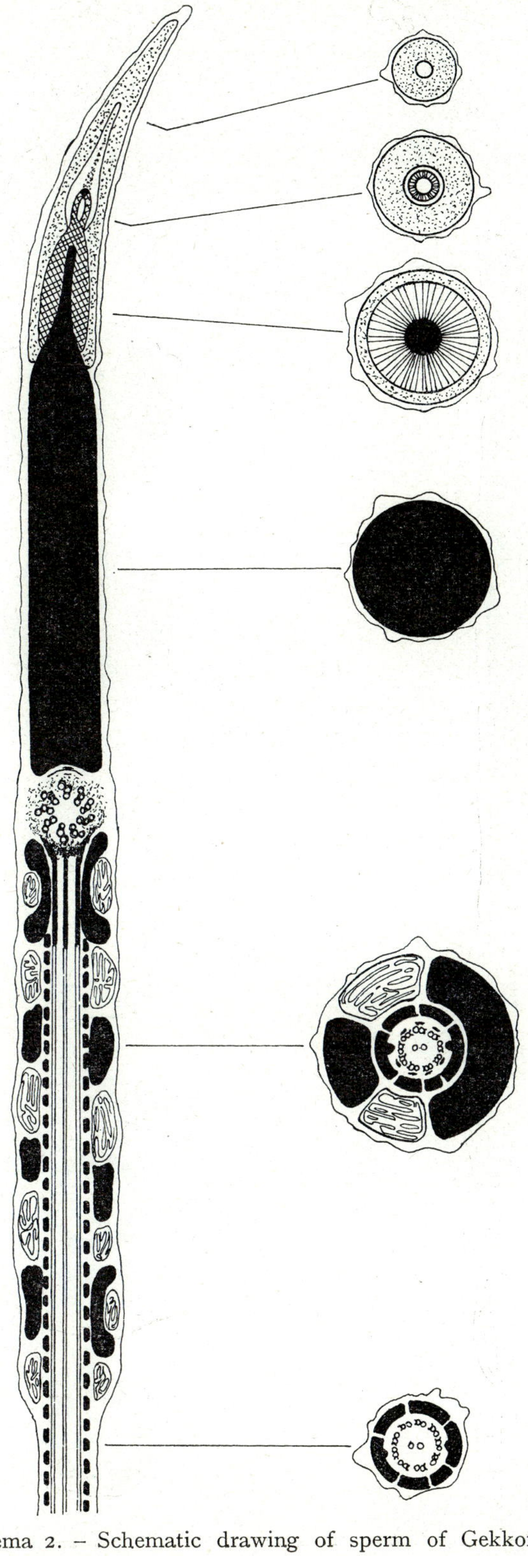

Schema 2. – Schematic drawing of sperm of Gekkonidae.

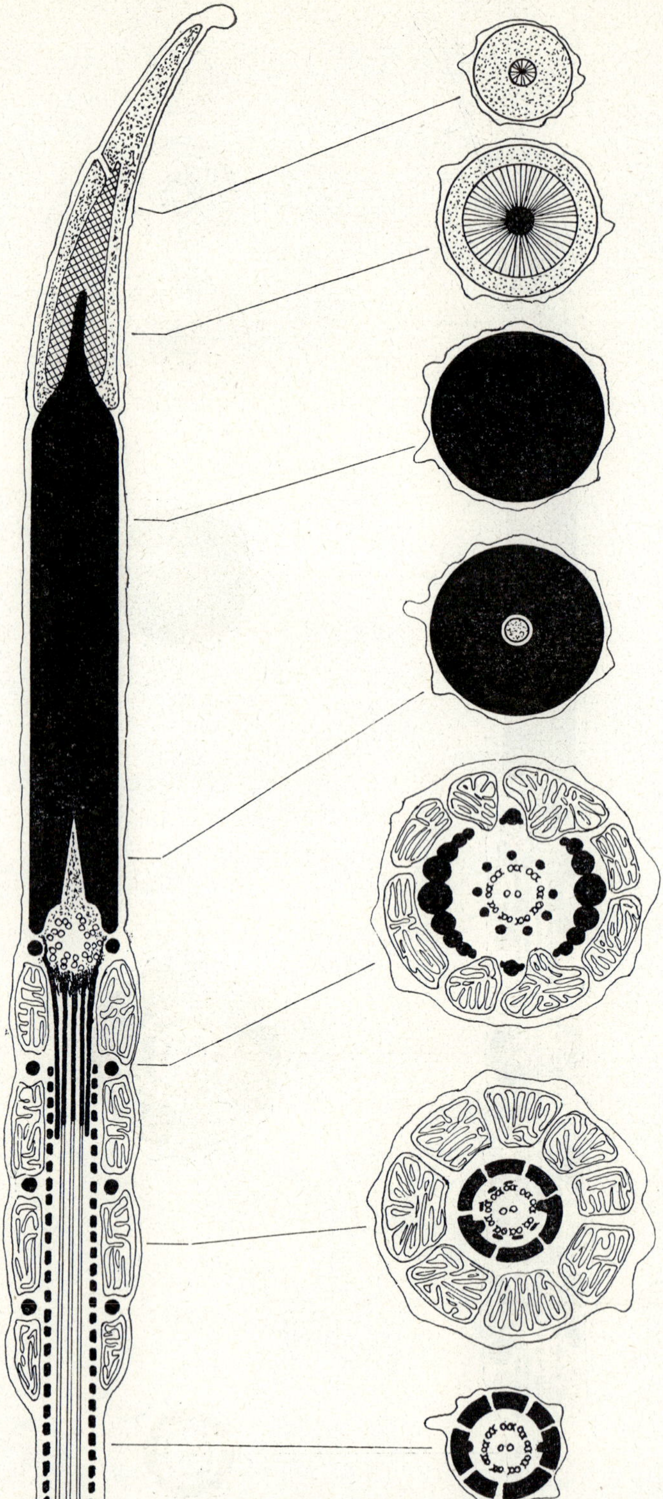

Schema 3. – Schematic drawing of sperm of Scincidae.

A final characteristic typical of this species is the presence of four rings formed by the juxtaposition of opaque spheroidal masses (Fig. 22). The first of these rings is immediately posterior to the nucleus, and the other three lie at equal distances along the mitochondrial sheath. The fibrous helix, which, as usual, envelops the flagellum almost to its tip, begins after the end of the connecting piece, between the second and third rings (Fig. 19). Since in *Chalcides*, as in all Squamata hitherto observed, the fibrous helix is at a more external level than the connecting piece, the suggestion I gave in 1967, that the former might derive from or be directly connected with the latter, no longer appears valid. In *Chalcides*, too, the fibers of the helix are supported by two longitudinal, parallel fibers lying within the helix and on a plane with doublets 3 and 8. I was not able to establish whether these two long longitudinal fibers proceed, like the other seven shorter and more slender fibers that flank the other peripheral doublets in the middle-piece, from the connecting piece.

The mitochondrial sheath is subdivided into four portions by the four opaque rings described above.

In *Chalcides* too, the internal cap of the acrosome consists of paracrystalline material.

Lacertidae.

I studied five species of this family belonging to two genera (Table I). The sperm of all these species are morphologically indistinguishable, and the diagramatic drawing of them is probably valid for the entire family (Schema 4). The general appearance of the various portions of this sperm is like that of the other families I have described, but here too the details are different. The inner cap of the acrosome is paracrystalline in structure, and the outer cap has a light cortex and a dark medulla (Fig. 25). The apical groove of the external cap is less axial than that of the Gekkonidae, but on less of a slant than in *Chalcides* (Fig. 24).

I shall not describe the nucleus, connecting piece, centrioles, and fibrous helix because they do not differ notably from those of other families, and, regarding flagellum I shall describe only the supporting fibers of the peripheral doublets.

The middle–piece, which in this family too is bounded by the mitochondrial sheath, is characterized by two particulars (Fig. 23): firstly, two opaque masses lie immediatly posterior to the nucleus. Their appearance and size varies from species to species but not clearly enough to be used as a defining characteristic. Secondly a large ring is inserted between the mitochondria in the most distal third of the sheath. It is homogeneous, electron–dense, and complicated in shape. In sagittal sections of the sperm it is seen as two large plaques between the mitochondria. The height of the two plaques is rarely the same, since the height of the ring varies greatly from point to point.

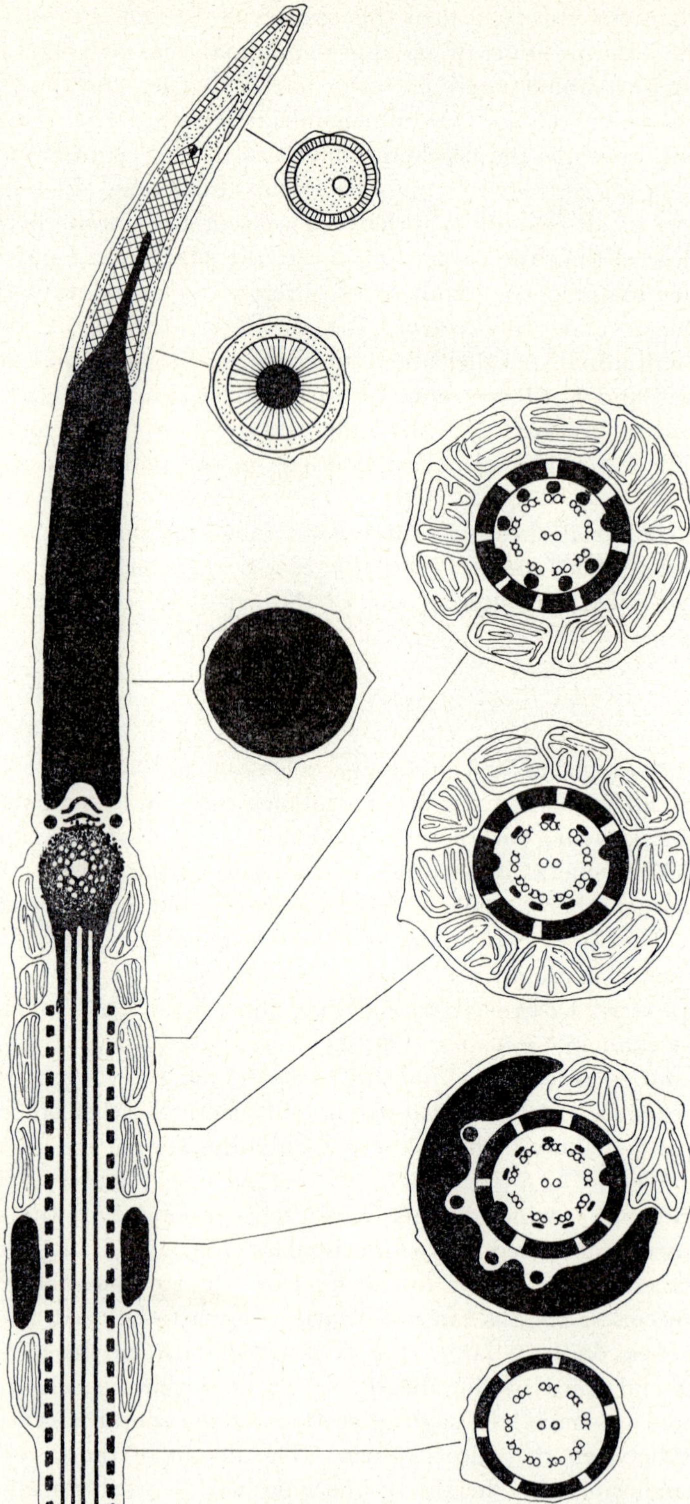

Schema 4. – Schematic drawing of sperm of Lacertidae.

Consequently, in cross sections, the ring sometimes appears complete and sometimes interrupted (Fig. 28). Its internal surface, especially about half way down, where the ring is thickest, is indented by numerous niches containing small masses of moderately opaque material.

In Lacertidae the nine dense fibers originating from the connecting piece are externally attached to the peripheral doublets and accompany them down to the opaque ring. Here too the fibers flanking doublets 3 and 8 are larger and are fused with the fibrous helix at each of its turns (Fig. 27).

Regarding the mitochondria of the sheath, they are filamentous and their cristae are not clearly delineated. Sections of the surface of the sheath show single mitochondria irregularity juxtaposed and not in a regular spiral as, for example, in mammals. Finally, the mitochondria anterior to the opaque ring are thicker than those posterior to it (Fig. 23).

Serpentes.

I studied two families of this sub-order, Colubridae (four species) and Viperidae (only one species, *Vipera aspis aspis* [FURIERI, 1965]) (Table I).

Although a great many anatomical differences divide these two families, their sperm are practically identical and I have made a single diagrammatic drawing for both of them (Schema 5).

Although snake sperm have much in common with those of Lacertilia, the differences are also substantial.

The sperm head in the two suborders is very similar: the nucleus is cylindrical and curved, the acrosome consists of two coaxial caps, with the tapered portion of the nucleus fitting into the internal paracrystalline cap. (Figs. 30, 31, 33). Snakes have the same furrow in the denser external cap holding the cylindrical structure that proceeds from the dense stopper of the inner cap. (Fig. 31).

The absence of a chamber between the anterior tip of the nucleus and the opaque tip distinguishes the sperm of snakes from those of Gekkonidae.

As in the Gekkonidae, the two centrioles are embedded in the opaque neck cylinder (Fig. 29). The posterior centriole is in direct connection with the flagellum and in this sub-family also the peripheral doublets are externally flanked by electron-dense supporting fibers (Fig. 36). However, they are considerably longer than in the Lacertilia, and we shall soon see why. As in previously described cases, the flagellum of snake sperm is almost entirely wrapped in a fibrous helix made of large fibers that spiral narrowly (Figs. 30, 33, 34), and at each turn the helix is attached to the two longitudinal fibers flanking doublets 3 and 8 (Fig. 36). The fibrous helix begins at a more cranial level in Serpentes than in Lacertilia (Fig. 35). All the opaque fibers that seem to reinforce the flagellar couplets gradually become more slender caudally.

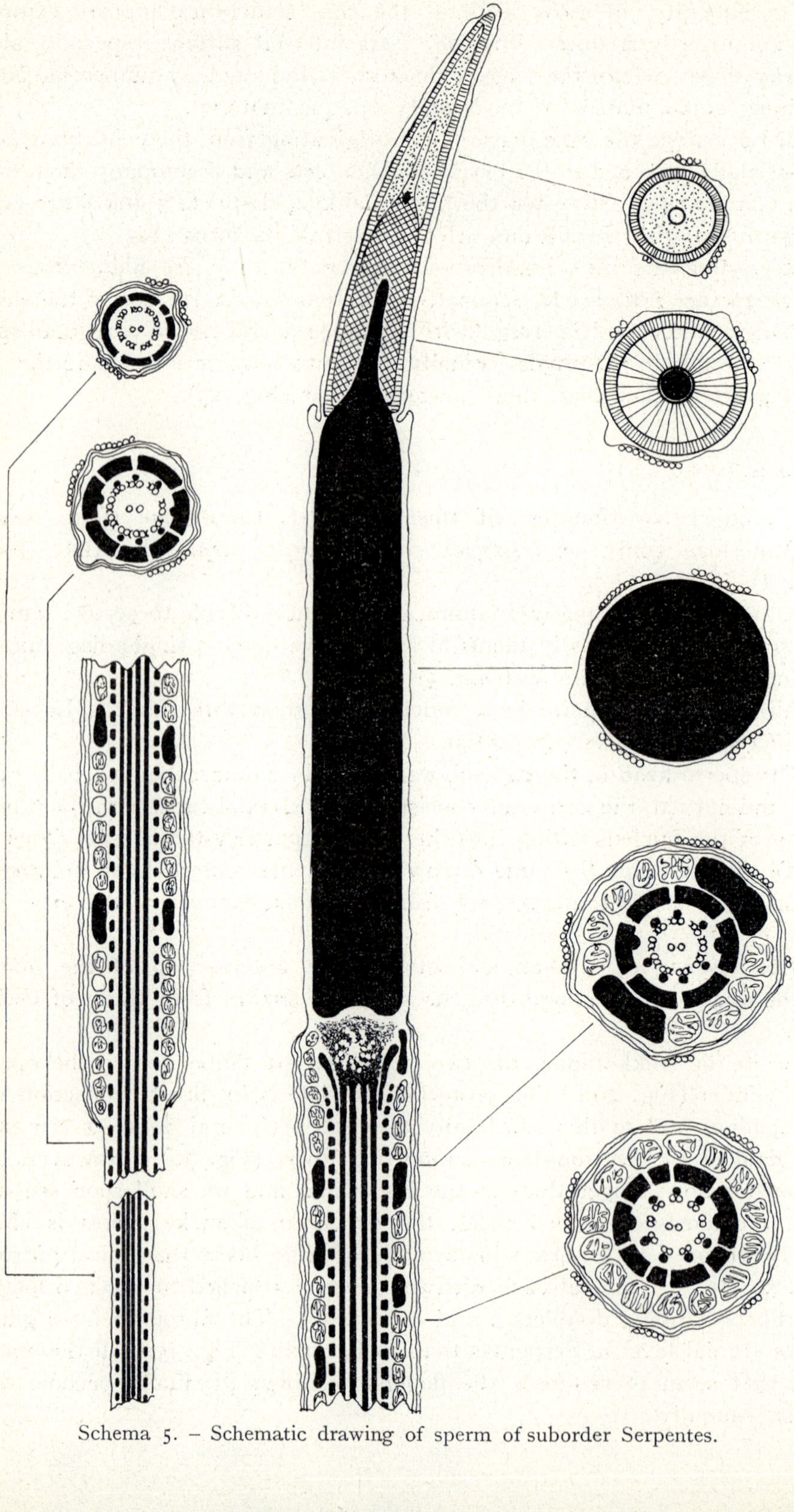

Schema 5. – Schematic drawing of sperm of suborder Serpentes.

A very obvious difference between the sperm of Serpentes and Lacertilia is found in the extraordinary length of the mitochondrial sheath in snake sperm, which covers almost two thirds of the flagellum. The outer dense fibers are present through most of this portion. Because of its exceptional length it seems more appropriate to refer to this part of the tail as the region of the mitochondrial sheath than as the middle-piece.

Irregularly interspersed among the mitochondria of the sheath, there are many clusters of four or five electron-dense plaques (Figs. 29, 30, 34).

The individual mitochondria are very slender and rather convoluted with cristae that are not well marked.

The electron density and intermitochondrial position of the plaques (already described by AUSTIN, 1965; HAMILTON & FAWCETT, 1968) suggest that they are homologous to the abundant material in the mitochondrial sheath in Gekkonidae, and the dense ring or rings in Lacertidae and *Chalcides*. Thus the same material in different arrangements permits us to recognize, without any doubt, different families, and, in the case of Gekkonidae, genera.

Regarding the cell membrane of snakes, it is clearly anchored to the structures it envelops at the level of the junction between acrosome and nucleus (Figgs. 30, 31, 35) and between the posterior pole of the nucleus and the beginning of the mitochondrial sheath. Furthermore, throughout the region of the mitochondrial sheath, it is pluristratified into 5 or 6 slightly irregular, coaxial membranes (Fig. 36).

In a previous work on the viper (1965), I described numerous microtubules forming a palisade around the sperm tail. (They were contemporaneously described by AUSTIN in 1965 and later by HAMILTON & FAWCETT in 1968). These microtubules run in the same direction as the sperm and are found along its whole length from acrosome to the tip of the tail. However, it is unusual to find a cross section of the sperm in which they form a complete ring around it (Fig. 36). In fact small portions of the microtubular palisade are dispersed in the sperm-duct fluid.

I think that the microtubules may be a residue of the "manchette" described by BOISSON, MATTEI and coll. as present during the spermiogenisis of the *Phython* and the Agamidae. However, it is noteworthy that the sperm I studied have lost almost all traces of cytoplasm, indicating that they are mature or almost so. In fact, the microtubules, which probably are of endocytoplasmatic origin, lie completely outside the sperm membrane. At this stage of sperm development, external microtubules are lacking in Gekkonidae, Lacertidae and Scincidae, and as far as I know they have never been observed in any animal but the snake.

To conclude, the relationship between systematic position and morphology of the mature sperm was examined in two orders of reptiles, Chelonia and Squamata. The differences are marked enough to permit certain recognition of the suborders and, in the suborder Lacertilia, it is also possible to distinguish families by their sperm. In the cases examined, morphological differences of the sperm permitted differentiation on a generic level only in three genera of Gekkonidae. In no case was it possible to identify a species by its sperm.

Acknowledgements. – Many thanks are due to Prof. S. RANZI, chairman of the " Istituto di Zoologia dell'Università di Milano " and Prof. G. LANZAVECCHIA for their hospitality and the use of the E. M. Hitachi H. U. 11S. E.; also Prof. E. ALLARA & Dr. T. BANI-SACCHI of the " Istituto di Istologia dell'Università di Firenze ", and Prof. B. BACCETTI and the personnel of the " Istituto di Zoologia di Siena " for the use of their E. M. Siemens Elmiskop 1.

I gratefully thank Prof. B. LANZA for specimens of *Algyroides*, *Lygodactylus*, *Hemidactylus* and *Chalcides* captured on the archipelago of Galita (Tunisia; 1967) and in Kenya (1968) during the " Mares " expedition (Scientific-research-and-underwater-techniques Group).

REFERENCES

AUSTIN C. R. (1965) – *Fine structure of the Snake Sperm Tail.* « J. Ultrastr. Res. », 12, 452–462.

BOISSON C. & MATTEI X. (1966) – *La spermiogenèse de* Python sebae *Gmelin observée au M. E.* « Ann. Sci. Nat. Zool. Paris », 12. S., T. VIII, 363–389.

CLARK A. W. (1967) – *Some aspects of spermiogenesis in a Lizard.* « Amer. J. Anat. », 121, 369–400.

CHARNIER M., BOISSON C. & MATTEI X. (1967) – *Ultrastructure de la manchette chromatique dans la spermatide d'*Agama agama (*Agamidae, Lacertilien*). « C. R. Soc. Biol. », T. CLXI, 4, 888–890.

HAMILTON D. W. & FAWCETT D. W. (1968) – *Unusual features of the neck and middle-piece of Snake spermatozoa.* « J. Ultrastr. Res. », 23, 81–97.

FURIERI P. & LANZAVECCHIA G. (1959). – *Studio al microscopio elettronico sull'ultrastruttura degli spermatozoi di* Lacerta sicula campestris. Atti II° Congr. Ital. Micr. Elettr. 155–163.

FURIERI P. (1962) – *Prime osservazioni al microscopio elettronico sulla ultrastruttura degli spermatozoi di* Tarentola mauritanica. « Boll. Soc. It. Biol. Sper. », 38, 32–35.

FURIERI P. (1965) – *Osservazioni ultrastrutturali sullo spermio di* Testudo hermanni *Gmelin.* « Boll. Soc. It. Biol. Sper. », 41, 144–146.

FURIERI P. (1965) – *Prime osservazioni al microscopio elettronico sulla ultrastruttura dello spermatozoo di* Vipera aspis aspis. « Boll. Soc. It. Biol. Sper. », 41, 478–480.

FURIERI P. (1967) – *Prime osservazioni sulla ultrastruttura dello spermio di* Chalcides ocellatus. « Boll. Soc. It. Biol. Sper. », 53, 782–784.

FURIERI P. (1968) – *La morfologia dello spermatozoo di* Lygodactylus picturatus. « Boll. Zool. », 35, 338.

MIRANTI J. P., KAPLAN H. M. & HIRANO T. (1964). – *The spermatozoon of the turtle* Pseudemys scripta elegans. « Copeia », 1, 209–211.

KAPLAN H. M. & GLACZENSKI S. S. (1966) – *Electron microscope study of Turtle sperm.* « Cytologia », 31, 99–104.

ROMER A. S. (1968) – *Notes and comments on Vertebrate Paleontology*. Univ. Chicago Press.

SUD B. N. (1961) – *Morphological and histochemical studies in the grassnake* Natrix natrix. « Quart. J. Micros. Sci. », 102, 51–58.

TATARINOV L. P. (1964) – *Lepidosauria.* In « Osnovy Paleontologij ». 5, 439–492 (in Russian, cited by ROMER).

Explanation of figures

List of abbreviations.

a = acrosome
at = apical tubules indenting the nucleus
ecc = groove in external acrosomal cap
icc = chamber of internal acrosomal cap
cp = connecting piece
ec = external acrosomal cap
f = flagellum
ef = fibrous helix
ias = stopper of internal acrosomal cap
ic = internal acrosomal cap
iom = electron opaque intermitochondrial material
m = mitochondrion
mm = residual microtubules of " manchette "
mp = middle-piece
mpr = intermitochondrial ring of the middle-piece
n = nucleus
ne = indentation of base of nucleus
nap = tapered apical process of nucleus
rf = reinforcing fibers of peripheral couplets of axial filament
sm = sperm membrane
t = end-piece of tail
tc = transverse centriole

Fig. 1. – *Emys orbicularis* 30,500×. Parasagittal section of mitochondrial sheath.

Fig. 2. – *Terrapene carolina* 56,000×. Longitudinal section of tapered apex of nucleus indented by two or three tubules and inserted into the acrosome, which consists of two coaxial caps. On the right, longitudinal section of a tail.

Fig. 3. – *Chrysemys picta picta* 60,000×. Tapered apex of nucleus indented by axial tubules. On the right, transverse section of middle-piece of sperm.

Fig. 4. – *Emys orbicularis* 56,000×. Transverse sections of nuclei at various levels, with two or three axial tubules.

Fig. 5. – *Chrysemys picta picta* 130,000×. Longitudinal section of a teratoid sperm with two flagella: the transverse centriole.

Fig. 6. – *Emys orbicularis* 76,000×. Transverse section of very anterior portion of middle-piece. The structure of the flagellum, reinforced by electron opaque material resembles the structure of the centriole; there seem to be three central fibrils.

Fig. 7. – *Chrysemys picta picta* 78,000×. Transverse section of more caudal portion of middle-piece than in Fig. 6. Here too the flagellum simulates the centriole; it is clear that there are only two central fibrils.

Fig. 8. – *Chrysemys picta picta* 70,000×. Transverse section of still more caudal portion of middle-piece. The electron-opaque supporting structures are considerably reduced.

Fig. 9. – *Emys orbicularis* 65,000×. Transverse section of very caudal portion of middle-piece. All the doublets of the axial filament are flanked by large electron-opaque fibers.

Fig. 10. – *Chrysemys picta picta* 57,000 ×. Parasagittal section of beginning of end-piece. The complicated fibrous helix.

Fig. 11. – *Lygodactylus picturatus* 13,000 ×. Parasagittal section of middle-piece.

Fig. 12. – *Lygodactylus picturatus* 13,000 ×. Section similar to preceding one, but more superficial. Several cross sections of sperm at different levels. The two micrographs give an idea of the substantial thickness of the opaque intermitochondrial material.

Fig. 13. – *Hemidactylus frenatus* 30,000 ×. The two acrosomal caps sectioned longitudinally.

Fig. 14. – *Tarentola mauritanica* 52,000 ×. Sagittal section of acrosome. Internal paracrystalline cap, chamber, and apical stopper.

Fig. 15. – *Lygodactylus picturatus* 48,000 × Longitudinal section of acrosome. The two caps, axial furrow in external cap, and cylinder originating from opaque stopper

Fig. 16. – *Tarentola mauritanica* 72,000 ×. Transverse section of middle-piece. The mitochondria are separated by opaque material, less abundant than in *Lygodactylus*.

Fig. 17. – *Tarentola mauritanica* 50,000 ×. Transverse section of middle–piece at a level where intermitochondrial material is more abundant.

Fig. 18. – *Hemidactylus frenatus* 38,000 ×. Parasagittal section of middle-piece. Scarse intermitochondrial material. On the lower right, transverse section of middle-piece still joined to a droplet of cytoplasm.

Fig. 19. – *Chalcides ocellatus* 48,000 ×. Parasagittal section of middle–piece. The sections of the four rings show up clearly.

Fig. 20. – *Chalcides ocellatus* 67,000 ×. Sagittal section of middle-piece. The base of the sperm head is deeply indented and the neck cylinder fits into it.

Fig. 21. – *Chalcides ocellatus* 38,000 ×. Longitudinal section of acrosome. The groove in the external cap is on a slant with respect to the sperm axis.

Fig. 22. – *Chalcides ocellatus* 67,000 ×. Transverse section of middle-piece at level of second ring.

Fig. 23. – *Lacerta lepida* 14,000 ×. Parasagittal section of nucleus and tail of sperm. At the upper left, an analogous section, but on a different plane. The moderately opaque masses are sections of proteic granules secreted by cells of epididymal duct.

Fig. 24. – *Lacerta sicula campestris* 43,000 × Sagittal section of acrosome embracing tapered nuclear process. The internal acrosomal cap is paracrystalline. The furrow in the external one is on less of a slant then in *Chalcides* but more than in the Gekkonidae.

Fig. 25. – *Lacerta laevis* 81,000 × Parasagittal section of external acrosomal cap: cortex and medulla are clearly distinguishable.

Fig. 26. – *Lacerta lepida* 72,000 ×. Transverse section of a nucleus and three tails at various levels.

Fig. 27. – *Lacerta lepida* 56,000 ×. Transverse section of middle-piece anterior to opaque ring.

Fig. 28. – *Lacerta laevis* 61,000 ×. Transverse section of middle-piece at level of opaque ring.

Fig. 29. – *Coronella austriaca* 7,500 ×. Longitudinal and oblique sections of the very long mitochondrial sheath.

Fig. 30. – *Coronella austriaca* 15,000 ×. Parasagittal section of two nuclei, one with acrosome. Mitochondrial sheath of two other sperm. Note that fibers of fibrous sheath are larger and the mitochondria are more slender than in other families. Irregularly interspersed among the mitochondria are plaques of opaque material.

Fig. 31. – *Natrix tessellata* 54,000×. Parasagittal section of acrosome showing paracrystalline wall of internal cap. The apical opaque stopper is clear, and the structured cylinder that lies in the furrow of the external cap seems to proceed from it.

Fig. 32. – 105,000×. Preceeding section at greater magnification. The sperm membrane, which is simple at the level of acrosome and the tail, is flanked by very long microtubules.

Fig. 33. – *Natrix natrix* 28,000×. Parasagittal section of mitochondrial sheath. Note convoluted mitochondria, five intermitochondrial plaques, and numerous microtubules.

Fig. 34. – *Vipera aspis* 50,000×. Sagittal section of sperm. Flagellum, fibrous helix, mitochondrial sheath with four opaque plaques, numerous surrounding membranes.

Fig. 35. – *Coronella austriaca* 37,000×. Parasagittal sections of sperm at various levels. At the center a nucleus with acrosome and a nucleus with attachment to structures below it. Note change from unit membrane of acrosome to pluristratified membrane of nucleus. Neck cylinder surrounds centrioles.

Fig. 36. – *Natrix tessellata* 60,000×. Transverse sections of mitochondrial sheath and end of tail. Here too, there are many membranes surrounding the sheath but only one surrounds the tail. The palisade of microtubules can be seen at all levels.

Discussion

MATTEI. – Nous avons décrit (BOISSON & MATTEI, 1966) la formation et la disparition de la manchette dans le spermatide d'un Serpent (*Python sebae*); comment expliquez-vous l'origine des microtubules que vous représentez à l'extérieur du spermatozoïde ?

FURIERI. – Evidemment les microtubules trouvent leur origine dans la manchette. À la fin de la spermiogénèse dans toutes les espèces d'animaux jusqu'ici connus, y compris les Ophidiens, la manchette se désagrège, mais dans ces derniers les microtubules ne se perdent pas dans le débris cellulaire, persistent et se disposent tout le long et autour des spermatozoïdes.

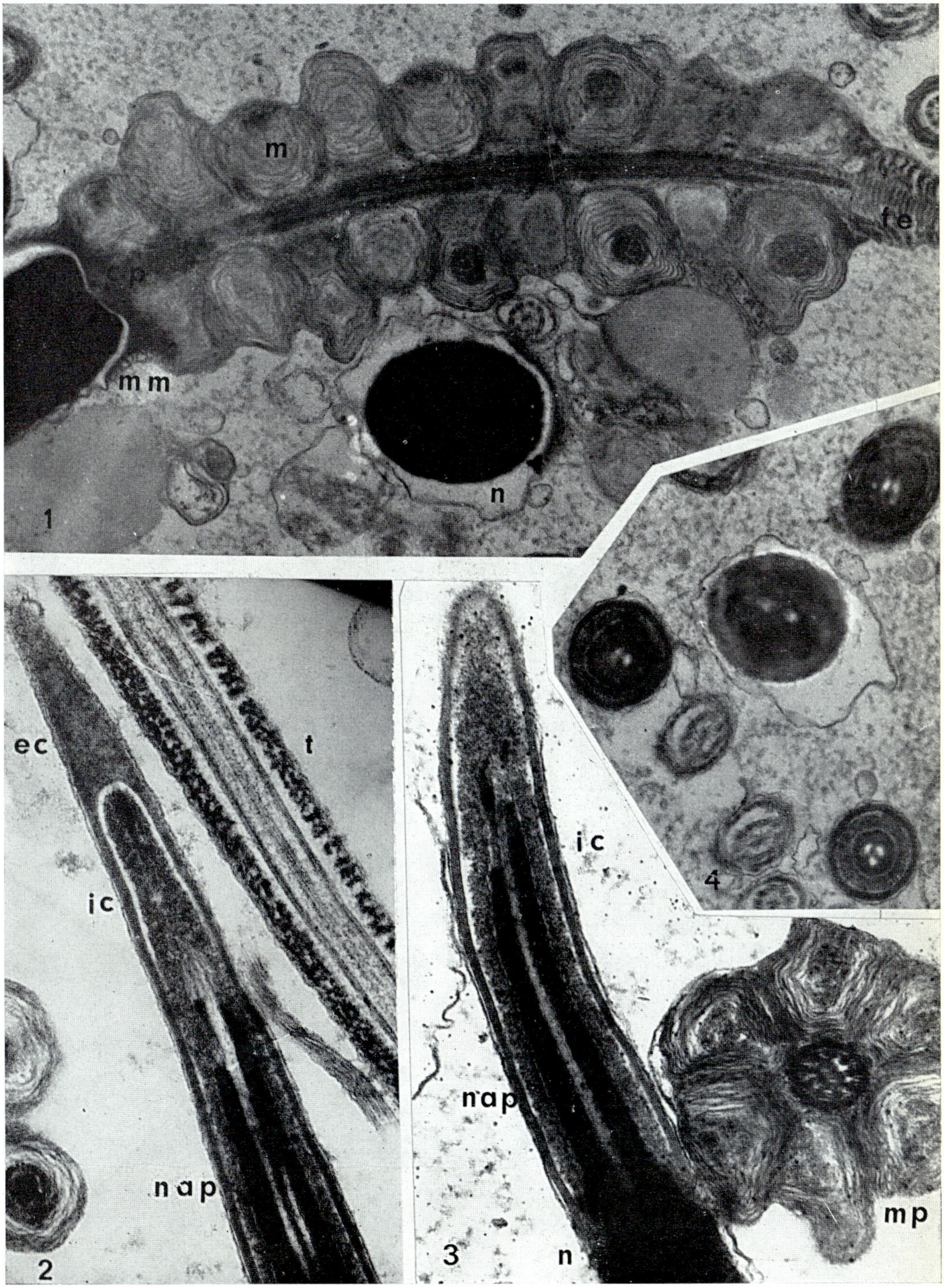
m
fe
mm
n
1
ec
t
ic
nap
2
ic
4
nap
mp
3
n

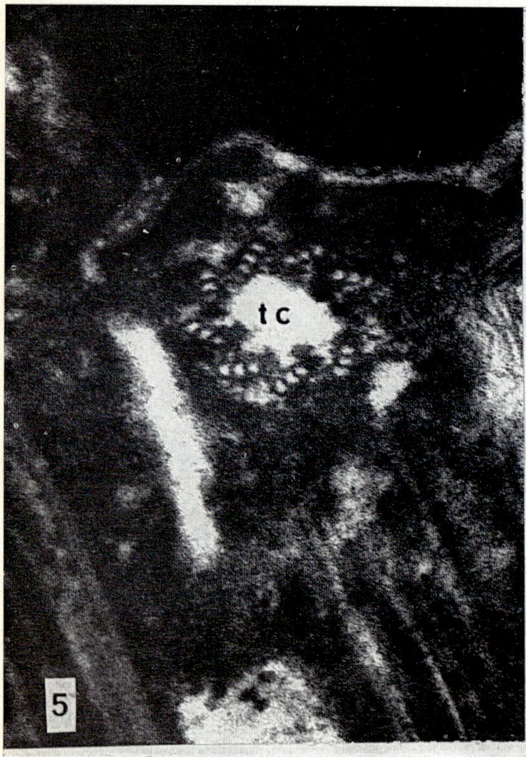
tc
5

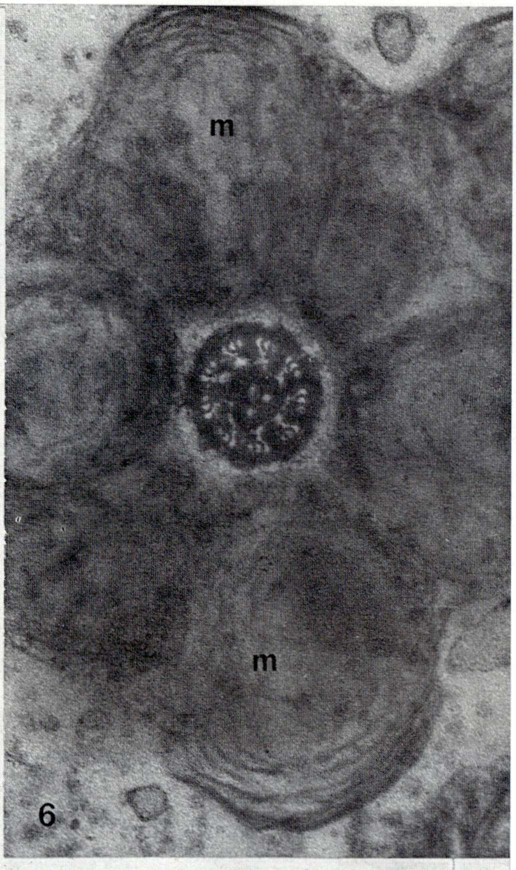
m
m
6

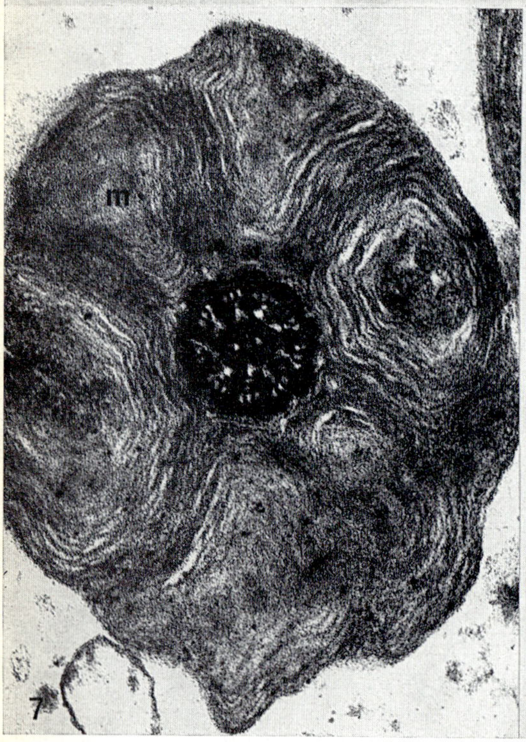
m
7

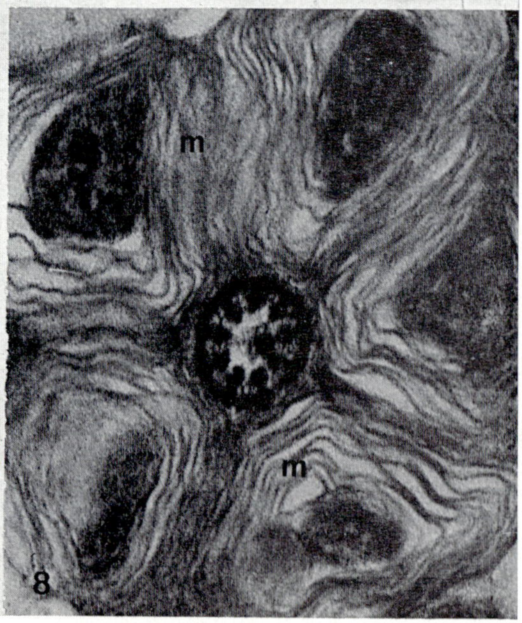
m
m
8

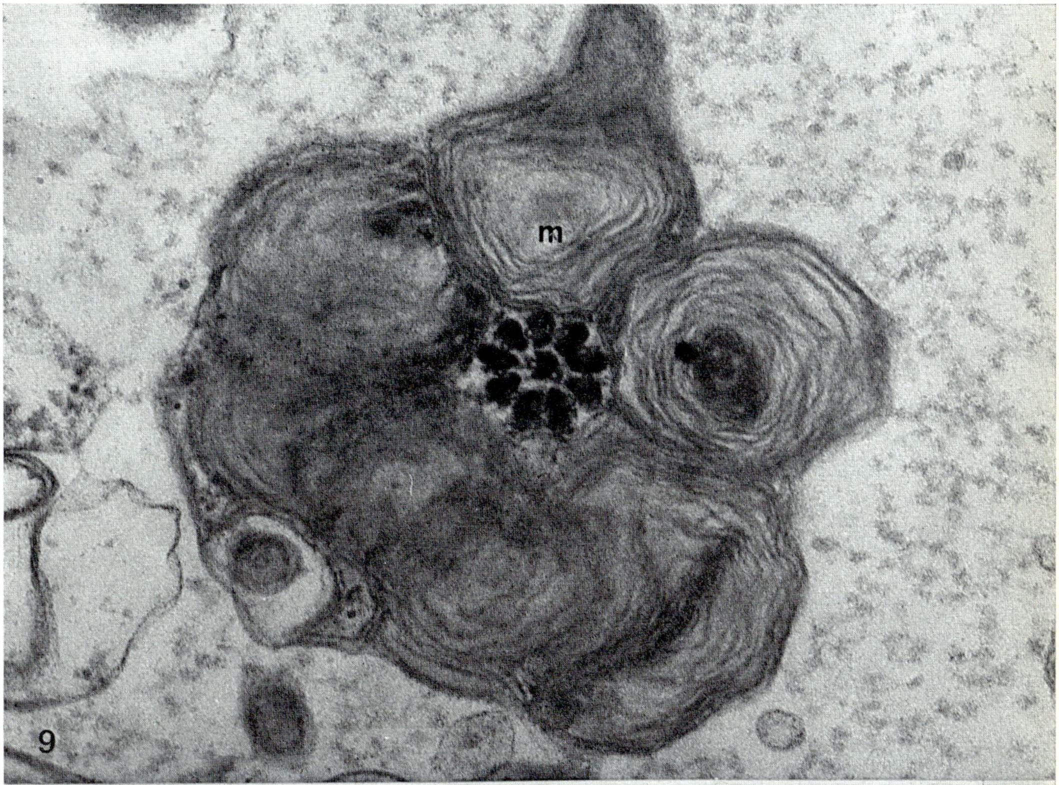
m
9

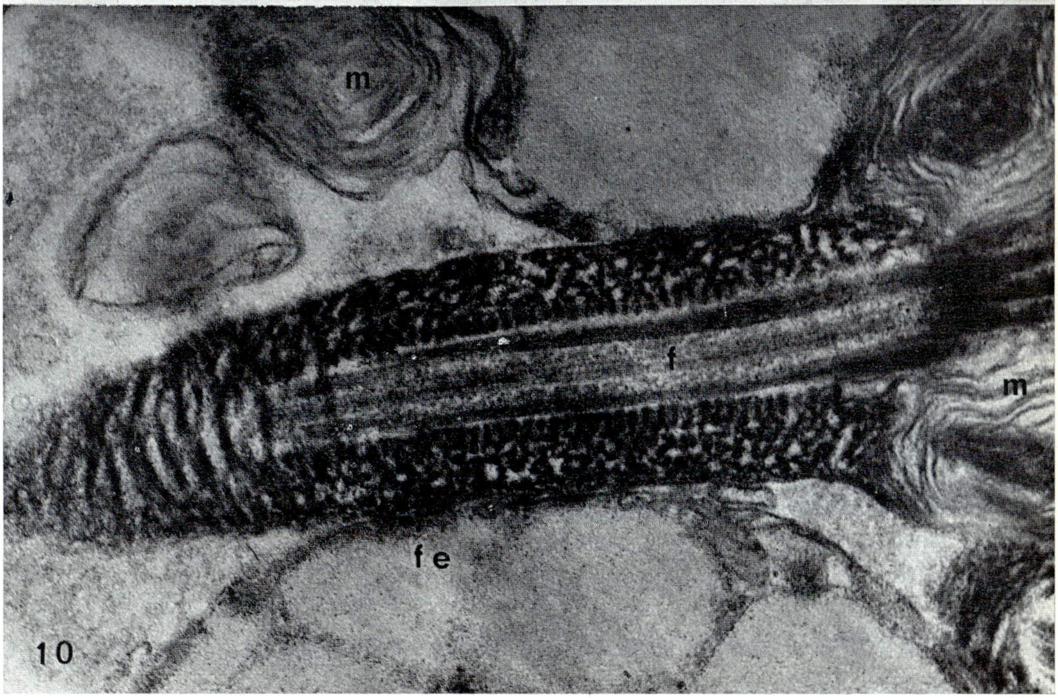
m
f
m
fe
10

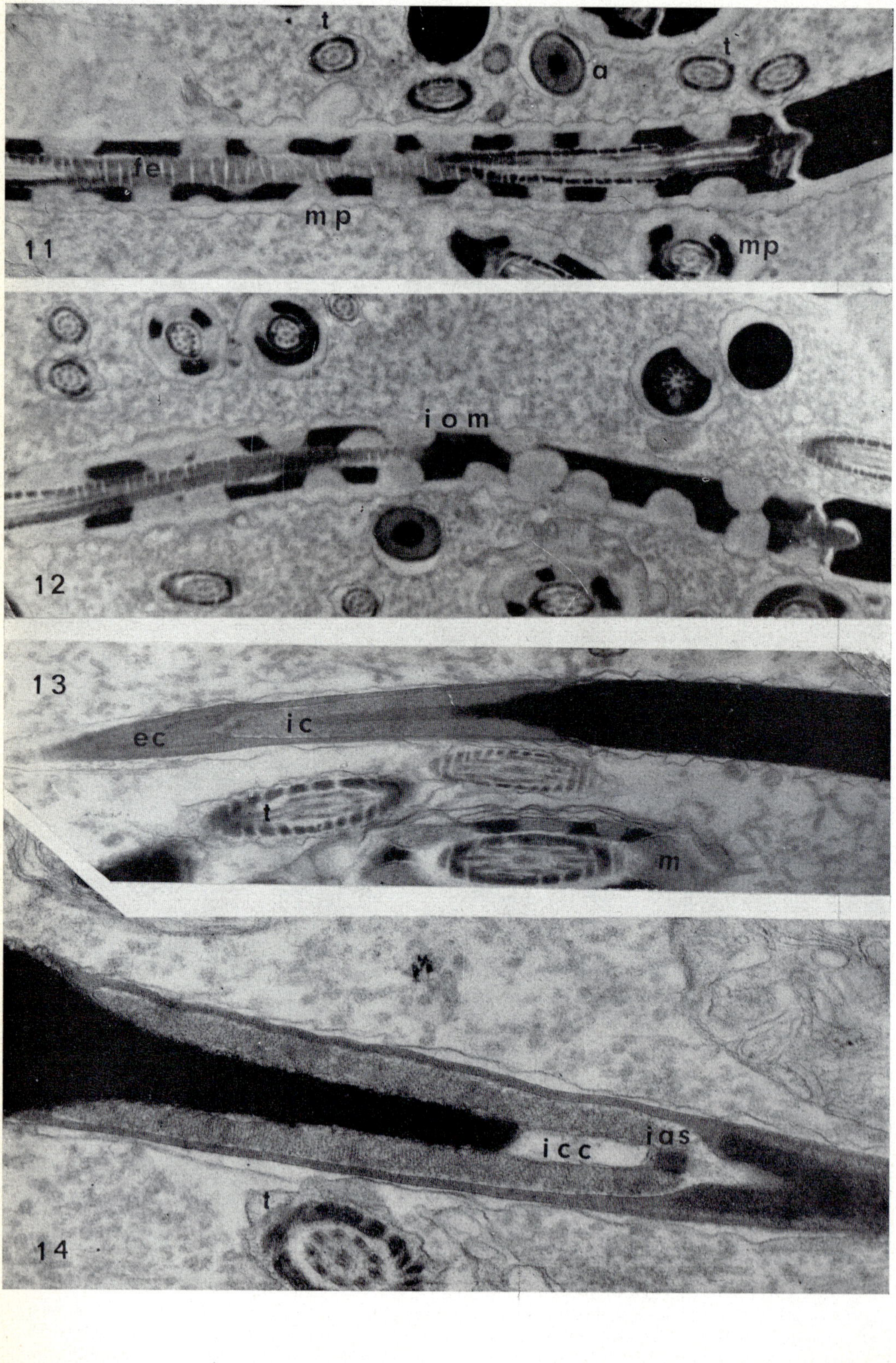
t
a
t
fe
mp
11
mp
12
iom
13
ec
ic
t
m
icc
ias
t
14

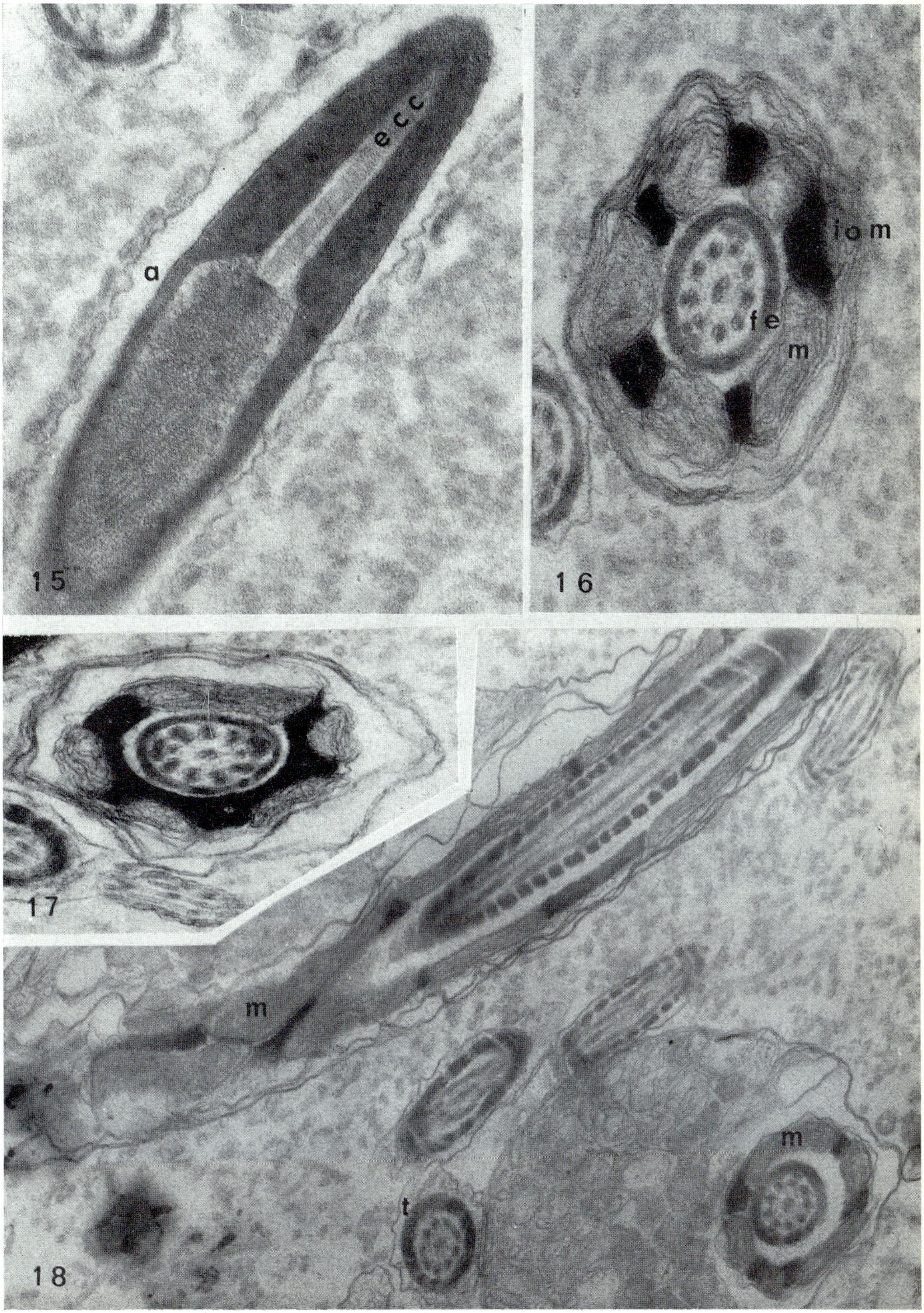
ecc
a
15
iom
fe
m
16
17
m
m
t
18

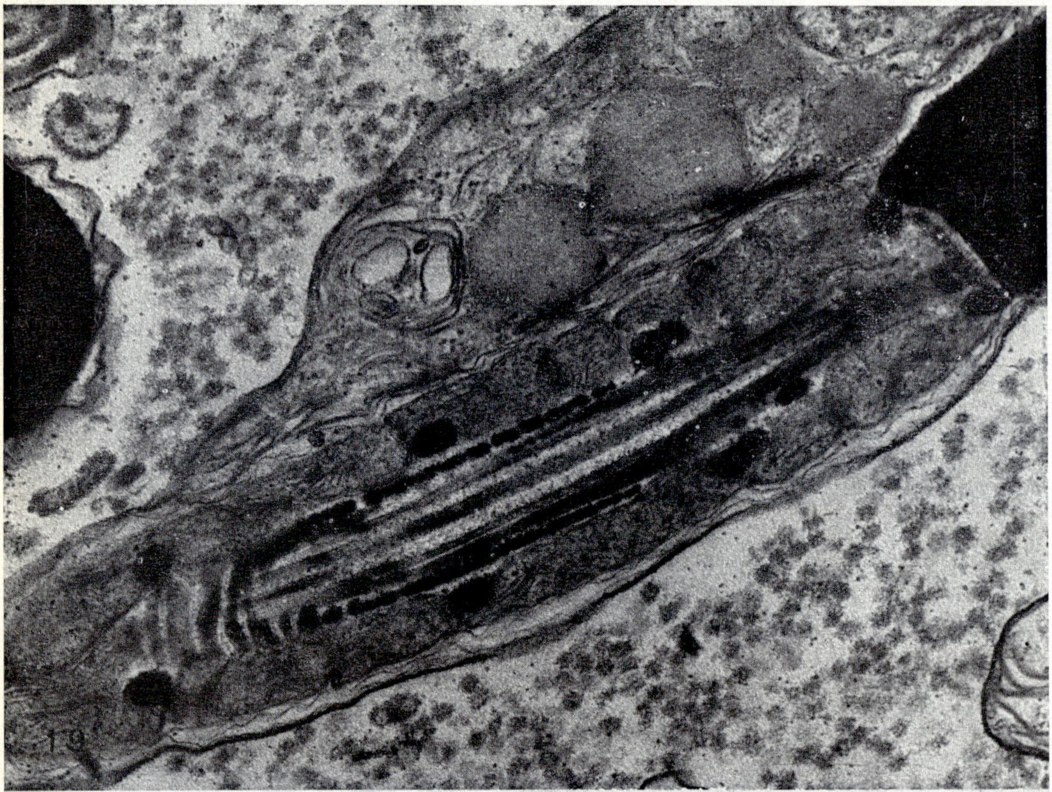
19

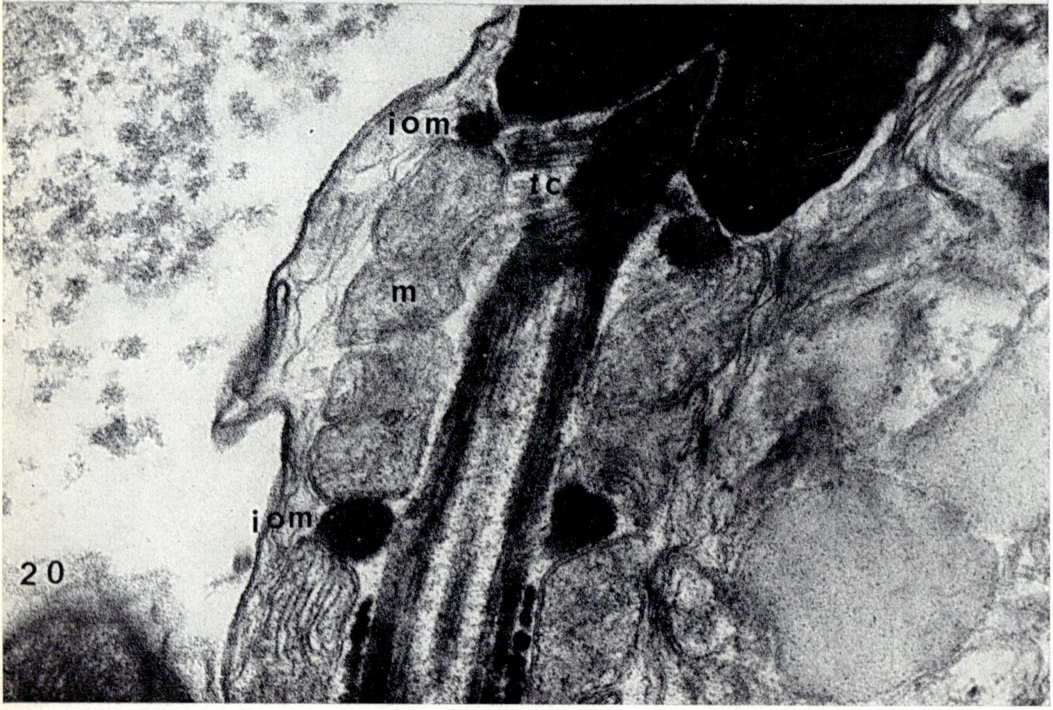
iom
tc
m
iom
20

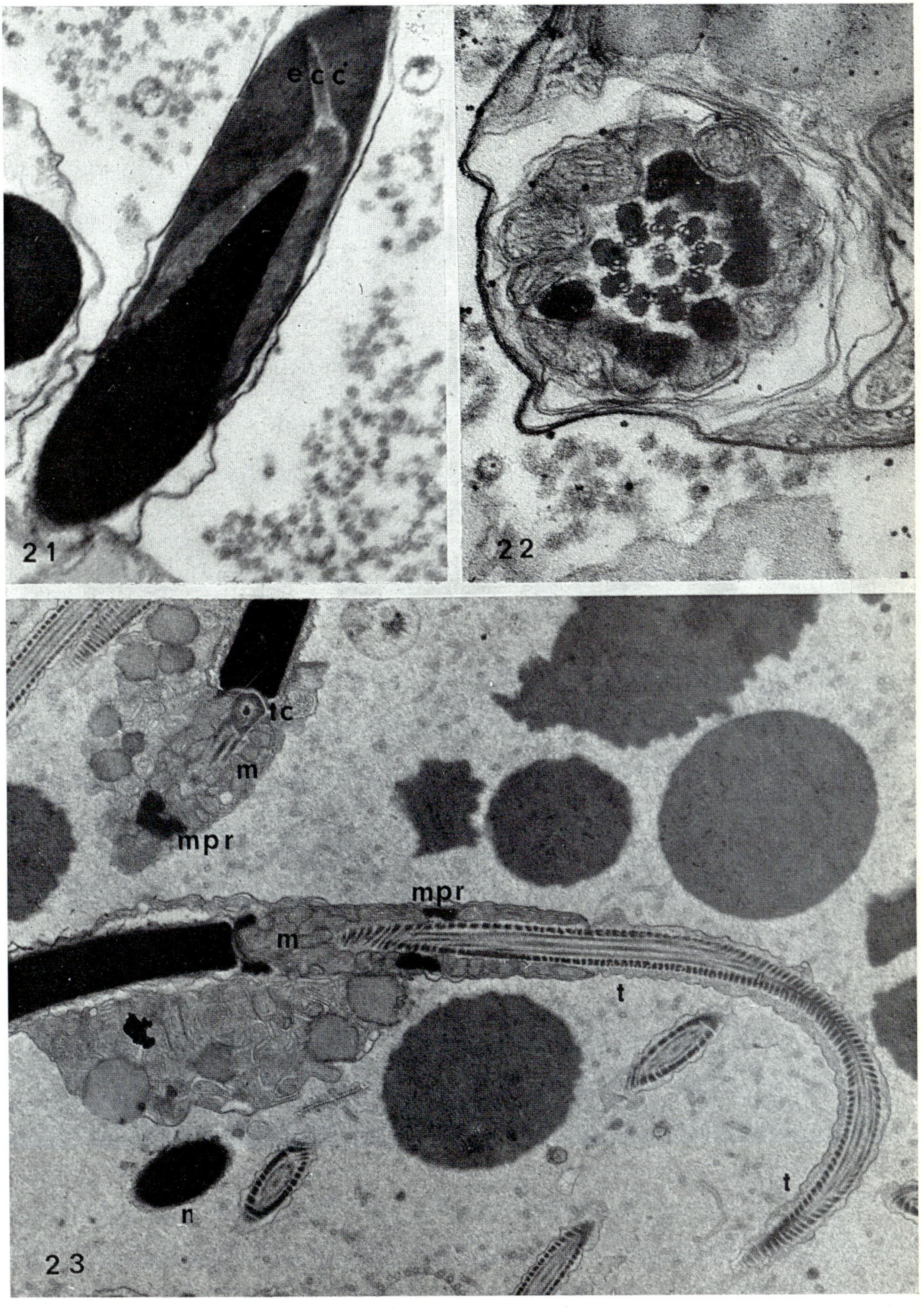
ecc
21
22
tc
m
mpr
mpr
m
t
t
n
23

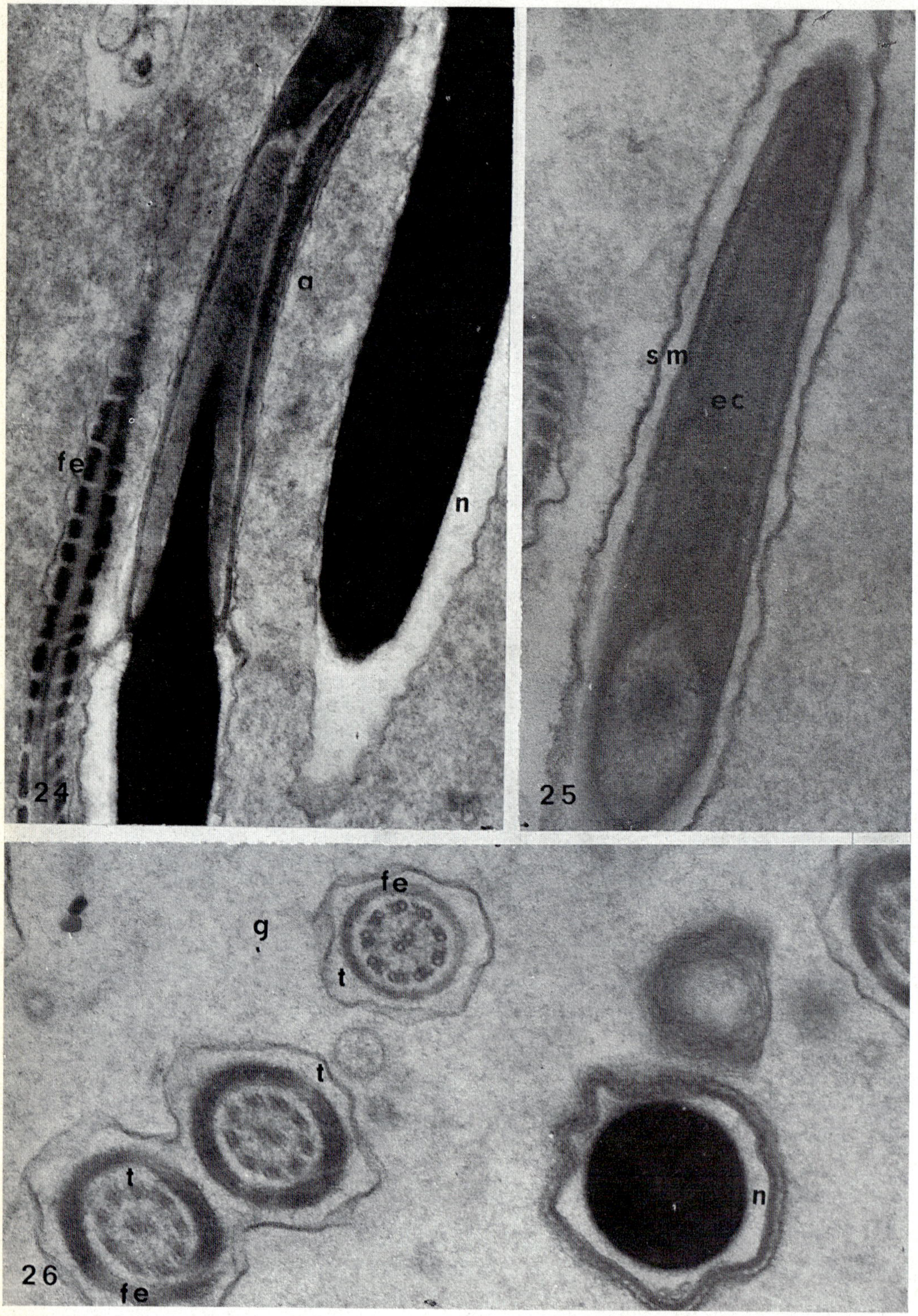
a
fe
n
24
sm
ec
25
fe
g
t
t
t
n
26
fe

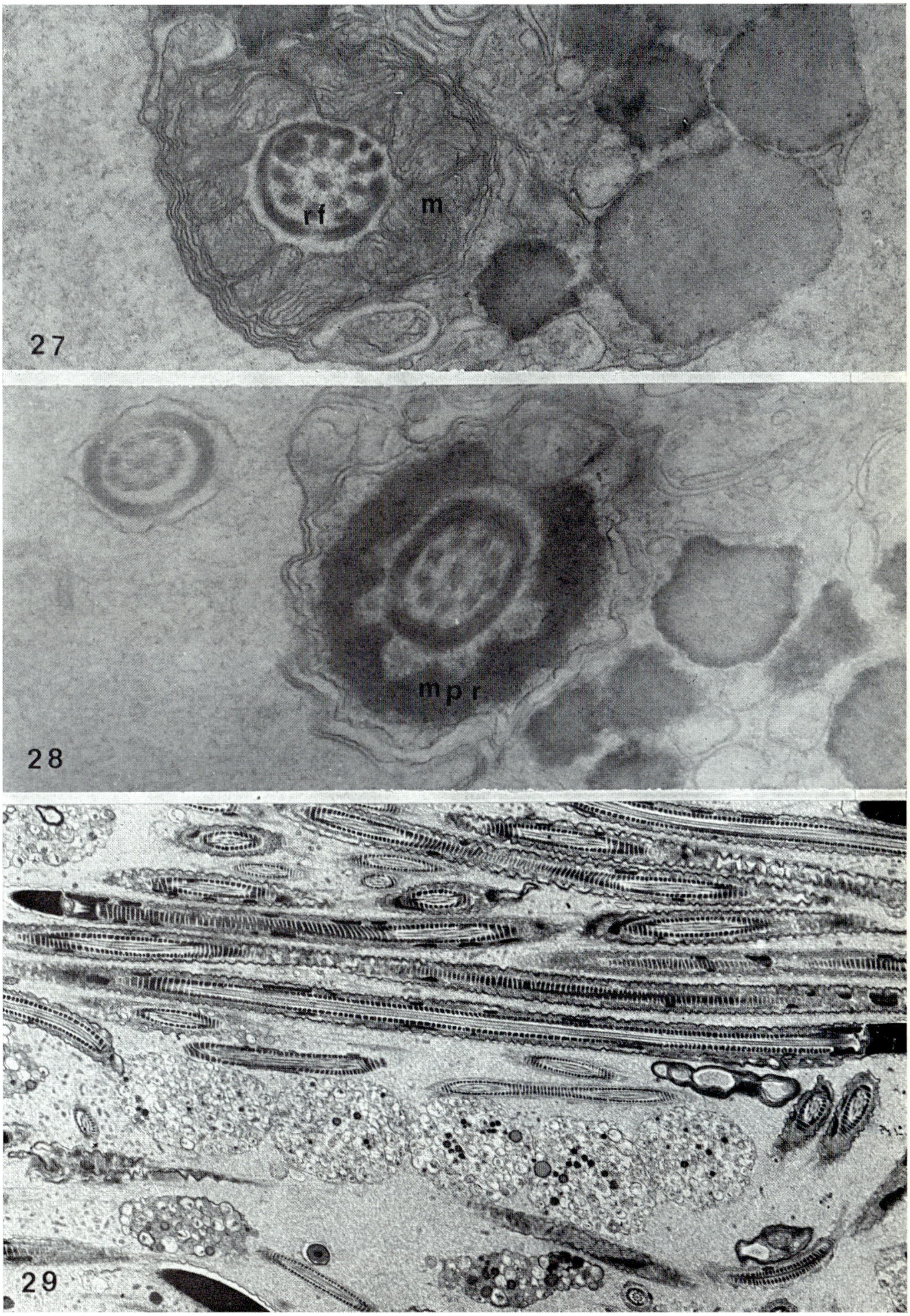
rf
m
27
mpr
28
29

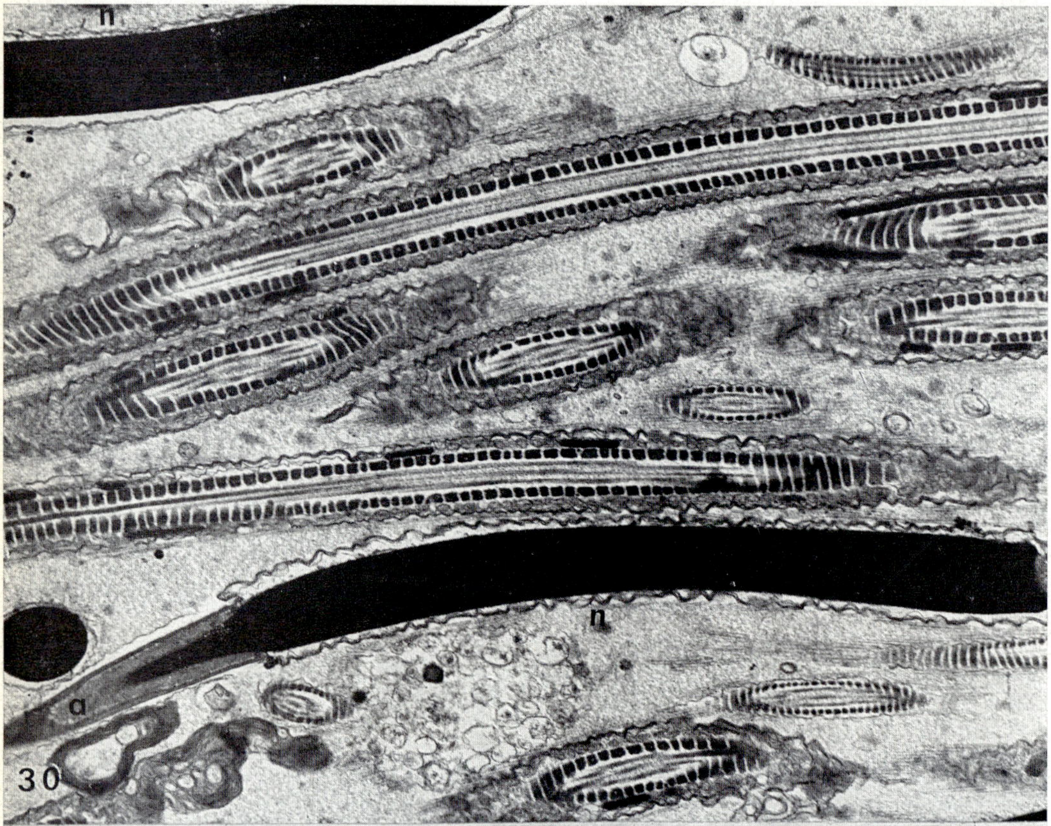
n
n
a
30

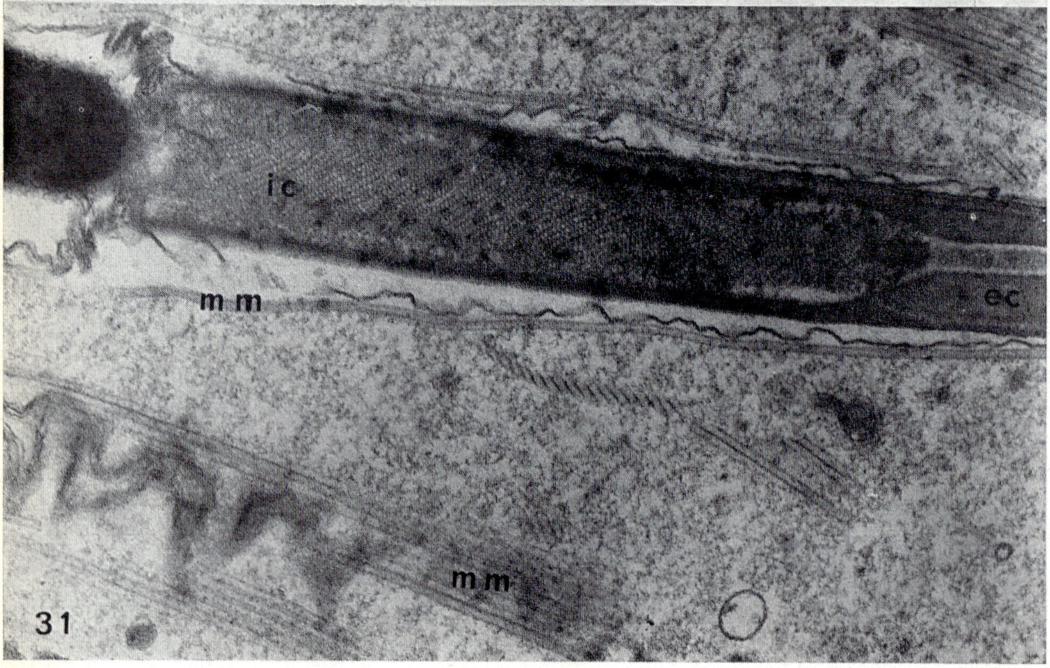
ic
mm
ec
mm
31

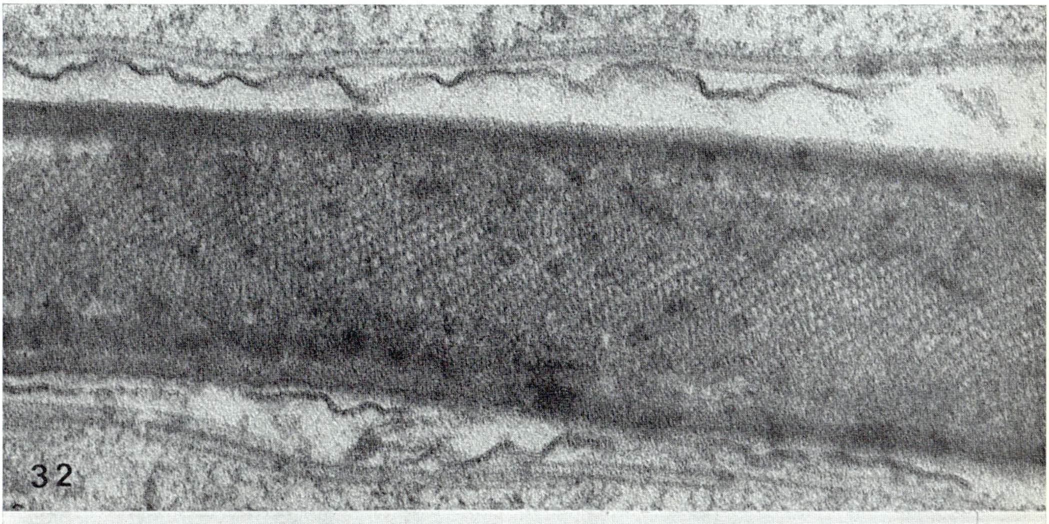

32

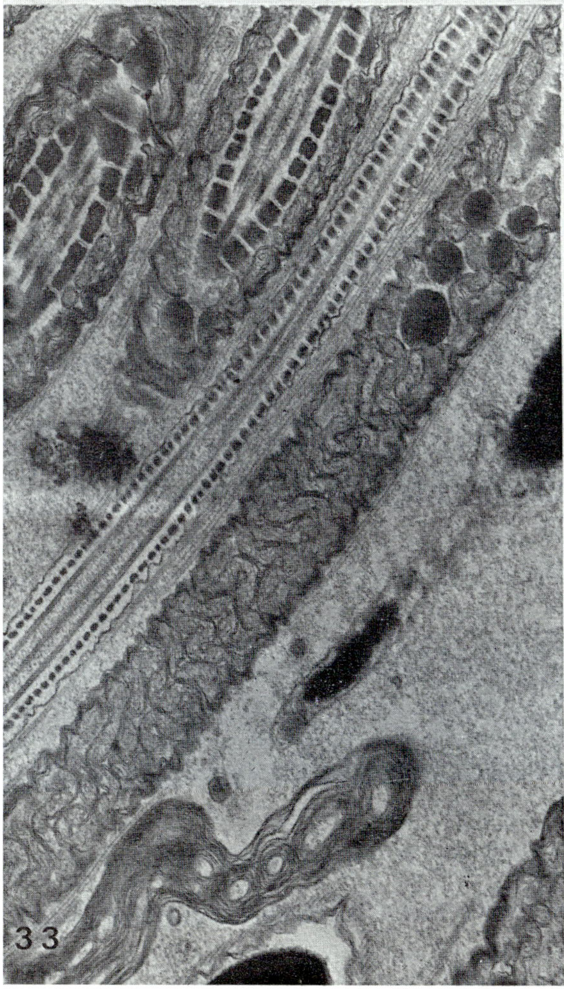

33

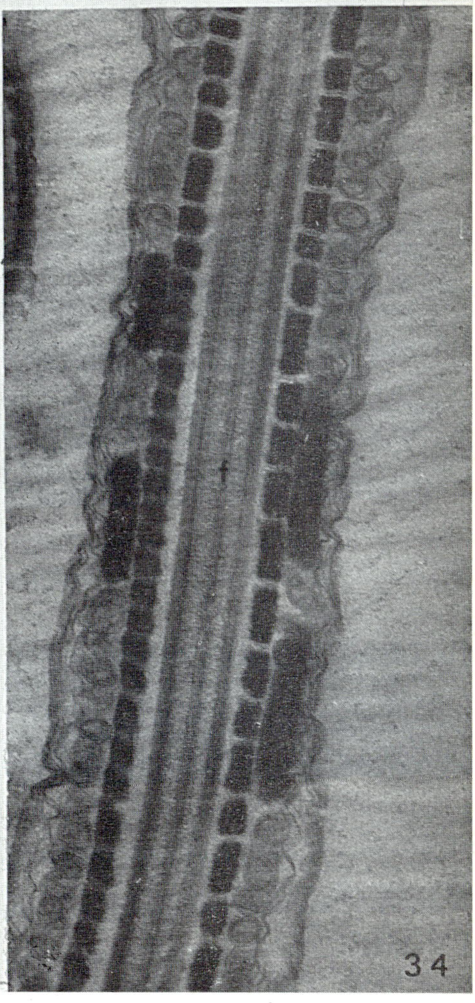

34

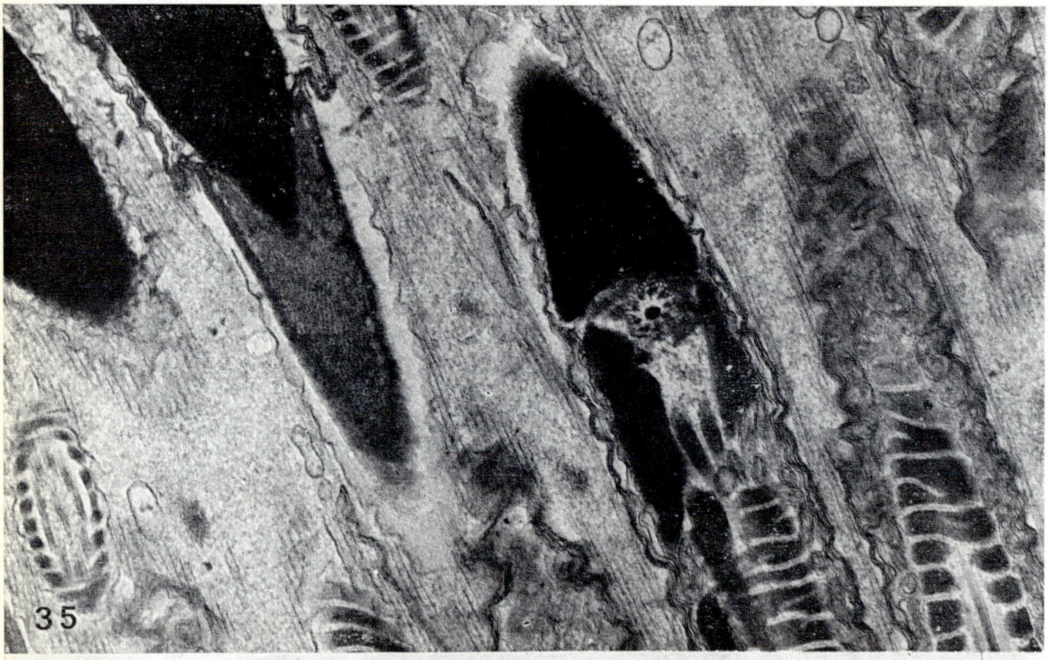
35

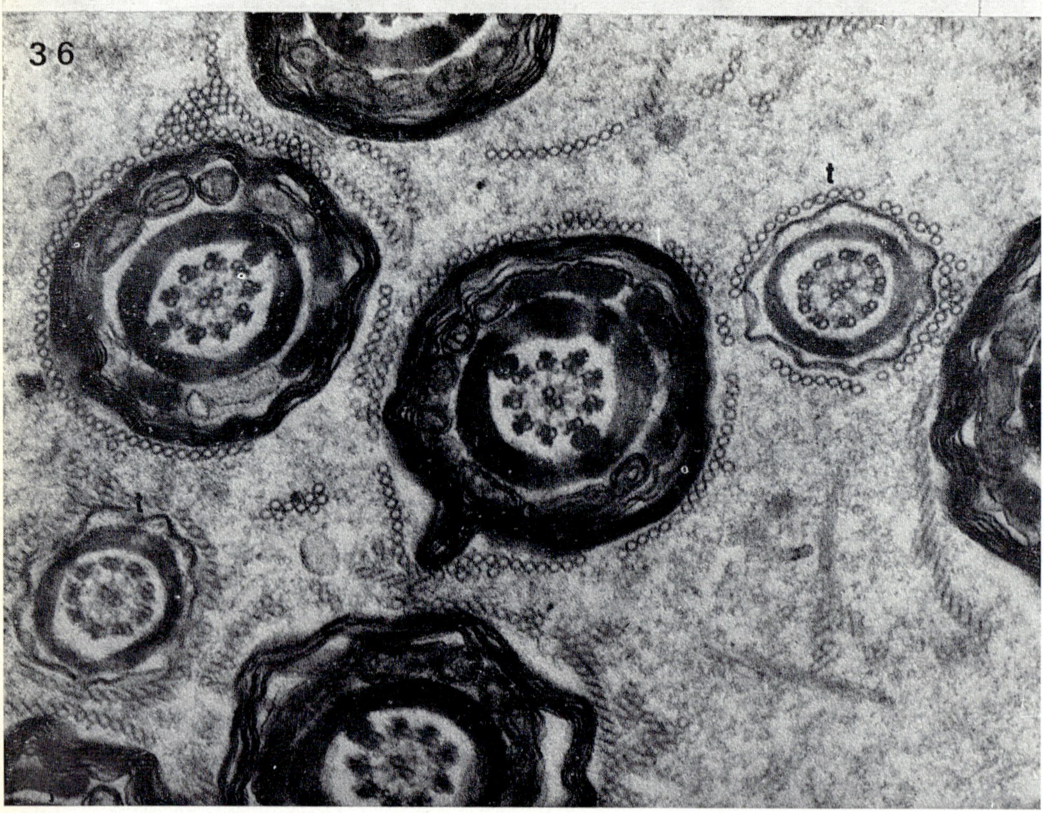
36
t
t

HENNING PEDERSEN (*)

ULTRASTRUCTURE OF THE EJACULATED HUMAN SPERM

SUMMARY. — The fine structure of the ejaculated human sperm follows the general pattern known from other mammalian sperms. The nucleus, often with granular chromatin, is anteriorly covered by the acrosome with an anterior, reactive and a posterior, stable equatorial segment, and posteriorly by a postnuclear cap. The connecting piece has a complicated and varying structure with an eccentrically placed proximal centriole. An inconspicuous annulus is found posterior to the mitochondrial helix, which is often disorderly arranged. In the anterior part of the principal piece semicircular, anastomosing ribs connect two longitudinal columns, which distally are replaced by overlapping of the ribs. Coarse fiber number 3 and 8 continue as thin laminae farthest distally, and the other fibers terminate in the following order in the antero-posterior direction: 4,2 and 7 followed by 5, 6 and 1, 9. In the distal part of the end piece the 9 + 2 pattern of the axial filament complex is changed by an uncoupling of the doublets and a successive termination of the tubular fibers.

RIASSUNTO. — La fine struttura degli spermi umani eiaculati segue lo schema generale conosciuto per gli spermi degli altri mammiferi. Il nucleo, spesso con cromatina granulare, è ricoperto anteriormente dall'acrosoma con un segmento anteriore reattivo e uno equatoriale stabile posteriore, e posteriormente da una calotta postnucleare. La parte intermedia ha una struttura varia e complicata con un centriolo prossimale posto eccentricamente. Un anello di debole consistenza è presente posteriormente all'elica mitocondriale che è spesso disposta disordinatamente. Nella parte anteriore del pezzo principale semicircolare delle coste che si anastomizzano connettono due colonne longitudinali che sono distalmente rimpiazzate dalla sovrapposizione delle coste. Le fibre numero 3 e 8 continuano come una sottile lamina fino all'estremo distale e le altre fibre terminano nell'ordine seguente in direzione antero–posteriore: 4,2 e 7 seguite da 5,6 e 1,9. Nella parte distale del pezzo finale la struttura 9+2 del filamento assile flagellare cambia a causa della disgiunzione dei doppietti e della successiva cessazione delle fibre tubulari.

The evaluation of human sperm morphology is complicated by a rather pleomorph cellular picture as compared to most other species, and it is difficult clearly to define the limits of normality (FREUND, 1966). In addition technical difficulties have contributed to the relative scarcity of knowledge of the spermatic fine structure. After introduction of sectioning techniques, electron microscopical studies of the human sperm are not substantial (ÅNBERG, 1957; SCHULTZ–LARSEN, 1958 and 1964; BAWA, 1963; CHRZANOWSKI, 1966; BEDFORD, 1967; ZAMBONI and STEFANINI, 1968; PEDERSEN, 1969) and many fundamental questions remain to be answered.

(*) Division of Electron Microscopy, Institute of Anatomy, University of Århus, Denmark.

Material and methods

Sperm samples from several men with demonstrated fertility were used. They contained more than 150 mill. cells pr. ml. of which less than 25% were immobile and less than 25% had abnormal head forms. At room temperature collidine buffered 4% glutaraldehyde with pH 7.3 – 7.5 was added to the liquefied sperm samples which were fixed for 1/2 hour. After centrifugation at 2000 r.p.m. for 20 min., the pellet was embedded in agar and this was followed by fixation in collidine buffered osmium tetroxide overnight. Dehydration in graded concentrations of ethyl alcohol and toluene was followed by embedding in Dow Epon (Lockwood and Langston, 1964). The sections were cut on LKB ultramicrotomes, stained by magnesium uranyl acetate (Frasca and Parks, 1965) and lead citrate (Venable and Coggeshall, 1965), and examined in a JEM–6C electron microscope.

Results

Head. In most cells the chromatin appears nearly homogenous, but very often it is more or less coarsely granulated. In no instances it has been possible to disclose any substructural details in the chromatin (Figs. 1–5). As a fairly constant feature small irregular vacuoles are found, preferably in the anterior end of the head. They are not membrane bounded and contain finely granulated matter and sometimes present irregular membranous structures. The nuclear membrane follows the chromatin closely but is separated from it by a light zone a few Å thick, except for the posterolateral part of the head. In this place it is separated from the chromatin forming a posterior nuclear space, and sometimes projects as a long evagination into the cytoplasm of the neck region. This space contains a light structureless matter (Fig. 1). With the technique of preservation available it has not been possible to establish, if the nuclear membrane contains normal nuclear pores except for the redundant nuclear membrane, where pore–like structures as a rule are found. In the posterior end of the head the nuclear membrane is modified corresponding to the implantation fossa. The thickened outer and inner membranes are separated by a 70 Å wide space and no nuclear pores are formed. As in other parts of the head the inner membrane is separated from the chromatin by a light space of a few Å. Apposed the outer surface of the outer membrane a thick electron dense layer is found, forming a concave basal plate (Figs. 4 and 5).

The anterior 2/3 – 3/4 of the head is covered by the acrosome which is composed of two different portions, an anterior comprising about 3/4 and a posterior 1/4 of the total length. It is bounded by a triple layered membrane, the outer and inner parts of which are parallel to each other with a distance of about 700 Å in the anterior and about 350 Å in the posterior portion. The content of the acrosome is homogenous and moderately electron dense, but there is a tendency of the content in the posterior, equatorial segment to be a little more dense than the content in the anterior portion. In the best preserved cells the outer and inner membranes of the acrosome have a straight and parallel course. For the equatorial segment this is maintained in most of the cells, but the anterior portion often presents a picture of progressive swelling, in the course of which the content is getting more light. In extreme cases the outer membrane is very irregular and shows a sort of vesiculation often involving the cell membrane. In most cells the subacrosomal space has a uniform, light appearance. However, this partly seems to be a preservation artefact, as at high magnification an electron dense material is found in this space, but the acrosome seems to be torn away from the nucleus. The outer nuclear membrane is often torn and irregular (Figs. 1, 2 and 3).

In the acrosome region the cell membrane is lying close and parallel to the surface of the acrosome with a thin layer of cytoplasm interposed. As shown in Fig. 3 this layer seems to be preserved in the same way as the subacrosomal space, in reality being a little more dense than is the general appearance. Posterior to the acrosome the cell membrane is parallel to the nuclear surface and is here apposed an about 175 Å thick layer of electron dense material but with an about 70 Å wide light zone in between. This layer is separated from the nuclear membrane by a few Å thick light zone. At the posterior border of this layer the cell membrane is retiring from the nuclear surface giving place to an upward extension of cytoplasm from the neck region. This event corresponds closely to the formation of the posterior nuclear space, as the anterior end of this is found exactly at the posterior end of the mentioned electron dense layer on the cell membrane (Fig. 1).

Neck region. In this morphologically ill defined region a spindle shaped accumulation of rather empty cytoplasm surrounds the complicated connecting piece. The central structure here is the proximal centriole, which is placed roughly in the horizontal plane in an angle of about 70 degrees with the longitudinal axis of the tail. It has an eccentrical position, often reaching outside the segmented columns (Fig. 4). On transverse sections it is placed centrally, and shows a structure typical of a centriole with nine tubular triplets evenly spaced as the wall of a cylinder (Fig. 5). From the basal plate the connecting piece tapers distally forming the segmented columns. The real three-dimensional structure of this organelle has not been unvailed, but probably it is variable, as for example the number of segments in the columns is found to vary. Anteriorly, around the proximal centriole, the segments change into rounded plates with irregular outlines, the most anterior of which, as the basal plate, is closely apposed the concave implantation fossa. As a rule the segmented columns look as proximal continuations of the outer coarse fibers, but sometimes the transition is not so smooth as would be expected, if the event was just a segmentation of the coarse fibers. Material of the same density is associated as well the outer as the inner aspect of the proximal centriole. Posteriorly the axial part of the connecting piece is occupied by the modified anterior end of the axial filament complex, the subfibers of which diverge and end close to the proximal centriole. The gamma fibers, are found in this region, too, with their connecting axis roughly perpendicular to the longitudinal axis of the proximal centriole (Fig. 6).

Axial filament complex. The structure of this closely follows the general pattern known from other mammalian sperms. On transverse sections alpha, beta end gamma fibers are recognized in the well known 9+2 arrangement (Figs. 10 and 11). The alpha fibers are nearly homogenous, about 210 Å thick and provided with two arms towards the beta fiber of the neighbouring doublet. The beta fibers are hollow with a diameter of about 250 Å and without evidence of crosstriation. This in contrast to the about 270 Å thick hollow gamma fibers, which on several sections are found to be finely crosstriated with a period of about 120 Å (Fig. 8). The cytoplasm within this complex is slightly more granulated than outside and with some evidence of organization. On transverse sections the two gamma fibers are interconnected by arc-like densities, and irregular irradiations are connecting these or the gamma fibers with the outer doublets, as a rule the alpha fibers. On longitudinal sections a regular periodicity in this cytoplasm sometimes is to be found (Fig. 9). The 9+2 pattern is withheld through most part of the tail including the end piece, but the arrangement of the fibers in the tip of the end piece is changed. In some sections the cell membrane encloses hollow tubules without evidence of doublet formation and in a decreasing number, indicating an uncoupling of the doublets and a successive termination of the single subfibers (Fig. 11).

Coarse fibers. These are extending from the connecting piece through the middle piece and a varying distance into the principal piece. The pattern of termination of the fibers is not exactly regular, but by examining many transverse sections involving these fibers, a general picture is disclosed. The first fiber to disappear is number 4 closely followed by number 2 and 7. Fiber number 5 and 6 then disappear as number 1 and 9 are left to terminate farthest posteriorly. Common to the mentioned fibers is their way of termination, as they are tapering and end as thin structures in close relation to the corresponding doublet of the axial filament complex. Fiber number 3 and 8 present a different picture. In the proximal end of the middle piece they become integrated into the longitudinal columns of the fibrous sheath, but distal to the termination of these the fibers are maintained as two thin laminae extending from the overlapping ribs to the alpha fibers of the corresponding doublets. These laminae are found distal to the termination of the outer fibers, but they terminate themselves before reaching the posterior end of the fibrous sheath (Fig. 11). The inner aspect of the coarse fibers has a motheaten appearance often with a little electron dense material separated from the fibers, but without evidence of substructural organization. On transverse sections fiber number 1, 5 and 6 are generally found to be larger than the others, but sometimes fiber number 7 and 9 are found to be large, too, as additional fibers are found occasionally.

Middle piece. In the middle piece the axial fibers are surrounded by a single layer of helix coiled mitochondria, the most anterior of which as a rule are found at the posterior end of the connecting piece (Figs. 4–7). Generally the mitochondria are arranged in a regular way, but often this regular pattern is disturbed by disorderly arranged mitochondria, especially in the anterior end. The size of the mitochondria is varying a great deal. They are flattened against the coarse fibers, from which they are separated by only a thin uniform layer of cytoplasm, and are in close contact with each other. The helix is closely enveloped by the cell membrane. The mitochondria have a complicated internal structure with a dense matrix, in which the cristae run a winding irregular course, often with slightly dilated intracristal spaces (Figs. 6, 7 and 10). Distal to the mitochondria an electron dense material is found apposed the cell membrane corresponding to the annulus of light microscopy. On longitudinal sections of the tail it is flattened or triangular, but as a rule not very conspicuous and without internal substructure (Fig. 7).

Principal piece. The anterior part of the fibrous sheath is formed by two longitudinal columns connected by semicircular anastomosing ribs, the transverse sections of which are varying and irregular. Posteriorly the longitudinal columns are gradually disappearing, as they are replaced by overlappings of the ribs. These are anteriorly at their inner aspect apposed the thin laminae which are in connection with the alpha fibers of fiber number 3 and 8. Distal to the laminae the overlapping areas continue to the posterior end of the principal piece becoming less conspicuous (Fig. 11).

End piece. The last few microns of the tail are composed of the axial filament complex surrounded by the cell membrane. As described the axial filament complex in this part of the cell is found to show the described 9+2 pattern, except for modifications in the most distal end (Fig. 11).

Conclusion

The chromatin of ejaculated mammalian sperms previously described has been found to be rather homogenous (Fawcett, 1958; Nicander and Bane, 1962 a and b; Hadek, 1963 b; Saacke and Almquist, 1964; Blom and Birch-Andersen, 1965; Fawcett, 1965; Fawcett and Ito, 1965). The same picture is found in human sperms, but a varying number of cells are found to have a more or less granular chromatin (Ånberg, 1957; Schultz-Larsen, 1958 and 1964; Bedford, 1967; Pedersen, 1969). This could be an expression of a varying degree of maturity, as a progressive condensation of the chromatin during spermiogenesis is known from several species including man (Ånberg, 1957; Horstman, 1961; Nagano, 1968). Cell death or degeneration are other possible explanations of this granularity, but this remains to be evaluated. In accordance with Bedford (1967) and Zamboni (1968) the chromatin is found to extend into the apical end of the nucleus, and no posterior nuclear compartment as described by Schultz-Larsen (1958) has been found. The general occurrence of intranuclear vacuoles in sperms of several species has been pointed out by FAWCETT (1958) and confirmed by many authors since then. In human sperms vacuoles as described are of general occurrence and might not be considered as degenerative (CHRZANOWSKI, 1966). The curled irregular membranous structures occasionally found in the nucleus are more likely to be degenerative, as the head form of these cells often is clearly abnormal. The nuclear membrane covering the posterior nuclear space is found to show pore-like structures as is the case with the same part of the membrane in the late spermatid (NAGANO, 1968). An occurrence of pores in the anterior parts of the membrane is uncertain (ANDRÉ, 1963; NICANDER and BANE, 1966 b) and the present technique of preservation does not allow to answer this question.

The structure of the acrosome with its anterior, reactive and posterior, stable part closely follows the pattern described for several mammalian species (BEDFORD, 1964; BLOM and BIRCH-ANDERSEN, 1965; NICANDER and BANE, 1966 a and b). No intranuclear extension of the acrosome has been found (SCHULTZ-LARSEN, 1958). Acrosome reactions have been related to the process of capacitation, but no morphological changes have been found (BEDFORD, 1964). The role of the acrosome in the process of fertilization is still not quite understood, but changes in the region are found very regularly (HADEK, 1963 a; BARROS, BEDFORD, FRANKLIN and AUSTIN, 1967; BEDFORD, 1968). The progressive swelling of the anterior part of the acrosome described in this work, could be seen in the light of this, but most probably it is merely a sign of different reactivity of the anterior and posterior parts of the acrosome to degeneration or preservation. A morphological feature as a sign of changes in maturity during passage through the excretory duct is a possibility, but this is at present largely unknown (FAWCETT and HOLLENBERG, 1963; BEDFORD, 1965; FAWCETT, 1966). The presence of two distinct portions of the acrosome seems to be a feature of the normal cell, and should not be considered a sign of degeneration (SAACKE and ALMQUIST, 1964 a) but the accentuation of this difference may be abnormal. The subacrosomal space has been found to be of a uniform density without regional accumulation of material as described for other mammals (NICANDER and BANE, 1966 a and b), but the appearance of this space may partly be a result of preservation difficulties, as the acrosome often has the appearance of being detached from the nuclear surface.

In earlier works on the human sperm nothing corresponding to the posterior nuclear cap has been found (ÅNBERG, 1957; SCHULTZ-LARSEN, 1958 and 1964), and in other species this part of the cell has been a matter of controversy (FAWCETT, 1965; NICANDER and BANE, 1966 b). In the present work a distinct electron dense material has been found in close apposition to the cell membrane, corresponding to a part of the postnuclear cap of light microscopy. This is in accordance with the findings of BEDFORD (1967), but no substructural organization as described by BLOM and BIRCH-ANDERSEN (1965) in the bull has been found. In the human spermatid the electron dense material in the nuclear ring is left at the cell membrane proximal to the ring, as it moves backwards, in this way forming the postnuclear cap (own unpublished observations).

The complex and perhaps varying structure of the connecting piece has not been fully evaluated. The electron dense material in this region is often found as columns along the triplets of the proximal centriole, imitating the coarse fibers of the tail. Also by forming the proximal centriolar rod (HORSTMANN, 1961) the properties of the proximal centriole to imitate the distal centriole is demonstrated. This complex seems to be formed by a collision of the two paracentriolar formations. Having the motheaten appearance of the inner aspect of the coarse fibers and the varying number of segments in the segmented columns in mind, it seems naturally to expect a varying picture of this structure. The existence of additional coarse fibers and variation in their size relations on transverse sections (BAWA, 1963) is confirmed, but the density of the fibers in the present preservation is rather uniform. The successive termination of the coarse fibers described by TELKKA, FAWCETT and CHRISTENSEN (1961) and later confirmed by SAACKE and ALMQUIST (1964 b) except for fiber number 3 and 8 deviates from the pattern found in the human sperm.

The general structure of the axial filament complex follows the pattern described by TELKKA, FAWCETT and CHRISTENSEN (1961) and FAWCETT and ITO (1965). A crossstriated appearance of axial fibers has been described in some works (SCHULTZ–LARSEN, 1958; ANDRÉ; 1962; PEASE, 1963). The crossstriation of the gamma fibers with a periodicity of 120 Å is in accordance with the findings of ANDRÉ (1962). The distal termination of the axial filament complex has not been fully evaluated, but seems to be largely in accordance with the descriptions of NICANDER and BANE (1966 a and b).

The significance of the progressive changes in mitochondrial internal structure during spermatogenesis is unknown (ANDRÉ, 1962). The mitochondrial structure found in this work is complicated and presumably as a result of preservation rather variable. A further evaluation of the membranous substructure (ELFVIN, 1968) has not been possible.

In earlier works on the human sperm the existence of longitudinal columns in the fibrous sheath was denied (ÅNBERG, 1957) and the sheath was considered as formed by spirally wrapped threads (ÅNBERG, 1957; SCHULTZ–LARSEN, 1958). The findings in this work are essentially in accordance with FAWCETT (1965). The longitudinal columns are not very conspicuous, however, and are not extending through the whole length of the fibrous sheath, as they distally are replaced by overlappings of the ribs. Most cells fit into the described general picture of the fibrous sheath, but it deserves notice that the picture is rather variable.

The difficulty of preservation of the cell membrane particularly in the anterior acrosome region (BEDFORD, 1964 and 1965) has been observed in this work too, and may be of functional significance, but the electron microscopical technique applied in this study is as yet far from perfect, and besides this problem several other morphological details remain to be fully evaluated.

References

Ånberg A. (1957) – *The ultrastructure of the human spermatozoon.* « Acta obstet. gynec. scand. », 36, suppl. 2.

André J. (1962) – *Contribution à la connaissance du chondriome.* « J. Ultrastruct. Res. », suppl. 2.

André J. (1963) – *Some aspects of specialization in sperm.* In: *The General Physiology of Cell Specialization.* Eds. Mazia D. and Tyler A. – McGraw–Hill.

Barros C., Bedford J. M., Franklin L. E. and Austin C. R. (1967) – *Membrane vesiculation as a feature of the mammalian acrosome reaction.* « J. Cell Biol. », 34, C1–5.

Bawa S. R. (1963) – *Outer coarse fibers of the mammalian sperm tail. An electron microscope study.* « J. Ultrastruct. Res. », 9, 475–483.

Bedford J. M. (1964) – *Fine structure of the sperm head in ejaculate and uterine spermatozoa of the rabbit.* « J. Reprod. Fertil. », 7, 228–221.

Bedford J. M. (1965) – *Changes in the fine structure of the rabbit sperm head during passage through the epididymis.* « J. Anat. », 99, 891–906.

Bedford J. M. (1967) – *Observations on the fine structure of spermatozoa of the Bush Baby (Galago senegalensis), the african green monkey (Cercopithecus aethiops) and man.* « Amer. J. Anat. », 121, 443–460.

Bedford J. M. (1968) – *Ultrastructural changes in the sperm head during fertilization in the rabbit.* « Amer. J. Anat. », 123, 329–358.

Blom E. and Birch–Andersen A. (1965) – *The ultrastructure of the bull sperm.* II. *The sperm head.* « Nord. Vet. Med. », 17, 193–212.

Chrzanowski S. (1966) – *Ultrastructure of human spermatozoon.* « Pol. Med. J. », 5, 482,–491.

Elfvin L–G. (1968) – *An ultrastructural difference between the outer and inner membrane of the middle piece mitochondria in rat spermatozoa.* « J. Ultrastruct. Res. », 24, 259–268.

Fawcett D. W. (1958) – *The structure of the mammalian spermatozoon.* « Int. Rev. Cytol. », 7, 195–234.

Fawcett D. W. (1965) – *The anatomy of the mammalian spermatozoon with particular reference to the guinea pig.* « Z. Zellforsch. », 67, 279–296.

Fawcett D. W. (1966) – *The ultrastructure of the spermatozoon.* « Proc. V. World Congr. Fertil. Steril. », 55.

Fawcett D. W. and Hollenberg R. D. (1963) – *Changes in the acrosome of guinea pig spermatozoa during passage through the epididymis.* « Z. Zellforsch. », 60, 276–292.

Fawcett D. W. and Ito S. (1965) – *The fine structure of bat spermatozoa.* « Amer. J. Anat. », 116, 567–610.

Frasca J. M. and Parks V. R. (1965) – *A routine technique for doublestaining ultrathin sections using uranyl and lead salts.* « J. Cell Biol. », 25, 157–165.

Freund M. (1966) – *A cooperative study on the rating of human sperm morphology.* « Proc. V. World Congr. Fertil. Steril. », 56.

Hadek R. (1963 a) – *Submicroscopic changes in the penetrating spermatozoon of the rabbit.* « J. Ultrastruct. Res. », 8, 161–169.

Hadek R. (1963 b) – *Study of the fine structure of rabbit sperm head.* « J. Ultrastruct. Res. », 9, 110–122.

Horstmann E. (1961) – *Elektronenmikroskopische Untersuchungen zur Spermiohistogenese beim Menschen.* « Z. Zellforsch. », 54, 68–89.

Lockwood W. R. and Langston L. L. (1964) – *A reliable and easily sectioned epoxy embedding medium.* « Anat. Rec. », 150, 129–140.

Nagano T. (1968) – *Fine structural relation between the Sertoli cell and the differentiating spermatid in the human testis.* « Z. Zellforsch. », 89, 39–43.

Nicander L. and Bane A. (1962 a) – *Fine structure of boar spermatozoa.* « Z. Zellforsch. », 57, 390–405.

NICANDER L. and BANE A. (1962 b) – *New observations on the fine structure of spermatozoa.* « Int. J. Fertil. », 7, 339–344.

NICANDER L. and BANE A. (1966 a) – *An electron microscopical study of the acrosome of some mammalian spermatozoa.* « Proc. V. World Congr. Fertil. Steril. », 597–601.

NICANDER L. and BANE A. (1966 b) – *Fine structure of the sperm head in some mammals with particular reference to the acrosome and the subacrosomal substance.* « Z. Zellforsch. », 72, 496–515.

PEASE D. C. (1963) – *The ultrastructure of flagellar fibrils.* « J. Cell Biol. », 18, 313–326.

PEDERSEN H. (1969) – *Ultrastructure of the ejaculated human sperm.* « Z. Zellforsch. », 94, 542–554.

SAACKE R. G. and ALMQUIST J. O. (1964 a) – *Ultrastructure of bovine spermatozoa.* I. *The head of normal, ejaculated sperm.* « Amer. J. Anat. », 115, 143–162.

SAACKE R. G. and ALMQUIST J. O. (1964 b) – *Ultrastructure of bovine spermatozoa.* II. *The neck and tail of normal, ejaculated sperm.* « Amer. J. Anat. », 115, 163–184.

SCHULTZ-LARSEN J. (1958) – *The morphology of the human sperm.* « Acta path. microbiol. scand. », suppl. 128.

SCHULTZ-LARSEN J. (1964) – *Spermatic ultrastructure* (*Homo*). In: Williams W. W., Sterility, 3, ed. Springfield, Mass.

TELKKA A., FAWCETT D. W. and CHRISTENSEN A. K. (1961) – *Further observations on the structure of the mammalian sperm tail.* « Anat. Rec. », 141, 231–245.

VENABLE J. H. and COGGESHALL R. (1965) – *A simplified lead citrate stain for use in electron microscopy.* « J. Cell Biol. », 25, 407–408.

EXPLANATION OF FIGURES

Fig. 1. – The nucleus with its nearly homogenous chromatin is covered by the anterior part of the acrosome (*aa*), the equatorial segment (*es*), the postnuclear cap (*pc*) and the redundant membrane around the posterior nuclear space (*ps*). The constant thickness of the equatorial segment is in contrast to the progressive swelling of the anterior part of the acrosome. ×35,000 and 60,000.

Fig. 2. – In the anterior pointed end of the head an intranuclear vacuole (*V*) is found. The granulated content is not limited by a membrane. ×62,000.

Fig. 3. – The subacrosomal space has a dense but uneven texture, as the acrosome seem to be torn away from the nuclear surface. The space between the outer acrosome membrane (*oa*) and the cell membrane (*cm*) has the same appearance. The outer part of the nuclear membrane (*nm*) is discontinuous. (*ia*) indicates the inner acrosome membrane. ×212,000.

Fig. 4. – In the neck region the nuclear membrane (*nm*) is modified. The inner membrane (*i*) is separated from the chromatin by a few Å wide light zone and the outer membrane (*o*) is on its outer surface apposed the basal plate (*bp*). The longitudinally sectioned proximal centriole (*pc*) is eccentrically placed. (*ps*) indicates the posterior nuclear space. ×72,000.

Fig. 5. – On transverse sections the proximal centriole is found in a midline position. ×116,000.

Fig. 6. – The gamma fibers (*gf*) continue through the region of the distal centriole with the connecting axis roughly perpendicular to the longitudinal axis of the proximal centriole (*pc*). ×65,000.

Fig. 7. – The annulus (*an*) is inconspicuous consisting of electron dense material apposed the cell membrane. ×80,000.

Fig. 8. – The gamma fibers appear crosstriated with a period of about 120 Å. ×145,000.

Fig. 9. – The intraflagellar cytoplasm shows a certain regularity indicated by white lines. ×33,000.

Fig. 10. – In this transverse section of the middle piece the axial filament complex is found in the traditional 9 + 2 pattern with alpha, beta and gamma fibers. Coarse fiber number 1, 5 and 6 tend to be a little larger than the others. ×206,000.

Fig. 11. – In the proximal end of the principal piece longitudinal columns (*lc*) have incorporated coarse fiber number 3 and 8. Farther distally the longitudinal columns are being replaced by overlappings of the ribs and these are connected with the alpha fiber by thin laminae (*lm*). The proximal part of the end piece shows the same 9 + 2 pattern, but distally the doublets are uncoupled and the hollow fibers terminate successively. ×76,000, 83,000, 83,000 and 115,000.

Discussion

AFZELIUS. – This question I have been asking for 15 years. Is it today possible to use the electron microscope as a diagnostic tool for cases of human sterility?

PEDERSEN. – I hope it should be, but until now the problems have been to understand fully the normal morphology. In the near future this technique may give valuable information in the evaluation of male fertility.

AFZELIUS. – May I then add: This is the answer I have received for 15 years.

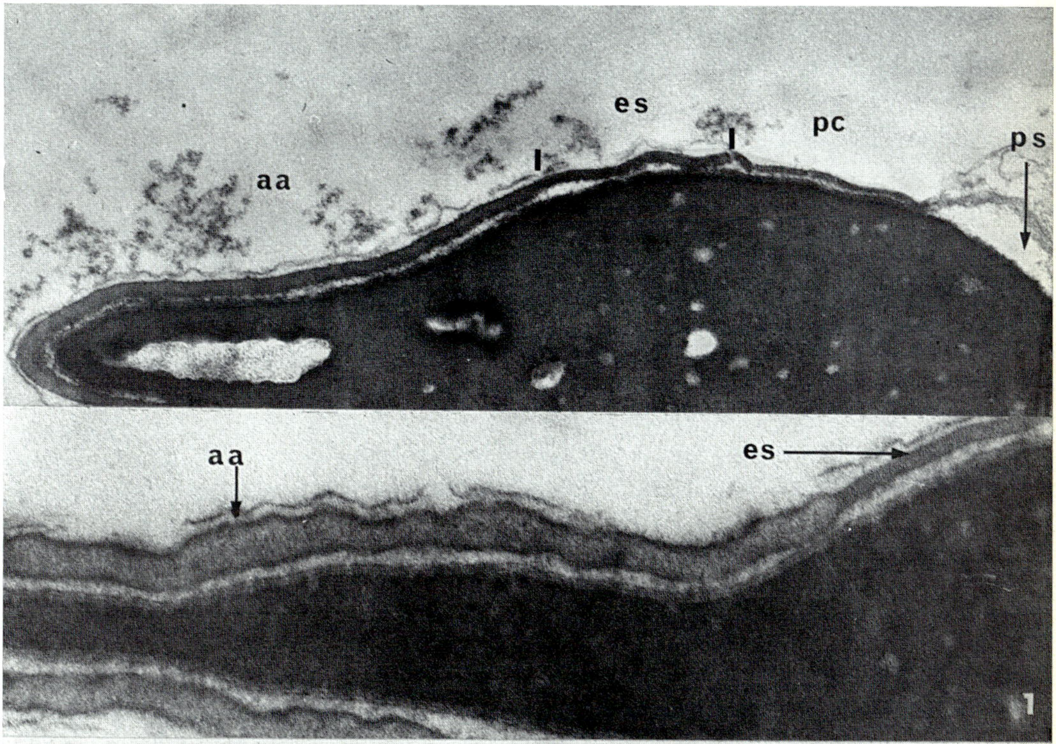
es
pc
ps
aa
aa
es
1

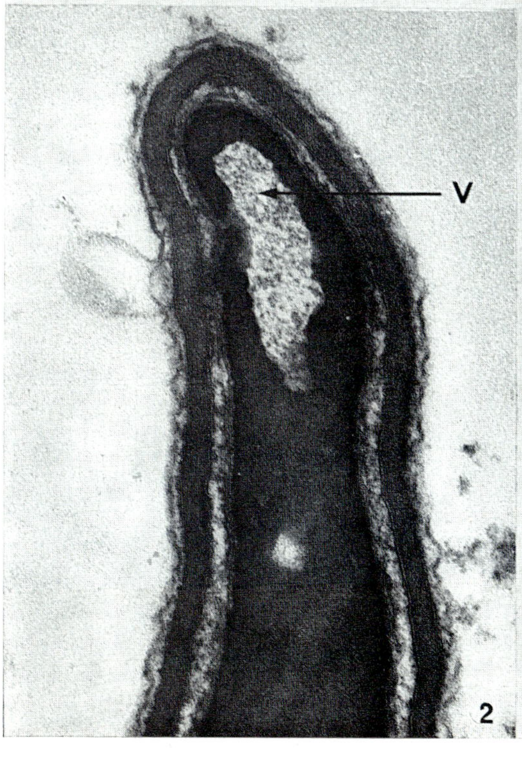
V
2

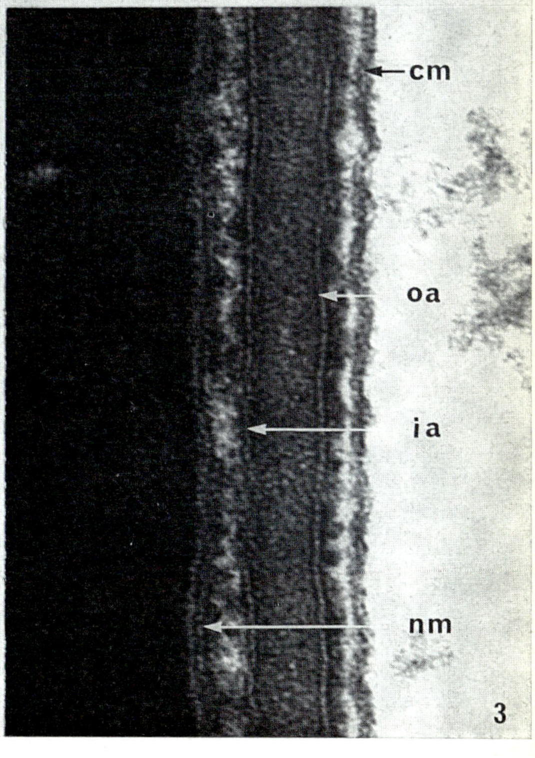
cm
oa
ia
nm
3

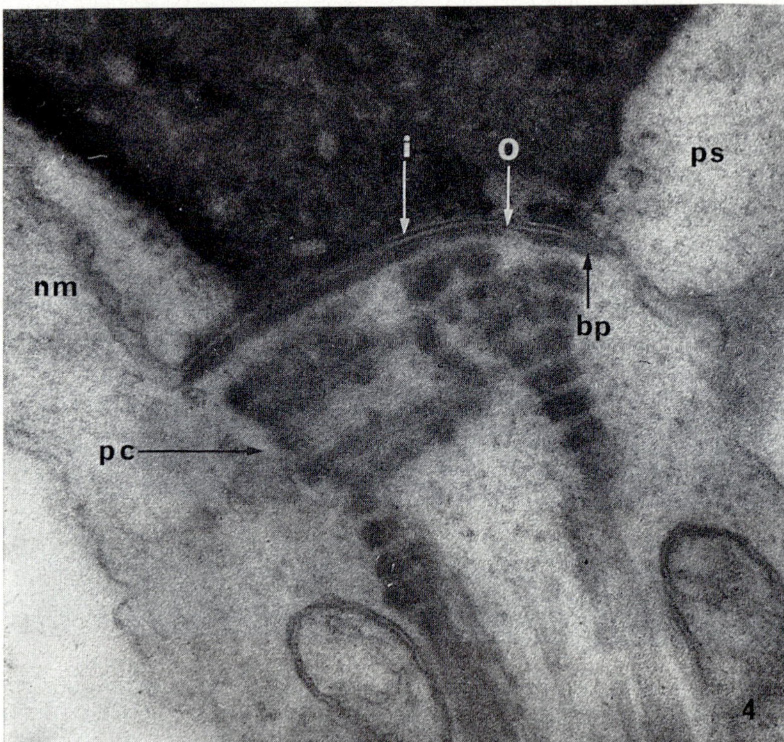
i
o
ps
nm
bp
pc
4

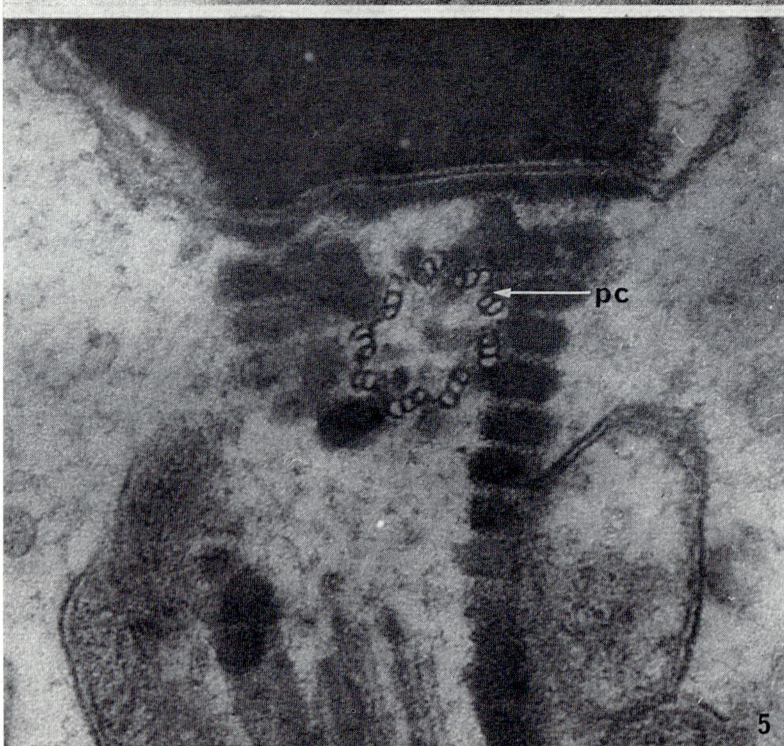
pc
5

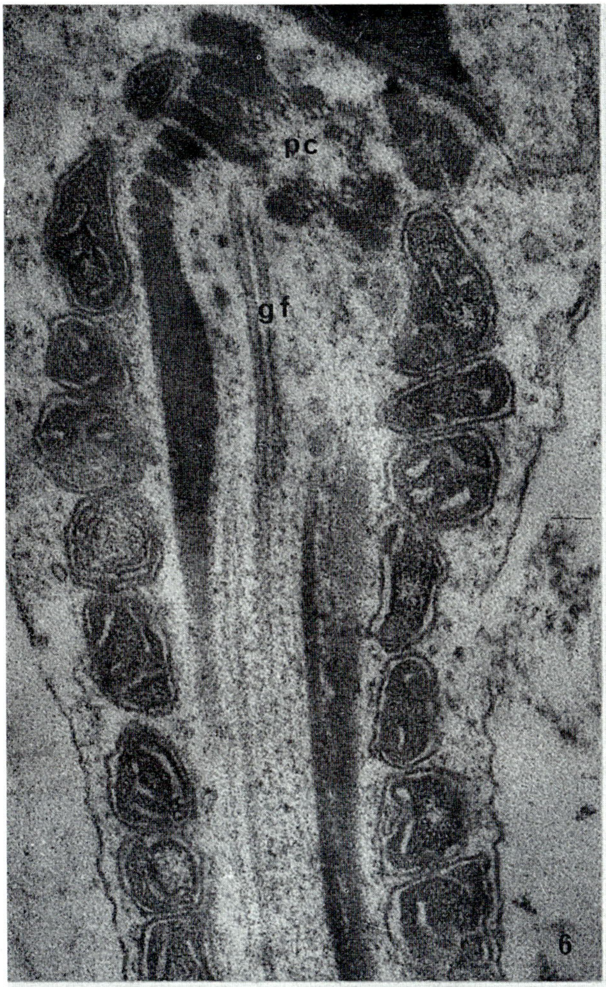
pc
gf
6

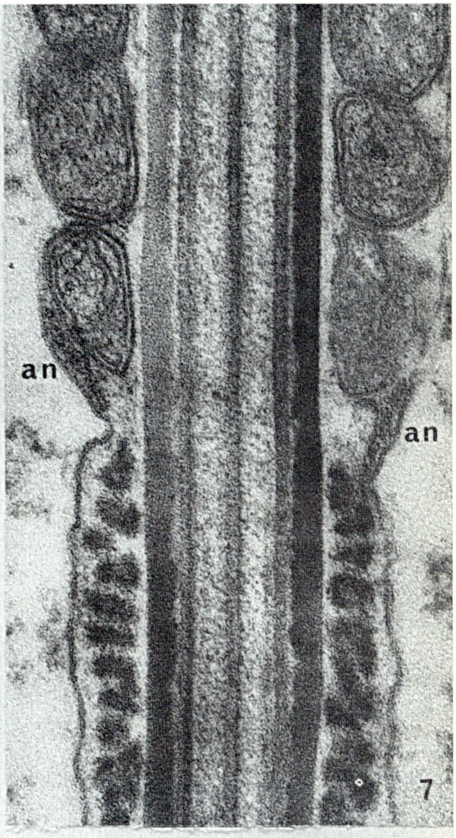
an
an
7

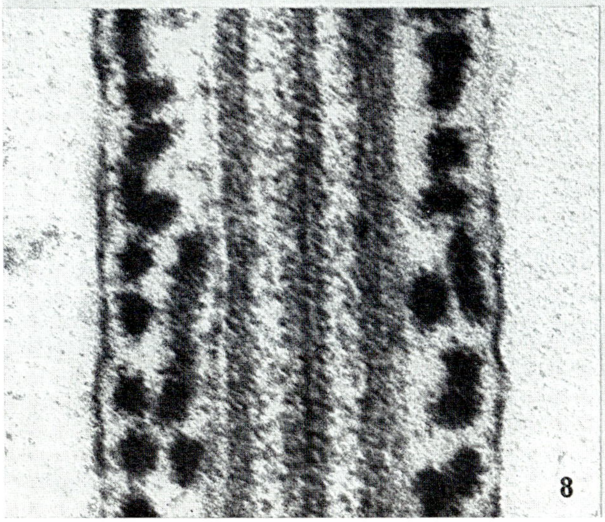
8

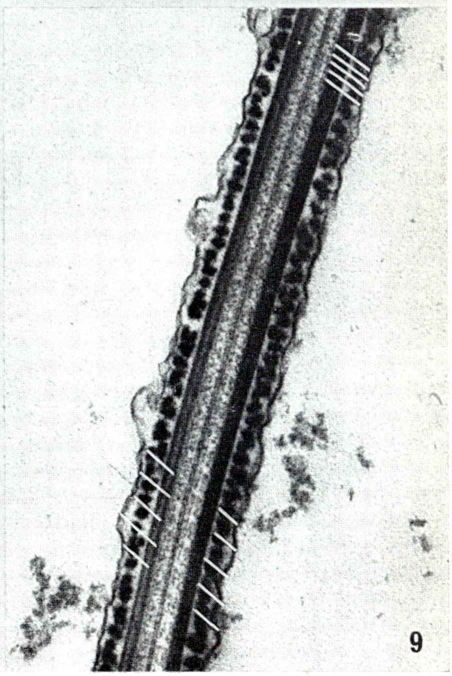
9

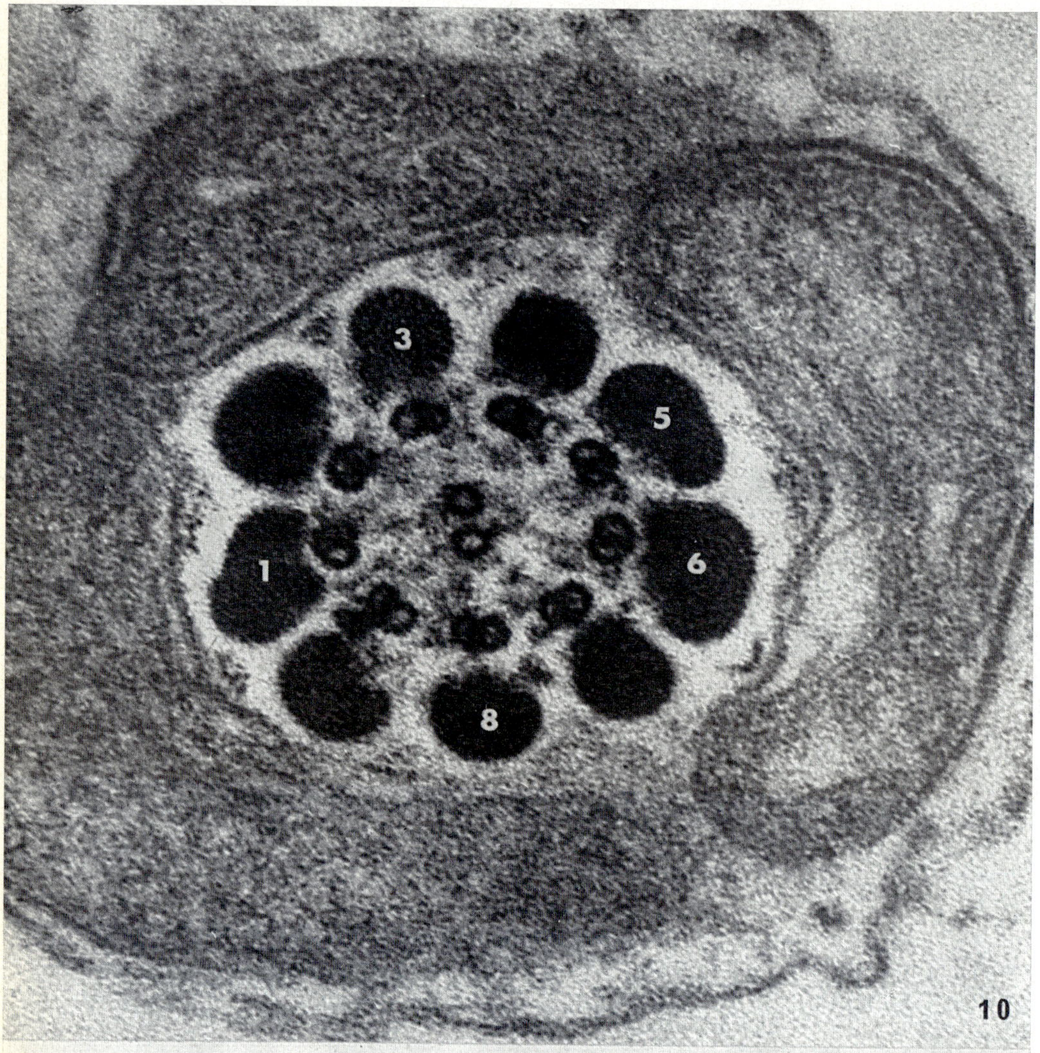

10

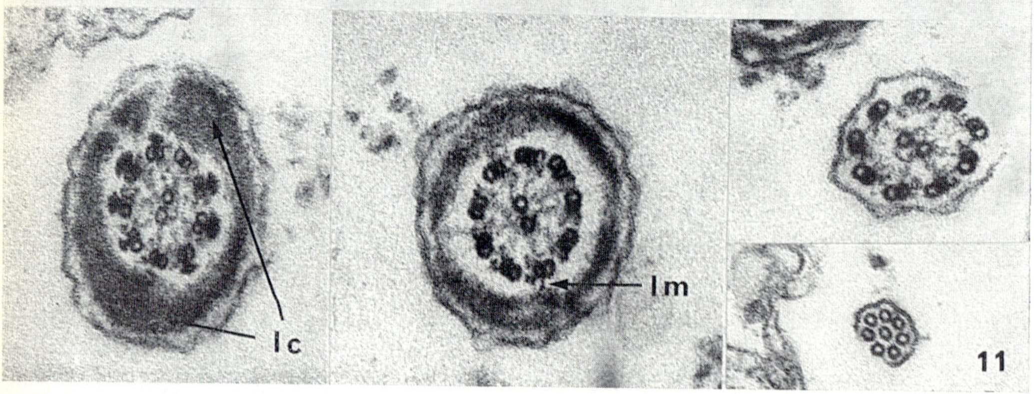

11

I. MANTON (*)

PLANT SPERMATOZOIDS

SUMMARY. — The paper reviews salient aspects of spermatozoid structure in plants, as revealed by electron microscopy, drawing mainly on the work of the author.

RIASSUNTO. — Il lavoro mette in evidenza gli aspetti salienti della struttura degli spermatozoi delle piante come rivelato con il microscopio elettronico, attingendo soprattutto al lavoro dell'autore.

Highly differentiated motile male gametes capable of fertilising much larger, non-motile, eggs are common but not universally present in plant life histories. The higher seed plants which at present constitute the dominant vegetation of the land have long ago eliminated dependence on water for swimming by simplifying their male gametes to such a degree that at present they consist merely of individual nuclei in a common cytoplasm, that of the pollen tube. In this case the major part of the problem of bringing the gametes of the two sexes into contact has been solved by harnessing external agents such as the wind, or animals (e.g. insects) able to cover much greater distances than can be attained by a swimming unicell. Growth of the pollen tube then completes the transfer of the male nucleus into the cytoplasm of the egg, after which syngamy, i.e. nuclear fusion, can proceed without impediment. Such gametes are nevertheless not spermatozoids in the strict sense and I shall therefore consider them no further here.

At earlier geological periods there must have been substantial differences since swimming spermatozoids are still in fact retained by two among the many groups of extant Conifer-relatives, namely in Cycads and Ginkgo the Japanese Maidenhair Tree. In these, swimming is still needed to bring the male gamete out of the pollen tube and onto the neck of the archegonium, a distance of less than a millimetre. Such male gametes are large and cumbersome but essentially comparable in structure with those encountered among the ferns and fern allies. There is no doubt therefore that the main groups of green land plants are phyletically all of a piece and that they have inherited oogamous reproduction, of the special type found in all the so-called archegoniates, from some earlier ancestor which must have been aquatic and which, if alive now, would have to be classed somewhere among

(*) Botany Department, The University, Leeds, England.

the green algae. Information on the origin of motile spermatozoids must therefore be sought among algae and not among land plants.

When such a search is made we find a much greater range of independently evolved reproductive structurestha n can be encountered among higher plants. There is no sexuality or perhaps one should say no obvious presence of differentiated gametes at the bottom of the evolutionary scale although the fairly recent detection of sexual potentialities in bacteria should warn us against a prematuraly negative attitude. Sex has not so far been positively demonstrated in Blue-green Algae or in many flagellates. On the other hand Red Algae, almost all of which are marine, have oogamous reproduction without motility of either gamete, the male gametes known as spermatia being small naked cells carried passively by water flow but able to adhere firmly and rapidly to part of the female gamete (the trichogyne) if they happen to hit it. This lack of flagella is thought e.g. by CHRISTENSEN (1962, 1966) to denote extreme antiquity for this group of plants, the flagellum with the now familiar 9+2 internal fibre pattern having evolved later. The name *Aconta* (meaning without flagella) has been proposed for the Red Algae to distinguish them from all other Eucaryotic plants, collectively designated *Contophora* (meaning flagella-bearing) although in most seed plants flagella have been secondarily lost. I shall exclude *Aconta* from this survey since spermatia also are not strictly spermatozoids.

Within the *Contophora* on the other hand, the algae and certain fungi give unique insight into early stages in the evolution of sex which cannot be matched among the lower animal groups; hence perhaps the importance of including botany in a symposium such as this. There can be little doubt that motility by means of flagella has preceded sexuality in many groups of pigmented organisms, and asexual zoospores are still produced by green, brown and yellow-green algae as well as in some of the lower fungi. In many life histories both zoospores and gametes occur in one and the same organism, in which case there may be a strong structural resemblance between the two types of cell in spite of their different functions. One of the more primitive manifestations of sex in both green and brown algae is isogamy i.e. the fusion of morphologically identical motile gametes in pairs (Fig. 1). In this case there is neither male nor female as such and potential gametes can sometimes germinate as if they were zoospores should syngamy fail to take place.

At a slightly higher level, differentiation of size (heterogamy) permits a clear distinction to be made between a larger female gamete and a smaller, otherwise similar, male gamete. Further specialisation in the same direction leads to loss of motility in the hypertrophied female, which becomes thereby an egg. This change has happened many times and I shall be able to show several entirely unrelated examples. Once oogamy has been established germination without syngamy is rarely possible for an egg and never for a spermatozoid which has given up too much of its normal cell structure. The degree of specialisation nevertheless varies enormously and in a very informative manner from species to species, the more primitive spermatozoids having a close resemblance to zoospores of the same or a related form while the more specialised spermatozoids may be so peculiar that their origin may be difficult or impossible to discover. This, as I shall show, presents some unsolved and perhaps insoluble problems concerning the origin of the land plants for which there are no extant zoospores suitable for acceptance as prototypes for the very peculiar and highly specialised spermatozoids characteristic of archegoniates (mosses, ferns etc.) and of one group of algae (*Characeae*).

Nevertheless plants are not animals and they show this clearly in the morphology of their motile cells. The familiar tadpole-like animal spermatozoid propelled by a single posterior flagellum is so rare in plants as to be virtually non-existent except in a few fungi. The water mould *Monoblepharis* has spermatozoids of this type but as far as I know these have not yet been examined fine structurally. I can however illustrate a comparable morphology in the zoospores of *Olpidium* (Fig. 3), a pathogen of cabbages and *Allomyces*, a tropical soil fungus (Fig. 4), though only with respect to their shope, since these micrographs, quoted from MANTON, CLARKE, GREENWOOD and FLINT, 1952, were taken before the advent of effective thin sectioning techniques. However the zoospores of *Allomyces* at least have subsequently been investigated by others (e.g. RENAUD and SWIFT, 1964) who record traces of a second flagellar base within the cell. A well developed second flagellar base (without a flagellum) was reported earlier for uniflagellate zoids of certain *Chytrids* (KOCH, 1956; see also KOLE, 1965), and *Olpidium* may be expected to be similar. These superficially animal-like zoids are therefore not likely to be primitive in any of these cases. Other examples of analogous reduction will be discussed below among certain uniflagellate algal spermatozoids (notably *Dictyota*).

Apart from these somewhat exceptional fungi the great majority of zoospores fall into one or other of two categories, namely, the isokont and the heterokont. In the former the flagella are equal in all respects and are symmetrically arranged at or near the anterior end of the cell (as in Fig. 1), regardless of whether their number is 2, 4 or many. In heterokont zoospores on the other hand (Fig. 2) the two flagella constituting a pair differ substantially from each other in length and in other ways. They are moreover attached to the cell laterally conferring a considerable degree of bilateral symmetry to the protoplast by this position. One flagellum is directed forwards and this one carries the two longitudinal rows of hairy appendages known as « Flimmer », while the other flagellum lacks Flimmer and is commonly directed either backwards or sideways. The length of the hind flagellum in heterokont zoids ranges from very short to longer than the front flagellum but it usually carries a photoreceptor near its base which is structurally orientated in relation to the eyespot. Heterokont zoids occur in Brown Algae, Yellow-green Algae, many flagellates (notably *Chrysophyceae*) and certain water moulds (Saprolegniaceae). Isokont zoids are characteristic of many Green Algae and a few peculiar brown flagellates (*Haptophyceae* sensu CHRISTENSEN, 1962, 1966). Both, as will be shown, provide prototypes for primitive spermatozoids and there is no means as yet of determining which type is the older.

With this introduction, a list of the more important categories of true spermatozoids about which some fine structure is known is appended below. I can show you at first hand examples of almost all although the degree of completeness of knowledge varies according to the date at which the work was carried out. As you will know, technical methods in electron microscopy have changed several times since 1950, the date at which I first examined the external morphology of the *Fucus* spermatozoid (MANTON and CLARKE, 1950; 1951). At that date the only known method was that of shadowcast whole mounts examined with a microscope which, in my case, was the Philips EM100 claiming a resolving power of no more than 70 Å. In spite of this limitation the high contrast of such preparations makes these early micrographs still acceptable in a way in which early sections are not. This applies event to the classic paper of FAWCETT and PORTER, 1954 in which the first effective sectioning technique, using methacrylate embedding and the old type of Porter Blum microtome, seemed, and indeed was, revolutionary at the time.

Plant spermatozoids for which some fine structure is known.

Uniflagellate:	*Diatoms*
	Dictyota
Isokont:	*Prasiola*
	Oedogonium
Heterokont:	*Fucoids*
	Vaucheria
Peculiar:	*Characeae*
	Bryophyta
	Pteridophyta
	Gymnosperms

Since 1962 the improvements initiated by the introduction, among other changes, of improved fixation (the use of aldehydes by SABATINI *et al.* 1963), better plastics, better microtomes, better stains and, last but not least, better electron microscopes has revolutionised the type of problem which can be effectively tackled. The special advantages of small naked cells, which most spermatozoids are, is no longer felt and the number of papers devoted to them using modern methods is correspondingly reduced. I must therefore ask for your forbearance if I sometimes have to draw on early sections carried out without these advantages, since in many cases examined before 1962 these may still be the only ones.

It will perhaps be sensible to begin with an unusual type of uniflagellate spermatozoid, namely that of the centric diatom *Lithodesmium*. Without the painstaking skill of Professor H. A. VON STOSCH of Marburg the prevalence of oogamy among centric diatoms might still not be known. His work was however summarised at the 1954 Botanical Congress in Paris, an occasion on which I also summarised the morphology and microanatomy of plant flagella including those of many spermatozoids. It has since been my privilege to visit Professor von Stosch's laboratory and with his assistance to take fixings and make preparations from specially prepared cultures. His diagram of the life history, amplified by photographs of the living cultures and micrographs of shadowcast and sectioned material, were published in 1966 (MANTON and VON STOSCH) while a more extended study of spermatogenesis from another point of view (that of the spindle) is in preparation or in the press as a series of four papers now.

Centric diatoms are exceptional among plants in the position of meiosis in the life cycle which is here part of gametogenesis as in many animals instead of remote from it as in almost all other plants. Whether this significantly influences spermatozoid structure may be doubted although perhaps it does so in one particular, namely the number of flagella which in this case is undoubtedly single. In other respects the cell structure of the male gamete seems primitive (Fig. 8) since it contains several small brown plastids and a nucleus attached to the flagellar base but not otherwise modified; if its origin were unknown this gamete could be mistaken for a zoospore or an independent naked monad.

It is important to notice that the single, forwardly directed flagellum of *Lithodesmium* is an apparently normal " Flimmergeissel " of the type already described with respect to the front flagellum of a heterokont zoid (Fig. 2). In the case of this diatom there is nevertheless no direct sign of a heterokont ancestry. If spermatogenesis is traced through the two meiotic divisions, each of which is accompanied by complete cytokinesis, the flagellar bases appear first at interkinesis as a single pair of bases attached together near the former spindle pole in each cell. As the new spindle develops during prophase of the second meiotic division the flagellar bases are forced apart until they come to occupy opposite ends of the cell, one being eventually incorporated in to each male gamete. This type of development is so unusual that phyletic interpretation will remain uncertain unless or until further evidence is obtained from other organisms which might prove to be related. It must be remembered that diatoms are geologically recent (BLACK *et al.* 1967). If their spermatozoids are primitive other examples of uniflagellate gametes of comparable type may yet be found. On the other hand if they are in fact reduced some signs of a precursor from which such reduction might have started may also turn up.

The spermatozoid of the brown alga *Dictyota*, also uniflagellate with an anteriorly directed " Flimmergeissel " betrays its ancestry more clearly. In this case a second flagellar base without a flagellum is present internally though, without the aid of sections, its existence could not be known (MANTON, CLARKE and GREENWOOD, 1952; MANTON, 1959). We have here an undoubtedly reduced type in which the hind flagellum of a former heterokont pair has been suppressed. Since zoospores of brown algae are normally heterokont with both flagella present, though the hind one is often short, the *Dictyota* spermatozoid cannot possibly be primitive and this conclusion is confirmed by the total elimination of the plastid and eyespot with which the hind flagellum is normally associated. This male gamete is insensitive to light. The functional flagellum is moreover embellished with a most unusual series of appendages namely a row of spines of unknown nature attached along one component of the 9+2. This position, it may be said in passing, was important in the early days as a means of determining the orientation of the central fibres with respect to the outer 9, an observation requiring a series of sections passing through a spine (MANTON, 1959). Though carried out with methacrylate embedding this has not yet been repeated with more modern methods though I hope shortly to do so.

In contrast, an example of a biflagellate spermatozoid in a relatively primitive condition, closely resembling an isokont zoospore, is presented by a small green seaweed *Prasiola stipitata* (MANTON and FRIEDMANN, 1960). In this organism both gametes contain a single chloroplast with a pyrenoid and starch, though the plastid of the spermatozoid is smaller than that of the egg. The arrangement of cell contents is so similar in the two gametes, in spite of the size difference that oogamy was not at first recognised, flagella being attributed to both (DREW and FRIEDMANN, 1957). Only when sections could be obtained indicating the position of the basal bodies was the suspicion aroused that the female was perhaps an egg and close study by means of a ciné film shown by Dr. FRIEDMANN at the 1959 Botanical Congress in Montreal confirmed this suggestion. The early stages of syngamy occur so rapidly that virgin eggs are virtually never encountered except at the moment of emergence from the thallus. Cytoplasmic union is mediated by means of an initial fusion between the plasmalemma of the egg and the membrane of one of the flagella of the male, the other flagellum continuing to propel the oblate zygote for some time before it rounds up. This very unusual morphology of young zygotes in the early stages explains the initial failure to detect oogamy. Nuclear fusion in this case is nevertheless slow, the nuclei and plastids introduced by each gamete remaining separated, even after the zygote has rounded up and secreted a wall rendering further study impossible with the older methods of fixation. This life history would therefore repay continued investigation with more modern methods.

The well known oogamous green alga *Oedogonium* is also descended from an isokont ancestor in which the number of flagella must have been greatly increased at an early date since this character is shared by both zoospores and spermatozoids. Each has a circle of flagella near the front end, the number of individual flagella being of the order of 120 in the large zoospores (HOFFMAN and MANTON, 1962) and c. 30 in the much smaller spermatozoids (HOFFMAN and MANTON, 1963). In other respects the two types of zoid are not dissimilar though the male is much smaller. I am indebted to Dr. HOFFMAN for lending a recent micrograph showing a spermatozoid within the oogonial wall just before entering the egg. As spermatozoids go this is not a specialised type although other aspects of cell structure and mode of growth in *Oedogonium* itself are so unusual among algae that this genus must have had a very long history.

Among Brown Algae heterokont zoospore-like spermatozoids occur among certain Fucoids notably *Himanthalia* and the *Cystoseiraceae* (MANTON, 1964 c). In these the only difference from a zoospore is the reduced size of the plastid which commonly retains a fully developed eyespot but little else. Occasional peculiarities such as the presence of a single spine in *Himanthalia* and *Xiphophora* (MANTON, 1956) stand out as unexplained oddities with no, as yet, ascertainable function. Apart from these features such gametes are replicas of zoospores and therefore relatively primitive.

The more advanced Fucoids on the other hand, notably *Fucus* (MANTON and CLARKE, 1951; 1956) *Ascophyllum* and *Pelvetia* (MANTON, CLARKE and GREENWOOD 1952) have highly specialised spermatozoids differing from any known zoospore in a great many details. The cell, including the nucleus within, is streamlined and flattened. The hind flagellum is enormously elongated, substantially exceeding the front one in length (Figs. 5 and 6). The anterior end of the cell is prolonged into a peculiar flattened structure with an internal framework of fibres or microtubules known as the " proboscis " derived from a modified flagellar " root " (MANTON, 1964 c). Finally the cell contents are so greatly reduced that the four large mitochondria which, apart from the eyespot, are virtually the only other cytoplasmic organelles, are pressed into a concavity in the surface of the nucleus, MANTON and CLARKE, 1956).

Somewhat unexpectedly the only parallel to the spermatozoid structure of the higher Fucoids (*Fucus*, *Ascophyllum* and *Pelvetia*) so far encountered is in the curious green coloured coenocytic alga *Vaucheria*. The spermatozoids of this were first described by PRINGSHEIM (1855) but studied fine structurally only quite recently. The presence of Flimmer on the anterior flagellum of the elongated bottle-shaped cells was demonstrated by KOCH (1951) using the Loeffler staining technique for light microscopy. The very beautiful observation by Ø. MOESTRUP recently carried out in my department amplify this in a most exciting manner. The *Vaucheria* spermatozoid is elongated (Fig. 9) and heterokont as first described, the front flagellum being a normal Flimmergeissel though shorter than the hind one, as in *Fucus*. The nucleus is elongated and indented to accommodate three or four enlarged mitochondria. There is no eyespot since all the plastids originally present in the antheridium are left behind in the enucleate residual cytoplasm after abstriction of the nucleated spermatozoids from the cytoplasmic surface, a mode of origin which is almost unique and perhaps a result of the coenocytic structure. Nevertheless most surprisingly, there is a proboscis (Fig. 9) containing a skeletal substructure derived from a modified flagellar " root " of a type very closely recalling that of *Fucus*.

Whether the so-called proboscis in *Fucus* and *Vaucheria* possesses acrosomal functions is unknown in either case. That the internal framework of microtubules derived from a modified flagellar " root " is homologous in the two can scarcely be doubted even though its modification and hypertrophy may have been independently acquired. These findings introduce a phyletic problem of considerable interest which cannot be adequately discussed here. The need for further observations on the functional significance of the various parts of these specialised spermatozoids can nevertheless perhaps usefully be stressed.

Somewhat similar problems are raised by the comparison between the spermatozoids of *Characeae* and those of Archegoniates. In this case however it will perhaps be best to begin with archegoniates since the degree of elaboration of some of these, notably the ferns, seems to be greater than anywhere else in the plant kingdom. The example best known to me personally is the bracken fern *Pteridium* (MANTON, 1959) though *Osmunda* and various species of *Dryopteris* were also looked at in the early days. In all these (and increasingly among Horsetails and the two groups of Gymnosperms already mentioned where the spermatozoids though similar to those of ferns are even larger) the elaborate shape can scarcely be understood from perusal of dried preparations without a great deal of preliminary guidance from careful light microscopy. Illustrations of undried cells taken with both light microscopy and ultraviolet microscopy will be found in MANTON, 1959. Each spermatozoid before liberation from the antheridium, has its nucleus coiled into a flat spiral which in *Pteridium* (the Bracken) consists of 2 1/2 turns, the anterior end being central. Once swimming starts, the shape becomes conical with the narrower front end occupying the apex of the cone (Fig. 14). The centre of the cone is filled with residual cytoplasm which includes a number of small plastids still containing starch. The nucleus itself, which is tapered as well as coiled is widest in the posterior gyre. Its position near the surface of the residual cytoplasm is maintained for much of its length by means of a cradle of microtubules slung to the lower edge of a more complex fibrous layer underlying the flagella (Fig. 15 arrows). The latter are numerous, *Pteridium* itself having about 40, but this number is greatly exceeded in the larger spermatozoids of *Equisetum* (MANTON, unpub) and Cycads (MIZUKAMI and GALL, 1965). On the inner face of the fibrous layer there are numerous scattered mitochondria (Fig. 15) which, along the forward edge, become united into a band all showing the distended cisternae characteristic of activated respiration. Swimming is rapid and accompanied by rotation, but it does not usually last for very long. In many hybridisation experiments carried out with ferns by members of my department it is usual to assume that swimming will have ceased within 30 min. of immersion of the antheridia in water (without which they do not open). Such spermatozoids are insensitive to light but respond directionally to certain chemicals notably the exudate from an opening archegonium containing an egg. In my own experience they are stimulated to swim more rapidly by a mild dose of alcohol added to their water although a concentration greater than 20 % is lethal. Under various chemical treatments, such as exposure to ammonia vapour or mild acids, the nucleus will readily become separated from the cytoplasm presumably by slight swelling; its elongated shape without any trace of spiral configuration can then be seen. The frontispiece to my book (MANTON, 1950) shows a good example of a spermatozoid in which this process has begun but the ciliated band is still attached, giving an elegant but quite unnatural appearance. Contact with the egg must undoubtedly exert the same effect since syngamy involves mainly the nucleus which in its elongated but not tightly coiled condition makes contact with the egg nucleus leaving the cytoplasmic organelles in the cytoplasm near the egg surface where they presumably degenerate.

Bryophytes and certain Pteridophytes, notably Lycopods possess apparently simpler spermatozoids in which the nucleus is commonly also elongated and coiled but locomotion is provided by only two long cilia. The spermatozoids of a very peculiar group of green algae are superficially similar and I propose to end by showing you examples of both kinds.

The first example of the spermatozoid of a moss to be investigated fine structurally was a species of bog moss, *Sphagnum*, about which we completed two papers in the early days, one without sections (MANTON and CLARKE, 1952) and a later one with sections (MANTON, 1957) though unfortunately only with methacrylate embedding after osmic fixation. The long snake-like nucleus is coiled in 1 1/2–2 turns and by fixing antheridia which had begun to open but had not yet emptied their contents I was able to obtain not only ready penetration of the fixative but also a large number of sections of mature spermatozoids still completely coiled. Unlike a fern there is no central cytoplasm but each gyre of the nucleus carries some cytoplasm, the shape of the whole being controlled by superficial microtubules (then termed fibres). A narrow band of more specialised fibrous construction accompanies the nucleus throughout its length and is associated at the anterior end with the attachment of the two flagella. The anterior end also contains what at that time appeared to be mitochondria in an imperfectly fixed condition.

An important detail which became clear to us on the first occasion (see Figs. 7 and 12) and was subsequently repeated with other objects was the fact that the two flagella are not attached at the same point, one being behind the other, and they are not in fact the same length. Since then a good deal of attention has been paid to the spermatozoid of one particular liverwort *Marchantia* (for obvious reasons since it is easy to obtain in large quantities at certain times of year). There is no doubt that in this also the flagella although arising closer together than in *Sphagnum* occur one behind the other. The fine structure of the fibrous band (since called "Vierergruppe" or spline by other workers) has been elucidated to a considerable extent both structurally and developmentally (see especially CAROTHERS and KREITNER, 1968).

In *Marchantia* itself the spermatozoid is fairly small relative to the enormous flagella (see MANTON, 1952). A different and perhaps more instructive situation occurs among liverworts of other, perhaps more primitive, kinds. *Pellia* for example and *Aneura* (Fig. 11) have relatively enormous spermatozoids with a snake-like nucleus coiled into as many as 3 1/2 gyres. Here again the two flagella are attached at different points near the front end of the protoplast and they may differ substantially in length, the one attached nearest to the tip being no more than 2/3rds the length of the more posteriorly attached flagellum.

When seen swimming (Fig. 11) the slow rotation and spiral form without central cytoplasm of the spermatozoid of *Aneura* or *Pellia* is at first sight as in *Sphagnum*. In sections within the antheridium however there is a substantial difference. In the thalloid liverworts (Figs. 10 and 13) the anterior surface of the coiled nucleus carries a vertical fibrous band which seems homologous with that underlying the flagellar suface of a fern spermatozoid. This structure produces such a peculiar appearance that my colleagues, accustomed to teaching *Pellia* to elementary classes of students, have one and all failed to identify such a section when first shown one. The presence of such a structure in this position nevertheless suggests strongly to me that the anacrogynous Jungermanniales are substantially closer to ferns than are the mosses and it is even possible that their gametes may be reduced from an ancestral type which had more than two flagella.

This brings us to the *Characeae*. The wonderful coiled snake-like spermatozoids are well-known objects (Fig. 16). They are almost as large as those of the liverworts discussed above and they have recently been investigated both in Australia (PICKET–HEAPS, 1968 on a species of *Chara*) and America (TURNER, 1968 on *Nitella missouriensis*). The work of TURNER is the more complete. He shows clearly, and it is not difficult to confirm this, that the two flagella of *Nitella* emerge to the surface a long way from the tip of the spermatozoid though they undoubtedly constitute a pair in the sense normal among algae. The flagellar bases are joined together in the usual way and the lengths of the two flagella differ by no more than about 10 %, a degree of resemblance which would be regarded as isokont if viewed with the light microscope. A derivation from a less specialised green algal type is therefore reasonable and some further guidance regarding what this ancestral type might or might not have been is provided by a very unexpected feature detected separately by both these authors, namely the presence of a covering of close-packed diamond-shaped scales all over the flagellar surfaces. We can confirm the exact resemblance of *Chara* in this respect (Fig. 17).

Now scaly flagella are well known in a large number of genera of green algae comprising the so-called *Prasinophyceae* (for literature see MANTON, 1965, 1968 etc.). The exact character of the scales in Characeae is not however as yet matched in any member of the Prasinophyceae in which very small flagellar scales often occur as an underlayer below large ones though they are not normally diamond-shaped but rounded (i.e. pentagonal or hexagonal) with a central hub. Unless and until diamond-shaped scales are encountered within this group it would be wrong to claim direct derivation of *Characeae* from *Prasinophyceae*. On the other hand recent evidence in America (MCBRIDE, personal communication) has shown that the flagella of the isokont asexual zoids of a sedentary green alga *Coleochaete* are also covered with diamond-shaped scales indistinguishable from those of *Nitella*. Such scales are however absent from many other green algae which might have been thought to be related to *Coleochaete* such as *Ulothrix*, *Draparnaldia* or *Stigeoclonium* (MANTON, 1965). Other examples can nevertheless scarcely fail to turn up and since the detailed character of scales, even more than their distribution, seem reliable and important as phyletic indicators we may confidently expect further light on this problem to accrue in the next few years.

It is thus probable that the resemblance between the spermatozoids of Characeae and Liverworts is not phyletic but convergent. If this is so we must ask what biological advantage can possibly be conferred by this curious development of a snake-like coiled nucleus, since natural selection can bring about convergence under no other conditions. During this symposium an impressive array of different animal groups possessing elongated spermatozoids have been introduced by other speakers to an extent excluding any possibility of phyletic relationships. If we are not to be trapped into absurdities, such as deriving the lung fish from mosses or vice versa, it is necessary to forget about phylogeny except within undoubtedly related groups. What is next required is an experimental follow-up of our present structural findings with special reference to the act of syngamy itself. The fine structural details of the nuclear fusion between gametes have been outside the terms of reference of almost all speakers. It may be, however, that it is here that the key to some of these remarkable convergent adaptations will be found.

REFERENCES

BARNARD J. E. and WELCH F. V. (1936) – *Practical Photomicrogaphy*. 3rd. ed. London.

BLACK M., DOWNIE C., ROSS R. and SARJEANT W. A. S. (1967) – *The Fossil Record. A symposium with documentation*. Chapter 2. Thallophyta Class Bacillariophyceae pp. 185 and 193–4. London (Geol. Soc.).

BOUCK G. B. (1969) – *Extracellular microtubules. The origin, structure and attachment of flagellar hairs in* Fucus *and* Ascophyllum *antherozoids*. « J. Cell Biol. » *40*, 446–460.

CAROTHERS Z. B. and KREITNER G. L. (1968) – *Studies of Spermatogenesis in the hepaticae*. II. *Blepharoplast structure in the spermatid of* Marchantia. « J. Cell Biol. », 36, 603–616.

CHRISTENSEN T. (1962) – *Alger. In Böcher, Lange and Sørensen: Botanik* Bd. 2, København (Edn. 2, 1966).

DREW K. M. and FRIEDMANN I. (1957) – *Occurrence of motile gametes in* Praisola stipitata *Suhr*. « Nature », 180, 557–8.

FAWCETT D. W. and PORTER K. R. (1954) – *A study of the fine structure of ciliated epithelia*. « J. Morph. », 94, 221–282.

HOFFMAN L. R. and MANTON I. (1962) – *Observations on the fine structure of the zoospore of* Oedogonium cardiacum *with special reference to the flagellar apparatus*. « J. Exp. Bot. », 13, 443–449.

HOFFMAN L. R. and MANTON I. (1963) – *Observations on the fine structure of* Oedogonium. II: *The spermatozoid of* O. cardiacum. « Amer. J. Bot. » 50, 455–463.

KOCH W. J. (1951) – *A study of the motile cells of* Vaucheria. « J. Elisha Mitchell Scient. Soc. », 67, 123–131.

KOCH W. J. (1956) – *Studies of the motile cells of chytrids.* I. *Electron microscope observations of the flagellum, blepharoplast and rhizoplast.* « Amer. J. Bot. », 43, 811–819.

KOLE A. P. (1965) – *Flagella. In Ainsworth G. C.* and *Sussman A. S. The Fungi* I. Chapter 4, p. 86, 91. Academic Press.

LEEDALE G., LEADBEATER B. and MASALSKI A. (1970) – *Intracellular origin of flagellar hairs in the Chrysophyceae and Xanthophyceae.* « J. Cell Sci. » (in the press).

MANTON I. (1949) – *Observations made with the ultraviolet microscope on the minor spiral of chromosomes in* Osmunda. « Biochim. Biophys. Acta », 3, 770–584.

MANTON I. (1950) – *Problems of cytology and evolution in the Pteridophyta.* Cambridge Press.

MANTON I. (1952) – *The fine structure of plant cilia.* « Symp. Soc. Exp. Biol. », 6, 306–319.

MANTON I. (1954) – *Microanatomy of cilia, flagella, etc.* 139. *Recent work on the internal structure of plant cilia.* « Proc. Int. Conf. Elec. Microscopy », London, 594–599.

MANTON I. (1956) – III. *Plant cilia and associated organelles. In Cellular Mechanisms in Differentiation and Growth.* ed. D. Rudnick, Princeton Univ. Press, New Jersey.

MANTON I. (1957) – *Observations with the electron microscope on the cell structure of the antheridium and spermatozoid of* Sphagnum. « J. exp. Bot. », 8, 382–400.

MANTON I. (1959 a) – *Observations on the internal structure of the spermatozoid of* Dictyota. « J. exp. Bot. », 10, 448–461.

MANTON I. (1959 b) – *Observations on the microanatomy of the spermatozoid of the Bracken Fern* (Pteridium aquilinum). « J. Biophys. Biochem. Cytol. », 6, 413–418.

MANTON I. (1964 a) – *Observations on the fine structure of the zoospore and young germling of* Stigeoclonium. « J. exp. Bot. », 15, 399–416.

MANTON I. (1964 b) – *The possible significance of some details of flagellar bases in plants.* « J. Roy. Microsc. Soc. », 82, 279–285.

MANTON I. (1964 c) – *A contribution towards understanding of « The Primitive Fucoid ».* « New Phytologist », 63, 244–254.

MANTON I. (1968) – *Observations on the microanatomy of the type species of* Pyramimonas (P. tetrarhynchus *Schmarda*). « J. Linn. Soc. », 179, 147–152.

MANTON I. and CLARKE B. (1950) – *Electron microscope observations on the spermatozoid of* Fucus. « Nature », 166, 973.

MANTON I and CLARKE B. (1951) – *An electron microscope study of the spermatozoid of* Fucus serratus. « Ann. Bot. N. S. », 15, 461–471.

MANTON I. and CLARKE B. (1952) – *An electron microscope study of the spermatozoid of* Sphagnum. « J. exp. Bot. », 3, 265–275.

MANTON I. and CLARKE B. (1956) – *Observations with the electron microscope on the internal structure of the spermatozoid of* Fucus. « J. exp. Bot. », 7, 416–432.

MANTON I., CLARKE B. and GREENWOOD A. D. (1952) – *Further observations with the electron microscope on spermatozoids in the Brown Algae.* « J. exp. Bot. », 4, 319–329.

MANTON I., CLARKE B., GREENWOOD A. D. and FLINT E. A. (1952) – *Further observations on the structure of plant cilia by a combination of visual and electron microscopy.* « J. exp. Bot. », 3, 204–215.

MANTON I. and FRIEDMANN I. (1960) – *Gametes, fertilisation and zygote development in* « Prasiola stipitata » Suhr. II. *Electron microscopy.* « Nova Hedwigia », 1, 22–42.

MANTON I. and VON STOSCH H. A. (1966) – *Observations on the fine structure of the male gamete of the marine centric diatom* Lithodesmium undulatum. « J. Roy. Microsc. Soc. », 85, 119–134.

MANTON I., RAYNS D. G., ETTL H. and PARKE M. (1965) – *Further observations on green flagellates with scaly flagella: the genus* Heteromastix *Korshikov.* « J. mar. biol. Ass. U.K. », *45*, 241–255.

MIZUKAMI I, and GALL J. (1966) – *Centriole replication II Sperm formation and the Cycad* Zamia *in the fern,* Marsilea. « J. Cell Biol. », *29*, 97–111.

MOESTRUP Ø. (1969) – *Observations on the fine structure and development of the spermatodozids of* Vaucheria sescuplicaria *Christensen.* « J. Cell Sci. » (in the press).

PICKETT–HEAPS J. D. (1968) – *Ultrastructure and differentiation in* Chara (fibrosa). « Australian J. Biol. Sci. », 21, 655–690.

PRINGSHEIM N. (1855) – *Über Befrüchtung und Keimung der Algen und das Wesen des Zeugungsactes.* Monatsber. d. Königl. Akad. Wiss. Berlin also in Gesammelte Abhandlungen *I.* 11–12. Jena 1895.

RENAUD F. L. and SWIFT H. (1964) – *The development of basal bodies and flagella in* Allomyces arbusculus. « J. Cell Biol. », 23, 339–361.

SABATINI D. D., BENSCH K. G. and BARRNETT R. J. (1963) – *Cytochemistry and electron microscopy. The preservation of cellular ultrastructure and enzymatic activity by aldehyde fixation.* « J. Cell Biol. », 17, 19–58.

VON STOCH H. A. (1954) – *Die Oogamie von* Biddulphia mobiliensis *und die bisher bekannten Auxosporenbildungen bei den Centrales.* « Rapp. Commn 8ieme Congr. int. Bot. », Sect. 17, 58.

TURNER F. R. (1968) – *An ultrastructural study of plant spermatogenesis. in* Nitella. « J. Cell. Biol. », 37, 370–393.

NOTE ON THE ILLUSTRATIONS

During the verbal communication some 80 micrographs were projected in 40 minutes. In selecting less than a quarter of these for reproduction allowance has been made for the fact that much of the early work, carried out between 1949 and 1955, was summarised in the proceedings of symposia or congresses in Manton 1952, 1954, 1956. These papers illustrate many types of spermatozoids that had been used in a survey of external morphology and internal structure of plant cilia and ciliated cells generally which dominated the early years of botanical electron microscopy . More recent work on flagellar morphology regardless of the type of cell will be found summarised in Manton 1965 to which a reader interested in discussion of topics such as the different types of flagellar hairs, or preliminary observations on flagellar scales, is referred.

The micrographs and photographs reproduced here in the four plates are selected to illustrate some of the range of diversity encountered among zoids, mainly spermatozoids with which I am acquainted personally without attempting to cover the whole field completely. Some micrographs (e.g. Fig. 6) are of historic importance as having been taken very early in the application of electron microscopy to plants. Other micrographs, notably Fig. 15 Pl. 4 are out of date technically but are reproduced in default of better to provide essential information required for the interpretation of other objects. A few, notably Fig. 9 and Figs. 16–17, draw on the as yet unpublished work of Øjvind Moestrup of Copenhagen who has spent the session 1968–69 in Leeds. Finally the bryophyte pictures on Plates 2 and 3 combine an early UV photograph of my own (Fig. 11) taken in 1949, a published micrograph (Fig. 12) of a different organism dating from 1952 and two sections of new material (Figs. 10 and 13) embedded shortly before the symposium and cut within a few days of it in 1969.

Regarding instrumentation, the light microscopy represented by Figs. 1 and 2, involves ordinary oil immerison observations on an unstained (Fig. 1) and a stained specimen (Fig. 2) respectively. Fig. 16 uses anoptral contrast by means of a Reichert Zetopan microscope fitted with a Polyphos condensor. Ultraviolet light microscopy is represented by Figs. 5, 7, 11 and 14. The instrument involved in this was made by Messrs. Cooke, Troughton and Simms of York modifying a design worked out at the National Institute for Medical Research in London (see Barnard and Welch 1936, Manton 1949). It carries quartz optical parts of pre-war Zeiss manufacture, computed for a wave length of 2750 Å supplied by a spark source with stationary cadmium electrodes, the cadmium spectrum being spread through two quartz prismus before entering the microscope. Fig. 11 was taken with a 6 mm quartz dry lens and a ×10 quartz occular. Figs. 5, 7 and 14 were taken with a 2 mm glycerine immersion quartz objective used with a $\times 5$ occular. This instrument was delivered to Leeds in 1949 and used intensively in preparation for electron microscopy which began in 1950 with delivery of the Philips EM100. Figs. 5 and 11 were taken in 1949 and the others somewhat later.

Among the electron micrographs three different instruments delivered to the department at different dates are represented. The Philips EM100, with a resolving power of no more than 70 Å, was used for all direct preparations, represented here by Figs. 3, 4, 6 and 12, up to 1958. In that year the Siemens Elmiskop I was installed, the sections illustrated in Figs. 8, 10, 13 and 15 being taken with it; that of Fig. 15 is unstained after methacrylate embedding while the other sections are stained after epon embedding. Finally Figs. 9, 16 and 17 were taken with the A.E.I. EM6B delivered to the Botany Department at Leeds in 1967, and currently in use side by side with the Siemens Elmiskop I.

Finally, thanks are due to the Oxford Press for permission to reproduce micrographs or photographs (Figs. 2–7 and Fig. 12) published in the Journal of Experimental Botany and Annals of Botany between 1951 and 1952, to the Rockefeller University Press for permission to reproduce Figs. 14 and 15 from a paper in the Journal of Biophysical and Biochemical Cytology (1959), to the Royal Microscopical Society for permission to use Fig. 8 (1966) and to Mr. Ø. Moestrup for providing the micrographs for Figs. 9, 16 and 17 from his, as yet, unpublished work.

Explanation of figures

Fig. 1. – *Chlamydomonas moewusii* at an early stage of isogamous sexual fusion; the two gametes morphologically identical, each with a pair of equal flagella (isokont). Oil immersion objective, blue filter, « pointolite » light source. $\times 2000$.

Fig. 2. – Asexual zoospore of *Saprolegnia ferax* (a water mould), stained by a modification of Kirkpatrick's method for bacterial flagella, showing the heterokont condition of the flagella, the anterior flagellum with two rows of lateral hairs and the posterior flagellum smooth. Reproduced from Manton, Clarke, Greenwood and Flint 1952. Light microscopy, oil immersion, exposure S 40.1. $\times 2000$.

Fig. 3. – Asexual zoospore of *Olpidium brassicae* showing a single posterior flagellum. Reproduced from Manton, Clarke, Greenwood and Flint 1952. Electron micrograph M 73.28. $\times 2000$.

Fig. 4. – Asexual zoospore of *Allomyces arbuscula* showing a larger example of a single posteriorly directed flagellum than that of Fig. 3 Reproduced from Manton, Clarke, Greenwood & Flint 1952. Electron micrograph M 59.10. $\times 2.000$.

Fig. 5. – Ultraviolet photograph of two spermatozoids of *Fucus serratus*, the upper one still coiled immediately after liberation from the antheridium, the lower one uncoiled and in a normal swimming attitude. Reproduced from Manton & Clarke 1951, 1957. UV series 207, exposure 3 a. $\times 3.000$.

Fig. 6. – A dried spermatozoid of *Fucus serratus*, the first published micrograph taken after delivery of the Philips EM 100 in 1950 (see Manton and Clarke 1950, 1951) showing body shrinkage as a result of drying (compared with Fig. 5) but no other obvious distortion; the " proboscis " and Flimmer visible even at this low magnification. Exposure M 7.3 $\times 3.000$.

Fig. 7. – Spermatozoid of a moss (*Sphagnum* sp.) partly uncoiled, showing a residual plastid in the centre and the two long flagella emerging at different points on the front end. Reproduced from Manton and Clarke 1952. Ultraviolet photograph, UV series 192, exposure 6 b, $\times 3.000$.

Fig. 8. – Median longitudinal section through the spermatozoid of a marine centric diatom (*Lithodesmium undulatum*) showing two plastids, a mottled spherical nucleus (*N*), mitochondria, vesicles, other inclusions and the single anteriorly directed flagellum, from Manton and von Stosch 1966. Micrograph D 240. ×10,000.

Fig. 9. – Longitudinal section through a spermatozoid of *Vaucheria sescuplicaria* showing the laterally attached flagella, the elongated nucleus (*N*) indented by some large mitochondria (*m*); the " proboscis " (*P*) visible at the anterior end. Micrograph M 922, ×15,000, from Moestrup 1969.

Fig. 10. – Parts of three spermatozoids of *Pellia epiphylla* from a section of an antheridium all with nuclei coiled into a spiral with 3 1/2 gyres; in the centre of the field two cells seen in median section in which the nucleus (N in one cell only) is transected 6 or 7 times, part of a similar cell seen in face view at the top of the field. Vesicles of fatty material which act as agents for spreading the coiled spermatozoids on a water surface after liberation here seen surrounding the coiled spermatozoids inside the antheridium. For more highly magnified details see Fig. 13. Micrograph D 9806. ×10,000.

Fig. 11. – Ultraviolet photograph of a recently killed spermatozoid of a thalloid liverwort, *Aneura pinguis*, showing the normal swimming attitude. UV photograph, 6 mm dry lens, ×10 eyepiece. Exposure, BC 4, ×2.000.

Fig. 12. – Front end of a coiled spermatozoid of a moss (*Sphagnum*) showing the two flagella (F1 and F2) attached at different points to the protoplast; the anterior end of the slender nucleus (*N*) terminating close to the point of attachment of the front flagellum at the tip of the cell, the hind flagellum showing fibrillar disintegration. Reproduced from Manton and Clarke 1952. Micrograph M 76.23. ×10,000.

Fig. 13. – *Pellia epiphylla* part of a coiled spermatozoid from the same antheiridum as that of Fig. 10 more highly magnified showing parts of three gyres each of which contains the nucleus (*N*) and a flange of cytoplasm containing microtubular substructure (arrows); part of a plastid with starch at right. For further description see text. Micrograph D 9803. ×60,000.

Fig. 14. – Ultraviolet photograph of a spermatozoid of a fern (*Pteridium aquilinum*, the Bracken) showing the coiled nucleus, central cytoplasm and many flagella. UV series 221, exposure 2 b, ×2,000.

Fig. 15. – Longitudinal section through part of a coiled spermatozoid of the Bracken (*Pteridium aquilinum*) passing through the two lower gyres of the coiled nucleus (*N*) but not quite median and therefore not including the anterior tip. Note the ridge of mitochondrial material forming the anterior edge above the nucleus with traces of the fibrous substructure (arrows) beneath the flagella visible laterally. Reproduced from Manton 1959 b. Micrograph H 4098 . ×10,000.

Fig. 16, – Spermatozoid of *Chara* (Characeae) showing the coiled body with the two cilia emerging together near the arrow. Courtesy Øjvind Moestrup. Anoptral contrast light microscopy. Micrograph L 25 a. ×1,000.

Fig. 17. – Tip of a flagellum of *Chara* showing the covering of small diamond-shaped scales from a shadowcast dried preparation. Courtesy Øjvind Moestrup. Micrograph M 819. ×30,000.

Discussion

KOEHLER. – Dr. MANTON, could you comment on the detailed relationship of the flagellar hairs (mastigonemes) to the rest of the flagellum, particularly with respect to the cell membrane?

MANTON. — As you may know, I regard " mastigoneme " as a most misleading word since hairs are of many kinds and what is true for one kind of flagellar hair is not necessarily at all true for another kind. For example, we know that the thick caducous hairs on green flagellates such as *Platymonas* or *Heteromastix* (MANTON, RAYNS, ETTL and PARKE, 1965) are formed in the Golgi cisternae as are the scales and both are deposited together when Golgi derivatives are liberated to the outside. On the other hand there is circumstantial, though not yet complete, evidence that the type of hair for which the word Flimmer was first used in the description of heterokont flagella (Phaeophyceae, Xanthophyceae, Chrysophyceae, and certain fungi) may be derived from ER in the sense that structures bearing a close morphological resemblance to this type of hair undoubtedly exist within parts of the ER system in a number of heterokont genera (see BOUCK, 1969 for *Fucus* and *Ascophyllum* and a forthcoming paper by LEEDALE, LEADBEATER and MASASLKI, 1970 for certain Chrysophyceae and Xanthophyceae) but the actual liberation process has not so far been seen in anything. Until this gap is filled the origin and mode of attachment of true Flimmer to the flagellar membrane will remain uncertain.

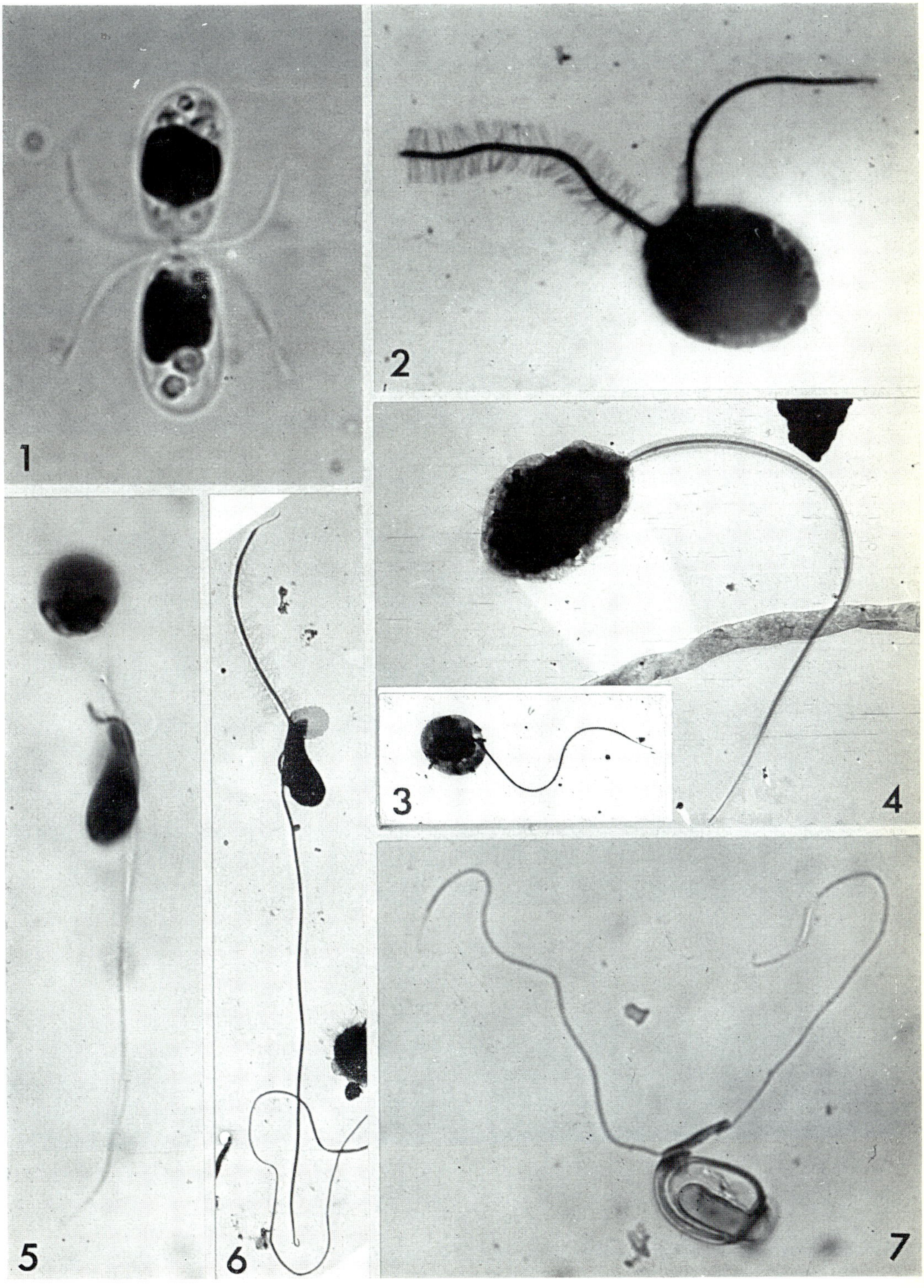
1
2
3
4
5
6
7

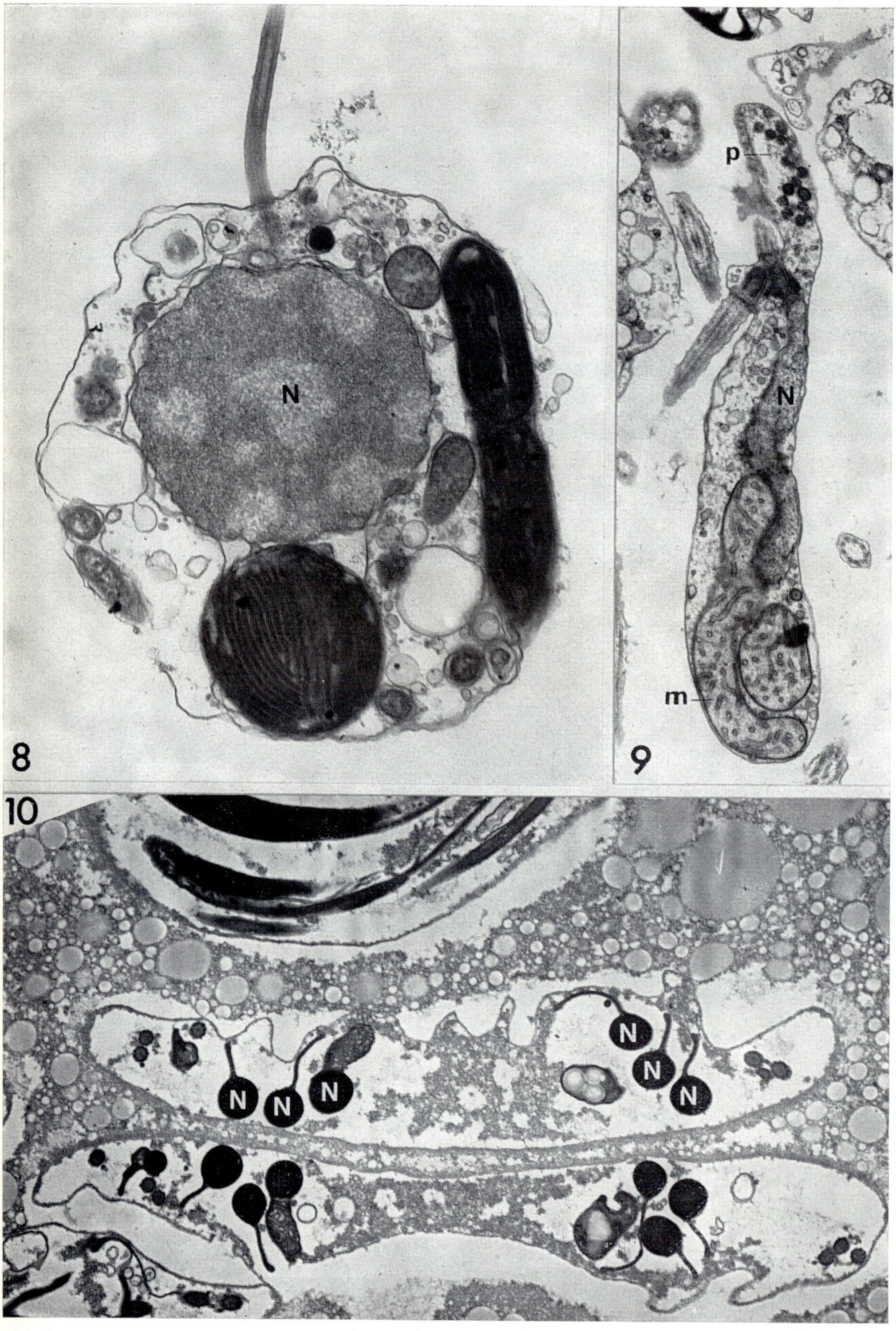
N
8
p
N
m
9
10
N
N
N
N
N
N

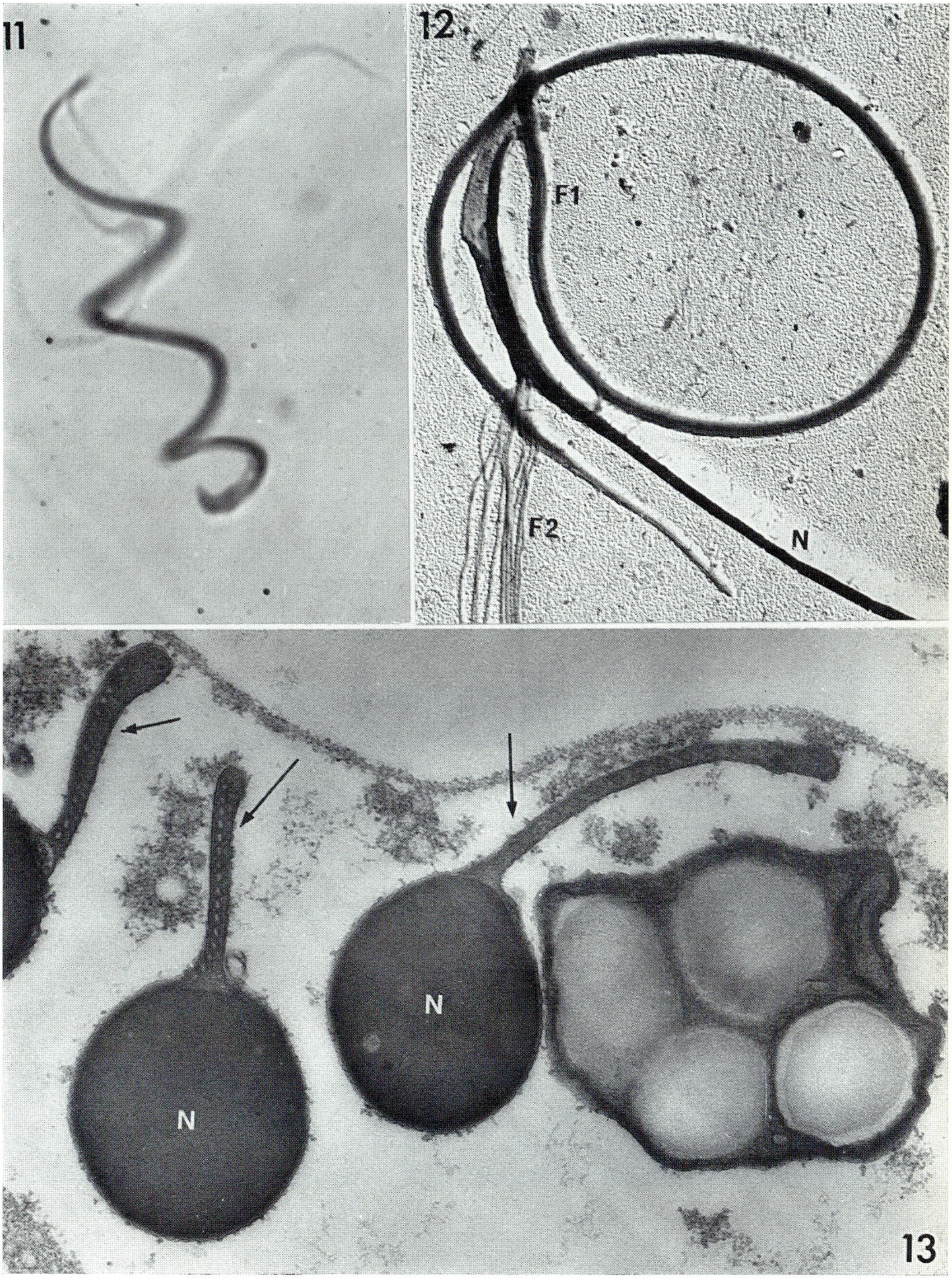
11
12
F1
F2
N
N
N
13

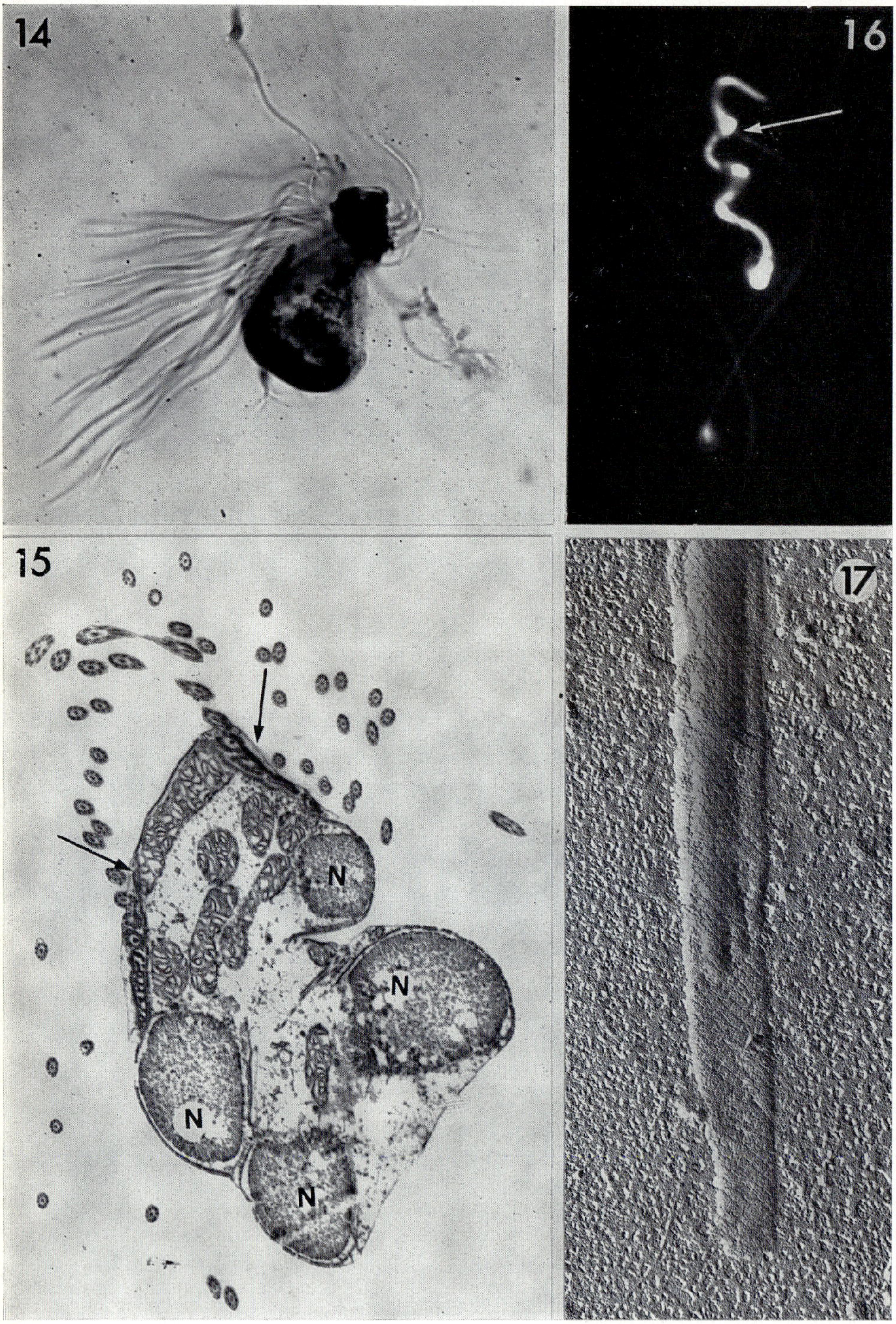
14
16
15
N
N
N
N
17

LOUIS GENEVES (*)

DIFFÉRENCIATION DE L'APPAREIL NUCLÉAIRE A L'ÉCHELLE INFRASTRUCTURALE, PENDANT LA SPERMATOGENÈSE, CHEZ UNE BRYOPHYTE (*POLYTRICHUM FORMOSUM*)

RÉSUMÉ. — Une étude évolutive de la différenciation de l'appareil nucléaire de *Polytrichum formosum* est réalisée à l'échelle infrastructurale dans la spermatide qui se transforme en spermatozoïde. Elle met en évidence la genèse de travées intranucléaires, qui évoluent en devenant moins nombreuses, plus épaisses et très osmiophiles. La formation de ces travées est liée intimement aux modifications du noyau, qui, d'abord sphérique et central, devient latéral; il s'allonge, il s'effile, puis acquiert une forme hélicoïdale.

Dans le gamète proche de la mâturité, le noyau est dense aux électrons, en sections ultrafines.

A aucun moment, au cours de l'élaboration de l'appareil nucléaire du gamète, on n'a pu caractériser de chromosomes semblables à ceux qui se forment au cours des mitoses du tissu spermatogène.

Au fur et à mesure que se forme l'appareil nucléaire où se localise l'ADN du spermatozoïde, la nucléole, les ribosomes, qui renferment de l'ARN régressent.

RIASSUNTO. — Viene realizzato a livello ultrastrutturale uno studio evolutivo sulla differenziazione dell'apparato nucleare di *Polytrichum formosum* nello spermatidio che si trasforma in spermatozoo. Tale studio mette in evidenza la genesi delle travate intranucleari che si evolvono diventando meno numerose, più spesse e molto osmiofile. La formazione di queste travate è legata alle modificazioni del nucleo, che, da sferico e centrale, diventa laterale, si allunga, poi acquista una forma elicoidale.

Nel gamete quasi maturo, in sezioni ultrasottili, il nucleo è denso agli elettroni.

In nessun momento, durante la formazione dell'apparato nucleare del gamete, si possono caratterizzare dei cromosomi paragonabili a quelli che si formano durante le mitosi del tessuto spermatogenico.

Man mano che si forma l'apparato nucleare, in cui si localizza l'ADN, il nucleo e i ribosomi che contengono l'ARN regrediscono.

INTRODUCTION

Le spermatozoïde constitue le vecteur des facteurs héréditaires, aussi plusieurs chercheurs ont ils tenté de connaître la structure de son appareil nucléaire.

Le noyau du spermatozoïde est le plus souvent très allongé. Puisqu'il renferme le matériel héréditaire correspondant au stock haploïde de chro-

(*) Faculté des Sciences, Paris, France.

mosomes, divers auteurs ont émis l'hypothèse que les chromosomes s'y disposaient d'une certaine manière. Selon REITBERGER (1964), le noyau du spermatozoïde d'une Hépatique, *Sphaerocarpos donnellii*, serait composé des huit chromosomes du génome, répartis linéairement. Au moment de l'individualisation des spermatides, ils se placeraient bout à bout en une file. Séparés temporairement les uns des autres, ils s'uniraient ensuite par leurs extrêmités. Ces observations ont été faites après coloration par la technique de FEULGEN.

Parmi les multiples travaux relatifs aux spermatozoïdes de la Drosophile, ceux de GOWEN et GAY (1933), sont de nature cytologique. Ils rapprochent la longueur de la tête du spermatozoïde (7,25 μ environ), de la longueur totale représentée par le lot des chromosomes métaphasiques, comprenant soit le chromosome X, soit le chromosome Y (7 μ environ). D'autre part, la largeur des chromosomes est analogue à celle de la structure chromatique du spermatozoïde. GOWEN et GAY, puis WOLF (1939) en déduisent que les chromosomes se disposeraient bout à bout, sur une ligne droite. C'est aussi l'opinion de COOPER (1952) qui aurait distingué les divers chromosomes dans des spermatozoïdes fixés à un état proche de la mâturité.

Cependant, RAPOPORT (1941), après coloration selon la technique de Feulgen, ne trouve aucune différence entre les catégories suivantes de spermatozoïdes: les uns normaux, d'autres privés de chromosomes X, d'autres encore avec un chromosome sexuel supplémentaire.

L'irradiation des spermatozoïdes par des neutrons rapides provoque des translocations chromosomiques, dont la fréquence varie linéairement avec la dose d'irradiation (MULLER et VALENCIA, 1951). Des chromosomes non homologues échangeraient des segments importants. Ce résultat impliquerait que, dans le spermatozoïde, ces chromosomes se trouvent superposés sur une longueur notable, au moment de l'irradiation (MULLER, 1954). Une étude statistique de la distribution des longueurs des masses chromatiques a été effectuée avec des spermatozoïdes normaux, des spermatozoïdes renfermant à la fois les chromosomes X et Y, et d'autres enfin dépourvus des chromosomes sexuels. Elle amène à infirmer l'hypothèse de chromosomes placés bout à bout en ligne droite; par contre, elle confirme l'idée que les chromosomes pourraient se recouvrir sur une partie de leur longueur, dans le gamète mâle (HERSKOWITZ et MULLER, 1954).

Par des méthodes complètement différentes, TAYLOR aboutit à des conceptions analogues sur un autre Insecte, la Sauterelle. Les études autoradiographiques qu'il utilise le conduisent à l'idée que les chromosomes du génome s'aligneraient d'abord bout à bout. Puis, ils glisseraient l'un sur l'autre à mesure que le spermatozoïde mûrit et s'allonge. Simultanément, le diamètre diminuerait, devenant inférieur à 0,5 μ.

L'étude ultrastructurale de divers spermatozoïdes végétaux a montré que les structures nucléaires restent difficiles à interpréter. C'est le cas pour les gamètes mâles de *Pteridium aquilinum* (MANTON, 1959). Le noyau est souvent constitué d'une substance osmiophile, apparemment homogène,

Ascophyllum, (CHEIGNON, 1964); *Nitella* (TURNER, 1968). *Sphaerocarpos* (DIERS, 1967).

Nous avons considéré l'appareil nucléaire des spermatozoïdes d'une Bryophyte, le *Polytrichum formosum*. Celui–ci est très différent du noyau de la cellule banale. L'analyse de sa différenciation progressive, au cours de la maturation du spermatozoïde, éclaire certains aspects de sa structure, dans le gamète mûr.

MATÉRIEL ET TECHNIQUES

L'évolution des spermatozoïdes a été suivie dans les anthéridies où ils se constituent. Les anthéridies ont été prélevées à l'extrêmité de rameaux de gamétophytes mâles de *Polytrichum formosum*, originaires de la forêt de Fontainebleau. Les récoltes ont eu lieu de Février à Mai. En début de saison, les corbeilles renferment beaucoup d'anthéridies jeunes, dont le tissu spermatogène prolifère, et quelques organes plus évolués. En fin de saison, les anthéridies jeunes se raréfient, bien qu'il en apparaisse encore quelques nouvelles. La plupart possèdent des spermatides en voie de différenciation, ou des spermatozoïdes constitués, plus ou moins proches de l'état de mâturité.

Les anthéridies ont été fixées par une solution de glutaraldéhyde tamponnée au cacodylate (1 h. à 0° C), puis postfixées par une solution de tétroxyde d'osmium tamponnée au véronal (1 h).

Chaque anthéridie était incluse à part, dans un bloc d'araldite. Sa longueur (1 mm. environ) rend difficile l'obtention des coupes ultrafines. Toutefois, si l'on sectionne les anthéridies avant la fixation ou avant l'inclusion, elles subissent des altérations, et le tissu spermatogène qu'elles renferment est mal conservé. Aussi a–t–il été nécessaire d'effectuer des coupes ultrafines intéressant des anthéridies entières.

Les coupes ont été contrastées par le permanganate de potassium, et observées avec les microscopes électroniques EMU 3 C et EMU 3 F du Laboratoire de Botanique de l'Ecole Normale Supérieure.

CARACTÈRES HISTOLOGIQUES DE L'ANTHÉRIDIE

L'anthéridie dérive d'une cellule superficielle du gamétophyte. Le tissu spermatogène, précocement différencié, prolifère pendant que l'assise superficielle s'accroît, les deux phénomènes étant harmonisés. A un certain stade, chacune des cellules spermatogènes engendre un massif, où les divisions se poursuivent d'une façon synchronique. Des parois plus épaisses séparent les massifs les uns des autres. A la fin de la phase de prolifération, chaque cellule constitue une spermatide, de forme polyédrique. La spermatide se transforme en spermatozoïde au cours de la phase de différenciation, qui sera analysée, après une brève étude de la structure des cellules spermatogènes en cours de prolifération.

LE NOYAU ET LES CHROMOSOMES DES CELLULES SPERMATOGÈNES

Les cellules spermatogènes, isodiamétriques, ont un noyau subcentral, sphérique (Fig. 1, n), et relativement volumineux (2 ou 3 μ de diamètre). Il renferme un gros nucléole (*nu*) qui possède une aire claire, incluse dans une masse essentiellement granulaire. Le nucléole atteint son diamètre maximum (1,5 μ), vers la fin de la phase de prolifération. La chromatine a l'aspect d'amas diffus, dont la structure est difficile à préciser avec les techniques employées (*c*). Une double membrane sépare le nucléoplasme, relativement clair aux électrons, du cytoplasme, qui possède des ribosomes abondants (*r*), et d'autres organites (mitochondries presque sphériques, plastes de type foliacé...).

Au cours de la prolifération, les cellules d'un secteur se divisent d'une façon synchronisée. On peut ainsi observer simultanément plusieurs plaques métaphasiques dans un groupe de cellules d'une section ultrafine. Dans le secteur voisin, les noyaux cellulaires peuvent être en interphase, ou à une autre phase de la mitose.

Les chromosomes, au nombre de six, ont des branches épaisses (0,6 à 0,8 μ) et allongées (1 à 3 μ) (Fig. 3, 4, ch). Sombres aux électrons, ils renferment de fines fibrilles, sinueuses, densément intriquées. Leur bord n'est pas clairement défini. Ils sont inclus dans le fuseau où l'on reconnaît des microtubules (mt) et des granules ayant les caractères des ribosomes.

L'ÉDIFICATION DES TRAVÉES NUCLÉAIRES OSMIOPHILES

Les caractères et l'évolution du noyau ont été précisés chez diverses Bryophytes en microscopie photonique (ALLEN, 1917; MOTTE, 1928; HAMANT, 1954). Quand la spermatide se transforme en spermatozoïde, le noyau, sphérique et subcentral, se déplace vers le bord de la cellule, et commence à s'allonger. Il devient complètement latéral alors que la cellule est encore globuleuse.

Dans le noyau s'édifient des travées osmiophiles (Figs. 5, 6, t), groupées en une masse qui s'accroît. D'une largeur assez constante (200 Å) dans un noyau donné, ces travées forment des filaments dont le profil est circulaire, en section transversale. Les divers aspects observés suggèrent que ces travées sont assez sinueuses et vraisemblablement réunies en un peloton serré.

Dans diverses sections favorables, des segments de travées sont sectionnés sur une longueur plus élevée (jusqu'à 0,8 μ) (Fig. 5, t).

Des travées osmiophiles se trouvent au voisinage immédiat du nucléole. (Fig. 6). Celui-ci a une structure granulaire analogue à celle du nucléole dans le noyau de la cellule spermatogène. Son diamètre (0,4 μ) s'est fortement réduit.

La genèse des travées osmiophiles commence quand le noyau change de forme, et se déplace vers le bord de la cellule. Dans une anthéridie, tous les noyaux sont au même stade de la différenciation. Même si quelques cellules se trouvent légèrement en avance ou en retard par rapport à l'ensemble, le décalage des phénomènes est à peine sensible. Le synchronisme presque parfait de l'évolution des noyaux dans l'ensemble de l'anthéridie s'oppose à la prolifération de type sectorial qui caractérise la phase de multiplication des cellules spermatogènes.

L'ÉVOLUTION DES TRAVÉES NUCLÉAIRES

La spermatide, isodiamétrique, s'aplatit et acquiert une forme lenticulaire. Elle se sépare des autres; des structures finement fibrillaires apparaissent dans les espaces intercellulaires.

Dans le noyau devenu latéral, les travées sont plus épaisses, légèrement plus denses aux électrons (Fig. 7, t). Selon leur orientation par rapport à la section, elles ont l'aspect de cercles ou de bâtonnets. Certaines sont accolées à la membrane nucléaire; les autres sont incluses dans le nucléoplasme.

A un stade plus avancé, dans les sections parallèles au plan équatorial de la spermatide, le noyau a l'aspect d'un fer à cheval; il est appliqué contre le bord de la cellule (Fig. 8). Il renferme d'épaisses travées osmiophiles, les unes situées dans la région axiale (*tc*), les autres en périphérie (*tp*).

Les travées axiales ont une section circulaire (800 à 1000 Å de diamètre); elles sont allongées en coupe longitudinale. Chacune semble constituer une hélice à pas très allongé (Fig. 9, *tc*). Les travées périphériques, étalées sous la membrane nucléaire, ont une section plutôt lenticulaire (Fig. 10, *tp*). En coupe tangentielle, elles se présentent à la manière de barreaux d'échelle, légèrement inclinés; elles paraissent former une structure hélicoïdale (Fig. 11).

Dans certaines travées, en particulier dans la région centrale, il est possible de reconnaître des structures fibrillaires, rectilignes sur une certaine longueur, et dont le diamètre est de l'ordre de 20 à 30 Å. Ces fibrilles sont enrobées dans une substance interstitielle dense, osmiophile.

L'existence de figures intermédiaires fait penser que les travées relativement épaisses dérivent des travées plus fines observées précédemment.

Les travées osmiophiles ont le même aspect dans les diverses régions du noyau. Elles s'accroissent à la même vitesse, leur différenciation étant harmonisée avec les transformations structurales du noyau qui s'allonge, s'amincit, et s'accole étroitement au bord de la cellule. Le nucléole n'a pas pu être caractérisé dans les noyaux à ce stade, dont il existe de nombreuses sections dans une seule coupe d'anthéridie. La membrane nucléaire a toujours la même structure. Son aspect sinueux en coupe transversale est vraisemblablement du à une rigidité plus grande des travées osmiophiles périphériques sur lesquelles elle se moule. Les substances du nucléoplasme subiraient une certaine rétraction au cours de la déshydratation qui suit la fixation; les replis de la membrane nucléaire correspondent aux intervalles séparant deux travées osmiophiles voisines. Le nucléoplasme présente de fines structures fibrillaires (*sf*) distribuées entre les travées osmiophiles.

LES CARACTÈRES STRUCTURAUX DE L'APPAREIL NUCLÉAIRE DIFFÉRENCIÉ

Dans diverses anthéridies, proches de la mâturité, les spermatozoïdes sont complètement séparés les uns des autres. Ils ont subi de profondes transformations; chaque cellule est limitée par une fine membrane (vésicule des auteurs) distincte de la pellicule ectoplasmique. Le noyau s'est allongé fortement. Il possède une enveloppe osmiophile épaisse et continue (Fig. 12). Dans la région centrale, se trouve une masse dense, composée de plusieurs travées accolées. Un espace clair aux électrons sépare l'enveloppe des masses internes. Le diamètre du noyau est plus faible qu'auparavant.

La membrane nucléaire n'est plus distincte. Il n'a pas été possible de savoir si elle s'accole intimement aux masses osmiophiles adjacentes, ou si elle disparaît.

Le nucléole, qui n'a pu être caractérisé, a vraisemblablement disparu au cours des stades précédents. L'amincissement du noyau, et le développement de structures fortement osmiophiles empêchent toutefois d'avoir une certitude complète à ce sujet.

Il est difficile de distinguer des structures fibrillaires fines analogues à celles définies précédemment dans le nucléoplasme.

Bien que nous n'ayons pas observé de spermatozoïdes mûrs, tels qu'ils se présentent dans le col de l'archégone, nous avons obtenu des images de gamètes très proches de cet état (Fig. 13). Les anthéridies prêtes à la déhiscence perdent une grande partie de leur contenu au cours de la fixation ou de la déshydratation. Elles renferment encore de rares spermatozoïdes, dont les structures nucléaires ne diffèrent guère de celles que l'on observe dans des anthéridies non déhiscentes.

Le noyau (*n*) est alors allongé, formant une hélice de un tour à un tour et demi. Il mesure environ 20 μ de longueur. Son diamètre, (0,2 à 0,3 μ), constant sur la plus grande partie de sa longueur, se réduit aux extrêmités qui sont effilées. Avec les techniques employées, le noyau apparaît dense, fortement osmiophile, presque homogène. Quelques espaces clairs apparaissent çà et là dans son épaisseur.

Les divers territoires typiques du noyau interphasique de la spermatide: membrane nucléaire, nucléole, travées chromatiques, nucléoplasme ne sont plus reconnaissables. L'aspect de la substance nucléaire est différent de celui des chromosomes de la même espèce, étudiés avec les mêmes techniques (comparer les Figs. 13 et 3).

La régression du nucléole et des ribosomes

Parmi les organites cellulaires, le comportement du nucléole et des ribosomes paraît être étroitement lié à celui de la genèse des travées osmiophiles intranucléaires.

La comparaison entre la section du nucléole d'une cellule spermatogène et celle d'un nucléole de spermatide au début de la différenciation montre que le volume de cet organite décroît beaucoup (de 13,3 μ^3 à 0,5 μ^3). Malgré cette importante réduction, le nucléole conserve une structure essentiellement granulaire. Certaines travées osmiophiles sont adjacentes au nucléole au début de leur développement. Elles apparaissent au moment où le nucléole, déjà considérablement réduit, va disparaître.

La régression du nucléole a été suivie chez *Polytrichum juniperinum* (ALLEN, 1912), où elle s'accompagne d'une disparition progressive de l'ARN qui entre dans sa constitution (CREPIN, 1968). Dans *Polytrichum formosum*, les ribosomes cytoplasmiques sont abondants dans les cellules spermatogènes en prolifération. Moins nombreux ensuite, ils forment des amas (polyribosomes) dans le cytoplasme des spermatides. Ils sont inclus dans une substance grise, dont la structure n'est pas distincte. Certains ribosomes sont groupés au voisinage des travées périphériques du noyau. Ils présentent quelquefois une disposition en spirale (Fig. 11, r).

Dans l'espèce voisine, *Polytrichum juniperinum*, le cytoplasme des cellules spermatogènes est riche en ARN; la teneur en ARN décroît au cours de la différenciation de la spermatide en spermatozoïde (CREPIN). Ces observations cytochimiques concordent avec le comportement des ribosomes, abondants dans les cellules spermatogènes, de plus en plus rares au fur et à mesure de la différenciation.

CONCLUSION

Une comparaison effectuée en microscopie photonique, entre les chromosomes des cellules en division et la masse chromatique nucléaire du spermatozoïde a conduit plusieurs auteurs à les rapprocher.

La réaction de Feulgen montre en effet que ces deux types de structures sont riches en ADN. D'autre part, une certaine concordance peut exister entre les dimensions de l'ensemble des chromosomes du génome et celles du noyau du gamète mâle.

Dans l'espèce *Polytrichum formosum*, l'emploi des techniques électroniques a permis de comparer les structures ultrafines des cellules qui prolifèrent et celles des spermatides qui se transforment en spermatozoïdes. Pendant la différenciation, des travées se constituent dans le nucléoplasme. D'abord abondantes, fines, sinueuses, et peu osmiophiles, elles deviennent moins nombreuses, plus épaisses, moins sinueuses et de plus en plus osmiophiles. Au début de leur évolution, elles ont un diamètre relativement faible (200 Å), le même dans les diverses régions du noyau. Elles se transforment simultanément, s'épaississant, devenant plus denses dans tout le nucléoplasme. Deux sortes de travées se différencient ensuite, les unes périphériques, plus larges et aplaties, les autres centrales, hélicoïdales, à section circulaire. Les travées périphériques confluent en une enveloppe continue, séparée des travées centrales par un espace clair qui s'amenuise. Enfin, l'appareil nucléaire apparaît constitué essentiellement par une substance dense aux électrons.

A mesure que les travées osmiophiles se développent, le noyau change de forme et de dimensions. Il s'allonge considérablement pendant que son diamètre se réduit.

Les travées intranucléaires observées sont à rapprocher des structures filamenteuses étudiées par EYME en microscopie photonique. Colorées par la technique de Feulgen, elles renferment de l'ADN. Le nombre, la disposition, et l'évolution des filaments riches en ADN au cours de la différenciation inclinent à penser que ces filaments et les travées osmiophiles ont la même nature.

L'ultrasctructure des travées osmiophiles est différente de celle des chromosomes, organites riches en ADN. A aucun moment, au cours de l'édification de l'appareil nucléaire du spermatozoïde, on ne voit apparaître de chromosomes typiques. La genèse et l'évolution des travées osmiophiles, liées étroitement aux transformations morphologiques du noyau, semble être un processus particulier, caractéristique de la différenciation du spermatozoïde de Polytric.

Les structures fibrillaires décelées dans certaines travées, en raison de leurs dimensions (20 à 30 Å de diamètre) pourraient renfermer de l'ADN. Toutefois, d'autres arguments seraient nécessaires pour l'assurer.

Le développement des travées osmiophiles paraît concorder avec celui des filaments de chromatine, définis par EYME (1954). Simultanément, le nucléole et les ribosomes, organites réputés riches en ARN, régressent plus ou moins complètement. Des rapports topographiques remarquables existent à certains moments, entre le nucléole et certaines travées nucléaires d'une part, entre les groupes de ribosomes et les travées osmiophiles d'autre part.

On ne peut concevoir l'appareil nucléaire du spermatozoïde de Polytric comme étant composé de chromosomes individualisés, placés bout à bout ou partiellement superposés. Les mécanismes de formation de l'appareil nucléaire du gamète différent de ceux de la division cellulaire banale.

Le problème de l'organisation des macromolécules d'ADN dans le spermatozoïde reste posé. On sait que dans les têtes de certains gamètes mâles, les molécules d'ADN pourraient être disposées parallèlement les unes aux autres, d'après des mesures de biréfringence (W. J. SCHMIDT), ou de dichroïsme dans l'ultraviolet (T. CASPERSSON). La distribution des macromolécules d'ADN n'est pas forcément la même dans le spermatozoïde et dans les chromosomes.

BIBLIOGRAPHIE

ALLEN C. E. (1912) – *Cell structure, growth and division in the Antheridia of* Polytrichum juniperinum *Willd.* « Arch f. Zellforsch », 8, 121–188.

ALLEN C. E. (1917) – The spermatogenesis of Polytrichum juniperinum. « Annals of Bot », 31, 269–291.

BRACHET J. (1947) – *Embryologie chimique*, ed. Desoer, Liège.

CASPERSSON T. (1940) – « Chromosoma », 5, 605.

CHEIGNON M. (1964) – *Ultrastructure du gamète mâle d'*Ascophyllum nodosum. « Comptes Rendus Ac. Sc. », 258, 676–678.

COOPER K. W. (1952) – *Studies on spermatogenesis in* Drosophila. « Yearb. Philos. Soc. », 1951, 146–147.

CREPIN D. (1968) – *Etudes cytochimiques de l'évolution du tissu spermatogène d'une Bryophyte:* Polytrichum juniperinum (*Polytrichacées*). « Rev. Gén. Bot. », 75, 481–492.

DIERS L. (1967) – *Der Feinbau des spermatozoids von* Sphaerocarpos donnellii *Aust.* (*Hepaticae*). « Planta (Berl.) », 72, 119–145.

EYME J. (1954) – *Recherches cytologiques sur les Mousses.* Thèse, Bordeaux, 1954.

GOWEN J. W. and GAY E. H. (1933) – *Gene number, kind and size in* Drosophila. « Genetics », 18, 1–31.

HAMANT C. (1954) – *Recherches cytologiques sur la reproduction chez quelques espèces du genre* Mnium. Thèse, Toulouse.

HERSKOWITZ I. H. and MULLER H. T. (1954) – *Evidence against a straight end–to–end alignment of chromosomes in* Drosophila *spermatozoa.* « Genetics », 39, 836–850.

MANTON I. (1959) – *Observations on the microanatomy of the spermatozoid of the Bracken Fern* (Pteridium aquilinum). « J. Biophysic and Biochem. Cytol. », 6, 413-418.

MOTTE J. (1928) – *Contribution à la connaissance cytologique des Muscinées.* « Ann. Sc. Nat. Bot. », 10, 293–543.

MULLER H. J. and VALENCIA J. I. (1951). – *The localisation of the mutagenic action of neutron–induced ionizations in* Drosophila (*Abstr.*). « Rec. Genet. Soc. Amer. », 20, 115–116 et « Genetics », 36, 567–568.

MULLER H. J. (1954) – *The relation of neutron dose to chromosome changes and point mutations in* Drosophila. I. *Translocations.* « Amer. Nat. », 88.

PELC S. R. (1957) – *On the connection between the synthesis of* RNA *and* DNA *in the testis of the mouse.* « Exp. Cell Res. », 12, 320–324.

RAPOPORT J. A. (1941) – *Mutations restituting the telomere.* « C. R. (Dokl.) Acad. Sci. U.R.S.S., N.S. », 31, 266–269.

REITBERGER A. (1964) – *Lineare Anordnung der Chromosomen in Kern des Spermatozoids des Lebermooses* Sphaerocarpus donnellii. « Naturwissenschaften », 16, 395–396.

SCHMIDT W. J. (1937) – *Die Doppelbrechnung von Karyoplasma,* Zytoplasma und Metaplasma, Berlin, 1937.

TAYLOR J. M. (1964) – *The arrangement of chromosomes in the mature sperm of the grasshopper.* « The Journ. of Cell Biol. », 21, 286–289.

TURNER F. R. (1968) – *An ultrastructural study of plant spermatogenesis. Spermatogenesis in Nitella.* « The Journ. of Cell Biol. », 37, 370–393.

WOLF E. (1939) – *Die Anordnung der chromosomen in Spermienkern von* Dicranomyia trinotata *Meig.* « Chromosoma », 1, 336–342.

LÉGENDES DES FIGURES

Cellules du tissu spermatogène dans l'anthéridie de *Polytrichum formosum.* Fixation, glutaraldéhyde – tétroxyde d'osmium. Inclusion, araldite. Contrastant, permanganate de potassium.

Fig. 1. – Fragment d'une cellule spermatogène, avec noyau (*n*), nucléole (*nu*), et chromatine (*c*) sous forme de travées ou d'amas. Le cytoplasme renferme des ribosomes (*r*). (G. ×25.000).

Fig. 2. – Détail d'un noyau de cellule spermatogène, montrant les structures granulaires du nucléole (*nu*), la chromatine (*c*). r, ribosomes cytoplasmiques. (G. ×51.000).

Fig. 3. – Partie d'une plaque métaphasique dans une cellule spermatogène. ch, chromosome; mi, mitochondrie. (G. ×25.000).

Fig. 4. – Chromosomes (*ch*) en plaque équatoriale, formés de fibrilles intriquées; *mt,* microtubules; *mi,* mitochondrie; *r,* ribosomes. (G. ×37.000).

Fig. 5. – Noyau d'une spermatide au début de la différenciation. *mn,* membrane nucléaire; *t,* travées en voie d'édification dans le nucléoplasme. (G. ×25.000).

Fig. 6. – Zone plus grossie d'un noyau au même stade. Les travées (*t*) se forment au voisinage du nucléole (*nu*), dont le diamètre est bien plus faible que dans la cellule spermatogène; *mn*, membrane nucléaire. (G. ×51.000).

Fig. 7. – Noyau d'une spermatide plus différenciée, renfermant des travées (*t*) plus denses que précédemment. *r*, ribosomes; *f*, fibrilles flagellaires. (G ×51.000).

Fig. 8. – Noyau plus étroit et plus long, dont les travées sont de deux sortes, les unes périphériques (*tp*), les autres centrales (*tc*); *r*, ribosomes; *f* fibrilles flagellaires. (G. ×21.000).

Fig. 9. – Section d'un noyau qui présente des travées centrales (*tc*), des travées périphériques (*tp*). Dans le nucléoplasme, apparaissent des structures fibrillaires fines (*sf*). (G. ×60.000).

Fig. 10. – Coupe transversale d'un noyau, dont la membrane (*mn*) suit le contour externe des travées périphériques osmiophiles (*tp*). Dans la partie centrale, travées à section circulaire (*tc*). *sf*, fibrilles dans le nucléoplasme. (G. ×60.000).

Fig. 11. – Disposition relative des ribosomes, groupés quelquefois en spirale (*r*) au voisinage de travées osmiophiles nucléaires. (G. ×51.000).

Fig. 12. – Coupe longitudinale d'un fragment de noyau dans un spermatozoïde à un stade plus avancé. Quelques espaces clairs existent encore entre l'enveloppe et la région centrale, toutes deux denses aux électrons. (G. ×89.000).

Fig. 13. – Section d'un spermatozoïde proche de la mâturité. Le noyau (*n*) encore entouré d'un étroit manchon cytoplasmique, est en grande partie osmiophile. (G. ×25.000).

L. GENEVES – *Différenciation de l'appareil nucléaire a l'échelle infrastructurale, pendant la spermatogenèse, chez une Bryophyte* (Polytrichum formosum).

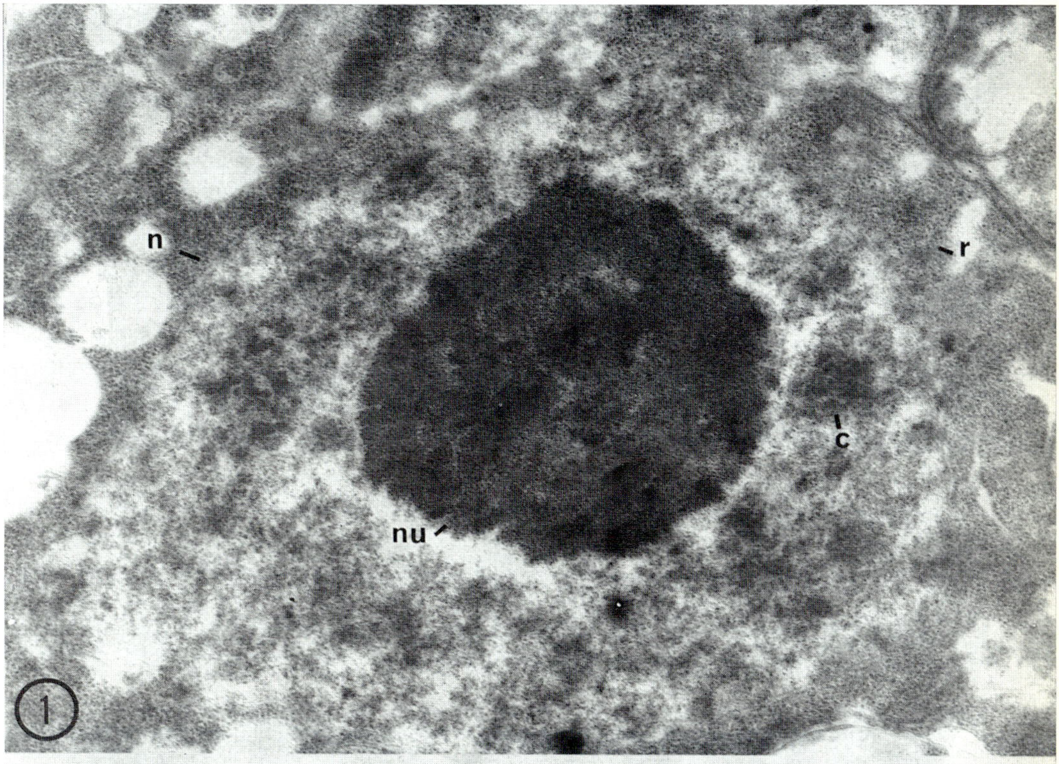

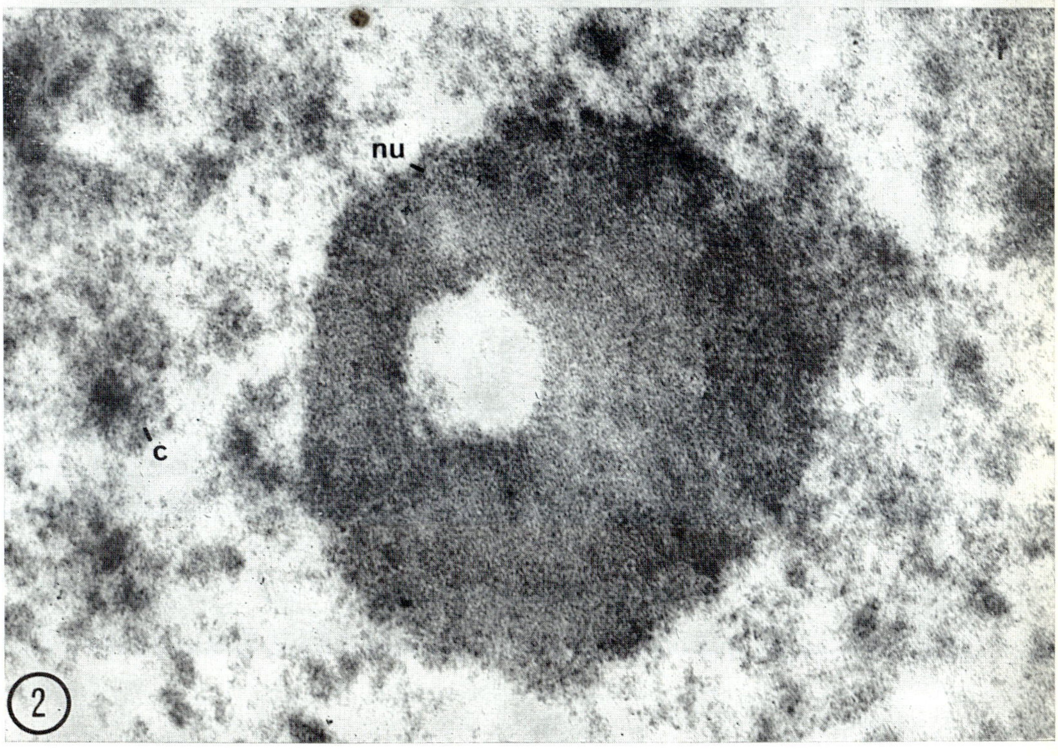

L. GENEVES – *Différenciation de l'appareil nucléaire a l'échelle infrastructurale, pendant la spermatogenèse, chez une Bryophyte* (Polytrichum formosum).

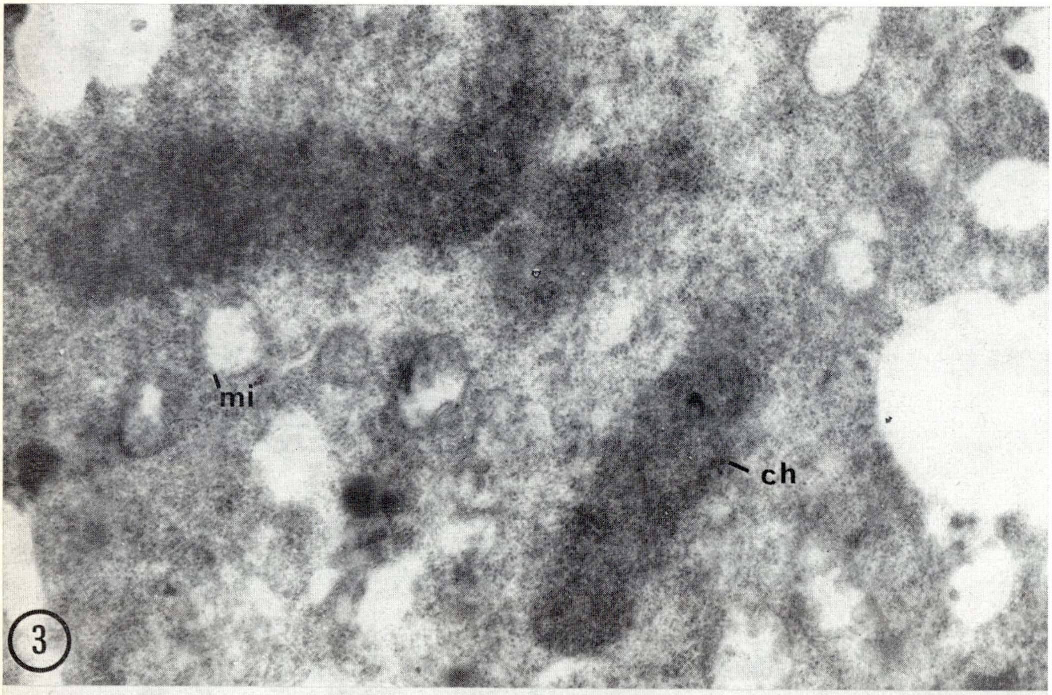

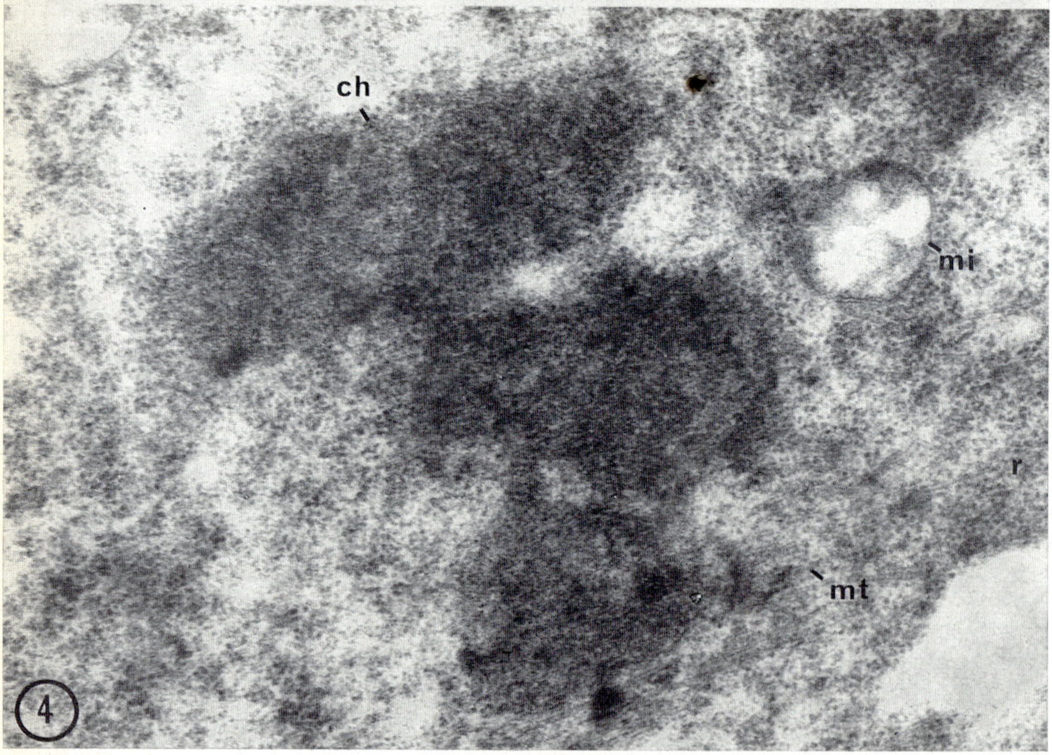

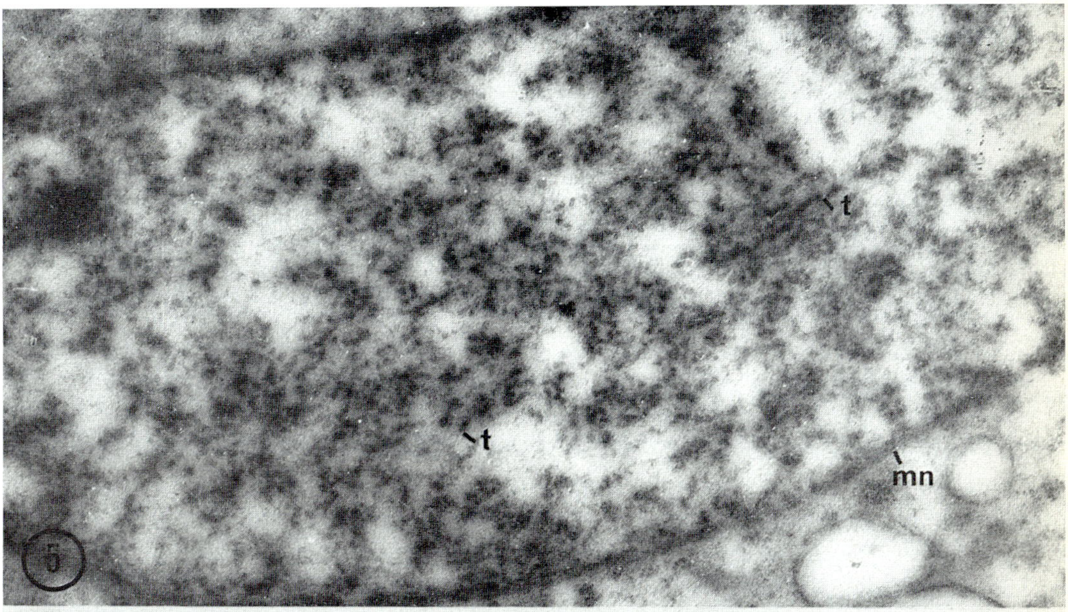
t
t
mn
5

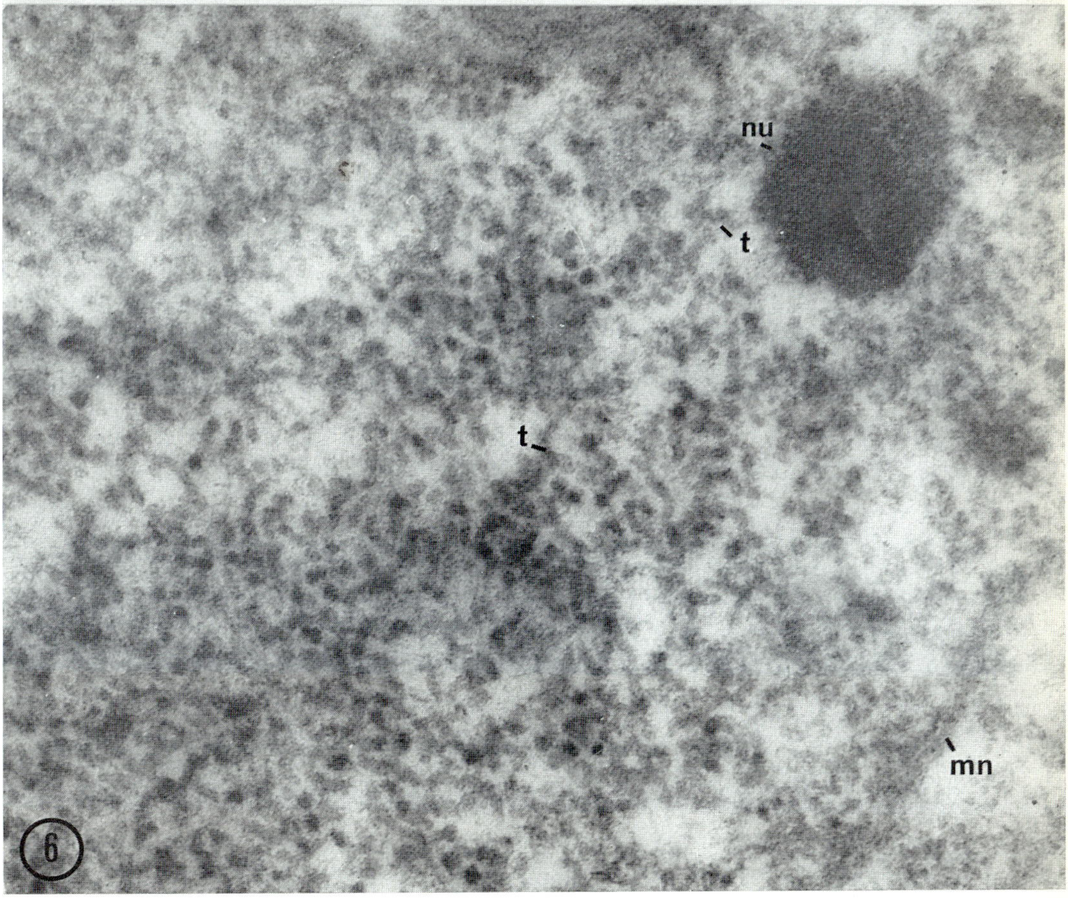
nu
t
t
mn
6

L. GENEVES – *Différenciation de l'appareil nucléaire a l'échelle infrastructurale, pendant la spermatogenèse, chez une Bryophyte* (Polytrichum formosum).

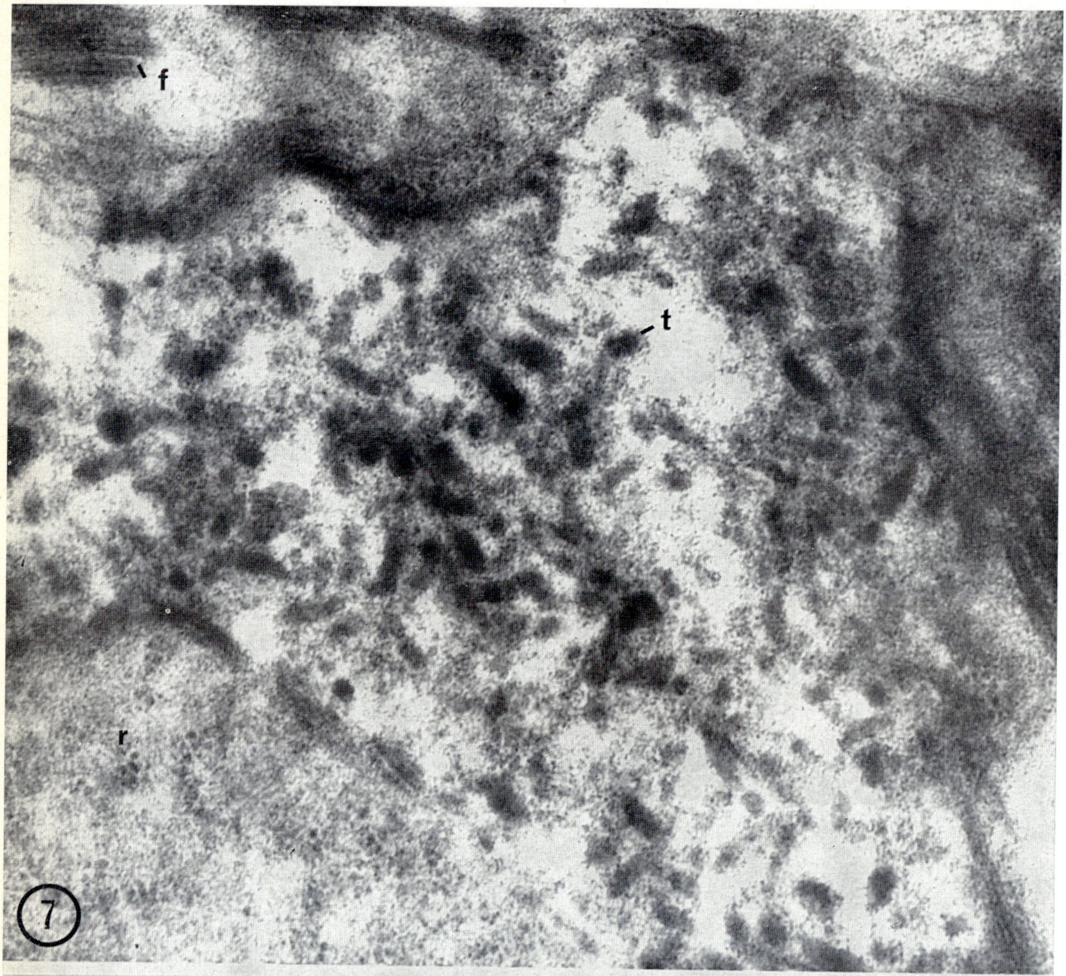

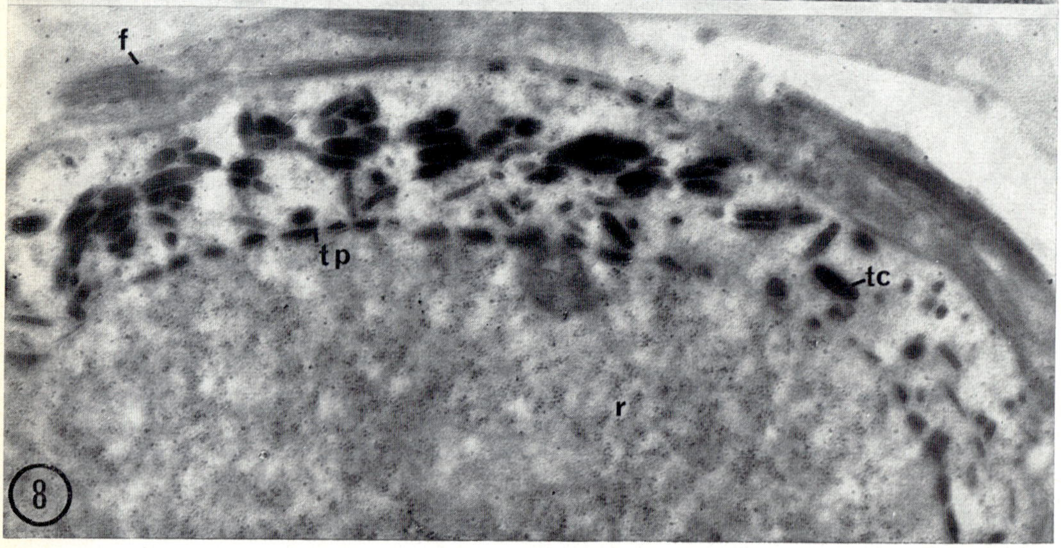

L. Geneves – *Différenciation de l'appareil nucléaire a l'échelle infrastructurale, pendant la spermatogenèse, chez une Bryophyte* (Polytrichum formosum).

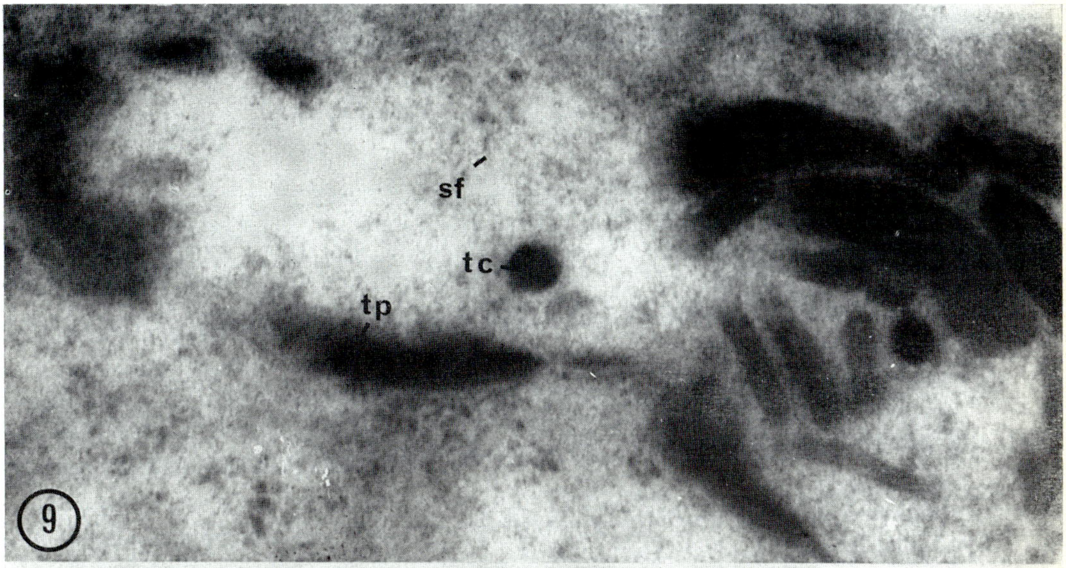

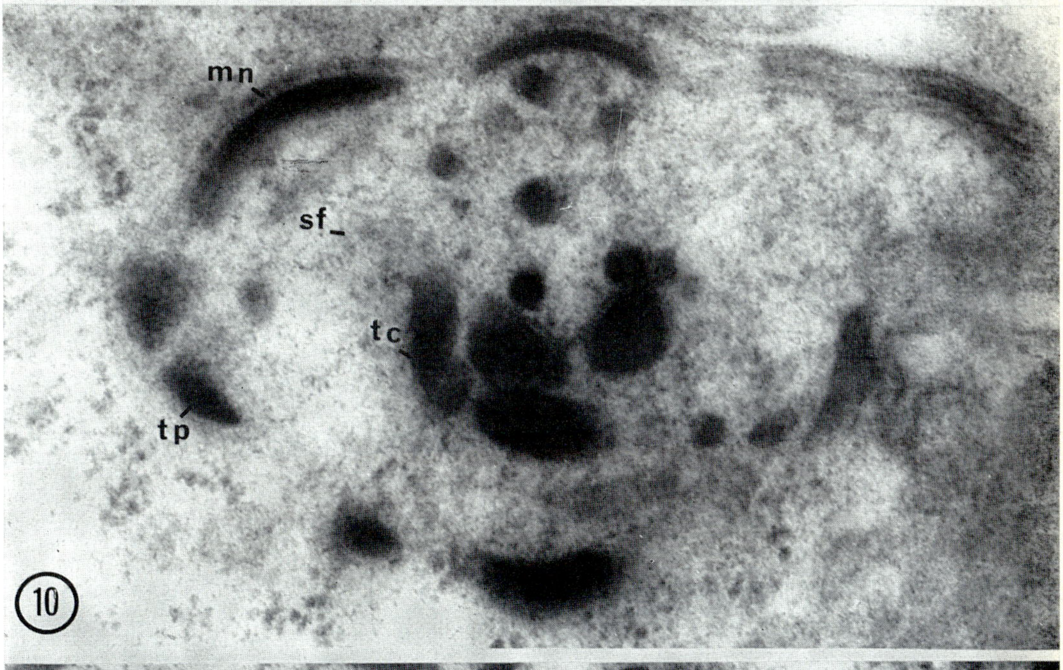

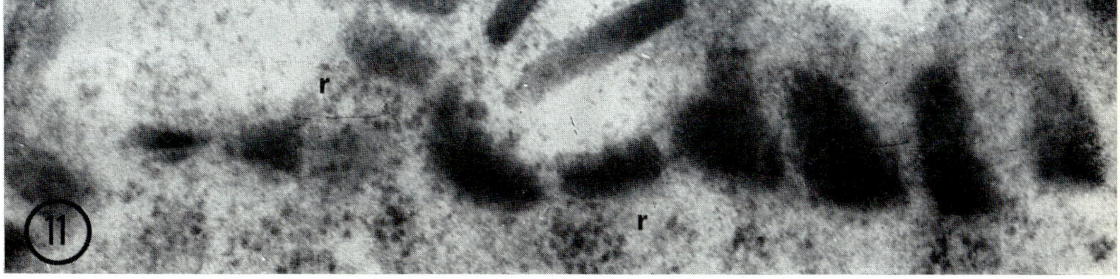

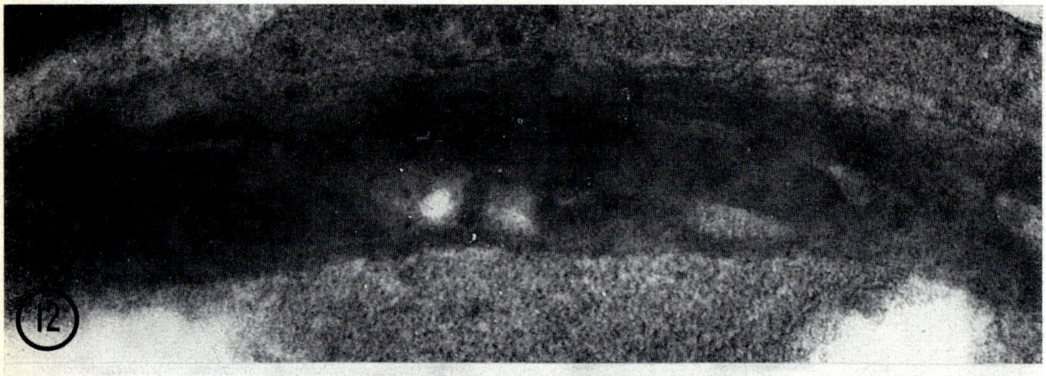
12

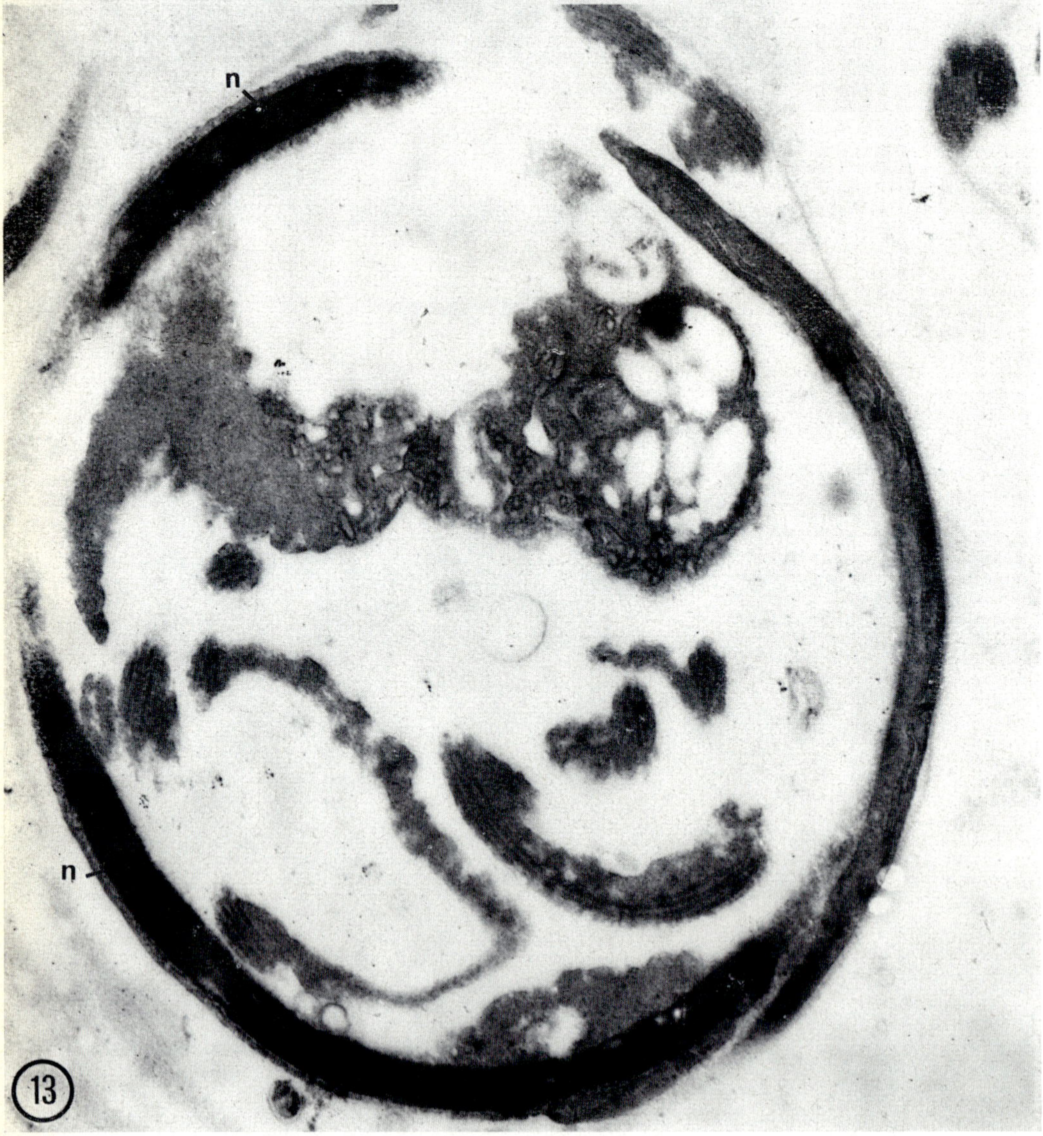
n
n
13

BACCIO BACCETTI (*)

THE SPERMATOZOON OF ARTHROPODA. IX. THE SPERM CELL AS AN INDEX OF ARTHROPOD PHYLOGENESIS

SUMMARY. — In this paper the author summarizes the actual knowledge on the fine morphology of Arthropod spermatozoon. A phylogenetical interpretation for the different sperm models is proposed, in good agreement with the usual classification of Arthropoda.

RIASSUNTO. — In questo lavoro l'Autore riassume le attuali conoscenze sulla fine struttura dello spermatozoo degli Artropodi e propone una interpretazione filogenetica per i diversi modelli di spermatozoo, in buon accordo con la usuale classificazione del phylum.

Throughout the phylum Arthropoda a conventional type of sperm is found which has the main characteristics of the sperm of the related phyla, *Annelida*, *Tardigrada* (unpublished: Fig. 1), and the primitive groups of the highly evolved major phyla, the *Mollusca* and *Chordata*. These characteristics are: head with concentrated chromatin, in a fibrillar, lamellar or homogeneous state; acrosome (originating from the Golgi complex) in form of a conical cap; two centrioles, sometimes fused, a tail containing an axial filament, and a mitochondrial complex. The axial filament has the basic 9+2 arrangement of tubular fibers. Prominent secondary and accessory fibers are present only in insects. Typical mitochondria in spermatids form a mitochondrial complex that exhibits varying degrees of evolution in the different classes.

The primitive model, with numerous unmodified mitochondria (ANDRÉ, 1963) and simple 9+2 axial filament complex (Fig. 2) devoid of secondary fibrils (BACCETTI, unpublished) is conserved only in *Merostomata*, where the head is complicated by an axial canal through which runs an elongated structure that perforates the acrosome. The class *Arachnida* shows a conspicuous evolution. In scorpions (ANDRÉ, 1959, 1963) the mitochondria become fused to form large bodies in which the cristae are anastomosed, forming a honeycomb, and the tail is of the primitive type. In pseudoscorpions (BOISSIN and MANIER, 1966, 1967) the tail filament (9+2) is coiled around an annular single mitochondrial derivative, and, in the head, an elongated acrosomal structure is coiled around the nucleus. This sperm is ejaculated in an encysted

(*) Institute of Zoology of the University of Siena, Italy.

form and it subsequently develops in the female ducts. In *Araneida* (ROSATI, BACCETTI and DALLAI, 1969) the evolution of the sperm is quite particular. The mitochondria which appear normal in spermatids, fuse to form an opaque, amorphous mass that disappears by the end of spermiogenesis. An acrosome is present. The flagellum consists only of a 9+3 filament complex

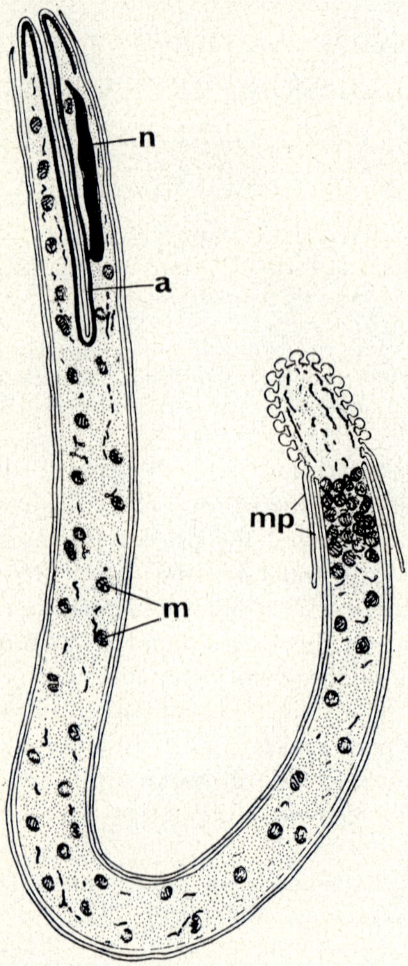

Diagram 1. – Schematic diagram of the mature spermatozoon in a Tick, *Amblyomma dissimili*. *a*, acrosome; *m*, mitochondria; *mp*, motile processes; *n*, nucleus (after Reger).

(Fig. 3), and the centriole is encircled by 9 opaque outer units similar to those described in *Lumbricus* by ANDERSON and ELLIS (1968). Spermatozoa of spiders also belong to the encysted category. In Opilionids (unpublished) the flagellum is absent and the sperms are encysted. *Acarina* (Diagram 1), the highest *Arachnida*, (REGER, 1963; BREUCKER and HORSTMANN, 1968) have nonflagellate, cylindrical sperm, with a U-shaped acrosome at an invaginated end, where a small nucleus is located. In addition, numerous cytoplasmic processes project from their surface; each process is composed of two motile filaments. The head trails and is not pushed forward. Thus,

Arachnida, a terrestrial class, have lower forms including encysted sperm with the 9+2 pattern of fibers, higher forms with 9+3, encysted spermatozoa, and highest forms with non-flagellate spermatozoa possessing highly specialized motile processes.

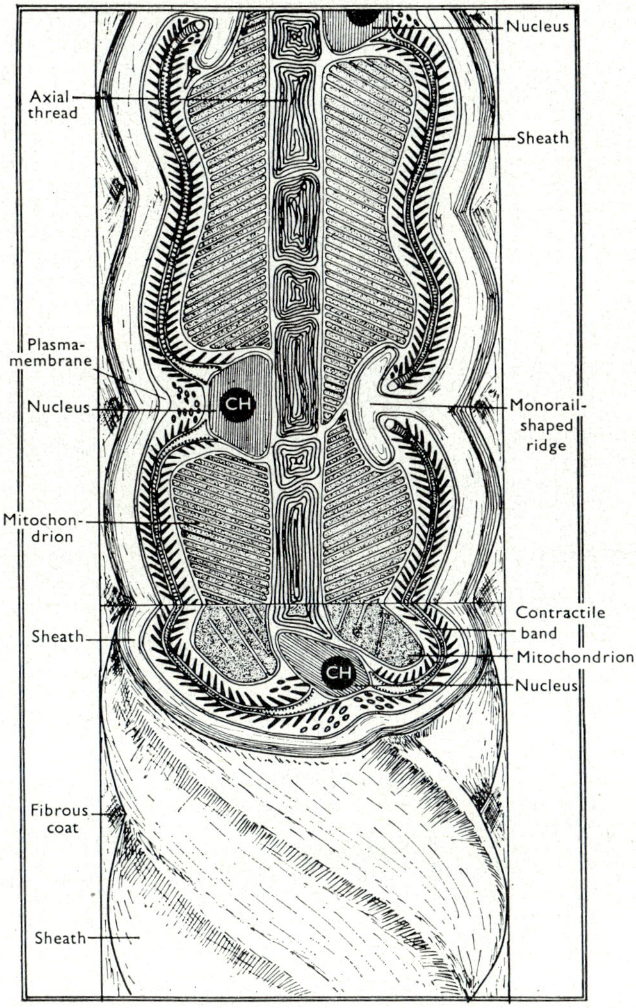

Diagram 2. – Diagram representing a three-dimensional visualization of one turn of the helix constituting the posterior thick part of the spermatozoon in an Ostracod, *Notodromas monacha* (after Gupta).

In *Crustacea* we observe a complicated evolution. Many papers in this Symposium are dedicated to them, and new findings can substantially modify the actual schema according to Brown (1966 a). There are: a group of primitive aquatic subclasses showing 9+2 flagellate elongated spermatozoa, where frequently the axial filament complex is coiled around the nucleus and mitochondria appear fused to form one or more units: these include the *Mysta-*

cocarida (BROWN and METZ, 1967), *Cirripedia*, and *Branchiura* (BROWN, 1966 b). From this primitive stock, many different evolutive lines of spermatozoa lacking an axial filament complex seem to be issued. *Copepoda*, strictly related to *Branchiura* (BROWN, 1966 a) have lost centriole, flagellum, acro-

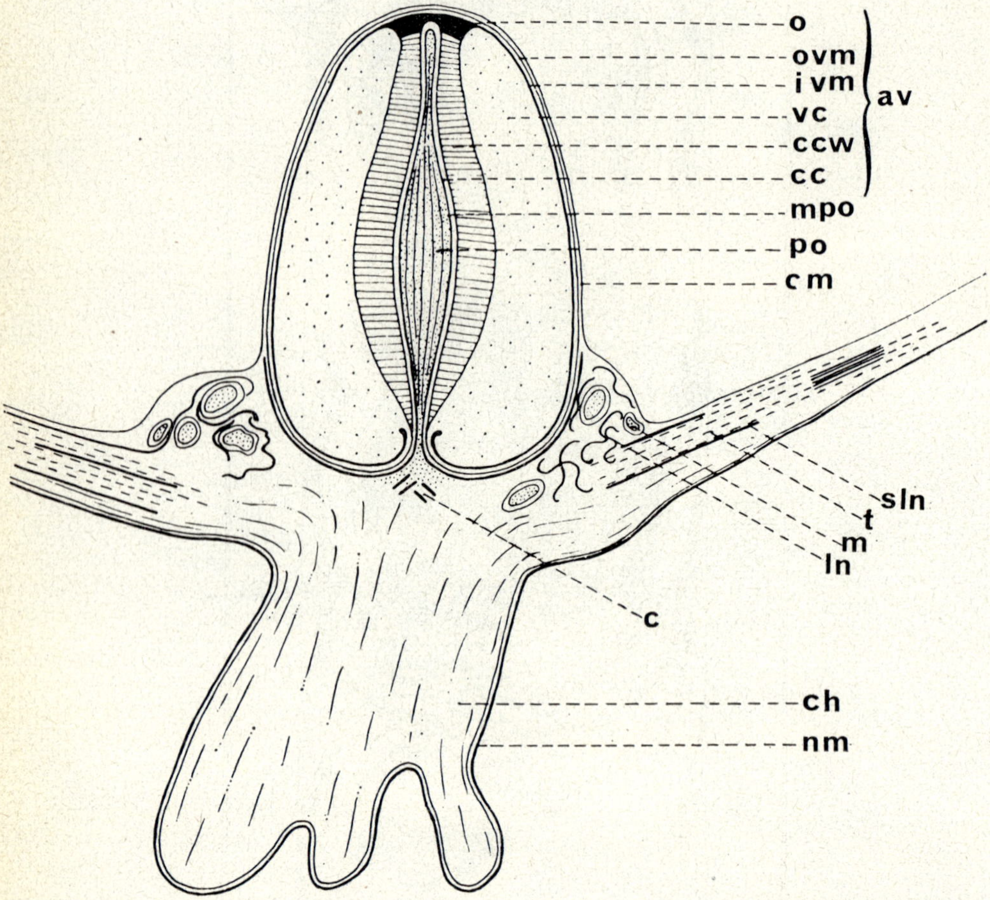

Diagram 3. – Diagram representing the mature spermatozoon of a Decapod: *av* acrosomal vesicle; *c*, centrioles; *cc*, central canal; *ccw*, central canal wall; *ch*, chromatine; *cm*, plasma membrane; *vc*, vesicular content; *ivm*, inner vesicular membrane; *ln*, laminae arising from the nuclear envelope; *m*, mitochondria; *mpo*, membrane of the percussive organ, *nm*, nuclear membrane; *o*, operculum; *ovm*, outer vesicular membrane; *sln*, sheat formed by the laminae arising from the nuclear envelope; *t*, tubule; *vc*, vesicular content (after Pochon-Masson).

some, but their sperm is probably not so simple. *Anostracha* (BROWN, 1966 a), a very primitive group, have nevertheless a particular spermatozoon, non-motile, spherical, with many arms and therefore " pin-cushion "-like. *Cephalocharida* (BROWN and METZ, 1967), too, have lost their flagellum, and they possess instead a rod-like immotile tail. Another substitution of the flagellum is present in *Ostracoda* (Diagram 2), where GUPTA (1968) and ZISSLER

(1969) observe an elongated nucleus surrounded by longitudinally arranged mitochondria and by two wing-like processes provided by numerous tubules, constituting a contractile structure.

The Peracarids *Misidacea, Isopoda* and *Amphipoda* (REGER, 1964 a and b, 1966; FAIN MAUREL, 1966) have whip-like sperm, with an immotile tail that is devoid of fibrils and mitochondria, and is cross striated. In the lowest Decapods, *Palaemonetes*, BROWN (1966 a) and METZ (1967) observed what is perhaps a comparable situation: centriole, flagellum and acrosome in the classic form are absent and a fibrous cross-striated tail is present. In the other Decapods many workers (MOSES, 1961; ANDERSON and ELLIS,

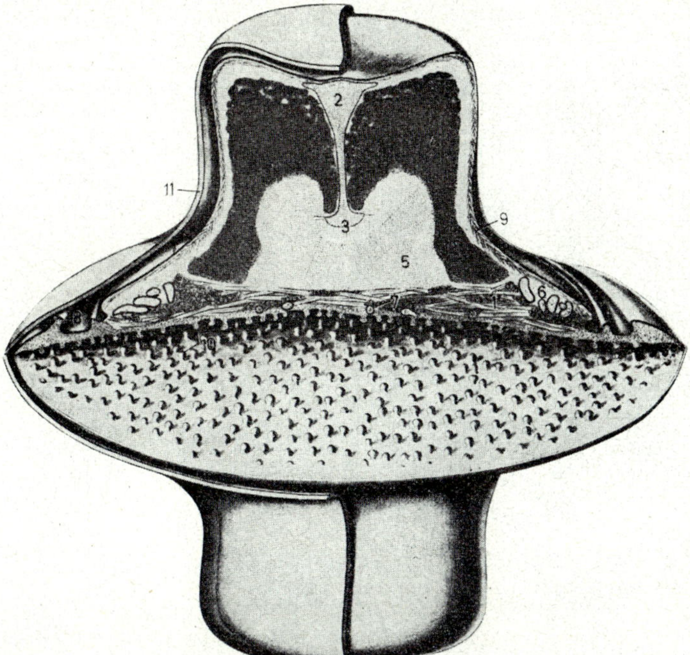

Diagram 4. – Diagram representing a spermatophore with two spermatozoa in a Myriapod, *Graphidostreptus*. 1, Caryoplasma; 2, acrosomal vacuole with 3, hemispheric calotte; 4, « M » bodies; 5, cristalloid; 6, circle of mitochondria; 7, utricles; 8, gutters; 9, mantle; 10, basal cytoplasmic protrusions; 11, wall of the spermatophore (after Horstmann and Breucker).

1967; YASUZUMI, 1960; BROWN, 1966, and above all POCHON–MASSON, 1968) observe a different structure. The sperm (Diagram 3) is non-flagellate, star-like with several arms penetrated by the nucleus. The mitochondria are transformed into laminae distributed into the mixed cytoplasm and nucleoplasm: the acrosome possesses the well known " explosive " properties, grouped by POCHON–MASSON (1968) in three different progressive categories.

In *Myriapoda* we find a situation different from that of the previously examined classes. A stock of primitive orders, *Pauropoda* (Fig. 4) and

Symphyla (Fig. 5) (ROSATI, BACCETTI and DALLAI, 1969) have spermatozoa with a conventional 9+2 flagellum, but well differentiated in other characteristics. For example a caudal U-shaped infolding, and prominent secondary fibrils an characteristic of sperm of the *Pauropoda* while highly differentiated acrosomes and mitochondria appear in the two types of the sperm of a same species of the *Symphyla*. In *Diplopoda* there exists a somewhat conventional

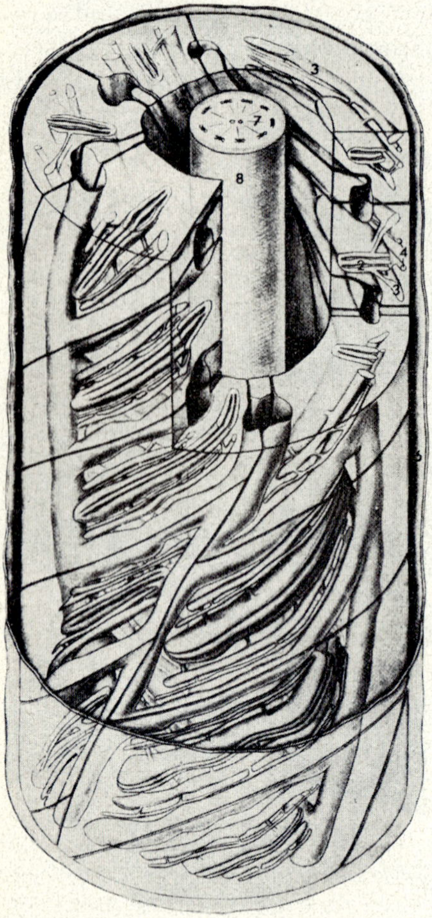

Diagram 5. – Diagram representing a segment of the spermatozoon of a Chilopod, *Geophilus linearis*: 1, spiral septa; 2, membranous bodies; 3, joints; 4, tubuli; 5, periaxial split; 6, submembranous split; 7, axial filament complex; 8, hollow cylinder (after Horstmann).

flagellate form which only develop in female ducts in *Polyxenus* (TUZET et MANIER, 1955). However, we do not know if a 9+2 complex is present in sperm of this species. In fact, the most numerous genera have the typical immotile spermatozoa (Diagram 4), combined two-by-two in the same spermatophore (REGER and COOPER, 1968; HORSTMANN and BREUCKER, 1969). These sperms possess a very complicated acrosome but they lack flagella or motile processes. The nucleus is nevertheless canaliculate and contains microtubules (HORSTMANN and BREUCKER, 1969). *Chilopoda* (Diagram 5) the class immediately above Myriapods in the phylogenetic schema, have conventional sperm where the 9+2 flagellum is encircled by a cylinder of transformed mitochondria, separated from each-other by transverse septa in which glycogen is located (HORSTMANN, 1968). Myriapods and *Chilopoda* appear now as a sufficiently homogeneous line, maintaining the classic characteristics observed in the highest forms, and with only a single deviation (highest Diplopods) to non-flagellarity. It is important to realize that other organs of movement substituting the typical flagellum are absent from this class. The maintained 9+2 axial filament appears the basis for the insect sperm evolution.

Collembola (DALLAI, 1967), the lowest insects examined, possess spermatozoa of the basic typical Arthropod form; however, secondary fibrils are now evident (Fig. 6). The mitochondrial derivative consists of two large tubular units running almost throughout the tail, plus several smaller units in the neck region. In all the orders of insects, with only few exceptions, the model of the spermatozoon is different because of the architecture of the tail. Usually there are two elongated mitochondrial derivatives. In the axial filament (ANDRÉ, 1961; BACCETTI and BAIRATI, 1964; KAYE, 1964; PHILLIPS, 1966; KESSEL, 1967) the classical two major central units are present with a sheath surrounding them. Nine " Afzelius rays " join this sheath to the 9 doublet fibers. Halfway along the rays, nine secondary, doublet fibers that are usually rich in glycogen-like material are present. The most important acquisition is a crown of nine outer fibers, each similar to the central pair, and sometimes embedded in an amorphous material. Limiting the count to the principal elements only, the structure is now of the model " 9+9+2 ". *Thysanura* have spermatozoa of such a model, in which, however, centrioles and acrosomes are juxtaposed (BAWA, 1964; WERNER, 1964). Their spermatozoa are twinned and function only in such a disposition. *Odonata* (KESSEL, 1966), *Blattoidea* (ROSATI, 1967), *Orthoptera* (KAYE, 1964; SHAY and BIESELE, 1968), *Phasmoidea* (BACCETTI, BIGLIARDI, DALLAI and ROSATI, 1969: Fig. 7), *Plecoptera* (BACCETTI, DALLAI and ROSATI, 1969) *Embioptera* (unpublished: Fig. 8) show the " 9 +9+2 " model, with two mitochondrial derivatives containing a crystalline protein.

Around the centriolar region, a ribonucleoprotein forms a particular " centriolar adjunct ". *Ephemeroptera* (BACCETTI, DALLAI and GIUSTI, 1969; PHILLIPS, 1969) show a particular mutation: the filament complex is of 9+9+0 pattern (Fig. 9). *Psocoptera* have a 9+9+2 pattern, but the 9 outer fibers are much more conspicuous and three of them are limited externally by an osmiophilic angular wall (BACCETTI, DALLAI and ROSATI, 1969). In each bundle of sperm numerous biflagellate units are constantly found. A complex of 9+9+1 central rod is described by PHILLIPS (1969) in a particular species. *Mallophaga* (BACCETTI, DALLAI and ROSATI, 1969), *Anoplura* (ITO, 1966) and *Heteroptera* (FURIERI, 1963 b; PAYNE, 1966; WERNER, 1966) have two axial filaments in the tail (Fig. 10). Two mitochondrial derivatives are always present. The " centriolar adjunct " is present. In *Heteroptera* this model of biflagellate sperm is not constant. Some species have two filaments of different lengths, others only one filament. In *Thysanoptera* (BACCETTI, DALLAI and ROSATI, 1969) the two basic 9+2 complexes are fused in a single 18+4 arrangement. In *Homoptera* there is typically only one filament, and biflagellarity is not apparent (LE MENN, 1966; HEROLD and MUNZ, 1967; FOLLIOT, 1968). Some species (*Ceresa*) have branched sperm tails (PHILLIPS, 1969). *Coccids* (ROBISON, 1966; ROSS and ROBISON, 1968) have lost all parts of the tail, and the spermatozoa are disposed in syncytial groups of a fixed number of units (16 in *Pseudococcus*, 32 in *Steatococcus*, 64 in *Eriococcus* and *Parlatoria*); in these species the nuclei are surrounded by several microtubules. Presumably microtubules are the only motile organelles.

Among the *Endopterygota* (the higher Insects) studied we find orders with a " 9+9+2 " axial filament complex and two orders with only " 9+2 " pattern. All have typically two mitochondrial derivatives, " centriolar adjunct " and acrosome. The first class of orders include *Neuroptera* (BACCETTI, DALLAI and ROSATI, 1969) in which the dense material embedding the 9 outer fibres is lacking (Fig. 11); *Coleoptera* (FURIERI, 1963 a; WERNER, 1966) but in Cicindelids the acrosome and centriole are juxtaposed; *Diptera* (Fig. 12) (BACCETTI and BAIRATI, 1964, 1965; MEYER, 1964; YASUZUMI, FUJIMURA and ISHIDA, 1958) in which sperm of some mosquitoes have a 9+9+1 pattern (BRELAND, GASSNER III, RIESS and BIESELE, 1966; PHILLIPS, 1969), and where a strong deviation is well known in the giant sperm of *Sciara* (PHILLIPS, 1966; 1967); and *Hymenoptera* (LORD ROTSCHILD, 1955; WILKES and LEE, 1965; THOMPSON and BLUM, 1967; HOAGE and KESSEL, 1968).

In this category, *Trichoptera* (Fig. 13) have the typical characteristics of the 9+9+2 axonemal pattern with outer accessory fibers, 200 Å thick, and composed of proteins and glycogen (BACCETTI, BIGLIARDI, DALLAI and ROSATI, 1969); *Lepidoptera*, a closely related order, have outer fibers of the same type (BACCETTI, BIGLIARDI, DALLAI and ROSATI, 1969), and 10–12 longitudinal cristae (ANDRÉ, 1962) produced by nuclear material (YASUZUMI and OURA, 1964, 1965) and surrounding the greater part of the sperm. Two species of *Trichoptera* have a curious, aberrant 9+7 spermatozoon, devoid of crystalline mitochondrial derivatives (PHILLIPS, 1969).

The " 9+2 " endopterygote class (Fig. 14) includes *Aphaniptera* (BACCETTI, 1968; PHILLIPS, 1969) and *Mecoptera* (BACCETTI, DALLAI and ROSATI, (1969). Both have coiled sperm, with only one well developed mitochondrial derivative. In *Panorpa* the flagellum arises cranially, under the acrosome and it is first coiled around the nucleus and subsequently around the mitochondrion.

In all these cases, differences between orders, families and species are also determined by the ratio of the lengths of the head and the tail, and by the evolution of the mitochondrial derivative (they are single not only in the 9+2 sperm, but also in some *Lepidoptera* and *Diptera* as well). It is very difficult to justify the 9+2 pattern in two close orders of *Endopterygota*; an independent origin from some 9+2 insect ancestors can be suggested. The difference between *Lepidoptera-Trichoptera* outer fibers, and these of the other *Endopterygota* orders, suggests, too, a particular evolution of the first two orders. Using some other important phylogenetical characteristics as the structure of the larvae, we suspect that *Trichoptera* and *Lepidoptera* originate from the Mecopteran stock. We can now propose an evolutive line from *Collembola*, through *Thysanura*, *Esopterygota* to *Neuroptera-Coleoptera* etc., and another from *Collembola* (or others ancestors) through *Mecoptera-Aphaniptera* to *Trichoptera-Lepidoptera*.

A general survey of the sperm structure in the phylum *Arthropoda* demonstrates some essential features. First: the basic 9+2 arrangement of the flagellum is not efficient for the internal fertilization out of the aqueous medium. Second: the penetration into the ovum requires very specific acrosome structures, which are absolutely different in all the species studied. The first proposition implies that in all the classes separate evolutionary lines arose from the primitive stock, encompassing the " encysted " situation in some sperm maintaining the " 9+2 " (or " 9+3 ") pattern (as in spiders, Myriapods, Collembols), or the acquirement of different motile processes, and progressive loss of axial filament complex (as, in different, ways, in the highest *Crustacea*, in *Acarina*, and in *Esopterygota* Insects, the Coccids), or the utilisation of particular spermathecae (as in the highest Diplopods, and in some insects) or, finally, the acquirement of the 9 outer accessory fibers, typical to the Arthropodan species better adapted to the life in the air, parallely acquired in other high animal phyla of similar ecological requirements.

The problem of acrosome evolution is more complicated and less clear. In all the classes we find several solutions, and it is very difficult (with the exception of Decapods sperms) to propose a phylogenetical interpretation. Acrosome evolution is surely linked to the evolution of the ovum, and the two points should perhaps be studied together.

References

Anderson W. A. and Ellis R. A. (1968) – *Acrosome morphogenesis in* Lumbricus terrestris. « Zeit. Zellforsch. », 85, 398–407.

André J. (1959) – *Étude au microscope électronique de l'évolution du chondriome pendant la spermatogenèse du Scorpion* Euscorpius flavicaudis. « J. Ultrastruct. Res. », 2, 288–308.

André J. (1961) – *Sur quelques détails nouvellemente connus de l'ultrastructure des organites vibratiles.* « J. Ultrastruc. Res. », 5, 86–108.

André J. (1962) – *Contribution à la connaissance du chondriome. Étude de ses modifications ultrastructurales pendant la spermatogénèse.* « J. Ultrastruct. Res. », supp. 3, 185 pgs..

André J. (1963) – *Some aspects of specialization in sperm.* « General Physiology of Cell Specialization » Mazia and Tyler Ed., McGraw Hill, 91–115.

André J. (1965) – *A propos d'une leçon sur la Limule.* « Ann. Sci. Clermont-Ferrand », 26, 27–38.

Baccetti B. (1968) – *Lo spermatozoo degli Artropodi. V. Aphaniptera.* « Redia », 51, 153–158.

Baccetti B. and Bairati jr. A. (1964) – *Indagini comparative sull'ultrastruttura delle cellule germinali maschili in* Dacus oleae *Gmel. ed in* Drosophila melanogaster *Meig* (*Ins. Dipt.*). « Redia », 49, 1–29.

BACCETTI B., BIGLIARDI E., DALLAI R. and ROSATI F. (1969) – *The outer «coarse» fibers in the axial filament complex of Insect spermatozoa.* « J. Microsc. », 8, 32 a–33 a.

BACCETTI B., DALLAI R. and GIUSTI F. (1969) – *The spermatozoon of Arthropoda.* VI. *Ephemeroptera.* « J. Ultrastruct Res. », 29, 343–349.

BACCETTI B., DALLAI R. and ROSATI F. (1969) – *The spermatozoon of Arthropoda.* III. *The lowest Holometabolic Insects.* « J. Microsc. », 8, 233–248.

BACCETTI B., DALLAI R. and ROSATI F. (1969) – *The spermatozoon of Arthropoda.* IV. *Corrodentia, Mallophaga and Thysanoptera.* « J. Microsc. », 8, 249–262.

BAIRATI jr. A. and BACCETTI B. (1964) – *Observations on the ultrastructure of the male germ cells of* Drosophila melanogaster *and* Dacus oleae. Electron Microsc., Proc. III. European Reg. Conf., Prague, B, 441–442.

BAWA S. R. (1964) – *Electron microscope study of spermiogenesis in a fire-brat insect,* Thermobia domestica *Pack.* « J. Cell Biol. », 23, 431–446.

BOISSIN L. and MANIER J. F. (1966) – *Spermatogenèse d'*Hysterochelifer meridianus (*L. Koch*) (*Arachnide, Pseudoscorpion, Cheliferidae*). II. *Étude de l'évolution du chondriome.* « Bull. Soc. Zool. France », 91, 697–706.

BOISSIN L. and MANIER J. F. (1967) – *Spermatogenèse d'*Hysterochelifer meridianus (*L. Koch*) (*Arachnide, Pseudoscorpion, Cheliferidae*). III. *Évolution de l'appareil de Golgi.* « Bull. de la Soc. Zoologique de France », 92, 705.

BRELAND O. P., GASSNER G., RIESS R. W. and BIESELE J. J. (1966) – *Certain aspects of the centriole adjunct, spermiogenesis, and the mature sperm of insects.* « Canad. J. Genet. Cytol. », 8, 759–773.

BREUCKER H. and HORSTMANN E. (1968) – *Die Spermatozoen der Zecken* Ornithodorus moubata (*Murr*). « Zeit. Zellforsch. », 88, 1–22.

BROWN G. G. (1966 a) – *Ultrastructural studies of sperm morphology and sperm–egg interaction in the Decapod* Callinectes sapidus. « J. Ultrastr. Res. », 14, 425–440.

BROWN G. G. (1966 b) – *Ultrastructural studies of crustacean spermatozoa and fertilization.* « Doctoral Diss. Univ. of Miami, Coral Gables, Florida », 239 pgs.

BROWN G. G. and METZ C. B. (1967) – *Ultrastructural studies on the spermatozoa of two primitive Crustaceans* Hutschinsoniella macrocantha *and* Derocheilocaris typicus. « Zeit. Zellforsch. », 80, 78–92.

DALLAI R. (1967) – *Lo spermatozoo degli Artropodi.* I. Anurida maritima (*Guérin*) *ed* Orchesella villosa (*Geoffroy*) (*Insecta, Collembola*). « Atti Accad. Fisiocritici, Siena », 16, 468–476.

FAIN-MAUREL M. A. (1966) – *Contribution a l'histologie et a la caryologie de quelques Isopodes. Spermiogenèse et infrastructure du spermatozoide des Oniscidés et des Cymothoïdés.* « Ann. Sci. Natur., Zool. », Paris, 12 ser. 8, 1–188.

FOLLIOT R. (1968) – *Les lamelles annelées intranucléaires des cellules du tissu germinal mâle avant la méiose chez* Philaenus spumarius *L.* (*Insecte Homoptère*). « Zeit. Zellforsch. », 92, 115–129.

FURIERI P. (1963 a) – *Aspetti morfologici della spermiogenesi di* Oryctes grypus *Illig.* « Redia », 48, 29–40.

FURIERI P. (1963 b) – *Osservazioni preliminari sulla ultrastruttura dello spermio di* Pyrrhocoris apterus *Fall.* (*Hemiptera, Pyrrhocoridae*). « Redia », 48, 179–187.

GUPTA B. L. (1968) – *Aspects of motility in the non-flagellate spermatozoa of fresh water ostracods.* In « *Aspects of Cell Motility* », 22, « Symp. Soc. Exp. Biology », 117–129.

HEROLD F. and MUNZ K. (1967) – *Ultrastructure of spermatozoa of* Peregrinus maidis (*Homoptera, Delphacidae*). « Zeit. Zellforsch. », 83, 364–374.

HOAGE T. R. and KESSEL R. G. (1968) – *An electron microscope study of the process of differentiation during spermatogenesis in the drone honey bee* (Apis mellifera *L.*) *with special reference to centriole replication and elimination.* « J. Ultrastr. Res. », 24, 6–32.

HORSTMANN E. (1968) – *Die Spermatozoen von* Geophilus linearis *Koch* (*Chilopoda*). « Zeit. Zellforsch. », 89, 410–429.

HORSTMANN E. and BREUCKER H. (1969) – *Spermatozoen und Spermiohistogenese von* Graphidostreptus *spec.* (*Myriapoda, Diplopoda*). I. *Die reifen Spermatozoen.* « Zeit. Zellforsch. », 96, 505–520.

ITO S. (1966) – *Movement and structure of louse spermatozoa.* « J. Cell. Biol. », 31, 128 A.

KAYE Y. S. (1964) – *The fine structure of flagella in spermatids of the house cricket.* « J. Cell Biol. », 23, 710–714.

KESSEL R. G. (1966) – *The association between microtubules and nuclei during spermiogenesis in the Dragonfly.* « J. Ultrastruc. Res. », 16, 293–304.

KESSEL R. G. (1967) – *An electron microscope study of spermiogenesis in the grasshopper with particular reference to the development of microtubular systems during differentiation.* « J. Ultrastruc. Res. », 18, 677–694.

LE MENN M. R. (1966) – *Observations sur la spermiogenèse et le spermatozoide des Psyllides (Homoptera Psylloidea).* « C. R. Acad. Sc. Paris », 262, 1731–1733.

METZ C. B. (1967) – *Gamete surface components and their role in fertilization.* In: C. Metz and A. Monroy: « Fertilization ». Academic Press, New York and London, 163–236.

MEYER G. F. (1964) – *Die parakristallinen koerper in der Spermienschwanzen von* Drosophila. « Zeit. Zellforsch. », 62, 762–784.

MOSES M. J. (1961) – *Spermiogenesis in the crayfish* (Procambarus clarkii). I. *Structural characterization of the mature sperm.* « J. Biophys. Biochem. Cytol. », 9, 222–228.

PAYNE F. (1966) – *Some observations on spermatogenesis on* Gelastocoris oculatus (*Hemiptera*) *with the aid of the electron microscope.* « J. Morph. », 119, 357–382.

PHILLIPS D. M. (1966) – *Fine structure of* Sciara coprophila *sperm.* « J. Cell Biology », 30, 499–517.

PHILLIPS D. M. (1966) – *Observations on spermiogenesis in the fungus gnat* Sciara coprophila. « J. Cell Biol. », 30, 477–497.

PHILLIPS D. M. (1967) – *Giant centriole formation in* Sciara. « J. Cell Biol. », 33, 73–92.

PHILLIPS D. M. (1969) – *Exceptions to the prevailing Pattern of Tubules* ($9 + 9 + 2$) *in the sperm flagella of certain insect species.* « J. Cell Biol. », 40, 28–43.

POCHON-MASSON J. (1968) – *L'ultrastructure des Spermatozoïdes vésiculaires chez les Crustacés Décapodes avant et au cours de leur dévagination expérimentale.* I. *Brachyoures et Anomoures.* « Ann. Sc. Nat., Zoologie, Paris », 10, 1–100.

POCHON-MASSON J. (1968) – *L'ultrastructure des Spermatozoïdes vésiculaires chez les Crustacés Décapodes avant et au cours de leur dévagination expérimentale* II. *Macroures. Discussion et conclusions.* « Ann. Sc. Naturelles, Zoologie, Paris », 10, 367–454.

REGER J. F. (1963) – *Spermiogenesis in the tick,* Amblyomma dissimili, *as revealed by electron microscopy.* « J. Ultrastruct Res. », 8, 607–621.

REGER J. F. (1964 a) – *The fine structure of spermatozoa from the Isopod* Asellus militaris *Hay.* « J. Ultrastruct Res. », 11, 181–192.

REGER J. F. (1964 b) – *A study on the fine structure of developing spermatozoa from the Isopod* Asellus militaris, *Hay.* « J. Microsc. », 3, 559–572.

REGER J. F. and COOPER D. P. (1968) – *Studies on the fine structure of spermatids and spermatozoa from the millipede* Polydesmus *sp.* « J. Ultrastruc. Res. », 23, 60–70.

ROBISON G. W. (1966) – *Microtubules in relation to the mobility of a sperm syncytium in an armored scale insect.* « J. Cell Biol. », 29, 251–265.

ROSATI F. (1967) – *Lo spermatozoo degli Artropodi.* II. Blaberus craniifer (*Insecta Blattoidea*). « Boll. Zool. », 34, 167.

ROSATI F., BACCETTI B. and DALLAI R. (1970) – *The spermatozoon of Arthropoda.* X. *Araneids and the lowest Myriapods. This Symposium.*

ROSS J. and ROBISON Jr. W. G. (1969) – *Unusual microtubular patterns and three-dimensional movement of mealybug sperm and sperm bundles.* « J. Cell Biol. », 40, 426–445.

ROTHSCHILD LORD (1955) – *The spermatozoa of the Honey-bee.* « Trans. R. Entom. Soc. London », 107, 289–294.

SHAY J. W. & BIESELE J. J. (1968) – *Ultrastructural observations on spermiogenesis in the cave cricket* Ceuthophilus secretus (*Scudder*). « La cellule », 67, 269–282.

THOMPSON T. E. and BLUM M. S. (1967) – *Structure and behavior of spermatozoa in the fire ant* Solenopsis laevissima (*Hymenoptera: Formicidae*). « Ann. Ent. Soc. America », 60, 632–642.

TUZET O. and MANIER J. F. (1955) – *Achèvement de la spermiogenèse dans les voies génitales femelles: cas de* Polyxenus lucidus *Chalande* (*Myriapode Diplopode*). « Ann. Sci. Nat., Zool. », 17, 351–356.

WERNER G. (1964) – *Untersuchungen ueber die Spermiogenese beim Silberfischen,* Lepisma saccharina *L.* « Zeit. Zellforsch. », 63, 880–912.

WERNER G. (1965) – *Untersuchungen ueber die Spermiogenese beim Sandlaufer,* Cicindela campestris *L.* « Zeit. Zellforsch. », 66, 255–275.

WERNER G. (1966) – *Untersuchungen ueber die Spermiogenese bei einem Laufkafer,* Carabus catenulatus *Scop., und der Skorpion–Wasserwanze,* Nepa rubra *L.* « Zeit. Zellforsch. », 73, 576–599.

WILKES A. and LEE P. E. (1965) – *The ultrastructure of dimorphic spermatozoa in the Hymenopteron* Dahlbominus fuscipennis (*Zett.*) (*Eulophidae*). « Canad. J. Genet. Cytol. », 7, 609–619.

YASUZUMI G., FUJMURA W. and ISHIDA H. (1958) – *Spermatogenesis in animals as revealed by electron microscopy. V. Spermatid differentiation of* Drosophila *and Grasshopper.* « Exper. Cell Res. », 14, 268–285.

YASUZUMI G. and OURA C. (1964) – *Spermatogenesis in Animals as revealed by Electron Microscopy.* XIII. *Formation of a tubular structure and two bands in the developing spermatid of the Silkworm,* Bombyx mori *L.* « Zeit. Zellforsch. », 64, 210–226.

YASUZUMI G. and OURA C. (1965) – *Spermatogenesis in animals as revealed by electron microscope.* XV. *The fine structure of the middle piece in the developing spermatid of the silkworm,* Bombyx mori *Linné.* « Zeit. Zellforsch. », 67, 502–520.

ZISSLER D. (1969) – *Die Spermiohistogenese des Subwasser–Ostracoden* Notodromas monacha *O. F. Müller. I. Die ovalen and spindelformigen Spermatiden.* « Zeit. Zellforsch. », 96, 87–105.

ZISSLER D. (1969) – *Die Spermiohistogenese des Subwasser–Ostracoden* Notodromas monacha *O. F. Müller* II. *Die Spindelformigen und schlauchformigen Spermatiden.* « Zeit. Zellforsch. », 96, 106–133.

EXPLANATION OF FIGURES

Fig. 1. – Cross section of the sperm tail in a Tardigrad, *Macrobiotus hufelandii.* ×30,000.

Fig. 2. – Cross section of the sperm tail in a Merostomata, *Xiphosura polyphemus.* ×90,000.

Fig. 3. – Cross section of different levels of head and tail in an encysted sperm of a Spider, *Pholcus phalangioides.* ×90,000.

Fig. 4. – Cross section of the sperm tail in a Pauropod, *Allopauropus* sp. ×60,000.

Fig. 5. – Cross section of the tail in the two kinds of spermatozoa in a Symphyle, *Symphylella vulgaris.* ×60,000.

Fig. 6. – Cross section of different levels of the tail in an encysted sperm of a Collembol, *Anurida maritima.* ×90,000.

Fig. 7. – Cross section of the sperm tail in a Phasmid, *Bacillus rossius.* ×60,000.

Fig. 8. – Cross section of the sperm tail in an Embiopterous, *Haploembia solierii.* ×60,000.

Fig. 9. – Cross section of the sperm tail in an *Ephemeroptera, Cloeon dipterum.* ×120,000.

Fig. 10. – Cross section of the sperm tail in a *Mallophaga, Menopon gallinae.* ×60,000.

Fig. 11. – Cross section of the sperm tail in a *Neuroptera, Chrysopa carnea.* ×90,000.

Fig. 12. – Cross section of the sperm tail in a *Diptera, Ceratitis capitata.* ×90,000.

Fig. 13. – Cross section of the sperm tail in a *Trichoptera, Mystacides azurea.* ×60,000.

Fig. 14. – Cross section of the sperm tail in a *Mecoptera, Panorpa annexa.* ×90,000.

Fig. 15. – Longitudinal section of the spermatozoon in an Opilionid, *Phalangium* sp. ×60,000.

Discussion

AFZELIUS. – This is a case of what IRENE MANTON yesterday called " sweeping generalizations based on sperm morphology " but it is surprising to see how well your data can be arranged. With respect to the situation of the *Mecoptera* I can add that I have looked on another species, *Boreus hiemalis*, and its spermatozoon has a 9+2 sperm tail, just as you would like it.

FRANZEN. – I would like to know what the term " normal mitochondria " among the lowest Arthropods means.

BACCETTI. – Mitochondria with cristae and without crystalline material.

FRANZEN. – Are there any indications of an aggregation of mitochondrial materials around the proximal part of the flagellum among the lowest Arthropods as in Annelids?

BACCETTI. – In very few cases, as *Limulus*.

FRANZEN. – Is it possible to speak about a middle piece among Arthropods?

BACCETTI. – No, in my opinion, because mitochondria are often present throughout the whole tail.

BROWN. – In my opinion the *Crustacea* should be split into two major groups with reference to the sperm structures. The Mystacocarid represent one group (*Mystacocarida*, *Cirripedia*, *Branchiura* and *Copepoda*) and the Cephalocarid another group (*Cephalocarida*, *Branchiopoda* and *Malacostraca*). Your work strongly supports that of FRANZÉN in the sense that a primitive sperm is found in conditions where gametes are shed into the medium. In all Arthropods, except *Limulus*, there is some form of accessory reproductive structures. This to me implies that in the Arthropod as the reproductive system becomes more complicated, so does the sperm.

MEYER. – Do you have any suggestions on the physiological significance of the transformation of the mitochondria into crystalline material? Is the transformation restricted to Insects?

BACCETTI. – We are studying this point by biochemical methods, but I have no ideas at present. I think that Molluscs have a comparable situation.

B. BACCETTI – *The spermatozoon of Arthropoda. IX. The sperm cell as an index of arthropod phylogenesis.*

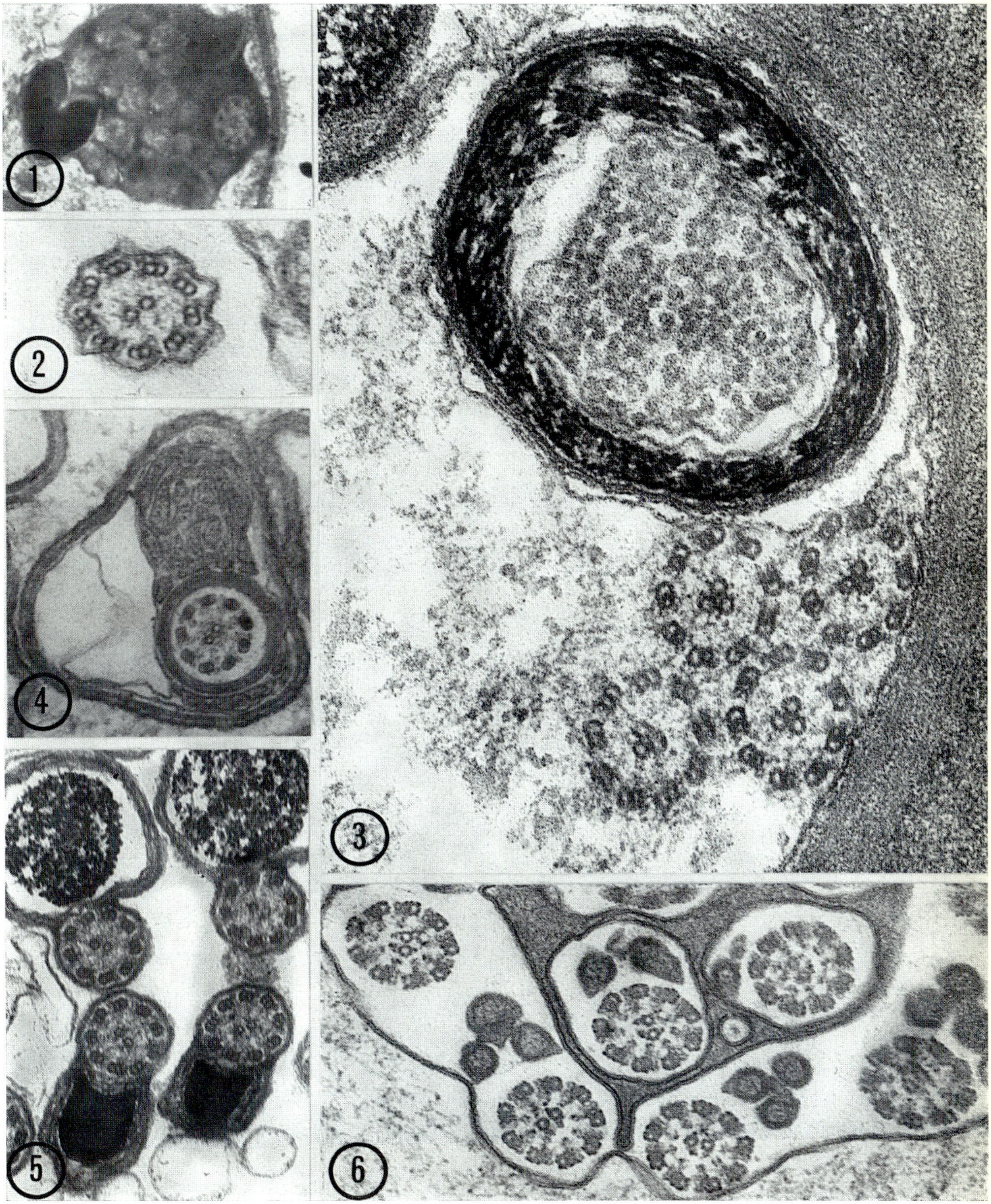

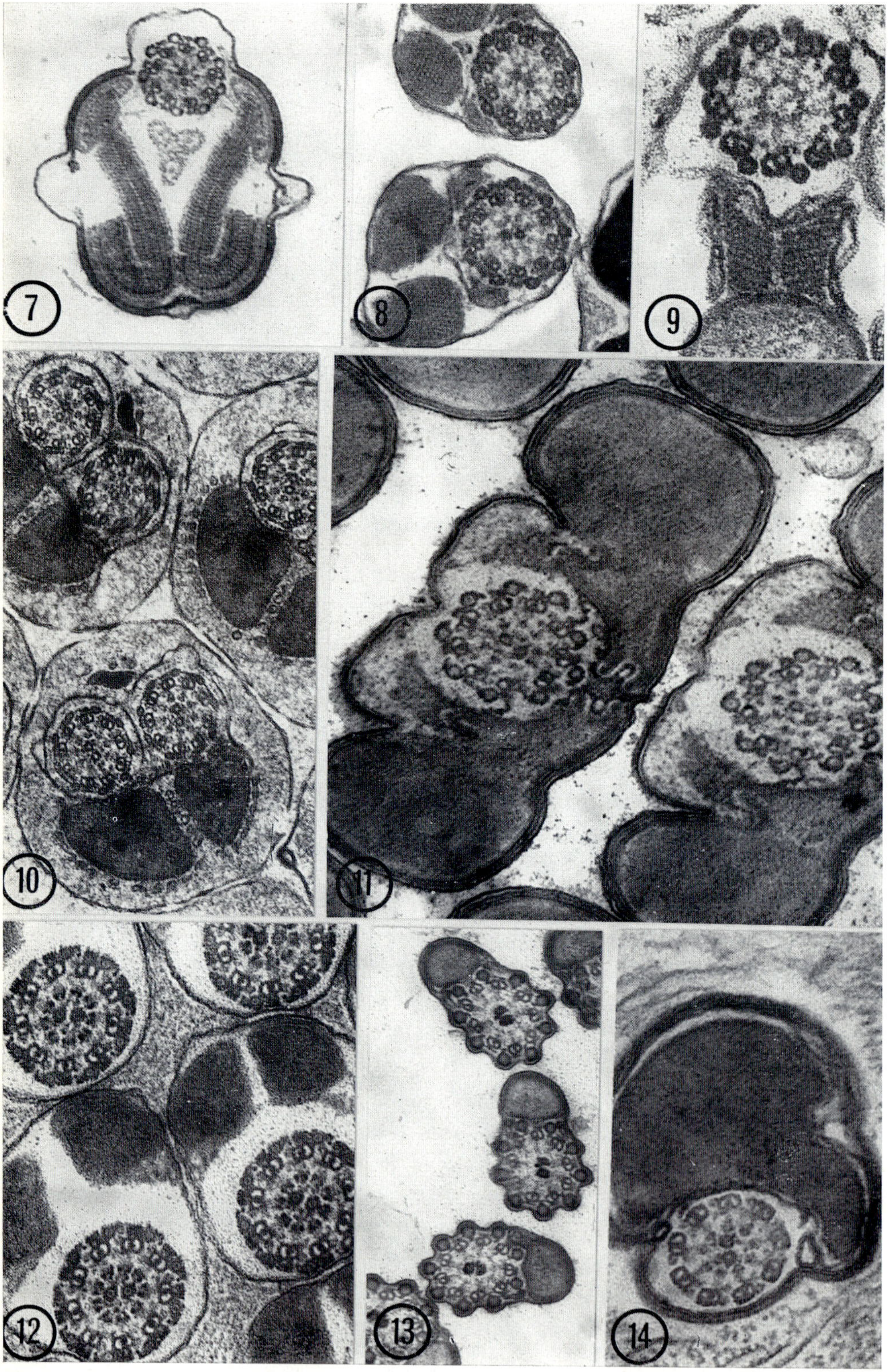
7
8
9
10
11
12
13
14

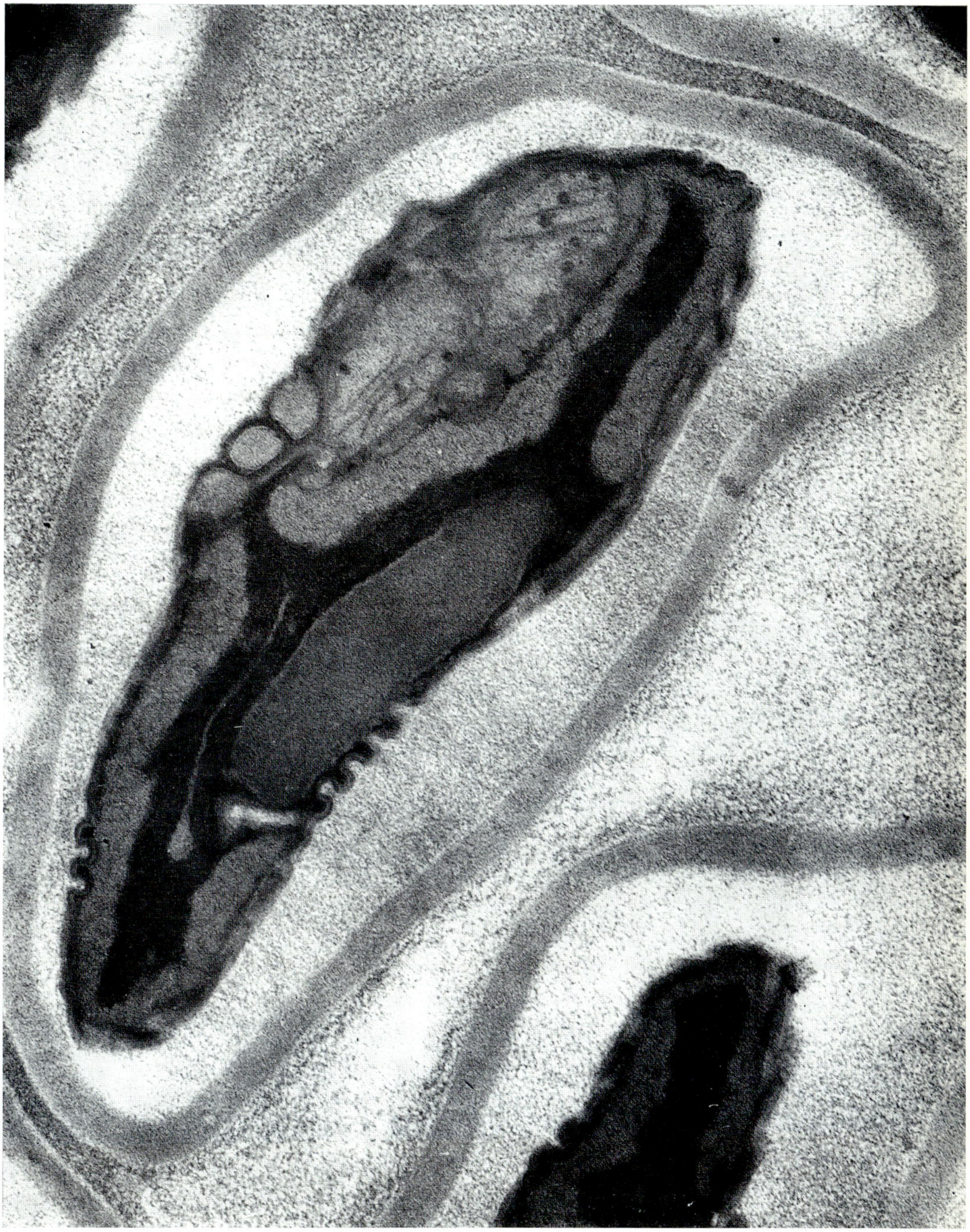

Fig. 15.

George Gordon Brown (*)

SOME COMPARATIVE ASPECTS OF SELECTED CRUSTACEAN SPERMATOZOA AND CRUSTACEAN PHYLOGENY

Summary. — The spermatozoa of five species, *Artemia salina*, *Chthalamus fragilis*, *Lepas sp*, *Calanus hyperboreus*, and *Argulus sp*, representing four crustacean subclasses were examined by light and electron microscopy, and by various cytochemical studies. This work plus the published accounts (and those in preparation) of crustacean sperm morphology, were combined in order to compare spermatozoa within and between subclasses. These studies revealed that each subclass is represented by unique spermatozoa.

This comparative study emphasizes the value of sperm morphology in determining phylogenetic relationships, based on the presence, absence, and modification of the sperm structures (acrosome, nucleus, mitochondrion, and flagellum). The Class Crustacea is separated into two groups with respect to flagellated and nonflagellated spermatozoa. Mystacocarida, Cirripedia, and Branchiura have flagellated spermatozoa. Those of Cephalocarida, Branchiopoda, and Malacostraca are nonflagellated. The Subclass Copepoda also has nonflagellated spermatozoa, but since the other copepod sperm structures appear similar to those of the first group, it is reasonable to include them. These groups fully agree with taxonomical separation.

Riassunto. — Gli spermatozoi di cinque specie, *Artemia salina*, *Chthalamus fragilis*, *Lepas* sp, *Calanus hyperboreus*, e *Argulus* sp, rappresentanti quattro sottoclassi di crostacei, sono stati esaminati con il microscopio ottico ed elettronico, e con varie analisi citochimiche. Questo lavoro, oltre a quelli pubblicati (e a quelli in preparazione) sulla morfologia degli spermatozoi dei crostacei, ha lo scopo di confrontare gli spermatozoi in e tra le sottoclassi. Questi studi rivelano che ciascuna sottoclasse è rappresentata da un unico spermatozoo.

Lo studio comparativo sottolinea il valore della morfologia degli spermi nella determinazione di relazioni filogenetiche, basate sulla presenza, assenza, e modificazioni delle strutture spermatiche (acrosoma, nucleo, mitocondri e flagello). La classe dei Crostacei è divisa in due gruppi rispetto agli spermatozoi flagellati e non flagellati. I Mistacocaridi, i Cirripedi, e i Brachiuri hanno spermatozoi flagellati. Quelli dei Cefalocaridi, Brachiopodi, e Malacostraci sono aflagellati. Anche la sottoclasse dei Copepodi ha spermatozoi aflagellati, ma poiché le altre strutture degli spermatozoi dei Copepodi sono simili a quelle del primo gruppo, è ragionevole includerli in questo. Questi gruppi concordano completamente con la separazione tassonomica.

Introduction

In general, the crustacean spermatozoa are atypical and bizarre (Retzius, 1909; Wilson, 1928). As a result in many instances these spermatozoa have been considered the exception to the conventional sperm and have been primarily ignored. This is particularly true since the voluminous studies of Retzius (1909) with the notable exceptions of the Decapoda (cf. Bloch,

(*) Department of Zoology and Entomology Iowa State University Ames, Iowa.

1935; NATH, 1942) and a few other groups (e.g. Branchiopoda, FAUTREZ–FIRLEFYN and FAUTREZ, 1955; Ostracoda, LOWNDES, 1936; Copopeda, HERBE-ERR, 1932, 1937, 1955). With the advent of the electron microscope, renewed interest has developed in the Crustacean spermatozoa. However, again the majority of the work has been with the Decapoda (cf. BROWN, 1966; POCHON–MASSON, 1968) with several exceptions (cfr. Isopoda, REGER, 1964; Copopeda, GUPTA, pers. comm.; Ostracoda, ZISSLER, 1969). Since an investigation of the spermatozoa of the various crustacean subclasses is needed the author has undertaken ultrastructural examination of spermatozoa from several representatives. These include species from each of the eight subclasses with the exception of the Ostracoda. Several of these studies have been published or are in preparation. They include a comparative investigation of spermatozoa of the two primitive subclasses Cephalocarida and Mystacocarida (BROWN and METZ, 1967) a study of the branchiopod *Artemia salina* sperm morphology (in preparation), and a comparative study of decapod spermatozoa (in preparation).

Interest in the crustacean spermatozoa began in the first part of the nineteenth century (HENLE, 1835; VON SIEBOLD, 1836, 1837; KOLLICKER, 1841, 1847). Although then as later, the greater emphasis was on the decapod spermatozoa, there were several observations made on other groups (cf. VON SIEBOLD, 1836; KOLLICKER, 1841). The filament shaped spermatozoa of certain of these groups (isopods, cirripeds, mysids) suggested to these workers that the flagellated sperm form was typical in the crustaceans. As a result, the stellate or " Strahlenzellen " forms of the decapod spermatozoa were considered immature. Not until the observations of LEUKART (1863) and OWSJANNIKOW (1869) were the stellate forms considered mature. These observations substantiated the concept of the unusual crustacean spermatozoa.

In the latter part of the nineteenth centure and early in the twentieth century, there was a major effort to further describe the various forms of crustacean spermatozoa by comparative and phylogenetic studies and to relate them to the more typical type of the animal sperm (SABATIER, 1897; GILSON, 1886; KOLTZOFF, 1906; GROBBEN, 1878, 1906). RETZIUS' (1909) well known and comprehensive works ended this very productive period.

Conventional spermatozoa have a basic form and consist of four components: acrosome, nucleus, mitochondrion, and flagellum (WILSON, 1928; TUZET, 1950; ANDRÉ, 1963). In the crustacean spermatozoa where one or more of these components may be absent (except nucleus) or radically changed from the conventional form, modification and specialization of the remaining organelles is observed. Thus in considering the crustacean spermatozoa in general, a complete array of forms and types exist. These include the amoeboid sperm of *Polyphemus pedicubes* (ZACHARIAS, 1884), the motile spermatozoa of the Cirripedia (KOLTZOFF, 1909), the non-motile filament-like sperm of isopods (REGER, 1964), the non-motile stellate forms of many decapods (cf. BLOCH, 1935), and the extremely long and large forms of ostracods (LOWNDES, 1936). Most of the studies have involved primarily descriptive aspects and very few functional aspects (e.g. sperm-egg interactions). Practically all functional studies treat the decapod " explosion " or acrosome reaction (cfr. BROWN, 1966). An exception is the " Physiologisher Spermiendualism " described by HERBERER (1955) in the copepod.

There are great varieties of crustacean spermatozoa and ultrastructural studies of modified organelles of some of these have already contributed to fertilization studies. For example, the specialized acrosomal region and the acrosome reaction of the *Callinectes* sperm have many features of spermatozoa of other phyla (BROWN, 1966). Ultrastructural studies of other crustacean spermatozoa may provide information on biological phenomena which are difficult to study with the conventional sperm.

With respect to phylogeny based on sperm morphology, attempts have been made in various groups (TUZET, 1950; FRANZEN, 1956; HUGHES, 1965; TOCHIMOTO, 1967; MCFARLANE, 1963). In this present study relationships are determined between the crustacean subclasses and other taxons based on the absence or presence, and modifications of such sperm organelles as nuclei, acrosomes, mitochondria, and flagella.

MATERIALS AND METHODS

The animals used in this study were obtained from the following sources:

Branchiopoda.

Specimens of *Artemia salina* Leach were raised from commercial cysts (Brine Shrimp Sales Company, Inc., Hayward, California).

Copepoda.

Specimens of *Calanus hyperboreus* were obtained from Dr. Robert Conover of the Woods Hole Oceanographic Institute. These were collected by Dr. Conover in the North Atlantic. Females were obtained in August, 1965, and males were obtained in November, 1965.

Branchiura.

Specimens of *Argulus sp* were collected from the surface of the garfish *Lepisosteus platyrhincus* Dekay kept in outdoor ponds at the Variety Childrens Research Center, Coral Gables, Florida, during Spring, 1967.

Cirripedia.

Specimens of *Chthalamus fragilis* Darwin were collected from rocks in the intertidal zone of Woods Hole, Massachusetts during the summer of 1965. Specimens of *Lepas sp* were collected from driftwood in Biscayne Bay, Dade County, Florida during November, 1965.

The testes and vas deferens were dissected from freshly killed males in the laboratory and when possible seminal receptacles were dissected from the female. These tissues were fixed for electron microscopical and paraffin studies. Additionally, squashed spermatophores, vas deferens, testes, or seminal receptacle were examined with phase-contrast optics to observe the living spermatozoa.

For electron microscopical studies the following fixation procedures were used:

1) 1% Osmium tetroxide (sea water) for one hour. pH 6.5.

2) 2.5% Glutaraldehyde and 2.5% acrolein (sea water) for one and a half hours and postfixed in 1% osmium tetroxide (sea water for one hour. pH 6.5.

3) 2.5% Glutaraldehyde (phosphate buffer and isotonically balanced in sodium chloride) for one to two hours and postfixed in 1% osmium tetroxide (phosphate buffer and isotonically balanced in sodium chloride) for one hour. pH 7.2.

4) Karnovshy's Formaldehyde–Glutaraldehyde (KARNOVSKY, 1965).

All tissues were dehydrated with ethyl alcohol, cleared with prophylene oxide, embedded in Araldite (Swiss, Fluka), sectioned on an LKB Ultrotome, counterstained with uranyl acetate (Watson, 1958) and lead citrate (REYNOLDS, 1963), and examined with the Philips 100 C, Philips 200, Hitaschi 11 C or Siemens Elmikskop Ia electron microscopes.

Tissues embedded for cytochemical studies were fixed with Carnoys Solution A (HUMASON, 1962, p. 16). The staining technique involved the Feulgen (HUMASON, 1962, p. 293) PAS (HUMASON, 1962, p. 298) and the Triple Stain (HIMES and MORIBER, 1956). Living spermatozoa were examined with Wild phase-contrast light optics.

OBSERVATIONS

Following are observations on spermatozoa of selected species from four crustacean subclasses: Branchiopoda, Cirripedia, Copepoda, and Branchiura. The accounts for the branchiopod *Artemia salina* sperm is notably brief since a more thorough work is in preparation.

Brachiopoda.

The spermatozoa of the anostracan *Artemia salina* were examined. In general the mature sperm is a non-motile spherical structure, approximately 5 micra in diameter, with a centrally located nucleus enclosed in a considerable amount of cytoplasm.

Spermatozoa were examined with phase-contrast in the vas deferens of the male animal in the dissected vas deferens, and finally in a free condition (Figs. 2 and 3). None were examined from the ovisac of the female. In the vas deferens the spermatozoa are packed in irregular shapes. From a dissected vas deferens, observed in the animal fluid on a microslide, the contraction of the vas deferens and gradual pressure on the coverslip forced spermatozoa free of this organ (Fig. 2). They were at first irregular in shape, but rapidly became more spherical. Also numerous arms or extensions were observed protruding from each sperm (Fig. 3). The highly refractive area is the periphery of the cell and stains positively for proteins (Napthol Yellow S). The central organelle is the nucleus since it is Feulgen positive. The diameter of the cell is approximately 5 micra and the arms have a length of approximately 5 to 10 micra. No motility was observed. No PAS positive structures were observed with cytochemical staining.

The complexity of the sperm structures certainly removed the *Artemia* sperm from the simple classification as is indicated by light optics on various branchiopods (RETZIUS, 1909; LONGHURST, 1956). The nucleus is irregularly shaped and possesses the typical nuclear envelope of double membranes (Fig. 1). A large proportion of the nucleus is heavily stained indicating a dense aggregation of nuclear material. Particularly unusual for mature spermatozoa is the large amount of cytoplasm found surrounding the nucleus. Scattered typical mitochondria, numerous endoplasmic reticula, and numerous vesicles (Fig. 1) are found within the cytoplasm. The slender arms observed with phase-contrast optics extend from the periphery of the cell. These are extensions of the cytoplasm and the plasma membrane. Their precise pattern around the cell is unknown but judging from the various micrographs and light optical studies, they appear to give the sperm a pin cushion effect. Since sperm-egg interactions were not studied, the functional aspects of the arms and other organelles can only be postulated.

Cirripedia.

The mature spermatozoa of the thoracian, *Chthalamus fragilis*, were examined with cytochemical and electron microscopical techniques. In addition, phase-contrast observations were made on the sperm of another thoracian, *Lepas sp.* In general, the sperm of these cirripeds is filiform and possesses a long head and a flagellum. The flagellum has an anterior origin, extends the length of the head, and projects posteriorly. Cytochemically, the long head is Feulgen positive, thus definitely the nucleus. There is no noticeable PAS–positive structure.

Phase-contrast observations were made on *Lepas sp* spermatozoa which were freed from a squashed vas deferens (Fig. 5). These were motile, but only in a vibratory manner. Occasionally, however, a sperm was observed moving rapidly across the field in a jerky but flagellated motion. The anterior end of such a sperm was usually folded back forming a loop (Fig. 6). The folded portion was usually the same length in the different spermatozoa observed, but this was not always the case. In some damaged spermatozoa, the flagellum was observed to be separated from the nucleus except at the anterior end of the sperm (Fig. 7).

Ultrastructurally, the nucleus, the flagellum, and the mitochondrial derivative of the *Chthalamus* sperm are examined (Fig. 4). No acrosomal structure is identified. The nucleus is quite large and occupies the bulk of the cell. The nuclear material is quite homogeneous in appearance. The nucleus is larger in diameter near the sperm anterior end and gradually tapers towards the posterior end (Fig. 4). The flagellum definitely has an axial unit tubular (9 plus 2) arrangement and extends the greater length of the sperm (Fig. 7). From the anterior attachment, the flagellum extends posteriorly on one side of the nucleus and becomes closely associated with the mitochondrial derivative near the posterior end of the nucleus (Fig. 4). The mitochondrial derivative extends parallel with the flagellum for a considerable distance.

Since the orientation of the flagellum based on the relationship of the cetral tubules has been considered in the mystacocarid sperm (Brown and

METZ, 1967) a brief observation will be included here. In various cross sections of the *Chthalamus* spermatozoa examined there is no exact orientation of the flagellum to the nucleus or mitochondrial derivative. This could indicate that the flagellum is spiral throughout the length of the sperm, a situation contrary to that found in the mystacocarid and branchiuran spermatozoa.

Several membranes can be resolved. The sperm plasma membrane is readily observed around the nucleus and flagellum. There appears to be a marked boundary on the nucleus but whether a nuclear envelope actually exists is not yet known. Membrane structures of the mitochondrian derivative have not been resolved. No centrioles or acrosomal structures were observed.

Copepoda.

Spermatozoa of the calanoid, *Calanus hyperboreus*, were examined with phase-contrast optics, cytochemical studies, and electron microscopy. Material was obtained from the male spermatophores and the female seminal receptacles. The nonmotile sperm is ovoid in shape (Fig. 10) and is approximately 5 to 6 micra in length.

Phase-contrast observations were made only on the intact and dissected seminal receptacle of the female. In the intact seminal receptacle the spermatozoa are observed packed together in an irregular fashion. Upon dissecting and squashing this organ, the spermatozoa were expelled into the medium. Unfortunately most ruptured, but several intact spermatozoa were examined. Released from the seminal receptacle, each sperm rounded into an ovoid shape (Fig. 10). These cells do not have any appendages and are not motile. There is a prominent organelle occupying the central bulk of the cell and several smaller organelles along the periphery. The prominent organelle is Feulgen positive, thus the nucleus.

In paraffin sections for cytochemical studies, the spermatophore in the male animal was thoroughly examined. This club shaped structure is approximately 200 micra in length and is similar to that of *Calanus finmarchius* (MARSHALL and ORR, 1955). The contents consist of an outer cylinder of densely packed spermatozoa and a central core of PAS positive material.

In ultrastructural studies, spermatozoa in the spermatophore and in the seminal receptacle were examined. Although these spermatozoa from both sources were very similar in structural aspects, those in the seminal receptacle were not satisfactorily fixed. As a result all ultrastructural examinations were made on the spermatozoa in the spermatophore.

The ultrastructure of this copepod sperm resembles no other crustacean sperm examined in this and other studies. Most of the organelles appear unique. Within the club shaped spermatophore the spermatozoa are packed in an orderly cylindrical fashion surrounding a PAS positive core composed of large granules. These spermatozoa have an irregular disc-shape with the large nucleus occupying the central bulk and the perimeter bounded with various organelles, particularly mitochondria (Figs. 8 and 9). The entire cell is uniformly bounded by a thick homogenous layer (Fig. 8). With osmium tetroxide the nuclear material has a diffused stranded pattern (Fig. 9) which appears very much like that of the crayfish, *Procambarus clarkii*, sperm (MOSES, 1961). However, with acrolein-glutaraldehyde fixation the nucleus has an extensive fibrous appearance (Fig. 8).

The perimeter of the disc contains an extensive array of membranes, many of which resembly mitochondria (Fig. 8). Also present in the perimeter is a thick dense staining, layer-like organelle which extends for a considerable distance (Figs. 9 and 10). A dense staining band which completely surrounds the entire cell lies adjacent to the nucleus and the described organelles. An outer unit membrane is resolved beyond this dense band. This represents the plasma membrane. There is no definitely resolved nuclear envelope. Finally, there is no evidence of a flagellum or centrioles. No defined acrosomal structures are present. It is quite obvious that spermatogenesis and fertilization studies must be carried out to determine the origins and functions of the various organelles.

Branchiura.

Spermatozoa of *Argulus sp.* were examined with phase-contrast optics, with certain cytochemical studies, and with electron microscopy. These examinations were made on sesticular, seminal vesicle, and seminal receptacle material. This branchiura sperm is filiform, thin, and approximately 350 micra in length.

Observations of mature spermatozoa from the seminal vesicle of the male and the seminal receptacle of the female were made with phase-contrast optics. The following observations are from a squashed seminal receptacle. The spermatozoa are motile and in some cases quite violently so but usually only a vibratory motion was observed. The sperm is thread-like with no noticeable structure such as a head. A spiral shape (Fig. 12) extends the entire length and frequently is more pronounced at one end. Whether the spiral is sinistral or dextral has not been determined. The motility is throughout the entire length. The general shape and action as described is not unlike that of several insect spermatozoa (WERNER, 1964, 1965; JACOB, 1959; WILKES and LEE, 1965; BAWA, 1964). No cytochemical studies were made.

Ultrastructurally, mature spermatozoa were examined primarily in the male seminal vesicle and testes, but those in the female seminal receptacle were also briefly examined. Various organelles such as the nucleus, mitochondria, and the flagellum are readily observed. Also resolved is a unique trough–shaped structure which extends the entire length of the sperm (Fig. 11). Presently no correlation of this structure can be made to an acrosome or any other sperm structure. In general, the arrangement of the mentioned organelles in cross sections is as follows: the nucleus, a row of three mitochondria, the flagellum, and the trough-shaped structure; adjacent to the mitochondrial row is a dorso-ventrally flattened organelle. All of the organelles extend for the greater part of the sperm.

The nucleus is an extremely narrow structure of approximately 0.3 micron at its widest point (Fig. 11). It extends almost the entire length of the sperm. The nuclear material contains light and dense areas.

Adjacent to the nucleus are three separate mitochondria aligned in a horizontal row. These structures each are enclosed by double membranes (Fig. 11) and typical mitochondrian cristae are resolved. In close proximity to the mitochondria is the flagellum with the axial unit tubular (9 plus 2) arrangement. This structure and the mitochondria extend the greater length of the sperm. The similarity and arrangement of these structures plus the nucleus also resembles that of several insect spermatozoa (WERNER, 1964, 1965). The parallel orientation of the two central flagellar microtubules with the row of mitochondria is the same throughout the various cross sections (Fig. 11).

The most obvious organelle is also the unique feature of the *Argulus* sperm. This structure is trough-shaped, homogenous appearing, and surrounds approximately half of the flagellum (Fig. 11). It extends the full length of the sperm and is the only organelle present at both ends of the sperm. Since studies of spermatogenesis and fertilization have not been made, the origin and function of this structure cannot be determined. Except for its length, the position of this structure is very similar to the acrosomes of *Lepisma* (WERNER, 1964) and *Cicindella* (WERNER, 1965) spermatozoa.

The lateral organelles are adjacent of each side of the mitochondria row (Fig. 11). They are homogenous, slab-like organelles approximately 0.5 micron at the greatest width and appear to extend a considerable length of each sperm. In several cases these lateral organelles are observed on both of the sperm, but in most cases only one is seen. This implies, however, that one of these organelles extends from each end of the sperm and is on opposite sides. Therefore in the sperm middle part, they overlap. This sperm certainly deserves more study, if for no other reason than its similarity to the spermatozoa of the primitive insects.

DISCUSSION AND CONCLUSIONS

Since this study covers a variety of biological aspects, the discussion is divided into two major portions. They are (1) sperm ultrastructure and comparative aspect of the crustacean spermatozoa and (2) sperm morphology and crustacean phylogeny.

Sperm Ultrastructure and Comparative Aspects of the Crustacean Spermatozoa.

The tremendous diversity of the forms of crustacean spermatozoa has been clearly shown in the preceding observations and other studies (BROWN and METZ, 1967). Comparing these with observations in other studies including light and electron microscopy, there are some interesting comparisons of spermatozoa within and between the various crustacean subclasses and with spermatozoa from other animal groups. In this section, some of these comparisons are indicated. Unfortunately, little comparative work on crustacean spermatozoa and only a few electron microscopical studies are recorded in the literature.

Cephalocarida.

Three genera of this subclass have been described. All are included in the same family. The only sperm observations are those presented in the study on *Hutchinsoniella macracantha* (BROWN and METZ, 1967). In view of the close relationship of the known cephalocarids, it is likely that their spermatozoa are similar to the *Hutchinsoniella* sperm. However, the few species and the primitiveness of this subclass (SANDERS, 1963) warrants examining the spermatozoa of the other genera. This is particularly true since the *Hutchinsoniella* sperm is nonflagellated and certain other crustacean spermatozoa are flagelated. With the exception of the flagellum and the absence of mitochondria, general features of the *Hutchinsoniella* sperm are roughly similar to several flagellated spermatozoa of various groups other than Crustacea, i.e., *Limulus* (ANDRÉ, 1963) and *Mytilus* (NIIJIMA and DAN, 1965).

Mystacocarida.

This subclass is presently represented by one genus and three species. Thus as in the cephalocarids the *Derocheilocaris typicus* sperm is probably a typical mystacocarid sperm.

The *Derocheilocaris* sperm is small and possesses the typical sperm organelles including acrosome, nucleus, mitochondria, and flagellum (BROWN and METZ, 1967). The general features, particularly the anterior origin of the flagellum and the elongated nucleus, are represented in spermatozoa of several groups, most notably, the cirripeds (*Chthalamus*) and the branchiurans (*Argulus*) examined in the present study, several insects (*Lepisma*, *Cicindela*, WERNER, 1964, 1965; *Thermobia*, BAWA, 1965), and in some flatworms (SILVERIA and PORTER, 1965).

Branchiopoda.

At present, there are four living orders of branchiopods: Conchostraca, Anostraca, Notostraca, and Cladocera (TASCH, 1963). Spermatozoa of representatives of three orders have been examined with light optical studies. These include an anostracan, *Artemia salina* (FAUTREZ-FIRLEFYN and FAUTREZ, 1955), a notostracan, *Triops cancriformis* (LONGHURST, 1954) and three cladocerans, *Podon intermedius* and *Daphnia pulex* (RETZIUS, 1909) and *Polyphemus pediculus* (ZACHARIAS, 1884). In general, these authors described a small spherical or oval sperm with one or more dense staining organelles. The anostracan, *Artemia salina*, as a result of the present study, is the only species in which the sperm has been examined ultrastructurally. Considering the various studies made, the *Artemia* sperm is similar to the other descriptions and could represent the general branchipod sperm. This sperm is certainly unique (Fig. 1) and is not comparable to either other crustacean or other animal spermatozoa.

Cirripedia.

Of the four cirriped orders, spermatozoa of representatives of only the Order Thoracica have been examined (BALLOWITZ, 1908; KOLTZOFF, 1909; RETZIUS, 1909). These observations resemble quite closely the spermatozoa of *Lepas sp* and *Chthalamus fragilis* examined in the present study.

Although the cirriped sperm has unique features, there are similarities with spermatozoa of other subclasses. The anterior origin of the flagellum is also observed in mystacocarid and branchiuran spermatozoa and, as previously mentioned, in other groups of animals. Additionally, the extension of the nucleus is a common feature with the branchiuran and certain copepod spermatozoa. The one quite unique feature of the *Chthalamus* sperm is the apparent absence of an acrosome.

Copepoda.

Spermatozoa of species representing four of the seven (Barnes, 1968) copepod orders have been examined in various degrees. These include studies of two free-living and two parasitic copepod groups. The observations on *Calanus hyperboreus* sperm (Fig. 8) reported here are the only electron microscopical study available.

By far the most thorough light optical studies are in the Order Calanoida, also represented by *Calanus*. These include the brief descriptions of spermatozoa by HERBERER (1932) on thirteen species, more thorough examinations of spermatozoa from *Paracalanus parva* and *Eurytemora velox* (RETZIUS, 1909), and general observations on the sperm of *Calanus finmarchius* (MARSHALL and ORR, 1955). In all these cases the spermatozoa are spherical, oval, or slightly oblong, but resemble the *Calanus hyperboreus* sperm quite closely. In other words the calanoids seem to possess a structurally uniform sperm.

In the Order Harpacticoida, FARHENBACH (1961) has presented a general account of the *Diarthrodes cystoecus* sperm. This sperm is 50–60 micra in length and 1 micron in width with a spiral form much like the *Argulus* sperm (Fig. 12). Features described by Farhenbach include an anterior acrosome and a nucleus extending nearly the entire length of the sperm. HERBERER (1955) has reported the sperm of *Trigriopus brevicornis* to be spindle shape.

Spermatozoa from two parasitic copepods have been examined. The two species are *Antheacheres dubenii* (RETZIUS, 1909) and *Pandarus sinuatus* (McCLENDON, 1907). The *Antheacheres* sperm is approximately 100 micra in length and appears to have a spiral nuclear structure which extends nearly the sperm length. Considering that this observation was made from fixed material and could be partially inaccurate, there does appear to be similarity between this sperm and the *Diarthrodes* sperm. One important comparison is the long extension of the nucleus, also demonstrated in spermiogenesis in the *Pandarus* sperm.

From this brief review, the indication is that the nonmotile *Calanus* sperm represents a common type and spermatozoa in the other orders are elongated forms of the same type. Certain unique features of the *Calanus* sperm are the lack of a flagellum and the presence of mitochondria. Whether the same features are found in the spermatozoa of the other orders awaits further investigations. In any case the copepod sperm represented by *Calanus* is unique among the other crustacean spermatozoa.

Branchiura.

This subclass consists of the Order Branchiura (GREEN, 1961). The earlier investigation of the spermatozoa of this group consists only of *Argulus foliaceus* sperm (RETZIUS, 1909). The observations of RETZIUS compare quite favorably with the present study on *Argulus sp* sperm. Spermatozoa of other genera should be examined, but most likely the motile *Argulus* sperm is quite typical to the branchiurans.

As with the spermatozoa of other crustacean subclasses, the *Argulus* sperm is quite unique with a few characteristics common to other crustacean groups. These include a typical flagellum, a characteristic of the mystacocarid and cirriped spermatozoa, and an extended nucleus similar to certain copepod and cirriped spermatozoa. Quite interesting is the apparent similarity of the *Argulus* sperm to various insect spermatozoa, particularly those of *Thermobia* (BAWA, 1964). *Lepisma* (Werner, 1964), *Cicindela* (WERNER, 1965), *Dahlbominus* (WILKES and LEE, 1965), and *Ptinus* (JACOB, 1959). This comparison includes similar general features, particularly the spiral form of the sperm. Ultrastructurally, this comparison consists of the precise arrangement of the nucleus, mitochondria, and flagellum and the extension of these organelles for nearly the entire length of the respective sperm. The unique structures of the *Argulus* sperm are the thick trough–shaped organelle (Fig. 11) which extends the entire length of the sperm and the lateral organelles. Certainly the presence of such a sperm in the bizarre array of crustacean spermatozoa is surprising unless it is considered primitive and even to resemble the ancestral insect-crustacean sperm. Unfortunately, spermatogenesis and fertilization studies are not available. Such studies could bring more information on the insect-crustacean similarity and on the functions of the unique trough-shaped structure which may possibly be an acrosome.

Malacostraca.

Within this subclass, the varied and bizarre decapod spermatozoa have been examined the most thoroughly. With the exception of the isopod sperm (REGER, 1964; BLANCHARD *et al.*, 1962; HOLLANDE and FAIN, 1964; FAIN–MAUREL, 1966), the only published electron micrographs of crustacean spermatozoa are from the decapods. This is probably true because of the abundance, availability, importance, and ease of study of this group. Such studies have included spermatogenesis (MOSES, 1961; POCHON–MASSON, 1968), cytochemistry (CHEVAILLIER and MAILLET, 1965; CHEVAILLIER, 1967; ANDERSON and ELLIS, 1967) and fertilization (BROWN, 1966).

Of twelve existing orders (GREEN, 1961) of Malacostraca (excluding the Decapoda), the spermatozoa in five orders have been examined in various details. These are the Orders Stomatopoda, Mysidacea, Cumacea, Amphipoda, and Isopoda. The isopod sperm of *Asellus militaris* has been thoroughly examined (REGER, 1964) by electron microscopical methods. The *Asellus* sperm consists of a long, thread-like nucleus which has a short cone-like acrosome at the anterior end. Extending at right angle from the acrosome is the " tail " which has a width of 0.5 micron and a length of 400 micra. This immotile " tail " is cross-striated with a major periodicity of 750 to 800 Å. A cross section of this structure does not resemble any form of flagellum. It is interesting to note that from light optical studies spermatozoa of species of the Orders Cumacea (*Diastylis*, RETZIUS, 1909), Mysidacea (*Mysis*, RETZIUS, 1909), and Amphipoda (*Gammarus*, RETZIUS, 1909, and GILSON, 1886) have the same general form as the isopod sperm. In a fifth order, the stomatopod, *Squilla mantis*, has a spherical sperm which from preliminary studies by Kerby (pers. comm.) appears unique to the Malacostracans.

Various aspects of the decapod spermatozoa have been described by numerous investigators. With regards to much of this work a sperm morphological comparison of the seven decapod tribes–Stenopodidea, Penaeidea, Caridea, Palinura, Astacura, Brachyura, and Anomura (from GREEN, 1961) is presently being prepared for publication. Therefore, this most intersting group is receiving only superficial attention in the present study.

Sperm Morphology and Crustacean Phylogeny.

An adequate approach to crustacean phylogeny with sperm morphology would require the investigation of numerous species from each order and most likely would have to be carried out on the family or generic level. However, major steps made in the evolutionary process should be distinguishable between various taxa, such as the loss or modification of a sperm structure. This could be in reference to Dollo's Law which states "Major evolutionary steps, once taken, are never reversed" (Dobson, 1960, pp. 153–54). Sperm structures should be considered major and any loss of these structures should constitute an irreversible evolutionary step. Also sperm phylogeny can be considered conservative since the typical sperm (possessing acrosome, nucleus, mitochondrion, and flagellum) is well represented in the animal kingdom (FRANZEN, 1956). When a major change does occur, this should be characterisitic of the group (Phylum, Class, Order, Family, etc.). For example the sperm of the teleost fishes lack a structural acrosome (GINSBERG, 1963; TYLER, pers. comm.) and the spermatozoa of the nematoda (LEE and ANYA, 1964), malacostracans (BROWN, 1966), and millipeds (REGER and COOPER, 1968), have no flagellum. However, caution in such interpretations is important. For example, if loss of the flagellum is a major evolutionary change, acquisition of an additional flagellum by the sperm as in the toadfish (HOFFMAN, 1963) and urodele *Pseudobranchous* (AUSTIN and BAKER, 1964) might be regarded as equally major. Yet these appear to be isolated cases of limited evolutionary significance.

The flagellar pattern found in three subclasses, Mystacocarida, Cirripedia, and Branchiura, is the characteristic axial unit tubular (9 plus 2) arrangement. In discussing the sperm flagellum the following aspects are considered: supplementary microtubules and orientation with respect to the cell organelles. In the *Derocheilocaris* sperm the flagellum possesses four to seven additional microtubules (BROWN and METZ, 1967). Such structures have also been described in the flagella of several insect spermatozoa (KAYE, 1964; WERNER, 1965). Their function or role in the flagellar motion is unknown. The orientation of the flagellum of the *Derocheilocaris* and the *Argulus* spermatozoa with respect to the other sperm organelles is exact. The two central microtubules of these flagella are in the same plane (in respect to the sperm organelles) thoughout the length of each sperm. The flagellum is not spiral. This correlates with several observations, particularly those from the primitive insect spermatozoa (cfr. *Lepisma*, BAWA, 1964). The orientation of the cirriped, *Chthalamus*, sperm flagellum has not been satisfactorially determined. The anterior position of the flagellum common in all three of these flagellated spermatozoa is of particular interest since the same is also found in various insect spermatozoa.

Considering only the primitive crustacean subclasses, Cephalocarida and Mystacocarida, the ultrastructural investigation reveals sperm structures which could conceivably represent primitive spermatozoa (BROWN and METZ, 1967). Flagellum, mitochondria, acrosome, and nucleus are present in *Derocheilocaris* sperm. The *Hutchisoniella* sperm contains an acrosome, a nucleus, and a posterior projection, but lacks a mitochondrion and flagellum. In reference to the primitiveness of these two animals (SANDERS, 1963 and HESSLER, 1964) and their simple sperm forms, the two sperm types could conceivably represent two major lines of crustacean phylogeny. In consideration of this, it is interesting that the Cirripedia (*Chthalamus*) and the Brachiura (*Argulus*) have flagellated spermatozoa also. Including the Copepoda (closely related to the Branchiura), the four subclasses (including Mystacocarida represent the Cohort Maxillopod, established by DAHL (1963). Further the Branchiopoda and the Malacostraca are considered to have closer relationship to the

Cephalocarida. These all have non-flagellated spermatozoa (as reported to the present). The Ostracoda (freshwater forms) which may possess the most bizarre spermatozoa have been examined by GUPTA (pers. comm.) but do not possess a flagellum.

A more meaningful approach appears within the Subclass Malacostraca in which spermatozoa of numerous species have been examined. The spermatozoa of species of Cumacea, Mysidacea, Isopoda, and Amphipoda have the same general type of sperm. These orders are all included in the Division Peracarida. The only other Order studied extensively in Decapoda. Within this order, the spermatozoa have been shown to be unique to each of seven tribes (BROWN, in preparation). The mature spermatozoa of each of the two primitive Tribes, Stenopodidea (*Stenopus*) and Penaeidea (*Peneus*) have been examined. The Tribe Caridea is well represented with the tacklike sperm (*Palaemonetes*) with no exceptions to date. The sperm of the Tribe Palinura represented by *Panulirus* is entirely unique. The Tribe Astacura consist of two major types of spermatozoa, those represented by *Astacus* (POCHON–MASSON, 1965) and *Procambarus* (MOSES, 1961) and those by *Homarus* (POCHON–MASSON, 1965) and *Nephrops* (CHEVAILLIER and MAILLET, 1965). The Tribe Brachyuran appears to consist of the same general sperm type with the exception of the *Dromidia antillensis* sperm. The Tribe Anomuran appears to consist of at least two major types of spermatozoa, those represented by *Pagurus bonairensis* and those represented by *Galathea* (KOLTZOFF, 1903) and *Petrolisthes*. It is of interest that the separation of these decapod groups based on sperm morphology agrees with the classification formed by BORRADAILE (1907).

Thus the possibility of sperm morphology as a tool in the phylogenetic study of Crustacea certainly seems practical and as indicated by other authors (ANDRÉ, 1963; TUZET, 1950; NATH, 1942; BLOCH, 1935) can be very useful as additional data to combine with preexisting information.

Acknowledgement. This work was initiated in the Institute of Molecular Evolution, University of Miami, and partially supported by Grant No. G. B. – 3899 from the National Science Foundation. Some studies were also done in the Fertilization and Gamete Physiology Program at the Marine Biological Laboratory in 1965 and 1967. This work was aided by Grant Tl HD–26–06 from National Institute of Health. Also this work was partially supported by a Postdoctoral Grant No. G. B. – 13027 from the National Science Foundation and through the facilities of Duke University Marine Laboratory.

REFERENCES

ANDERSON W. A. and ELLIS R. A. (1967) – *Cytodifferentiation of the crayfish spermatozoon: Acrosome formation, transformation. Of mitochondria and development of microtubules.* « Z. Zellforsch. », 77, 80–94.

ANDRÉ J. (1963 a) – *A propos d'une leçon sur la limule.* «Ann. Sci. Clermont», 26, 27–38.

ANDRÉ J. (1963 b) – *Some aspects of specialization in sperm.* In: *The General Physiology of Cell Specialization.* D. Mazia and A. Tyler, Eds. McGraw–Hill Book Co., New York, 91–115.

AUSTIN C. R. and BAKER C. L. (1964) – *Spermatozoon of* Pseudobranchus striatus ananthus. « J. Reprod. Fertil. », 7, 123–125.

BALLOWITZ E. (1908) – *Die Kopflosen Spermien der Cirripedien* (Balanus). « Zeit. f. wiss. Zool. », 91, 421–426.

BARNES R. D. (1963) – *Invertebrate Zoology*. W. B. Saunders. Philadelphia.

BAWA S. R. (1964) – *Electron microscope study of spermiogenesis in a firebrat insect,* Thermobia domestica *Pack.* I. *Mature spermatozoon.* « J. Cell Biol. », 23, 431–446.

BLANCHARD R. E., LEWIN R. A. and PHILPOTT D. E. (1961) – *Fine structure of sperm tails of isopods.* « Crustaceana », 2, 16–20.

BLOCH F. (1935) – *Contribution à l'étude des gamètes et de la fécondation chez les Crustacés Décapodes.* « Trav. St. Zool. Wimereux. », 12, 185–279.

BORRADAILE L. A. (1907) – *On the classification of the Decapod Crustaceans.* « Ann. Mag. N. Hist. », 19, 457–486.

BROWN G. G. (1966) – *Ultrastructural studies of sperm morphology and sperm egg interaction in the decapod* Callinectes sapidus. « J. Ultrastruct. Res. », 14, 425–440.

BROWN G. G. and METZ C. B. (1967) – *Ultrastructural studies on the spermatozoa of two primitive crustaceans* Hutchinsoniella macracantha *and* Derocheilocaris typicus. « Z. Zellforsch. », 80, 78–92.

CHEVAILLIER P. and MAILLET P. L. (1965) – *Structure fine et constitution cytochimique du spermatozoïde de la langoustine* Nephrops norvegicus *L.* (*Crustacé Décapode*). « J. Microscopie », 4, 679–700.

CHEVALLIER P. (1967) – *Mise en evidence et étude cytochimique d'une proteine basique extranucleaire dans les spermatozoïdes des crustacés décapodes.* « J. Cell Biol. », 32, 547–556.

DAHL E. (1963) – *Main evolutionary lines among recent Crustacea. Phylogeny and Evolution of Crustacea.* A. H. B. Whittington and W. D. I. Rolfe, Eds., Museum of Comparative Zoology, Cambridge, Mass., 1–15.

DOBSON E. O. (1960) – *Evolution: Process and Product, Reinhold Publishing Corp.*, New York.

FAHRENBACH W. H. (1961) – *The Biology of a Harpacticoid Copepod.* « La Cellule », 62, 303–376.

FAIN-MAUREL M. A. (1966) – *Contribution à l'histologie et à la caryologie de quelques Isopodes. Spermiogenèse et infrastructure du spermatozoïde des Oniscidés et des Cymothoïdés.* « Ann. Sci. Natur. »; Zool. et Biol. Animale, 8 (1), 187.

FAUTREZ-FIRLEFYN N. and FAUTREZ J. (1955) – *Étude cytologique et cytochimique du spermatozoïde d'*Artemia salina *L.* Seconde Partie: *Le noyau, l'acrosome, le grain, les microgranules.* « Arch. Biol. », 66, 195–222.

FRANZÉN Å. (1956) – *On spermiogenesis, morphology of the spermatozoon, and biology of fertilization among invertebrates.* « Zool. Bidr. Upsala. », 31, 355–482.

GILSON G. (1886) – *Étude comparée de la spermatogenèse chez les arthropodes.* « La Cellule », 2, 83–239.

GINSBURG A. S. (1963) – *Sperm-egg association and its relationship to the activation of the egg in salmonid fishes.* « J. Emb. Exp. Morph. », 11, 13–33.

GREEN J. (1961) – *A Biology of Crustacea, Quadrangle Books,* Chicago.

GROBBEN C. (1878) – *Beitrage zur Kentniss der Mannlichen Geschlechtsorgane der Dekapoden.* « Arb. Zool. Inst. Univ. Wien u. Zool. Stat. Triest », 16, 57–150.

GROBBEN C. (1906) – *Zur Kenntniss der Dekapodenspermien.* « Arb. a. d. Zool. Inst. Wien. », 16, 1–8.

GUPTA. B. L. – *Unpublished observations.*

HENLE (1835) – *Ueber die Gattung* Branchiobdella *und uber die Deutung der inneren Geschlechtstheile bei den Anneliden und hermaphroditischen Schnecken.* Muller's Archiv. 603.

HERBERER G. (1932) – *Untersuchungen uber Bau und Funktion der Genitalorgane der Copepoden.* I. *Der mannliche Genitalapparat der calanoiden Copepoden.* « Zeit. mikr. anat. Forsch. », 31, 250–424.

HERBERER G. (1937) – *Weither Ergebnisse uber Bildung und Bau der Spermatophoren und Spermatophoren Koppelapparate bei calanoiden Copepoden.* « Verh. Deutsch. Zool. Ges. », 39, 86–93.

HERBERER G. (1955) – *Physiologischer Spermiendualismus bei harpacticoiden Copepoden.* « Naturwiss. », 42, 261–262.

HESSLER R. R. (1964) – *The Cephalocarida: comparative skeletal musculature.* « Mem. Conn. Acad. Arts *and* Sci. », 16, 1–97.

HIMES M. and MORIBER L. (1956) – *A triple stain for deoxyribonucleic acid, polysaccharides, and proteins.* « Stain Technol. », 31, 67–00.

HOFFMAN R. A. (1963) – *Gonads, spermatic ducts, and spermatogenesis in the reproductive system of male toadfish,* Opsanus tau. « Chesapeake Sci. », 4, 21–29.

HOLLANDE A. and FAIN M. (1964) – *Structure and ultrastructure du spermatozoide des Cymothoides.* « C. R. Acad. Sc. », 258, 5063–5066.

HUGHES R. L. (1965) – *Comparative morphology of spermatozoa from five marsupial families.* « Aust. J. Zool. », 13, 533–543.

HUMASON G. L. (1962) – *Animal Tissue Techniques,* W. H. Freeman, San Francisco and London.

JACOB J. (1959) – *A peculiar type of spermateleosis in the Spider Beetle* Ptinus hirtellus *Sturm.* « Cytologia », 24, 76–80.

KARNOVSKY M. J. (1965) – *A Formaldehyde-Gluteraldehyde Fixative of High Osmolality for use in Electron Microscopy.* « J. Cell Biol. », 27, 137 A–138 A.

KAYE J. S. (1964) – *The fine structure of flagella in spermatids of the house cricket.* « J. Cell Biol. », 22, 710–714.

KERBY C. – *Unpublished observations.*

KOLLICKER A. (1841) – *Observations pour servir à l'histoire des organes sexuels et du liquide seminal des Crustacés et des Cirrhipèdes.*

KOLLICKER A. (1847) – *Die Bildung der Samenfaden in Blaschen als allgemeines Entwicklungsgesetz.* Neue Denkschriften d. allg. schweiz. Gesellsch. fur die Gesammt. – Naturwiss., Bd. 8.

KOLTZOFF N. K. (1903) – *Untersuchungen über Spermien und Spermiogenese bei Decapoden.* « Anat. Anz. », 24, 83–95.

KOLTZOFF N. K. (1906) – *Studien über die Gestalt der Zelle. Untersuchungen über die Spermien der Dekapoden, als Einleitung in das Problem der Zellengestalt.* « Arch. Mikr. Anat. », 67, 364–572.

KOLTZOFF N. K. (1909) – *Studien über die Gestalt der Zelle.* « Arch. Zellforsch. », 2, 1.

LEE D. L. and ANYA A. O. (1967) – *The structure and development of the spermatozoon of* Aspiculuris tetraptera (*Nematoda*). « J. Cell Sci. », 2, 537–544.

LEUKART R. (1843) – *Artikel « Zeugung » in Wagner's Handworterbuch der Physiologie,* 4.

LONGHURST A. R. (1955) – *The reproduction and cytology of the Notostraca.* « Proc. Zool. Soc. Lond. », 125, 671–680.

LOWNDES A. G. (1953) – *The sperm of freshwater ostracods.* « Proc. Zool. Soc. Lond. », 35–48.

MARSHALL S. M. and ORR A. P. (1955) – *The Biology of a Marine Copepod.* – Oliver and Boyd, Edinburgh.

MCCLENDON J. F. (1907) – *The spermatogenesis of* Pandarus sinuatus *Say.* – « Biol. Bull. », 13, 114–120.

MCFARLANE R. W. (1963) – *The taxonomic significance of avian sperm.* Proc. 13th Intern. Ornith. Congress, 91–102.

MOSES M. J. (1961) – *Spermiogenesis in the crayfish* (Procambarus clarkii). II. *Description of stages.* « J. Biophysic. Biochem. Cytol. », 10, 301–333.

NATH V. (1942) – *The Decapod Sperm.* « Trans. Natl. Inst. Sci. India », 2, 87–135.

NIIJIMA L. and DAN J. (1965) – *The acrosome reaction in* Mytilus edulis. I. *Fine Structure of the Intact Acrosome.* « J. Cell Biol. », 25, 243–248.

OWSJANNIKOW (1869) – *Ueber die Entwicklung und den Bau des Samenkorperchen der Fische.* « Bull. Acad. Saint Petersbourg », 13, 247.

POCHON-MASSON J. (1965) – *Schema general du spermatozoïde vesiculaire des Décapode*. «C. R. Acad. Sc.», 260, 5093-5095.

POCHON-MASSON J. (1968) – *L'ultrastructure des spermatozoïdes vésiculaires chez les crustacés décapodes auant et au cours de leur dévagination experimentale.* I. *Brachyoures et Anomoures.* «Ann. Sci. Natur.», 10, 1-100.

REGER J. F. (1964 b) – *A study on the fine structure of developing spermatozoa from the isopod,* Asellus militaris (*Hay*). «J. Microscopie», 3, 559-572.

REGER J. F. and COOPER D. P. (1968) – *Studies on the fine structure of spermatids and spermatozoa from the millipede* Polydesmus sp. «J. Ultrastruct. Res.», 23, 60-70.

RETZIUS G. (1909) – *Die Spermien der Crustacean.* «Biol. Untersuch.», 14, 1-54.

REYNOLDS E. S. (1963) – *The Use of lead citrate as an electron dense stain in electron microscopy.* «J. Cell Biol.», 17, 208-212.

SABATIER A. (1893) – *De la spermatogenèse chez les Crustacés décapodes.* «Trav. Inst. Zool. Montpellier», 2, 393.

SANDERS H. L. (1963) – *The Cephalocarida: functional morphology, larval development, and comparative external anatomy.* «Mem. Connecticut Acad. Arts, Sci.», 15, 1-80.

VON SIEBOLD (1836) – *Ueber die Spermatozoen der Crustaceen, Insecten, Gasteropoden und ciniger anderer wirbellosen Thiere.* «Muller's Archiv.», 26.

VON SIEBOLD (1837) – *Fernere Beobachtungen über die Spermatozoen der wirbellosen Thiere.* «Muller's Archiv».

SILVEIRA M. and PORTER K. R. (1964) – *The Spermatozoids of flatworms and their microtubular systems.* «Protoplasma», 59, 240-265.

TASCH P. (1963) – *Evolution of the Branchiopoda.* In: *Phylogeny and Evolution of Crustacea.* H. B. Whittington and W. D. I. Rolfe, Eds. – Museum of Comparative Zoology. Cambridge, Mass., 145-157.

TOCHIMOTO T. (1967) – *Comparative histochemical study on the dimorphic spermatozoa of the prosobranchia with special reference to polysaccharides.* «Tokyo Kyoiku Daigaku», 13, 75-109.

TUZET O. (1950) – *Le spermatozoïde dans la série animale.* «Rev. Suisse Zool.» 57, 433-451.

TYLER P. J. – *Unpublished observations.*

WATSON M. L. (1958) – *Staining of tissue sections for electron microscopy with heavy metals.* «J. Biophys. Biochem. Cytol.», 4, 475-478.

WERNER G. (1964) – *Untersuchungen über die Spermiogenese beim Silberfischen,* Lepisma saccharina *L.* «Z. Zellforsch.», 63, 880-912.

WERNER G. (1965) – *Untersuchungen über die Spermiogenese beim Sandlaüfer,* Cicindela campestris *L.* «Z. Zellforsch.», 66, 255-275.

WILKES A. and LEE P. E. (1965) – *The Ultrastructure of Dimorphic Spermatozoa in the Hymenopteron* Dahlbominus fuscipennis (*Zett.*) (*Eulophidae*). «Can. J. Genet. Cytol.», 7, 609-619.

WILSON E. B. (1928) – *The Cell in Development and Heredity.* The Macmillan Co., New York.

ZACHARIAS O. (1884) – *Uber die Amoeboiden Bewegungen der Spermatozoen von* Polyphemus pediculus (*de Geer*). «Zeit. f. wiss. Zool.», 61, 252-258.

ZISSLER D. (1969) – *Die Spermiohistogenese des Susswasser Ostracoden* Notodromas monacha *O. F. Müller.* «Zeit. Zellforsch.», 96, 87-133.

Explanation of figures

Fig. 1. – A section of an *Artemia salina* sperm in the vas deferens. Resolved are the nucleus (*N*), mitochondria (*M*), endoplasmic reticula (*ER*), and cytoplasmic arms (*CA*). The nucleus contains dense staining material and is bounded by a nuclear envelope (*NE*). Karnovsky's Glutaraldehyde. Electron Micrograph. ×17,700.

Fig. 2. – *Artemia salina.* Field of sepmatozoa forced from dissected vas deferens. No fixation. Phase-contrast. ×895.

Fig. 3. – *Artemia salina.* Mature sperm from vas deferens with some of the numerous cytoplasmic arms present. No fixation. Phase-contrast. ×1,730.

Fig. 4. – *Chthalamus fragilis.* Sections of several spermatozoa in the vas deferens. Present are the three major components, nucleus (*N*), mitochondrial derivative (*MD*), and flagellum (*F*). Acrolein-glutaraldehyde followed by osmium tetioxide. Electron micrograph. ×19,200.

Fig. 5. – *Lepas sp.* Field of mature spermatozoa from squashed vas deferens. No fixation. Phase – contrast. ×180.

Fig. 6. – *Lepas sp.* Higher magnification of anterior end of motile sperm. The anterior end is foled back forming a loop. Numerous motile spermatozoa were found in this condition. No fixation. Phase-contrast. ×2,100.

Fig. 7. – *Lepas sp.* A damaged mature sperm showing the separation of the flagellum (*F*) from the elongated nucleus (*N*). This indicates that the flagellum origin is near the sperm anterior end (arrow). No fixation. Phase-contrast. ×2,100.

Fig. 8. – Cross section of a disc-shaped *Calanus hypergoreus* sperm showing the fibrous nucleus (*N*) and the mitochondrial material (*M*). Covering the nuclear material is a dense staining band (*DB*) and adjacent to this is the sperm plasma membrane (*SPM*). Completely surrounding the surface of the sperm is a homogeneous layer (*HL*). Acroleinglutaraldehyde. Electron micrograph. ×20,600.

Fig. 9. – *Calanus hyperboreus.* Cross section of the perimeter of several disc-shaped spermatozoa. Some relationships of the large dense staining organelle which may be an acrosome (*A*) are noticeable. Osmium tetroxide (sea water). Electron micrograph. ×10,300.

Fig. 10. – *Calanus hyperboreus.* Two spermatozoa from a squashed seminal receptacle. The irregular shaped spermatozoa freed become oval shaped in the medium. The large bulk of each sperm is the nucleus. In the sperm at the top of the figure, a thin layer of organelles is observed at each end of the long axis, while in the sperm at the bottom of the figure, such a thin layer of organelles is completely around the periphery. This indicates that there is a band of organelles passing around the nucleus. These two spermatozoa are thus in different orientations. No fixation. Phase-contrast. ×2,810.

Fig. 11. – *Argulus sp.* Cross sections of mature spermatozoa in the testes. The major components of each sperm are the trough-shaped organelle (*TO*), the flagellum (*F*), the mitochondria (*M*), the nucleus (*N*), and the lateral organelle (*LO*). The flagella have the typical axial unit (9 plus 2) tubular arrangement. The mitochondria are aligned in a row (arrows 1 and 2) and have typical mitochondrian features such as double membranes (*dm*) and cristae (*c*). The lateral organelles are slab like and in several cases are on opposite sides of the same sperm (arrows 3 and 4). Acrolein-glutaraldehyde followed by osmium tetroxide. Electron micrograph. ×35,800.

Fig. 12. – *Argulus sp.* One of the ends of a mature sperm showing the spiral form. No fixation. Phase-contrast. ×1,300.

Addendum

In reference to the cirriped spermatozoa (*Chthalamus*, *Lepas*), the author wishes to acknowledge an error. As a result of the excellent study by Dr. Jacqueline Pochon–Masson on the development of the cirriped sperm, I have definitely labeled two organelles incorrectly. In Figure 4, the organelle labeled " mitochondrial derivative " should be " nucleus " instead. Also the organelle labeled " nucleus " is an unique vesicle and most likely will eventually be shown to have acrosomal functions.

Discussion

Note by author: During my oral presentation, I included some research studies which are not incorporated in the above paper. These involved ultrastructural investigations of initial sperm-egg interactions in the horseshoe crab, *Limulus polyphemus* (in preparation for publication, R. L. Shoger and G. G. Brown). Several of the following questions are directly related to this work.

EDDLEMAN. – Does the " trough structure " extend the entire length of the spermatozoon?

BROWN. – In the *Argulus* sperm this structure does extend the entire length and is the definitive organelle at each end.

REGER. – Does your data indicate that the intranuclear rod is delimited from the nucleus by the nuclear membrane and also where it penetrates the acrosome or infolds its surface by the acrosome membrane. In other words these rods of invertebrate sperm where seen are sub-acrosomal or perforatorial in fact.

BROWN. – In the *Limulus* sperm, the axial rod extends from the acrosomal vesicle through the nucleus and coils around the nucleus base. It is delimited by the nuclear envelope and acrosomal membrane. However, André (1963) has reported the coiled portion lying in the space between the two membranes of the nuclear envelope. In my opinion, the *Limulus* axial rod in accordance with Austin (*Ultrastructure of Fertilization*, 1968) is subacrosomal. Also I prefer to consider conclusively the acrosomal vesicle and the axial rod as the acrosomal complex or acrosomal region.

AFZELIUS. – Dr. Brown, when you modify the scheme on the reacted *Limulus* sperm by André by adding a membrane to the outside of the reacted acrosome filament, did you do this based on actual findings or because you want a membrane to be there? I ask this question because there is a fundamental difference, I think, between the case of the lamprey shown to you by Nicander on Tuesday and the *Limulus*. The preformed acrosome of the *Limulus* seems to perforate the entire nucleus, transforming it to a topological torus, a doughnut if you wish, whereas the lamprey nuclear membrane topologically is a sphere, an unbroken ballon although the preformed filament pushes a long canal into it.

BROWN. – During sperm-egg interactions the *Limulus* sperm attaches to the egg surface and undergoes the acrosome reaction projecting the acrosomal filament. This filament passes through the egg envelope (50 μ thick) to the egg plasma membrane. It is in this egg envelope that the membrane is observed surrounding the axial rod (thus forming the acrosomal filament). We have not studied the sperm acrosome reaction free from the egg. In answer to your question there is definitely a membrane present.

The topography of the nucleus is an interesting question. In my opinion the axial rod perforates the nucleus thus causing the formation of a torus. However, a study of spermiogenesis should be performed for proof.

DAN. – The *Mytilus* is also totally perforated by the filament, like the *Limulus*.

ANDRÉ. – In my work on *Limulus*, I never saw a membrane enclosing the axial rod after the acrosomal reaction. This can be due either to the fact that there is indeed no membrane in this species, or to the fact that it was not preserved by the experimental conditions that I used. In the latter case, we should have to explain a difficult problem of membrane biogenesis. In fact, on the one hand the acrosomal reaction is explosive, on the other the axial rod is long, longer than the whole cell. Therefore, we should have to explain how the cell could more or less double the surface of its membrane in a very short fraction of a second. As far as I know, such a mobility of biological macromolecules is not known at present.

BROWN. – We have only investigated the reacted sperm on the egg. A membrane is definitely present. In reference to the acrosomal reaction and the formation of this membrane, DAN has described a situation in starfish sperm where the membrane of the acrosomal " process " is formed from nonmembranous precursors. In this species, the acrosome reaction takes 20 seconds which can allow time for membrane biogenesis. In *Limulus*, I do not know the time period of the acrosome reaction although I agree it is " explosive ". Thus two alternatives could be a *de novo* membrane formation from precursor substances or a stretching or extension of the acrosomal membrane. As a personal opinion, I suspect the latter is true in *Limulus*, although this needs more investigation for proof.

FAVARD. – Have you shown that the membrane which appears around the axial filament at the time of acrosomal reaction is really a phospholipidic membrane?

BROWN. – No, I have not shown this. I have used the term " membrane " somewhat literally. There is a possibility it is a precipiting layer, but I doubt this.

NICANDER. – Is there any decrease in the thickness of the plasma membrane of the crustacean spermatozoon in connection with the acrosome reaction, similar to the membrane transformation during the acrosome reaction in lampreys?

BROWN. – I do not know. We have considered mainly an event which has occurred. Unfortunately, our observations have primarily concerned the reacted sperm with little comparison to the unreacted sperm. Since there are so many problems and so much interest on the formation of the acrosomal filament membrane, I will definitely investigate this in the future. Next time I will have the results.

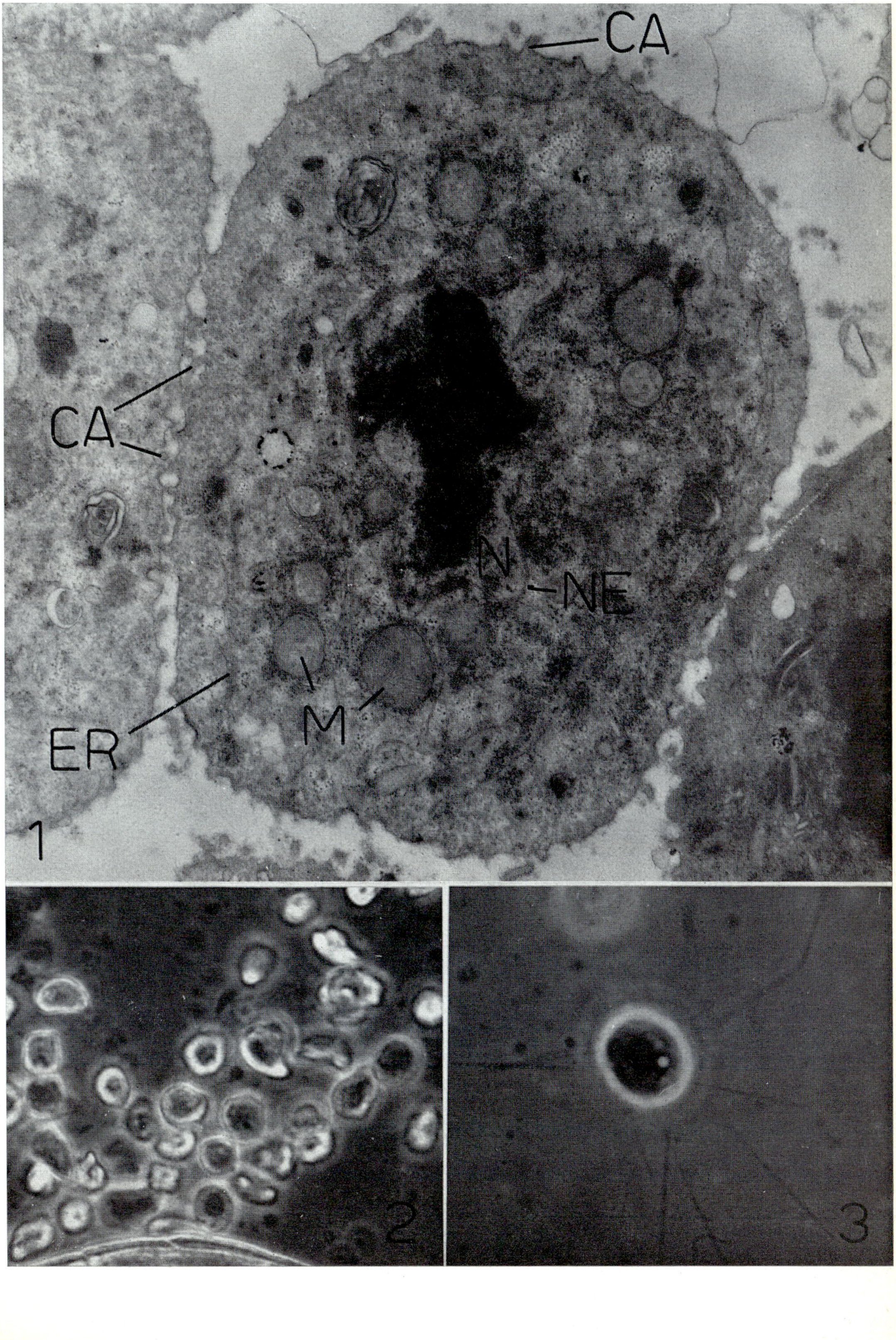
CA
CA
N
NE
ER
M
1
2
3

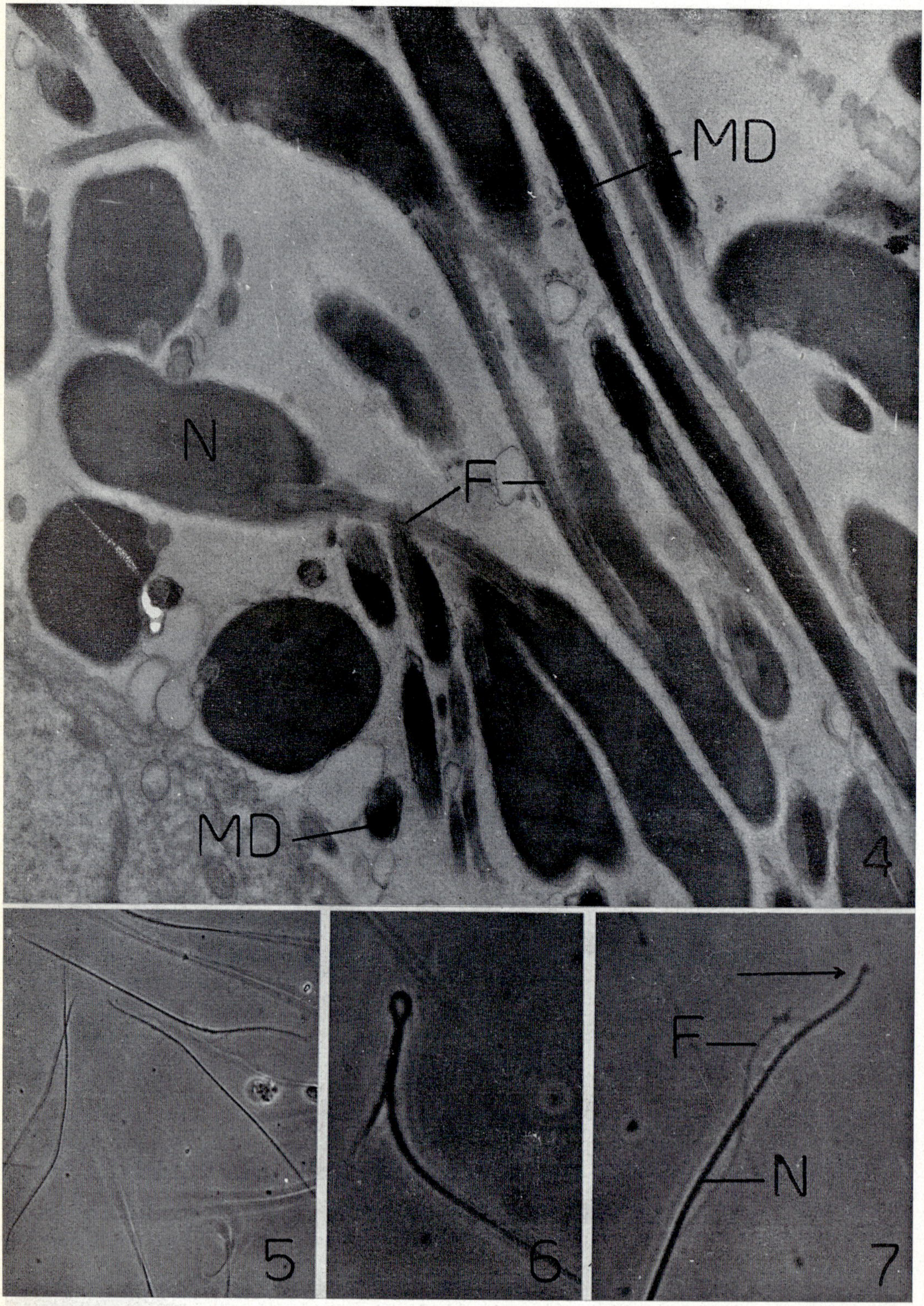
MD
N
F
MD
4
5
6
F
N
7

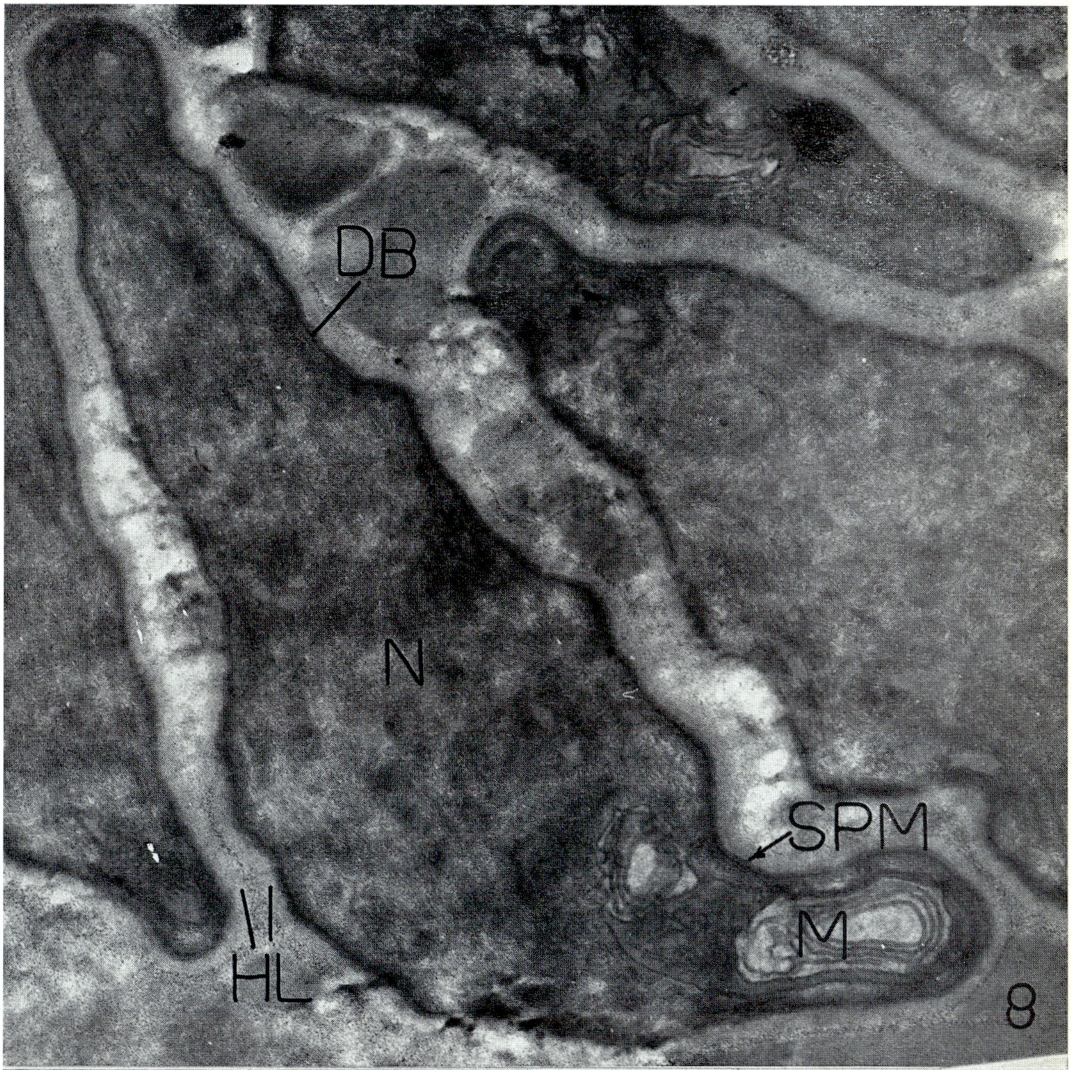
DB
N
SPM
M
HL
8

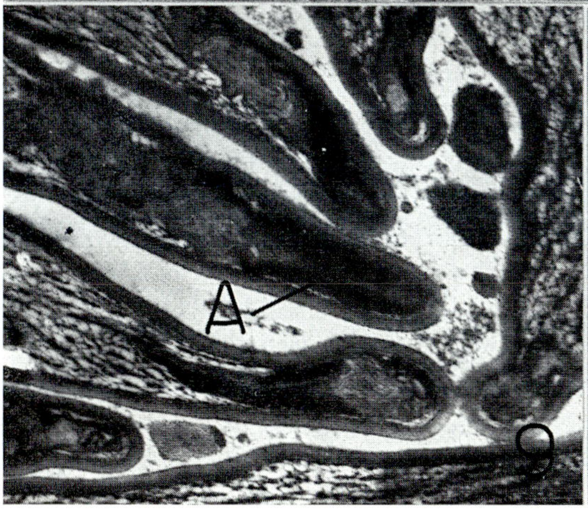
A
9

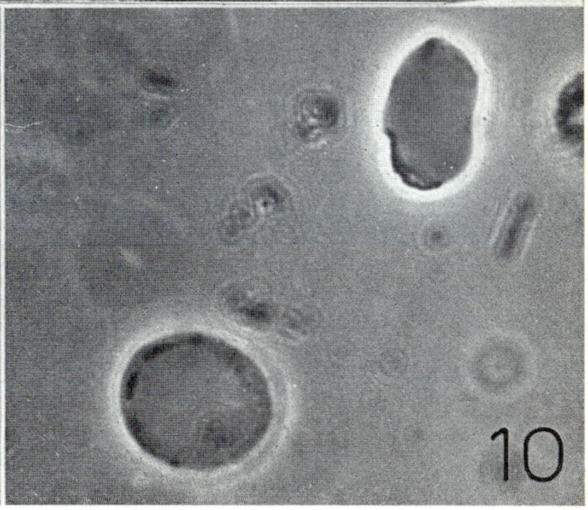
10

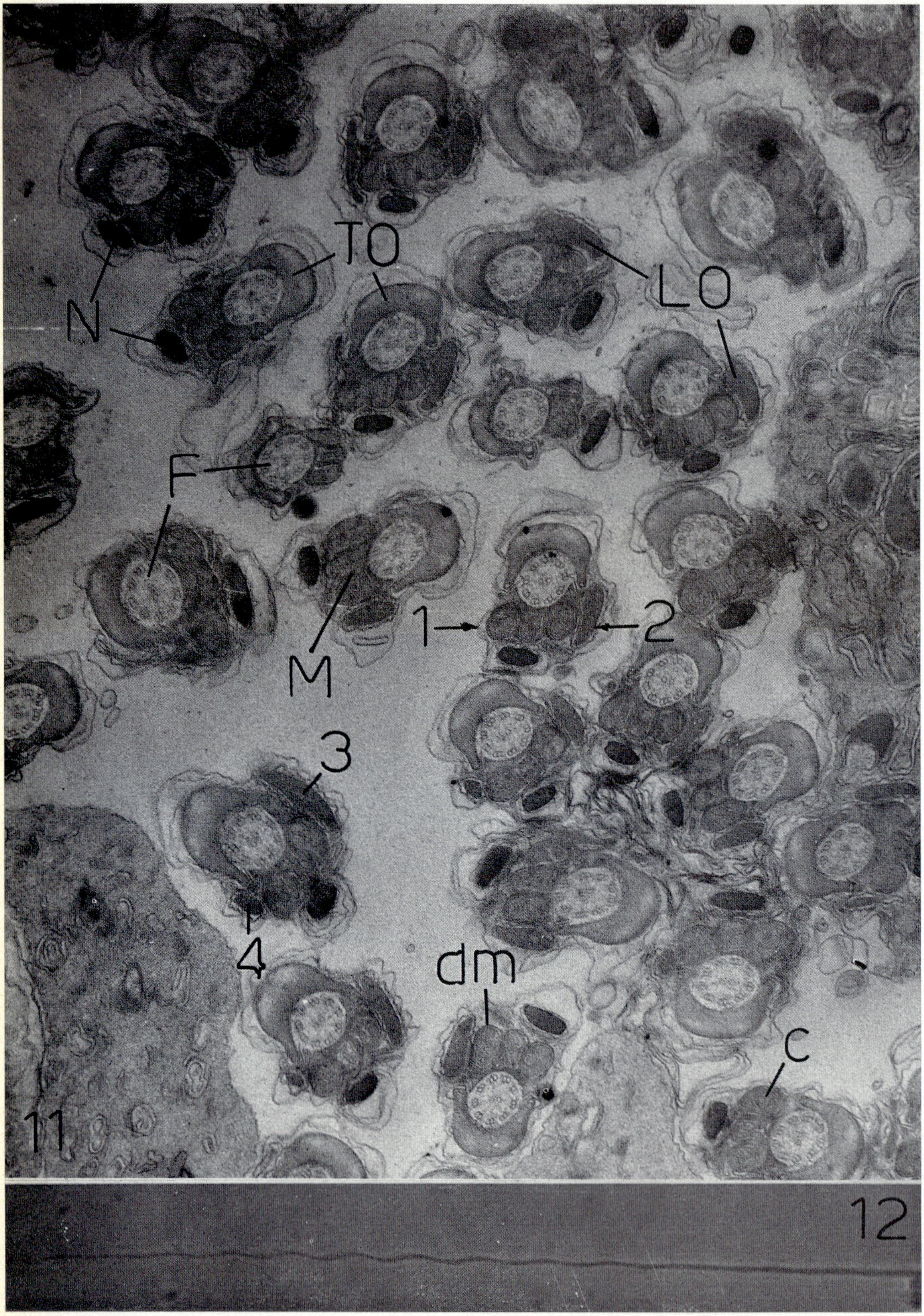
TO
LO
N
F
M
1
2
3
4
dm
c
11
12

J. POCHON-MASSON (*), J. BOCQUET-VÉDRINE (*) et Y. TURQUIER (*)

CONTRIBUTION A L'ÉTUDE DU SPERMATOZOÏDE DES CRUSTACÉS CIRRIPÈDES

RÉSUMÉ. — Le spermatozoïde des Cirripèdes est du type flagellé, mais présente certaines particularités que nous pouvons préciser à l'aide de la microscopie électronique. Nos observations concernent des Cirripèdes appartenant à des groupes différents. L'étude de la spermiogenèse de *Balanus perforatus* (Thoracique Operculé) et celle de *Trypetesa nassarioides* (Acrothoracique) montre la formation de la structure acrosomienne, la position antérieure du centriole porteur du flagelle, l'écoulement du noyau le long du flagelle, la présence d'une gaine flagellaire glycoprotéique comportant des cordons sinueux, le nebenkern réduit à une seule mitochondrie, et enfin la présence provisoire d'une vésicule APS – négative appendue au noyau dans sa région antérieure. Une gamme d'aberrations peut affecter les spermatozoïdes qui, dans ce cas présentent toujours une polyflagellarité.

Le plan d'organisation du spermatozoïde des Cirripèdes, effectué d'après une vue comparative des différents groupes, est discuté en fonction de nos connaissances sur les gamètes mâles des autres Crustacés et principalement des Décapodes.

RIASSUNTO. — Lo spermatozoo dei Cirripedi è flagellato, ma presenta certe caratteristiche che noi possiamo precisare con l'aiuto della microscopia elettronica. Le nostre osservazioni riguardano Cirripedi appartenenti a gruppi differenti. Lo studio della spermiogenesi di *Balanus perforatus* (Toracico Operculato) e di *Trypetesa nassarioides* (Acrotoracico) mostra la formazione dell'acrosoma, la posizione anteriore del centriolo distale, lo scorrimento del nucleo lungo il flagello, la presenza di una guaina flagellare glicoproteica con cordoni sinuosi, il nebenkern ridotto a un solo mitocondrio, e infine la presenza provvisoria di una vescicola PAS – negativa appesa al nucleo nella sua regione anteriore. Possono verificarsi delle aberrazioni negli spermatozoi che in tal caso si presentano sempre poliflagellati.

Il piano d'organizzazione dello spermatozoo dei Cirripedi, effettuato dopo uno studio comparativo dei differenti gruppi, viene discusso in funzione delle nostre conoscenze sui gameti maschili degli altri Crostacei e principalmente dei Decapodi.

INTRODUCTION

L'interprétation du spermatozoïde des Cirripèdes a donné lieu à de nombreuses controverses dont GRASSÉ et TUZET (1928 et 1932) ont rendu compte dans leur étude fondamentale sur la spermatogenèse de *Balanus perforatus* BRUG. A la même époque, SALHEANU (1932) a établi une comparaison entre la spermiogenèse des Operculés et celle des Pédonculés. D'autre part, chez

(*) Faculté des Sciences, Laboratoire d'Evolution des Etres Organisés et C.N.R.S., Laboratoire de Microscopie Electronique appliqué à la Biologie, 105, Bd Raspail, Paris, France.

les Rhizocéphales, la spermatogenèse a fait l'objet de travaux surtout anciens (notamment ceux de DELAGE, 1884, de GIARD, 1873 et de DUBOSCQ, 1901). Plus récemment, l'un de nous a étendu cette étude au genre *Chthamalophilus*, représentant du groupe très remarquable des Akentrogonides (BOCQUET–VÉDRINE, 1961).

L'observation en microscopie électronique pouvait seule, cependant, permettre de compléter les résultats apportés par ces divers auteurs. Aucune recherche approfondie n'a pourtant été entreprise dans ce domaine, en dehors d'une étude générale du spermatozoïde des Crustacés due à BROWN (1966). Les problèmes soulevés par les observations faites en microscopie photonique dans les divers groupes de Cirripèdes nous ont incités à essayer d'établir un schéma–type du spermatozoïde de ces Crustacés à l'aide d'une étude ultrastructurale comparée. Notre analyse récente de l'infrastructure du gamète mâle de *Trypetesa* (= *Alcippe*) (Cirripède Acrothoracique) souligne en effet l'originalité d'une organisation et l'existence de certains constituants, dont il était intéressant de connaitre le degré de généralisation au sein de la sous–classe des Cirripèdes (TURQUIER et POCHON–MASSON, 1969).

En fait, le spermatozoïde des Cirripèdes (quel que soit l'ordre auquel ils appartiennent) est flagellé et renferme les éléments fondamentaux d'un gamète banal. Par contre, son plan architectural est original: la tête, fort longue, est munie d'un unique centriole en position sous–acrosomienne, et le flagelle chemine le long du noyau. D'autre part, la présence d'un matériel périflagellaire et l'adjonction d'une vésicule transitoire dont nous avons suivi la cytodifférenciation chez *Balanus* (BOCQUET–VÉDRINE et POCHON–MASSON, sous presse) sont des particularités qui semblent caractériser le gamète mâle des Cirripèdes.

MATÉRIEL ET MÉTHODES

Les animaux qui ont permis de réaliser ce travail appartiennent aux espèces suivantes:

– *Balanus perforatus* BRUGUIÈRE et *B. crenatus* BRUG., (Thoraciques Operculés);
– *Scalpellum scalpellum* (L.), (Thoracique Pédonculé);
– *Trypetesa lampas* (HANCOCK) et *T. nassarioides* TURQUIER, (Acrothoraciques);
– *Sacculina carcini* THOMPSON et *Chthamalophilus delagei* BOCQUET–VÉDRINE, (Rhizocéphales).

Certaines d'entre elles ont fait l'objet d'une étude plus approfondie au niveau ultrastructural.

1) *Microscopie photonique.*

Un éventail très large de techniques (« squashes », frottis humides, coupes classiques), de fixations et de colorations a été utilisé afin de faciliter l'interprétation du matériel.

– Fixateurs employés: Bouin 15 d'Allen, Helly, Gendre, Carnoy, formol neutre à 10% dans l'eau de mer.

– Colorations réalisées: orcéine lacto–propionique et orcéine acétique, hématoxyline de HEIDENHAIN ou de REGAUD, Mann biacide, Feulgen, vert de méthyle–pyronine, fuchsine d'Altmann.

– Recherche des composés APS–positifs (méthodes à l'acide périodique–Schiff et à l'azur –SO2, précédées ou non par l'action de la ptyaline ou du dimédon); recherche des protéines totales (méthode à l'alloxane-Schiff) ou basiques (méthodes d'ALFERT et GESCHWIND, 1953; BLOCH et HEW, 1961).

2) *Microscopie électronique.*

Des fragments d'appareil génital ont été inclus dans l'épon 812 ou bien étalés en frottis sur lame d'épon (technique de ZAGURY, ZYLBERBERG et ZEITOUN, 1966).

Fixateurs employés à froid pendant 45 minutes à 1 heure:

- acide osmique à 1% dans le tampon Palade ou dans l'eau de mer filtrée;
- glutaraldéhyde, suivi d'une post-osmification appropriée, à 2,3 ou 4%, soit dans le tampon mono-et disodique 0,1 M à, pH 7,2 (avec 5% de sucrose dans le cas des 3%), soit dans le tampon cacodylate de Na 0,1 M à pH 7,2 (comportant ou non 5% de sucrose ou 37% d'eau de mer)
- glutaraldéhyde à 2,5%, avec 2% de paraformaldéhyde dans le tampon cacodylate enrichi d'eau de mer à 40%. Le paraformaldéhyde seul à 4% a été également utilisé dans le tampon cacodylate-eau de mer 50%.

Après le passage des blocs au microtome REICHERT OMU 2, les coupes ont été contrastées par une double coloration à l'acétate d'uranyle et au citrate de plomb et ont été examinées à l'aide des microscopes Hitachi de type HU 11 A et HU 11 B, ou Philips du type EM 300.

VUE COMPARATIVE DES SPERMATOZOÏDES

1°) *Morphologie générale.*

Les spermatozoïdes des Cirripèdes étudiés sont mobiles et filiformes; leur diamètre est d'un demi μ environ et leur longueur varie selon les groupes (un peu plus de 20 μ chez les Rhizocéphales jusqu'à une centaine de μ chez les Acrothoraciques).

En général, on distingue la tête (comportant un acrosome court et effilé, et un noyau allongé accompagné d'une languette chromatique), la pièce intermédiaire, plus ou moins développée, et la queue. Une gouttelette protoplasmique est appendue au tiers antérieur du gamète immature sauf chez *Lepas* où SALHEANU (1932) observe seulement une structure très ténue dans cette région. Ces observations correspondent, au niveau ultrastructural, à la présence:

- d'une vésicule acrosomique encapuchonnant le bâtonnet axial,
- du noyau que longe le flagelle (celui-ci est issu du centriole distal situé en position sub-acrosomienne et est accompagné d'une gaine).
- d'une goutte de sécrétion logée sous la membrane cytoplasmique,
- enfin, d'une simple mitochondrie située en arrière du noyau et qui permet de situer la pièce intermédiaire.

Le matériel périflagellaire persiste dans la partie principale de la queue du spermatozoïde et disparaît dans la partie terminale ou ne subsiste que le flagelle.

D'autre part une polymégalie se manifeste fréquemment dans les spermatides et les spermatozoïdes. La microscopie électronique nous a permis de proposer une interprétation morphologique de ce phénomène.

2°) *Structure de la tête.*

La tête du spermatozoïde des Cirripèdes présente un allongement remarquable. En arrière de l'acrosome le flagelle chemine le long du noyau très étiré.

a) *Acrosome.*

Il est constitué de 2 éléments essentiels: la vésicule acrosomique, d'origine golgienne et APS-positive, et le bâtonnet axial entièrement coiffé par la vésicule (Fig. 18). Le matériel du bâtonnet axial repose sur une lame nucléaire dont il semble provenir (Fig. 10), et qui est coincée entre l'acrosome et le centriole distal.

Deux d'entre nous ont donné une description détaillée de ce complexe acrosomien relativement classique et de sa formation chez *Trypetesa nassarioides* (TURQUIER et POCHON-MASSON, 1969).

On notera cependant que la structure fine du bâtonnet axial, d'aspect homogène au moment de sa formation, a la particularité d'évoluer en une série de strates hautes de 350 Å comportant des filaments sinusoïdaux d'un diamètre de 70 Å environ.

b) *Complexe centriolaire et flagelle.*

Le spermatozoïde des Cirripèdes semble ne conserver qu'un centriole qui porte le flagelle. La position antérieure de ce centriole est très remarquable et entraîne un bouleversement important de la topographie du gamète par rapport à celle du type flagellé classique. Le centriole n'est séparé de l'acrosome que par un mince disque nucléaire épais de 100 à 200 Å. Chez *Trypetesa*, il présente des différenciations particulières, sous forme d'anneaux, que l'on ne retrouve pas chez la Balane.

Le flagelle, dans tous les cas observés, possède une structure du type 9 + 2 (défini par BACCETTI, DALLAI et ROSATI, 1968). Cette structure reste identique sur la majeure partie de sa longueur, et ne se désorganise qu'à son extrémité postérieure où les microtubules sont disposés irrégulièrement et disparaissent peu à peu.

c) *Noyau*

Il se présente sous la forme d'une bande large de 0,4 à 0,5 μ et épaisse d'environ 0,2 μ chez *Balanus*, *Trypetesa* et *Sacculina*. Il est animé d'un mouvement hélicoïdal à grand pas. Sa position, parallèle à celle du flagelle, est évidemment liée à l'emplacement du centriole précédemment décrit. Sa silhouette, en section transversale, est caractéristique de chaque genre étudié (Figs. 15 à 17): réniforme chez les Balanes, au contour biconcave chez *Trypetesa*. Des modifications de détail s'observent d'une espèce à l'autre dans la silhouette et la structure de la région antérieure du spermatozoïde. Chez *Balanus perforatus*, par exemple, le disque nucléaire situé entre les complexes acrosomien et centriolaire est moins réduit que chez *Trypetesa*, et encapuchonne l'extrémité antérieure du centriole et du flagelle sur une longueur de 0,5 μ environ. Feulgen-positif et pourvu de protéines basiques, il devient intensément osmiophile au cours de la spermiogenèse. Corrélativement l'enveloppe nucléaire se modifie.

Les actions inductrice et polarisatrice du flagelle sur l'évolution nucléaire sont manifestes, mais s'expriment différemment suivant les cas.

Chez les Balanes, la chromatine des spermatozoïdes ne présente pas, au cours de son remaniement, comme chez *Trypetesa*, l'aspect d'une frange osmiophile, située à proximité du flagelle. Elle se condense au contraire et s'amasse le long de celui-ci, l'osmiophilie n'apparaissant que tardivement. L'aboutissement du phénomène est le même, mais sa réalisation dans le temps est très différente.

D'autre part, la transformation concomitante de l'enveloppe nucléaire se manifeste par un ensemble de caractères: disparition des pores nucléaires, augmentation de l'osmiophilie des feuillets constitutifs, réduction possible de l'espace périnucléaire (notamment au niveau du disque nucléaire sous-acrosomien), enfin accolement du feuillet interne à la chromatine. Le remaniement morphologique du noyau, sphérique chez la spermatide jeune, qui aboutit à la longue baguette nucléaire du spermatozoïde, entraîne également celui de l'enveloppe nucléaire. Cette dernière subit un simple allongement chez les Acrothoraciques, mais, chez la Balane, le phénomène est plus complexe: la région opposée à celle où se condense la chromatine est destinée à être éliminée en se détachant du noyau nouvellement formé. En définitive, elle acquiert le même aspect légèrement plissé dans les gamètes mûrs.

d) *Manchette.*

Les microtubules constitutifs de la manchette entourent l'acrosome, le noyau et les mitochondries dans la spermatide âgée. Ils apparaissent d'abord dans le champ périflagellaire puis envahissent peu à peu la périphérie du noyau. D'un diamètre de 270 Å, ils s'étendent dans le cytoplasme résiduel parallèlement à l'axe du gamète. Il est classique de leur attribuer un rôle dans l'allongement du spermatozoïde et une fonction cytosquelettique. D'autre part, chez la Balane, leur progression est liée à celle de l'enveloppe nucléaire modifiée (Fig. 4). Cette évolution est actuellement étudiée par deux d'entre nous (BOCQUET-VÉDRINE et POCHON-MASSON). L'existence de cette manchette paraît éphémère puisque les microtubules ne s'observent plus à des niveaux homologues dans le spermatozoïde.

e) *Matériel périflagellaire.*

Le spermatozoïde des Cirripèdes se caractérise, de façon constante, tout au moins dans le champ de notre investigation, par la présence d'un matériel remarquable localisé à proximité du flagelle. Ce matériel occupe l'espace laissé libre de part et d'autre de l'axonème entre l'enveloppe nucléaire et la membrane cytoplasmique. Dans les coupes longitudinales, il apparaît immédiatement en arrière du niveau centriolaire, puis accompagne l'axonème jusqu'à la fin de la pièce principale, sans présenter de modification structurale. Il est constitué de cordons pleins, moyennement osmiophiles, d'un diamètre de 250 Å, qui s'entortillent plus ou moins sur eux-mêmes. Aucune membrane ne semble limiter l'ensemble de ces cordons qui peuvent se répartir de façon variable; parfois ils se groupent sur un côté du flagelle, dont la surface en section transversale n'est guère plus grande que la leur. Vraisemblablement composés de protéines non basiques selon les résultats obtenus en microscopie photonique, ils contiennent aussi des éléments polysaccharidiques.

Leur apparition est tardive dans tous les cas et s'effectue dans une zone cytoplasmique étroite qui borde le flagelle et qui contient des ribosomes libres et quelques cisternes de reticulum endoplasmique lisse.

f) *Vésicule.*

Alors que le spermatozoïde quitte le testicule et paraît acquérir la maturité pour l'ensemble de ses constituants, il conserve une structure insolite qui, interprétée de façons variées par les auteurs anciens, évoque un reliquat cytoplasmique persistant. En fait, la microscopie électronique montre l'originalité de cette formation qui correspond à une inclusion sécrétée par la spermatide. Cette vésicule, logée sous la membrane cytoplasmique, est généralement accolée aux baguettes nucléaire et flagellaire au niveau de leur tiers antérieur. La cytodifférenciation et l'évolution de cette structure font l'object d'une étude particulière (Bocquet-Védrine et Pochon-Masson) chez *Balanus perforatus*.

Suivant les cas, la taille de la vésicule varie considérablement. Il ne faut cependant pas attribuer à cette variation une valeur taxonomique très grande puisque, à l'intérieur d'un même genre, les différences de taille sont relativement importantes: chez *Balanus perforatus*, par exemple, la vésicule atteint un développement considérable (Fig. 6) alors qu'elle est beaucoup plus discrète chez *B. crenatus* (Fig. 7). Celle des Acrothoraciques ne mesure que quelques μ de long et un demi μ de large. Chez les Rhizocéphales, elle est plus volumineuse; par contre le spermatozoïde des Pédonculés ne présente aucune protubérance décelable en microscopie ordinaire bien que cette structure soit décelable à l'échelle infrastructurale (communication personnelle de Brown).

De forme variable, elle est limitée par une membrane unique qui peut présenter certaines différenciations (striations, épaississements). Son contenu diffère quelque peu selon l'espèce considérée: finement fibrillaire chez *Trypetesa*, il est nettement plus homogène chez la Balane. Il se modifie aussi avec l'âge de la cellule germinale; ainsi, les traces de la lobulation initiale (Fig. 12) ou l'aspect réticulé de la substance d'origine disparaissent dans le spermatozoïde.

La vésicule prend naissance, dans la spermatide moyennement âgée, par la confluence de cisternes du reticulum endoplasmique. Celles–ci sont gonflées d'une sécrétion de nature protéique (dont des protéines basiques) et plus vraisemblablement lipo–protéique. En raison de sa faible coloration à l'APS, la vésicule ne peut contenir qu'une petite quantité de composés polysaccharidiques. Si la spermatide comporte encore un cytoplasme riche en ribosomes, le noyau est déjà en voie d'allongement au moment de l'édification de cette vésicule qui résulte d'un phénomène de sécrétion tardive et non pas d'un processus de dégénérescence et d'élimination retardée.

Cette vésicule, limitée par une membrane simple, est susceptible de présenter des particularités remarquables. On observe, chez *Balanus perforatus*, au sein du contenu vésiculaire osmiophile, la différenciation d'une substance plus claire qui entoure un long axe rigide et dense aux électrons, ainsi que la formation d'un corpuscule long de un à deux μ et composé d'un peloton d'éléments d'aspect tubulaire. Ces microtubules ont une paroi très épaisse de 400 Å et une lumière centrale réduite à 120 Å de diamètre (Figs. 9 et 10). Lorsque le spermatozoïde est en attente dans le canal déférent, la vésicule subit des remaniements: vacuolisation et perte de substance sous forme de grains vraisemblablement lipo–protéiques (Fig. 8). Cette diminution de la densité vésiculaire apparait également dans les cas de spermatozoîdes anormaux en dégénerescence.

3°) *Pièce intermédiaire.*

La pièce intermédiaire du spermatozoïde des Cirripèdes est obligatoirement incomplète par rapport au type flagellé banal puisqu'elle est privée de la présence centriolaire. Elle est donc principalement définie par le chondriome qui n'est représenté ici que par une unique mitochondrie, longue de quelques μ. Celle–ci suit parallèlement le flagelle et sa gaine, à l'arrière du noyau. Elle conserve ses crêtes transversales plus ou moins nombreuses sans qu'aucune métamorphose ne semble intervenir. Parfois, dans les spermatides en cours de différenciation, le flagelle est accompagné d'une structure énigmatique. Cette dernière, composée de deux lames osmiophiles distantes de 150 Å environ et reliées entre elles par de nombreux filaments ténus, n'est plus visible dans le spermatozoïde mûr.

4°) *Queue.*

La queue comprend deux parties, la pièce principale, courte en général, définie simplement par le prolongement du matériel périflagellaire autour de l'axonème, et la pièce terminale, composée uniquement du flagelle recouvert de la membrane cytoplasmique. L'extrémité postérieure ne contient plus que quelques microtubules de moins en moins nombreux provenant de la désorganisation du flagelle.

Cas anormaux et polymégalie

Deux séries d'aberrations doivent être distinguées:

a) d'une part, des cellules plus ou moins sphériques qui correspondent à des spermatozoïdes dont les constituants fondamentaux, différenciés, sont enroulés au sein d'un hyaloplasme entouré de la membrane cytoplasmique. Le déroulement du gamète semble être inhibé par un comportement aberrant de la membrane cytoplasmique et par la présence de ce hyaloplasme.

b) d'autre part, des cellules allongées qui correspondent à des spermatozoïdes ayant atteint un développement normal mais affectés à des degrés divers d'une duplication des structures. Cette duplication peut aller d'une simple biflagellarité à un dédoublement total, caractérisé par la répétition de chaque structure, l'ensemble étant entouré d'une membrane cytoplamique commune. Toutes les étapes intermédiaires sont possibles. En particulier le gamète peut rester mononucléé et présenter toutefois une charge double en chromatine sous la forme de deux masses distinctes incluses dans une même enveloppe. Enfin, il arrive aussi que s'installe un état polyflagellaire: certaines images nous ont permis d'observer des gamètes pourvus vraisemblablement de plusieurs flagelles.

Le nombre de spermatozoïdes en duplication est plus élevé chez *Balanus* que chez *Trypetesa* mais, dans le deux cas, la polyflagellarité s'observe dès le début de la spermiogenèse et paraît être la condition *sine qua non* du dédoublement des autres structures.

Conclusions

Les résultats conjugués de la microscopie photonique et de la microscopie électronique montrent qu'il est maintenant possible d'établir un schéma-type du spermatozoïde des Cirripèdes (Schéma 1) en raison de l'agencement très parallèle des structures homologues.

Ce spermatozoïde est fondamentalement caractérisé:

– par la présence de tous les éléments d'un gamète flagellé (acrosome, noyau, flagelle et chondriome);

– par la présence d'éléments qui lui sont propres (matériel périflagellaire, vésicule de sécrétion);

– par la disposition particulière de ses constituants (remontée du centriole distal dans la tête; disque nucléaire d'une extrême minceur, pincé entre l'acrosome et ce centriole, tandis que le reste du noyau s'étire vers l'arrière le long du flagelle).

L'originalité du spermatozoïde des Cirripèdes est donc suffisante pour être caractéristique du groupe mais, en fait, elle réside bien plus dans la façon dont s'est réalisé l'aspect filiforme que dans la structure propre de chacun de ses constituants.

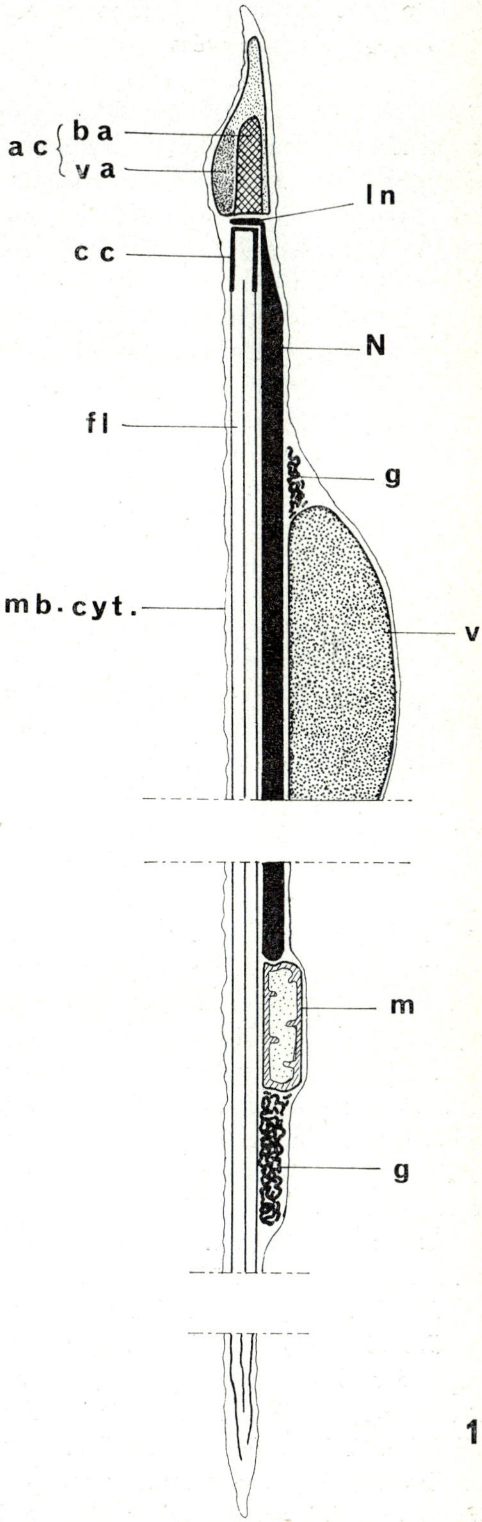

Schéma I. – Schéma-type d'un spermatozoïde de Cirripède.

ac.: acrosome; *b.a.*: bâtonnet axial; *c.c.*: complexe centriolaire; *fl.*: flagelle; *g.*: gaine périflagellaire; *l.n.*: lamelle nucléaire; *m.*: mitochondrie; *mb.cyt.*: membrane cytoplasmique; *N.*: noyau; *v.*: vésicule; *v.a.*: vésicule acrosomique.

On peut établir une graduation dans la valeur significative des variations morphologiques observées.

En premier lieu, le spermatozoïde comporte des caractéristiques telles que la structure particulière en strates du bâtonnet axial, la fine striation de la membrane acrosomienne, l'aspect du contenu de l'acrosome, les différenciations annulaires du centriole de *Trypetesa*, qui ne représentent que des variations légères d'ordre simplement cytologique.

Le spermatozoïde de Cirripède regroupe un certaine nombre de particularités qui lui confèrent une originalité par rapport au type banal, mais qui se retrouvent néanmoins isolément dans d'autres gamètes, principalement chez les Arthropodes. La position antérieure du centriole a déjà été décrite chez le Mystacocaride *Derocheilocaris typicus* (Brown et Metz, 1967), chez les Insectes *Lepisma* et *Cicindela* (Werner, 1964 et 1965) et *Panorpa* (Baccetti, Dallai et Rosati, 1969). Notons que, chez les Cirripèdes, la situation centriolaire respecte cependant la contigüité de l'enveloppe nucléaire et du bâtonnet axial par l'intermédiaire du disque nucléaire. La disparition d'un des éléments du diplosome a été signalée dans des groupes zoologiques plus variés: chez les Nématodes (Favard, 1961), chez une Annélide (Fallon et Austin, 1963) et chez la Limule (Philpott et Shaw, 1959; André, 1963).

Un chondriome peu développé appartient en général à des spermatozoïdes aflagellés (Ascaris, Iule et Crustacés Décapodes). Ce caractère morphologique est en corrélation avec la faible consommation en oxygène de cette cellule (Barnes, 1962). Le besoin énergétique du flagelle est peu élevé, ce qui s'expliquerait par le fait que les modes de fécondation ne nécessitent pas de grands déplacements du gaméte.

L'évolution du noyau au cours de la spermiogenèse et le remaniement de son enveloppe rappellent les phènomènes observés par Werner (1966), chez la Nèpe et le Carabe; chez ces espèces on assiste à une élimination, tout au moins partielle, de l'enveloppe initiale, à la disparition des pores nucléaires et à une augmentation de son osmiophilie au fur et à mesure de la progression périphérique de la manchette.

Le flagelle de type 9+2 est commun aux gamètes flagellés des Crustacés et à ceux des Insectes inférieurs (Baccetti, Dallai et Rosati, 1968). La formation bilamellaire qui l'avoisine occupe un emplacement identique à celui de la lamelle annelée des cellules germinales mâles de l'Abeille (Hoage et Kessel, 1968).

Deux caractères morphologiques semblent caractériser plus particulièrement le spermatozoïde des Cirripèdes; il s'agit de la vésicule transitoire de sécrétion et du matériel périflagellaire.

La vésicule est en fait un grain de sécrétion d'origine ergastoplasmique, emporté temporairement par le spermatozoïde sous sa membrane cellulaire, dans le canal déférent. Elle doit jouer un rôle de réserve dans le métabolisme cellulaire. A la différence des Décapodes, les spermatides ne sont pas environnées de cellules intercalaires qui peuvent leur apporter des éléments nutritifs. Les possibilités sécrétrices d'une cellule germinale mâle sont donc susceptibles de devenir importantes et de donner lieu à des inclusions volumineuses par rapport à la taille des gamètes.

Le matériel périflagellaire qui engaine de façon assez lâche le flagelle est d'origine vraisemblablement ribosomique. Pour cette raison, il ne nous apparaît pas assimilable au « centriolar adjunct » rencontré surtout chez les Insectes. Il évoque plutôt la gaine fibreuse du spermatozoïde des Mammifères. Il doit être impliqué dans un contrôle mécanique du complexe noyau–flagelle, légèrement spiralé, et plus particulièrement dans celui du mouvement flagellaire réduit à des ondulations de faible amplitude, dans les parties céphalique et intermédiaire du gamète. Une étude histochimique approfondie permettrait de déceler comment il intervient dans le métabolisme (substances de réserve, enzymes). Le spermatozoïde des Cirripèdes est, enfin, l'objet d'anomalies qui, en raison de la bi–ou polyflagellarité obligatoire, de la duplication variable de ses structures (vésicule et noyau) semblent provenir d'un ensemble de perturbations affectant les mitoses de maturation. Le cas de biflagellarité dans un spermatozoïde à noyau haploïde peut résulter d'une retenue accidentelle du deuxième centriole habituellement disparu chez les Cirripèdes.

Lors de l'étude de l'un d'entre nous sur la spermiogenèse des Crustacés Décapodes (POCHON–MASSON, 1968 a et b, 1969), nous avions essayé de rechercher comment s'effectuait le passage d'une cellule germinale flagellée à celle d'un type aberrant, immobile et aflagellé, en fonction des connaissances acquises sur les spermatozoïdes des divers Crustacés. Les Malacostracés ne conservent pas la structure typique du flagelle dans leurs gamètes; par contre, chez les Entomostracés, si les spermatozoïdes des Phyllopodes sont amiboïdes, ceux des Copépodes, des Cirripèdes et des Mystacocarides possèdent un flagelle du type 9+2 que l'on retrouve également chez certains Arachnides et chez les Insectes inférieurs (BACCETTI, DALLAI et ROSATI, 1968). Le spermatozoïde des Cirripèdes représente certainement, au sein des Crustacés, un type cellulaire primitif; c'est pourquoi il est particulièrement intéressant d'y déceler, au niveau ultrastructural, des caractères morphologiques comparables à ceux des gamètes vésiculaires des Décapodes. Certains de ces caractères, comme la réduction du chondriome, correspondent peut–être simplement à un phénomène de convergence physiologique; mais la position centriolaire sous–acrosomienne et la présence d'une vésicule de sécrétion d'origine ergastoplasmique (présente également chez les Isopodes) témoignent d'un bouleversement très original de l'organisation du gamète. Cependant, les homologies que l'on peut établir entre les constituants du spermatozoïde des Cirripèdes et des Crustacés les plus évolués restent modestes. Les lacunes de nos connaissances, dans ce domaine, se comblent peu à peu et les informations récentes permettent de mieux comprendre l'évolution très remarquable de la cellule germinale mâle chez les Crustacés.

Bibliographie

ALFERT M. et GESCHWIND I. (1953) – *A selective method for the basic proteins of the cell nuclei.* « Proc. Nat. Acad. Sci. », 39, 991–999.

ANDRÉ J. (1963) – *Existence d'un axe nucléairé dans le spermatozoïde de la Limule: ses relations avec la réaction acrosomienne.* « J. Microscopie », 2, 21.

BACCETTI B., DALLAI R. et ROSATI F. (1968) – *Sur la structure du flagelle dans le spermatozoïde des Arthropodes.* « J. Microscopie », 7, 4, 20 a.

BACCETTI B., DALLAI R. et ROSATI F. (1969) – *The spermatozoon of Arthropoda.* III. *The lowest holometabolic Insects.* « J. Microscopie », 8, 2, 233–248.

BARNES H. (1962) – *The oxygen uptake and metabolism of* Balanus balanus *spermatozoa.* « J. Exp. Biol. », 39, 353–358.

BLOCH D. P. et HEW H. Y. C. (1961) – *Methods for the cytochemical characterization of nuclear basic proteins and their application to problems of development.* « Ann. Histoch. », 6, 497–500.

BOCQUET-VÉDRINE J. (1961) – *Monographie de* Chthamalophilus delagei *J. Bocquet-Védrine, Rhizocéphale parasite de* Chthamalus stellatus (*Poli*). « Cahiers Biol. Mar. », 2, 455–595.

BOCQUET-VEDRINE J. et POCHON-MASSON J. – *Cytodifférenciation de la vésicule au cours de la spermiogenèse chez* Balanus perforatus *Brug.* (*Crustacé Cirripède*). « Arch. Zool. exp. géné. », (sous presse).

BROWN G. G. (1966) – *Ultrastructural studies of crustacean spermatozoa and fertilization.* « Doct. Diss. Univ. Miami ».

BROWN G. G. et METZ C. B. (1967) – *Ultrastructural studies of the spermatozoa of two primitive crustaceans* Hutchinsoniella macracantha *and* Derocheilocaris typicus. « Z. Zellforsch. mikr. Anat. », 80, 1, 78–92.

DELAGE Y. (1884) – *Evolution de la Sacculine* (Sacculina carcini), *Crustacé endoporasite de l'ordre nouveau des Kentrogonides.* « Arch. Zool. exp. géné. », 2, 415–736.

DUBOSCQ O. (1901) – *Sur l'évolution du testicule chez la Sacculine.* « Arch. Zool. exp. géné. », 3. 9, XVII–XXIX.

FALLON J. F. et AUSTIN C. R. (1963) – *Fine structure of* Nereis limbata *spermatozoa.* « Biol. Bull. », 125, 362.

FAVARD P. (1961) – *Evolution des ultrastructures cellulaires au cours de la spermatogenèse de l'Ascaris.* « Ann. Sci. Nat., Zool. Biol. animale », 3, 53–152.

GABE M. (1968) – *Techniques histologiques.* Masson et Cie éd., Paris, 1968, 733 p.

GIARD A. (1873) – *Sur les Cirripèdes Rhizocéphales.* « C. R. Acad. Sci. Paris », 77, 945–948.

GRASSÉ P. P. et TUZET O. (1928) – *Le spermatozoïde de la Balane,* Balanus perforatus *Brug.* « C. R. Soc. Biol. », 99, 1543–1545.

GRASSÉ P. P. et TUZET O. (1932) – *Recherches sur la spermatogenèse de* Balanus perforatus *Brug.* « Arch. Zool. exp. géné. », 73, 9–21.

HOAGE T. R. et KESSEL R. G. (1968) – *An electron microscope study of the process of differenciation during spermatogenesis in the Drone Honey Bee* (Apis mellifera *L.*) *with special reference to centriole replication and elimination.* « J. Ultrastr. Res. », 24, 6–32.

PHILPOTT D. E. et SHAW W. N. (1959) – *An electron microscopic study of the sperm of* Limulus polyphemus. « Biol. Bull. », 117, 423–424.

POCHON-MASSON J. (1968 a) – *L'ultrastructure des spermatozoïdes vésiculaires chez les Crustacés Décapodes avant et au cours de leur dévagination expérimentale.* I. *Brachyoures et Anomoures.* « Ann. Sci. Nat. », 12, 10, 1, 1–100.

POCHON-MASSON J. (1968 b) – *L'ultrastructure des spermatozoïdes vésiculaires chez les Crustacés Décapodes avant et au cours de leur dévagination expérimentale.* II. *Macroures. Discussion et Conclusions.* « Ann. Sci. Nat. », 12, 10, 3, 367–454.

POCHON-MASSON J. (1969) – *Infrastructure du spermatozoïde de* Palaemon elegans (*De Man*), (*Crustacé Décapode*). « Arch. Zool. exp. gené. », 110, 3 (sous presse).

SAHLEANU E. (1932) – *Spermatogenese und Spermien bei Cirripedien.* « Bull. Fac. Sti. Cernauti », 5, 229–259.

TURQUIER Y. et POCHON–MASSON J. (1969) – *L'infrastructure du spermatozoïde de* Trypetesa (= Alcippe) nassarioides *Turquier* (*Cirripède Acrothoracique*). « Arch. Zool. exp. géné », 110, 3 (sous presse).

WERNER G. (1964) – *Untersuchungen über die Spermiogenese beim Silberfischchen,* Lepisma saccharina *L.* « Z. Zellforsch. », 63, 880–912.

WERNER G. (1965) – *Untersuchungen über die Spermiogenese beim Sandlaüfer,* Cicindela campestris *L.* « Z. Zellforsch. », 66, 255–275.

WERNER G. (1966) – *Untersuchungen über die Spermiogenese bei einem Laufkäfer,* Carabus catenulatus *Scop., und der Skorpion–wasserwanze,* Nepa rubra *L.* « Z. Zellforsch. », 73, 576–599.

ZAGURY D., ZYLBERBERG L. et ZEITOUN P. (1966) – *L'inclusion en lamelle d'Epon pour l'étude en microscopie photonique. Application à la mise en évidence des phosphatases alcalines.* « C. R. Acad. Sci. Paris », 269, 2166–2168.

LÉGENDES DES FIGURES

Spermiogenèse comparée de *Balanus perforatus* et de *Trypetesa nassarioides.*

Fig. 1. – Spermatides moyennement âgées de *T. nassarioides.*

Les ribosomes (*r.*) sont abondants le long du noyau (*N.*) qui s'allonge et devient osmiophile. La vésicule (*v.*) est ébauchée. La membrane cytoplasmique (*m.c.*) perle. Les reliquats cytoplasmiques restent unis par des ponts persistants (*p.c.*). ×21.000.

Fig. 2. – Spermiogenèse de *Balanus perforatus.*

Stade moins avancé que celui de la fig. 1. L'aspect du noyau est plus homogène; (*m.t.*): microtubules de la manchette. ×13.000.

Fig. 3. – Spermiogenèse de *B. perforatus.*

Stade jeune; le noyau, encore sphérique, est bordé partiellement par les microtubules de la manchette (*m.t.*). Entre la mitochondrie (*m.*) et le flagelle, présence d'une lamelle paraflagellaire (*l.f.*). ×54.000.

Fig. 4. – Spermiogenèse de *B. perforatus.*

Stade plus évolué: l'évolution nucléaire est relativement avancée et l'enveloppe nucléaire (*e.n.*) très modifiée. ×55.000.

Comparaison des spermatozoïdes de *Balanus perforatus* et de *B. crenatus.*

Fig. 5. – Spermatides âgées et spermatozoïdes de *B. perforatus.*

Dans les spermatides la vésicule est en cours d'élaboration; son cristalloïde n'est pas encore présent, mais une enclave hyaloplasmique claire indique son emplacement futur.
Certains spermatozoïdes sont sectionnés à un niveau très antérieur: région sous-acrosomienne, centriole (flèche). ×16.000.

Fig. 6. – Spermatozoïdes de *B. perforatus.*

Noter, sur les sections transversales, la forme du noyau, la présence de la gaine périflagellaire (*g.*). La vésicule (*v.*), dont le cristalloïde (*cr.*) est constitué, se présente sous des aspects très variés (en trame, homogène vacuolisée). ×16.000.

Fig. 7. – Spermiogenèse avancée de *B. crenatus.*

Noter l'aspect très différent de la vésicule. (×16.000).

La vésicule du spermatozoïde des Cirripèdes.

Fig. 8. – Frottis de spermatozoïdes de *Balanus perforatus*.

Le contenu vésiculaire a été fortement remanié: élimination de granules osmiophiles, substance hétérogène renfermant un axe dense aux électrons (flèche). ×7.500.

Fig. 9. – Détail du corpuscule cristalloïde et du contenu vésiculaire. ×50.000.

Fig. 10. – Section transversale des éléments du corps cristalloïde. ×25.000.

Figs. 11 et 12. – Spermatozoïde de *Trypetesa nassarioides*.

La vésicule est appendue au noyau à quelque distance de l'acrosome (*ac.*) et du compl exe centriolaire (*c.c.* ×32.000 et ×20.000.

Les autres constituants du spermatozoïde des Cirripèdes.

Fig. 13. – Section longitudinale des spermatozoïdes de *Balanus perforatus* montrant la structure de la gaine (*g*), du flagelle et de l'enveloppe nucléaire. ×32.000.

Fig. 14. – Coupes transversales de spermatozoïdes de *B. crenatus* au niveau de la vésicule (*v.*) et de la pièce intermédiaire. (*m.*): mitochondrie. ×64000.

Fig. 15. – Coupes transversales de spermatozoïdes de *Trypetesa nassarioides*.

Noter la silhouette biconcave du noyau, la gaine, l'unique mitochondrie; l'astérisque souligne un cas de gamète dédoublé. ×22.000.

Fig. 16. – Coupes transversales de spermatozoïdes de *B. crenatus*.

La membrane cytoplasmique (*m.c.*) est en cours d'élimination. La flèche montre la désorganisation du flagelle dans sa partie tout-à-fait postérieure. ×32.000.

Fig. 17. – Coupes transversales de spermatozoïdes de *B. perforatus* montrant de nombreux cas de gamètes biflagellés (astérisque). Une section intéresse la région antérieure d'un spermatozoïde: centriole et lame nucléaire (flèche). ×13.500.

Fig. 18. – Coupes longitudinale et transversale de l'acrosome chez *T. nassarioides*.

(*b.a.*): bâtonnet axial; (*v.a.*): vésicule acrosomique; la flèche souligne la présence du disque nucléaire sous-acrosomien. ×50.000.

Fig. 19. – Coupe longitudinale de l'acrosome chez *T. nassarioides*.

(*c.c.*): anneaux du complexe centriolaire. ×64.000.

Fig. 20. – Formation de l'acrosome chez *T. nassarioides*.

La vésicule acrosomique, qui renferme le grain acrosomien, coiffe la substance initiale du bâtonnet axial. ×12.000.

Discussion

BACCETTI. – Je vous demande quelques précisions sur l'origine de la vésicule et du matériel de la gaine entourant le flagelle.

POCHON–MASSON. – La vésicule s'édifie au cours de la spermiogenèse à partir de cisternes qui s'accroissent et se gonflent de sécrétion avant de fusionner entre elles. Les spermatides âgées de *Trypetesa* conservent les contours des éléments qui viennent grossir la vésicule, ce qui lui confère un aspect lobulé tardif. Par contre le matériel périflagellaire est une production de dernière heure. Les cordons, non limités par une enveloppe commune, s'édifient dans la mince languette cytoplasmique périflagellaire pourvue auparavant de ribosomes et de quelques petites cisternes de reticulum endoplasmique.

PERSONNE. – Votre matériel périflagellaire est probablement constitué de particules de glycogène. Nous avons, avec ANDERSON, observé un tel matériel périflagellaire de nature glycogénique chez le *Lepas*. La positivité à l'APS plaide en cette faveur.

POCHON–MASSON. – La positivité à l'APS plaide en la faveur d'une nature glycoprotéique du matériel périflagellaire. Le glycogène n'étant pas morphologiquement décelable à ce niveau, et la ténuité des structures rendant difficile l'observation en microscopie ordinaire, seule une réaction élective du glycogène à l'échelle ultrastructurale peut définir s'il s'agit effectivement de ce sucre. Etant donné la réaction positive que vous avez obtenue chez le *Lepas*, nous vérifierons la généralisation de ce résultat au sein du groupe des Cirripèdes.

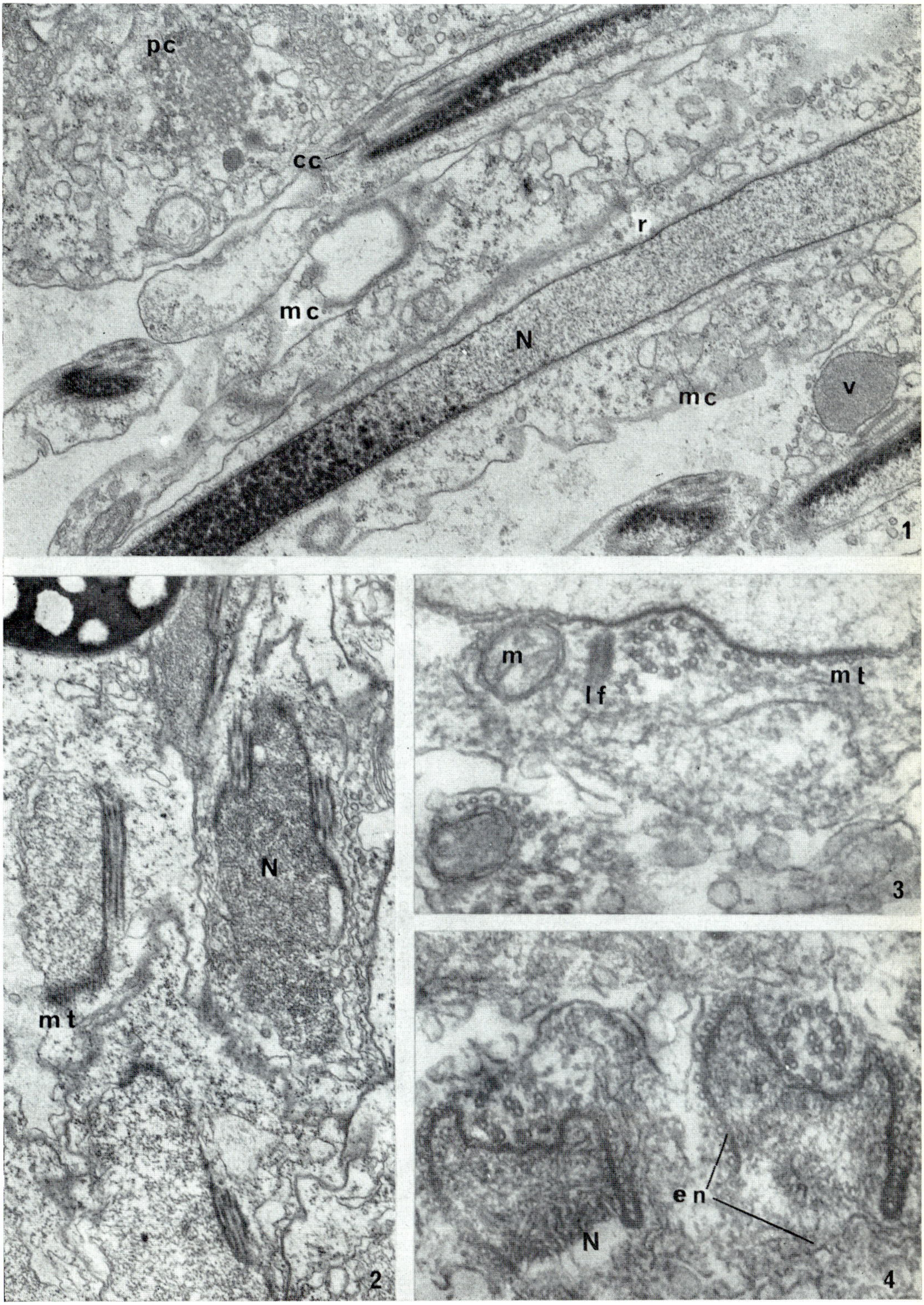
pc
cc
r
mc
N
mc
v
1
mt
N
2
m
lf
mt
3
en
N
4

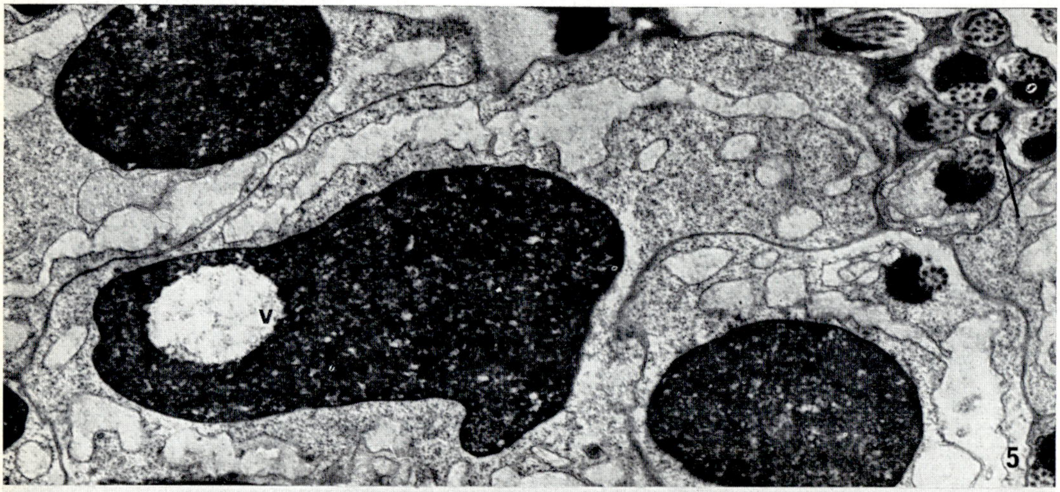
v
5

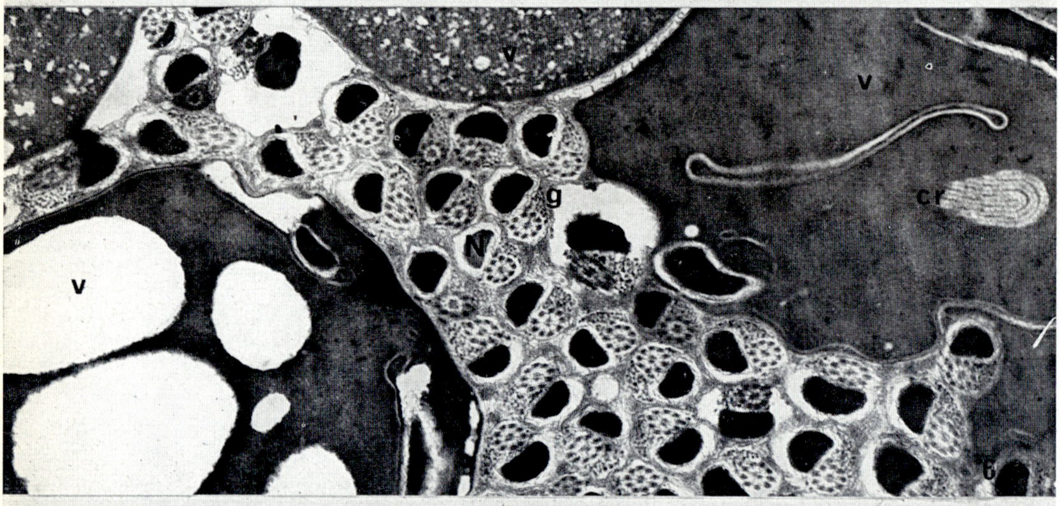
v
v
g
N
cr
v
6

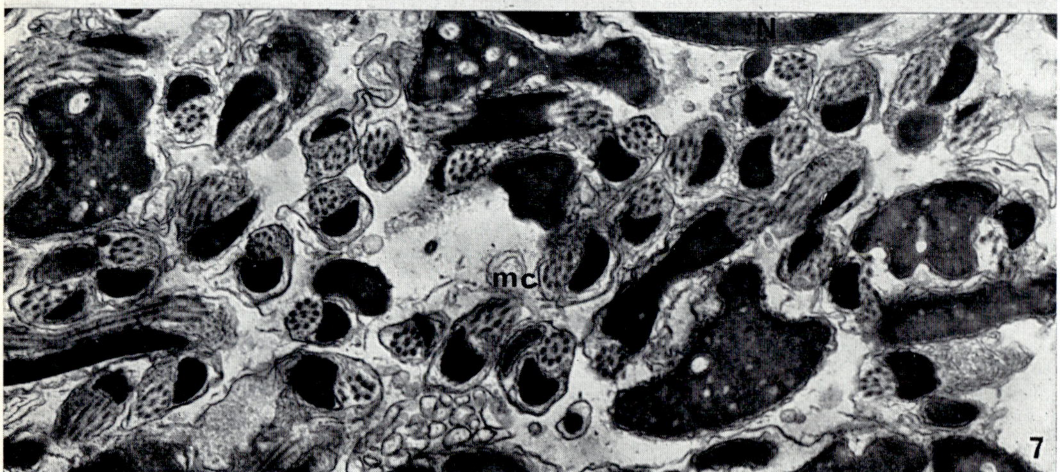
N
mc
7

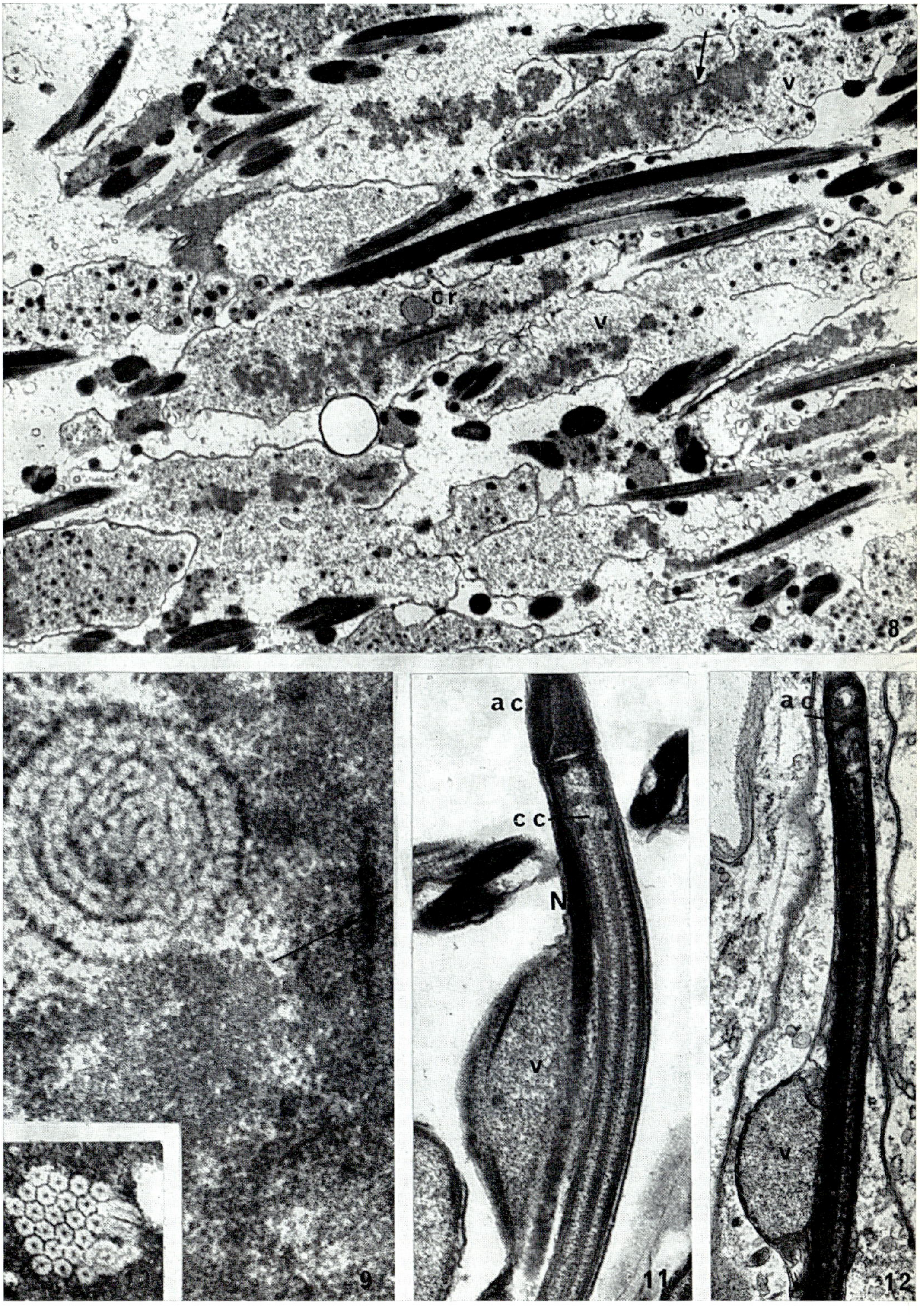

cr
v
v
8
9
10
ac
cc
N
v
11
ac
v
12

J. Pochon – Masson et al. – *Contribution à l'étude du spermatozoïde des Crustacés Cirripèdes.*

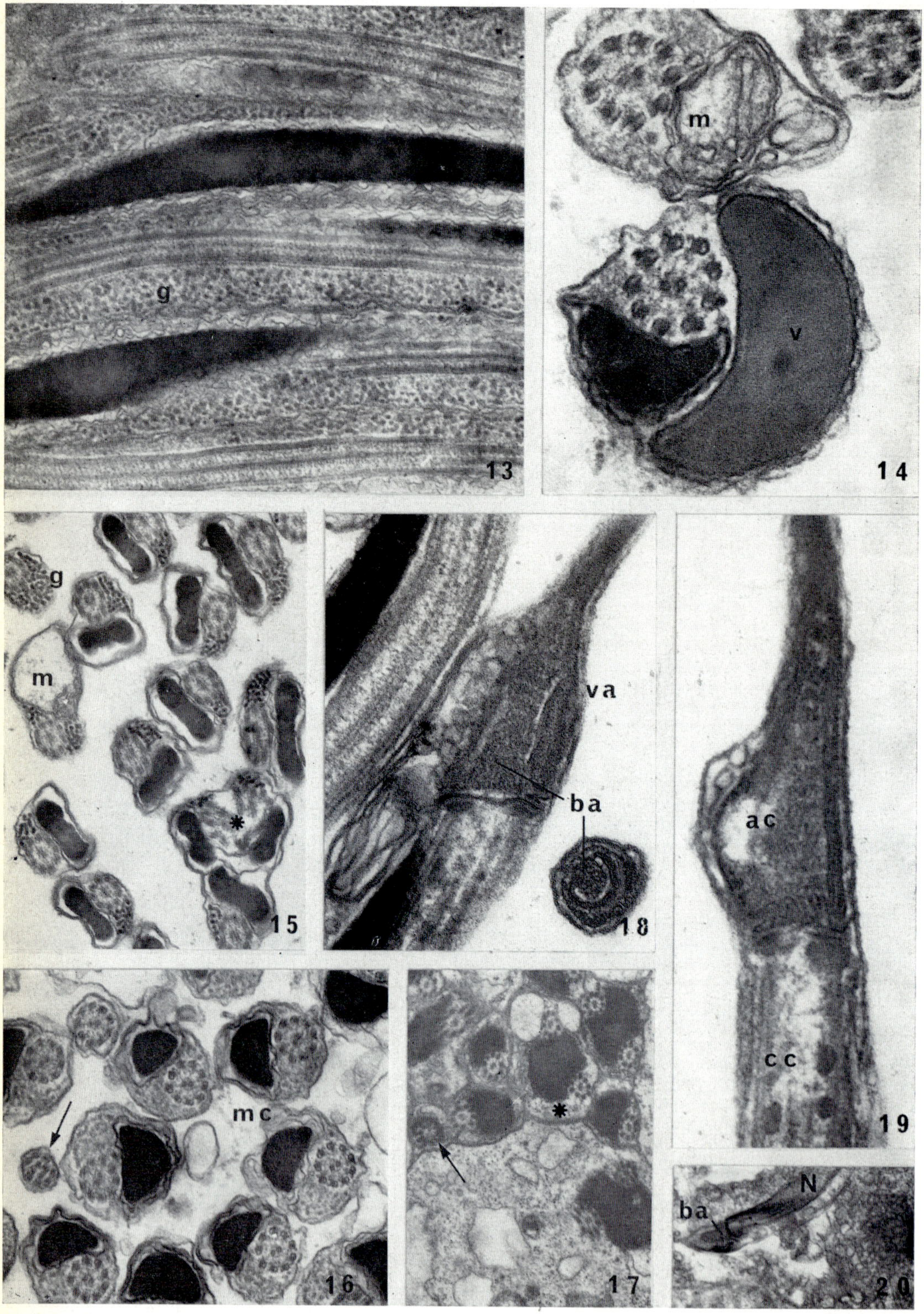

M. A. FAIN-MAUREL (*)

LE SPERMATOZOÏDE DES ISOPODES

RÉSUMÉ. — Les spermatozoïdes des Isopodes, libres ou parasites, associés en spermatophores, sont des gamètes immobiles et coudés; au sommet d'une longue hampe est suspendue une courte lanière contenant le noyau et un filament, la cresta. Ces gamètes présentent, en outre, la particularité de se scinder en deux parties au niveau d'une formation vésiculaire de la lanière dans laquelle est encastrée la base de la hampe.

Ces gamètes sont dépourvus de flagelle, de pièce intermédiaire et d'acrosome normalement constitués. Cependant, la localisation du complexe golgien à l'extrémité libre de la lanière qui contient le noyau désigne le pôle antérieur du spermatozoïde. Le diplosome situé dans une échancrure nucléaire à l'autre extrémité de la lanière marque donc le pôle postérieur du noyau. La hampe, pourvue d'une striation transversale périodique caractéristique de chaque espèce, sans avoir la structure d'un flagelle, en occupe l'emplacement et correspond également à une évagination cytoplasmique qui se forme près du centrosome. La cresta, structure tubulaire entourée d'un manchon plurilamellaire, pourrait représenter un type particulier de pièce intermédiaire comme en témoigne la localisation des mitochondries à son niveau. Les spermatozoïdes des autres Péracarides (Amphipodes, Mysidacés et vraisemblablement Cumacés) appartiennent au même type morphologique.

RIASSUNTO. — Gli spermatozoi degli Isopodi, liberi o parassiti, riuniti in spermatofore, sono dei gameti immobili e caudati; alla sommità di una lunga asta è sospeso un corto bastoncello contenente il nucleo e un filamento. Questi gameti presentano inoltre la particolarità di scindersi in due parti a livello di una formazione vescicolare del bastoncello in cui è incastrata la base dell'asta.

Questi gameti sono sprovvisti di flagello, di regione intermedia e di acrosoma normalmente costituiti. L'asta è provvista di una striatura trasversale periodica caratteristica di ciascuna specie e occupa il posto del flagello, pur non avendone la struttura. Il filamento è una struttura tubolare circondata da un manicotto plurilamellare e potrebbe rappresentare un tipo particolare di regione intermedia, come testimonia la localizzazione dei mitocondri a questo livello. Gli spermatozoi degli altri Peracaridi (Anfipodi, Misidacei e Cumacei) appartengono allo stesso tipo morfologico.

Chez les Isopodes, les spermatozoïdes sont dépourvus de mobilité propre. Ils appartiennent tous à un type morphologique insolite: ils sont coudés; au sommet d'une longue hampe filamenteuse (900 μ), apparemment rigide, est suspendue une courte lanière fusiforme (20 à 30 μ) ou rubanée (200 μ) contenant le noyau et un filament, la cresta.

Ce type de gamète présente, en outre, la particularité de se scinder en deux parties au niveau de la zone de jonction qui relie la lanière à la hampe.

(*) Laboratoire d'Évolution des Êtres Organisés et Laboratoire de Microscopie électronique appliquée à la Biologie, C.N.R.S. Paris, France.

La fragilité de cette zone d'articulation explique le fait qu'au siècle dernier ZENKER (1854) chez *Asellus* et MAYER (1879) chez *Nerocila* aient décrit deux types de spermatozoïdes, les uns longs et filamenteux, les autres courts, en forme de massue, fixés aux précédents par leur extrémité caudale. SARS (1867) et HERMANN (1883) suggérèrent, à cette époque, que les deux types de spermatozoïdes décrits devaient représenter la tête et la queue du gamète mâle de ces Isopodes. Cette conception, ultérieurement admise par GILSON (1884), NICHOLS (1902) et VANDEL (1928), récemment infirmée par TUZET et BESSIÈRE (1952) et par REGER (1964 *a* et *b*), peut être – semble-t-il – partiellement étayée par l'étude infrastructurale de la morphologie et de la morphogenèse de ces gamètes (HOLLANDE et FAIN-MAUREL, 1964, 1965; FAIN-MAUREL, 1966).

En fait, la structure des spermatozoïdes des Isopodes pose trois problèmes:

– En fonction de l'absence de motilité de ces gamètes, quelle signification peut-on attribuer aux deux appendices flagelliformes, la hampe et la cresta?

– Existe-t-il des données morphologiques expliquant la scission de ces gamètes au niveau d'une zone dont la structure est caractéristique de chaque espèce?

– Peut-on sans ambiguité orienter ces gamètes coudés? Doit-on localiser le pôle antérieur du gamète à l'extrémité libre de la hampe, à l'extrémité libre de la lanière ou au point de jonction de ces deux éléments?

RESULTATS

I. – *La morphologie du spermatozoïde des Isopodes.*

Chez tous les Isopodes les spermatozoïdes sont groupés en spermatophores; de nombreux microtubules, issus des cellules folliculeuses polyploïdes qui tapissent la paroi des ampoules testiculaires, s'immiscent entre les éléments germinaux (Figs. 8, 9). L'existence des spermatophores est liée à la disposition des jeunes spermatides qui, dans la gonade, forment des îlots (Fig. 1 a) séparés par des expansions cytoplasmiques émises par les cellules folliculeuses périphériques (Fig. 13). Dans chaque îlot, les spermatides, contigües, radiairement orientées autour d'une lumière centrale, subissent une évolution synchrone (Fig. 1 b); à la fin de la spermiogenèse, les gamètes groupés en îlots sont expulsés dans la vésicule séminale sous forme de spermatophores et remplacés par les éléments germinaux du cycle spermatogenétique suivant.

Les spermatozoïdes des espèces d'Isopodes étudiées présentent certes des caractères spécifiques bien individualisés. Ainsi chez les Cymothoïdés, Isopodes parasites hermaphrodites, les spermatophores sont volumineux, dissociés en forme de gerbe (Fig. 2); les lanières sont courtes (20 à 30 μ), fusiformes ou en massue; la cresta, autonome, s'enroule autour du noyau

(Fig. 3 b). Chez les Isopodes libres (Oniscidés, Sphéroïdés, Idothéïdés, Asellidés), les spermatophores sont moins volumineux, les hampes sont groupées en faisceaux (Fig. 4); les lanières sont longues (200 μ) et rubanées (Fig. 5 b); la cresta est courte, accolée au noyau. Cependant tous les gamètes des Isopodes répondent au même type infrastructural.

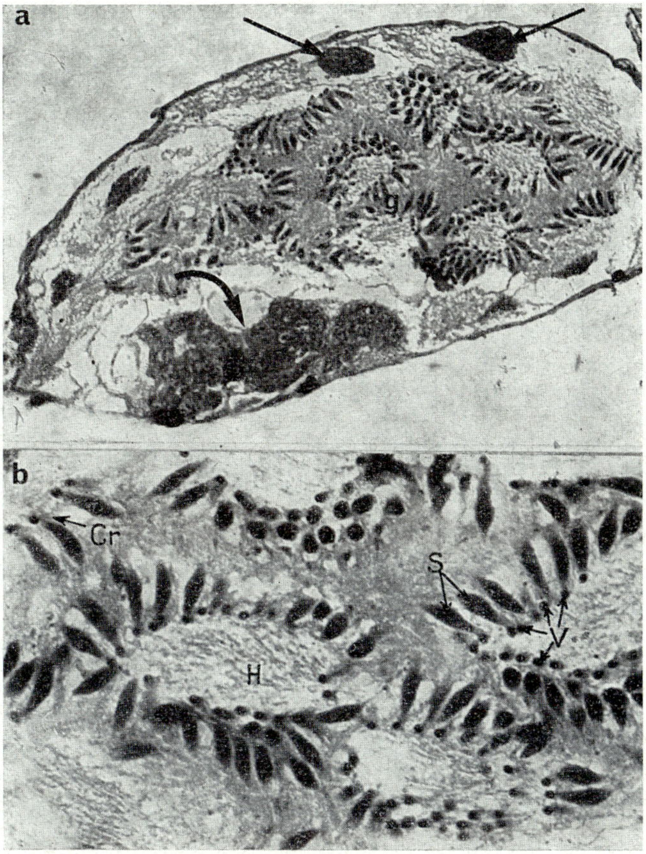

Fig. 1. – *Ampoule testiculaire de Anilocra physodes*. Les jeunes spermatides sont groupées en ilôts et radiairement orientées autour d'une lumière centrale. Les vésicules (V) qui se différencient à l'un des pôles nucléaires saillent dans la lumière; les hampes (H) s'y assemblent en faisceaux; la cresta (Cr) longe le noyau. Des cellules folliculeuses à noyau polyploïde (flèches droites) tapissent la paroi de la gonade. Un lot de spermatogonies (flèche courbe) assure une activité spermatogénétique cyclique.

1°) *La hampe*, correspondant à la queue du spermatozoïde décrite par les Auteurs du siècle dernier, ne possède pas la structure multifibrillaire d'un flagelle (Fig. 18). Cette longue tige éosinophile, tubulaire, est limitée par la membrane cellulaire et par une épaisse paroi sous-jacente pourvue d'une striation périodique transversale; la lumière centrale est parcourue par une baguette axiale, homogène, opaque aux électrons. La période de la striation transversale est caractéristique de chaque espèce (BLANCHARD et coll., 1961; HOLLANDE et FAIN-MAUREL, 1964, 1965; REGER, 1964 a, b, 1966; FAIN-MAUREL, 1966).

La hampe est acuminée et obturée par une substance médullaire à son extrémité libre; au niveau de la zone de jonction avec la lanière, elle présente, en particulier chez les Cymothoïdés (FAIN-MAUREL, 1966) et chez les Amphipodes (observation personnelle), un épaississement nettement mis en évidence lors de la dissociation par pression des deux parties constitutives du sperma-

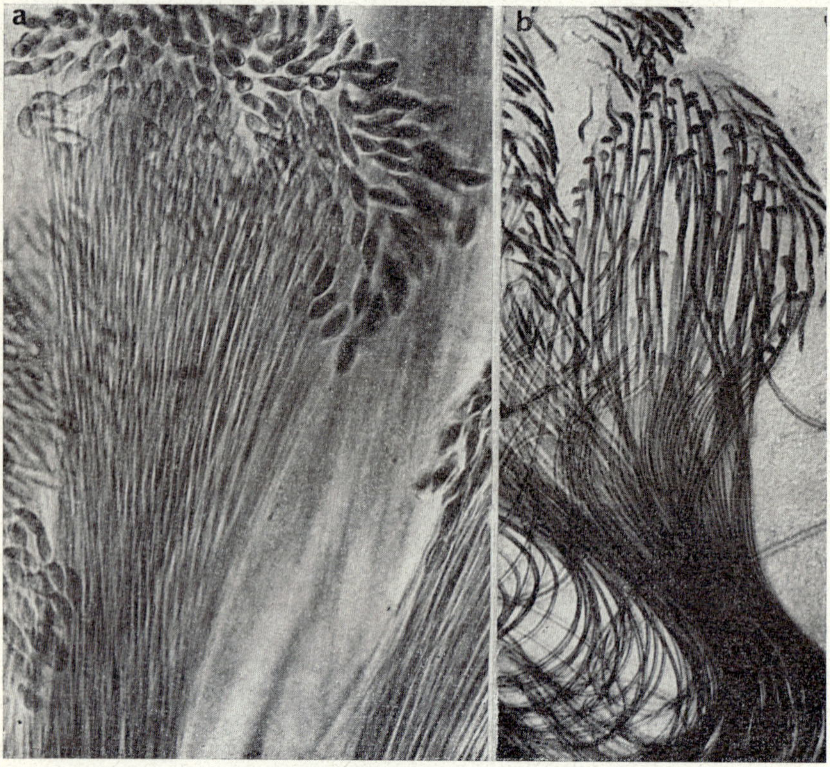

Fig. 2. – *Spermatophores des Isopodes parasites.* a. *Anilocra physodes*; b. *Nerocila bivittata.*

tozoïde. Cet épaississement est volumineux, hémisphérique chez *Nerocila bivittata* RISSO (Fig. 2 a), petit et globuleux chez *Anilocra physodes* L. (Fig. 3 a), chez *Anilocra frontalis* M. EDW. et chez *Meinertia oestroides* RISSO, tronconique chez *Orchestia gammarella* PALLAS et chez *Orchestia mediterranea* COSTA.

2°) *La lanière*, courte et renflée chez les Cymothoïdés (Fig. 2 et 3), longue (200 µ) et rubanée chez les Isopodes libres (Fig. 5 b), contient le noyau et la cresta. Elle est reliée à la hampe par l'intermédiaire d'un bec d'insertion court, épais, arqué chez *Nerocila* (Fig. 6); chez *Anilocra physodes*, une petite formation en capuchon coiffe la zone de jonction entre hampe et lanière; chez *Armadillidium vulgare* LATR., chez *Oniscus asellus* L. et chez les Amphipodes du genre *Orchestia*, un rostre effilé, prismatique triangulaire à sa base, surmonte la zone de jonction entre les deux parties constitutives du gamète (Fig. 4).

Le noyau dont l'élongation a entrainé celle de la lanière, est, dans le spermatozoïde mûr, homogène et opaque aux électrons. A proximité de la zone de jonction entre la hampe et la lanière, le pôle nucléaire présente une échancrure contenant une sphérule fuschinophile constituée d'un matériel granuleux, dense aux électrons, qui entoure le diplosome; les deux élements du diplosome sont parallèles chez les Oniscidés (Fig. 15), situés dans deux plans orthogonaux chez les Cymothoïdés. Un ensemble de tubules divergents (150 Å de diamètre) issus de la région péricentriolaire entoure le noyau.

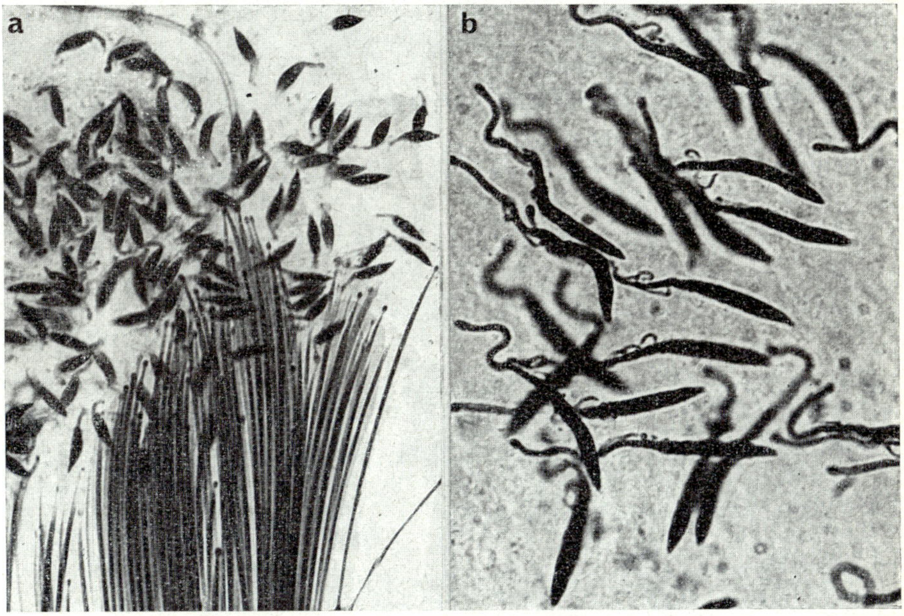

Fig. 3. – *Spermatophores soumis à un écrasement ménagé.* a. *Anilocra physodes:* hampes et lanières dissociées; b. *Nerocila bivittata:* après dissociation, la cresta reste enroulée autour des lanières en forme de massue.

Tous les stades des modifications nucléaires classiques du déroulement de la spremiogenèse peuvent être observés chez les Isopodes. Les microfibrilles (100 Å de diamètre) contenues dans les noyaux des jeunes spermatides (Figs. 8, 10) se réunissent en faisceaux qui s'anastomosent en certains points délimitant ainsi des alvéoles clairs. Des structures lamellaires parallèles au grand axe du noyau se forment ensuite par coalescence des faisceaux fibrillaires (Fig. 9).

Chez *Armadillidium*, les noyaux à structure lamellaire se présentent avec une grande netteté dans les spermatides au stade dit « en grappe » (GILSON) (Fig. 5 a et c). En effet, ce stade est caractérisé par l'existence de sphérules cytoplasmiques reliées par un long pédoncule à un axe multifibrillaire qui représente le faisceau de hampes (Fig. 5 a); à ce stade les structures nucléaires, lamellaires, alignées dans le pédoncule, décrivent des ondulations régulières et sont au niveau de la sphérule repliées sur elles-mêmes (Fig. 5 c).

Chez *Oniscus asellus*, dans les spermatides agées, les noyaux présentent une torsion hélicoïdale (Fig. 4). Chez ces deux espèces la disparition de la torsion du noyau ou de son enroulement dans la sphérule cytoplasmique entraine son élongation et lui confère son aspect rubané définitif (Fig. 5 b). Les structures nucléaires lamellaires confluent alors en une masse homogène opaque aux électrons.

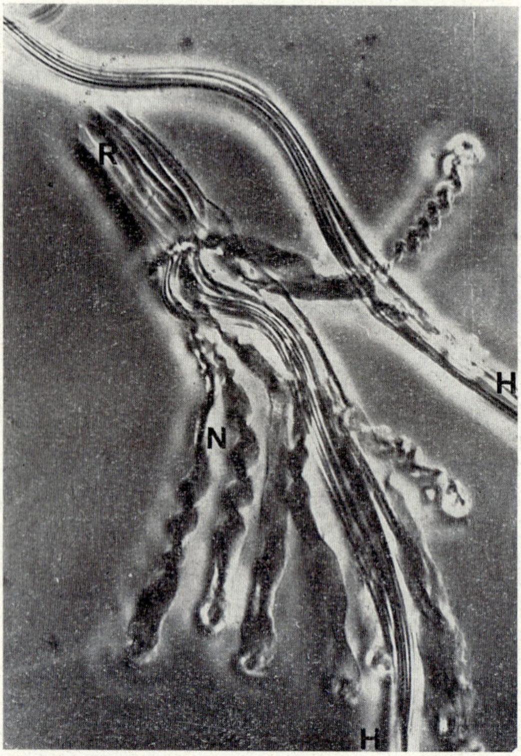

Fig. 4. – *Spermatophore d'un Isopode non parasite*. Spermatides agées de *Oniscus asellus* (en contraste de phase). H = faisceaux de hampes; N = noyaux enroulés hélicoïdalement sur eux-même; R = rostre effilé reliant la lanière à la hampe.

La cresta, comme la hampe, ne possède pas la conformation multifibrillaire d'un flagelle (Figs. 8, 10); c'est une structure tubulaire (300 Å de diamètre chez les Oniscidés, 1500 Å chez les Cymothoïdés) à paroi épaisse, opaque aux électrons, entourée d'un manchon plurilamellaire le long duquel des mitochondries sont régulièrement alignées (Figs. 9, 10).

La cresta, issue de la zone de jonction entre hampe et lanière (Figs. 15, 16), est parallèle au noyau dans la spermatide (Figs. 8, 9); elle reste incrustée dans le noyau des spermatozoïdes des Isopodes non parasites mais devient autonome chez les Cymothoïdés (Fig. 3 b).

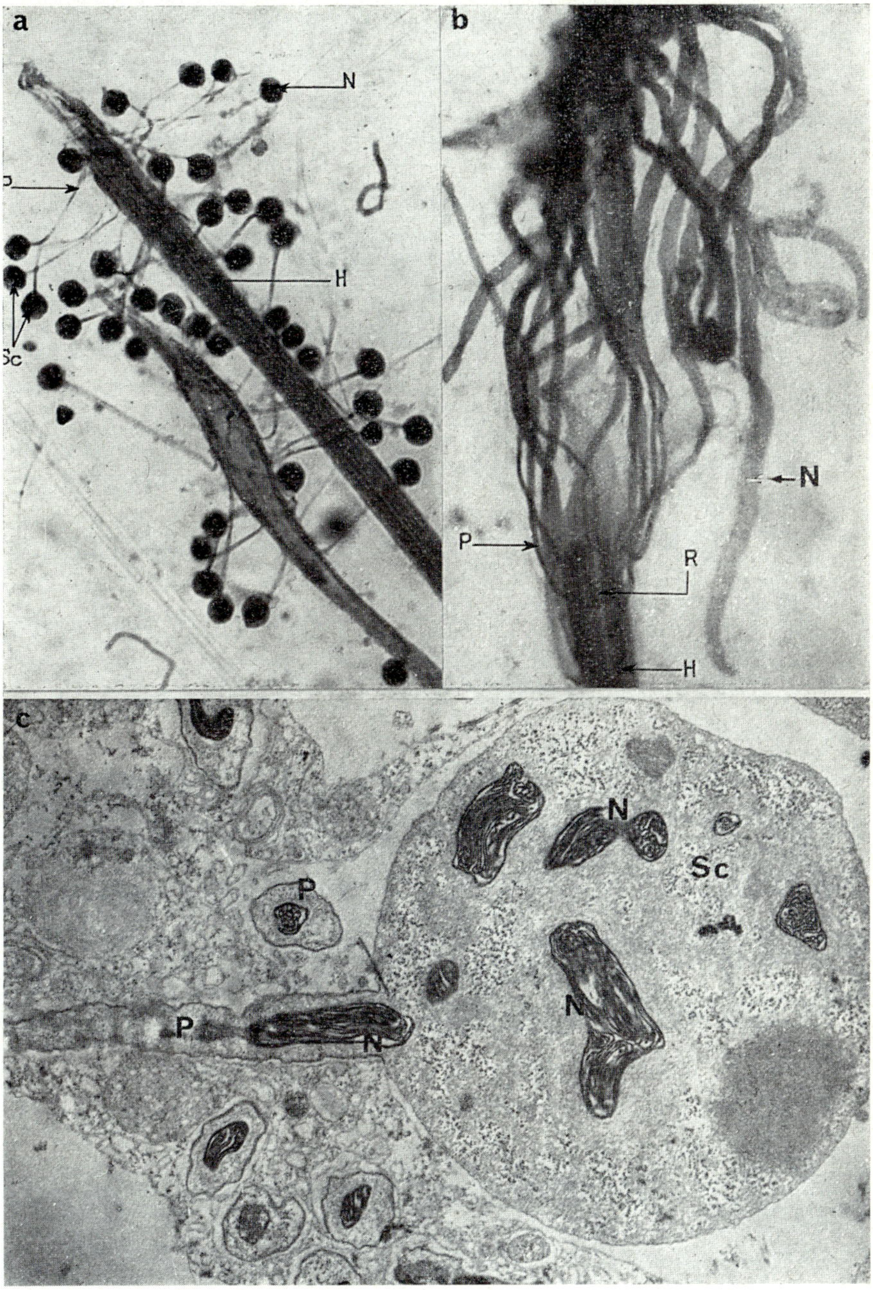

Fig. 5. – *Spermiogenèse chez les Isopodes non parasites.*

a, c – « stade en grappe » chez *Armadillidium vulgare*. Des sphérules cytoplasmiques (Sc), observées au microscope photonique (Fig. 5 a) et électronique (Fig. 5 c), contiennent le noyau rubané (N), replié sur lui-même, et sont reliées par un long pédoncule (P) à un axe multifibrillaire qui représente l'ensemble des hampes (H).

b. – spermatozoïdes de *Oniscus asellus* associés en spermatophore, avec leur noyau (N) long et rubané.

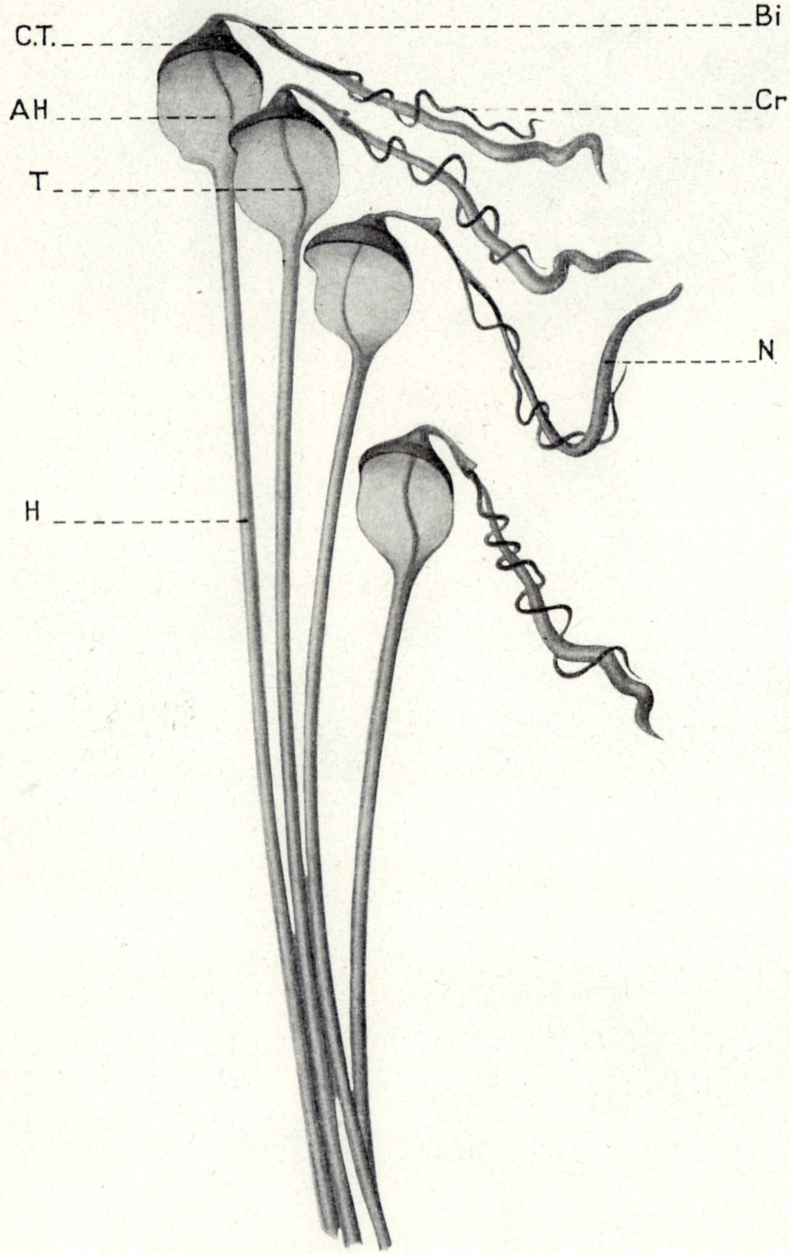

Fig. 6. – *Nerocila bivittata*: spermatides agées. La hampe (H) est dilatée à sa base en une formation ampullaire (AH) parcourue par une tigelle axiale (T). Un bec d'insertion (BI) relie la lanière constituée du noyau (N) et de la cresta (Cr) à la base de la hampe qui sera réduite dans le spermatozoïde mûr à l'épaississement hémisphérique en « tête de champignon » (CT).

En résumé, chez les Isopodes, le noyau du gamète mâle subit au cours de la spermiogenèse une évolution comparable à celle de nombreux spermatozoïdes. En revanche, les deux appendices flagelliformes de ces gamètes immobiles, la hampe et la cresta, ne présentent pas la structure multifibrillaire classique d'un fouet. Le problème de la signification de ces formations tubulaires différenciées reste donc posé en relation avec celui de leur origine au niveau de la zone d'articulation des deux parties dissociables du gamète.

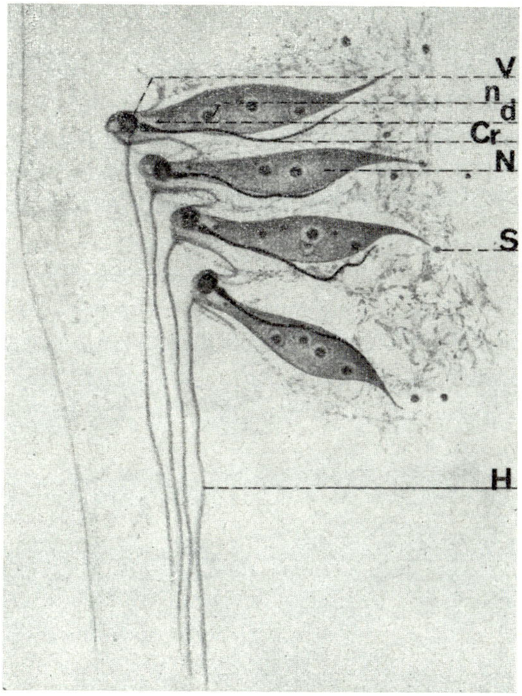

Fig. 7. – *Nerocila bivittata*: spermatides jeunes. Le noyau (N) contenant 2 ou 3 nucléoles (n) est surmonté d'une vésicule (V) d'ou émergent à proximité du diplosome (d) la hampe (H) et la cresta (Cr). A l'autre extrémité siège une sphérule (S) identifiable au grain acrosomien.

II. – *La dissociation du spermatozoïde des Isopodes.*

La dissociation, sous l'effet de la moindre pression, des deux parties constitutives de ce type de gamète peut être expliquée par l'étude des transformations morphogénétiques affectant au cours de la spermiogenèse une formation vésiculaire qui se différencie à l'un des pôles de la jeune spermatide. Cette vésicule d'où émergent la hampe et la cresta constituera la charnière d'articulation entre la hampe et la lanière.

En effet, lorsque les jeunes spermatides groupées radiairement en îlots (Fig. 1) ont acquis une forme ovoïde, une vésicule se différencie au pôle de la spermatide saillant dans la lumière centrale de l'îlot (Fig. 1 b). Cette vésicule apparait en microscopie photonique formée d'une partie chromophile et d'une partie chromophobe. Aux dépens ou au contact de la vésicule s'individualisent deux filaments (Fig. 7); l'un, colorable par la fuschine d'Altmann, longe le noyau; il représente donc la cresta; l'autre, éosinophile, naît à la manière d'un fouet en un point diamétralement opposé et constitue la hampe du gamète. Les hampes se groupent en faisceaux à l'intérieur de l'espace libre ménagé au centre de chaque îlot (Fig. 1 b) et poursuivent leur élongation dans la cavité de l'ampoule testiculaire.

1°) *L'individualisation de la vésicule.*

Le premier indice de la différenciation de la vésicule peut être décelé, au microscope électronique, sous la forme d'une lame dense aux électrons qui apparemment s'individualise dans un saccule ergastoplasmique accolé, dans la région centrosomienne, à la membrane cellulaire (Figs. 11, 12, 13). Cette lame d'un côté s'épaissit en un gros nodule dense aux électrons (Figs. 12, 14, 15), de l'autre émet un diverticule (Fig. 15) qui obture le cône cytoplasmique saillant dans la lumière de l'ampoule testiculaire. La vésicule ainsi formée comprend donc deux parties d'origine et de structure différentes: une partie homogène, dense aux électrons, qui correspond à la partie chromophile observée en microscopie photonique et représente une différenciation de la lame dense aux électrons; une partie chromophobe, dépourvue d'opacité aux électrons, qui correspond au cytoplasme séquestré dans le cône cellulaire obturé par le diverticule de la lame dense.

2°) *L'individualisation de la hampe et de la cresta.*

La hampe et la cresta s'individualisent au niveau de deux zones épaissies de la membrane limitant le compartiment cytoplasmique de la vésicule (Fig. 14).

Aux dépens de l'un de ces épaississements s'édifie à l'extérieur de la vésicule une formation réniforme homogène, opaque aux électrons, qui reste encastrée dans la partie chromophobe de la vésicule dont elle est séparée par une mince couche cytoplasmique (Figs. 14 et 15). Cette formation réniforme constitue le sommet de la hampe (Fig. 14); la baguette axiale de la hampe est incrustée dans la partie médiane de la formation réniforme chez les Cymothoïdés (Fig. 14), dans la partie latérale chez les Isopodes libres (Fig. 15, 17). La membrane cellulaire qui circonscrit la formation réniforme s'évagine avec le feuillet dense aux électrons qui la tapisse pour former la paroi de la hampe (Fig. 14); le feuillet dense, pourvu à ce niveau de la striation transversale périodique caractéristique de chaque espèce, s'épaissit au cours du déroulement de la spermiogenèse (Fig. 18).

Le second épaississement de la membrane limitant la partie cytoplasmique de la vésicule est localisé à proximité du diplosome logé dans l'échancrure nucléaire. Cet épaississement est associé au manchon périphérique de la cresta (Fig. 14), la structure tubulaire axiale étant reliée à la partie de la vésicule opaque aux électrons (Fig. 15).

3°) *Le mode de dissociation de la hampe et de la lanière.*

Les modifications morphologiques qui affectent la vésicule à la fin de la spermiogenèse contribuent à assurer à la zone de jonction une structure caractéristique de chaque espèce; cependant les mécanismes permettant la dissociation des deux parties constitutives du gamète sont identiques chez tous les Isopodes.

Chez les Isopodes non parasites, chez *Armadillidium vulgare* par exemple, la vésicule s'allonge en un rostre étroit (Fig. 17); la partie chromophile opaque aux électrons s'amenuise en un petite lame apicale; la partie cytoplasmique chromophobe constitue seule la partie basale du rostre dans laquelle est encastrée la formation réniforme, base de la hampe. Par simple pression, à la façon d'une tête osseuse qui sortirait de sa cavité articulaire, la formation réniforme peut être séparée du rostre qui demeure solidaire de la lanière contenant le noyau et la cresta.

Chez les Isopodes parasites, chez *Nerocila bivittata* en particulier, les modifications morphologiques qui se produisent à la fin de la spermiogenèse affectent conjointement la vésicule et la base de la hampe.

En effet, la distension des replis cytoplasmiques qui, dans la jeune spermatide, circonscrivent le tubercule réniforme (Fig. 14) provoque l'apparition d'une formation ampullaire (Figs, 6, 16) qui ultérieurement acquiert son aspect hémisphérique en « tête de champignon » (Fig. 2 b).

Le développement spectaculaire du sommet de la hampe est accompagné d'un aplatissement de la partie chromophobe de la vésicule et d'un étirement de la partie chromophile qui relie ainsi la lanière contenant le noyau et la cresta au sommet de la hampe (Fig. 16). La séparation des deux parties constitutives du spermatozoïde s'effectue, comme chez les Isopodes libres, au niveau du tubercule réniforme, base de la hampe, encastré dans la fragile partie cytoplasmique de la vésicule.

A la fin de la spermiogenèse, la cresta solidaire de la partie chromophile de la vésicule devient chez les Cymothoïdés autonome dans sa partie distale. Elle est alors incluse dans une mince couche cytoplasmique contenant des chondriosomes et limitée par la membrane cellulaire.

En résumé, la hampe et la cresta représentent des différenciations d'un feuillet dense aux électrons qui tapisse la membrane cellulaire dans la région centrosomienne. Ce feuillet participe à l'édification d'une vésicule assurant l'articulation entre la hampe et la lanière. La séparation de la hampe et de la lanière s'effectue par déboitement d'une formation réniforme, base de la hampe, encastrée dans la vésicule. Ces données s'avèrent néanmoins insuffisantes pour attribuer une orientation à ce type de spermatozoïde coudé.

III. – *L'orientation du spermatozoïde des Isopodes.*

Aucun acrosome morphologiquement bien défini n'a pu être mis en évidence dans le spermatozoïde des Isopodes libres et parasites et n'a permis d'orienter ces gamètes de manière indiscutable.

Cependant, dans les jeunes spermatides, de nombreux documents révèlent la présence d'un complexe golgien au pôle cellulaire opposé à celui où siègent la vésicule et le diplosome (Figs. 11, 13). Le complexe golgien est donc situé à l'extrémité libre de la lanière et, à ce niveau, l'espace périnucléaire est fréquemment dilaté.

L'aire golgienne contient un petit nombre de dictyosomes constitués de quelques saccules courts et souvent dilatés, de vacuoles claires polymorphes, de petites vésicules à contour épaissi et de granules denses aux électrons. Ultérieurement, ces granules denses fusionnent pour former un gros grain (1 μ) fréquemment entouré de citernes ergastoplasmiques. Ce grain qui, par sa taille et sa localisation, correspond à une volumineuse sphérule éosinophile observée en microscopie photonique à l'extrémité libre de la lanière (Fig. 7), pourrait donc être assimilé à un grain acrosomien.

En résumé, si l'orientation de ce type aberrant de gamète ne peut être fondée sur la localisation d'un acrosome et d'un flagelle normalement constitués, du moins peut-elle être présumée par la présence du complexe golgien à l'extrémité libre de la lanière et discutée en fonction des données relatives aux spermatozoïdes des autres Péracarides.

Conclusions

La structure du spermatozoïde des Isopodes, gamète immobile et coudé, dépourvu de flagelle, de pièce intermédiaire et d'acrosome morphologiquement bien définis, devrait inciter à le considérer comme un spermatozoïde atypique et aflagellé. Cependant des analogies peuvent être établies entre la structure de ce type de gamète et celle des spermatozoïdes flagellés typiques.

– *La localisation du complexe golgien à l'extrémité libre de la lanière qui contient le noyau désigne, a priori, le pôle antérieur du spermatozoïde.*

De plus, une étude comparative du spermatozoïde des Isopodes et de celui des Mysidacés fournit un argument supplémentaire susceptible d'étayer une telle présomption.

Le spermatozoïde des Mysidacés, celui de *Praunus flexuosus* en particulier, étudié par Labat (1962), présente en effet d'évidentes analogies avec celui des Isopodes. Il est immobile et coudé. La hampe, très longue, est reliée à la lanière par un rostre identique à celui des Isopodes. Cependant, chez les Mysidacés, la lanière contient un acrosome localisé à son extrémité libre, un noyau, et une pièce intermédiaire. L'acrosome se présente sous la forme d'une large lame cytoplasmique festonnée, animée de lents mouvements ondulatoires; il contient un granule acrosomien situé à proximité du noyau, identique à celui du gamète des Isopodes. La pièce intermédiaire a la forme d'une longue gouttière qui renferme un cordon mitochondrial. Le cytoplasme résiduel est éliminé, comme chez les Isopodes, à l'extrémité antérieure de la spermatide.

Il semble donc qu'une telle analogie structurale puisse permettre d'identifier le granule élaboré par l'appareil de Golgi à l'extrémité libre du gamète des Isopodes au grain acrosomien du gamète des Mysidacés.

Enfin, l'origine de la vésicule qui se différencie chez les Isopodes aux dépens d'un feuillet dense aux électrons, accolé à la membrane cellulaire ne permet pas d'assimiler cette vésicule, selon la conception de REGER (1964 a, b) et sur le seul critère de son APS–positivité, à un acrosome dont la hampe et la cresta seraient des dépendances.

– *Le diplosome, localisé dans une échancrure nucléaire à l'autre extrémité de la lanière, serait alors, conformément aux données classiques, situé au pôle postérieur du noyau.* L'ensemble de tubules (150 Å) issus de la région péricentriolaire et divergeant en direction du noyau pourrait être homologué à la manchette du spermatozoïde des Mammifères.

– *La hampe, sans avoir la structure et la motilité d'un flagelle, pourrait être considérée comme un fouet modifié*; en effet, elle en occupe l'emplacement car elle correspond, comme un flagelle, à une évagination du corps cytoplasmique qui se forme à proximité du centrosome.

– *La cresta, organite permanent du spermatozoïde des Isopodes, pourrait correspondre à un type particulier de pièce intermédiaire* comme en témoigne la localisation de mitochondries régulièrement alignées à son niveau en particulier dans la partie comprise entre le noyau et la vésicule; fréquemment des connexions microtubulaires semblent même s'établir entre les chondriosomes et le manchon plurilamellaire de la cresta.

En conclusion, il semble donc que des analogies puissent être effectivement faites entre l'organisation type du spermatozoïde et celle de ces gamètes immobiles, coudés et dissociables en deux parties. Cette conception peut même être généralisée au spermatozoïde des Mysidacés et des Amphipodes. De plus, si l'étude du spermatozoïde des Cumacés – actuellement en cours – révèle que ce gamète appartient au même type morphologique, la réunion de tous ces Crustacés dans l'ordre des Péracarides sera justifiée par un argument supplémentaire.

BIBLIOGRAPHIE

BLANCHARD R. E., LEWIN R. M. and PHILPOTT D. E. (1961) – *Fine structure of sperm tails of Isopods.* «Crustaceana», 2, 16–20.

FAIN–MAUREL M.-A. (1966) – *Contribution à l'histologie et à la caryologie de quelques Isopodes. Spermiogenèse et infrastructure du spermatozoïde des Oniscidés et des Cymothoïdés.* «Ann. Sci. Nat., Zoologie», Paris, 8, 1–188.

GILSON G. (1884) – *Etude comparée de la spermatogenèse chez les Arthropodes.* «La Cellule», 1, 16–188.

GILSON G. (1885) – *Etude comparée de la spermatogenèse chez les Arthropodes.* «La Cellule», 2, 83–239.

HERMANN G. (1833) – *Sur la spermatogenèse chez les Crustacés Edriophtalmes.* « C. R. Acad. Sci. », Paris, 97, 958–961.

HOLLANDE A. et FAIN-MAUREL M. A. (1964) – *Structure et ultrastructure du spermatozoïde des Cymothoïdés.* « C. R. Acad. Sci. », Paris, 258, 5063–5066.

HOLLANDE A. et FAIN-MAUREL M. A. (1965) – *Nouvelles observations sur l'infrastructure du spermatozoïde des Isopodes. Origine et évolution de la vésicule spermatique d'*Armadillidium vulgare. « C. R. Acad. Sci. », Paris, 261, 787–789.

LABAT R. (1962) – *La spermatogenèse chez* Praunus flexuosus (*Crustacé Mysidacé*) « Bull. Soc. Hist. Nat. », Toulouse, 97, 51–60.

MAYER P. (1879) – *Ueber den Hermaphroditismus bei einigen Isopoden.* « Mittheil. aus der Zoolog. Station zu Neapel », 1, 165–179.

NICHOLS M. L. (1902) – *The spermatogenesis of* Oniscus asellus *Linn. with special reference to the history of the chromatin.* « Proceed. Americ. Philos. Soc. », 41, 77–112.

REGER J. F. (1964 a) – *The fine structure of Spermatozoa from the Isopod* Asellus militaris *Hay.* « J. Ultrastruct. Res. », 11, 181–192.

REGER J. F. (1964 b) – *A study on the fine structure of developing spermatozoa from the Isopod* Asellus militaris *Hay.* « J. Microscopie », France, 3, 559–572.

REGER J. F. (1966) – *A comparative study on the fine structure of developing spermatozoa in the Isopod,* Oniscus asellus, *and the Amphipod,* Orchestoidea *sp.* « Zeit. fur Zellf », 75, 579–590.

SARS G. O. (1867) – *Histoire naturelle des Crustacés d'eau douce de Norvège.* « Les Malacostracés », Tome 1, Jonhsen édit., Christiana.

TUZET O. et BESSIERE C. (1952) – *Recherches sur la spermatogenèse et les cellules bordantes des follicules et canaux testiculaires des Isopodes.* « Ann. Sci. Nat., Zoologie », Paris, 13, 453–465.

VANDEL A. (1928) – *La parthénogenèse géographique.* 1. *Contribution à l'étude biologique et cytologique de la parthénogenèse naturelle.* « Bull. Biol. », 62, 164–281.

ZENKER D. (1854) – *Ueber Asellus aquaticus.* « Archiv. f. Naturgeschichte », 20 103–138.

LÉGENDES DES FIGURES 8–18

Fig. 8. – Coupe longitudinale d'une jeune spermatide de *Nerocila bivittata*, entourée de microtubules (Mt). La cresta (Cr) longe le noyau (N) contenant, à ce stade, des microfibrilles orientées selon son grand axe. ×24.000.

Fig. 9. – Coupe longitudinale d'une spermatide âgée de *Armadillidium vulgare.* Des mitochondries sont régulièrement alignées le long de la cresta (Cr), plus grêle chez les Isopodes non parasites que chez les Cymothoïdés. Le noyau, à ce stade, contient des structures lamellaires. × 18.000.

Fig. 10. – Coupe transversale de la cresta (Cr) dans une jeune spermatide de *Nerocila* avec sa structure tubulaire axiale à paroi épaisse, son gros manchon périphérique plurilamellaire et les mitochondries (M) qui l'accompagnent sur toute sa longueur. ×43.000.

Fig. 11. – Première manifestation de la différenciation de la vésicule sous forme d'un feuillet (F), dense aux électrons, sous-jacent à la membrane cellulaire de la jeune spermatide G = appareil de Golgi (*Armadillidium*) ×215.000.

Fig. 12. – Epaississement d'une partie du feuillet dense aux électrons (F) et formation du cône cytoplasmique saillant dans la lumière de l'ampoule testiculaire. Les membranes cellulaires des spermatides adjacentes sont généralement accolées et doublées de reticulum endoplasmique sacculaire. ×20.500.

Fig. 13. – Localisation de la jeune vésicule (V) et du complexe golgien (G) en deux points diamétralement opposés par rapport au noyau. Les cellules folliculeuses périphériques émettent des expansions cytoplasmiques (CF) qui s'immiscent entre les jeunes spermatides (Sp). ×16.000.

Fig. 14. – *La vésicule chez les Isopodes parasites* (*Nerocila bivittata*) B = baguette axiale de la hampe incrustée dans la partie médiane du tubercule réniforme. CC = limites du cône cytoplasmique saillant dans la lumière de la gonade. Cr = manchon de la cresta en rapport avec un des 2 épaississements de la membrane limitant la vésicule. D = substance granuleuse entourant les 2 éléments du diplosome. F = feuillet dense aux électrons, sous-jacent à la membrane cellulaire, origine de la vésicule. H = hampe limitée par la membrane cellulaire et le feuillet sous-jacent pourvu de la striation transversale périodique. T = tubercule réniforme, base de la hampe, encastré dans la vésicule au niveau d'une portion épaissie de la membrane. V_1 = compartiment chromophile, dense aux électrons, de la vésicule. V_2 = compartiment chromophobe de la vésicule ×19.000.

Fig. 15. – *La vésicule chez les Isopodes libres* (*Armadillidium vulgare*) B = point d'émergence de la baguette axiale de la hampe. CC = limites du cône cytoplasmique saillant dans la lumière de la gonade. Cr = cresta en relation avec la partie chromophile de la vésicule. D = les 2 éléments du diplosome logés dans une échancrure nucléaire (N) sont parallèles chez les Isopodes libres. Di = diverticule du feuillet dense qui obture à sa base le cône cytoplasmique, formant ainsi la vésicule. T = tubercule réniforme, base de la hampe. V_1 = compartiment chromophile de la vésicule. V_2 = compartiment cytoplasmique de la vésicule au niveau duquel le feuillet dense présente une structure paracristalline. ×44.500.

Fig. 16. – *Spermatide agée de Nerocila bivittata.* La base de la hampe (H) est dilatée en une formation ampullaire traversée par la baguette axiale (B). La cresta (Cr) est reliée au compartiment chromophile (V_1) de la vésicule qui s'est étiré et rattache la lanière à la base de la hampe. Le compartiment chromophobe (V_2) forme un fragile pont d'union entre la hampe et le lanière. ×14.000.

Fig. 17. – *Spermatide agée de Armadillidium vulgare.* Le compartiment chromophile de la vésicule (V_1) forme la partie apicale du rostre effilé. La baguette axiale (B) de la hampe est incrustée dans la partie latérale du tubercule réniforme (T) qui reste encastré dans le compartiment cytoplasmique (V_2) de la vésicule. D = localisation du diplosome. ×60.000.

Fig. 18. – *La hampe.* Chez *Nerocila,* la période de la striation transversale est de 650 Å environ; les bandes sombres sont constituées de 3 stries élémentaires séparées par un espace clair; les bandes claires sont subdivisées en 3 compartiments inégaux par 2 stries sombres. ×45.000.

Discussion

REGER – What is the origin of extracellular tubules situated between spermatozoa and nurse cells?

FAIN-MAUREL. – Certaines observations inciteraient à penser que les microtubules sont issus de la partie chromophile de la vésicule; en effet, au début de la spermiogenèse, cette partie de la vésicule est, de manière transitoire, hérissée de courtes protubérances dont le diamètre est identique à celui des microtubules. Cependent, il n'et pas exclu que les microtubules correspondent à ceux qui sont élaborés dans les cellules folliculeuses; ils constitueraient alors les seuls vestiges des expansions de ces cellules qui s'étaient immiscées entre les éléments germinaux.

BROWN. – What is the origin and function of the striated structures?

FAIN MAUREL. – Les structures striées (hampes des spermatozoïdes) représentent une différenciation locale et un épaississement du feuillet dense aux électrons, sous jacent à la membrane cellulaire au niveau du cône cellulaire saillant dans la lumière de la gonade. Cette structure apparemment pourvue d'une certaine rigidité pourrait servir de support et de véhicule à ce type de spermatozoïde immobile.

MATTEI. – J'ai observé chez un Sélacien une baguette de même type qui présente cepandant une structure différente; elle est constituée d'un empilement de disques. Cette formation se développe à partir des centrioles, en direction du noyau et insère sa portion antérieure dans la fossette nucléaire, (emplacement réservé généralement au centriole).

Chez les Téléostéens de la famille des *Chaetodontidae*, une courte baguette de même structure est associée au centriole proximal et deux baguettes sont visibles chez un Pomadasyidae.

Chez les Sélaciens la baguette peut être considérée comme une attache reliant le centriole au noyau. Ceci n'est pas valable pour les Téléostéens, cités precédemment car leurs spermatozoides sont de type II (d'après la classification donnée le premier jour de ce Symposium) et le centriole et la baguette sont placés en dehors de la dépression nucléaire.

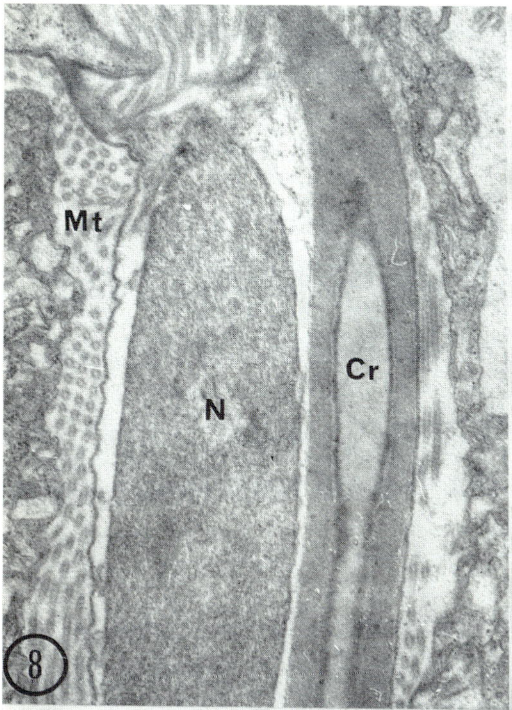
Mt
Cr
N
8

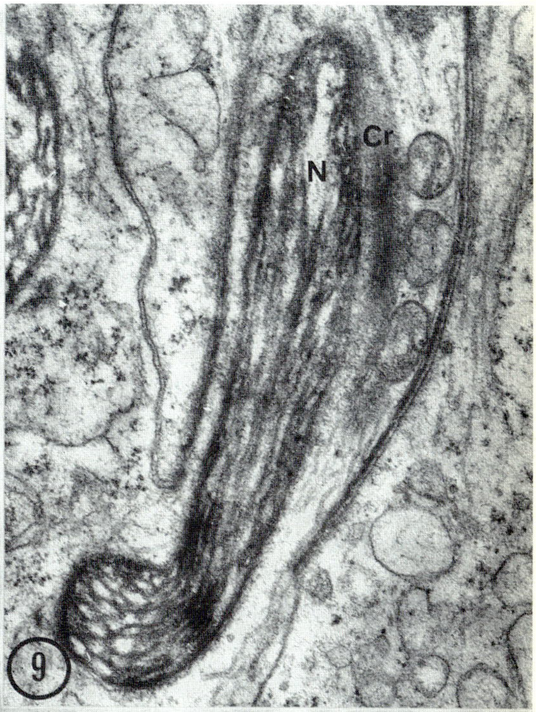
Cr
N
9

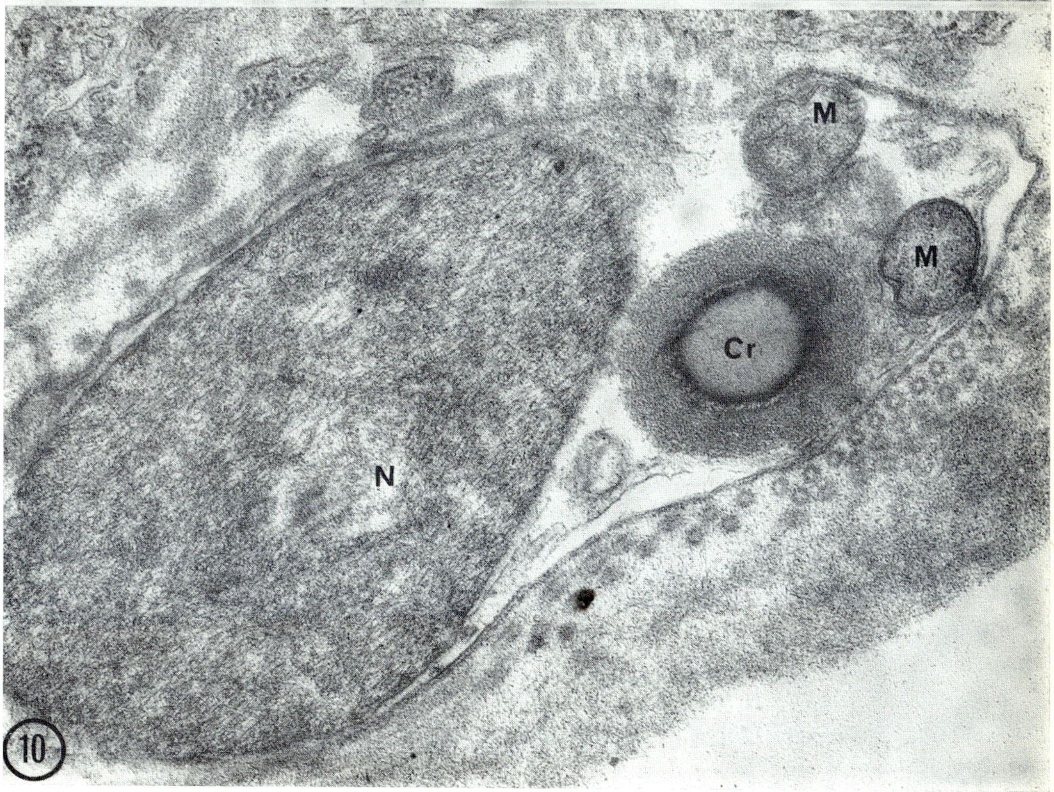
M
M
Cr
N
10

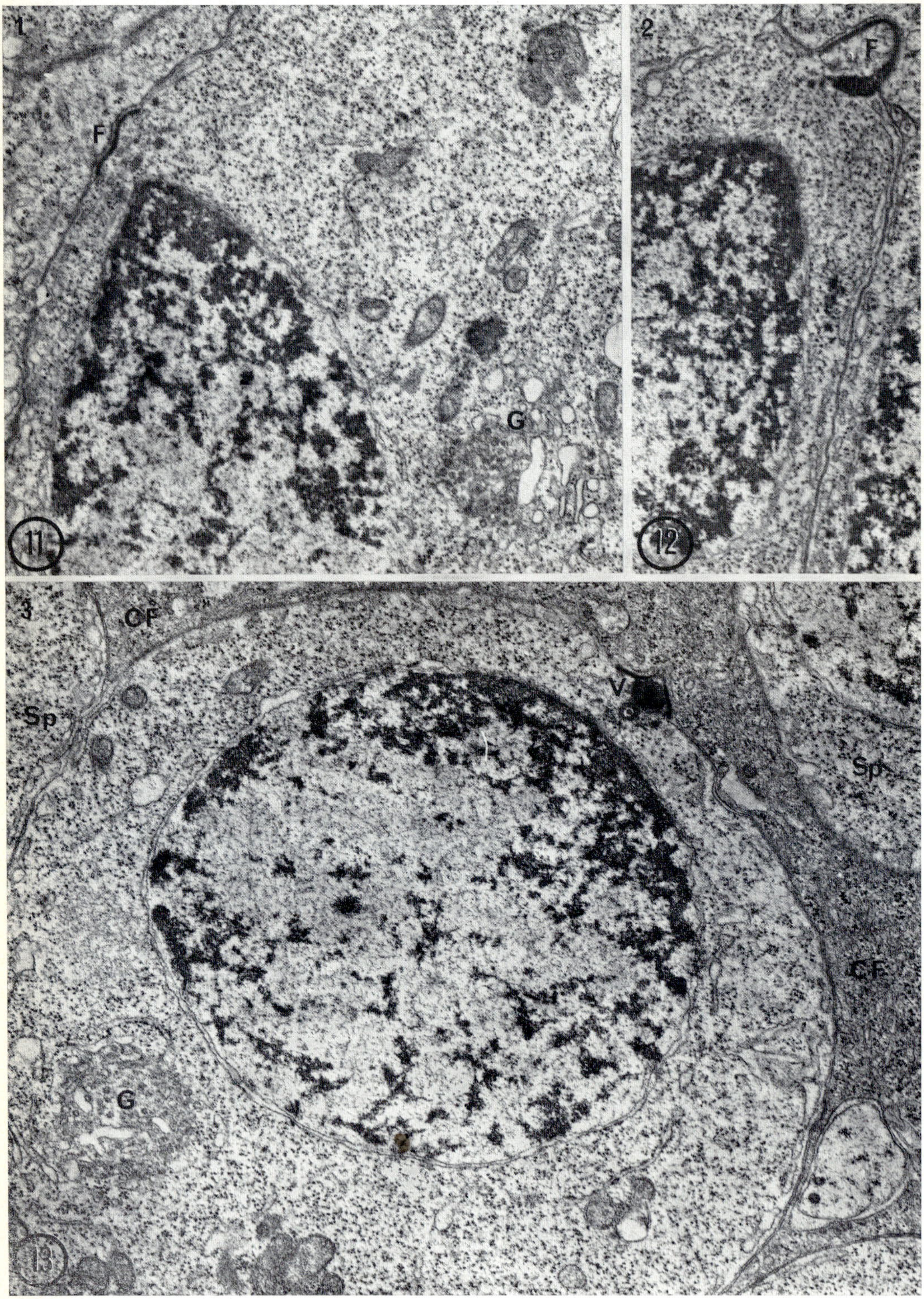
1
F
G
11
2
F
12
3
CF
Sp
V
Sp
CF
G
13

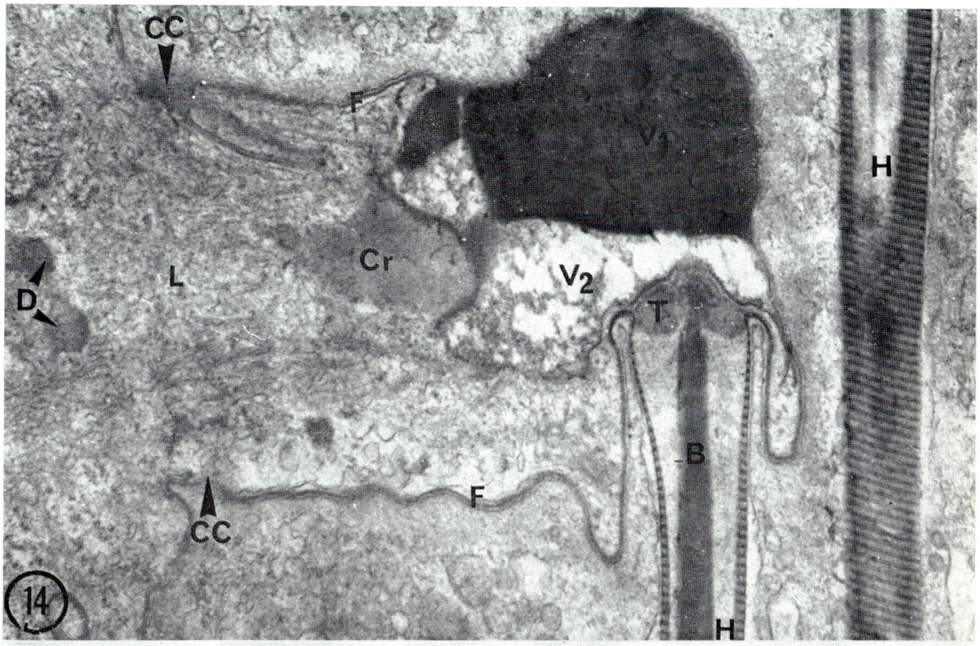
CC
F
V1
H
Cr
L
D
V2
T
B
F
CC
14
H

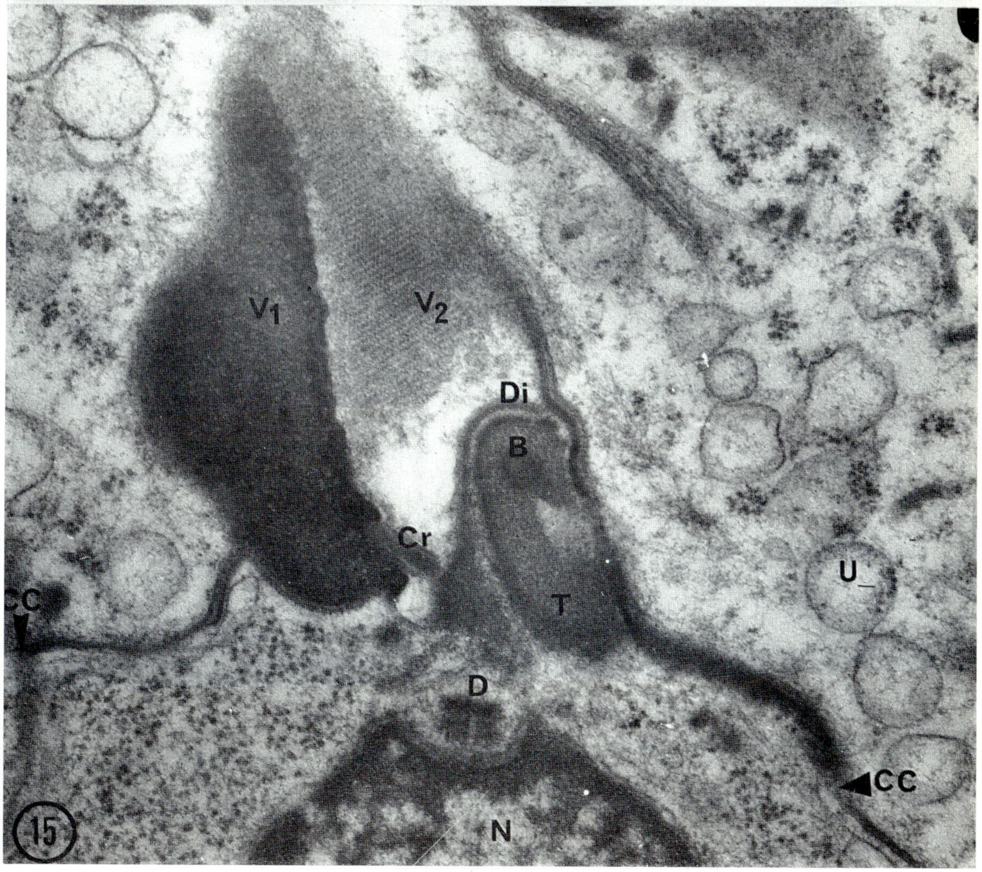
V1
V2
Di
B
Cr
U
CC
T
D
CC
15
N

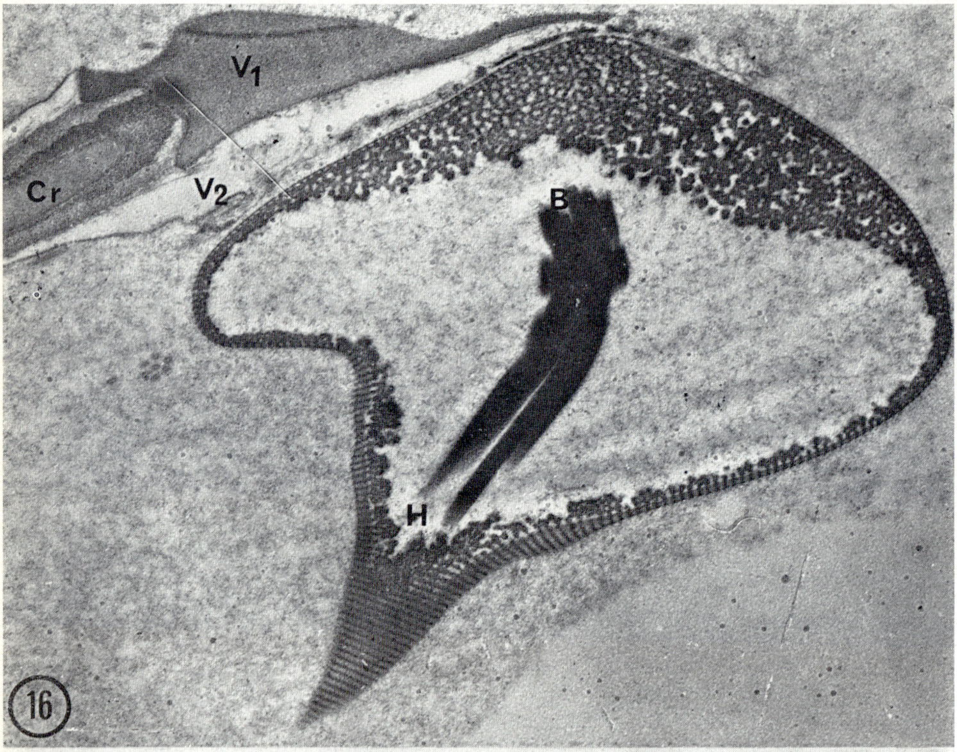
V1
Cr
V2
B
H
16

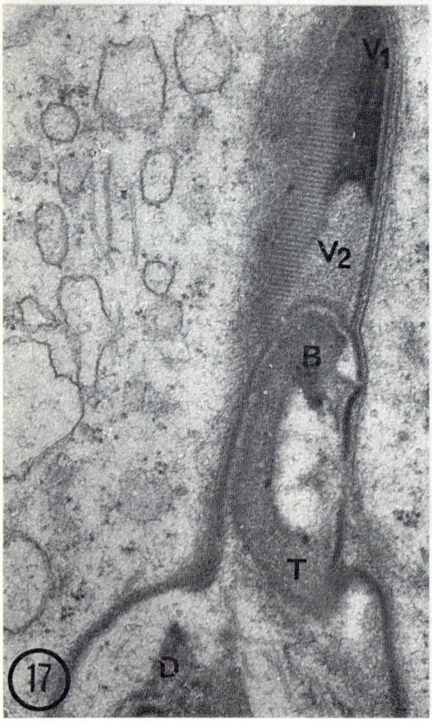
V1
V2
B
T
D
17

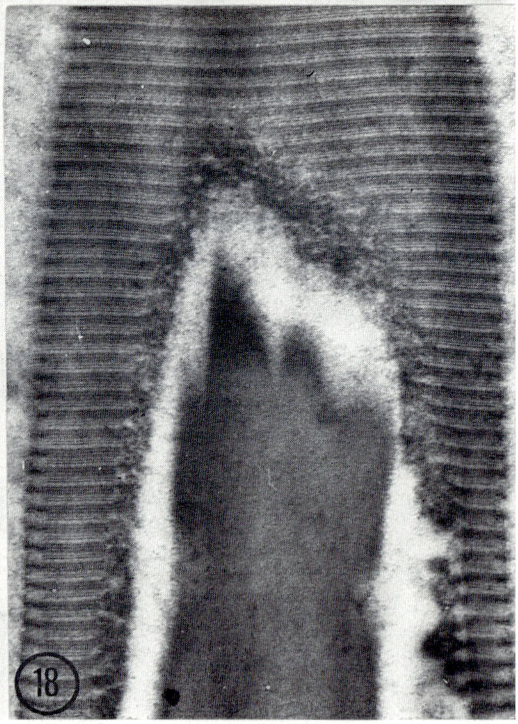
18

James F. Reger (*)

SOME ASPECTS OF THE FINE STRUCTURE OF FILIFORM SPERMATOZOA (OSTRACOD, *CYPRIDOPSIS* SP.) LACKING TUBULE SUB-STRUCTURE [1]

Summary. — Observations on spermatids and spermatozoa of the Ostracod, *Cypridopsis* sp. demonstrate several differences from typical, flagellate spermatozoa. The nucleus elongates concomitantly with the formation of a surface invagination which assumes a cylinder-like shape within the center of the nucleus. Paired mitochondria, with tubular-shaped cristae containing 40–60 Å-sized filaments, become spirally aligned along three-fourths the length of the mature spermatozoon. Paired elements of endoplasmic reticulum, in continuity with the outer nuclear membrane, give rise to bilateral membranous organelles that extend three-fourths the length of the mature spermatozoon on either side of the nucleus and mitochondria. Multiple vesicles from the Golgi complex become aligned in repeat order along lateral and longitudinal extents of the membranous organelle. Possible correlates of this unusual fine structure with that of more typical spermatozoa are made.

Riassunto. — Osservazioni condotte su spermatidi e spermatozoi di *Cypridopsis* sp. (Ostracoda) hanno messo in evidenza parecchie differenze rispetto ai tipici spermatozoi flagellati. Contemporaneamente all'allungamento del nucleo, si osserva la formazione di una invaginazione nucleare che assume una forma cilindrica. I due mitocondri, con creste tubulari contenenti filamenti di 40–60 Å, sono disposti a spirale per 3/4 della lunghezza dello spermatozoo. Elementi appaiati del reticolo endoplasmico in continuità con la membrana nucleare esterna danno origine ad organuli membranosi bilaterali che si estendono per 3/4 della lunghezza dello spermatozoo maturo ai lati sia del nucleo sia dei mitocondri. Molteplici vescicole originate dal complesso del Golgi sono disposte ordinatamente longitudinalmente e lateralmente agli organuli membranosi. Vengono proposte possibili correlazioni tra questa inconsueta fine struttura e quella dei più tipici spermatozoi.

Introduction

Many of the structural-functional correlates drawn from fine structure studies of typical filiform, flagellate spermatozoa are known. For example, on the basis of several lines of evidence (Fawcett, '62; Gibbons, '68) it is generally concluded that the two-plus-nine, the two-plus-nine-plus-nine tubule substructure, or some variation thereof underlies motility. This conclusion

(*) Department of Anatomy, The University of Tennessee Medical Units, Memphis, Tennessee, U.S.A.

(1) Supported by U.S.P.H.S. Grant No. NB-06285.

is particularly strengthened by the fine structural similarity between sperm flagella and motile cilia.

Some filiform spermatozoa lack the two-plus-nine tubule substructure. These include spermatozoa from the ticks, *Ornithodorus moubata* (ROTHSCHILD, '61; BREUCKER and HORSTMANN, '68) and *Amblyomma dissimili* (REGER, '61, '62, '63), certain species of Isopods (REGER, '64, '66; HOLLANDE and FAIN, '65; FAIN–MAUREL, '66), the fungus gnat, *Sciara coprophilia* (PHILLIPS, '66), the armored scale insect, *Parlatoria oleae* (ROBISON, '66) and the Ostracods *Cypria ophthalmica* (ZISSLER, '66), *Candona candida* (TETART, '67) and *Cypridopsis* sp. (REGER and FLORENDO, '69 a, b). Neither motility nor fertilization capacity has been demonstrated in all of these atypical, filiform spermatozoa, but motility has been shown in some species of ticks (CASTEEL, '17; ROTHSCHILD, '61) and Ostracods (LOWNDES, '35).

The following study on *Cypridopsis* sp. spermatids and spermatozoa is presented to determine possible analogies of their fine structure with more typical spermatozoa and to broaden our knowledge on the possible sub-structure which may underly motility in these atypical, filiform spermatozoa.

MATERIALS AND METHODS

Because of the small size of Ostracod, *Cypridopsis* sp., whole animals isolated from fresh water ponds were immersed directly into cold (0–5°) 4% glutaraldehyde (*p*H 7.6; 0.1 M phosphate buffer) and subsequently sectioned in the mid-line for rapid penetration of fixative. After fixation in glutaraldehyde for 1 hour the animals were washed for an hour in cold (0–5°) phosphate buffer (*p*H 7.6; 0.1 M phosphate) and postfixed for an hour in cold (0–5°) buffered OsO_4 (*p*H 7.6; 0.1 M phosphate buffer). After fixation the tissue was dehydrated in 5-minute changes of successive 10% grades of ethanol (beginning with 50%), and embedded in Epon 812. Sections 1–2 μ thick were made of the Epon-embedded tissue and stained with Mallory Azure II–Methylene blue for purposes of identification of spermiogenic tissue and spermatozoa in males.

Thin sections were cut with a diamond knife fitted to an LKB Ultrotome II, floated on distilled water, mounted on carbon-coated grids, stained with uranyl acetate and lead citrate, and examined with a Hitachi 11 A electron microscope. Micrographs, at initial magnifications of 7500–40,000 at exposures of 3–5 seconds, were made on Cronar, Ortholitho, Type A sheet film and were photographically enlarged up to 10 times.

OBSERVATIONS (1)

The early spermatid of *Cypridopsis* sp. (Fig. 1) contains a nebenkern (Ne, Fig. 1), nucleus (N, Fig. 1), endoplasmic reticulum (ER, Fig. 4) and Golgi complex (G, Figs. 4, 6). As spermiogenesis proceeds, the spermatid elongates. During elongation a nuclear invagination (arrows, Fig. 2) occurs

(1) Portions of this data are concurrently being published in the Journal of Ultrastructure Research.

which eventually extends as an intranuclear cylindrical rod (Figs. 4, 7). Two mitochondria (M, Fig. 4) come to lie along the longitudinal axis of the elongating spermatid. Microtubules (Mt, Figs. 5 a, b) are closely apposed to the nucleus and the mitochondria of the elongating spermatid.

The elongating nucleus of the early spermatid (Figs. 4, 7–9) contains scattered electron opacities (EO, Figs. 4, 9). The nucleus comes to extend the full length of the spermatozoon (N, Fig. 14, Diag. 1) and takes on a uniform electron opacity. It is the only element found in the tail-end of the mature spermatozoon (T, Fig. 14, Diag. 1). The nuclear invagination (arrows, Fig. 2) initially contains microtubules (Mt, Fig. 3) and scattered electron opacities. In the later spermatid the invagination assumes a central position within the nucleus (IC, Figs. 4, 7) and contains electron opacities (EO, Fig. 9).

The spermatid contains abundant amounts of granular endoplasmic reticulum (Fig. 4). As spermiogenesis proceeds portions of the endoplasmic reticulum are found as paired elements (arrows, Figs. 4, 5 a, b), at the juncture of juxtaposed nucleus and mitochondria. These elements are continuous with the external leaflet of the outer nuclear membrane (arrow, Figs. 5 a, b), are C-shaped, and exhibit high electron opacity at their point of apposition (EO, Figs, 5 a, b). During spermatid elongation these endoplasmic reticulum derivatives widen laterally (Figs. 7, 8) and longitudinally (Fig. 9) to form two, laterally placed, membranous organelles (MO, Figs. 7, 8). Vesicles (V_1, V_2, V_3, Fig. 6), derived from the Golgi complex (G, Fig. 6), become aligned along the lateral and longitudinal surfaces of the membranous organelles (V, Figs. 8, 9). In the late spermatid the organelles become arched and C-shaped (MO, Fig. 12).

Paired mitochondria (M, Fig. 4) become spirally situated along three-fourths the length of the mature spermatozoon (Figs. 12–14). They maintain close appositional contact (arrows, Fig. 8) with the nucleus during spermatid elongation and are found in the mature spermatozoon lateral to the nucleus (N, Fig. 12). The mitochondrial cristae (C, Figs. 9–11) are tubule-shaped and contain a centrally situated filament (F, Figs. 9–11). The filaments are 40–60 Å in diameter and when seen in favorable sections exhibit a spiral pattern.

The mature spermatozoon of *Cypridopsis* sp. is a filiform, spiral-patterned cell (Figs. 12–15) and approximately 1.0 mm long. The spiral pattern results from a pair of grooves (G_1, G_2, Figs. 13, Diag. 1) indenting the surface of the spermatozoon. The spiral pitch of the grooves increases from approximately 3 microns at the head-end (H, Diag. 1) to approximately 7 microns at the tail-end (T, Diag. 1). The spiral tilt-angle of the two grooves is approximately 45°. The grooves (G_1, G_2, Diag. 1) are staggered 180° to each other. Nucleus (N, Fig. 12), mitochondria (M, Fig. 12) and membranous organelles (MO, Fig. 12) follow the spiral course of the surface grooves.

The mature spermatozoon is enveloped by a spermatophore sheath (S, Fig. 14) which originates as a secretory product of the spermatic-duct nurse cells (NC, Fig. 12).

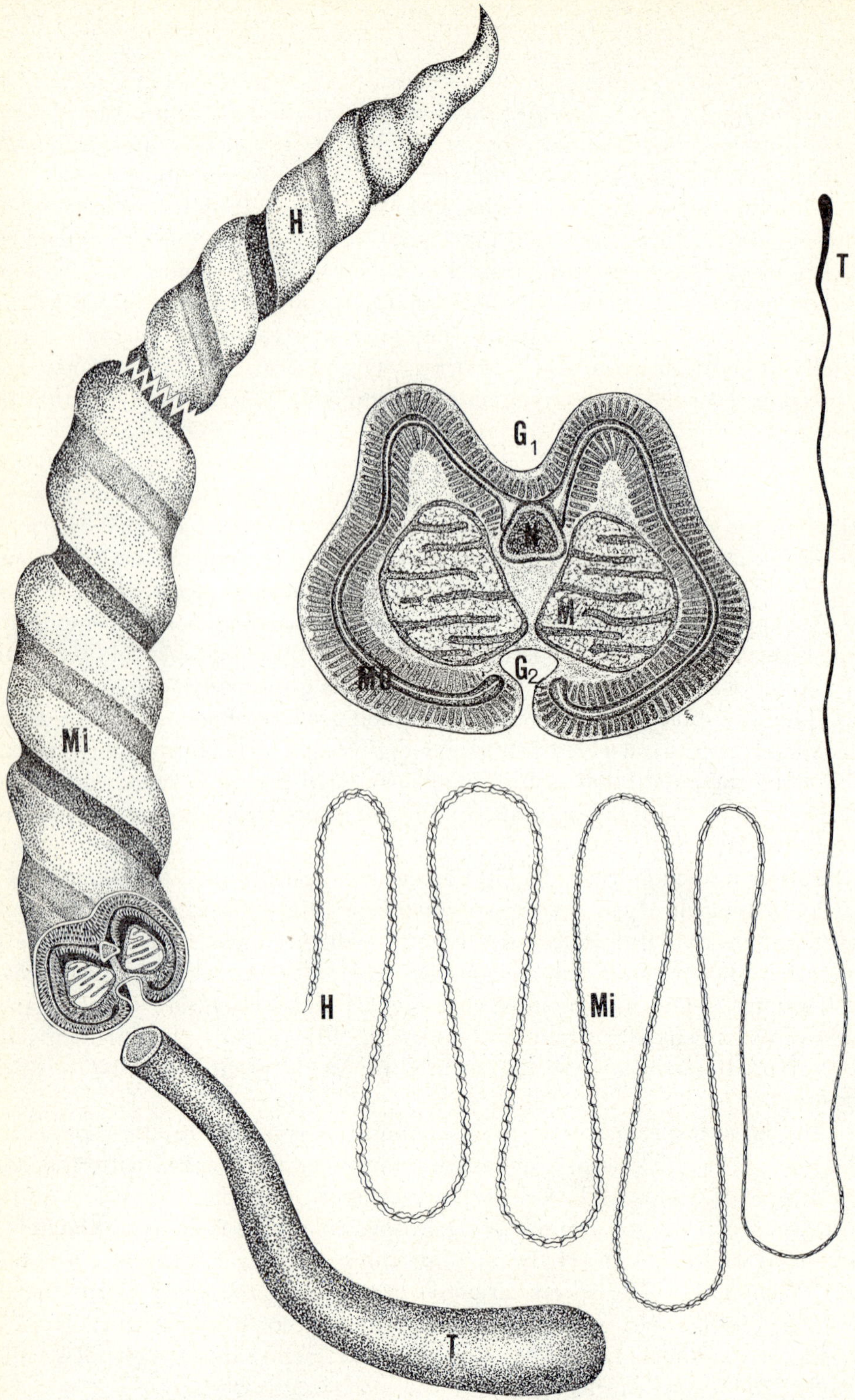

Diag. 1. – Schematic drawing of enlarged head (H), middle (Mi) and tail (T) segments of *Cypridopsis* sp. spermatozoon taken from complete spermatozoon shown in middle lower right of figure. Enlarged cross section taken from middle region of spermatozoon is shown in middle portion of figure. Two grooves (G_1, G_2) present on surface of spermatozoon are staggered 180° with respect to each other and exhibit a pitch angle of approximately 45°. (N) Nucleus. (M) Mitochondrion. (MO) Membranous organelle.

Conclusion

The fine structure of spermatids and spermatozoa of the Ostracod *Cypridosis* sp. seen here is unusual, and it is therefore difficult to draw functional analogies with typical spermatozoa. However, certain aspects of development and fine structure lend support to the following conclusions.

The nuclear invagination, found as a cylindrical structure in spermatids of *Cypridopsis* sp. is similar in location to perforatoria, or subacrosomal material, of more typical spermatozoa. Perforatoria of other spermatozoa are closely associated in development with the nucleus. They are either found as an invaginated, central, rod-like structure within the nucleus (Reger, '63; Nijima and Dan, '65), embedded in a surface groove of the nucleus (Nagano, '62) or situated between closely apposed nucleus and acrosome (Nicander and Bane, '66). The function of perforatoria is still obscure, but a possible role in egg activation and/or induction of the formation of the division apparatus of egg cytoplasm following fertilization has been suggested (Austin, '68).

The mode of formation of the membranous organelle and its association with the closely apposed, Golgi-derived vesicles suggests an analogy with typical acrosomes. Although acrosomes generally are derived from a single or multiply-fused acrosomal vesicle, there are many variations in the structure of mature acrosomes. Further, a close relationship between the endoplasmic reticulum and Golgi complex in typical acrosome production is implied by the known structural-functional relationship which exists between the endoplasmic reticulum and Golgi complex generally.

The paired mitochondria observed to extend three-fourths the length of the mature spermatozoon raises interesting questions about their possible role in motility. It is generally believed that mitochondria found in the midpiece of typical motile spermatozoa only serve as an ATP-energy source (Gibbons, '68). In this connection many non-motile spermatozoa are known to lack mitochondria. This has been demonstrated in several species of Isopods (Reger, '64, '66; Hollande and Fain, '64), Amphipods (Reger, '66), a Cephalocarida (Brown and Metz, '67) and a millipede (Reger, '68).

The functional significance of the 40–60 Å thick filaments found in mitochondrial cristae of Ostracod sperm is not known. However, for the sake of speculative argument these filaments are within the size range of filaments of actin (Hanson and Lowy, '65), filaments in contractile regions of amoeba (Wohlfarth–Bottermann, '64), filaments thought to be contractile found on the inner aspect of trypsinized, guinea-pig red cell ghost membranes (Marchesi and Palade, '67) and filaments found to bind heavy meromyosin in cultured, chick myogenic, chondroblastic and fibroblastic cells (Ishikawa, '68). Further, it has been observed (Frederic, '58) that configurational and volumetric changes occur in mitochondria of cultured fibroblasts where a role in cellular motility was suggested. Finally, it is well known that isolated mitochondria undergo cyclic conformational changes in vitro (HACKENBROCK, '66). However, these latter movements are of a type not easily reconcilable with the synchronized translational movements usually observed in motile spermatozoa. Thus although it is tempting to associate mitochondria in spermatozoa of *Cypridopsis* sp. with a more direct role in motility than merely serving as an ATP source, evidence to date is too meagre and indirect to warrant such a conclusion.

In final conclusion the observations presented here and on other atypical spermatozoa serve to emphasize the diversity of biological organization present in living systems.

REFERENCES

AUSTIN C. R. (1968) – *Ultrastructure of fertilization.* Holt, Rinehart and Winston, New York.

BREUCKER H. und HORSTMANN E. (1968) – *Die spermatozoen der zecke* Ornithodorus moubata *(Murr).* « Z. Zellforsch. », 88, 1–22.

BROWN G. G. and METZ C. B. (1967) – *Ultrastructural studies on the spermatozoa of two primitive crustaceans* Hutchinsoniella macracantha *and* Derocheilocaris typicus. « Z. Zellforsch. », 80, 78–92.

CASTEEL D. B. (1917) – *Cytoplasmic inclusions in male germ cells of the fowl tick,* Argas miniatus, *and histogenesis of the spermatozoon.* « J. Morphol. », 28, 643–683.

FAIN-MAUREL M. A. (1966) – *Thesis: Contribution a l'histologie et a la caryologie de quelques Isopods. Spermiogenèse et infrastructure du spermatozoïd des Oniscidés et des Cymothoïdés.* – Masson e Cie, Éditeurs, Paris.

FAWCETT D. W. (1962) – *Sperm tail structure in relation to the mechanism of movement.* in D. W. BISHOP ed., Spermatozoon motility. – American Association for the Advancement of Science, Publication No. 72, Washington, D. C. 147–169.

FREDERIC J. (1958) – *Recherches cytologiques sur le chondriome normal ou soumis à l'expérimentation dans des cellules vivantes cultivées in vitro.* « Archiv. Biologie », 69, 169–349.

GIBBONS I. R. (1968) – *The biochemistry of motility.* « Annual Rev. Biochem. », 37, 521–546.

HACKENBROCK C. R. (1966) – *Ultrastructural basis for metabolically linked mechanical activity in mitochondria.* I. *Reversible ultrastructural changes with change in metabolic steady state in isolated liver mitochondria.* « J. Cell. Biol. », 30, 269–298.

HANSON J. and LOWY J. (1965) – *Molecular basis of contractility in muscle.* « Brit. Med. Bull. », 21, 264–271.

HOLLANDE M. A. et FAIN M. (1964) – *Structure et ultrastructure du spermatozoïde des Cymothoïdés.* « C. R. Acad. Sci. », 258, 5063–5066.

ISHIKAWA H. (1968) – In situ *demonstration of heavy meromyosin-bound filaments in sectioned preparations.* « J. Cell Biol. », 39, 65 a.

LOWNDES A. G. (1935) – *The sperms of freshwater Ostracods.* « Proc. Zool. Soc. London. », 1, 35–48.

MARCHESI V. T. and PALADE G. E. (1967) – *Localization of ATPase activity in red cell ghost membranes.* « Proc. Natl. Acad. Sci. », 58, 991–995.

NAGANO T. (1962) – *Observations on the fine structure of the developing spermatid in the domestic chicken.* « J. Cell Biol. », 14, 193–205.

NICANDER L. and BANE A. (1966) – *Fine structure of the sperm head in some mammals, with particular reference to the acrosome and the subacrosomal substance.* « Z. Zellforsch. », 72, 496–515.

NIIJIMA L. and DAN J. (1965) – *The acrosome reaction* in Mytilus edulis. I. *Fine structure of the intact acrosome.* « J. Cell Biol. », 25 243–248.

PHILLIPS D. M. (1966) – *Fine structure of* Sciara coprophila *sperm.* « J. Cell. Biol. », 30, 499–518.

REGER J. F. (1961) – *The fine structure of spermatids from the tick,* Amblyomma dissimili. « J. Ultrastruct. Res. », 5, 584–599.

REGER J. F. (1962) – *A fine structure study on spermiogenesis in the tick,* Amblyomma dissimili, *with special reference to the development of motile processes.* « J. Ultrastruct. Res. », 7, 550–565.

REGER J. F. (1963) – *Spermiogenesis in the tick, Amblyomma dissimili, as revealed by electron microscopy.* « J. Ultrastruct. Res. », 8, 607–621.

REGER J. F. (1964) – *A study on the fine structure of developing spermatozoa from the Isopod,* Asellus militaris. « J. de Microscopie », 3, 559–572.

REGER J. F. (1966) – *A comparative study on the fine structure of developing spermatozoa in the Isopod* Oniscus asellus, *and the Amphipod,* Orchestoidea *sp.* « Z. Zellforsch. », 75, 579–590.

REGER J. F. and COOPER D. P. (1968) – *Studies on the fine structure of spermatids and spermatozoa from the millipede* Polydesmus *sp.* « J. Ultrastruct. Res. », 23, 60–70.

REGER J. F. and FLORENDO N. T. (1969 a) – *Studies on motile, non-tubule containing, filiform spermatozoa of the Ostracod,* Cypridopsis *sp.* I, *Spermiogenesis.* « J. Ultrastruct. Res », 28, 235–249.

REGER J. F. and FLORENDO N. T. (1969 b) – *Studies on motile, non-tubule containing, filiform spermatozoa of the Ostracod,* Cypridopsis *sp.* II. *Mature Spermatozoa.* « J. Ultrastruct. Res. », 28, 250–258.

ROBISON W. G. (1966) – *Microtubules in relation to the motility of a sperm syncytium in an armored scale insect.* « J. Cell Biol. », 29, 251–265.

ROTHSCHILD LORD (1961) – *Structure and movement of tick spermatozoa* (Arachnida, *Acari*). «Quart. J. Micr. Sci. », 102, 239–247.

TÉTART J. (1967) – *Étude de l'ultrastructure des spermatozoïdes des Ostracodes du genre* Candona. «C. R. Acad. Sci. », Series D., Paris., 265, 419–422.

WOHLFARTH-BOTTERMANN K. E. (1964) – *Differentiation of the ground cytoplasm and their significance for the generation of the motive force of amoeboid movement,* In: *Primitive motile systems in Cell Biology* (Eds. R. D. ALLEN and N. KAMIYA), pp. 79–110, Acad. Press, New York and London.

ZISSLER D. (1966) – *Zur feinstruktur der Ostracoden-Spermien.* « Die Naturwissenschaft », 21, 561–562.

EXPLANATION OF FIGURES

Fig. 1. – Early spermatid prior to cellular elongation and following nebenkern (Ne) formation. Nucleus (N) juxtaposed to nebenkern exhibits a low electron opacity ×8,000. (Reger and Florendo, 1969 a).

Fig. 2. – Longitudinally oriented portion of early spermatid to show beginning formation of inner (IC) and outer (OC) nuclear compartments by nuclear invagination (arrows). ×16,000.

Fig. 3. – Oblique section of early spermatid. Notice inner nuclear compartment (IC) contains microtubules (Mt) and electron opacities (EO). (OC) Outer compartment. ×32,000. (Reger and Florendo, 1969 a).

Fig. 4. – Elongated spermatid seen in cross-section to show bilateral elements of endoplasmic reticulum (arrows) apposed to the nucleus (N). These give rise to membranous organelles (MO, Fig. 7) of later spermatids. (ER) Endoplasmic reticulum. (IC) Inner compartment. (EO) Electron opacities. (M) Mitochondrion. (G) Golgi complex. ×16,000.

Figs. 5 a, b. – Similar to Fig. 4, but at higher magnification to show continuity of endoplasmic reticulum (ER) with outer nuclear membrane (arrow) (Mt) Microtubules. (EO) Electron opacities. ×64,000. (Reger and Florendo, 1969 a).

Fig. 6. – Portion of obliquely sectioned spermatid at a somewhat later stage than Figs. 4 and 5 to demonstrate the vesicles (V_1, V_2, V_3) which originate from the Golgi complex (G) and become longitudinally and laterally aligned along the membranous organelle (MO). ×64,000. (Reger and Florendo, 1969 a).

Fig. 7. – Cross-section through later spermatid than previous figures. Note the membranous organelle (MO) widens laterally. (IC) Inner compartment. ×16,000.

Fig. 8. – As spermiogenesis proceeds spermatids flatten and the membranous organelle widens and arches laterally. (Arrows) Appositional contact between nucleus and mitochondrion. (V) Vesicles. (N) Nucleus. Bar indicates level of section shown in figure 9 transverse to section plane here. ×32,000. (Reger and Florendo, 1969 a).

Fig. 9. – Longitudinal section of spermatid at stage similar to figure 8. Plane of section indicated by bar (Fig. 8). Note filaments (F) in the tubule-shaped, mitochondrial cristae. Also note repeat order of aligned vesicles (V) and the electron opacities (EO) within the condensing nucleus. (Mt) Microtubules. ×64,000. (Reger and Florendo, 1969 a).

Figs. 10 and 11. – High mgnification micrographs showing tubule-shaped mitochondrial cristae (C) with contained 40–60 A filaments (F).

Fig. 10. – ×96,000. Fig. 11. – (Reger and Florendo, 1969 b). ×48,000.

Fig. 12. – Cross-section of nearly mature spermatozoon embedded in nurse cell (NC) of spermatic duct. (N) Nucleus. (M) Mitochondrion. Note almost completed arching of lateral membranous organelles (MO). ×32,000. (Reger and Florendo, 1969 b).

Fig. 13. – Longitudinal section of portion of spermatozoon showing almost one complete pitch of the spiral. (G_1, G_2) Two grooves in surface of sperm. See also schematic diagram 1. ×16,000. (Reger and Florendo, 1969 b).

Fig. 14. – Cross-section of several mature spermatozoa in female genital tract. Note the head (H), middle (Mi) and tail (T) ends. (N) Nucleus. (G_1, G_2) Grooves. (S) Spermatophore sheath. ×9,600.

Discussion

ROBISON. – From your very elegant micrographs it appears that the intramitochondrial fibers that you reported are limited to the intracristal spaces. Do you ever find these fibers in the matrix region? Do you have evidence that they are really fibers? Some appeared to be trilaminar and therefore to resemble membranes.

REGER – Yes, the filaments are limited to intracristal spaces. No, I do not ever find the filaments in the matrix. Evidence that they are actually filaments comes from observations of them in cross-section, where they appeared as 40–60 Å dots.

BACCETTI. – 1) The vesicles of the arms appear now to be not endoplasmic reticulum derivatives but Golgi elements. This is very important: but are they contractile as previous authors supposed?

2) And, what is the significance of the alternance of more or less osmiophilic masses inside the nucleus longitudinally sectioned?

REGER – Yes, the vesicles are no doubt Golgi derivatives, but I have no evidence on their possible contractile properties. Remember also that the vesicles apposed to the lateral arms are Golgi derivatives, but the arms themselves, are derived from the endoplasmic reticulum. I do not know what the significance of the alternate electron opaque and electron lucent regions in the nuclear invagination is, other than to say that in position and origin this material would appear to be analogous to perforatoria seen in other spermatozoa.

PRATT. – The mitochondrial body you showed on an early spermatid is remarkably similar to the early nebenkern of insect spermatids. Is the differentiation of this body before it forms two mitochondrial derivatives similar to that of the insect nebenkern? Also, when do the two centrioles you showed in a lateral position move to that position?

REGER – Yes, the mitochondrial nebenkern comes from two mitochondrial derivatives as your work has shown in some insect species. I do not know in what stage of spermiogenesis the centrioles move to their lateral positions.

ANDRÉ. – Did you try the Thiéry staining for polysaccharides, and, if so, what are the results?

REGER. – Yes. Negative results.

ANDRÉ. – What results did you got for–SH groups and acid proteins?

REGER. – Positive.

BROWN. – Could you describe the motility of ostracod spermatozoa. I have always been of the opinion that LOWNDES description of sperm movement was due to tension as a result of a coiled condition.

REGER – Gupta is in a better position to answer this than I am since he has recently published more detailed observations (GUPTA B. J., *Aspects of Cell Motility*, XXIInd Symposium, Soc. Exp. Biol., 1968). I will say that the movements I have observed are somewhat suggestive of an uncoiling of a previously coiled structure under tension, but that this movement continues and appears to reverse direction which should not occur if uncoiling under previous tension were the only motive force for movement.

J. F. Reger – *Some aspects of the fine structure of filiform spermatozoa (Ostracod,* Cypridopsis *sp.) lacking tubule sub-structure.*

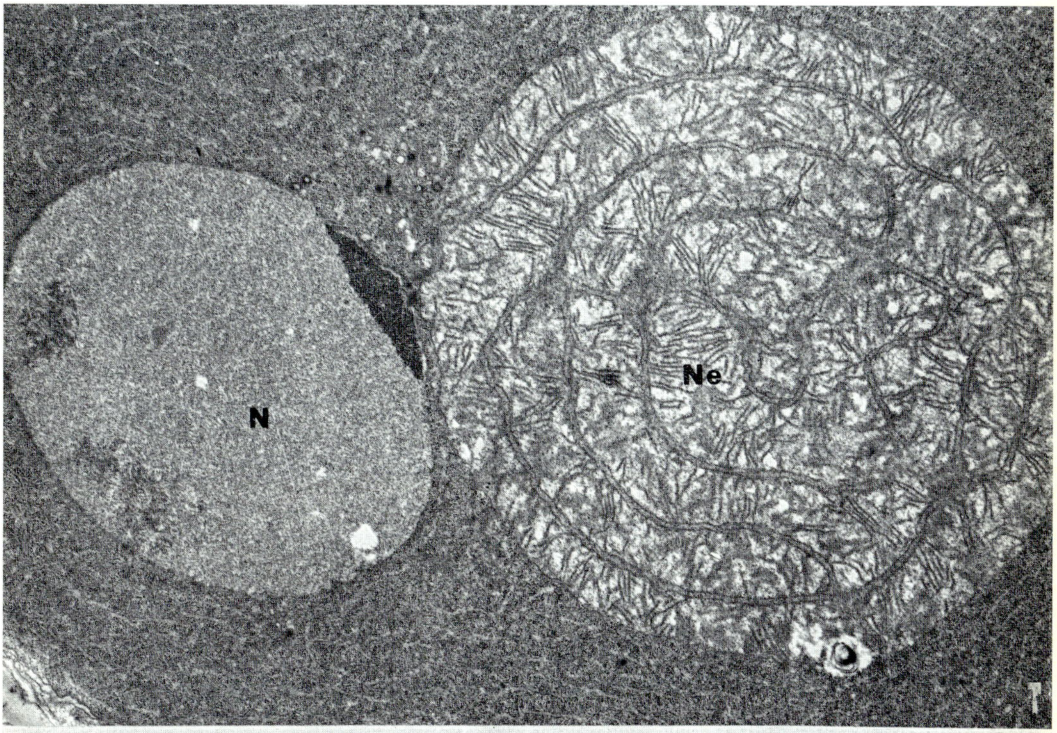

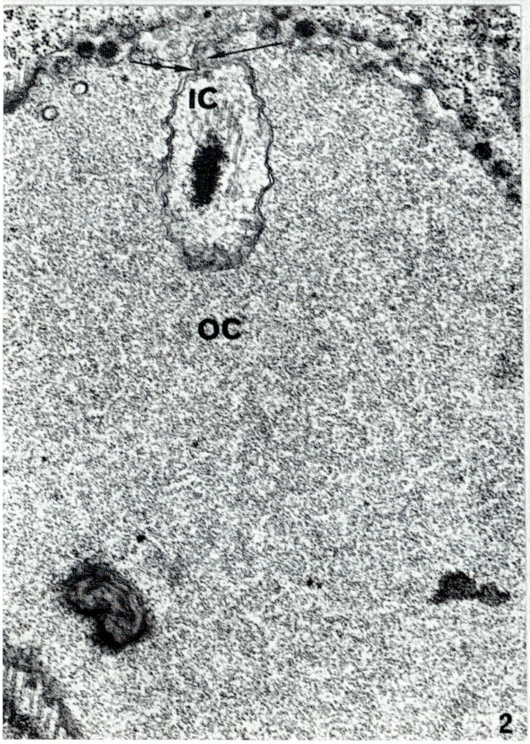

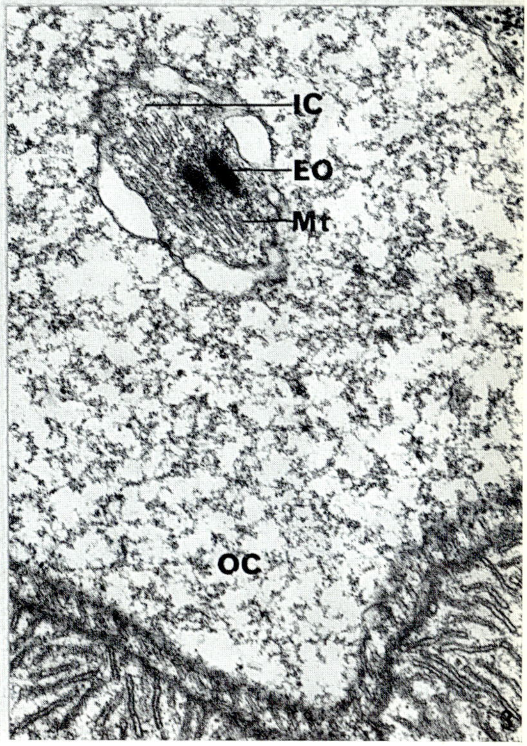

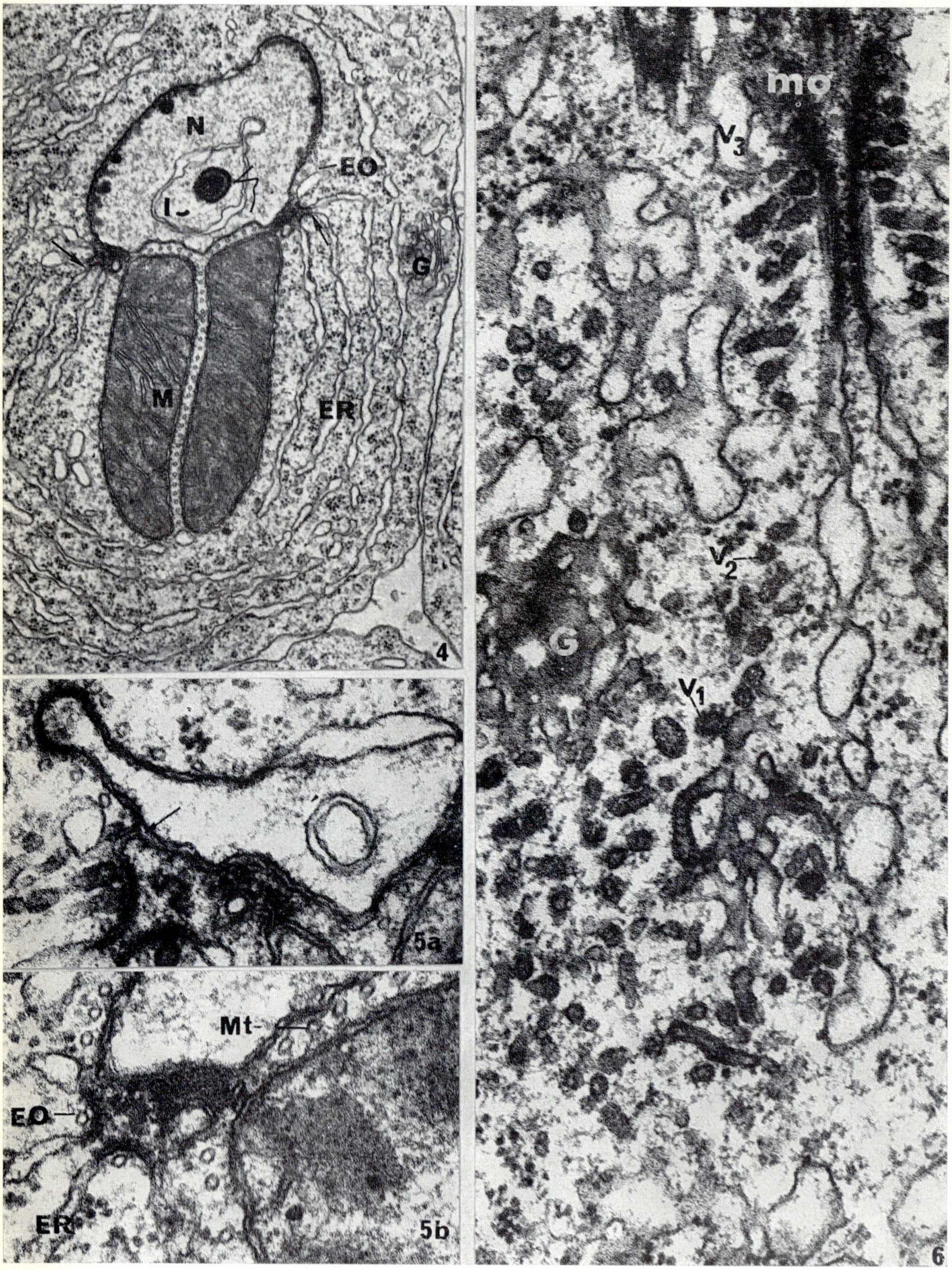
N
EO
I
G
M
ER
4
5a
Mt
EO
ER
5b
mg
V_3
V_2
G
V_1
6

J. F. Reger – *Some aspects of the fine structure of filiform spermatozoa (Ostracod,* Cypridopsis *sp.) lacking tubule sub-structure.*

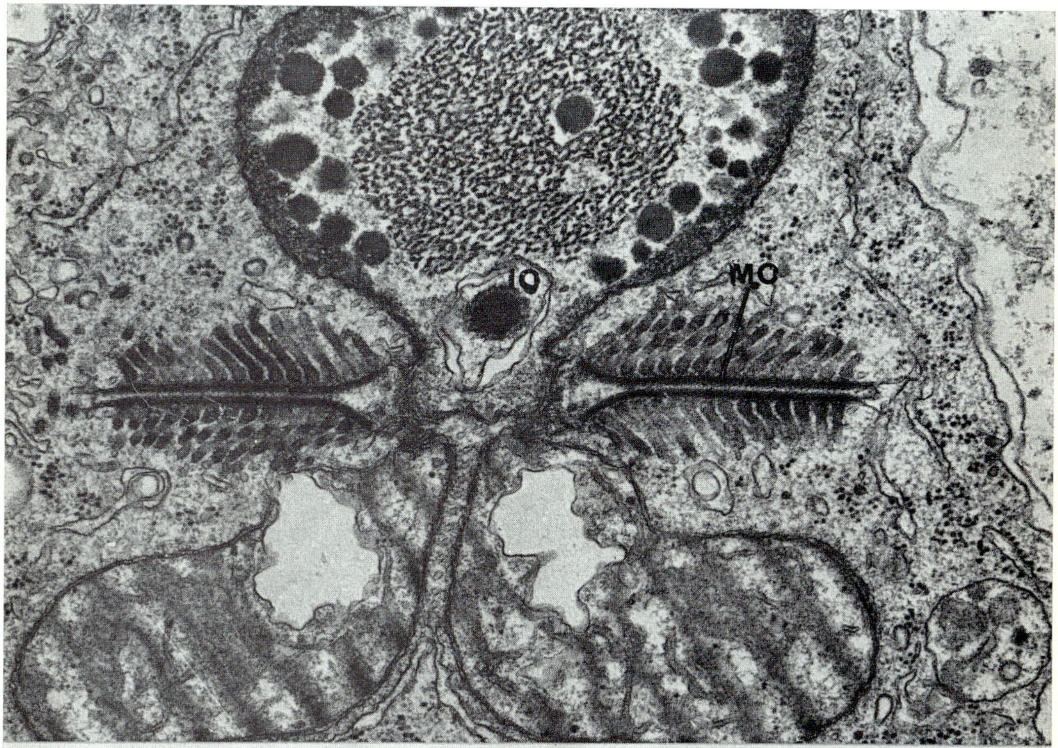

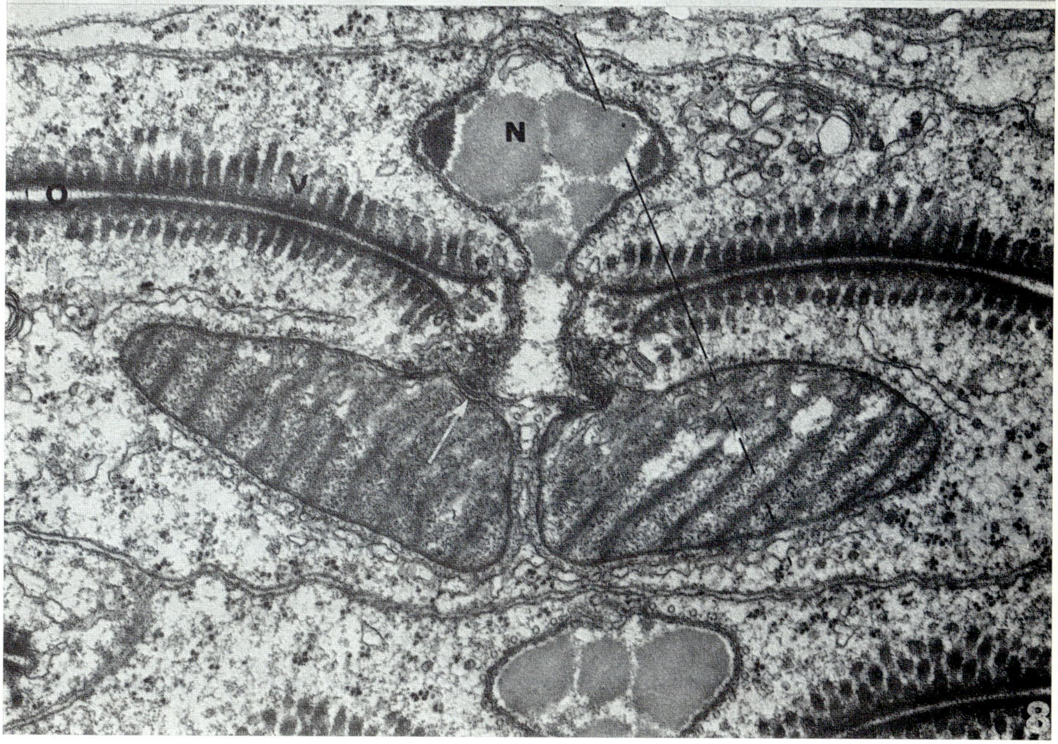

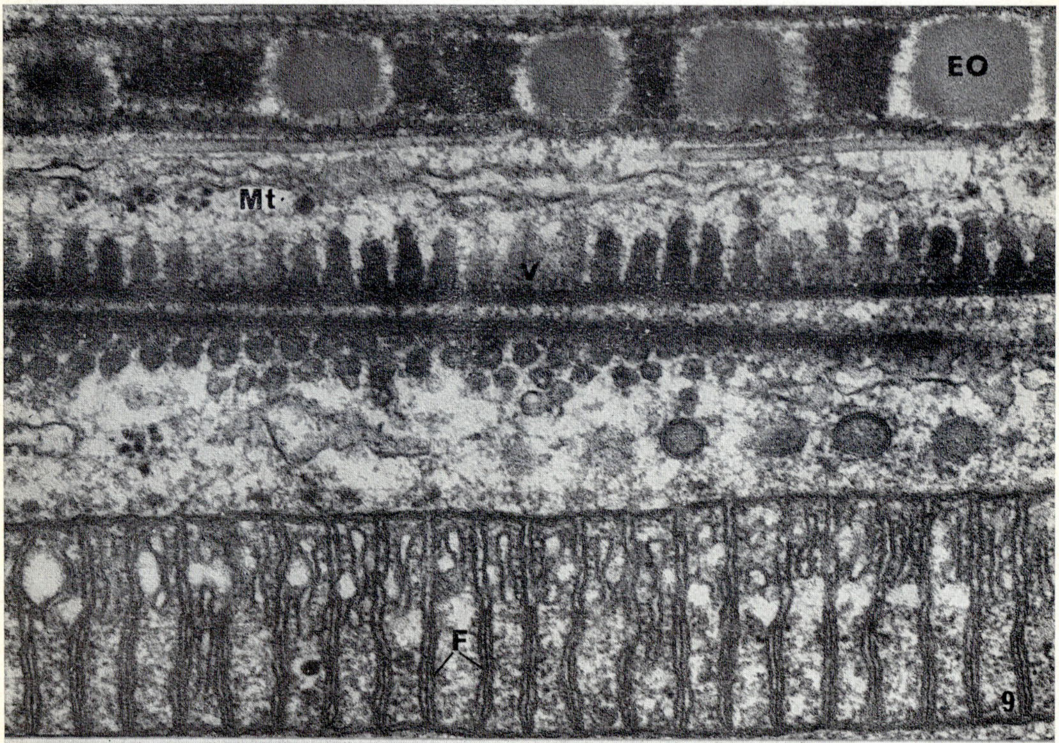
EO
Mt
V
F
9

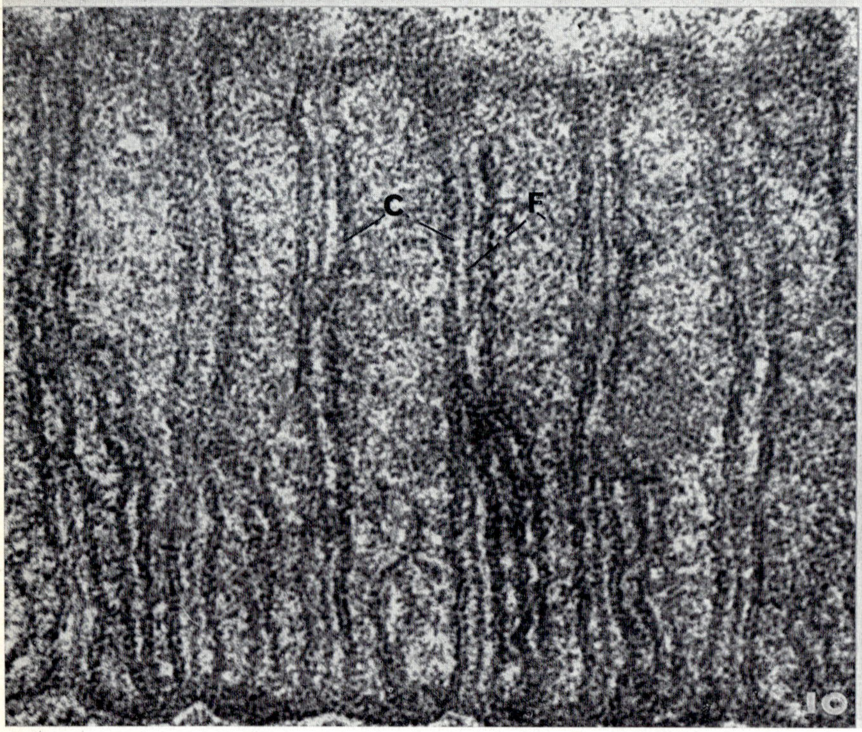
C
F
10

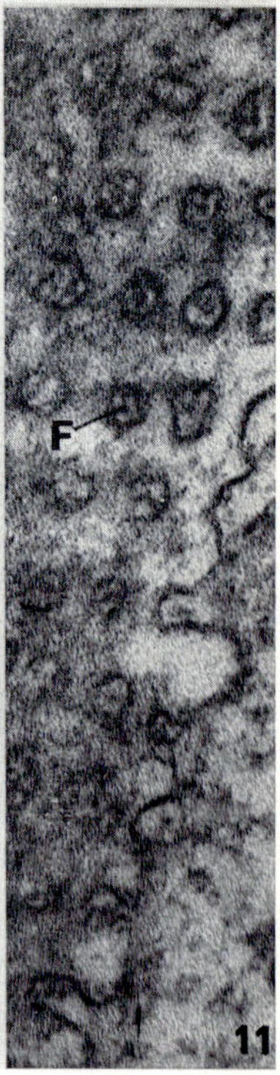
F
11

J. F. Reger – *Some aspects of the fine structure of filiform spermatozoa (Ostracod,* Cypridopsis *sp.) lacking tubule sub-structure.*

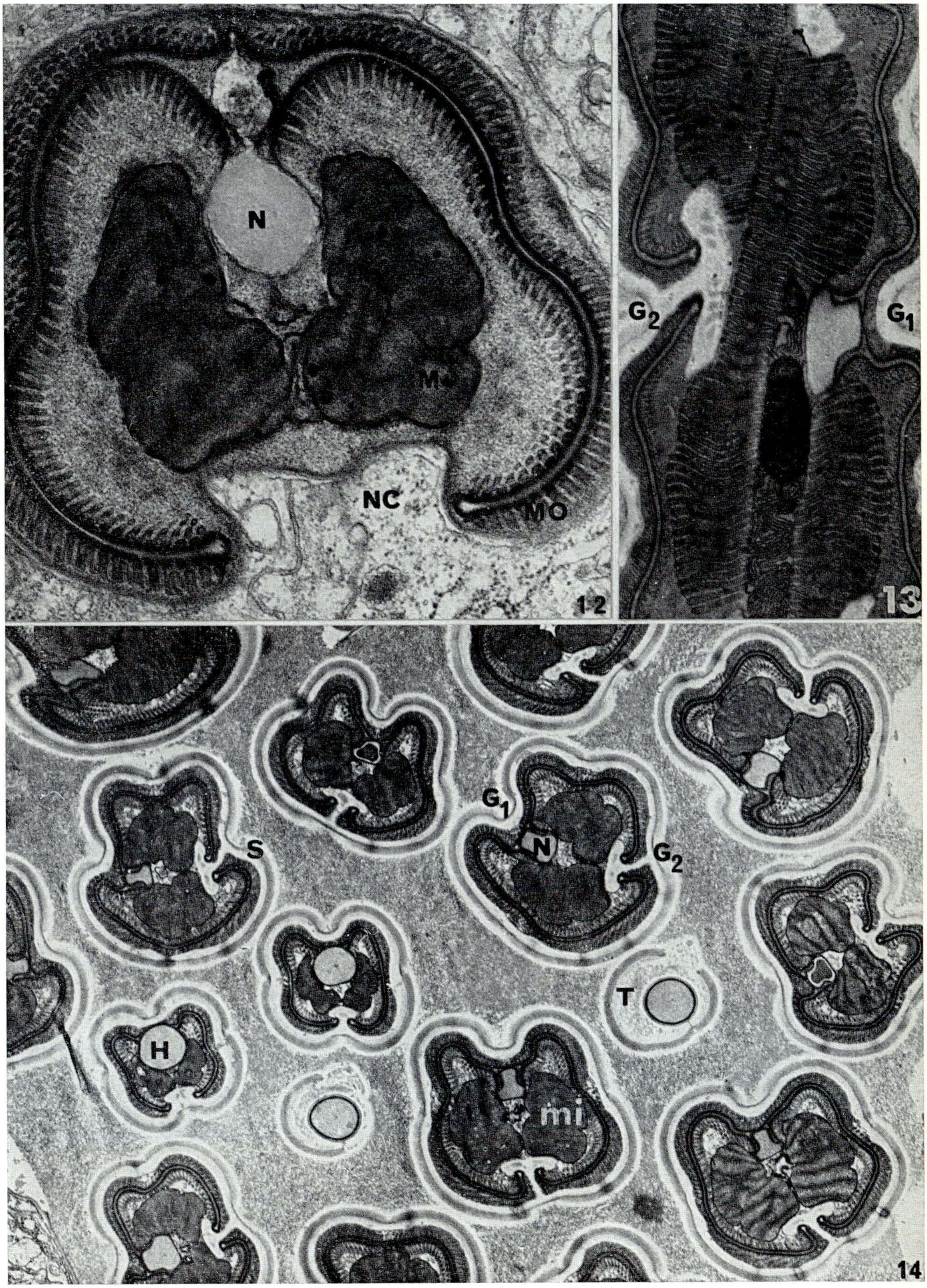

FLORIANA ROSATI (*), BACCIO BACCETTI (*) and ROMANO DALLAI (*)

THE SPERMATOZOON OF ARTHROPODA. X. ARANEIDS AND THE LOWEST MYRIAPODS

SUMMARY. — In this research the sperms of Araneida and of the most primitive stock of myriapods, Symphyla and Pauropoda, are examined.

The sperm of the spiders present particular characteristics: it is rolled up, mitochondria degenerate during maturation, secondary fibrils are not evident, a third central microtubule is present throughout the whole length of the tail, conditioning " 9+3 " pattern. In Symphyla two different kinds of spermatozoa are present: a smaller model and an atypical gigantic model in which the nucleus is caudal to the flagellum and the head is lacking.

The sperms of Pauropoda have two principal characteristics: constant absence of acrosome and presence of a caudal opened cylinder full of extracellular material.

Symphyla and Pauropoda belong to the " 9+2 " pattern of axial filament complex.

RIASSUNTO. — In questa ricerca sono stati esaminati gli spermatozoi degli Araneidi e dei più primitivi gruppi dei Miriapodi, Sinfili e Pauropodi.

Lo spermatozoo dei Ragni presenta particolari caratteristiche: è arrotolato, i mitocondri degenerano durante la maturazione, le fibrille secondarie non sono evidenti, un terzo microtubulo centrale è presente per l'intera lunghezza della coda condizionando il modello « 9 + 3 ».

Nei Sinfili sono presenti due diversi tipi di spermatozoi: un modello più piccolo e un modello atipico gigante nel quale il nucleo è caudale al flagello e la testa è assente.

Gli spermatozoi dei Pauropodi hanno due caratteristiche principali; la costante assenza dell'acrosoma e la presenza di un cilindro caudale aperto pieno di materiale extracellulare.

Sinfili e Pauropodi appartengono al modello di complesso assile flagellare « 9 + 2 ».

INTRODUCTION

In the comparative spermatology of Arthropods, Myriapoda and Arachnida present two puzzling problems. In the first, the highest class, Diplopoda, is well known for the presence of unmotile sperms, but nothing is known about the most primitive stock, Symphyla and Pauropoda. In the second, we know a lower stock with normal 9 + 2 flagellum (scorpions and pseudoscorpions) and the highest order (Acarina) with non-flagellate sperms, but nothing is known about the most important middle order, Araneida, whose sperm is entirely unknown in its ultrastructure. In this work we will try to answer both the questions.

(*) Institute of Zoology of the University of Siena, Italy.

Material and methods

The present research was carried out on three species of araneids (*Pholcus phalangioides, Agelena labyrinthica* and *Pardosa vittata*), one species of Symphyla (*Symphylella vulgaris*) and two of Pauropoda, one belonging to the genus *Allopauropus*, but hitherto undescribed, and one undetermined. The identification of the spiders is due to Dr. P. Tongiorgi (Pisa), that of the symphyle to Dr,. L. Juberthie—Jupeau (Moulis, Ariège), that of the pauropode to Dr. W. Huther (Saarbrucken).

The testes were fixed in vivo in 2.5 Hoyle-buffered, *p*H 7.2, glutaraldheyde for 30', postfixed for 5'–10' in 1% osmium tetroxide in Hoyle buffer, *p*H 7.2 dehydrated and embedded in Epon. Sections cut on LKB II and Reichert ultramicrotomes were collected on grids and usually stained with 1.5% uranyl acetate and lead citrate. For visualization of some chemical components several enzymic digestions were performed on ultrathin sections of the same material. For protein research 700–800 Å sections were floated for 10' on 10% H_2O_2 solution, thoroughly rinsed in distilled water, and floated for 5'–10'–30' on 0.5% pepsin in 0.1 N HCl at 37° C, according to the method of Behnke and Forer (1967). In all instances, after digestion, the sections were rinsed with distilled water, and finally stained with uranyl acetate and lead citrate. Undigested sections have been always examined for control. The subcellular localization of polysaccharides was investigated by the periodic thyosemicarbazide acid-silver protein method (Thiéry, 1967). For a confirmation of the polysaccharides distribution the sections previously floated on 10% H_2O_2 solution were treated with 0.1% phosphate-buffered *p*H 6,9 amylase at 20' for 1 h. Carbon coated sections were examined in a Siemens Elmiskop 1A kw of the Institute of Zoology of Siena.

Observations

1. – The spermatozoon of the spiders.

While contained in the male reproductive organs, the sperm of *Pholcus phalangioides*, is six times rolled on itself, forming six circumferences of about 2.5 μ in diameter. This rolled spermatozoon is incysted in a 0.1 μ thick sheath formed by an electron dense homogeneous extracellular material (Fig. 7), stratified on the cell membrane during the maturation of the spermatid. The mature spermatozoon, incysted or, after ejaculation, developed, is about 50 μ long, 20 of them occupied by the head (Fig. 1). The head is a spindle-shaped, elongated structure, with a longitudinal central canal. The head is encircled by a very thin membrane that, near the cranial apex, enlarges into two opposing wing-like protrusion devoid of chromatin. The whole nucleus, in the spermatid, is surrounded by several microtubules. A small cylinder of moderately osmiophilic material is contained in the cranial half of the canal of the mature spermatozoon. This cylinder penetrates into the acrosome, a brief osmiophilic organelle placed over the tip of the nucleus, basally located in a nuclear concavity and apically lanceolate (Fig. 4). In the nucleus the chromatin, osmiophilic material is concentrated at the periphery (Figs. 7, 8). The central canal becomes larger near the tail, and there it is occupied by a granular substance, in the center of which the centriole is located (Fig. 6). The centriole and the cranial part of the axial filament complex, are therefore intranuclear. This situation is very clear in the spermatid too, where a small channel is invaginated into the still spherical nucleus, and it is occupied by a centriole structure that, in longitudinal section, seems to be the result of two aligned units, i.e. two coaxial parallel centrioles (Fig. 3). Inside the nucleus the axial filament complex starts. In this region it bears an absolutely unusual pattern of fibrils.

The basic model is constantly 9 + 3, and in this region 9 osmiophilic longitudinal units encircle the 9 doublets, with each osmiophilic longitudinal unit closely corresponding to a doublet (Figs. 2, 5). It is important to remark that this 9 + 9 + 3 pattern is not homologous to the 9 + 9 + 2. The outer units are, in the spiders, very brief coarse deposits of osmiophilic homogeneous material, devoid of microtubules and recall the 9 outer units observed in the same region of *Lumbricus* by ANDERSON and ELLIS (1968).

The sperm tail starts immediately after the nucleus. It bears throughout almost its whole length the 9 + 3 pattern (Fig. 8). The aspects of the 9 peripheral doublets is the normal one with short arms and the A subfiber slightly opaque. Afzelius rays, secondary fibrils and a central sheath are not evident; the 3 central tubules, disposed in triangle, are wide and closely similar to the B subfiber. The extreme region of the tail is devoid of outer doublets. Only the three central tubules constitute the terminal region of this sperm. In the developed sperm mitochondria are entirely lacking. In the spermatid, 3 or 4 of them with normal structure are present around the nucleus. In the incysted spermatozoon they occupy the central region and are limited by the circumferences described by the head and the tail. But at a later stage in development the mitochondria degenerate (Fig. 2), lose the cristae and fuse into a unique, opaque mass that becomes dispersed in the cytoplasm where the sperm develops.

This structure, with some insignificant variations, remains the same in other families of spiders. We have constantly found a 9 + 3 pattern in the flagella of *Pardosa vittata* (Licosidae) and *Agelena labyrintica* (Agelenidae).

2. – The two spermatozoa of a symphyle.

In the testes and in the male ducts of *Symphylella vulgaris* studied by us, two different kinds of spermatozoa are regularly found: a smaller model, and a gigantic model (Fig. 9). The second is less numerous, and is interpreted by us as an atypical sperm class. Atypical gigantic sperms have already been observed in a class very close to myriapods, the chilopods by BOUIN (1925, 1934) and ANSLEY (1954) recently revised by FAIN-MAUREL (1968).

The smaller sperms are curious guitar-like organisms constituted by an enlarged head region and a narrow tail region only 4 μ long (Fig. 10). The former in dorsal view is 2.5 μ long and 2 μ large; in lateral view (Fig. 14) it appears 1 μ high. In the head, three consecutive structures can be found: a cranial system of concentric membranes, enveloping a unique central, great mitochondrion, a central system of tortuous tubules externally opened and, near the origin of the tail, an opaque, homogeneous, flattened, discoidal nucleus (Fig. 10). The mitochondrion has an elliptical form 1 μ×0.5 μ in diameter and a normal structure, with deep inner cristae and an opaque matrix (Fig. 17). The system of membranes enveloping it has a Golgian origin (Fig. 14) and is entirely proteinaceous. After pepsin digestion it is electively removed, when the other parts of the sperm are unaffected (Fig. 11). In our opinion it is an acrosome. The tubular system is a very concentrated endoplasmic reticulum. The single tubules appear to open at the outer surface of the sperm cell (Fig. 17). The nucleus is, in dorsal view, 1.2 μ in diameter and 0.1 μ high. In the mature sperm it is absolutely electronopaque. The tail arises at the level of the caudal portion of the nucleus (Fig. 12), causing a small concavity in its profile. In a ondulate membrane only the axial filament is contained. The others organelles are, in fact, in the head anterior to the nucleus. In the cranial half of the tail, 2 μ long and 0.5 μ thick, the axial filament has a simple 9 + 2 pattern (Fig. 13), with evident doublets and singlets, but no Afzelius arms and secondary fibrils. The caudal half of the tail is smaller in diameter (1/4 of μ) and contains only the two longest central units of the axial filament complex (Fig. 13).

The gigantic sperms are filiform organisms 60 μ long and with a somewhat, constant diameter of 0.5 μ. Only in the extreme apical tip do we find a vesicular irregular enlargement (Fig. 15); in the other part of the sperm three elongated components are helicoidally coiled with a pitch of about 10 μ. The apical enlargement of the sperm is a head recalling that of the smaller sperms. There we find a large empty vesicle with small system of concentric membranes near the centre and, in the basal position, a moderate concentration of endoplasmic tubules (Fig. 15). The nucleus elongated and compactly osmiophylic, arises with the axial filament complex, at the base of this apical enlargement that has the position of a head but not its significance. The tail is therefore constituted by a coiling of nucleus and axial filament in the cranial segment of the elongated sperm. The substructure of the nucleus is more or less filamentous (Fig. 16), that of the axial filament follows the classic 9 + 2 pattern (Fig. 16), without secondary fibrils and Afzelius rays. Near the middle region of the sperm its diameter is increased by the addition of a coiled, elongated mitochondrial derivative. This organelle has a strongly osmiophilic matrix, and several cristae longitudinallly arranged. In this region the diameter of the nucleus is greater and its content less compact. Near the end of the sperm the axial filament terminates and the paired nucleus and mitochondrial derivative reach the tip devoid of organelles of motility.

3. – The spermatozoon of Pauropoda.

In the two species of pauropods studied by us, many characters are held in common and only few details can distinguish them. In both cases the spermatozoon is a cylindrical moderately elongated flagellated organism (Fig. 18).

The head contains only the elongated and osmiophilic nucleus, the acrosome always being absent. The caudal part of the nucleus is plain and after it a centriole is located. The axial filament complex is of the 9 + 2 pattern (Fig. 21). It is encircled by mitochondrial derivatives (Fig. 21), has an helicoidal arrangement and finishes at the tip of the sperm tail. The limiting membrane of the sperm determines in both species a curious modification of the end region. In a deep cylindrical infolding, a loose wall extends some micra backwards, it contains a cylinder of compact osmiophilic extracellular material, which is trailed the sperm (Fig. 20). Differences between the two species are in the fact that the first has around the nucleus a pleated limiting membrane determining, in longitudinal section, an ondulate profile of the sperm head (Fig. 19). The second species has a smooth head (Fig. 23), but shows a crown of long microtubules (absent in the first) arising from the border of the caudal infolding (Fig. 22).

The nuclear material and the mitochondrial derivative are more concentrated in the first species than in the second one. The nucleus is compactly osmiophilic in the first, granular in the second. The mitochondrial material is very compact, homogeneous, with narrow longitudinal cristae in the first species, constituted by several small mitochondrial units forming a chain around the axial filament in the second.

CONCLUSIONS

The most important aim of this research was to ascertain whether, in some Arthropodan groups commonly considered, at the basis of highly evolved orders with non flagellate sperms, the spermatozoon maintains the conventional characteristics. Spiders do not possess any characteristics common to Acarina. In the attitude of the spermatozoon before ejaculation they are close to other 9 + 2 terrestrial Arthropods, (i.e. pseudoscorpions, diplopods, collembols) and have incysted spermatozoa.

This sperm, which develops in the male ducts immediately before ejaculation, has particular characteristics. It is devoid of mitochondria (according to the old cytological data of SHARMA 1950; SHARMA & GUPTA 1956, and to the more recents histochemical findings of KANWAR, 1967) and in the axial filament complex shows the most important following characters.

Secondary fibrils are not evident (at least not in the typical fashion of other insects).

A third central microtubule is present throughout the whole length of the tail, forming a " 9 + 3 " pattern, a fact absolutely new for all cilia and flagella, because only in cilia of Ctenophora and Mollusca did AFZELIUS (1961) and GIBBONS (1961) demonstrate the presence of a third central unit, which was linear rather than tubular. The region of the axial filament near the centriole region bears 9 outer coarse units, there reaching a 9 + 9 + 3 pattern. This accessory range of coarse paracentriolar fibers, very distinct from the normal microtubules, is new for arthropods, where only insects have the 9 + 9 + 2 pattern by accessory microtubules, and it recalls the situation of *Lumbricus* (ANDERSON & ELLIS 1967).

The classes showing a 9 + 9 (+ 0 or 1 or 2 or 3) pattern are eight: Oligochaeta, Gastropoda, Arachnida, Insecta, Cyclostomata, Reptilia, Aves, Mammalia. The myriapods studied have given some unsurprising results. The most important point is that both Symphyla and Pauropoda have a conventional flagellum with a 9 + 2 pattern.

The two kinds of sperms in *Symphylella* extend to myriapods the presence of atypical gigantic sperms, up till now considered a characteristic peculiar to Chilopoda. A curious fact is that in these last spermatozoa the nucleus is caudal to the flagellum, and the head is lacking. Typical sperms of *Symphylella* have the main characteristic of a single mitochondrion enveloped in acrosomial membranes; the relatively simple sperms of pauropods have the constant absence of acrosome and presence of a caudal opened cylinder full of extracellular material. But these are particular characteristics whose evolutive significance is very difficult to evaluate.

REFERENCES

AFZELIUS B. A. (1961) – *The fine structure of the cilia from ctenophore swimming plates.* « J. Biophys. Biochem. Cytol. », 9, 383–394.

ANDERSON W. A. and ELLIS R. A. (1968) – *Acrosome Morphogenesis in* Lumbricus terrestris. « Zeit. Zellforsch. », 85, 398–407.

ANSLEY H. R. (1954) – *A cytological and cytophotometric study of alternative pathways of meiosis in the house centipede* (Scutigera forceps *Rafinesque*). « Chromosoma », 6, 656–695.

BEHNKE O. and FORER A. (1967) – *Evidence for four classes of microtubules in individual cells.* « J. Cell Biol. », 2, 169–192.

BOUIN P. (1925) – *Les cinèses de maturation et la double spermatogènèse chez* Scolopendra cingulata. « La Cellule », 35, 373–421.

BOUIN P. (1934) – *L'évolution d'un chromosome spécial* (*hétérochromosome*) *au cours de la double spermatogenèse chez* Scutigera coleoptrata. « Arch. Zool. Exper. », 75, 595–613.

FAIN-MAUREL M. (1966) – *Acquisitions récentes sur les spermatogenèses atypiques.* « Ann. Biol. ». Fasc. 11–12, 513–564.

GIBBONS I. R. (1961) – *The relationship between the fine structure and direction of heat in gill cilia of a lamellibranch mollusc.* « J. Biophys. Biochem. Cytol. », 11, 179–205.

KANWAR U. (1907) – *Histochemistry of spermatogenesis in the spider,* Lycosa chaperi. « Res. Bull. Panjab Univ. N. S. », 18, 95–108.

SHARMA G. P. (1950) – *Spermatogenesis in the spider,* Plexippus paykulli. « Res. Bull. East Panjab Univ. Zool. », 5, 67–80.

SHARMA G. P. and GUPTA B. L. (1956) – *Cytological studies on the male germ cells of the spider,* Pardosa *sp. with observations under the phase contrast microscope.* « Res. Bull. Panjab Univ. », 84, 1–5.

THIÉRY J. (1967) – *Mise in evidence des polysaccharides sur coupes fines en microscopie électronique.* « J. Microscopie », 7, 987–1019.

Explanation of figures

Fig. 1. – Longitudinal section of the head in developed spermatozoon of *Pholcus phalangioides*. ×16.000.

Fig. 2. – Cross section of the centriole region of immature spermatozoon of *Pholcus phalangioides*. 9 osmiophilic units (*u*) encircle the 9 doublets. At left degenerating mitochondria are evident. ×60.000.

Fig. 3. – Longitudinal section of the centriole region. (*n*) nucleus. ×30.000.

Fig. 4. – Longitudinal section of the acrosome. The intranuclear cylinder penetrates into the acrosome (*a*). (*n*) nucleus. ×30.000.

Fig. 5. – Cross section of the caudal centriole region. Only five osmiophilic units are present around the doublets. ×60.000.

Fig. 6. – Centriole region (*cr*) of the spermatid of *Pholcus phalangioides*. (*n*) nucleus. ×30.000.

Fig. 7. – Cross section of the rolled spermatozoon incysted in a sheath of electron dense material. (*f*) filament complex; (*n*) nucleus. ×30.000.

Fig. 8. – High magnification of the nucleus (*n*) and filament complex (*f*). ×90.000.

Fig. 9. – Electron micrograph of isolated sperms of *Symphylella vulgaris*. A smaller spermatozoon and a gigantic one are present. ×2.500.

Fig. 10. – Longitudinal section of the smaller model of spermatozoon. A system of concentric membranes (*mc*) and of tortuous tubules (*t*) is present in the cranial region. (*n*) nucleus; (*f*) tail. ×30.000.

Fig. 11. – The cranial region of the same spermatozoon after pepsin digestion. The concentric membranes (*mc*) are quite removed. The tubules (*t*) and the central mitochondrion (*m*) are conserved. ×30.000.

Fig. 12. – Sections of the head of the smaller spermatozoon of *Symphylella vulgaris*. A centriole (*c*) is present between the concentric membranes (*mc*) and the nucleus (*n*). ×30.000.

Fig. 13. – Cross section of filament complex of the same spermatozoon. At left a caudal section of the tail: only the central units are evident. ×60.000.

Fig. 14. – Lateral view of the head of the smaller model of spermatozoon. (*m*) mitochondrion; (*mc*) concentric membranes; (*t*) tubules; (*n*) nucleus. ×60.000.

Fig. 15. – The cranial region of the gigantic sperm of *Symphylella vulgaris*. A small system of concentric membranes (*mc*) is located in an empty, terminal vesicle. (*t*) tortuous tubules; (*n*) nucleus. ×30.000.

Fig. 16. – Cross sections of sperm of the gigantic model. The more or less filamentous structure of the nucleus (*n*) is evident. (*f*) filament complex. ×60.000.

Fig. 17. – A high magnification of the cranial region of the smaller model of spermatozoon of *Symphylella vulgaris*. ×60.000.

Fig. 18. – A longitudinal section of entire spermatozoon of undeterminated pauropod. (*n*) nucleus; (*f*) tail; (*c*) terminal cylinder. ×12.000.

Fig. 19. – A longitudinal section of the nucleus and centriole region of the same spermatozoon. ×30.000.

Fig. 20. – Longitudinal section of the terminal region of the same spermatozoon. The opened cylinder trailed by the tail is seen. ×30.000.

Fig. 21. – Cross section of the tail of spermatozoon of *Allopauropus*. (*m*) mitochondria; (*f*) filament complex. ×60.000.

Fig. 22. – The terminal region of the cylinder trailed by the tail of the spermatozoon of *Allopauropus*. Microtubules (*mi*) arising from the border of the caudal infolding are seen. ×60.000.

Fig. 23. – Longitudinal section of the spermatozoon of *Allopauropus*. (*n*) nucleus; (*f*) tail. ×30.000.

Discussion

ANDERSON. – I am impressed by your excellent presentation on this most difficult subject. I would like to know the substructure of the centriole that is associated with the "9 doublets + 3 central tubular complex" that forms the axoneme.

ROSATI. – The centriole bears the normal structure of 9 triplets.

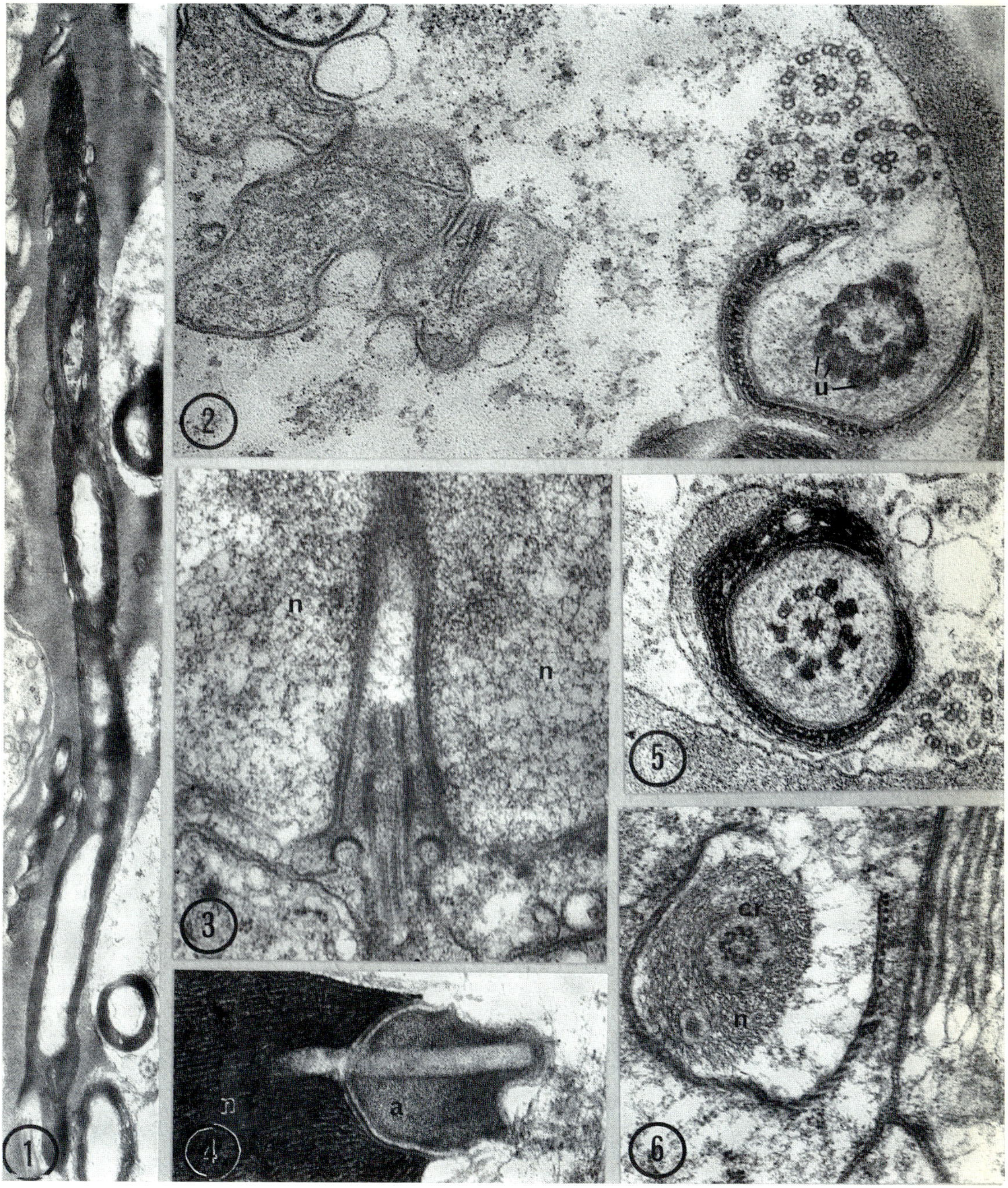
1
2
u
3
n
n
4
n
a
5
6
cr
n

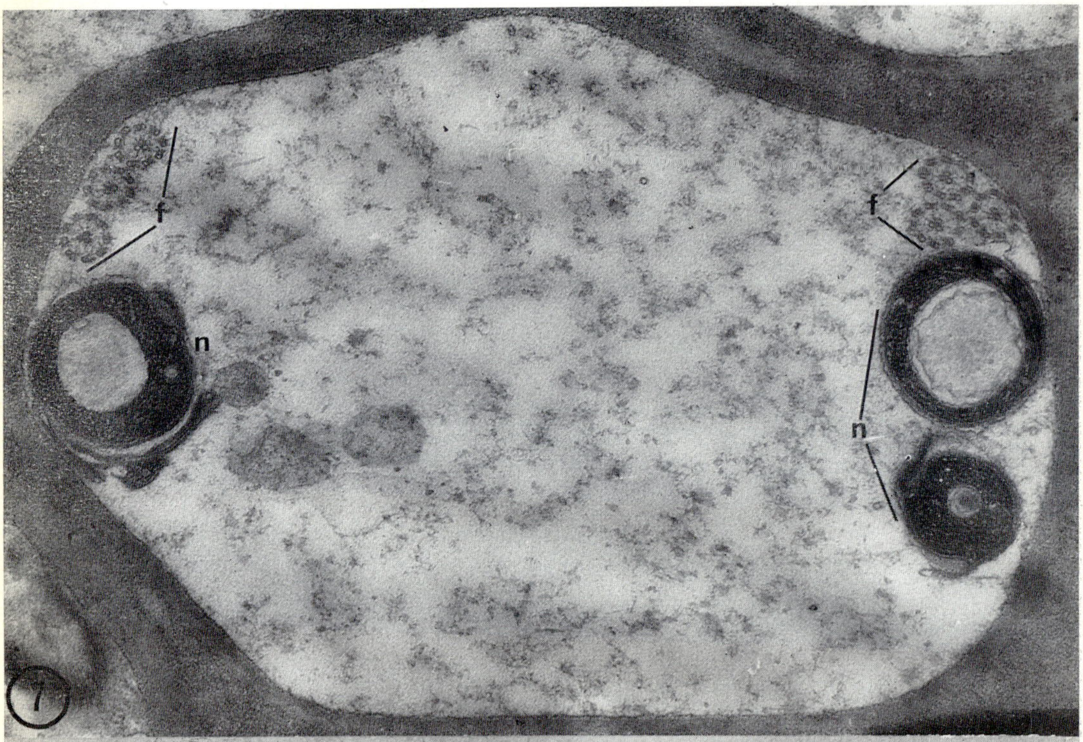

7

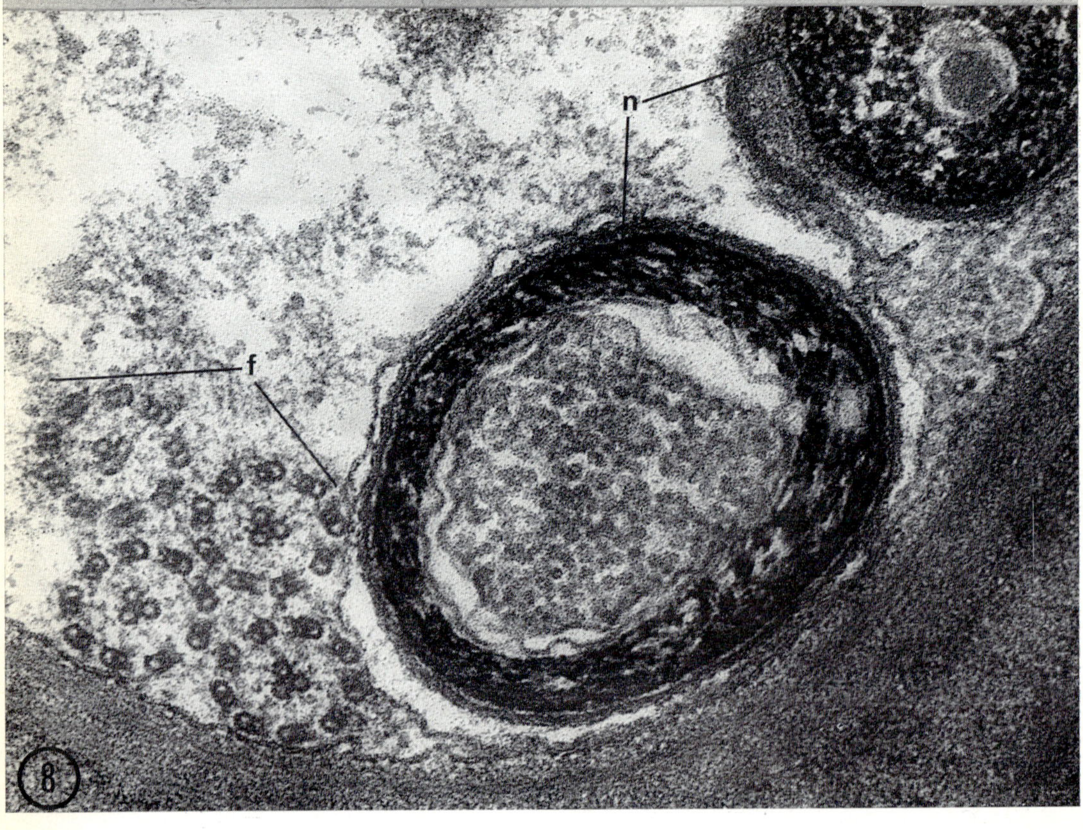

8

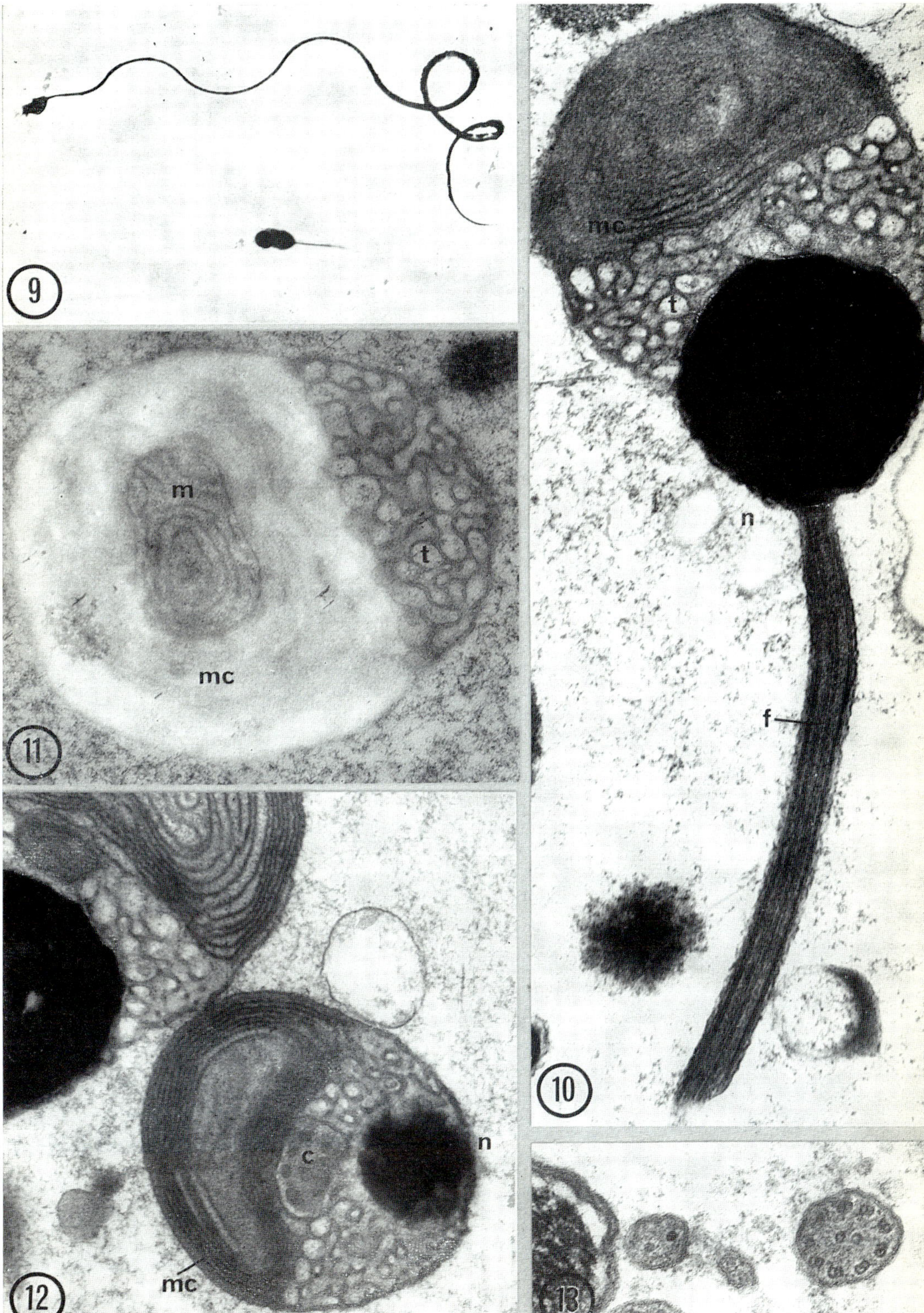
9
mc
t
n
f
10
m
t
mc
11
c
n
mc
12
13

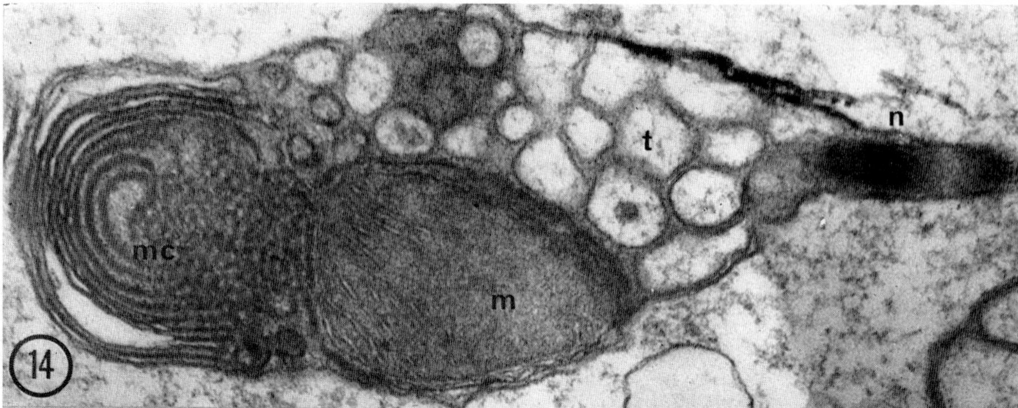
n
t
mc
m
14

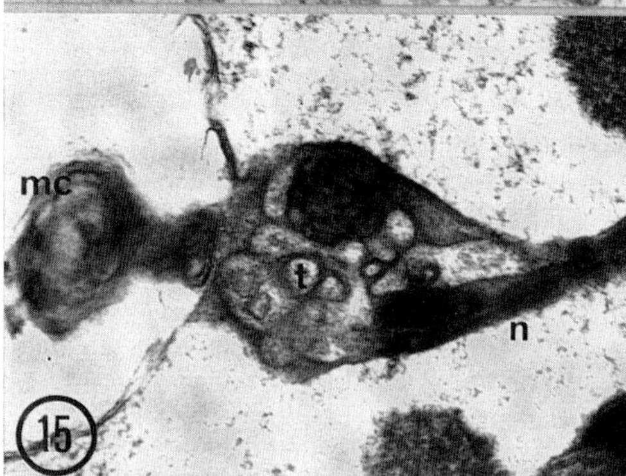
mc
t
n
15

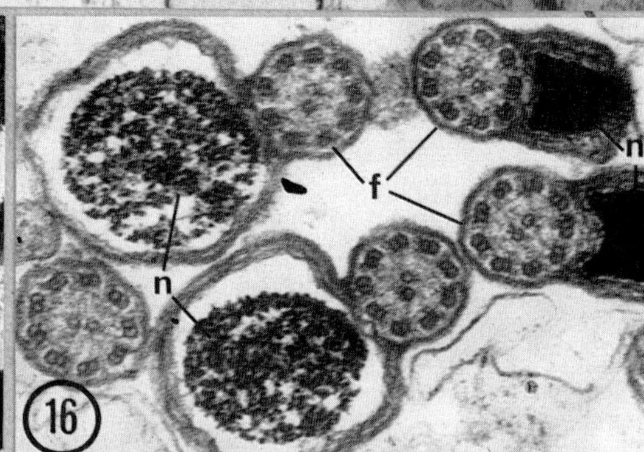
n
f
n
n
16

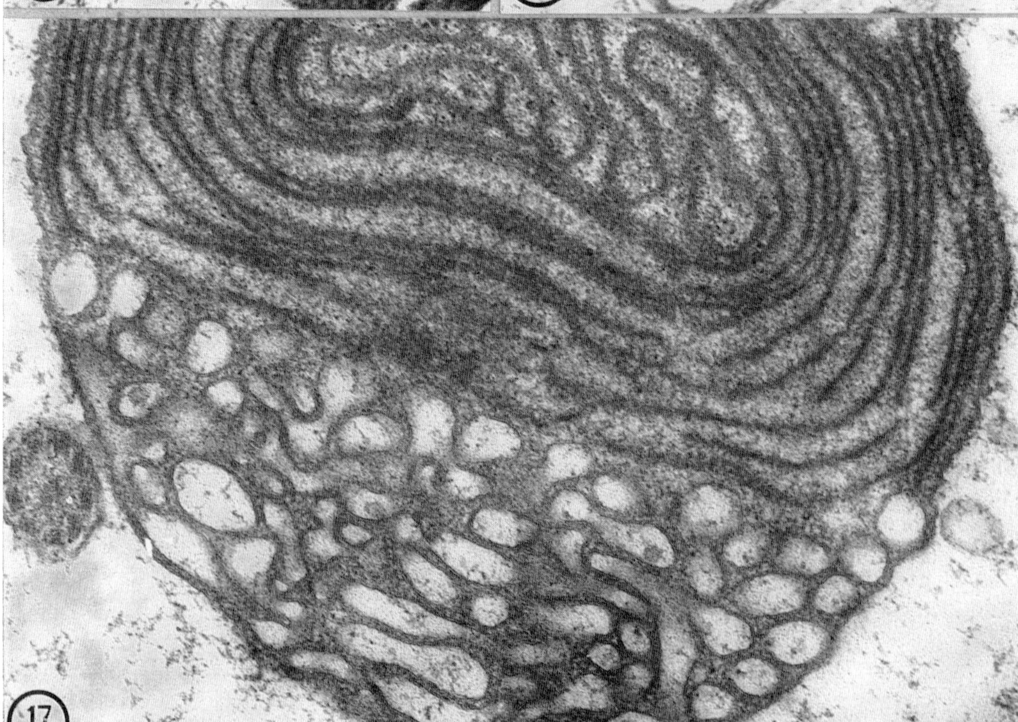
17

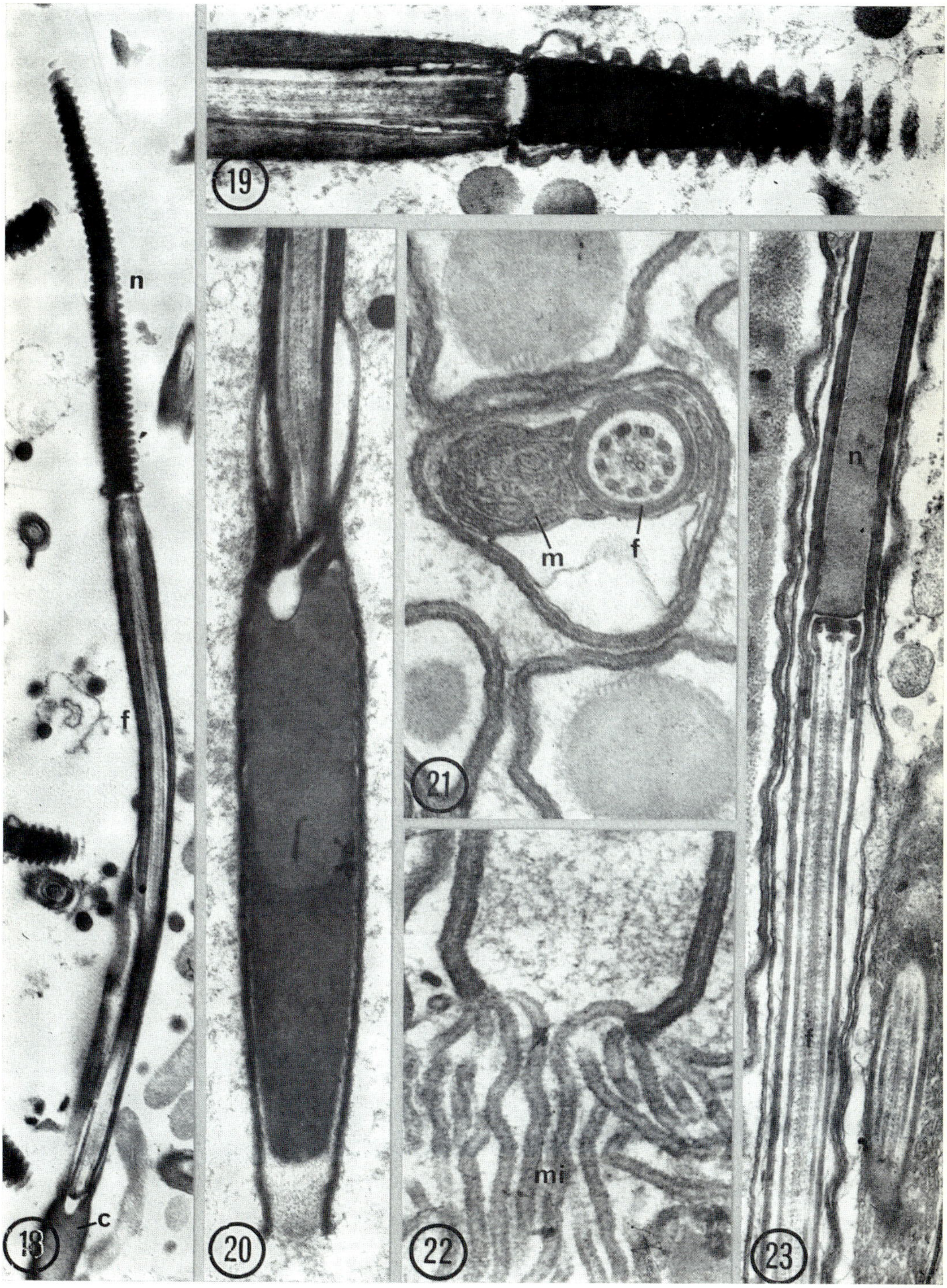
n
f
c
18
19
20
21
m
f
22
mi
23
n
f

E. HORSTMANN (*)

THE ACROSOME COMPLEX OF THE DIPLOPODE *SPIROSTREPTUS SP.*

SUMMARY. — The acrosome complex of the diplopode *Spirostreptus sp.* consists of the acrosome vacuole, the calotte, the cristalloid, the M – body and the envelope. The fine structure and the differentiation of these compartments are described and compared with the acrosome complex of diplopodes and other animals. The special relationship between the nucleus and the acrosome structure is demonstrated.

RIASSUNTO. — Il complesso acrosomiale del diplopode *Spirostreptus sp.* è formato dal vacuolo acrosomiale, dalla calotta, dal cristalloide, dal corpo M e dall'involucro. Viene descritta la fine struttura e la differenziazione di questi organuli e viene confrontata con il complesso acrosomiale dei diplopodi e di altri animali. Vengono mostrate le speciali relazioni tra il nucleo e la struttura acrosomiale.

The spermatozoa of most species transform their cell organelles into special structures, evolving specialized mitochondria, flagella, the acrosome and other additional structures. In this respect they differ from the soma cells and are of cytological interest.

Exceptionally specialized spermatozoa are those of the *Diplopoda* which were first observed by GILSON in 1886, and described in more detailed form by Mme. TUZET and MANIER (1956).

Together with Dr. BREUCKER I have studied the spermatozoa and the spermiogenesis of *Spirostreptus sp.* We have described the mature spermatozoon using the name *Graphidostreptus*. A new classification by an expert, Prof. O. KRAUS, Hamburg, resulted in the exact name. I want to show you the structures we call "Akrosomkomplex". Studying these forms we found several remarkable points.

At the beginning I shall describe briefly the mature spermatozoon and thereafter the histogenesis of the acrosome. The hat-like spermatozoon of *Spirostreptus* consists of a disk and a cylindrical body (Schema 1). The basal disk, containing besides the nucleus only little, but very dense PAS–positive cytoplasm (Fig. 2 b), is drawn out thinly. This fine drawn space is filled by cytoplasm only (Fig. 1). The nucleus—recognized in the light microscope by the positive Feulgen-reaction (Fig. 2 a)—is distinguished by high electron density and consists of closely packed tubules. These tubules

(*) Hamburg, Germany.

consist of an outer layer which does not give any contrast (Fig. 3). Along their axis they contain an electron-dense cylinder which in turn exhibits an optically empty space in the middle of which runs an electron-dense threadlike core.

The acrosome complex is composed of five different portions. In the axis of the apical half of the cylindrical body the PAS–positive acrosome vacuole is situated. It is formed like a nail with a large head and a point which is thickened to a hemisphere. The thickened point is surrounded by a calotte of neatly arranged material. Basally and laterally of the calotte the cristalloid is found. These three central structures (acrosome vacuole, calotte and cristalloid) are enveloped by a M–shaped ring. The short sides of this M–body are perforated by the nail-like acrosome vacuole. They cover the cristalloid. The long sides surround the periphery of the cristalloid; their basis broadens particularly towards the periphery. The M–body is

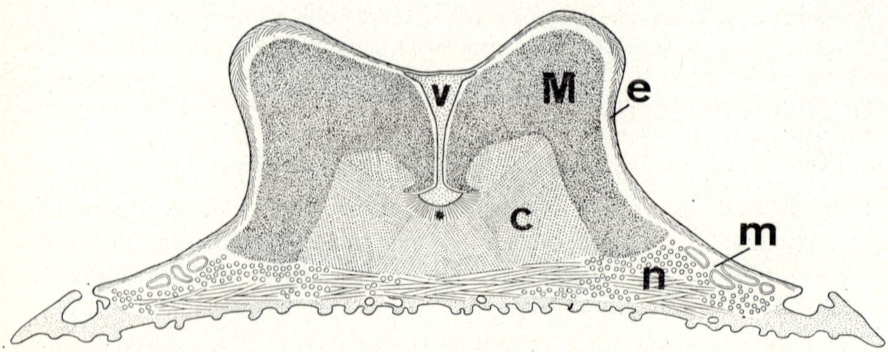

Schema 1. - Schema of a mature sperm of *Spirostreptus sp.*; (*n*) nucleus, (*v*) acrosome vacuole, (*) calotte, (*c*) cristalloid, (*M*) M–body, (*e*) envelope, (*m*) ring of mitochondria.

covered by the so-called " envelope ". This envelope is lying just beneath the cell membrane and extends to the border of the hat-like sperm. Where the head of the hat passes over into the border, a ring of mitochondria surrounds the boundary between nucleus and M–body. In the mature spermatozoa of our species we never saw a centriole.

Next I shall demonstrate these five compartments of the acrosome complex and their cytogenesis one after another. The *acrosome vacuole* is surrounded completely and permanently by a membrane (Fig. 5). Like a well bred acrosome vacuole it originates in vesicles of the Golgi-complex (Fig. 4). Its position markes the apical pole of the spermatid. Initially the vacuole is globular and dents the nucleus. While the M–body is appearing, the membrane of the vacuole forms fine processes extending into the M–body (Fig. 7). These processes do not disappear until the end of spermiogenesis. In their neighbourhood the substance of the M–body condenses, and apparently material of the vacuole drops into the M–body. The acrosome vacuole gives a positive PAS–reaction (Fig. 2 b), also after treatment with amylase. When the vacuole dents the nucleus a clear layer, the " *calotte* ", arises between the nucleus and the vacuole (Fig. 6). From the beginning the calotte shows radial and concentric streaks. The radial streaking results from radial approximately hexagonal prisms which compose the calotte. The length of the prisms corresponds to the thickness of the calotte.

The whole size of the calotte is enclosed by the *cristalloid*, consisting of seven to ten sectors (Fig. 8); they have already been described and demonstrated by TUZET and MANIER (1956) in light microscopy. Its ultrastructure shows a characteristic and periodical composition which induced us to term it " cristalloid " (Fig. 12). Tubules of a thickness of 100 to 120 Å are deposited exactly linear and strictly parallel. The direction or the arrangement

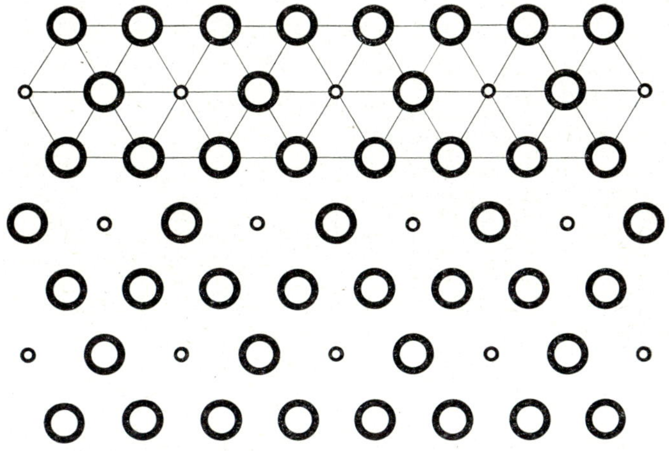

Schema 2. – Schema of the rhombic arrangement of the tubules in the cristalloid. In the center of the rhombs are the thin tubules, at the top dense material between the tubules is indicated.

of the tubules is different in every sector. In cross sections they are arranged hexagonally (Schema 2). Moreover the hexagons are arranged in such a manner that only two sides of adjacent tubules are common. So they need more room than a honey comb pattern, and three-cornered spaces exist between the hexagons. This arrangement is realy a rhombic pattern. The angels of the rhombs are 60°, respectively 120°. The rhombs are limited by 8 tubules. In the center of every rhomb lies a thin tubule of 60 Å in diameter. Neighbouring tubules are connected with one another by bridges of dense material. This strictly cristalloid composition is identical in all sectors, only the direction of the tubules is different.

The cristalloid arises shortly after the onset of differentiation of the M–body (Fig. 6). It grows as long as the M–body increases in size. There is no relation between the formation of the calotte or the cristalloid with any known cell organelle.

The *M–body* of the mature spermatozoa is of high electron density. The material of the long sides is finely granulated and homogeneous, that of the short sides is spotted or brightened by irregular stripes (Fig. 1). This material stems from the nucleus. With the beginning of the formation of the acrosome complex the double membrane of the nucleus becomes interrupted (Fig. 6). The interruption is limited to the contact area between M–body and nucleus. Within reach of the acrosome vacuole and later on of the calotte and of the cristalloid the pores of the nucleus disappear. In relation to the growing cristalloid the contact area of M–body and nucleus moves to the periphery. The circular contact area becomes wider and wider. In this area the gap between nucleus and plasm is interrupted (Fig. 9). Peripheral to the circular contact zone and at the basal surface of the nucleus membrane and pores remain. The interruption of the contact area does not form the well known nuclear pores, instead there is a wide communication or several interruptions of the nucleus membrane. Granular material will be delivered by the caryoplasm up to the M–body. This material reacts basophilic in microscopical preparations.

The *envelope* of the hat consists of a double layer of fine parallel stripes (Fig. 10 a). The stripes in both layers are orientated perpendicular to each other. As far as we know they consist of ribbon-like profiles. Only at an advanced stage of differentiation of the M–body the envelope appears. Initially it consists of tubules which are circular in cross section (Fig. 10 b). subsequently the tubules flatten. We know no more about this structure.

At the end of the differentiation of the acrosome complex the changes within the caryoplasm set in. At first the gap of membrane disappears at the entire surface of the nucleus. The split is replaced by a dense complex of membranes. After some changes of the structure of caryoplasm the membrane complex also disappears. Now the nuclear area might be recognizable only by its structure. This structure changes once more fundamentally into the tubulus structure, described above. When the nucleus membrane disappears the increase of the M–body stops and the delivery of material of the nucleus ceases too.

A few weeks ago we have got a living specimen of a new species of the genus *Alloporus* (PORAT) (see ATTEMS 1928), enabling us to study the spermiogenesis and the mature spermatozoa. This genus belongs to the same subfamily as *Spirostreptus* (1). As expected from earlier light microscopic studies, the spermatozoa of *Julimorpha* are constructed according to the same scheme. The outside and also the form of the particular structures differ a little but the structures themselves are the same (Fig. 13). The acrosome vacuole is somewhat clumsier corresponding to the lower hat. The M–body

(1) I thank Prof. Dr. O. KRAUS, Hamburg, for classification.

is formed like a simple ring and the cristalloid is more flattened. There is a calotte too and a structure which you can compare with the envelope. The differentiation of these structures follows the same schema (Fig. 14). In the light microscope the nucleus has the form of a ring, because the central parts of the disk are very thin. The structure is the same. The mitochondria are arranged in a peripheral ring in which the centriole is situated. Here too the free border of the spermatozoon is drawn out very thin, but a little modified in its contours. It is not round, but three-cornered; such forms have already been observed in other species by light microscopy (TUZET et MANIER, 1956). There is indeed an extensive correspondence in building and structure. This conforms with the evidence obtained in other groups of animals.

In the electron microscope, as far as I know, only REGER and COOPER (1968) investigated the spermatozoa of the diplopode *Polydesmus sp. Polydesmus* belongs to the suborder of *Proterandria* and to the group of *Eugnatha*, like *Spirostreptus*, but to another subcohors; therefore it is not very closely

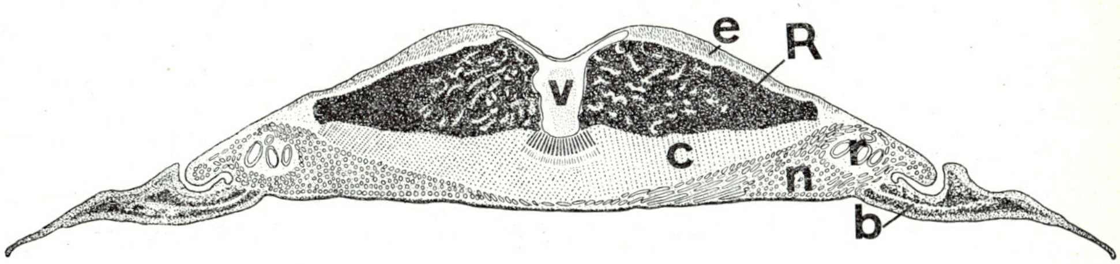

Schema 3. – Schema of a mature sperm of the new species of the genus *Alloporus*. (*n*) Nucleus, (*v*) acrosome vacuole, (*c*) cristalloid, (*R*) ring-body, (*e*) envelope, (*r*) ring of mitochondria, (*b*) basal cytoplasm, especially in the thinly drawn border.

related to our species. The spermatozoa of *Polydesmus* are small (ca. 2 μ diameter). The nucleus occupies the whole basal plate and a part of the hat. The acrosome vacuole is situated at the same place. REGER and COOPER did not say anything about the other parts, but I think, looking at their pictures, a structure like the cristalloid is found there.

Many spermatozoa of *Diplopodes*, described by TUZET and MANIER (1956), show the acrosome vacuole, the cristalloid and a structure corresponding to the M–body, especially in *Spirostreptus castaneus* and *Sp. ibanda*, also in *Scaphiostreptus* and *Brachyspirobolus*. Also among the forms described by BESSIÈRE (1948) there are some spermatozoa structurally similar to the spermatozoa of *Spirostreptus*. An observation of the acrosome reaction is never mentioned. The spermatozoa of all *Diplopodes* seem to belong to one type of sperms although it is difficult to identify homologous details of composition in the light microscope.

Complex structures of the acrosome are described in different groups of animals. I might call to your mind the spermatozoa of mussels, for instance *Barnea* (demonstrated by PASTEELS and DE HARVEN, 1962), of the oyster *Crassostrea* (by GALTSOFF and PHILPOTT, 1960), of the polychaeta *Nereis japonica* (by R. and Y. TAKASHIMA, 1963), and of the decapode *Callinectes sapidus* (by BROWN, 1966). Of the two latter it is known that the whole complex structure participates in the acrosome reaction. This has also been demonstrated for the acrosome complex of *Astoterias amurensis* by HAGIWARA, DAN and SAITO (1967).—In our objects we could not elicit the acrosome reaction till now.

Regarding the spermatozoa and the spermiogenesis of *Spirostreptus* several remarkable facts exist. The most striking features are the relations between the nucleus and the formation of the acrosome.

Firstly there is a chromosomal structure at the apical pole of the nucleus below the acrosome vacuole, connected with the nucleus membrane (Fig. 11). Such structures were observed within the nuclei of spermatocytes and spermatids of several species of arthropods. Their meaning is not yet clarified. When the calotte is appearing the chromosomal structure passing to the periphery remains closely bound up with the nucleus membrane in the neighbourhood of the M–body until it disappears. Such a clear relation between a nuclear and a cytoplasmatic structure during differentiation is remarkable, especially because there are no ribosomes or endoplasmatic reticulum in this part of spermatids.

Secondly basophilic material leaves the nucleus and takes part in the formation of the M–body, as I have demonstrated.—It has been observed in all spermatozoa that nuclear material passes into the cytoplasm not only by the normal way through pores, but also by delamination of nucleus membrane and adjacent material. All this material disappears during maturation of spermatids. In the first phase of spermiohistogenesis of *Spirostreptus*, however, this kind of delivery of nuclear material can be observed at the basal side of the nucleus membrane. On rising of the M–body its material is augmented by the nuclear substance at the apical side in the periphery of the acrosome complex respectively of the cristalloid. This material forms the M–body and persists still in the mature spermatozoa.

In these two relations between nucleus and acrosome complex we see a cytological particularity of general interest.

REFERENCES

BESSIÈRE CL. (1948) – *La spermatogénèse de quelques Myriapodes Diplopodes.* « Arch. Zool. exp. », 85, 149–236.

BROWN G. G. (1966) – *Ultrastructural studies of sperm morphology and sperm-egg interaction in the decapod* Callinectes sapidus. « J. Ultrastruct. Res. », 14, 425–440.

DAN J. C. and HAGIWARA Y. (1967) – *Studies on the acrosome.* IX. *Course of acrosome reaction in the starfish.* « J. Ultrastruct. Res. », 18, 562–579.

GALTSOFF P. S. and PHILPOTT D. E. (1960) – *Ultrastructure of the spermatozoon of the oyster,* Crassostrea virginica. « J. Ultrastruct. Res. », 3, 241–253.

GILSON G. (1886) – *Étude comparée de la spermatogénèse chez les arthropodes.* « Cellule », 2, 83–239.

HAGIWARA Y., DAN J. C. and SAITO A. (1967) – *Studies on the acrosome.* VIII. *The intact starfish acrosome.* « J. Ultrastruct. Res. », 18, 551–561.

HORSTMANN E. and BREUCKER H. (1969) – *Spermatozoen und Spermio-histogenese von* Graphidostreptus spec. (*Myriapoda, Diplopoda*). I. *Die reifen Spermatozoen.* « Z. Zellforsch. », 96, 505–520.

PASTEELS J. J. and DE HARVEN E. (1962) – *Étude au microscope électronic du spermatozoide d'un mollusque bivalve,* Barnea candida. « Arch Biol. (Liège) », 73, 445–463.

REGER J. F. and COOPER D. P. (1968) – *Studies on the fine structure of spermatids and spermatozoa from the millipede* Polydesmus sp. « J. Ultrastruct. Res. », 23, 60–70.

TAKASHIMA R. and TAKASHIMA Y. (1963) – *Electron microscope studies on the fine structure of Nereis spermatozoa before and after the acrosomal reaction.* « Tokushima J. Exp. Medicine », 10, 117–123.

TUZET O. and MANIER J. F. (1956) – *Recherches sur la spermatogénèse de neuf Myriapodes Diplopodes de l'ordre des Spirostreptidae et des Spirobolidae.* « Bull. Inst. roy. Sci. nat. Belg. », 32, 1–38.

EXPLANATION OF FIGURES

Fig. 1. – Spermatozoon of *Spirostreptus.* (*n*) Nucleus, (*v*) acrosome vacuole, (*ca*) calotte, (*c*) cristalloid, (*M*) M–body, (*e*) envelope, (*m*) ring of mitochondria, (*b*) basal cytoplasm. 8000×.

Fig. 2 a, b. – Spermatophores including two spermatozoa. (*a*) Feulgen-reaction. (*b*) PAS–reaction; note the acrosome vacuole. 2000×.

Fig. 3. – Structure of caryoplasm (*n*). (*b*) Basal cytoplasm 50,000×.

Fig. 4. – Apical part of an early spermatid. (*n*) Nucleus, (*v*) acrosome vacuole, (*g*) Golgi–complex. 10,000×.

Fig. 5. – The acrosome vacuole (*v*), (*M*) M–body, (*c*) cristalloid. 30,000×.

Fig. 6. – Acrosome complex of a spermatid. (*n*) Nucleus, (*v*) acrosome vacuole, (*M*) M–body. Between nucleus and acrosome vacuole the calotte. (*c*) The arising cristalloid, centriole (arrow). 20,000×.

Fig. 7. – Spermatid. (*v*) Acrosome vacuole with processes which extend into the M–body (*M*), (*c*) cristalloid, (*n*) flattened nucleus, (*b*) basal cytoplasm. 20,000×.

Fig. 8. – Cross section of a late spermatid. The cristalloid is divided into sectors and surrounded by the M–body. In the center the acrosome vacuole, below the cristalloid. 20,000×.

Fig. 9. – Contact (|——|) between nucleus (*n*) and M–body (*M*). The gap of the nucleus membrane is interrupted. 20,000×.

Fig. 10 a, b. – The envelope (*a*) of a late spermatid, (*b*) of an earlier spermatid. (*o*) Outer, (*i*) inner layer, (*M*) M–body. (*a*) 40,000×, (*b*) 25,000×.

Fig. 11. – Apical part of an early spermatid (*Spirostreptus*). (*n*) Nucleus with (*a*) chromosomal structure, (*M*) M–body starting. 20,000×.

Fig. 12. – Cristalloid. Cross section of the tubules. conf. schema 2. 100,000×.

Fig. 13. – Spermatophore including two sperms of the new species (genus *Alloporus*). 12,000×.

Fig. 14. – Sperm of the new species. (*n*) Nucleus, (*v*) acrosome vacuole, (*ca*) calotte, (*R*) ring–body, (*c*) cristalloid, (*e*) envelope, (*m*) ring of mitochondria, (*b*) basal cytoplasm, especially in the thinly drawn border. 24,000×.

Discussion

BROWN. – I am greatly impressed by the development of the acrosome, structure and the basic structure of the sperm and the relationship to decapod spermatozoa (Brachyura). I would think that the acrosome reaction would be similar also. Have you attempted such studies?

HORSTMANN. – We tried to induce the acrosomal reaction by bringing mature sperms to eggs from living females bloated in physiological solution for insects and arachnoids, but without any effect.

MEYER. – The body you demonstrated in spermatids could mean a chromocenter or a heterochromatic chromosome. There is little doubt that the lamines represent synaptinemal complexes which are known to be formed in some cases in spermatids.

EDDLEMAN. – I have observed in the early spermatids of several cockroaches, during early development of acrosome, a localization of dense material within the nuclear membrane and apposite the forming acrosome. Often, there are one or two synaptineural complexes in close association with the dense material within the nucleus.

HORSTMANN. – I thank dr. EDDLEMAN for this information. Our findings demonstrate the general relationship between the nucleus and the acrosome of nearly all spermatozoa in a more specialized form.

ANDERSON. – Based on morphological findings, it is difficult to determine whether the opaque material adjacent to the nuclear envelope represents an out-flow of material from the nucleus to the cytoplasm or an in-flow of cytoplasmic material to the nucleus.

HORSTMANN. – The extrusion of nuclear material into the M–body is concluded from the following facts: During differentiation the M–body increases, while the nucleus decreases. Secondly, at the end of the differentiation of the acrosome complex the nuclear membrane disappears, and a small portion of granulated material is delivered and is added to the M–body.

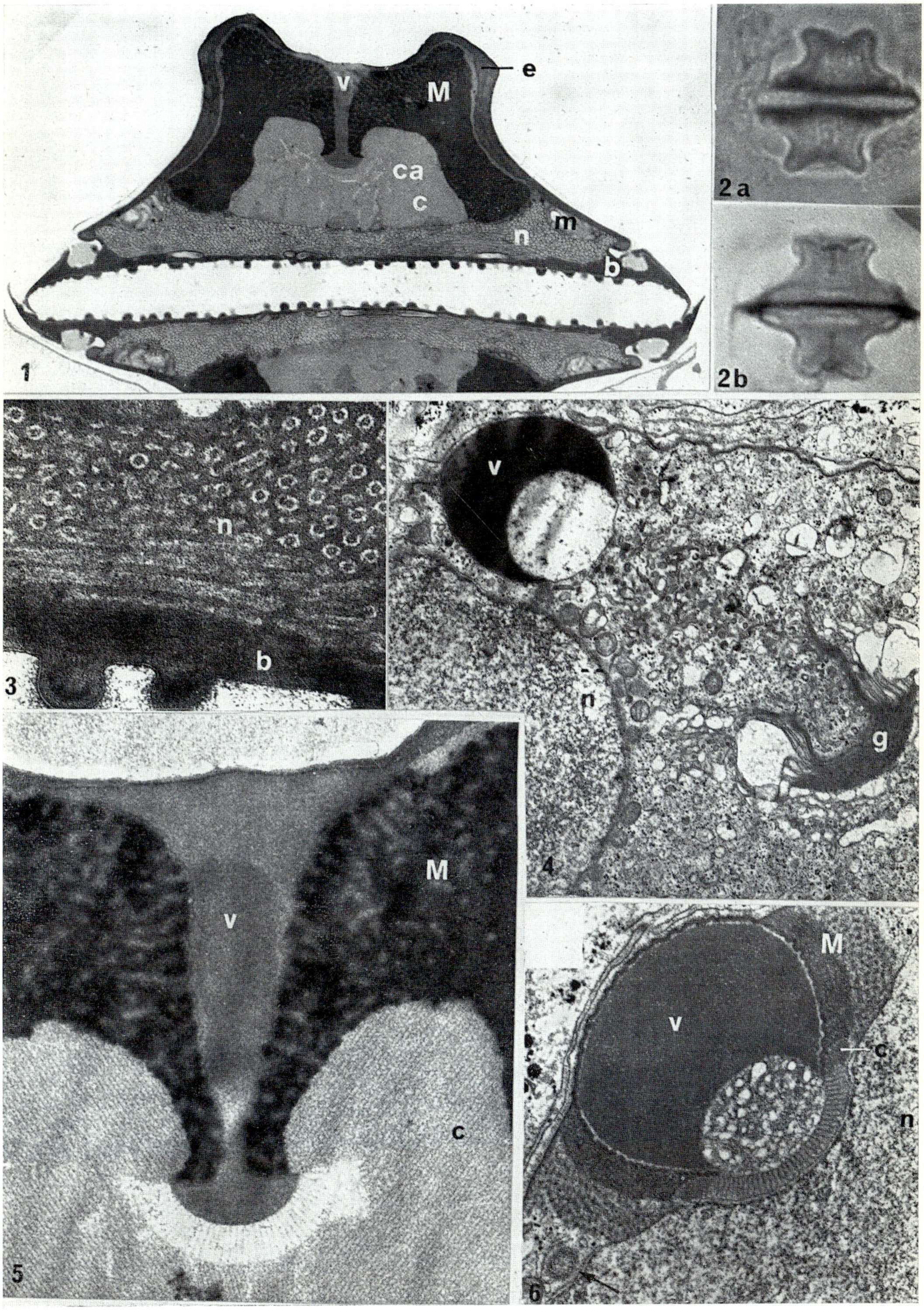
e
v
M
ca
c
m
n
b
1
2 a
2 b
n
b
3
v
n
g
4
M
v
c
5
M
v
c
n
6

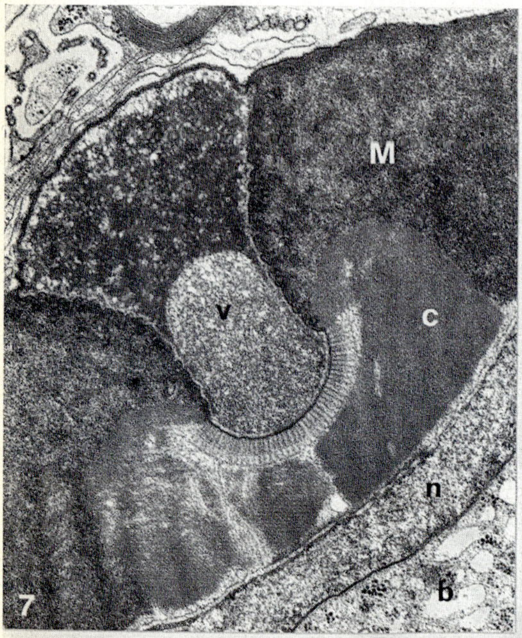
M
v
c
n
b
7

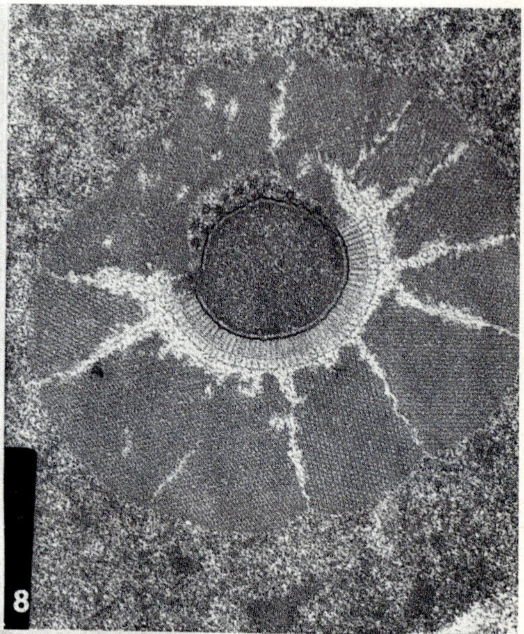
8

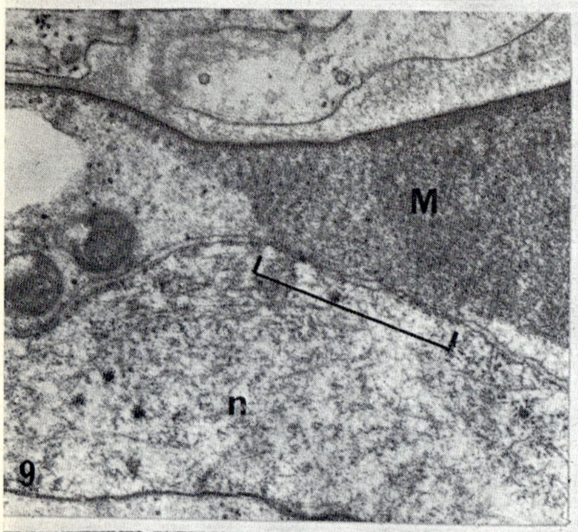
M
n
9

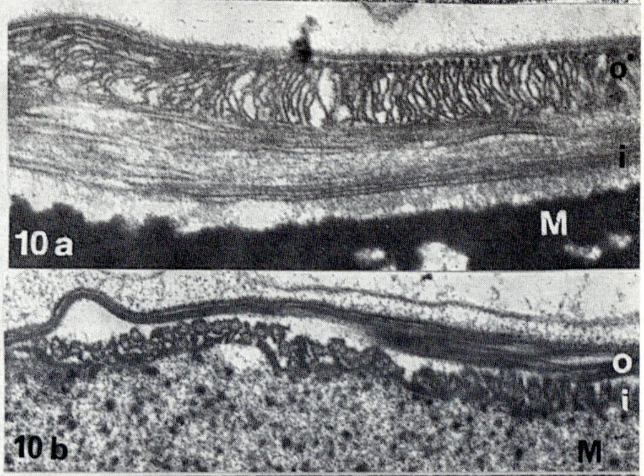
o
i
M
10 a
o
i
10 b
M

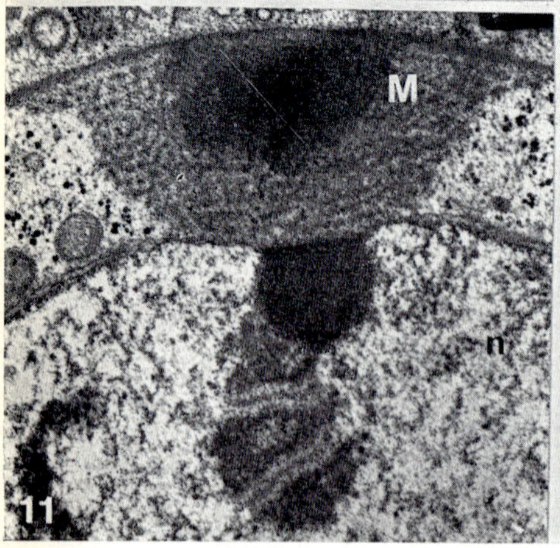
M
n
11

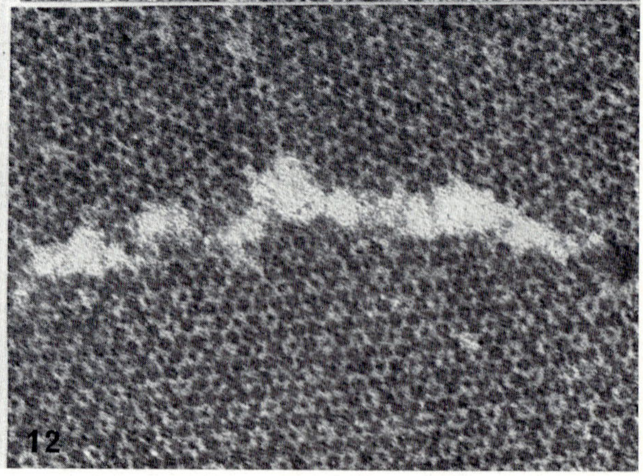
12

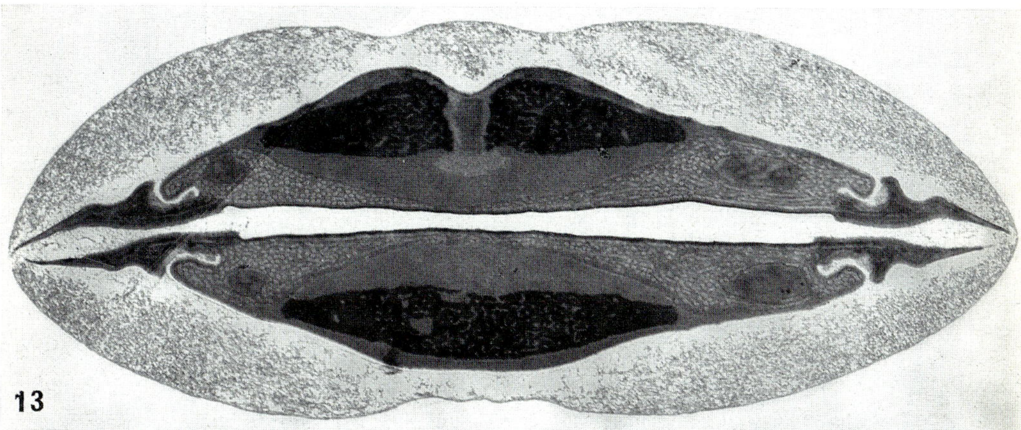
13

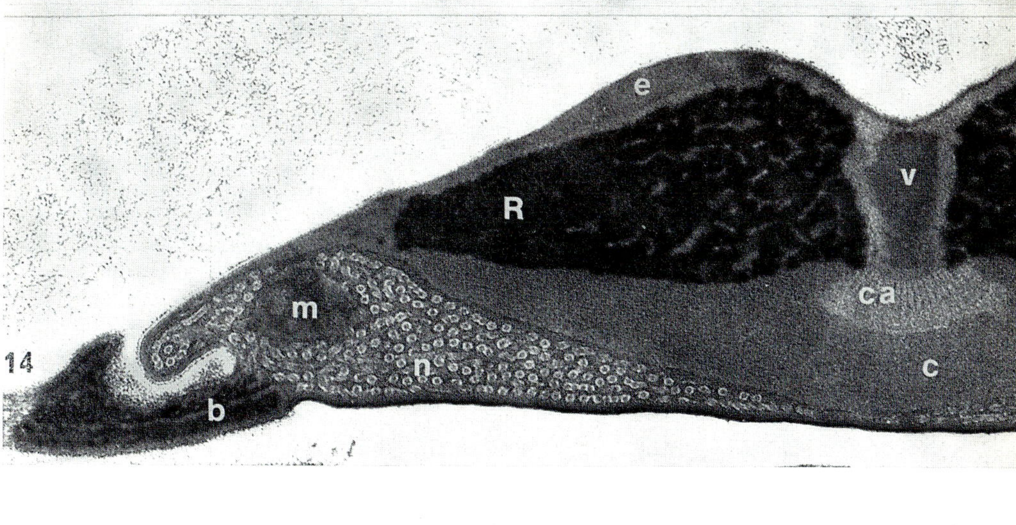
e
v
R
ca
m
14
n
c
b

DAVID M. PHILLIPS (*)

INSECT FLAGELLAR TUBULE PATTERNS THEME AND VARIATIONS (**)

SUMMARY. — This paper summarizes the results of a broad comparative survey of the structure of insect sperm flagella. The typical insect sperm flagellum has 9 singlet accessory tubules peripheral to the 9 doublets of the flagellum. Most insect sperm flagella have a central pair of singlet tubules which are similar in morphology to the 9 peripheral accessory tubules. However, caddisfly flagella have 7 central tubules; a mycetophilid was found to have 3 central tubules; mosquitoes and the psocid *Psocus* possess a single central element; and mayfly spermatozoa apparently lack central tubules entirely. The 9 doublets and 9 accessory fibers of the flagellum of *Psocus* sperm are distinctive in that they are not straight but describe a long-pitched helical course. Even more peculiar is the flagellum of the cat flea where the doublets also describe a helical course and, in addition, the entire flagellar tubule array spirals around a thick, extraflagellar shaft. Treehoppers also have a unique type of sperm flagellum. In treehopper species the flagellum branches regularly into 4 long tails, each of which contains 2 or 3 of the 9 flagellar doublets and like numbers of the peripheral singlets. The most peculiar flagella occur in sperm of *Sciara.* These flagella have approximately 70 doublet and 70 accessory singlet tubules in a spiral array.

RIASSUNTO. — Questo lavoro riassume i risultati di un vasto studio comparativo sulla struttura dei flagelli degli spermi degli insetti. Il tipico flagello spermatico degli insetti possiede 9 tubuli accessori periferici ai 9 doppietti. La maggior parte dei flagelli degli insetti possiede un paio di tubuli centrali che sono simili morfologicamente ai 9 tubuli accessori esterni. Tuttavia, i flagelli del tricottero hanno 7 tubuli centrali; è stato trovato un micetofilide con 3 tubuli centrali; le mosche e lo psocide *Psocus* hanno un solo elemento centrale; e gli spermatozoi dell'Efemera mancano completamente di tubuli centrali. I 9 doppietti e le 9 fibre accessorie del flagello di *Psocus* sono caratteristici perché non sono diritti ma descrivono un'elica. Ancora più caratteristico è il flagello della pulce del gatto in cui anche i doppietti descrivono un'elica e, inoltre, l'intero flagello è disposto a spirale intorno ad uno spesso fusto extraflagellare. Anche le Cicaline hanno un solo tipo di flagello. In essi il flagello si ramifica regolarmente in 4 lunghe code, ciascuna delle quali contiene 2 o 3 dei 9 doppietti e uguale numero di tubuli periferici. Il flagello più peculiare si trova negli spermi di *Sciara.* Questi flagelli hanno circa 70 doppietti e 70 tubuli accessori disposti a spirale.

INTRODUCTION

For the past few years I have been looking at the testes from various insect species. This work has admittedly been motivated in part by my interest in driving out to the country on sunny summer days and swinging a net

(*) Department of Biology, Washington University St. Louis, Missouri, USA.

(**) Supported by Research Grant GM–06927, and Anatomical Sciences Training Grant 406 from The National Institutes of Health and by Research Grant GB–8069 from The National Science Foundation.

as I stroll through the fields, but motivations aside, it has resulted in a broad comparative survey of the fine structure of insect sperm in some 200 insect species representing 15 orders. The insects were collected in the fields and woods around Boston, Massachusetts, Chicago, Illinois and St. Louis, Missouri.

In spite of the wonderful diversity in appearance among insect species, the sperm of most insects are quite similar to each other. In this paper I shall present a summary of the general appearance of the typical insect testis and typical insect spermatozoan. However, I am more intrigued with those insect spermatozoa which are not typical, particularly ones which are exceptional in their flagellar tubule arrays, since flagellar tubule arrays are constant in appearance not only among insects, but among most other organisms as well. I feel that careful examination of the exceptional tubule arrays which are found in flagella of occasional insect species may provide some indication of the roles in motility of the various tubular elements common to most cilia and flagella. Thus, in this paper I shall give most attention to the flagella of typical insect sperm and the deviations from the typical flagellar form which occur naturally in some insect species.

Materials and methods

The testes of 195 insect species representing fifteen orders have been examined. Testes were dissected in cold fixative, usually within a few hours after the insects were collected. Testes were usually fixed 2 to 6 hours in 3 to 6% glutaraldehyde (Eastman-Rochester, New York) buffered with 0.2 M, 24, 6–Trimethylpyridine (Eastman) at pH 7.2–7.6. Testes were then transferred through several changes of cold buffer (5 to 30 min) and postfixed 1 to 4 hours in 1% collidine-buffered OsO_4. After dehydration in alcohol, tissues were embedded in Epon (LUFT, 1961) sectioned on a Serval MT–1 ultramicrotome with a diamond knife (DuPont) and stained in 3% aqueous uranyl acetate (12 to 16 hrs) and lead citrate (VENABLE and COGGESHALL, 1965). Sections were examined on a Siemens Elmiskop I.

Results

The Typical Insect Testis.

Generally the testes of insects are paired organs, each of which consists of a number of follicles enclosed by a layer of simple, often pigmented, epithelium. The number of follicles within each testis varies greatly from one insect group to another. Each follicle is itself delimited by an epithelial layer and is filled with cysts. The cysts are actually clones of germinal cells embedded in large polytene epithelial cells. The number of spermatids per cyst is generally approximately equal to an integral power of 2. It may be 2^5, 2^6, 2^7 or 2^8, depending on the species. This results from the fact that gonial and meiotic divisions occur synchronously in all the germ cells of a given cyst. In fact, since cytoplasmic bridges remain between cells after these divisions, the cells of a given cyst are not merely a clone, but functionally a synsyctium.

The cysts elongate with the elongation of the spermatids and the developing sperm come to be alligned side by side in nearly perfect register. This makes it possible to cut transverse sections through a cyst containing late spermatids such that all of the spermatids are transected at the same level (Fig. 1).

The Typical Insect Spermatozoon.

Although the size and shape of various components of insect spermatozoa show wide interspecies variation, the organelles present and their topological relationship to one another are rather constant. Anteriorly, an acrosome overlies the nucleus. The acrosome may be huge or so small that its presence could easily be missed. The most anterior portion of the flagellum is juxtaposed to the nucleus and is embedded in electron dense material refered to as the centriolar adjunct. No centrioles persist in mature insect spermatozoa. One or two (depending on the species) long, thin mitochondrial derivatives occupy a position adjacent to the flagellum and extend almost to the caudal end of the cell. These mitochondria are filled with proteinaceous crystalline material and crystae are found only at the edges of these large organelles. In spermatozoa of some species, most of the volume of the cell is occupied by the mitochondrial derivative.

The Typical Insect Flagellum.

The flagella of most insect sperm possess a tubule array which is slightly more complex than the basic tubule pattern of most cilia and flagella.

Peripheral to the familiar 9 + 2 array of tubules, insect sperm flagella generally possess 9 additional singlet tubules, each located just distal and to one side of subfiber B of a flagellar doublet. These singlet tubules, which are sometimes referred to as accessory fibers (KAYE, 1964; CAMERON, 1965) usually extend further anteriorly and terminate sooner posteriorly than do the doublet tubules or the central pair of singlets (PHILLIPS, 1966 b; 1966 c). In cross section, these accessory tubules appear in some species as hollow tubes; in other species they enclose a central rod or tubule (Fig. 2); and in others they appear completely solid. Depending on the species, they may larger or smaller than, or similar in size to the flagellar doublets, which do not vary in size from one species to another. Interestingly, we find that the particular morphology characterizing the accessory tubules of a given species is usually repeated in the central pair of tubules in that species. For example, in the black scavenger fly *Sepsis*, the accessory tubules and the central pair of tubules enclose a central tubule.

The walls of all tubules of insect flagella appear to be composed of subunits. In cross sections of sperm flagella of *Sepsis*, we have been able to count 13 evenly spaced subunits in the walls of the central pair and the accessory tubules. Each subunit is approximately 70 Å in diameter and, in transverse section, is seen to possess an electron lucid center 30 to 40 Å across (PHILLIPS, 1966 c).

Exceptions to the Typical 9 + 9 + 2 Tubule Pattern

Variations in the 9 + 2 Tubule Array.

The 9 radially arranged doublet tubules common to most animal and plant cilia and flagella appear to be the most constant and unchanging feature of insect sperm flagella. In one ephemerid, *Tricarythodes* sp., subfiber A of each doublet is slightly smaller and more irregularly shaped than subfiber A of other insect sperm flagella. This is the only case we have encountered of any detectable variation in the doublets of insect sperm.

The two central singlet tubules, however, are subject to considerable variation among species. Not only have we found variations in their morphology, as discussed in the previous sections, but we have also encountered variations in the number of central elements. Mature sperm of the 3 species of mayflies we have examined (*Pentagenia villigera*, *Hexagenia* sp., and *Tricarythodes* sp.) lack the central tubules entirely (Phillips, 1969). Encircling the area where the central pair is generally situated is a single faintly staining cylinder about 600 Å in diameter which has 9 arms radiating out to meet subfiber A of each doublet (Fig. 3 a). The two mosquito species we have examined (*Culex* sp. and *Aedes canadensis canadensis*) possess but a single central tubule which is slightly larger than the accessory tubules and contains a central rod (Fig. 3 b). Mature spermatozoa of the psocid *Psocus* also possess a single rod or fiber rather than a tubule. The rod is about 300 Å in diameter and rather irregular in shape (Fig. 3 d).

We found flagella with 3 central tubules disposed in a triangle in sperm of one species of fungus gnat (Mycetophilidae) (Fig. 3 c). Unfortunately the specimen to whom these interesting 9 + 3 flagella originally belonged was so damaged in dissection that we were unable to determine its genus.

Flagella with 7 central tubules in place of the usual 2 characterize two of the twelve caddisfly (Trichoptera) species we have examined. In these 2 species (*Hydropsyche* sp. and *Polycentropus* sp.), 6 of the tubules are symmetrically arranged around the centrally located seventh tubule (Fig. 3 c) (Phillips, 1969).

Spiraling of Flagellar Tubules.

In longitudinal sections of sperm of the psocid *Psocus*, the flagellar tubules are found to form an angle of about 8° with the long axis of the flagellum (Phillips, 1969). In sections which cut the sperm in near transverse section, the flagellar tubules appear in true cross section on one side of the flagellum while those on the opposite side are obliquely cut (Fig. 3 d). These observations indicate that the doublet tubules and accessory fibers of *Psocus* sperm describe a long pitched helix around the central rod.

The sperm flagellum of the cat flea *Ctenocephalides felis* is even more peculiar. In these sperm, which lack accessory tubules, the flagellar doublets describe a spiral around the central pair (Fig. 3 f) as just described in sperm of *Psocus*. In addition, the entire flagellar tubule array spirals around a thick (0.5 μ in diameter) central shaft, somewhat as climbing vines twine around tree trunks.

Flagellar Branching.

In squash preparations of treehopper (Membracidae) testis viewed in the light microscope, the sperm appear to have the form of minute cat-o-nine tails with a long handle and four stiff tails. When the sperm are swimming (e.g. in saline) the " handle " portion leads and the four tails trail behind. Only the anterior portion undulates; the four straight tails do not bend (PHILLIPS, 1969). We have examined the testes of 4 species of treehoppers in the electron microscope: *Ceresa sp.*, *Ceresa diceros*, *Stictocephala sp.* and *Telamona sp.* The anterior part of sperm of these species has the typical 9 + 9 + 2 pattern. (Fig. 4). Where sperm are transected further posteriorly we find groupings of 4 tails, three of which contain two doublet and two singlet tubules and one of which contains three doublet and three singlet tubules. This indicates that posteriorly the tubules are parceled out in a very regular manner. Three of the four flagellar branches contain two doublet and two singlet tubules and the fourth contains three doublet and three singlet tubules. This regular segregation of the flagellar components in a ratio of 3 : 1 between transversely sectioned tails with two doublet and two singlet tubules and those with three doublet and three singlet tubules (Fig. 4) (PHILLIPS, 1969).

Sciara.

Perhaps the most unusual flagellum that has been described is the giant flagellum of the fungus gnat *Sciara* (MAKIELSKI, 1966; PHILLIPS, 1966 a; 1966 b). The flagellum in mature spermatozoa is made up of about 70 doublet tubules and 70 peripheral accessory tubules arranged in a spiral configuration. Although this tubule array bears little superficial resemblance to the typical 9 + 9 + 2 insect flagellar form, it must, on the basis of certain similarities, be considered a true flagellum. The doublet tubules of the giant flagellum of *Sciara* sperm have a subfiber A and B as do typical flagella. The giant flagellum of *Sciara*, like other flagella, arises from a centriole. The centriole which serves as basal body for the giant flagellum is also unusual in that it is composed of 70 singlet tubules arranged in an oval (Fig. 5). However, it is clearly a true centriole; it arises at right angles to preexisting centrioles and serves as a center for mitotic and meiotic divisions. In young spermatids the forming flagellum, reflecting the tubule pattern of its unusual basal body, is composed of about 70 doublet tubules arranged in an oval (Fig. 6). Arms are observed on subfiber A which, as in other flagella (GIBBONS and GRIMSTONE, 1960), are directed clockwise when the mature flagellum is viewed from base to tip (PHILLIPS, 1966 b). The accessory fibers bear the same spatial relationship to the doublets as they do in other insect flagella (KAYE, 1966; CAMERON, 1965) and, as in other insect flagella, form after the doublets have formed (PHILLIPS, 1966 a).

CONCLUSIONS

A 9 + 9 + 2 tubule array characterizes sperm flagella of the large majority of insect species we have examined. This arrangement has also been observed by other investigators in the orders Apterygota (BAWA, 1964; WERNER, 1964), Odonata (KESSEL, 1966), Orthoptera (YASUZUMI *et al.*, 1958; KAYE, 1964; BASSOT and MARTOJA, 1966; SHAY and BIESELE, 1968; BRELAND *et al.*, 1968; KESSEL, 1967), Mellophaga (ITO, 1966), Hemiptera (FURIERI, 1963 b; BARKER and RIESS, 1966; TANDLER and MORIBER, 1966), Homoptera (HEROLD and MUNZ, 1967), Neuroptera (BACCETTI *et al.*, 1968), Coleoptera (FURIERI, 1963 a; CAMERON, 1964), Lepidoptera (YASUZUMI and OURA, 1965; ANDRÉ, 1961, 1962), Diptera (YASUZUMI *et al.*, 1958; NUNEZ, 1963; BACCETTI and BAIRATI, 1964; BAIRATI and BACCETTI, 1964; BRELAND *et al.*, 1966; ANDERSON, 1967; HESS and MEYER, 1968; MEYER, 1968) and Hymenoptera (ROTSCHILD, 1965; WILKES and LEA, 1965; THOMSON and BLUM, 1967; HOAGE and KESSEL, 1968). Only two insect orders have been studied in which this basic 9 + 9 + 2 array has not been found: Ephemera (mayflies), which in the 3 species we have examined display a 9 + 9 + 0 pattern, and Ctenochephalides (fleas) of which 3 species are now known to have a 9 + 2 array of helically disposed tubules (S. ITO, personal communication; M. ROTHSCHILD and B. GUPTA, personal communication). Thus the basic pattern of insect flagellar tubules is 9 + 9 + 2. The wide distribution of insects with exceptional flagella and the observation that, in many of the orders which contain exceptional forms, most species examined possess typical flagella suggests that the several types of exceptional flagella observed in insects evolved independently.

What can we learn from the naturally occurring variations in the flagellar tubule array? The most stable components of the insect flagellum are the nine doublet tubules. Subfiber A and subfiber B never possess central rods or tubules as do the accessory tubules and central pair. They do not (with one minor exception) vary in size as do accessory tubules or in number (with the exception of *Sciara*) as do the central elements, and they are never absent. Even in the highly unconventional flagellum of *Sciara* sperm, the doublets, though there are 60 to 90 of them, are identical in morphology to doublets in other cilia and flagella.

Accessory elements, though they are quite different in appearance in flagella of insect and mammalian sperm, share certain similarities and may play a similar role in motility. In both insect and mammalian sperm the accessory elements are located just peripheral to the nine doublets. In both cases the accessory elements arise after the 9 + 2 flagellum has formed as apparent outgrowths of the 9 doublets. Accessory tubules or other elements are, of course, absent from most cilia and flagella, and their role in sperm motility, in either insects or mammals, is not understood. Accessory tubules are lacking in some exceptional insect sperm flagella, i.e. in fleas and some caddisflies, and are apparently not essential for motility.

Central tubules are absent in the sperm flagella of mayflies and from the giant flagellum of *Sciara*, and other arrangements of tubules replace the central pair in exceptional flagella of other species. The existence of natural variation in the number and arrangement of central tubules may prove useful in analyzing how these elements function in motility.

References

ANDERSON W. A. (1967) – *Cytodifferentiation of Spermatozoa in* Drosophila melanogaster: *the effect of elevated temperature on Spermiogenesis.* «Molec. Gen. Genetics», 99, 257.

ANDRÉ J. (1961) – *Sur quelques détails nouvellement connus de l'ultrastructure des organites vibratiles.* « J. Ultrastr. Res. », 5, 86.

ANDRÉ J. (1962) – *Contribution à connaissance du chandriame. Etude de ses modifications ultrastructurales pendant la spermatogénès.* « J. Ultrast. Res. », Suppl. 3.

BACCETTI B. and BAIRATI A. (1964) – *Indagini sull'ultrastruttura delle cellule geminali maschili in* Dacus oleae Geml. « Redia », 49, 1.

BACCETTI B., DALLAI R. and ROSATI F. (1968) – *An Unusual 9+2 Spermatozoan in a Pterygote Insect.* – Fourth European Regional Conference on Election Microscopy. Rome 1968, 345.

BAIRATI A. and BACCETTI B. (1964) – *Observations on the ultrastructure of the male germ cells of* Drosophila melanogaster *and Dacus oleae.* – Proc. European Regional Conf. Electron Micr., Prague. 1964, B 44.

BARKER K. R. and RIESS R. W. (1966) – *An Electron Microscope Study of Spermateleosis in the hemiploran* Oncopeltus fasciatus. « La Cellule », 66, 41.

BASSOT J. M. and MARTOJA R. (1966) – *Données histologiques et ultrastructurales sur les microtubules cytoplasmiques du canal éjaculateur des insectes Orthoptères.* « Z. für Zellforsch. », 74, 145.

BAWA S. R. (1964) – *Electron microscope study of spermiogenesis in a fire-brat insect,* Thermobia domestica I. *Mature spermatozoan.* « J. Cell Biol. », 23, 431.

BRELAND O. P., EDDLEMAN C. D. and BIESELE J. J. (1968) – *Studies of insect spermatozoa.* I. « Entomological News », 79, 197.

BRELAND O. P., GASSNER G., RIESS R. W. and BIESELE J. J. (1966) – *Certain aspects of the centriole adjunct, spermiogenesis, and the mature sperm of insects.* « Can. J. Genet. Cytol. ».

CAMERON M. L. (1965) – *Some details of the ultrastructure in the development of flagellar fibers of the tenebrio sperm.* « Canad. J. Zool. », 43, 1005.

FURIERI P. (1963 a) – *Aspetti morfologici della spermiogenesi di* Oryctes grypus *Illig.* « Redia », 48, 29.

FURIERI P. (1963 b) – *Osservazioni preliminari sulla ultrastruttura dello spermio di* Pyrrhocoris aptecus *Fall. Hemiptera, Pyrrhocoridae.* « Redia », 48, 179.

GIBBONS I. R. and GRIMSTONE A. V. (1960) – *On flagellar structure in certain flagellates.* « J. Biophys. Biochem. Cytol. », 7, 697.

HEROLD F. and MUNZ K. (1967) – *Ultrastructure of Spermatozoa of* Peregrinus maidis. « Z. für Zellforsch. », 83, 364.

HESS O. and MEYER G. (1968) – *Genetic Activities of the – chromosome in* Drosophila *during spermatogenesis.* « Advances in Genetics », 14, 171.

HOOGE T. R. and KESSEL R. G. (1968) – *An electron microscope study of the process of differentiation during spermatogenesis in the Drone honey bee* (Aphis mellifera *L.*) *with special reference to centriole replication and elimination.* « J. Ultrastruct. Res. », 24, 6.

ITO S. (1966) – *Movement and structure of louse spermatozoa.* « J. Cell Biol. », 31, 128 A.

KAYE J. S. (1964) – *The fine structure of flagella in spermatids of the house cricket.* « J. Cell Biol. », 22, 710.

KESSEL R. G. (1966) – *The association between microtubules and nuclei during spermiogenesis in the dragonfly.* « J. Ultrastruct. Res. », 16, 293.

KESSEL R. G. (1967) – *An electron microscope study of spermiogenesis in the grasshopper with particular reference to the development of microtubular systems during differentiation.* « J. Ultrastruct. », 18, 677.

LUFT J. H. (1961) – *Improvements in epoxy resin embedding methods.* « J. Biophys. Biochem. Cytol. », 9, 409.

MAKIELSKI S. K. (1966) – *The structure and maturation of the spermatozoa of* Sciara coprophila. « J. Morphol. », 11, 118.

MEYER G. F. (1968) – *Spermiogenese in normalen und – defizienten Mannchen von* Drosophila melanogaster *and* D. hydei. « Z. für Zellforsch. », 84, 141.

NUNEZ J. A. (1963) – *Über den Feinbau des Speimienschwanzes von* Culex pipiens. « Biol. Zentr. », 82, 1.

PHILLIPS D. M. (1966 a) – *Observations on spermiogenesis in the fungus gnat* Sciara coprophila. « J. Cell Biol. », 30, 477.

PHILLIPS D. M. (1966 b) – *Fine structure of* Sciara coprophila *sperm.* « J. Cell Biol. », 30, 499.

PHILLIPS D. M. (1966 c) – *Substructure of flagellar tubules.* « J. Cell Biol. », 31, 635.

PHILLIPS D. M. (1967) – *Giant centriole formation in* Sciara. « J. Cell Biol. », 33, 73.

PHILLIPS D. M. (1969) – *Exceptions to prevailing pattern of tubules (9+9+2) in the sperm flagella of certain insect species.* « J. Cell Biol. », 40.

ROTHSCHILD L. (1955) – *The spermatozoa of the Honey-bee.* « Trans. Royal Soc. London », 107, 289.

SHAY J. W. and BIESELE J. J. (1968) – *Ultrastructural observations on spermiogenesis in the cave cricket* Ceuthophilus secretus (*Scudder*). « La Cellule », 67, 269.

TANDLER B. and MORIBER L. G. (1966) – *Microtubular structures associated with the acrosome during spermiogenesis in the water-strider,* Gerris remigis (*Say*). « J. Ultrastr. Res. », 14, 391.

THOMPSON T. E. and BLUM M. S. (1967) – *Structure and behavior of spermatozoa of the fire ant* Solenopsis saevissima. « Ann. Entomological Soc. of Am. », 60, 632.

VENABLE J. G. and COGGESHALL R. G. (1965) – *Simplified lead citrate stain for use in electron microscopy.* « J. Cell. Biol. », 25, 407.

WERNER G. (1964) – *Untersuchungen uber die spermiogenese beim silberfischen* Lepisma saccharinal. « Zeitsch. f. Zellforsch. », 63, 880.

WILKES A. and LEE P. E. (1965) – *The ultrastructure of dimorphic spermatozoa in the hymenopteran,* Dahlbominus fuscipennis (*Zelf.*) (Eulophidae). « Can. J. Genet. Cytol. », 7, 609.

YASUZUMI G. and OURA C. (1965) – *Spermatogenesis in animals as revealed by electron microscopy.* XV. *The fine structure of the middle piece in the developing spermatid of the silkworm,* Bombyx mori *Linné.* « Zeitsch. f. Zellforsch. », 67, 502.

YASUZUMI G., FUJIMURA W. and ISHIDA H. (1958) – *Spermatogenesis in animals as revealed by electron microscopy.* V. *Spermatid differentiation of* Drosophila *and grasshopper.* « Exp. Cell Res. », 14, 268.

EXPLANATION OF FIGURES

Fig. 1. – Transversely sectioned cyst of the Caddisfly *Neuronia.* Dense material fills the cyst lumen. In addition to the 9+2 flagellar tubule pattern, insect sperm possess 9 singlet tubules (accessory fibers) disposed peripheral to and between the 9 doublets. In the species shown the accessory tubules are somewhat larger than the other tubules. The cell membrane in this caddisfly is scalloped and follows the contour of the large accessory fibers. Such scalloped cell membranes also characterize spermatozoa of other insect species we have studied, notably several four species of fungus gnats (Mycetophilidae, Diptera) and some other caddisfly species. Cells of cyst wall (cyst) ×33,000.

Fig. 2. – Some typical insect flagella, (*a*) Lacewing, *Chrysoptera,* (*b*) black scavenger fly, *Sepsis,* (*c*) Leafhopper, *Draeculacephala,* (*d*) Caddisfly, *Neuronia,* (*e*) Dragonfly, *Libellula,* (*f*) Grasshopper, *Melanoplus.* ×100,000.

Fig. 3. – Exceptions to the typical 9+9+2 tubule pattern. (*a*) Mayfly, *Pentagenia,* (*b*) Mosquito, *Culex,* (*c*) Fungus gnat, (*d*) Psocid, *Psocus,* (*e*) Caddisfly, *Polycentropus,* (*f*) flea, *Ctenocephalides.* ×100,000.

Fig. 4. – Transversely cut spermatid tails of the treehopper *Telamona.* ×62,000.

Fig. 5. – Transversely and longitudinally transected giant centrioles from a spermatogonial cell of *Sciara.* ×64,000.

Fig. 6. – Transversely cut spermatid flagellum of *Sciara.* ×52,000.

Discussion

MEYER. – There seems to be no centriole present in *Lepidoptera* sperm. In one cell in a moth we observed two dictyosomes at both poles and membraneous material connecting the dictyosomes with the chromosomes and surrounding them. However, there are centrioles in somatic tissues. *Lepidoptera* belong to the organisms with a diffuse centromere. That would be a possible explanation why in spermatids a centriole is not present. Did you observe centriole in spermatogonia of *Lepidoptera*?

PHILLIPS. – We have never looked at spermatogonia of lepidopterans since we've only examined imaginal testes and they don't contain spermatogonia. I imagine that they do contain centrioles since the sperm develop a normal 9 + 2 flagellum which originally probably had an ordinary 9–membered basal body. I would expect organisms with diffuse centromeres to have centrioles, for instance, Schrader figured centrioles in several Hemipterins. But this is aside from my point. I find no centrioles in mature spermatozoa of other insect orders either, and I feel that absence of a centriole is a general characteristic of mature insect sperm.

AFZELIUS. – Your beautiful micrograph certainly shows a pronounced bilateral symmetry, you also use this term " bilateral symmetry ". This poses a problem, because a perfect bilateral symmetry is theoretically impossible on a molecular or macromolecular level. This impossibility is due to the indisputable fact that the biological structures all consist of asymmetrical molecules, proteins and carbohydrates. You cannot have right-handed alfa helices on one side, and left handed alfa helix protein on the other. Hence a construction of perfect bilateral symmetry is impossible, still your micrographs show this type of symmetry quite well. And this will be difficult feature to explain by specialists on macromolecules and symmetries.

EDDLEMANN. – Have you observed adjunct in most of the Insect spermatozoa that you have examined?

PHILLIPS. – Yes. In all species in which we have studied spermiogenesis carefully we find centriole adjuncts. However, during spermiogenesis the adjunct material disappears entirely in some species and is greatly reduced in others.

EDDLEMANN. – Would you care to speculate on the origin and the function of the centriole adjunct?

PHILLIPS. – The material appears to form in association with the basal body as do the columns of the connecting piece in mammalian spermatozoa. It has been suggested that the columns secure the axial filament complex of mammalian spermatozoa to the base of the head, and this seems pretty reasonable. The centriole adjunct might also perform such a function.

ANDRÉ. – It is difficult to say a word after this exceedingly good presentation...

I would like to come back to my comment of this morning's session relative to the force necessary to bend a straight rod on the one hand, and the same rod, but helical in shape, on the other. As I said, the force to be applied in order to obtain a given amount of bending, is much less in the latter case. The exceptionally clear pictures shown by DAVE PHILLIPS allows us to distinguish three helical arrangements of decreasing size. First, if we look at these Insect sperm with the light microscope, we already see a general helical shape. What we are looking at is a rod of roughly 5,000 Å in diameter. Then, DAVE PHILLIPS deducted trom the clear appearance of some neighbouring microtubules of the axoneme and from the blurred appearance of the diametrally opposite tubules, that these tubules follow a helical course along the axoneme. What we are looking at this time measures 200 Å in diameter. And, finally, I believe I have noticed in an exceptionally good high resolution picture that the protofibrils, in the walls of the tubules, are also clear on one side, blurred in the opposite. This means that they also are in helical arrangement, the helix being probably very long pitched. This time, the rod we are looking at is 30 Å in diameter, that is to say, is of molecular size. It is tempting to hypothesize that this last helical arrangement is a morphogenetic expression of the general lack of symmetry of protein molecules. We can summarize the situation in saying that the sperm tails of large size are coils of coils, an architecture favourable to bending.

PHILLIPS. – There is, as you know, evidence for helical arrangement of subunits from negative stained data. However, the pitch of a helix would have to be very gentle or one wouldn't be able to count protofibrils in thin sections at all. In the micrographs I've shown, the protofibrils do sometimes appear more obscured on one side of the tubule than on the other, but in other tubules I think they appear blurred on two opposite sides. Although your interpretation is quite possible; differences could also be due to preparative or staining differences.

AFZELIUS. – Remark to remark by ANDRÉ: Jean, look on it this way. The role of these filaments may be to be stiff and rigid, rather than flexible. Hence straight subfilaments would be expected.

WALKER. – There have been reports of microtubules associated with the centriolar adjunct in Insects, e.g. grasshopper or dragonfly (KESSEL 1966, 1967). These microtubules subsequently surround the developing nucleus. Could you make any comments on the speculation that the centriolar adjunct is a site or store of monomer for microtubule formation?

PHILLIPS. – It's true that some microtubules are in close association with the centriole adjunct in some insect species. For one to say that the centriolar adjunct is a site or store of microtubular subunits is, I think, speculating a bit more than is warranted on the basis of this observation alone.

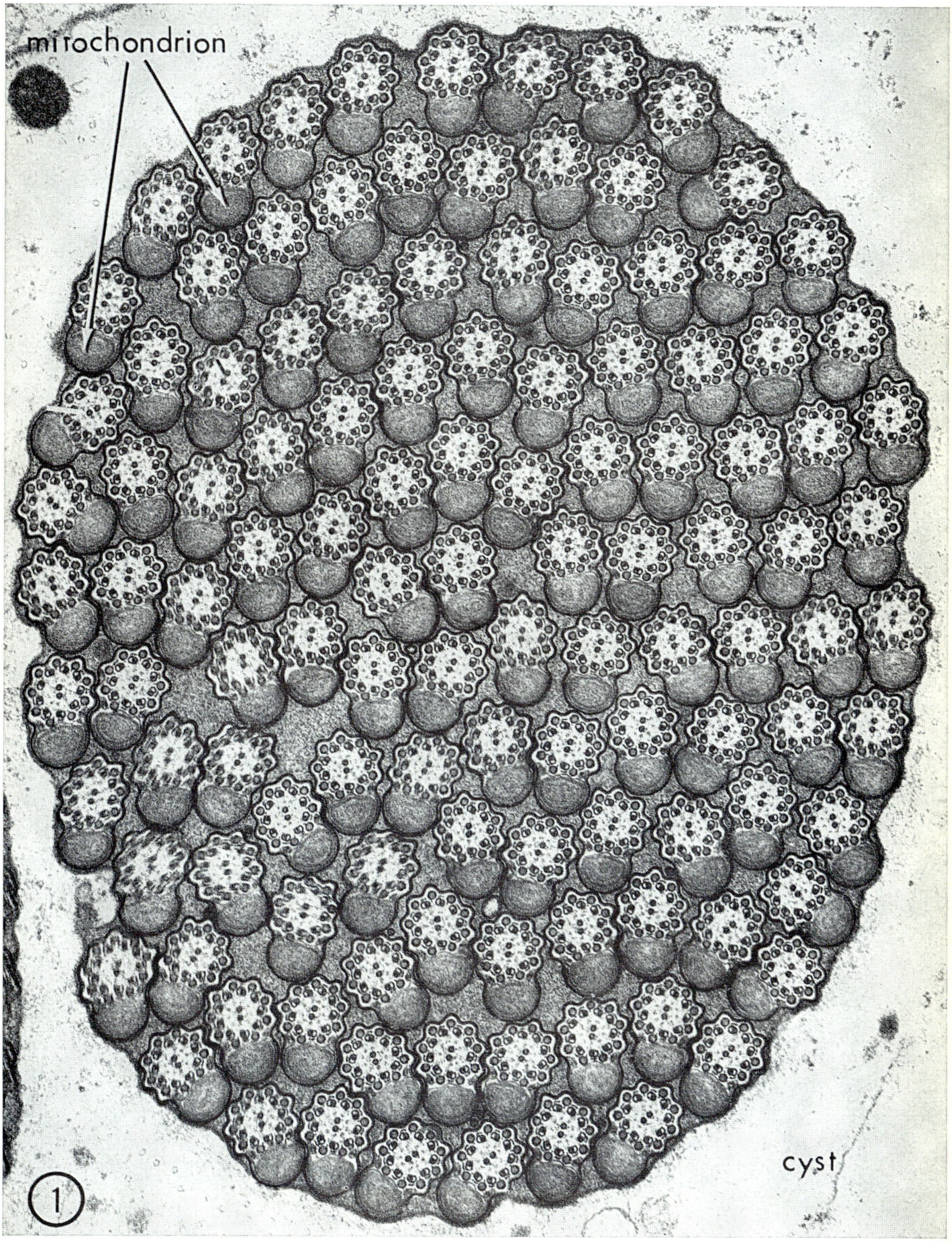
mitochondrion
cyst
1

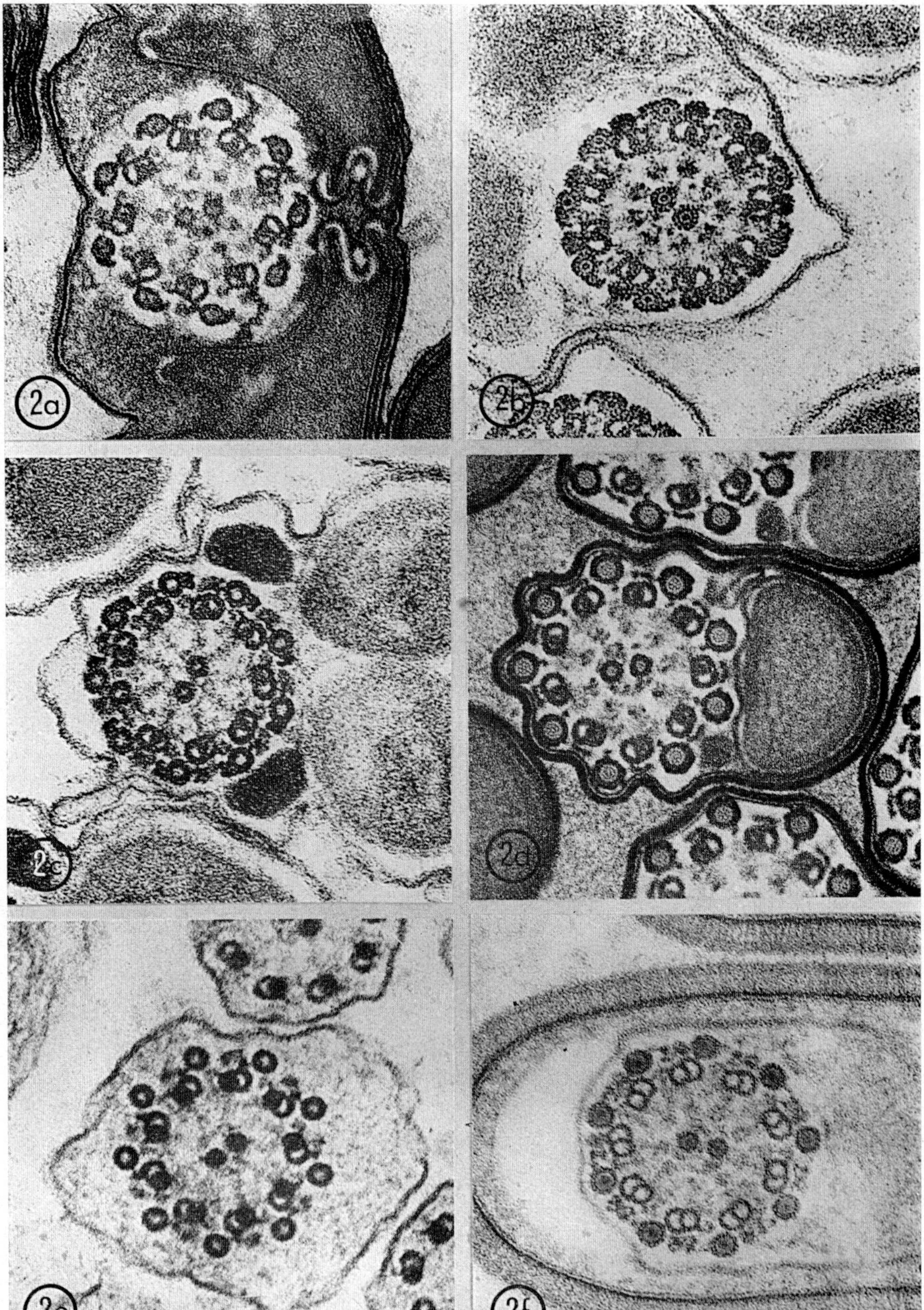
2a
2b
2c
2d
2e
2f

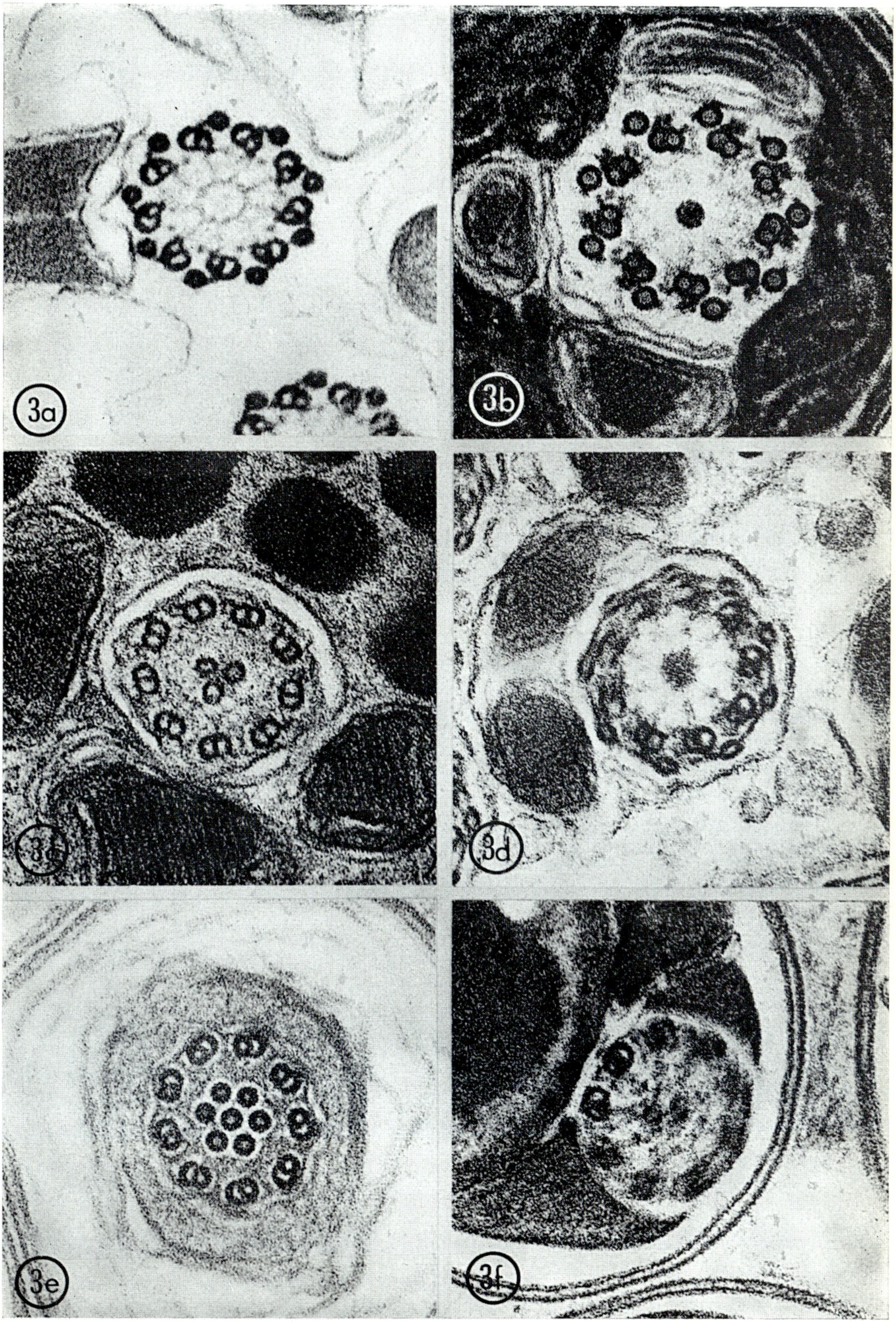
3a
3b
3c
3d
3e
3f

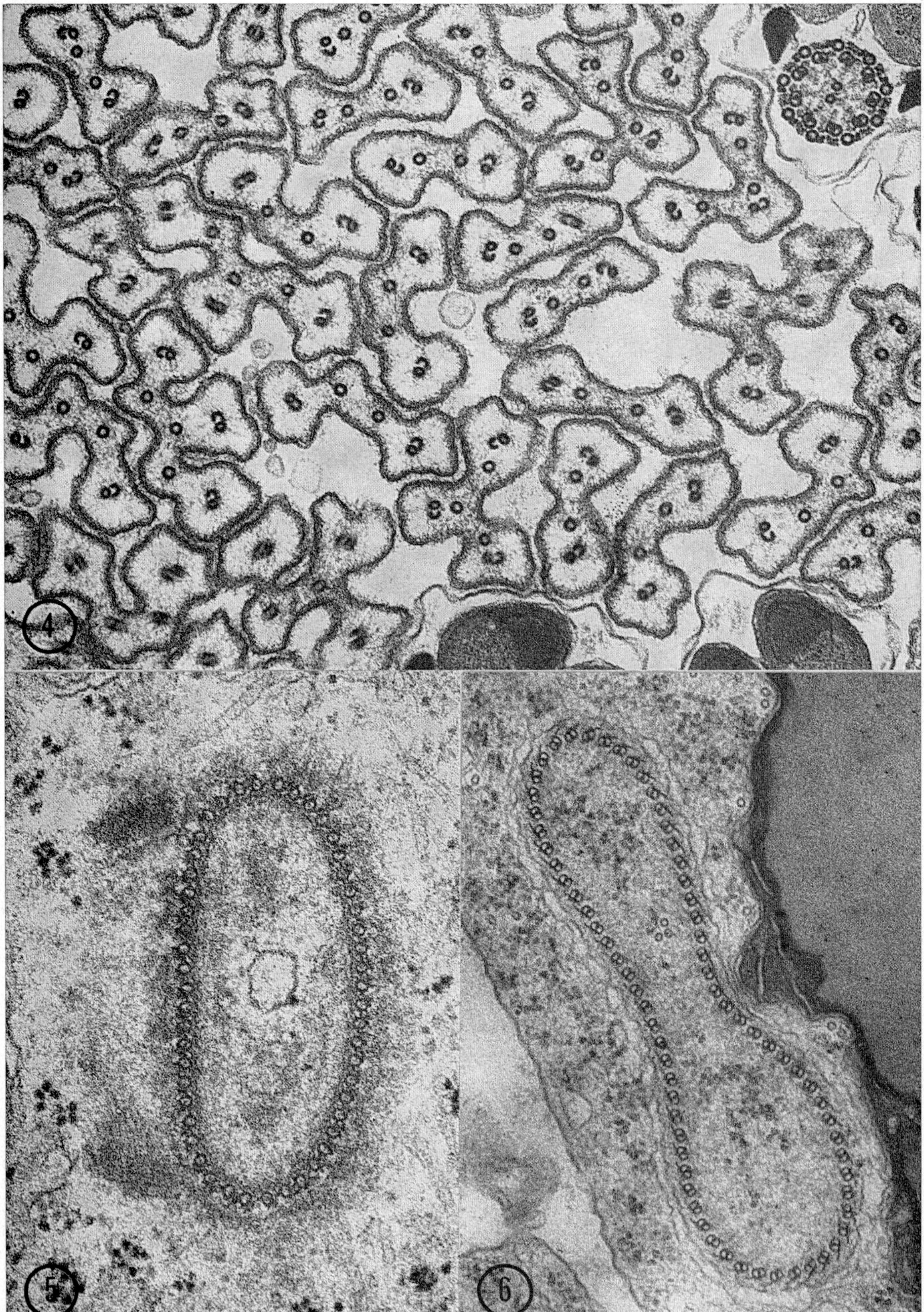
4
5
6

ROMANO DALLAI (*)

THE SPERMATOZOON OF ARTHROPODA. XI. FURTHER OBSERVATIONS ON COLLEMBOLA

SUMMARY. — The principal phases of the spermiogenesis of certain *Collembola* (*Anurida maritima, Orchesella villosa, Dicyrtoma melitensis*) are described and the curiously rolled-up arrangement of the sperm near the end of the ductus deferens is noted.

RIASSUNTO. — Nel presente lavoro sono descritte le principali fasi della spermiogenesi di alcuni Collemboli (*Anurida maritima, Orchesella villosa, Dicyrtoma melitensis*) e viene messo in evidenza il particolare aspetto dello spermatozoo, arrotolato su se stesso, in prossimità del canale deferente.

Recent papers (KRZYSZTOFOWICZ and BYCZKOWSKA-SMYK, 1966; DALLAI, 1967) have described the fine structure of the sperm of certain Collembola, emphasising, above all, the 9 + 2 pattern of the axial flagellar filament, which had not previously been found in insects.

Since then, I have continued to study the spermiogenesis of these insects and have found other traits that, as far as I know, have never been observed in other insect orders.

It will be noticed that certain phases of spermiogenesis remain insufficiently explained in this work; this is because the maturation of the germinal cells in Collembola, unlike other insects, occurs almost synchronously throughout the gonad and even when one collects the material periodically, it is still very difficult to trace the transformation of the various cellular components.

MATERIAL AND METHODS

Specimens of *Anurida maritima* (Guérin), *Orchesella villosa* (Geoffroy) and *Dicyrtoma melitensis* Stach, were dissected *in vivo*. The male reproductive organs were extracted, prefixed in 2,5% gluteraldehyde in a Hoyle buffer with 8% sucrose, fixed in 1% osmium tetroxide and embedded in Epon. BEHNKE and FORER's method (1967) was used to indicate the presence of proteic substances. The material was observed in a Siemens Elmiskop 125 Kv electron microscope.

OBSERVATIONS

The young, roundish spermatid (3 μ in diameter) has a nucleus that is 1.3 μ in diameter, in the center of which the chromatin appears to be concentrated in the form of short fibers (Fig. 1). To the side of the region

(*) Institute of Zoology of the University of Siena, Italy.

of contact between nucleus and mitochondria, masses of vesicles and elongated, smooth-walled cisternae are gathered (Fig. 2). These are homologous to a Golgi complex and presumably produce the material that constitutes the acrosome. In longitudinal sections only two mitochondria can be observed posterior to the nucleus (Fig. 1), but a third one is revealed in the cross sections of this region. The three mitochondria, which are of normal appearance, surround the centriole and the beginning of the flagellum.

At a more advanced stage of maturation the spermatid is elongated, and the acrosome, with its typical concentric layers, is already clearly visible (Figs. 4, 5). At the level of the attachment between acrosome and nucleus, the external membrane of the acrosome invaginates, forming a cylindrical cavity (Fig. 5). Amorphous material lies within this cavity, which extends a good way down into the axial region of the nucleus (Figs. 3, 4, 5). The nucleus is now elliptic and its chromatin is condensed into slender lamellae (150 Å thick). Posterior to the nucleus there is a mass of slightly electron-dense amorphous material that may be considered homologous to the adjunct centriole (Fig. 3). The mitochondrial derivatives are more elongated than in the previous stage, but their cristae are still recognizable (Figs. 3, 4).

At a still more advanced stage of maturation, the spermatid becomes extremely elongated. The nucleus is cylindrical throughout, except for its posterior pole, which is wedge shaped (Fig. 6). Its chromatin is arranged in concentric 150-200 Å–thick lamellae. In certain sections of the anterior portion of the nucleus, the axis of amorphous material that extend from the acrosome is present. There are no traces of cristae in the almost cylindrical mitochondria, but the mitochondrial matrix is more opaque (Fig. 7). In transverse section, the three mitochondria lie at the corners of a triangle and surround electron-opaque material (Fig. 7). The flagellum begins to one side of the nucleus; frequently, in sections at the level of the junction between nucleus and flagellum, a ring of less than nine peripheral doublets complemented by a few single tubules that sometimes have arms appears. Two further micro-tubules of those surrounding the nucleus migrate towards the center of the axial filament complex (Fig. 8). The axial filament complex is of the $9 + 2$ pattern (central tubules, central sheath and Afzelius rays, secondary fibrils, peripheral doublets). Immediately below the centriole, the nine peripheral doublets appear completely empty, but more posteriorly, when the nucleus no longer appears in the sections, they are filled with electron-opaque material so that it is difficult to distinguish subfibers A and B (Figs. 7, 8). The fact that when the sections are treated with pepsin for 8 minutes, both the material surrounded by the mitochondria and that within the doublets is removed, suggests that in both cases, it is proteic (Fig. 9).

The nucleus and mitochondria are surrounded by a series of microtubules that direct the elongation of these structures (Figs. 6, 7, 8). As the nucleus continues to elongate, its chromatin becomes more and more condensed, assuming a homogeneously dense appearance. At this point the spermatozoon is an extremely elongated cell (as much as 60 μ long). It is constituted by a 24 μ-long head with the 0.85-μ-long tapered acrosome at its top. Immediately under the acrosome is the nucleus, cylindrical except at its posterior pole, were it is shaped like the mouthpiece of a flute. The cylinder filled with amorphous material traverses the axis of both acrosome and nucleus. The one side of the nucleus the flagellar axial filament begins.

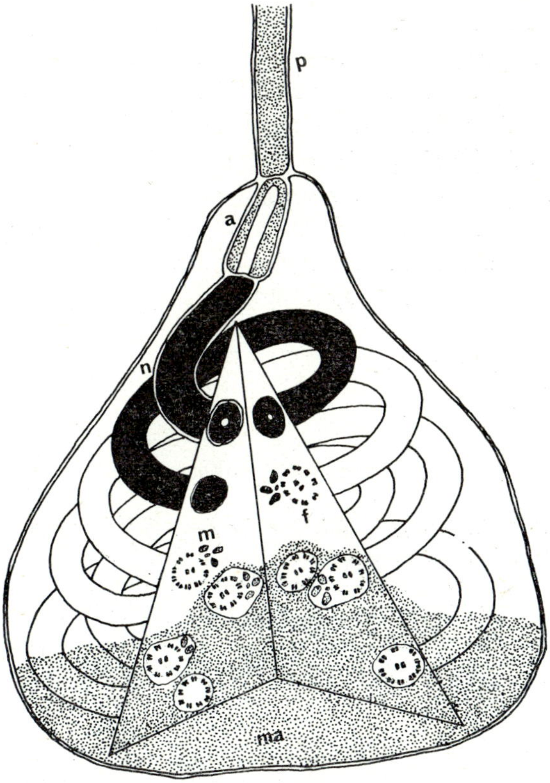

Schema 1. – Schematic drawing of spermatozoon of *Anurida maritima*. (*a*) acrosome; (*f*), flagellum; (*m*) mitochondria; (*ma*) granular material; (*n*) nucleus; (*p*) peduncle.

The three mitochondrial derivatives lie immediately under the nucleus, still arranged in a triangle and surrounding amorphous material. More caudally, one of the mitochondrial derivatives, the one opposite the flagellum, disappears leaving the other two to accompany the flagellar filament complex for a good part of its course. The 9 + 2 axial filament complex has no external accessory fibres; the peripheral doublets are filled with proteic material.

The spermatozoon leaves the cell wall that has held it up to this stage and enters the ductus deferens. Here it is more filiform and the " manchette " of microtubules that surrounded it disappears (Fig. 12). But the most curious fact is that it is rolled around itself six times with a bit of granular cytoplasm in the middle (Figs. 10, 11). The outer four turns are within the external membrane of the cyst, whereas the inner two turns of the tail are wrapped in their own membrane and run towards the center of the granular cytoplasmic mass (Figs. 10, 11 and schema).

The spermatozoon is anchored to the cells of the testicle wall by a long peduncle, 0.20 μ in diameter (Fig. 10). The peduncle consists of finely granulated material surrounded by a thick wall (Fig. 14) and is attached to the sperm membrane at the apex of the acrosome (Fig. 13). The function of the peduncle is not clear.

The above description applies in particular to *Anurida maritima*, a Collembola belonging to the family *Poduridae*, but it is likely that it fits the entire order. In fact the spermatozoa found in the ductus deferens of *Dicyrtoma melitensis* (*Sminthuridae*) seem to be exactly the same as those of *Anurida* (Fig. 16), and in *Orchesella villosa* (*Entomobryidae*) there are no substantial differences. However, in this species, the peduncle that attaches the sperm to the testicle wall has a different structure; it is composed of numer ous closely packed fibers running longitudinally to the peduncle (Fig. 17). In transverse section it can be seen that they are in hexagonal array forming a paracrystalline pattern (Fig. 15).

References

BEHNKE O. and FORER A. (1967) – *Evidence for four classes of microtubules in individual cells.* « J. Cell Science », 2, 169–192.

DALLAI R. (1967) – *Lo spermatozoo degli Artropodi.* I. Anurida maritima (*Guérin*) *ed* Orchesella villosa (*Geoffroy*) (*Insecta, Collembola*). « Atti Accad. Fisiocritici, Siena », 17, 468–476.

KRZYSZTOFOWICZ A. and BYCZKOWSKA-SMYK W. (1966) – *Preliminary investigations on the fine structure of spermatozoa of* Tetrodontophora bielanensis (*Waga*) (*Collembola*). « Acta Biol. Cracov. », 9, 551–558.

Explanation of figures

Fig. 1. – Section of young spermatid of *Anurida maritima:* (*m*), mitochondria; (*n*) nucleus. ×40,000.

Fig. 2. – Section of young spermatid of *Anurida maritima:* (*f*), flagellum; (*g*), Golgi complex (*n*). nucleus. 40,000.

Fig. 3. – Sagittal section of *Anurida maritima* spermatid: (*c*), intranuclear cylinder; (*cg*), adjunct centriole; (*f*), flagellum; (*m*), mitochondrion; (*n*) nucleus. ×30,000.

Fig. 4. – Parasagittal section of *Anurida maritima* spermatid: (*a*), acrosome; (*c*) intranuclear cylinder; (*f*), flagellum; (*m*), mitochondria; (*n*), nucleus. ×30,000.

Fig. 5. – Longitudinal section of the zone of attachment between acrosome and nucleus; in *Anurida maritima* spermatid. The amorphous material that fills the axial zone of the acrosome continues within the intranuclear cylinder, (*a*) acrosome; (*n*) nucleus. ×60,000.

Fig. 6. – Sagittal section of nearly mature spermatid of *Anurida maritima.* The posterior region of the nucleus (*n*) is shaped like the mouthpiece of a flute. (*f*) flagellum; (*m*) mitochondria; (*mi*) microtubules. ×60,000.

Fig. 7. – Transverse section at level of nucleus and flagellum of spermatids of *Anurida maritima*. Only slightly posterior to the centrioles the peripheral doublets seem to be completely empty, but more posteriorly they are filled with electron–opaque material; (*f*) flagellum; (*m*) mitochondria; (*n*) nucleus. ×60,000.

Fig. 8. – Transverse section of nearly mature spermatid of *Anurida maritima* at level of centriole. (*f*), flagellum; (*m*) mitochondria; (*mi*) microtubules; (*n*) nucleus. ×60,000.

Fig. 9. – Same section of micrograph 7 after 8–minute digestion with pepsin. Note removal of material within peripheral doublets and of that surrounded by the three mitochondria. ×60,000.

Fig. 10. – Spermatozoa of *Anurida maritima* near end of ductus deferens. ×24,000.

Fig. 11. – Spermatozoa of *Anurida maritima* near end of ductus deferens. (*f*), flagellum; (*m*), mitochondria; (*ma*), granular material; (*n*) nucleus. ×30,000.

Fig. 12. – Detail of micrograph II at greater magnification. (*f*), flagellum; (*m*), mitochondria. ×60,000.

Fig. 13. – Detail of zone of attachment of sperm to peduncle in *Anurida maritima*. (*a*) acrosome; (*p*) peduncle. ×90,000.

Fig. 14. – Transverse section of peduncle of spermatozoon in *Anurida maritima*. ×90,000.

Fig. 15. – Transverse section of peduncle of spermatozoon in *Orchesella villosa*. ×50,000.

Fig. 16. – Spermatozoon of *Dicyrtoma melitensis* near end of ductus deferens. ×20,000.

Fig. 17. – Spermatozoon of *Orchesella villosa* showing the structure of the peduncle in longitudinal section. ×30,000.

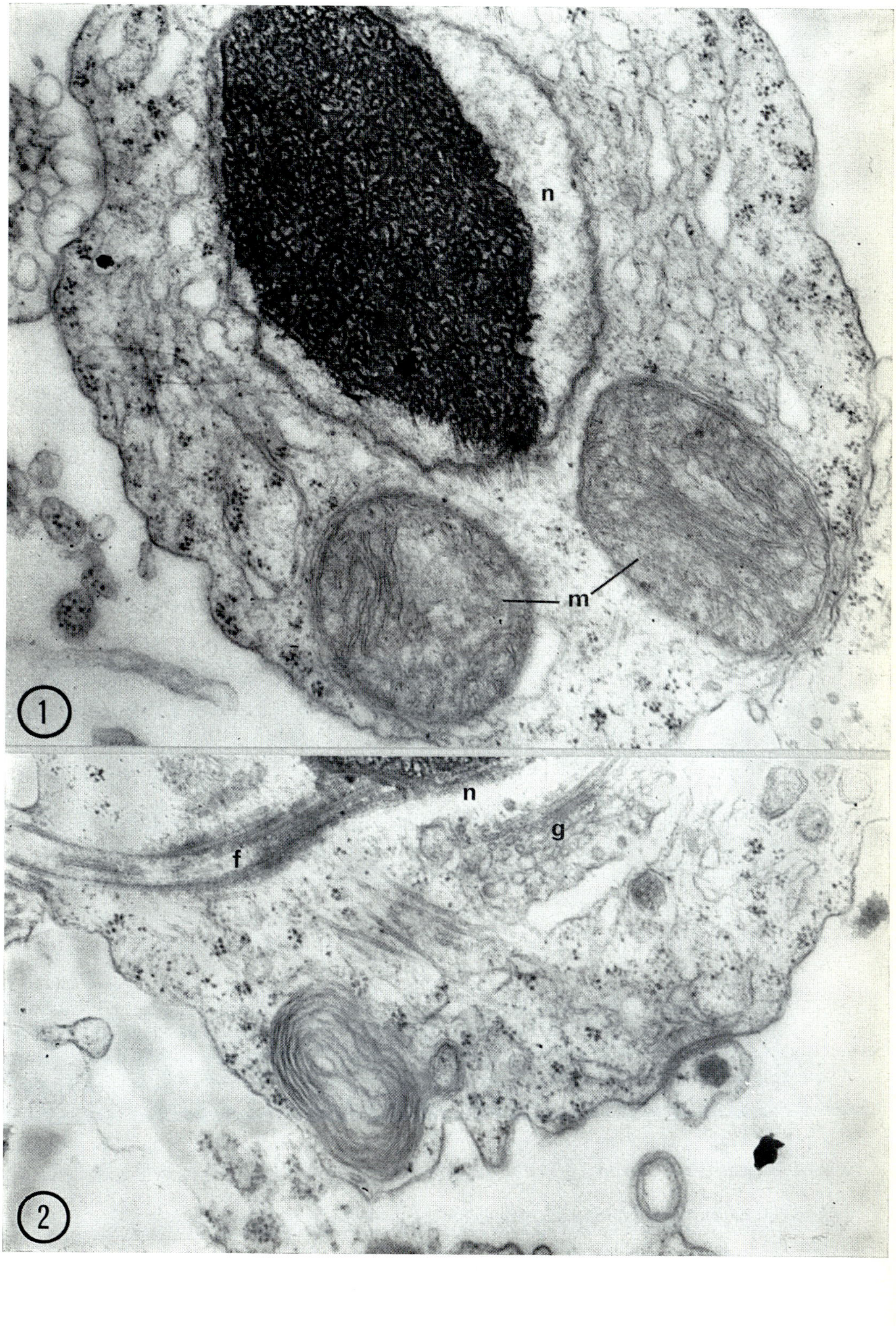
n
m
1
n
g
f
2

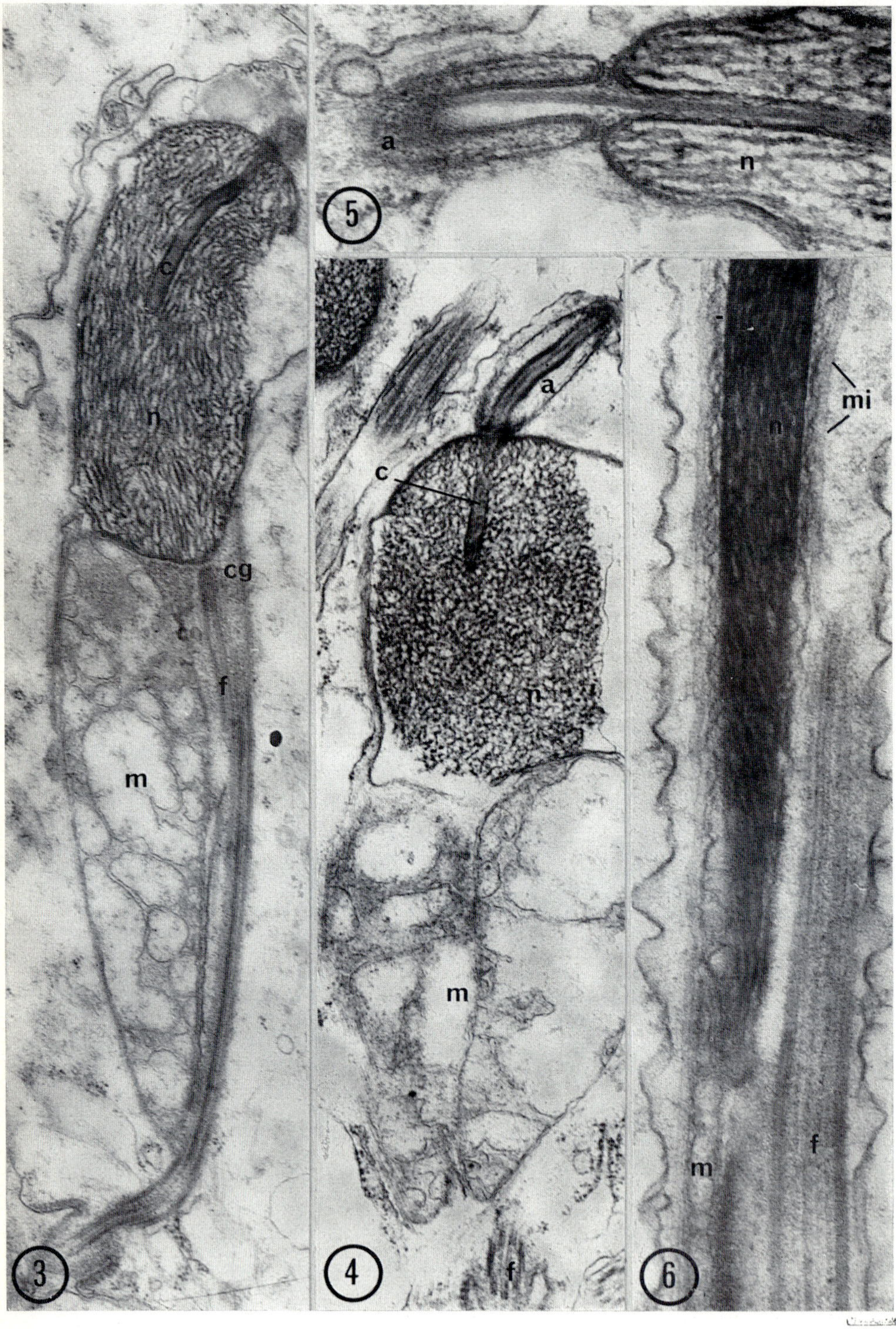

5
a
n
3
c
n
cg
f
m
4
a
c
n
m
f
6
mi
n
m
f

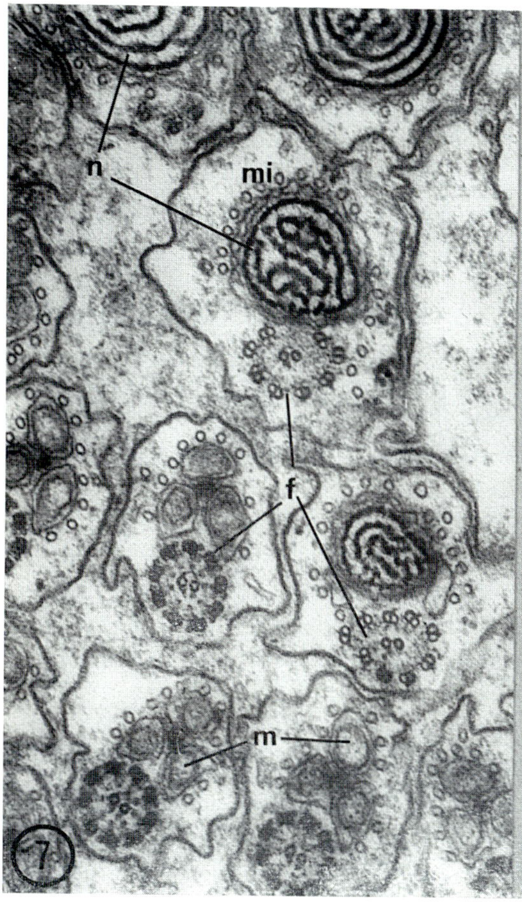
n
mi
f
m
7

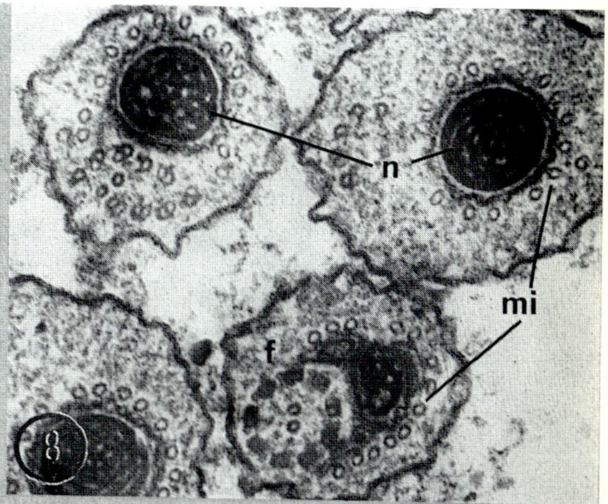
n
mi
f
8

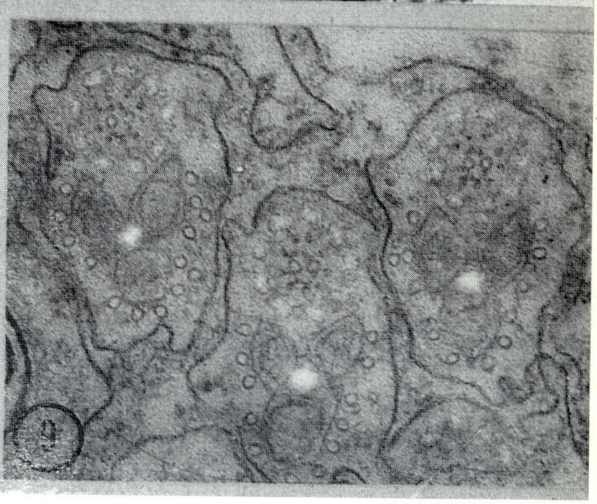
9

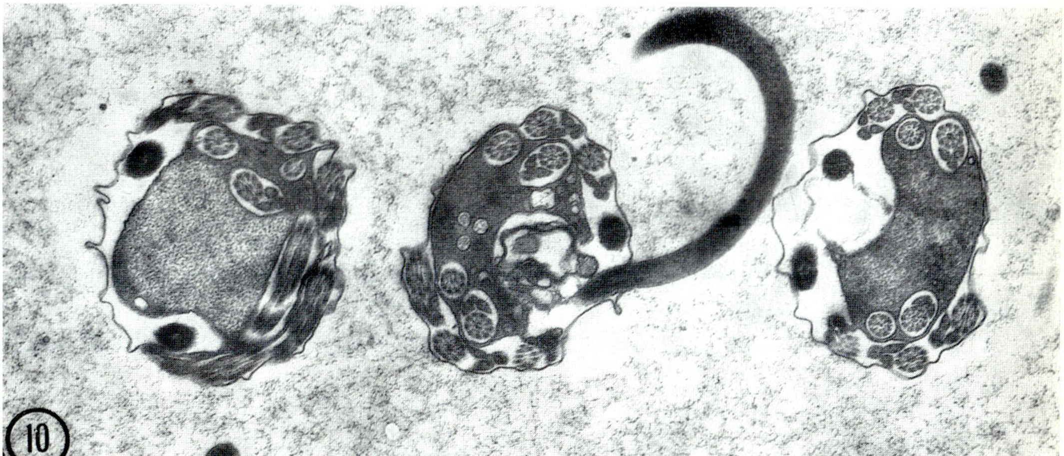
10

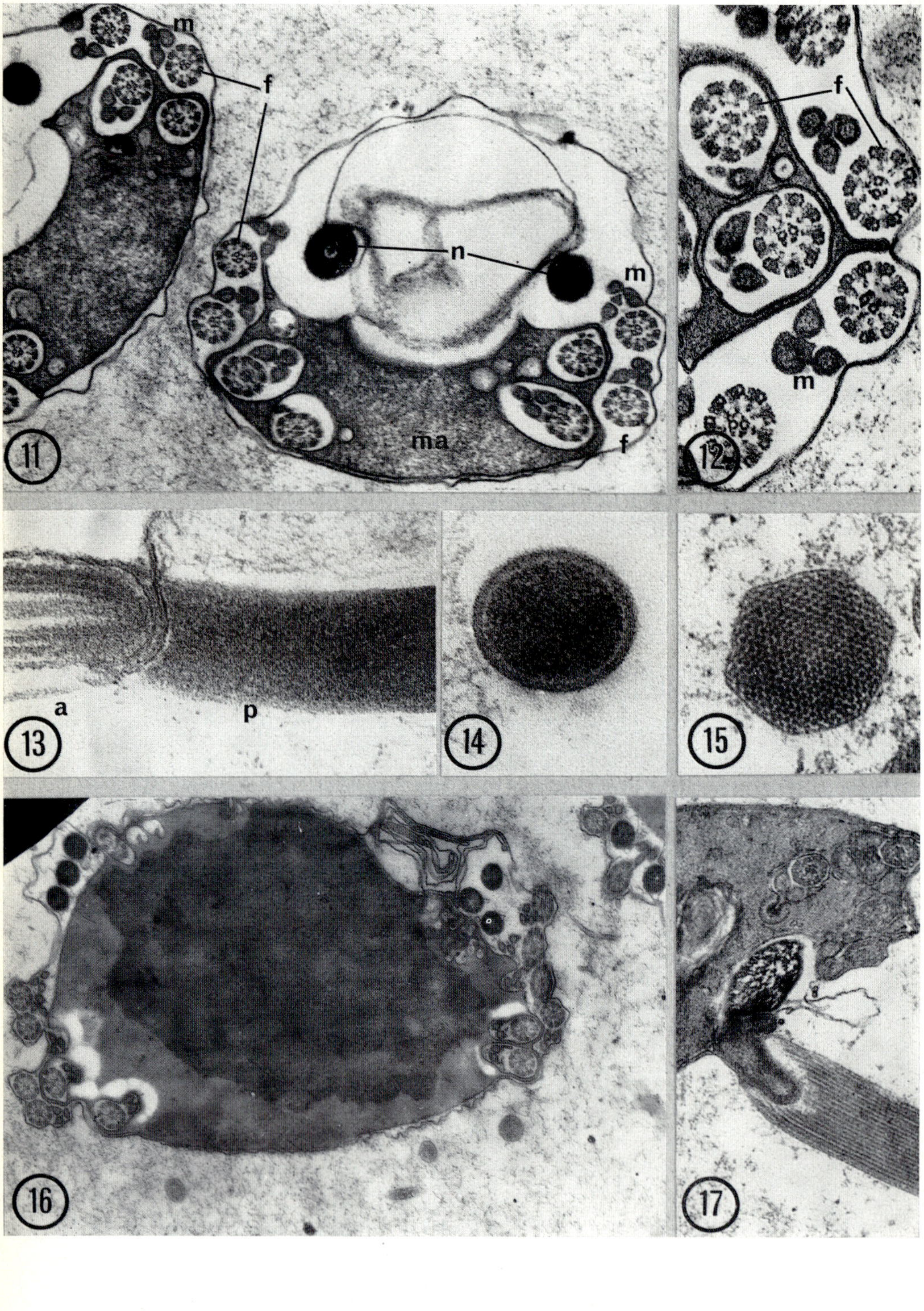
m
f
n
m
ma
f
11
f
m
12
a
p
13
14
15
16
17

C. D. EDDLEMAN [1], O. P. BRELAND [2]
and J. J. BIESELE [2]

A THREE-DIMENSIONAL MODEL OF THE ACROSOME IN THE AMERICAN COCKROACH, *PERIPLANETA AMERICANA* [3]

SUMMARY. — The acrosome of *Periplaneta americana* has been reconstructed. The acrosome is platyleiform, and in general outline resembles a duckbill. It is homogeneous and of medium electron density, and possesses an axial chamber which is u-shaped. Within the chamber and conforming closely to its outline is a 2–ply complex of fuzzy, laminated rod-like structures. This complex has been identified as the axial rod.

A highly transparent, broadly expanded area surrounding the acrosome is cytoplasmic in nature, and is termed the periacrosomal material. The acrosomal base forms a cup-like concavity which receives the dome-shaped anterior tip of the nucleus.

RIASSUNTO. — È stato ricostruito l'acrosoma di *Periplaneta americana*. L'acrosoma è piatto e come schema generale rassomiglia a un becco di anatra. È omogeneo, di media densità elettronica e possiede una camera assiale a forma di U. Nella camera, addossato alle pareti è presente un complesso bistratificato di strutture bastoncellari increspate e laminate. Questo complesso viene interpretato come bastone assiale.

Una grande area trasparente che circonda l'acrosoma è di natura citoplasmica, ed è definita materiale periacrosomiale. La base dell'acrosoma forma una concavità a forma di tazza che ospita il polo anteriore del nucleo conformato a cupola.

The acrosome of *Periplaneta americana* (L.) was first described from phase-contrast studies by NATH, GUPTA and SEHGAL (1957). According to their report the acrosome consisted of 2 main regions: an inner, dense area, surrounded by a broad, flat leaf-like portion having extremely low contrast (Diag. 1). The denser area was in turn seen to be composed of two different materials. One part, an inner core, was extremely dark and ensheathed by a thick cap of lower contrast, but nonetheless having considerably higher contrast than the outer flattened " leaf-like " part.

The anterior tip of the nucleus is described by these same authors as dome-shaped. It was seen to fit rather loosely into a cup-shaped concavity

(1) Present address: Department of Biology, Union College, Lincoln, Nebraska, 68506, U.S.A.

(2) Department of Zoology, The University of Texas at Austin, Austin, Texas, 78712, U.S.A.

(3) This research was supported in part by the following grants: No. 4644, Penrose Fund, American Philosophical Society; Research Career Award 5–K6–CA–18366 from the National Cancer Institute, National Institutes of Health; and The University of Texas Research Institute.

at the base of the acrosome. In vivo, the acrosome was often separated completely from the nucleus. NATH *et al.* (1957) state that it was common for living spermatozoa to become glued to the surface of the slide by the broad " leaf-like " portion of the acrosome.

MATERIALS AND METHODS

The present work is based on specimens from cockroach colonies maintained in the laboratory. One colony was started from individuals captured within the city limits of Austin, Texas. Another colony was derived from specimens trapped in Yucatan, Mexico, by Mr. DAVID SIMON, a graduate student in the Department of Zoology, The University of Texas at Austin. A third colony is descended from stocks maintained by Dr. LOUIS M. ROTH, Pioneering Research Division, U. S. Army Natick Laboratories, Natick, Massachusetts, and generously provided through Dr. ROBERT H. BARTH, Department of Zoology, The University of Texas at Austin. No variations in material were observed which could be attributed to the different sources of the insects.

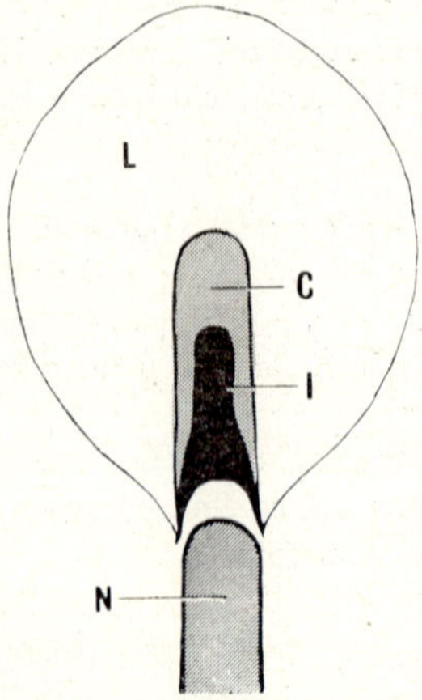

Diag. 1. – Acrosome, frontal view, as reported by NATH *et al.*, 1957.

Techniques for phase contrast microscopy are reviewed in detail by BRELAND, EDDLEMAN and BIESELE (1968). These consisted essentially of the following steps:

1) Dissection of the testes, seminal vesicles or spermathecae after anaesthetizing the specimen with CO_2 in a cold dry ice chest.

2) Preparation of a temporary wet mount with Belar's saline as a medium.

3) Application of a cover glass which was sealed or partially sealed with Krönig cement prior to observation.

The preparative procedure has also been previously stated for electron microscopy (BRELAND, GASSNER, RIESS and BIESELE, 1966). Testes, seminal vesicles or spermathecae were fixed in chilled 2.5% gluteraldehyde, buffered to *p*H 7.2 with 0.05 M Sorensen's buffer. Duration of fixation varied from 1 to 2 hours. Post-fixation was accomplished with 1% osmium tetroxide for 2 hours at 4° C. at *p*H 7.2. This was followed by staining with uranyl acetate for from 18 to 20 hours at room temperature. Dehydration with serial ethanols preceded embedding in a plastic mixture of Epon, Araldite and DDSA. Sections cut on a Porter–Blum ultramicrotome with a DuPont diamond knife were floated on water, applied to uncoated grids and post-stained with lead citrate. Observation was with a Siemens Elmiskop I and exposures were made on either Kodak Contrast Process Ortho Film or Kodak Projector Slide Plates Contrast.

Observations

In the present work, spermatozoa observed with phase contrast light microscopy afforded very little acrosomal detail. At phase magnifications of from 600 to 1,200 diameters, the acrosome usually appeared to consist of a homogeneously dark, cylindrical " core " invested by a lighter, translucent bleb or bubble (Fig. 1). Several variations in shape and disposition of the buble were observed. In some, the " bubble " was symmetrical, with a round or " tear-drop " shape (Figs. 1, 2). However, the " bubble " was irregular and asymmetrical in other specimens (Figs. 3, 4). Whereas some spermatozoa exhibited a complete ensheathing of the core, on others the bubble seemed attached only at the terminal tip, and in living preparations, was seen to shift from side to side, as if capable of rolling back and forth around the end of the acrosome. Finally, some acrosomes were completely devoid of the " bubble " (Fig. 5).

Examination of spermatids at successive stages of elongation (e.g., from early nymphal testes, adult testes, seminal vesicles, inseminated spermathecae) revealed that the younger stages possessed larger " bubbles ". As elongation proceeded, the " bubble " diminished in size and moved forward to the acrosome tip, from which it was eventually shed. This " blebbing off " of the " leaf-like " portion of the acrosome (NATH *et al.*, 1957) resembles cytoplasmic exfoliation, and we applied the term " cytoplasmic bleb " to this area.

With electron microscopy, two distinct types of acrosomal transverse sections were observed (Figs. 6–9). Both were roughly oblong in general outline, with horizontal dimensions ranging from 0.80 to 1.90 micron. The vertical dimensions vary from 0.3 to 1.0 micron. The lateral aspects of the acrosome are always rounded. The dorsal and ventral surfaces are either flat, bulge slightly outward (Figs. 6, 7), or curve inward (Figs. 8, 9), the last two situations presenting biconvex and biconcave outlines, respectively. The outer surface of the acrosome is composed of an electron-dense, double membrane. The bulk of the acrosome is moderaely dense, and in some specimens has a granular appearance (Fig. 8).

Some transverse sections (Figs. 6, 8) reveal a pair of cavities or acrosomal lumens. Each cavity is located laterally and is lined with a dense membrane that appears identical to the external membrane.

The other distinct type of transverse section differs in having a single, oblong cavity or lumen which occupies most of the section (Figs. 6, 7). Within the lumen is a dense, irregularly shaped mass that is fuzzy in appearance. In some cases, it exhibits a 2–ply structure. All transverse sections of the acrosome are surrounded by an extensive, usually irregularly shaped mass of cytoplasm confined within a cell membrane.

Two mediosagittal sections are shown in Figs. 10 and 11. The length of such sections ranges from 1.15 to 2.43 micra. The base or proximal end of the acrosome is thickest, ranging from 0.50 to 0.75 micron. The acrosome tapers toward the anterior, attaining a minimum measurement of 0.25 to 0.32 micron a short distance posterior to the tip. There is a bulbous swelling near the tip, within which the lumen is located. It contains the same dense fuzzy material seen in transverse sections. The cup-like socket of the base invaginates anteriorly to form a deep axial pocket. Both the outer covering of the acrosome and inner lining of the lumen consist of a double membrane.

Figs. 12 and 13 are parasagittal sections of the acrosome. The length and thickness are comparable to the dimensions found in the mediosagittal sections, although some are slightly shorter than the latter. The main difference in outline is attributable to a less abrupt taper along the length and a smaller swelling at the tip. Internally, the lumen (cavity) extends the entire length of the acrosome and communicates through a narrow passage with the space between the nuclear tip and the face of the acrosome socket. Thus, the acrosomal cavity is continuous, through this channel, with the cytoplasm of the spermatozoon. Some sections reveal within the cavity a moderately dense amorphous material that is identical to the dense material of the cytoplasm (Figs. 10, 12). A dense, fuzzy, 2–ply rod-like structure fills most of the length of the lumen.

In frontal section, the acrosome is bilaterally symmetrical (Figs. 14, 15). It is roughly platyleiform, with a broadly-rounded anterior tip. The greatest breadth of the acrosome in this aspect is attained in the anterior 1/3, ranging from 1.0 to 1.37 micron. Posterior to this point, the sides taper gradually inward to the base where the acrosome attains its narrowest breadth of 0.50 to 0.83 micron. Proceeding posteriorly, the sides abruptly flare outward and accommodate the nucleus within the basal cup or acrosomal socket.

Viewed in frontal plane, the cavity is U–shaped or horseshoeshaped. Within the confines of the cavity and conforming closely to its shape, is an electron dense structure composed of up to six parallel laminated rods. The surfaces of the rods are covered with short, minute projections which cause the laminated complex to have a fuzzy, brushy appearance.

A broad, flat, leaf-like expanse of cytoplasm completely envelops the acrosome. This cytoplasm is surrounded by the plasma membrane, which is clearly continuous along the entire length of the spermatozoon.

Interpretation and Conclusion

Electron microscopy shows definitely that the " leaf-like " portion described by Nath *et al.*, (1957) is not acrosomal material *per se*, but an anterior extension of the cytoplasm.

Richards (1963), on the basis of light microscopy, described the acrosome of *P. americana* as of a " duck-bill " shape. Whereas the true acrosome is actually this shape, it was probably not evident at the level of magnification at which he worked. It is believed that the duck-bill material in Richards' micrographs is actually adhering cytoplasm conforming generally to the outline of the acrosome.

We are not aware of other reports of spermatozoa or acrosomes retaining such a large amount of cytoplasm in these advanced stages of spermiogenesis. It has been shown in some species (AUSTIN, 1968) that anteriorly, the plasma

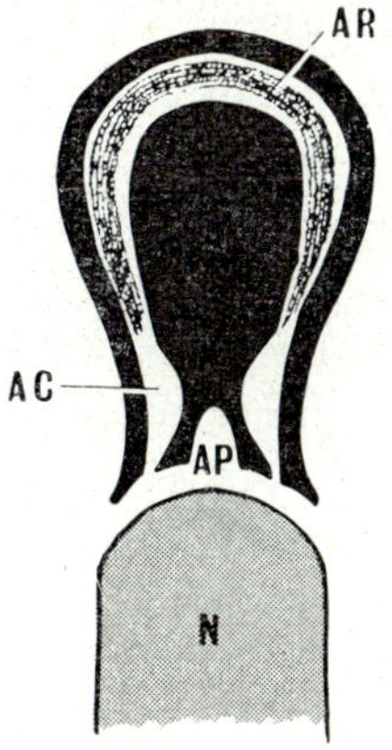

Diag. 2. – Acrosome, frontal section, reconstructed from electron micrographs of transverse, mediosagittal, parasagittal, and parafrontal sections.

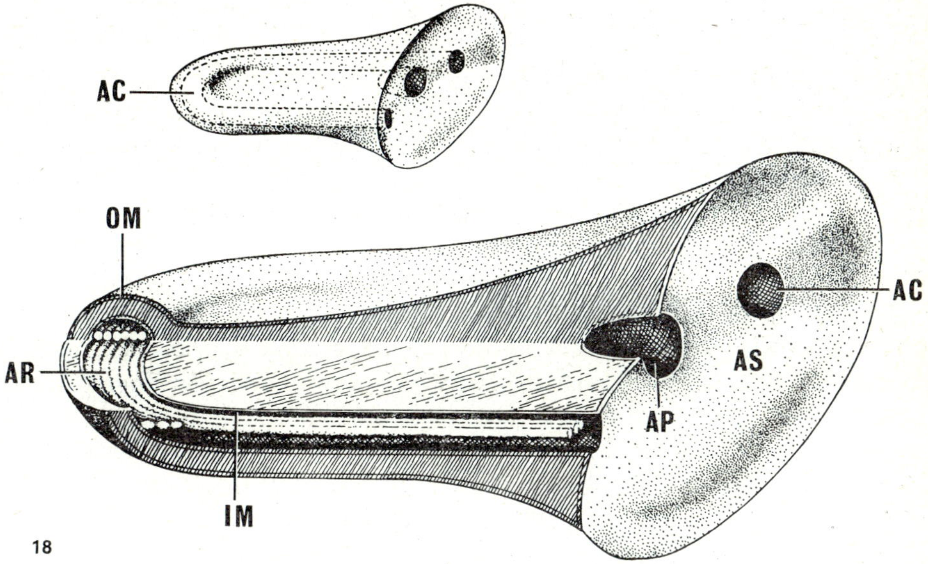

Diag. 3. – Cut-away diagram, showing external and internal structure of acrosome.

membrane is very closely applied to the acrosomal membrane. However, we have not found this to be true in all cases. Of fifteen cockroaches that we have examined, the following resemble *P. americana* by retaining excess acrosomal cytoplasm late in spermiogenesis: *P. australasiae*, *P. brunnea*, *P. fuliginosa*, *P. japonica*, and *Blatta orientalis*.

The reconstruction of the acrosome from transverse, sagittal and frontal sections reveals a very complex morphology (Diag. 2, 3). A clear understanding of this structure is further complicated by confusing terminology in the literature. This has been pointed out by BRELAND *et al.*, (1968). The main difficulty stems from the fact that in the past, investigators have attempted to apply mammalian terminology to all spermatozoa; this practice is untenable in view of what appears to be fundamental differences between insect spermatozoa and mammalian spermatozoa.

However, in an effort to minimize further confusion, we have attempted to use, as far as feasible, the terminology set forth by AUSTIN (1968). In applying this terminology, the large volume of anterior cytoplasm should be called periacrosomal material, as it is interposed between the plasma membrane and the outer acrosome membrane. By the same precedence, that which we have called the acrosomal cavity or lumen is designated as the axial chamber, and the membrane lining it, the inner acrosome membrane. This latter term is also applicable to the membrane covering the surface of the basal " cup-like " concavity.

The laminated complexn ested within the axial chamber is the axial rod, and is apparently the same as the structure termed " perforatorium " in the past.

Its fuzziness seems due to a periodic cross-striation. The axial rod, as the term is used here, should not be confused with the " axial rod " of NATH *et al.*, (1957) (Diag. 1). KAYE (1962) describes in *Acheta domesticus*, the house cricket, the development of a structure, the inner cone, which may be homologous with the axial rod of the cockroach.

KAYE describes the acrosome of the house cricket as consisting of two parts, an inner cone and an outer cone. The inner cone occurs within a space formed by an invagination of the base of the outer cone. The outer cone is derived from the proacrosomal granule, but Kaye suggests that the inner cone develops from amorphous material that appears during early stages of invagination. The author thus concludes that the fully developed acrosome is derived from two distinct sources.

It is a clear possibility that the axial rod in *P. americana* has its origin from a mass of material similar to that which forms the inner cone in *Acheta*. Material which may be remnants of this substance, exhibiting the same approximate electron-density as the axial rod, is to be seen adhering to the polar surface of the nucleus (Figs. 10, 12). Although we feel that the axial rod in *P. americana* and the inner cone of *Acheta domesticus* are homologous, this conclusion may be questioned, as Kaye's micrographs do not show the laminated construction of this complex as viewed in *P. americana* (Figs. 13, 14).

SHAY (1968) and SHAY and BIESELE (1968), in working with another Orthopteran, the cave cricket *Ceuthophilus secretus* (Scudder), suggest that the perforatorium (= axial rod) probably arises from a mass of dense material that can be identified during the early stages of spermiogenesis. The material occurs between the nuclear and proacrosomal granule membranes when these two bodies are in close apposition. As the acrosome base invaginates this material seems to move into the axial chamber before it is closed off by subsequent fusion of the base.

An important difference in the acrosomes of *P. americana* and the crickets cited above, is the presence in the cockroach of the massive amount of acrosomal material called " axial rod " by NATH *et al.*, (1957) (Diag. 1). This area of the acrosome appears to result from a second invagination of the acrosome base. After primary invagination creates the axial chamber, the acrosomal material fuses across the base and the inner membrane invaginates secondarily to produce this area. The deep axial pocket visible in mediosagittal section is probably a vestige of this secondary invagination.

We know of no previous reports that describe the secondary invagination of the acrosome mentioned above. Hence, no term has been suggested for this region which occurs in *P. americana*. We are therefore using the term " acrosomal core " for this region of the acrosome.

Acknowledgments. - We wish to thank Mrs. Pauline West who drew the cut-away diagram and mounted the photographs. We also wish to express our appreciation to Miss Priscilla M. Smith and Mr. Bill Records who assisted with some of the photography, and to Mr. Everett Simmons who gave technical assistance in the laboratory.

References

AUSTIN C. R. (1968) – *Ultrastructure of Fertilization.* Holt Rinehart and Winston, New York.

BRELAND OSMOND P., EDDLEMAN CHARLES D. and BIESELE JOHN J. (1968) – *Studies of insect spermatozoa.* I. « Entomological News », 79, 197–216.

BRELAND OSMOND P., GASSNER GEORGE III, RIESS ROBERT W. and BIESELE JOHN J. (1966) – *Certain aspects of the centriole adjunct, spermiogenesis, and the mature sperm of insects.* « Can. J. Gen. and Cytol. », 8, 759–773.

KAYE J. S. (1962) – *Acrosome formation in the house cricket.* « J. Cell Biol. », 12, 411.

NATH VISHWA, GUPTA B. L. and SEHGAL P. (1957) – *Mitochondria and Golgi bodies in the spermatogenesis of* Periplaneta americana *as studied under the phase contrast microscope.* « Res. Bull. Panjab Univ. », 112, 317–326.

RICHARDS A. GLENN (1963) – *Giant sperm in the cockroach,* Periplaneta americana. « Ent. News », 74, 57–61.

SHAY JERRY W. (1968) – *Ultrastructural observations on spermiogenesis in the cave cricket,* Ceuthophilus secretus (*Scudder*). Unpublished Master's Thesis, Department of Zoology, The University of Texas at Austin.

SHAY JERRY W. and BIESELE JOHN J. (1968) – *Ultrastructural observations on spermiogenesis in the cave cricket* Ceuthophilus secretus (*Scudder*). « La Cellule », 67, 269–282.

Explanation of figures

Abbreviations.

A = Acrosome
AC = Axial chamber (= acrosomal cavity or lumen)
AP = Axial pocket
AR = Axial rod (= perforatorium or laminated complex)
AS = Acrosomal socket (= cup-like concavity)
C = Outer core
CM = Cell membrane
I = Inner core

IM = Inner acrosome membrane
L = Leaf-like portion
N = Nucleus
OM = Outer acrosome membrane
PM = Periacrosomal material (= cytoplasm).

Figs. 1–5. – Phase micrographs of spermatozoa of *P. americana*, showing variations in the acrosomal " Bubble ".

Fig. 1. – From testis of 8th nymphal stage, *ca.* 1,700×.

Fig. 2. – Same as above.

Fig. 3. – From seminal vesicle, *ca.* 1,600×.

Fig. 4. – Same as above.

Fig. 5. – From spermatheca of inseminated female, *ca.* 1,700×.

Figs. 6–7. – Electron micrographs, transverse sections of the acrosome.

Fig. 6. – From testis of 9th nymphal stage, *ca.* 35,000×.

Fig. 7. – From seminal vesicle, adult male, *ca.* 44,500×.

Figs. 8–15. – Electron micrographs, various planes of section, of the acrosome. All from seminal vesicle except Fig. 9.

Fig. 8. – Transverse section, *ca.* 32,000×.

Fig. 9. – Transverse section, from testis, 9th nymphal stage, *ca.* 32,000.×

Fig. 10. – Mediosagittal section, *ca.* 24,000×.

Fig. 11. – Mediosagittal section, *ca.* 20,000×.

Fig. 12. – Parasagittal section, *ca.* 20,000×.

Fig. 13. – Parasagittal section, *ca,* 20,000×.

Fig. 14. – Parafrontal section, *ca.* 18,000×.

Fig. 15. – Parafrontal section, *ca.* 18,000×.

Discussion

BARKER. – Have you ever studied, seen, or induced an acrosomal reaction in insect sperm?

EDDLEMAN. – Electron microscopic studies of *P. americana* spermatozoa that were pre-treated *in vitro* with an extract of eggs removed from females suggest the possibility of an acrosome reaction. Certain changes in the acrosome, as well as in the nuclear contents, are observed in the treated specimens. This work has not extended beyond the initial states.

BACCETTI. – Can the differences between the three layers of the cockroach acrosome be related to chemical differences?

EDDLEMAN. – We assume that differences in density and texture, observable with the electron microscope, are due, in part, to chemical differences. However, we have not approached this problem in terms of chemical analysis or cytochemical techniques so we are not able to elaborate on this aspect at the present time.

C. D. EDDLEMAN et AL. – *A three-dimensional model of the acrosome in the american cockroach*, Periplaneta americana.

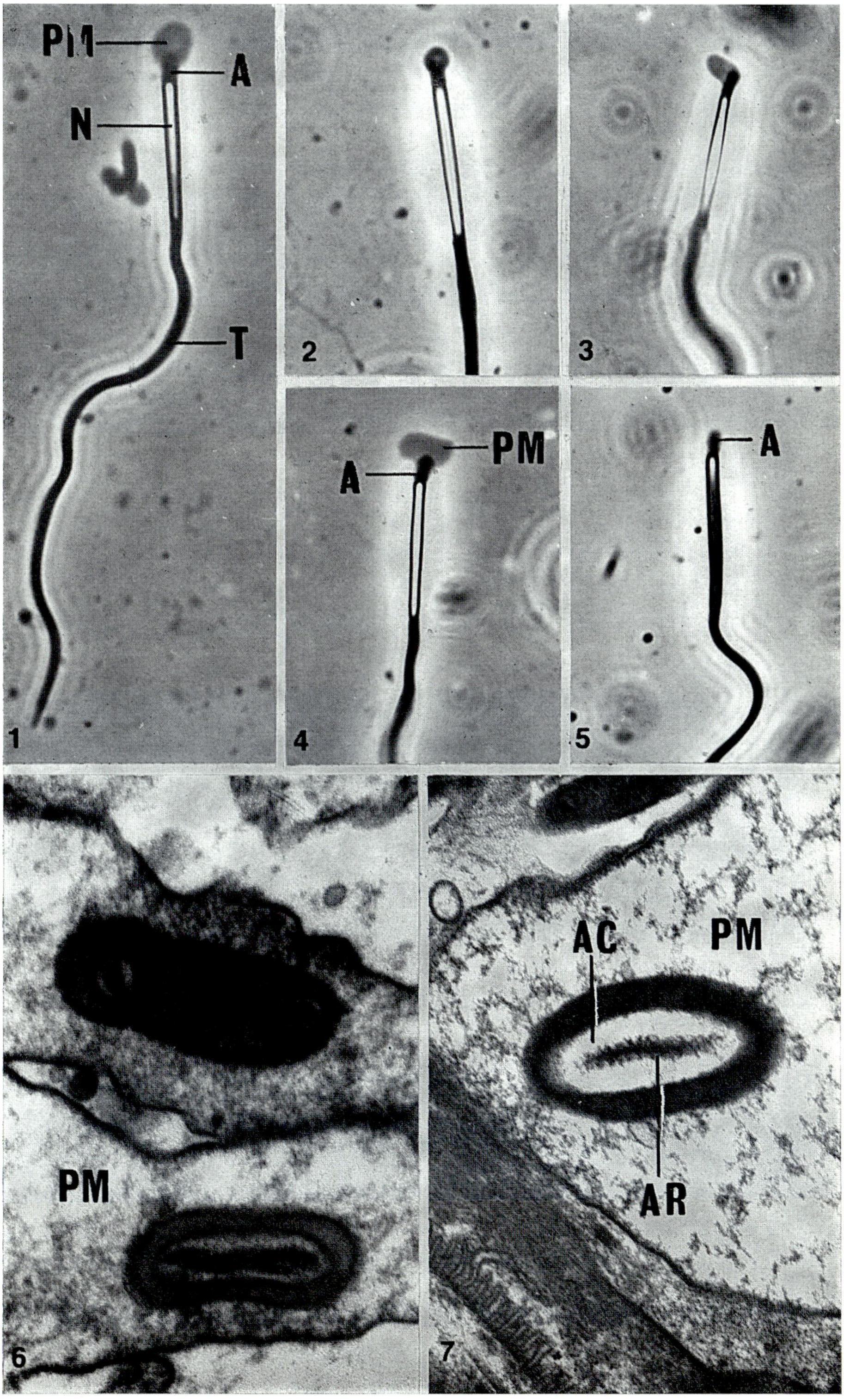

C. D. Eddleman et al. – *A three-dimensional model of the acrosome in the american cockroach,* Periplaneta americana.

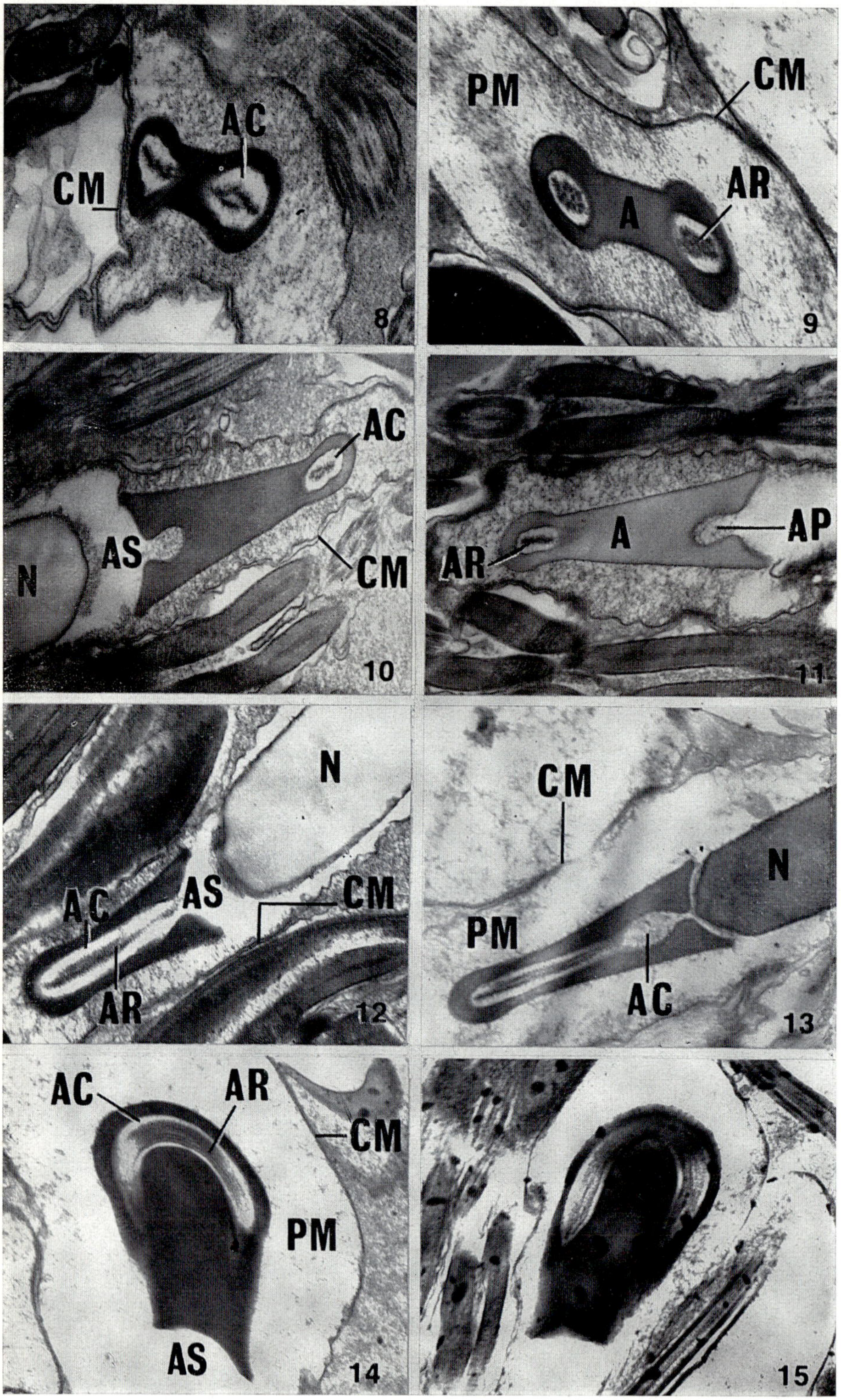

ROGER FOLLIOT (*) (**) et PIERRE-L. MAILLET (*) (**)

ULTRASTRUCTURE DE LA SPERMIOGENÈSE ET DU SPERMATOZOÏDE DE DIVERS INSECTES HOMOPTÈRES

SUMMARY. — The species used in this study belong to several families of the suborder *Auchenorhyncha: Cicadidae, Cercopidae, Cicadellidae, Typhlocybidae, Ulopidae, Cixiidae, Delphacidae.*

At the end of its differentiation, the acrosome is a bilaterally symmetric fibrous structure with a hollow cavity along one face. In most species studied, the acrosome is not at the very tip of the spermatozoon, for there is an anteacrosomal cytoplasmic bleb as long as the acrosome itself. This happens in species where the spermatozoa are packed in large bundles. The tail is also bilaterally symmetric. It consists of two mitochondrial bodies, each with an outer paracrystalline material and the flagellum with peripheral structures in addition to the typical 9+2 pattern. The plane of symmetry, as that which was described in the guinea-pig spermatozoon by FAWCETT (1968). In some families, two additional structures are seen along the flagellum. They originate certainly from the pericentriolar matrix. In sperm-bundle forming families, the anteacrosomal cytoplasmic vesicles of mature spermatozoa lie in a groove between special glandular cells of the testicular cysts walls. Here, they are embedded in a protein material, secreted through the intercellular spaces.

Transverse and complete sagittal sections permit the reciprocal orientation of the different components of this type of bilaterally symmetric spermatozoon. Furthermore this orientation can be compared with that of the mammalian spermatozoon.

Otherwise, the families *Typhlocybidae* and *Cicadidae* display the following unique biological fact: rickettsia-like microorganisms are often present in the spermatozoon nucleus, and by this way, can be transported into the female genital duct.

RIASSUNTO. — Le specie usate in questo studio appartengono a diverse famiglie del sottordine *Auchenorhyncha: Cicadidae, Cercopidae, Cicadellidae, Typhlocybidae, Ulopidae, Cixiidae, Delphacidae.*

Alla fine della sua differenziazione, l'acrosoma è una struttura fibrosa a simmetria bilaterale con una cavità vuota lungo una faccia. Nella maggior parte delle specie studiate, l'acrosoma non è proprio in cima allo spermatozoo, perché c'è una vescicola citoplasmica antiacrosomiale lunga come l'acrosoma stesso. Questo accade nelle specie in cui gli spermatozoi sono riuniti in grossi fasci. Anche la coda è a simmetria bilaterale.

Essa è formata da due corpi mitocondriali, ciascuno con materiale paracristallino esterno e dal flagello con strutture periferiche in aggiunta al modello tipico 9 + 2. Il piano di simmetria è quello descritto negli spermatozoi di cavia da Fawcett (1968). In alcune famiglie lungo il flagello sono presenti due strutture addizionali. Esse si originano certamente

(*) Avec la collaboration technique de Melle G. BOGUAIS et de Mr. B. MORILLE.

(**) Groupe de Recherches de Biologie cellulaire, (Equipe de recherche associée au C.N.R.S. «Cytologie ultrastructurale» n°. 129). Faculté des Sciences, Université de Rennes, France.

dal materiale pericentriolare. Nelle famiglie che formano fasci di spermi, la vescicola antiacrosomale degli spermatozoi maturi giace in un solco tra le cellule ghiandolari della parete delle cisti testicolari. Qui esse sono incluse in un materiale proteico, secreto attraverso gli spazi intercellulari. Sezioni trasversali e completamente sagittali permettono la reciproca orientazione dei differenti componenti di questo tipo di spermatozoo a simmetria bilaterale. In più, questo orientamento può essere confrontato con quello degli spermatozoi dei mammiferi.

D'altra parte, le famiglie *Typhlocybidae* e *Cicadidae* presentano questa unica caratteristica biologica: organismi simili a rickettsie sono spesso presenti nel nucleo dello spermatozoo, e, in questo modo, possono essere trasportati nel dotto genitale femminile.

La spermatogenèse des Homoptères Auchenorhynches a été l'objet de divers travaux consacrés tout d'abord au déroulement de la méïose. Mais l'attention des chercheurs a été retenue ensuite par un phénomène qui, sans leur être exclusif, reste assez curieux: l'agrégation des spermatozoïdes en un spermatodesme. La mise en évidence de ce fait dans ce groupe d'Insectes a été réalisée par ROBERTSON et GIBBS (1937) chez le Cercopide *Philaenus spumarius* L. Depuis, l'un d'entre nous a retrouvé cette particularité dans certaines autres familles du même groupe (MAILLET, 1959). Toujours dans le même laboratoire, la genèse du spermatodesme a fait l'objet d'une étude cytochimique (CHEVAILLIER, 1962, 1963; CHEVAILLIER et MAILLET, 1965). Nous avons entrepris ensuite l'étude ultrastructurale de la spermatogenèse chez les Homoptères Auchenorhynches. La structure fine des cellules germinales avant la méïose (FOLLIOT, 1968) et les problèmes posés par les complexes synaptonématiques chez *Philaenus spumarius* (MAILLET et FOLLIOT, 1965; FOLLIOT et MAILLET, 1966) ont déjà fait l'objet de publications.

Nous nous proposons, dans le cadre du présent article, d'étudier la spermiogenèse et le spermatozoïde, éventuellement le spermatodesme, en insistant sur les traits les plus originaux et en comparant les représentants de diverses familles d'Auchenorhynches. Nous tiendrons compte du travail publié récemment sur une espèce de ce groupe par HEROLD et MUNZ (1967).

MATERIEL ET METHODES

Les espèces examinées appartiennent aux familles suivantes:

Cicadidae	*Cicada orni* L.
	Lyristes plebejus Scop.
Cercopidae	*Philaenus spumarius* L.
	Cercopis sanguinea Geoffr.
Cicadellidae	*Cicadella viridis* L.
Typhlocybidae	*Typhlocyba douglasi* Edw.
Ulopidae	*Ulopa reticulata* Fabr.
Cixiidae	*Cixius nervosus* L.
Delphacidae	*Muellerianella fairmairei* Perris.

Chez les Cigales (*Cicadidae*), les stades précoces de la spermiogenèse se déroulent en grande partie dans les larves de dernier stade. Celles-ci étant très difficiles à récolter, ces stades seront surtout décrits dans les autres espèces.

Les deux dernières familles appartiennent à la superfamille des *Fulgoroïdea*, les précédentes, à celle des *Cicadoïdea*.

Pour l'examen au microscope électronique, les testicules ou vésicules séminales sont fixés le plus souvent, soit par le tétroxyde d'osmium à 2% dans un tampon cacodylate de *p*H 7,2 soit par la glutaraldéhyde à 2% ou 3% dans le tampon Millonig à *p*H 7,2, suivie d'une post–fixation par le tétroxyde d'osmium à 2%. L'inclusion est faite dans l'araldite. Les coupes sont contrastées à l'acétate d'uranyle–citrate de plomb (exceptionnellement à l'acide phosphotungstique).

Observations

Pour faciliter la descriptions et la comparaison de différents spermatozoïdes contruits selon un même plan fondamental, nous définirons une orientation. Le spermatozoïde mûr des Homoptères Auchénorhynches montre une symétrie bilatérale de la queue, de l'acrosome et souvent du noyau. Dans

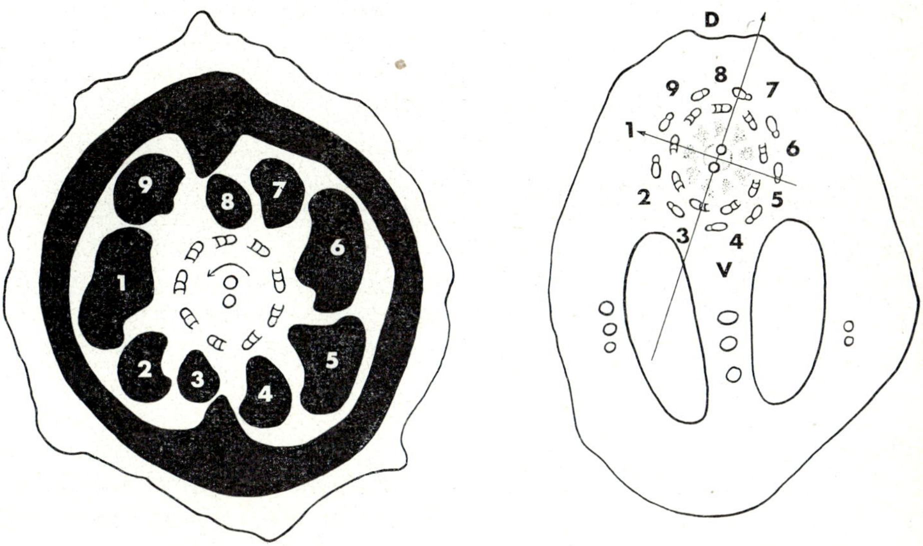

Diag. 1. – Orientation comparée de la queue du spermatozoïde d'un Homoptère et de celle du spermatozoïde d'un Mammifère. A gauche, coupe transversale de la pièce principale du spermatozoïde de Cobaye (d'après FAWCETT, The Cell, Fig. 236). La partie supérieure correspond à la face dorsale du spermatozoïde. A droite, coupe transversale de la pièce intermédiaire du spermatozoïde de *Lyristes plebejus*; *D*, face dorsale. *V*, face ventrale. Dans les deux cas, le point de vue est celui d'un observateur regardant de l'extrémité du flagelle vers la base.

la queue, cette symétrie résulte de l'existence de deux dérivés mitochondriaux juxtaposés au flagelle (Fig. 5 par exemple). Nous pouvons donc définir, dans la queue, une face « mitochondriale » et une face « antemitochondriale ». Une section longitudinale sub–sagittale complète d'un spermatozoïde, comme celle de gauche dans la Fig. 1, nous permet d'appliquer les mêmes dénominations à tous les niveaux du spermatozoïde.

L'acrosome et sa formation.

Les premières manifestations de cette formation s'observent, par exemple chez *Philaenus spumarius* dans les spermatocytes I. A un pôle de la cellule, où sont aussi rassemblés la plupart des mitochondries, près d'un diplosome, les corps de Golgi se montrent enveloppés par des citernes ergastoplasmiques dont la face interne bourgeonne des vésicules à intervalles réguliers. Ces vésicules se pédiculisent et se détachent selon le processus décrit chez une libellule par KESSEL (1966). L'appareil de Golgi environné sur tout son pourtour d'une auréole de ces vésicules offre un aspect très caractéristique. Dans les spermatides, on peut observer des relations semblables entre le réticulum endoplasmique et les lamelles golgiennes de l'acroblaste. (Le même phénomène se poursuit encore dans les reliquats cytoplasmiques éliminés le long du flagelle du spermatozoïde en voie d'achèvement).

Le grain acrosomien, sécrété souvent au voisinage du centriole flagellaire, migre au pôle opposé du noyau de la spermatide et s'applique sur celui–ci. Cependant un matériel granuleux s'interpose entre lui et le noyau. D'abord sphérique, le grain acrosomien se déforme en s'étalant sur la surface antérieure du noyau, puis en devenant conique. Parallèlement, il se creuse d'une dépression interne. Le matériel granuleux se rassemble à la base de cette dépression. Les caractères de la membrane nucléaire et certaines images de ce matériel, amènent à imaginer que ce dernier pourrait provenir du noyau. Chez *Cicadella viridis*, il est concentré en une boulette dense aux électrons.

La dépression formée à l'intérieur de l'acrosome va être à l'origine d'un canal intraacrosomien dont la section transversale se montre, selon le niveau, circulaire ou aplatie (Fig. 14, A_2 et A_1) contre la face « antemitochondriale » de l'acrosome (Fig. 2, *Fa*). La substance même de l'acrosome présente une texture variable. Initialement, l'acrosome sphéroïdal présente une zone périphérique foncée et une zone interne, basale, plus claire. Plus tard, au contraire, c'est la région antérieure de l'acrosome, dilatée, qui se montre plus claire. L'acrosome allongé, d'aspect fibreux, est parcouru par des tubules longitudinaux de 150 Å environ de diamètre (Fig. 2, *Ta*) comparables à ceux de l'hémiptère *Gerris remigis* décrits par TANDLER et MORIBER (1966).

Finalement l'acrosome se trouve implanté obliquement sur le sommet du noyau. Celui–ci est encadré par deux « racines » acrosomiennes latérales (Fig. 14, A_3).

L'ampoule ante–acrosomienne.

Si la genèse de l'acrosome se déroule d'une façon relativement classique, un fait supplémentaire rend le spermatozoïde assez original dans plusieurs des familles étudiées. En effet l'acrosome ne va pas être entièrement au contact de la membrane plasmique du spermatozoïde. Lors de la phase de différenciation de la spermatide, une zone de cytoplasme, dense à sa périphérie, subsiste en avant de l'acrosome. Celui–ci ne se trouve donc pas à l'extrémité antérieure de l'acrosome, mais en retrait derrière une ampoule de cytoplasme (Figs. 1, 2, *Aa*). Celle–ci renferme l'extrémité des microtubules longitudinaux qui entourent la tête du spermatozoïde. Elle peut être aussi longue que l'acrosome lui–même. L'existence d'une telle ampoule cytoplasmique préacrosomienne a été trouvée dans les familles des *Cicadidae*, *Cercopidae*, *Cicadellidae*, *Typhlocybidae* et *Ulopidae*.

Le noyau.

La différenciation du noyau de la spermatide s'accompagne initialement d'un important rejet de matériel dont l'étude cytochimique chez *Philaenus spumarius* a montré la nature essentiellement ribonucléique (MAILLET et GOURANTON, 1965). Cette élimination assez spectaculaire s'effectue par les pores nucléaires d'une région localisée au voisinage du centriole flagellaire donc du nebenkern. Dans cette région d'échanges avec l'extérieur, la paroi nucléaire est particulièrement osmiophile (voir dans ce meme ouvrage, l'article de PH. CHEVAILLIER, Pl. IV).

Par la suite, le noyau en voie d'allongement prend une symétrie bilatérale. Celle–ci se réalise d'abord dans la structure interne. Alors que la région médiane du noyau est occupée par de nombreuses fibres, des mottes de matériel dense de plusieurs certaines d'Å de diamètre se répartissent sur les côtés (Fig. 4). Cette symétrie bilatérale s'accentue par la formation d'expansions latérales ou côtes où se concentre le matériel dense. Les faits concernant l'évolution du contenu nucléaire durant la spermiogenèse de *Philaenus spumarius* sont incorporés à l'article sus–dit de PH. CHEVAILLIER (Pl. III) auquel le lecteur est prié de se reporter.

Autour du noyau (comme autour de l'acrosome), on observe de nombreux microtubules durant la phase de différenciation du spermatozoïde. Ils sont répartis le long des faces mais non le long des côtes latérales. Leur diamètre est de l'ordre de 280 Å. On peut y mettre en évidence un corpuscule central osmiophile (Fig. 4, *mt*). La masse des microtubules se montre parfois enveloppée extérieurement par une citerne ergastoplasmique. Chez les *Cicadidae*, les microtubules, particulièrement nombreux sur la face « mitochondriale » du noyau, paraissent enrobés dans un stroma cytoplasmique dense.

Notons enfin que dans deux familles au moins, *Cicadidae* et surtout *Typhlocybidae*, le noyau du spermatozoïde peut contenir des microorganismes de type rickettsien (Fig. 4) transmissibles à la femelle par ce moyen (MAILLET et FOLLIOT, 1964 et 1967).

La région du cou.

Dans le spermatozoïde différencié, près de la base du noyau, sur la face « mitochondriale » déprimés, en avant des dérivés mitochondriaux, on observe un amas de matériel creusé de cavités (Fig. 3, *Mc*). En face de cet amas, les pores de la paroi nucléaire du noyau sont particulièrement exaltés, indiquant une origine nucléaire possible de ce matériel.

A la base du noyau, le centriole unique est situé au sein d'un matériel péricentriolaire dense, lui-même en rapport avec quelques amas irréguliers de même aspect disposés au voisinage (Fig. 3, *Mp*).

Les dérivés mitochondriaux.

Dans la spermatide en différenciation, les mitochondries constituent un nebenkern de configuration classique, qui donne naissance à deux dérivés mitochondriaux parallèles au flagelle. Les remaniements internes aboutissent à l'empilement alterné de crêtes de contenu clair et d'espaces matriciels sombres. Au centre de chaque dérivé se développe une formation de texture cristalline (Fig. 3, *Cm*). En coupe longitudinale, les éléments constitutifs du « cristal » montrent une disposition d'allure sinusoïdale.

L'appareil flagellaire.

Comme il est régulier chez les Insectes, un seul centriole est repérable à la base du flagelle. Au début de sa différenciation, le flagelle comporte seulement les deux doublets centraux et la couronne de neuf doublets périphériques. Plus tard, un prolongement de la sous-fibre B de chaque doublet périphérique donne naissance à une couronne supplémentaire de tubules selon le processus décrit chez *Tenebrio molitor* par CAMERON (1965).

Finalement la structure du flagelle est particulièrement complexe (Fig. 5). Elle montre au total les deux doublets centraux, la gaine centrale, un matériel radiaire représentant les fibres secondaires et rayons d'AFZELIUS, neuf doublets périphériques, à l'extérieur, en face de ceux-ci une double densification, et toujours à l'extérieur des doublets mais en face des intervalles entre ceux-ci, une fibre tubulaire complexe composée en fait de deux sous-fibres de tailles inégales. Dans la plus large de ces sous-fibres, un axe osmiophile peut être mis en évidence comme dans les microtubules ordinaires de la tête du spermatozoïde.

Le flagelle s'achève par une « pièce terminale » (Fig. 14, *Q3*) où les tubules centraux disparaissent les premiers. La paroi des doublets périphériques s'ouvre ensuite, en prélude à la disparition de toute structure. Chez *Ulopa reticulata*, l'extrémité du flagelle, très dilatée, de section rectangulaire, montre 20 à 18 filaments dispersés.

Les microtubules et les formations accessoires de la queue.

Dans le nebenkern en voie d'allongement, on observe quelques microtubules épars. Plus tard les microtubules sont observés à proximité des dérivés mitochondriaux et du flagelle. Certaines espèces (Fig. 5) montrent la coexistence de microtubules de deux diamètres différents (environ 220 Å et 150 Å).

Dans certaines familles, la queue montre une organisation plus complexe. Ainsi chez *Typhlocyba douglasi*, *Ulopa reticulata* et *Cicadella viridis* (Figs 6, *C* et 14, *Q1*), deux formations denses, chacune annexée à un dérivé mitochondrial, encadrent le flagelle. Elles s'achèvent avant la fin de la pièce intermédiaire (Fig. 14, *Q2*). D'après les sections observées en Fig. 6, ces formations semblent dériver du matériel péricentriolaire. Des formations accessoires beaucoup plus importantes encore, existent chez les *Cixiidae* (Figs. 7 et 8) et les *Delphacidae*. Dans cette dernière famille, elles ont été signalées par HEROLD et MUNZ. Elles nous paraissent correspondre aux formations plus réduites des familles précédentes. D'ailleurs chez le Delphacide que nous avons étudié, les formations accessoires sont de taille semblable à celle des cas précédents. Lorsque la différenciation est assez avancée, les formations accessoires des *Cixiidae* (Fig. 9) et *Delphacidae*, montrent une structure interne tubulaire. Pour HEROLD et MUNZ, ce fait prouverait que les formations accessoires correspondent aux faisceaux de microtubules des autres spermatozoïdes. Nous ne pouvons partager ce point de vue car des microtubules typiques existent indépendamment des formations accessoires (Fig. 7). De plus, alors que les microtubules disparaissent en règle générale, à l'achèvement de la maturation, les formations accessoires persistent dans le spermatozoïde mûr (observé dans les voies génitales femelles, par exemple chez *Typhlocyba douglasi*). Enfin les formations accessoires semblent avoir leur origine dans le matériel péricentriolaire.

Le corps central observé chez *Cixius nervosus* (Fig. 7) et *Muellerianella fairmairei* (mais non chez les *Typhlocybidae* et *Cicadellidae*) entre les deux dérivés mitochondriaux, est peut-être l'homologue de la formation inter-mitochondriale observable chez *Cicadella viridis* très près du centriole (Fig. 6, *B*). Dans ce cas, il serait aussi d'origine péricentriolaire.

En résumé, si le flagelle proprement dit et les dérivés mitochondriaux ont une structure semblable dans les diverses familles étudiées, l'organisation complète de la queue est variable. Chez les *Cicadidae* et *Cercopidae*, on n'observe pas de formations accessoires. Il en existe deux de taille réduite chez les *Ulopidae*, *Typhlocybidae* et *Cicadellidae*. Chez les *Delphacidae* et *Cixiidae*, ces formations sont très développées.

Notons enfin que, chez *Cixius nervosus*, le spermatozoïde assez évolué est entouré de nombreux tubules longitudinaux de grand diamètre (700 Å environ). Ces tubules, extérieurs à la cellule (Fig. 8) ont une origine énigmatique. Certains documents amènent à penser qu'ils pourraient résulter d'une sorte de bourgeonnement de la membrane plasmique (?). Des tubules, d'origine également mystérieuse, environnent les spermatozoïdes de serpents décrits par AUSTIN (1965) et par HAMILTON et FAWCETT (1968).

Le spermatodesme.

Dans les espèces de plusieurs familles, les spermatozoïdes sont agglomérés en un spermatodesme. Dans les cystes testiculaires, certaines cellules de la paroi, les « cellules-satellites », président à la formation de ce spermatodesme. Les spermatozoïdes entrent en contact avec ces cellules par leur ampoule cytoplasmique anteacrosomienne dont la zone périphérique est alors particulièrement osmiophile. Ce contact s'établit dans une zone particulière de la paroi du cyste, en forme de gouttière, où convergent les limites cellulaires de nombreuses « cellules–satellites ». Par les espaces intercellulaires, un matériau protéique dense est déversé autour des ampoules anteacrosomiennes (Fig. 10). Celles–ci se trouvent insérées dans un amas commun qui constitue le spermatodesme (Fig. 12). Les ampoules cytoplasmiques sont séparées, à l'intérieur du spermatodesme par des travées lamellaires (Figs. 13 et 14, *L*).

Dans certaines espèces (*Typhlocybidae*, *Cicadellidae*, *Ulopidae*), seules l'ampoule anteacrosomienne et une partie très antérieure de l'acrosome de chaque spermatozoïde se trouvent insérées dans un spermatodesme et de plus, d'un même côté de celui–ci (Figs. 13 et 14). Par contre dans d'autres espèces (*Cercopidae*, *Cicadidae*), chaque spermatozoïde est inséré par la tête presque entière et cette insertion peut se réaliser tout autour du spermatodesme (Fig. 12).

Complètant et modifiant nos précédentes observations (MAILLET, 1959), nous constatons l'existence de spermatodesmes dans toutes les familles étudiées des *Cicadoidea*. Par contre cette formation n'existe pas chez les *Delphacidae* et *Cixiidae* examinés.

CONCLUSION

En dehors de certains aspects assez classiques et en dehors aussi des phénomènes proprement nucléaires étudiés ailleurs, les spermatozoïdes des divers Homoptères présentent quelques traits particuliers intéressants.

La présence d'une ampoule cytoplasmique anteacrosomienne est certainement un fait en corrélation avec l'agglutination des spermatozoïdes en spermatodesmes. Cette ampoule existe dans la famille où se forme un spermatodesme, mais elle n'a pas été retrouvée dans les autres familles, en particulier chez les *Delphacidae* (PRIGENT, 1969). Peut–être joue–t–elle un rôle dans l'évolution biochimique montrée par le spermatodesme au cours de sa progression dans les voies déférentes? Notons qu'une structure semblable nous semble exister dans les spermatozoïdes de *Locusta* étudiés par CANTACUZENE (1968), qui sont aussi agrégés en spermatodesmes.

Le matériel de la région du cou et celui de la région péricentriolaire posent divers problèmes et tout d'abord celui de leur similitude éventuelle. Ce problème ne sera pas aisément résolu. S'ils étaient identiques, ils ressortiraient ensemble au « centriole adjunct » observé chez divers Insectes. Le matériel du cou est d'aspect très voisin par exemple de celui du « centriole adjunct » de *Culex molestus* décrit par BRELAND et Coll. (1966). Toutefois nous ne sommes pas convaincus de l'identité, chez les Homoptères, des deux types de matériel en question. Le matériel péricentriolaire proprement dit est en effet plus osmiophile que l'autre.

De toute manière, ce matériel péricentriolaire nous semble à l'origine des formations accessoires de la queue du spermatozoïde présentes dans certaines familles et parfois si développées. Une étude cytochimique ultrastructurale sera nécessaire pour préciser la nature et l'origine de ces formations ainsi que leur homologie éventuelle avec des formations annexes de la queue signalées également chez d'autres Insectes (ANDRÉ, 1961; WERNER, 1965 et 1966 par exemple) et peut-être dans d'autres groupes.

Le flagelle, s'il est conforme au plan général des Insectes Ptérygotes (BACCETTI et Coll., 1968), montre cependant une complexité particulière des neuf tubules surnuméraires extérieurs. D'autre part, le plan passant par les deux tubules centraux est oblique par rapport au plan de symétrie de la queue (donc du spermatozoïde) comme cela a été signalé chez les Mammifères par FAWCETT (1965 b) et chez des Insectes par PHILLIPS (1967). Nous avons essayé de comparer à ce point de vue le cas du cobaye (FAWCETT, 1968) et celui des Insectes que nous étudions. Si on oriente de façon semblable le flagelle de cobaye et celui d'un Insecte Homoptère, après repérage du doublet n° 1 selon la méthode D'AFZELIUS (1959), on constate (Fig. 15) que les plans des tubules centraux sont inclinés de la même façon dans les deux cas. (Il reste que diverses sections peuvent montrer une certaine variabilité de cette disposition).

Notons enfin que cette comparaison nous permet aussi de mettre en parallèle les orientations générales de ces deux spermatozoïdes. Dans la queue du spermatozoïdes de cobaye, on peut définir d'après les documents de FAWCETT (1968) une face dorsale et une face ventrale, dénommées ainsi arbitrairement par rapport aux descriptions de WALDEYER et MEVES rapportées par FAWCETT (1965 a). Il en résulte que, dans le spermatozoïde d'Homoptère, la face « mitochondriale » correspond à la face ventrale du spermatozoïde de cobaye et la face opposée, à la face dorsale. Une telle méthode devrait permettre, dans de nombreux autres cas, la recherche des orientations homologues des permatozoïdes, là où un autre élément d'asymétrie n'existe pas et dans la mesure où l'identification du doublet n° 1 n'est pas trop aléatoire.

BIBLIOGRAPHIE

AFZELIUS B. (1959) – *Electron microscopy of the sperm tail.* « J. Biophys. and Biochem. Cytol. », 5, 269–278.

ANDRÉ J. (1961) – *Sur quelques détails nouvellement connus de l'ultrastructure des organites vibratiles.* « J. Ultrastr. Res. », 5, 86–108.

AUSTIN C. R. (1965) – *Fine structure of the snake sperm tail.* « J. Ultrastr. Res. », 12, 452–462.

BACCETTI B., DALLAI R. and ROSATI F. (1968) – *An unusual « 9+2 » spermatozoon in a pterygote insect.* – Fourth European Regional Conference on Electron Microscopy, Rome, II, 345.

BRELAND O. P., GASSNER G. III., RIESS R. W. and BIESELE J. J. (1966) – *Certain aspects of the centriole adjunct, spermiogenesis, and the nature sperm of insects.* « Can. J. Genetics and Cytology », 8, 759–773.

CAMERON M. L. (1965) – *Some details of ultrastructure in the development of flagellar fibers of the* Tenebrio *sperm.* « Can. J. Zool. », 43, 1005–1010.

CANTACUZENE A. M. (1968) – *Recherches morphologiques et physiologiques sur les glandes annexes mâles des Orthoptères* (III). « Z. Zellforsch. », 90, 113–126.

CHEVAILLIFR PH. (1962) – *Sur la genèse et la constitution histochimique du spermatodesme des* Cercopidae. « C. R. Acad. Sc., Paris », 254, 1148–1149.

CHEVAILLIER PH. (1963) – *Le spermatodesme des* Cercopidae. « Bull. Biol. Fr. Belg. », 97, 553–571.

CHEVAILLIER PH. et MAILLET P. L. (1965) – *Sur quelques aspects du métabolisme des « cellules-satellites » du testicule des Homoptères Auchenorhynches et en particulier de* Cicada orni. « C. R. Acad. Sc., Paris », 260, 1255–1258.

FAWCETT D. W. (1965 a) – *The anatomy of the mammalian spermatozoon with particular reference to the guinea-pig.* « Z. Zellforsch. », 67, 279–296.

FAWCETT D. W. (1965 b) – « J. Cell Biol. », 27, 28 A.

FAWCETT D. W. (1968) – *The topographical relationship between the plane of the central paeir of flagellar fibrils and the transverse axis of the head in guinea-pig spermatozoa.* « J. Cell Sc. », 3, 187–198.

FOLLIOT R. et MAILLET P. L. (1966) – *Sur l'indépendance des complexes synaptonématiques à l'égard des chromosomes au cours de la méïose de* Philaenus spumarius *L. mâle.* « C. R. Acad. Sc. », Paris, 262, 394–396.

FOLLIOT R. (1968) – *Les lamelles annelées intranucléaires des cellules du tissu germinal mâle avant la méïose chez* Philaenus spumarius *L.* « Z. Zellforsch. », 92, 115–129.

HAMILTON D. W. and FAWCETT D. W. (1968) – *Unusual features of the neck and middle-piece of snake spermatozoa.* « J. Ultrastr. Res. », 23, 81–97.

HEROLD F. and MUNZ K. (1967) – *Ultrastructure of spermatozoa of* Perigrinus maidis (Homoptera, Delphacidae). « Z. Zellforsch. », 83, 364–374.

KESSEL R. G. (1966) – *The relationship between the sudoplasmic reticulum and the Golgi complex in spermatids of the Dragonfly.* « J. Cell Biol. », 31, 148 A.

MAILLET P. L. (1959) – *Sur la reproduction des Homoptères Auchénorhynches.* « C. R. Acad. Sc., Paris », 249, 1945–1947.

MAILLET P. L. et FOLLIOT R. (1964) – *Sur le transport de corpuscules d'allure rickettsienne par un spermatozoïde.* « C. R. Acad. Sc., Paris », 259, 2717–2720.

MAILLET P. L. et FOLLIOT R. (1965) – *Sur les ultrastructures chromosomiques de la méïose chez* Philaenus spumarius *L. mâle.* « C. R. Acad. Sc., Paris », 260, 3486–3489.

MAILLET P. L. et FOLLIOT R. (1967) – *Nouvelles observations sur le transport de microorganismes intranucléaires appelés particules Phi par les spermatozoïdes chez des insectes homoptères.* « C. R. Acad. Sc., Paris », 264, 965–968.

PHILLIPS D. M. (1967) – *Comparative fine structure of insect sperm.* « J. Cell Biol. », 35, 156 A.

PRIGENT J. P. (1969) – En préparation.

ROBERTSON A. and GIBBS A. J. (1937) – *Spermatogenesis and fertilization in* Philaenus spumarius. « J. Trop. Med. Hygiene », 40, 257–262.

TANDLER B. and MORIBER L. G. (1966) – *Microtubular structures associated with the acrosome during spermiogenesis in the water-strider,* Gerris remigis. « J. Ultrastruct. Res. », 14, 391–404.

WERNER G. (1965) – *Untersuchungen über die spermiogenese beim sandläufer,* Cincindela campestris *L.* « Z. Zellforsch. », 66, 255–275.

WERNER G. (1966) – *Untersuchungen über die spermiogenese bei einem laufkäfer,* Carabus catanulatus *Scop. und der skorpion-wasserwanze,* Nepa rubra *L.* « Z. Zellforsch. », 73, 576–599.

Légendes des figures

Fig. 1. – *Cercopis sanguinea*. Sections longitudinale sub–sagittale (à gauche) et frontale (à droite) de spermatozoïdes. *A*, acrosome. *Aa*, ampoule cytoplasmique anteacrosomienne. *F*, flagelle. *M*, microtubules. *Mc*, matériel du cou. *Mi*, dérivé mitochondrial. *Ms*, membrane plasmique du spermatozoïde. *N*, noyau. ×10.000.

Fig. 2. – *Cercopis sanguinea*. Sections sub–sagittales de l'avant de la tête du spermatozoïde. *Aa*, ampoule anteacrosomienne. *Cs*, membrane plasmique de la « cellule–satellite ». *Fa*, fente intraacrosomienne. *Ta*, tubules acrosomiens. ×23.000.

Fig. 3. – *Cercopis sanguinea*. Section sub–sagittale de la base de la tête du spermatozoïde. *Cm*, cristal intramitochondrial. *Mc*, matériel du cou. *Mp*, matériel péricentriolaire. ×30.000.

Fig. 4. – *Typhlocyba douglasi*. Sections transversales de noyaux de spermatides en voie d'évolution avec mottes latérales et fibres médianes. *Mt*, microtubule avec axe osmiophile. *P*, particule de type rickettsien. ×37.500.

Fig. 5. – *Lyristes plebejus*. Section transversale de la pièce intermédiaire. Mc, dérivé mitochondrial. Mt_1 et Mt_2, microtubules de diamètres différents. Pour le flagelle voir texte. ×200.000.

Fig. 6. – *Lyristes plebejus*. (*A*) et (*B*), sections transversales respectivement au niveau du centriole et un peu en dessous. (*C*) section de la pièce intermédiaire. *Ce*, centriole, flèches, matériel péricentriolaire ou formations accessoires. ×39.000.

Fig. 7. – *Cixius nervosus*. Section transversale de la pièce intermédiaire. *Cc*, corps central. *Cm*, cristal intramitochondrial. *F*, formation accessoire. *Mt*, microtubules. × 35.000.

Fig. 8. – *Cixius nervosus*. Spermatozoïde plus évolué qu'en Fig. 7. *Te*, tubules externes. ×25.000.

Fig. 9. – *Cixius nervosus*. Fragment de la formation accessoire. *T*, tubule. ×64.000.

Fig. 10. – *Cicada orni*. Spermatozoïde au contact des cellules sécrétrices du spermatodesme. *Aa*, ampoule anteacrosomienne. *Cs*, membrane plasmique de « cellules–satellites ». *S*, spermatozoïde, flèche, matériel sécrété dans un espace intercellulaire. ×25.000.

Fig. 11. – *Cicada orni*. *Aa*, ampoule anteacrosomienne. *Se*, sécrétion des « cellules–satellites ». ×25.000.

Fig. 12. – *Cercopis sanguinea*. Spermatodesme en coupe longitudinale. *A*, acrosome. *Aa*, ampoule anteacrosomienne. *N*, noyau. *Q*, queue. ×8.500.

Fig. 13. – *Cicadella viridis*. Spermatodesme en coupe longitudinale. *A*, acrosome. *Aa*, ampoule anteacrosomienne. *L*, lamelle de matériel entre deux ampoules anteacrosomiennes. ×12.000.

Fig. 14. – *Cicadella viridis*. Spermatodesme en coupe transversale. A_1, A_2, A_3, niveaux progressivement postérieurs de l'acrosome. *L*, lamelle de matériel entre ampoules anteacrosomiennes. *Mc*, matériel du cou. *N*, noyau. Q_1, Q_2, Q_3, niveaux progressivement postérieurs de la queue. *Sp*, spermatodesme. ×22.000.

Discussion

BACCETTI. – Voulez–vous nous donner quelques détails supplémentaires sur l'importance des microtubules dans la queue des Homoptères (qui évoluent jusqu'à la structure aflagellée des Coccides), et sur les connaissances actuelles sur la transmission des viroses au moyen du spermatozoïde?

FAIN–MAUREL. – En réponse à la remarque du PR. BACCETTI sur la richesse en microtubules des spermatozoides d'Homoptéres, on peut signaler que de nombreux tissus chez les Insectes sont très riches en microtubules, par exemple les oenocytes, les glandes ventrales ou les corpora allata de *Locusta migratoria*.

ANDRÉ. – Vous démontrez ici la transmission verticale par le mâle d'un microorganisme apparemment non pathogène pour le vecteur animal. Que sait–on du cycle du parasite?

Je voudrais rapprocher ce cas de transmission verticale d'un autre cas qui est étudié dans mon laboratoire par DANIÈLE TENINGES. Il s'agit du virus nommé sigma par PH. L'HÉRITIER et qui est responsable de la sensibilité au gaz carbonique de la Drosophile. Ici la particule virale infectante bourgeonne à la surface de la spermatide et est émise dans le liquide séminal. La fonction vectrice du sperme est donc moins parfaite que dans le cas que vous avez présenté où, apparemment, la cellule fécondante porte encore le germe infectant au moment de la fécondation.

R. FOLLIOT et P. L. MAILLET – *Ultrastructure de la spermiogenèse et du spermatozoïde de divers insectes homoptères.*

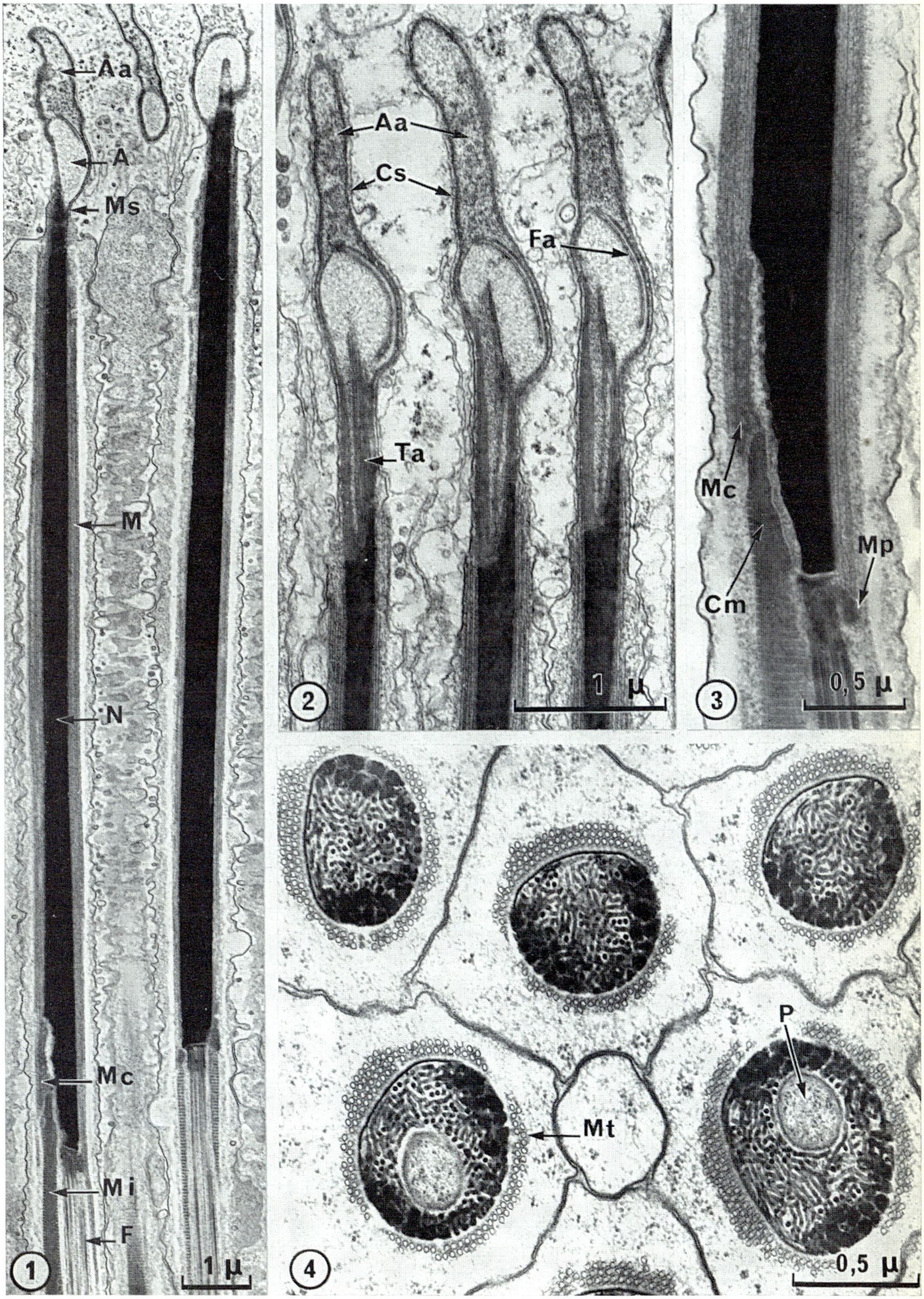

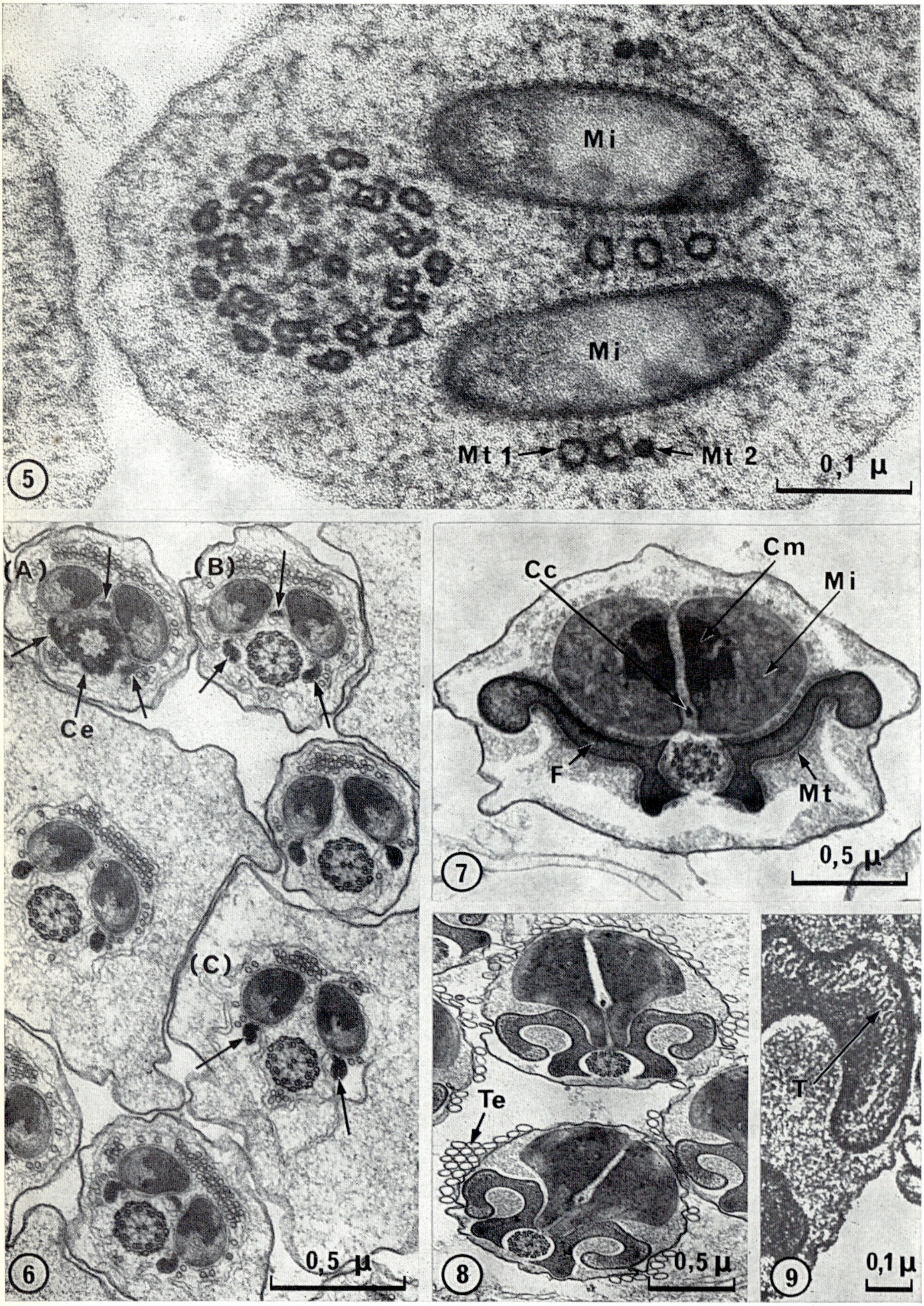
Mi
Mi
Mt 1
Mt 2
0,1 μ
5
(A)
(B)
Ce
(C)
0,5 μ
6
Cc
Cm
Mi
F
Mt
0,5 μ
7
Te
0,5 μ
8
T
0,1 μ
9

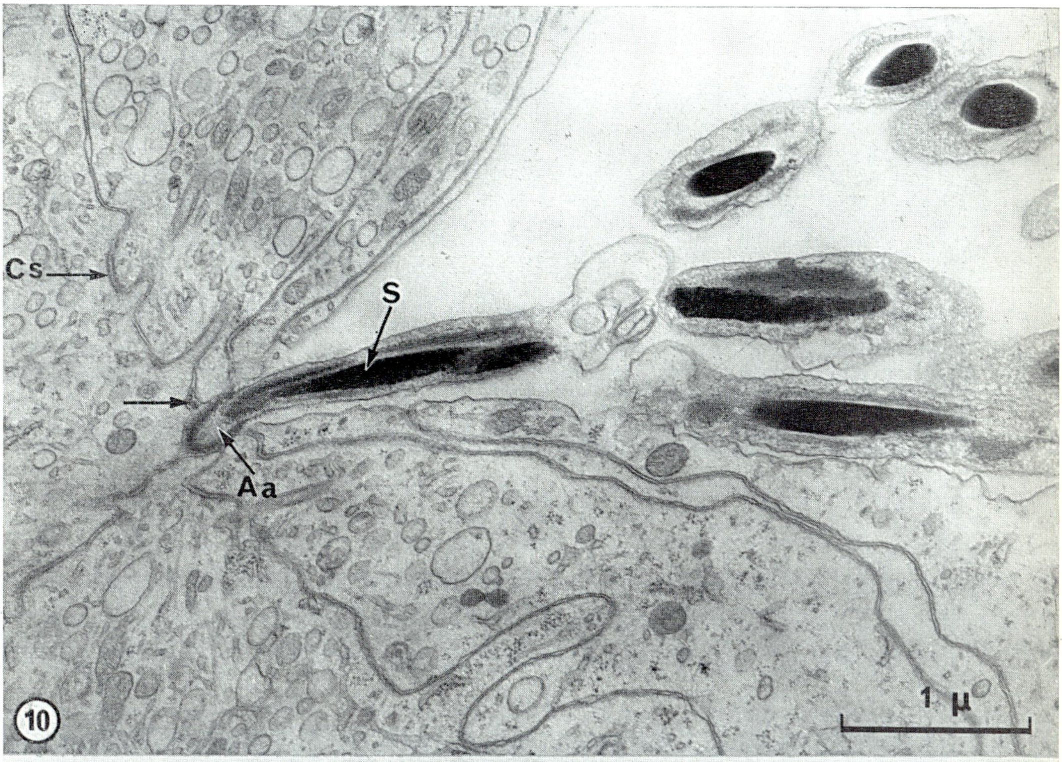
Cs
S
Aa
1 μ
10

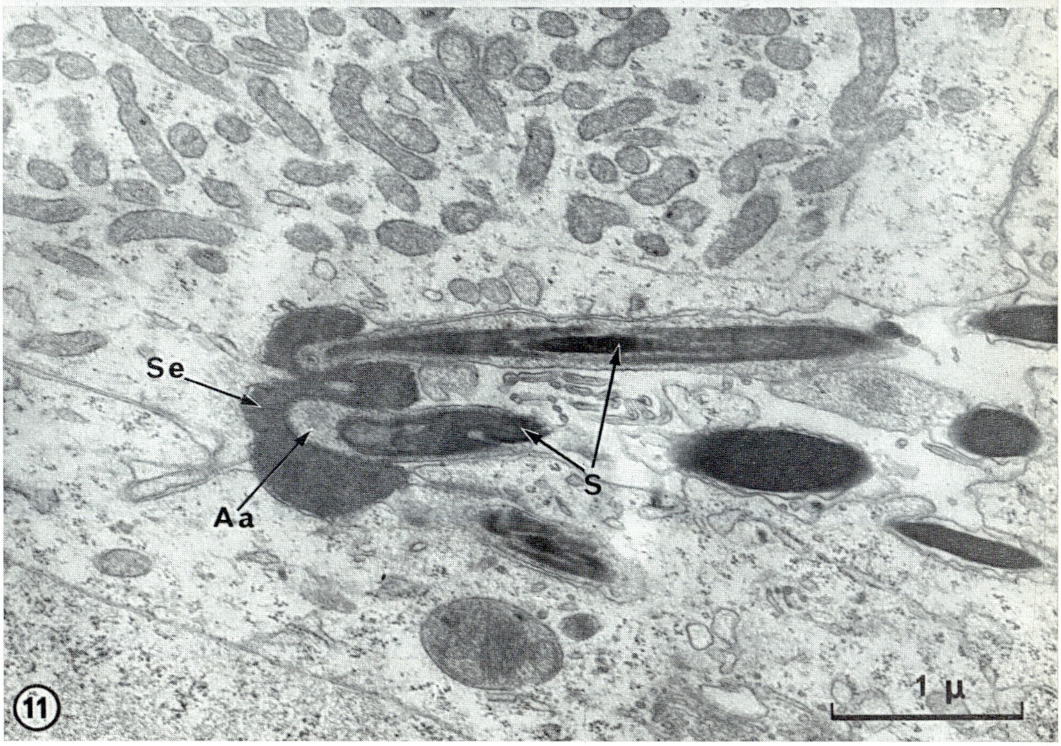
Se
Aa
S
1 μ
11

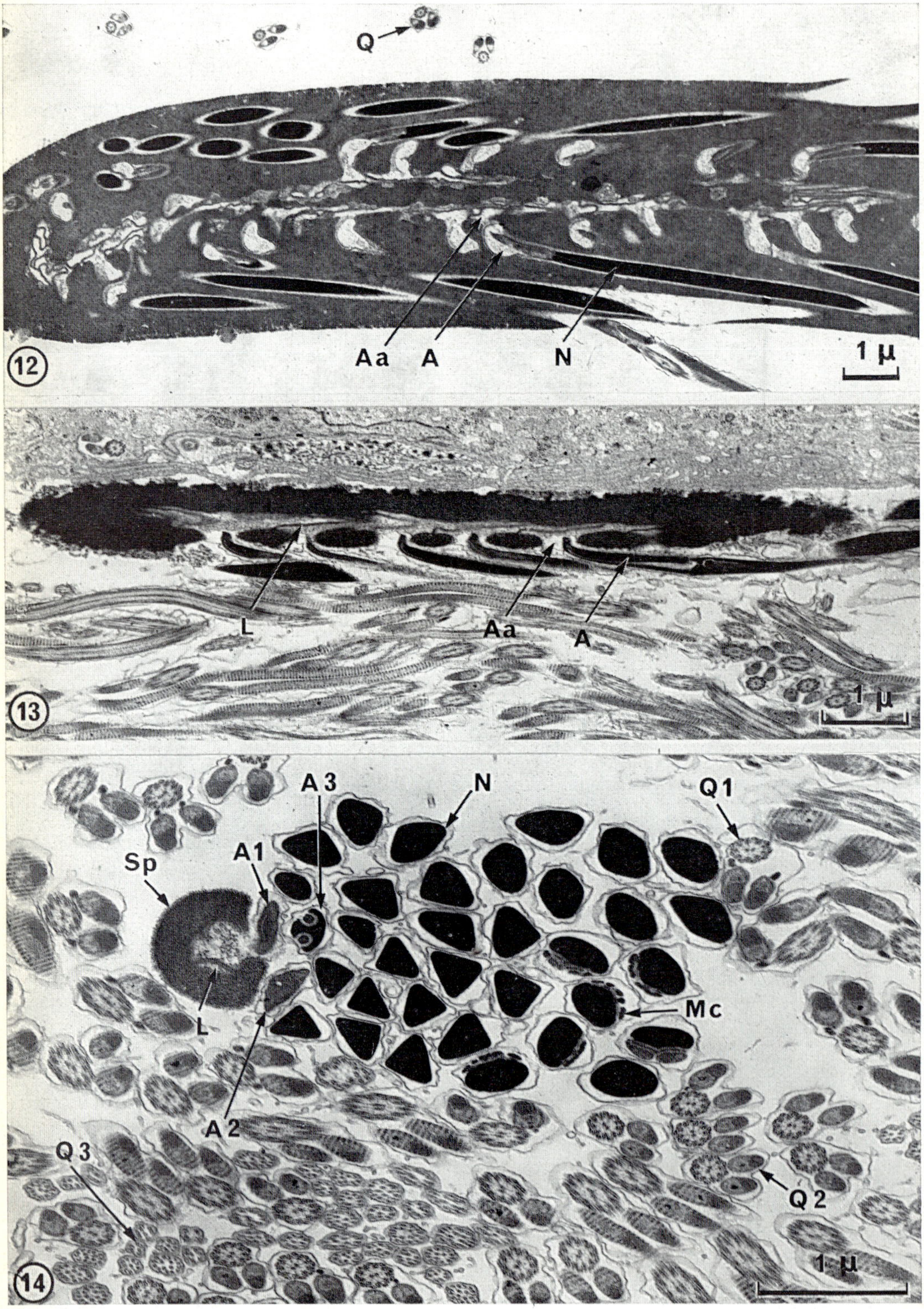
Q
Aa
A
N
1 µ
12
L
Aa
A
1 µ
13
A 3
N
Q1
Sp
A1
Mc
L
A2
Q 3
Q 2
1 µ
14

S. PRATT (*) (**)

FORMATION AND DIFFERENTIATION OF THE NEBENKERN IN SPERMATIDS OF AN HEMIPTERAN INSECT, *MURGANTIA HISTRIONICA* (***)

SUMMARY. — Nebenkerns of *Murgantia histrionica* were examined in serial sections to determine how the mitochondria in early spermatids form the nebenkern and how the nebenkern later divides. The study shows that the mitochondria fuse with each other to form a nebenkern made of one piece. Some segments of the newly formed nebenkern are organized into networks of rings. The networks are interlocked, but they are also connected with each other by other nebenkern segments. Later the nebenkern becomes bipartite and its segments form two unconnected and completely interlocked networks of rings. Segments connecting different networks probably break as the nebenkern becomes bipartite. Subsequently, the nebenkern appears to remain bipartite, but the shape of its parts changes and the amount of interlocking gradually decreases. Each network is transformed into a set of sheets producing a nebenkern made of four concentric layers. The three outer layers are each made of two curved sheets and they surround a bipartite core. Alternate sheets are joined by rod-like segments. The number of layers then decreases to three and later to two. These nebenkerns resemble the four-layered nebenkern, but fewer connections between alternate segments are present. The two parts of the nebenkern probably separate after most of the latter connections disappear. It is suggested that the decrease in interlocking is due to many breaks in segments of each nebenkern part.

RIASSUNTO. — Vengono esaminate sezioni in serie di « nebenkern » di *Murgantia histrionica* per determinare come nei giovani spermatidi i mitocondri formino il « nebenkern » e come il « nebenkern » più tardi si divida. Lo studio dimostra che i mitocondri si uniscono l'uno all'altro a formare un « nebenkern » fatto di un solo pezzo. Alcuni segmenti del « nebenkern » sono anastomizzati a formare anelli che sono connessi l'uno all'altro a formare delle reti. Queste reti sono isolate, ma sono anche connesse l'una all'altra da segmenti dell'altro nebenkern.

Più tardi il nebenkern diventa bipartito e i suoi segmenti formano due reti di anelli completamente isolate e non connesse. I segmenti che uniscono reti differenti probabilmente si rompono non appena il nebenkern diventa bipartito. Ciascuna rete si trasforma in una serie di lamine formando un nebenkern fatto di quattro strati concentrici. I tre strati esterni sono formati ciascuno da due lamine curve e circondano un cuore bipartito. Lamine alternate sono unite da segmenti simili a bastoncelli. Il numero di lamine decresce poi a tre e più tardi a due. Questi nebenkern rassomigliano a quelli a quattro strati, ma sono presenti meno connessioni tra segmenti alternati. Le due parti del nebenkern probabilmente si separano dopo che la maggior parte delle connessioni scompare.

(*) Department of Anatomy, School of Medicine, University of New Mexico, Albuquerque, New Mexico.

(**) Present address: 2860 Preston Street, Salt Lake City, Utah 84106, U.S.A.

(***) This study was performed in the Department of Biology, University of Rochester, Rochester, New York and was supported by a National Institutes of Health Predoctoral Fellowship, 1 F1 GM-20, 188-01.

Mitochondria in early spermatids of many insects aggregate and form a round body, the nebenkern. Later the nebenkern divides into two separate bodies (MEVES, 1900; GATENBY, 1917; BOWEN, 1922 abc; POLLISTER, 1930). In single sections viewed with the electron microscope, newly formed nebenkerns appear to be made of several mitochondria (TAHMISIAN *et al.*, 1956; DE ROBERTIS and RAFFO, 1957; YASUZUMI and OURA, 1965). However, by examining short series of sections with the electron microscope, ANDRÉ (1959, 1962) and PRATT (1962) obtained evidence that nebenkerns are bipartite before they divide.

In the present study, nebenkerns at several stages of formation and differentiation were reconstructed from electron micrographs of serial sections to determine how the several mitochondria in early spermatids of insects

---

Fig. 1. – Part of an aggregate near the nucleus of an early spermatid. The drawing shows about 0.5 μ of depth and was made using serial sections. Some of the mitochondria bend around each other and three are branched (*a, d, g*). (from Fig. 10, S. A. PRATT, « J. Morph. », 126, 47). ×10,000.

Fig. 2. – A reconstruction made from serial sections of a newly formed or early cluster nebenkern and showing about 0.4 μ of depth. Two networks, each made of ring-like structures, occupy part of this region of the nebenkern (heavy and light stippling). The networks are interlocked, but they are also connected with each other by other segments of the nebenkern (arrows). (From Fig. 20, S. A. PRATT, « J. Morph. », 126, 53). ×15,000.

Fig. 3. – A reconstruction made from serial sections of a mid cluster nebenkern and showing about 0.4 μ of depth. Most of this part of the nebenkern is occupied by two interlocked networks of ring-like structures (stippled and unstippled). Arrows indicate a segment which connects the two networks. The same segment bends around other segments and then passes close to itself. (From Fig. 22, S. A. PRATT, « J. Morph. », 126, 53). ×15,000.

Fig. 4. – A reconstruction made from serial sections of a late cluster nebenkern. About 0.4 μ of depth are shown. This part of the nebenkern is made of two unconnected and completely interlocked networks (stippled and unstippled). (From Fig. 24, S. A. PRATT, « J. Morph. », 126, 53). ×15,000.

Fig. 5. – A drawing of part of a nebenkern with two small sheets at its surface. About 0.4 μ of depth are shown in the interior and about 1.5 μ of depth at the surface. Part of the nebenkern surface is occupied by two small sheets (*a, b*) while the rest of the surface and the interior are occupied by networks of rings. Rod-like extension from the edges (*c, d*) and inner sides (*e*) of the surface sheets join the networks. Free ends occur at the nebenkern surface (*g*). The nebenkern is made of two pieces (stippled and unstippled). (From Fig. 26, S. A. PRATT, « J. Morph. », 126, 55). ×16,000.

Fig. 6. – A drawing of a nebenkern with larger sheets at its surface than in the previous figure. About 0.4 μ of depth are seen in the interior and about 0.6 μ of depth at the surface. The two surface sheets (*a, b*) meet at a furrow in the nebenkern surface (*F*). There extensions from the edges of the sheets pass into the interior (*c, d*). Other extensions arise from the inner sides of the sheets (*e, f, g, h*). The extensions are continuous with interlocked networks in the interior of the nebenkern. The nebenkern is bipartite (stippled and unstippled). (From Fig. 29, S. A. PRATT, « J. Morph. », 126, 57). ×16,000.

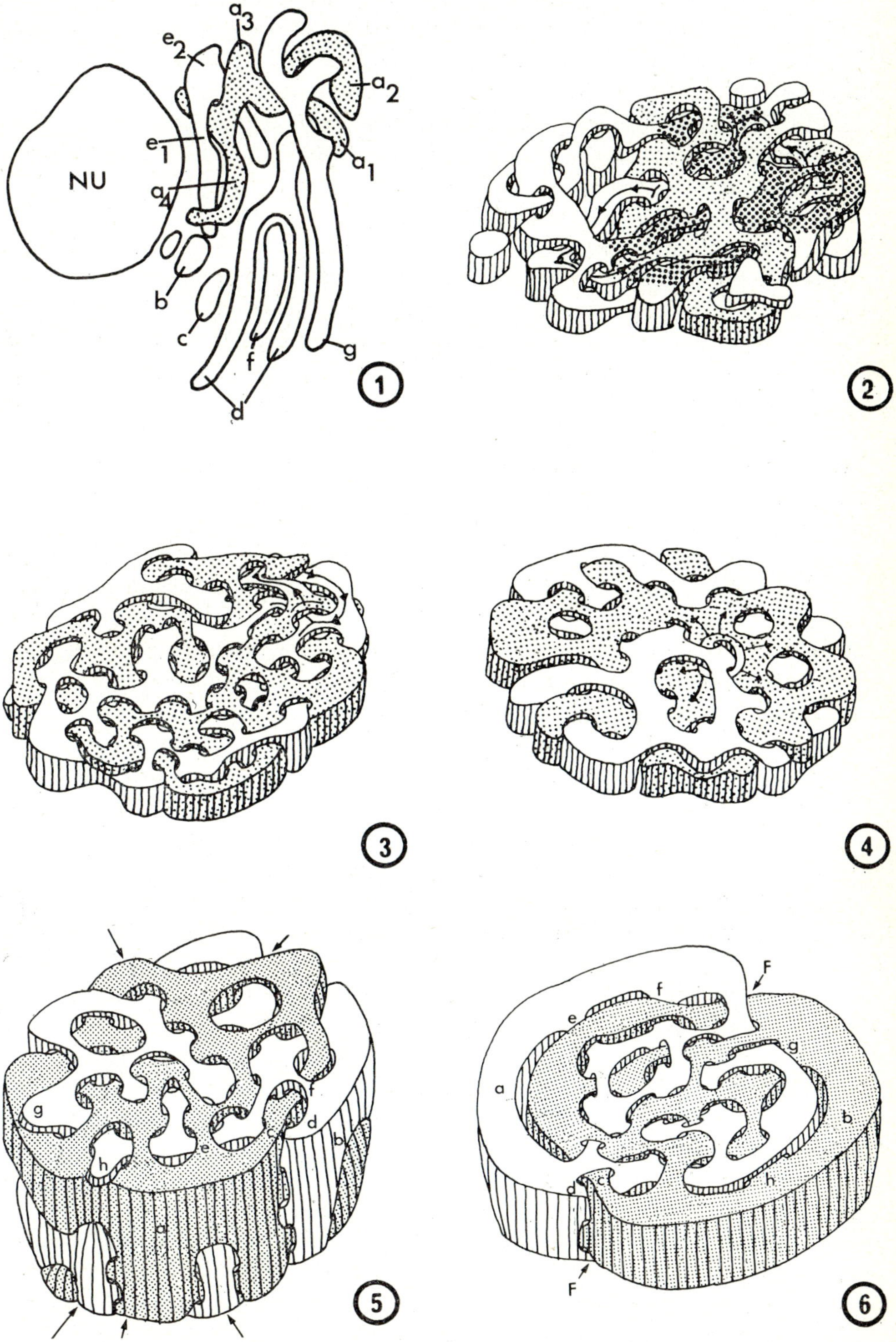

Figs. 1–6.

transform into the two separate bodies in later spermatids. *Murgantia histrionica* was chosen because its nebenkern is only about 3 μ in diameter. The study is summarized here; details of the methods and data have appeared earlier (PRATT, 1967, 1968).

During telophase II, mitochondria in *Murgantia histrionica* are filaments which lie at the edge of the spindle and extend between the cleavage furrow and the chromosome plate. A few mitochondria are branched, but the frequency of branching is low and segments of mitochondria up to 5 μ long in the serial sections examined showed no branches.

Mitochondria aggregate near the nucleus of early spermatids. Fig. 1 shows part of an aggregate reconstructed from serial sections. The mitochondria bend around each other and some are branched. Examination of parts of four aggregates indicated that the frequency of branching during aggregation is greater than at telophase II.

A newly formed or early cluster nebenkern is a complicated anastomosis of rod-like segments. In single sections it appears to be made of several mitochondria with various shapes (Figs. 13 and 14), but the early cluster nebenkern is actually made of only one piece. Segments which are separate in one section are continuous in nearby sections. In parts of seven early cluster nebenkerns examined in this study, all segments joined into one piece. In parts of three other nebenkerns, a few small profiles occurred near the end of each series; these probably joined the larger piece in other regions of the nebenkern. Thus the mitochondria fuse with each other as the nebenkern forms. Furthermore, segments of the early cluster nebenkern branch about every 0.4 μ along their length suggesting that the mitochondria fuse with each other at many small regions of their surfaces (GATENBY and TAHMISIAN, 1959).

The late cluster nebenkern resembles the early cluster nebenkern in single sections (Fig. 15). It is made, however, of two pieces as indicated in this study by the examination of parts of ten late cluster nebenkerns in serial sections. Thus the nebenkern becomes bipartire between the early and late cluster stages.

Knowledge of the three dimensional structure of cluster nebenkerns provides some information concerning how the nebenkern becomes bipartite. Reconstructions of parts of three cluster nebenkerns are illustrated in Figs 2 to 4. Each drawing shows about 0.4 μ of depth and is drawn approximately to scale. Some segments in the interior, however, have been distorted to illustrate structure.

The early cluster nebenkern is an anastomosis of segments, some of which form rings (Fig. 2). The so-called rings are not planar, however, as can be seen in models constructed out of Balsawood. The term ring is used only for convenience. Rings are connected with each other to form networks. Some segments passing through rings of one network are segments of a second similar network. The two networks are interlocked. Such interlocked networks occupied small regions of each early cluster nebenkern examined.

In the early cluster nebenkern, networks which interlock are connected with each other by other segments of the nebenkern (arrows, Fig. 2). Later at a mid cluster stage, interlocked networks occupy a larger volume of the nebenkern, but the networks are still connected with each other and the nebenkern is made of one piece (Fig. 3). The late cluster nebenkern is made of two unconnected and completely interlocked networks (Fig. 4).

For the nebenkern to become bipartite, connections between different networks in early and mid cluster nebenkerns must break. How the rings and networks form, however, is unclear. In early and mid cluster nebenkerns, some segments pass through the centers of rings and then bend so as to pass close to themselves (Figs. 3 and 14). Fusion into rings may occur where these segments pass close to each other.

Since the parts of the late cluster nebenkern are interlocked, breaks must occur before they can separate. As the breaks occur, the shape of the parts changes, but the nebenkern appears to remain bipartite. Initially, rings at the surface of the late cluster nebenkern transform into sheets. At first small sheets cover part of the nebenkern surface (Fig. 5). In single sections, such sheets appear as elongate profiles extending over part of the nebenkern surface (Fig. 16). Later two large surface sheets are present and each covers about one-half of the nebenkern surface (Fig. 6). Interlocked networks occur in the interior of the nebenkern at both stages. The surface sheets are connected with the networks by rod-like extensions that arise from the edges and inner sides of the sheets. As the surface sheets enlarge, a furrow becomes apparent in the surface of the nebenkern where the surface sheets meet (arrows, fig. 6). There extensions from the edges of the sheets alternate with each other.

A possible explanation for the formation of surface sheets is that rings of a network at the surface of the late cluster nebenkern break and the free ends remaining retract into the interior. Segments of the other network at the nebenkern surface then fuse to form solid sheets. Free ends did occur at the surface of a nebenkern intermediate in surface sheet formation (Fig. 5).

Next curved sheets form in the interior of the nebenkern until four concentric layers are produced (Fig. 17). The three outer layers are each made of two curved sheets and they surround a core made of two segments. Reconstructions showing the nebenkern surface indicate that the surface sheets cover most of the nebenkern (Fig. 7). Omitting a surface sheet from a reconstruction permits a surface view of a sheet in the second layer (Fig. 8) while reconstructions of small parts near the center of the nebenkern show the core and the sheets in each layer viewed on edge (Fig. 9). The surface sheets meet at a furrow which extends around the entire circumference of the nebenkern. There rod-like extensions from the edges of each surface sheet join segments in the interior. In Fig. 8, the extensions from one sheet are seen in cross section and those from the other sheet in side view. Similar extensions arise from the inner sides of the surface sheets, pass through channels in the second layer and join segments in the third layer. Only alternate segments of four-layered nebenkerns are continuous with each other.

Sheets within the nebenkern may form as extensions from the inner sides of the surface sheets break and retract and channels remaining in the second layer close to form solid segments. Sheets in the third layer may form similarly as extensions from the second layer break and retract. In this hypothesis, the layers form progressively from the outside towards the inside of the nebenkern as observed by light microscopists (HENKING, 1891; BOWEN, 1922 b; POLLISTER, 1930).

Next the number of layers constituting the nebenkern decreases from four to three and later to two. Three-layered (Figs. 10 and 11) and two-layered nebenkerns (Figs. 12 and 18) resemble four-layered nebenkerns. However, many connections between alternate segments of the nebenkern disappear as layers disappear. Thus in some three-layered nebenkerns, only one extension from the inner side of each surface sheet was observed (Fig. 10) while in some two-layered nebenkerns none were present. Also the number of extensions from the edges of the surface sheets at the furrow decreases

---

Figs. 7–9. – Three reconstructions of a four-layered nebenkern. The drawings show about 2.6 μ, 2.0 μ and 0.5 μ of depth at the nebenkern surface, respectively. The three outer layers of this nebenkern are each made of two curved sheets and they surround a bipartite central core. Fig. 7 shows parts of the two surface sheets (1 and 8) and the tops of the two sheets in the second layer (2 and 7). Extensions from the edges of each sheet pass into the interior (*a, b, c, d*). In Fig. 8, one surface sheet has been omitted to permit a surface view of a sheet in the second layer (2). The extensions from the edges of the missing surface sheet are seen in crosssection (*a, c*) and those from the other surface sheet in side view (*b, d*). The extensions alternate with each other. Other extensions arise from the inner sides of the surface sheets (*g*) and pass through channels in the second layer (*e, f*). In fig. 9, reconstructed from sections near the center of the nebenkern, the latter extension (*f*) joins a sheet in the third layer (3). Also in this drawing, the extensions from the edges of the surface sheets join alternate segments in the interior (*c*). The sheets in the three outer layers are viewed on edge (1 and 8, 2 and 7, 3 and 6) and they surround the central core (4 and 5). (From Figs. 37–40, S. A. PRATT, « J. Morph. », 126, 61). ×14,000.

Figs. 10–11. – Drawings of two adjacent parts of a three-layered nebenkern reconstructed from serial sections. Each drawing shows about 0.5 μ of depth. The two outer layers are each made of two curved sheets (1 and 6, 2 and 5) and they surround a bipartite core (3 and 4). As in the four-layered nebenkern, many extensions from the edges of the surface sheets join alternate segments in the interior (*b, c, d*). One extension from the inner side of each surface sheet is continuous with a core segment (*n, m*, Fig. 10). (From Figs. 42–43, S. A. PRATT, « J. Morph. », 126, 63). ×14,000.

Fig. 12. – A drawing showing about 0.6 μ of depth of a two-layered nebenkern. Two curved sheets (1 and 4) surround a core made of two segments (2 and 3). The core segments and sheets are connected with each other by extensions that come from the edges (*c, d, f, g*) and inner sides of the sheets (*n*). CS indicates a vacuole in one surface sheet. (From Fig. 45, S. A. PRATT, « J. Morph. », 126, 63). ×14,000.

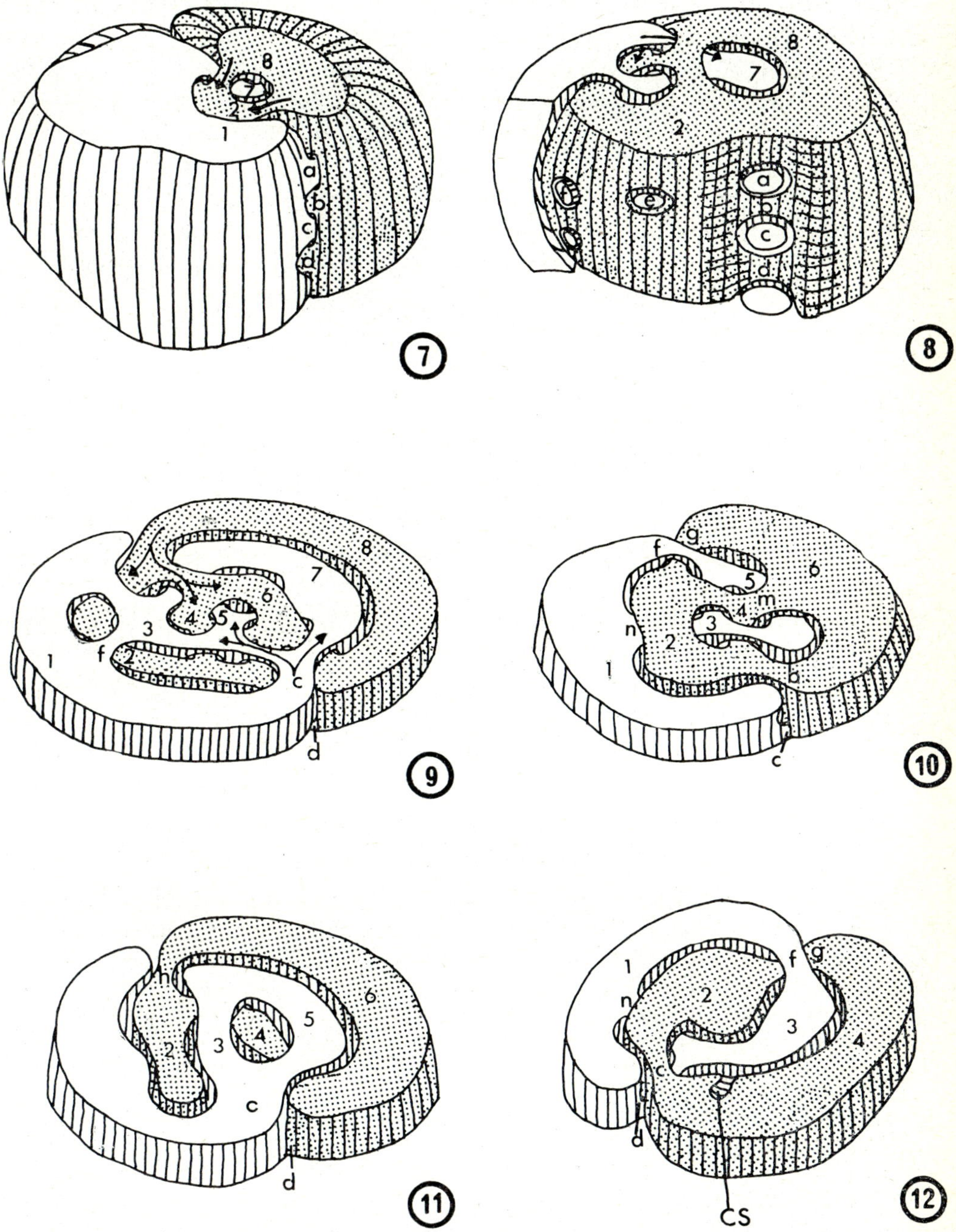

Figs. 7–12.

between the four-layered and two-layered stages. Presumably the extensions break. Furthermore, material must be redistributed among the remaining nebenkern segments as the breaks occur since the volume of the nebenkern remains approximately constant (MORIBER, 1956).

The parts of the two-layered nebenkern are still interlocked at the surface furrow. The nebenkern probably divides after all but one extension from each surface sheet to an inner core segment break so that the two parts can separate.

This study has demonstrated that mitochondria in early spermatids of *Murgantia histrionica* fuse with each other to form a nebenkern made of one piece. Soon, however, the nebenkern becomes bipartite and its segments form two completely interlocked networks. During subsequent nebenkern differentiation, the amount of interlocking gradually decreases until the two parts are able to separate from each other. Breaks in segments of the nebenkern appear to explain how the nebenkern becomes bipartite and how the amount of interlocking decreases. The breaks may represent a form of mitochondrial division. Each division of a mitochondrion, however, usually produces additional mitochondria. In contrast, many breaks apparently occur within the nebenkern between the early and late cluster stages and yet only two pieces result. After the late cluster stage, the number of pieces constituting the nebenkern remains unchanged even though many breaks apparently occur as nebenkern differentiation proceeds further. The breaks which occur within the nebenkern thus appear to function in the organization of the mitochondrial parts for their role in the developing spermatid.

REFERENCES

ANDRÉ J. (1959) – *Étude au microscope électronique de l'évolution du chondriome pendant la spermatogénèse du Pappilon du Chou,* Pieris brassicae. « Ann. des Sc. Nat., Zool. », 12, 283–307.

ANDRÉ J. (1962) – *Contribution à la connaissance du chondriome. Étude de ses modifications ultrastructurales pendant la spermatogénèse.* « J. Ultrastruct. Research », suppl., 3, 1–185.

BOWEN R. H. (1922 a) – *Studies on insect spermatogenesis.* II. *The components of the spermatid and their role in the formation of the sperm in Hemiptera.* « J. Morph. », 37, 79–193.

BOWEN R. H. (1922 b) – *Studies on insect spermatogenesis.* III. *On the structure of the nebenkern in the insect spermatid and the origin of nebenkern patterns.* « Biol. Bull. », 42, 53–85.

BOWEN R. H. (1922 c) – *Studies on insect spermatogenesis.* V. *On the formation of the sperm in Lepidoptera.* « Quart. J. Micr. Sci. », 66, 595–626.

DEROBERTIS E. and RAFFO F. (1957) – *Submicroscopic organization of the mitochondrial body and other cytoplasmic structures of insect testes.* « Exp. Cell Research », 12, 66–79.

GATENBY J. B. (1917) – *The cytoplasmic inclusions of the germ cells.* Part. I. *Lepidoptera.* « Quart. J. Micr. Sci »., 62, 407–463.

GATENBY J. B. and TAHMISIAN T. N. (1959) – *Centriole adjunct, centrioles, mitochondria, and ergastoplasm in Orthopteran spermatogenesis, An electron microscope study.* « La Cellule », 60, 103–134.

HENKING H. (1891) – *Untersuchungen uber die ersten Entwicklungsvorgange in den Eiern der Insekten.* II. *Ueber Spermatogenese und deren Beziehung zur Entwicklung bei* Pyrrochoris. « Z. fur wiss. Zool. », 51, 685–736.

MEVES F. (1900) – *Ueber den von v. la Valette St. George entdecken Nebenkern (Mitochondrienkorper) der Samenzellen.* « Arch. fur Mikr. Entwick. », 56, 553–606.

MORIBER L. G. (1956) – *A cytochemical study of Hemipteran spermatogenesis.* « J. Morph. », 99, 271–327.

POLLISTER A. W. (1930) – *Cytoplasmic phenomena in the spermatogenesis of* Gerris. – « J. Morph. Physiol. », 49, 455–507.

PRATT S. A. (1962) – *An electron microscope study of nebenkern differentiation in the spermatogenesis of an Hemipteran insect.* M. Sc. Thesis, University of Rochester, Rochester, New York.

PRATT S. A. (1967) – *An electron microscope study of nebenkern formation and differentiation in spermatids of* Murgantia histrionica (*Hemiptera, Pentatomidae*). Ph. D. Thesis, University of Rochester, Rochester, New York.

PRATT S. A. (1968) – *An electron microscope study of nebenkern formation and differentiation in spermatids of* Murgantia histrionica (*Hemiptera, Pentatomidae*). « J. Morph. », 126. 31–66.

TAHMISIAN T. N., POWERS E. L. and DEVINE R. L. (1956). – *Light and electron microscope studies of morphological changes of mitochondria during spermatogenesis in the grasshopper.* « J. Biophys. Biochem. Cytol. », 2 suppl., 325–330.

YASUZUMI G. and OURA C. (1965) – *Spermatogenesis in animals as revealed by electron microscopy.* XV. *The fine structure of the middle piece in the developing spermatid of the silkworm,* Bombyx mori *Linne.* « Z. fur Zellforsch. Mikr. Anat. », 67, 502–520.

EXPLANATION OF FIGURES 13–18

Fig. 13–14. – Two sections of one early cluster nebenkern. In single sections, the nebenkern appears to be made of several mitochondria with various shapes: round, oval, elongate and curved, and branched. Many profiles which are separate in one section, however, are continuous in the other section (small arrows). One segment bends so as to lie next to itself (large arrow, Fig. 14), a distinguishing feature of early cluster nebenkerns in single sections. ×18,000.

Fig. 15. – A section of a late cluster nebenkern. This nebenkern resembles the early cluster nebenkern in single sections and also appears to be made of several mitochondria. Examination of serial sections, however, shows that this nebenkern is actually made of two pieces. ×16,000.

Fig. 16. – One section from a series of sections through a nebenkern with a small sheet at its surface. The sheet (arrow) has been cut on edge and appears as an elongate profile extending over part of the nebenkern surface. The rest of the surface is occupied by smaller profiles which are actually segments of two networks of rings at the surface of this nebenkern (see Fig. 5). ×17,000.

Fig. 17. – A section cut approximately through the center of a four-layered nebenkern. The three outer layers are each made of two curved sheets which are viewed on edge in this micrograph (1 and 8, 2 and 7, 3 and 6). They surround a bipartite core (4 and 5). The surface sheets meet at a furrow in the nebenkern surface (arrows). There extensions from the edges of one sheet are continuous with alternate segments in the interior (*a*, *b*). The sheets in each layer are roughly symmetrical with each other about the plane in which the furrow lies. (From Fig. 31, S. A. PRATT, « J. Morph. », 126, 59). ×16,000.

Fig. 18. – A section of a two-layered nebenkern. Two sheets cover the surface of the nebenkern and surround a bipartite core. The edge of each sheet is connected with a core segment. The surface of the nebenkern is furrowed where the surface sheets meet (arrows), as seen in other layered nebenkerns. ×17,000.

Discussion

ANDRÉ. – You demonstrated beautifully how precise and invariant for a given species are the morphogenetic movements of the mitochondria involved in the formation of the nebenkern. Most evidently these movements and modifications are the morphologic expression of what could be called the specialization of the mitochondria in the germ cell line. In other words some genes, whose target is the chrondriome, are derepressed and become transcribed. It would be most interesting to know if these genes are part of an eventual mitochondrial genome or part of the more general nuclear genome. In this direction, have you any information on the DNA content of spermatid mitochondria? More specifically, have you any idea of what happens to the mitochondrial " nucleoids " when all the mitochondria of the cell become connected in one single body and then become separated into two halves? This unique process of fusion and division may have some important bearing on the DNA content of the mitochondrial derivative and the translation of their eventual genome, since it is known after W. ANDERSON and J.-J. CURGY'S work, that the mitochondrial derivative still synthesizes RNA in the aged spermatid.

PRATT. – I have not studied the DNA content of the nebenkern. The techniques used in this study were not the best for revealing mitochondrial " nucleoids " and I have not looked for them using more appropriate methods. In regard to a genome within the nebenkern and its expression, it appears from Dr. MEYER's work that the nucleus has some control over nebenkern formation or differentiation in *Drosophila*. Thus in his experiments, when the Y chromosome is altered in certain ways, mitochondria either fail to aggregate and fuse properly in some early spermatids or else the nebenkern is formed but then " falls apart " into many separate pieces. This does not exclude the possibility, however, that a mitochondrial genome controls other changes in nebenkern structure which occur later in spermiogenesis.

SUSAN PRATT – *Formation and differentiation of the nebenkern in spermatids of an hemipteran insect,* Murgantia histrionica.

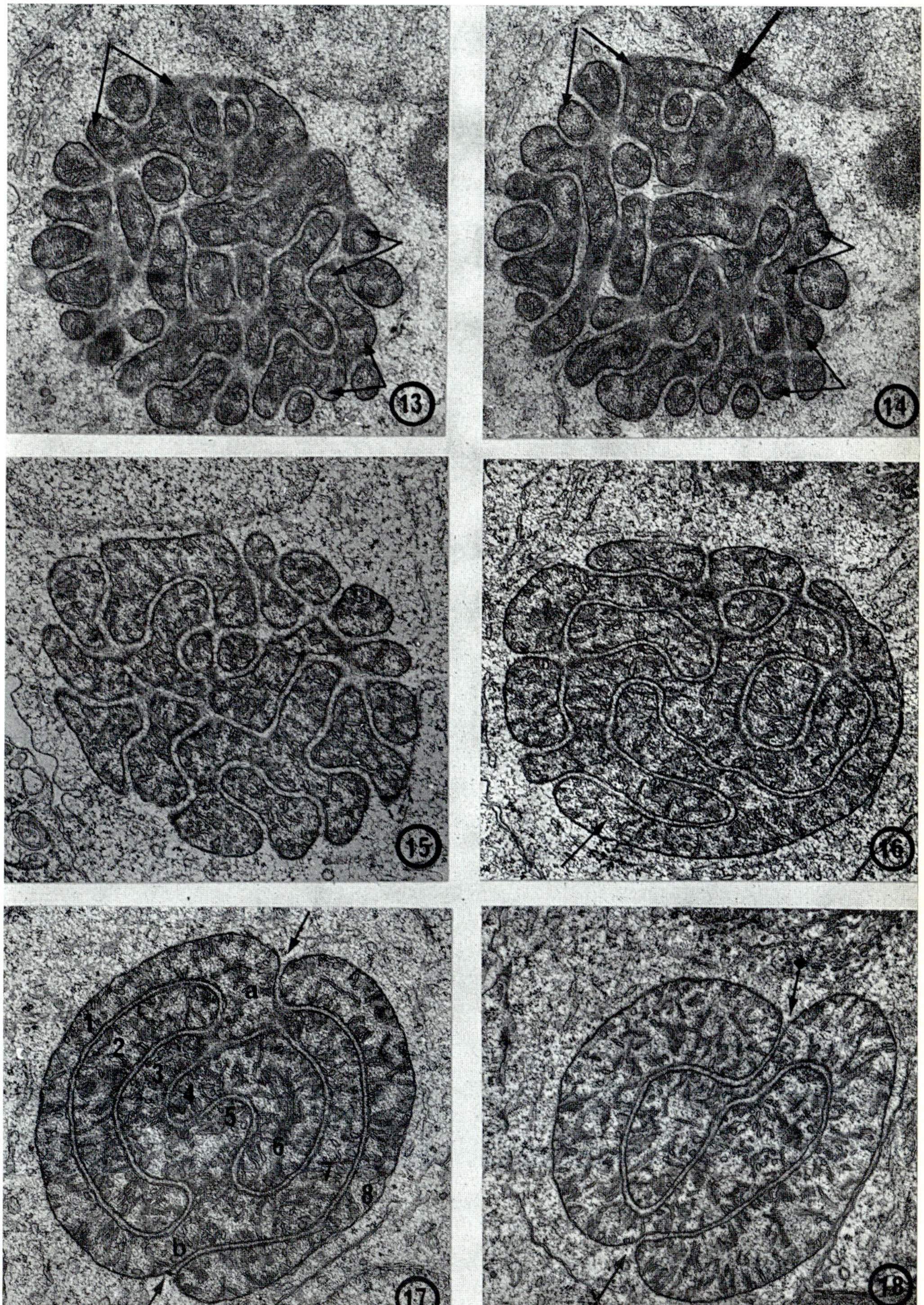

W. GERALD ROBISON, JR. (*)

UNUSUAL ARRANGEMENTS OF MICROTUBULES IN RELATION TO MECHANISMS OF SPERM MOVEMENT (**)

SUMMARY. — New information regarding the indispensible elements of the ultrastructure of motile filaments was derived from studies of flagella-like motion in the structurally aflagellate spermatozoa of coccid insects.

These spermatozoa are filamentous and indistinguishable from a long, "headless" flagellum in external morphology and motile behavior. However, they have a putative motile apparatus surrounding their threadlike core of chromatin, which is composed of unusual arrays of singlet microtubules in lieu of a typical axial filament complex composed of nine doublet microtubules surrounding a pair of singlets. The spermatozoon of *Parlatoria oleae* has a simple spiral of 1 1/2 turns with 45–50 microtubules and other species have 1 1/2, 2 1/2, 3 1/2 and 7–8 concentric rings of 20–250 microtubles. Most of these microtubular patterns appear to be related to each other and to the 9+2 pattern in that they have an inner, partial row of microtubules which disrupts their radial symmetry in somewhat the same manner as the two central microtubules disrupt that of a typical flagellum. Two-dimensional bending occurs, as in the 9+2 motile apparatus, in a plane approximately perpendicular to a reference plane which divides the patterns into "halves" with unequal numbers of microtubules. Three-dimensional motion appears to arise intrinsically. The structural basis for flagellar and flagella-like motility appears to be microtubules organized in "asymmetric" patterns.

RIASSUNTO. — Lo studio del moto di tipo flagellare negli spermatozoi strutturalmente aflagellati degli Insetti Coccidi consente nuove informazioni riguardanti gli elementi indispensabili dell'ultrastruttura dei filamenti mobili.

Questi spermatozoi sono filamentosi e indistinguibili, nella morfologia esterna e nel comportamento in moto, da un lungo flagello privo di testa. Tuttavia essi hanno attorno ad un asse centrale di cromatina, un ipotetico apparato motile che è composto di un insolito sistema di microtubuli isolati al posto di un tipico filamento assile 9+2. Lo spermatozoo di *Parlatoria oleae* ha una semplice spirale di 1,5 giri con 45–50 microtubuli ed altre specie hanno 1,5, 2,5, 3,5 e 7–8 anelli concentrici da 20 a 250 microtubuli. Molte di queste organizzazioni microtubulari appaiono collegabili l'una con l'altra, e perfino con il modello 9+2, in quanto esse hanno una interna, parziale rosa di microtubuli che interrompe la loro simmetria radiale, così come fanno, nel flagello tipico, le due unità centrali. Come nell'apparato motile 9+2, anche in questo caso si realizza una curvatura bidimensionale in un piano approssimativamente perpendicolare al piano di riferimento che divide il modello in due metà con un numero

(*) Department of Biology University of Virginia, Charlottesville, Virginia., U.S.A.

(**) This study was supported by research grants from the National Science Foundation (GB–5850 and GB–8481) and the United States Public Health Service (FR 07094–01 and FR 07094–02) and by the Air Force Office of Scientific Research and the National Academy of Sciences through an NAS–NRC Postdoctoral Research Fellowship.

ineguale di microtubuli. Il moto tridimensionale sorge così intrinsecamente. La base strutturale per una motilità flagellare o di tipo flagellare appare dunque essere l'organizzazione dei microtubuli in modelli asimmetrici.

Introduction

Most analyses of flagellar and flagella-like motion have been based on the activities of filaments which are cell appendages and possess an axial filament complex composed of a ring of nine doublet microtubules surrounding a pair of singlets. Cilia and flagella have an axial filament alone (FAWCETT, 1961; GIBBONS, 1967), whereas the sperm tails of several insect species possess an additional, outer ring of nine single microtubules (PHILLIPS, 1969) and those of mammals and certain other species have an outer ring of nine coarse (dense) fibers (FAWCETT, 1962, 1965). In some respect, our understanding of motility has been handicapped by the fact that all but a few motile cell processes (AFZELIUS, 1962; BURTON, 1966, 1967; PHILLIPS, 1969; SILVEIRA, 1969) have a common 9 + 2 or 9 + 9 + 2 pattern of organization.

The numerous investigations available on the motilities of cilia, flagella and sperm tails (BISHOP, 1962; FAWCETT, 1961, 1962; HOLWILL, 1966; KINOSITA and MURAKAMI, 1967; PARDUCZ, 1967; SATIR, 1968) suggest that they all demonstrate a basic, two-dimensional component and varying degrees and types of three-dimensional characteristics. The two-dimensional bending correlates well with the structural evidence in that it occurs in a plane approximately perpendicular to that formed by a line drawn to connect the two central microtubules of the axial filament complex (FAWCETT, 1962, 1968; FAWCETT and ITO, 1965; FAWCETT and PORTER, 1954; GIBBONS, 1961). On the other hand, the three-dimensional motion is more variable than what might have been predicted from the structural uniformity observed, leaving us with no completely satisfactory explanation. Questions regarding basic units of motility and the significance of the 9 + 2 organization have been difficult to approach without comparative material of novel structural organization.

Recently, filamentous spermatozoa ("headless sperm"), which are indistinguishable from long flagella in their diameter, length and motile activity (HUGHES-SCHRADER, 1946, 1948) have been shown to lack the typical ultrastructure of a flagellum (MOSES and COLEMAN, 1964; ROBISON, 1966, 1968 a, 1968 b; ROSS and ROBISON, 1969). Because the entire sperm cell exhibits flagella-like activity, its ability to effect the three-dimensional component of the motion must be intrinsic and not a characteristic endowed to an appendage by the shape or control of a "parent cell". The evidence to be presented in this report suggests that the two-dimensional bending maintains a fixed topographical relationship with respect to the unusual patterns of microtubules seen in transections of these spermatozoa. The contributions to our understanding of flagellar motion provided by this new, comparative material will be discussed.

Motility of filamentous spermatozoa

The spermatozoa of coccid insects, unlike many spermatozoa, have no distinguishable head, middle piece, or tail, (Hughes-Schrader, 1946, 1948; Moses and Coleman, 1964; Robison, 1966; Robison and Moses, 1970; Ross and Robison, 1969). They are filamentous, have approximately the diameter of a flagellum (0.15 to 0.45 microns) and are 200–300 microns long (Fig. 1). They have a thread-like, central core of chromatin which extends from half to most of their length but have no centrioles, mitochrondria or typical flagellum (Figs. 2 and 3).

Although coccid spermatozoa may be classified as aflagellate, they exhibit flagella-like motility throughout essentially all of their length (Robison, 1966; Ross and Robison, 1969). Three-dimensional motion is demonstrated by the fact that forward movement in a viscous solution involves rotation around the axis of propagation as well as anterior-to-posterior undulations (Ross and Robison, 1969). Two-dimensional bending is inferred from the spermatozoon's ability to form a coil in buffered saline and during two stages of its ontogeny (Robison, 1966, 1968 a). Targioni–Tozzetti (1867) and Berlese (1893) drew coccid spermatozoa with loops near their ends, which could be interpreted to demonstrate two-dimensional bending. Such loops are not static, but are rapidly formed and reformed (Fig. 1).

Unusual patterns of microtubules

The small diameter of coccid spermatozoa and the presence of motile activity as well as chromatin throughout most of their length predict the occurrence of a different type of motile apparatus. This could not be, what might be classified, a *postnuclear* type such as that common to most spermatozoa or a *paranuclear* type like that observed in firebrats by Bawa (1964) and in spider beetles by Dlugosz and Harrold (1952). Neither could it be the *intranuclear* type reported for certain amphibians, insects and molluscs (Champy, 1913; Hickman, 1931; Hyman, 1923; Tuzet, 1930; Walker and McGregor, 1968). It must be *perinuclear*, accomodating the chromatin within the motile apparatus.

Indeed, the spermatozoa of coccid insects have no 9 + 2 or closely related arrangements of microtubules; nor do they have doublet microtubules. Apparently the only structural elements which could provide a coccid spermatozoon with motile ability are numerous (20–250) microtubules which surround its thread-like core of chromatin and run approximately parallel to the longitudinal axis. These perinuclear microtubules are arranged in several completely novel patterns as viewed in transection (Moses, 1966; Moses and Coleman, 1964; Nebel, 1956, 1957; Robison, 1966, 1968 a, 1968 b; Robison and Moses, 1970; Ross, 1967; Ross and Robison, 1969).

The spermatozoa from approximately eight species of coccid insects have been examined with the electron microscope and these have presented some six new patterns. In spermatozoa of *Parlatoria oleae* (Figs. 2 and 3) there is a simple spiral of about 1 1/2 turns with 45–50 microtubules, whereas there are approximately 1 1/2 concentric rings with 20–30 microtubules in *Stomaccocus plnatani* (Fig. 4), 1 1/2 to 2 1/2 concentric rings with 50–60 microtubules in *Kermes sp.* (Fig. 5), 2 1/2 concentric rings with 55–60 microtubules in *Pseudococcus obscurus*, 2 1/2 to 3 concentric rings with 80–90 microtubules in *Steatoccus tuberculatus*, and 2 1/2 to 3 1/2 rings with 95–100 microtubules in *Puto yuccae* and *Puto albicans* (Fig. 6). Perhaps the most unorthodox pattern is exhibited by the spermatozoa of *Matsucoccus bisetosus* (Fig. 7), which have an array of 200–250 microtubules in seven to eight concentric rings. All but the outer ring have about 25 microtubules. These are staggered from one row to the next with a slight bias so that 25 whorled radii of six to seven microtubules can be followed from the center to near the periphery of each spermatozoon. The outer ring consists of 50 tubules which appear to be connected.

Microtubules and direction of bending

Whether microtubules are directly involved in cell movement or not, their patterns of organization appear to influence motile behavior. Except for a few possible deviations (Ringo, 1967), the two-dimensional component of ciliary, flagellar, and sperm tail movements occurs in a plane approximately perpendicular to a reference plane which connects the two central microtubules of the 9 + 2 motile apparatus (Fawcett, 1961, 1962, 1968; Fawcett and Ito, 1965; Fawcett and Porter, 1954; Gibbons, 1961, 1967).

The unusual patterns of microtubules discovered in the spermatozoa of coccid insects can be related to spermatozoan motility also. A straight line drawn to connect the two end microtubules of the spiral pattern in *Parlatoria oleae* (Figs. 2 and 3) divides the spermatozoon into one " half " (sector) with two rows of microtubules and another with one (Robison, 1968 a). The microtubular patterns involving 1 1/2, 2 1/2, and 3 1/2 concentric rings (Figs. 4–6) can be divided similarly, into sectors with unequal numbers of microtubules, if a straight line is drawn between the two ends of their inner, partial row of microtubules. Such lines define reference planes which can be used in comparing the direction of spermatozoan bending to the orientation of these unusual microtublar patterns. No such reference line could be drawn for *Matsuccocus bisetosus* (Fig. 7).

The spermatozoa of *Parlatoria oleae* express two-dimensional bending best when, during two stages of their ontogeny, they form flattened coils. During the formation of sperm bundles each sperm cyst within the testis becomes disc-shaped as its 32 spermatozoa bend in one plane and form its thickened rim by coiling around themselves two to four times (Fig. 8). The spermatozoa remain in this naturally bent, rather quiescent state for many hours, thus permitting chemical fixation while bent in one plane. A section passing perpendicular to the disc-shaped cyst and through its center transects the rim of the cyst twice, once on each side of the cyst center. The rim is populated with transections of bundled spermatozoa which are cut once for each of their revolutions of the cyst (Fig. 9). The plane of bending is known since it must coincide with a line drawn to connect the two transections of the rim, and the direction of bending is towards the center of the cyst, or the midpoint of this line. Thus the orientation of the reference line of the microtubular pattern in every spermatozoon can be compared with the plane and direction of bending. As seen in Fig. 10 the spermatozoa do not bend at random, but rather in a plane essentially perpendicular to the reference plane which divides them into halves with unequal numbers of microtubles; and they bend towards the side with fewer microtubules.

The second stage in which the spermatozoa of *Parlatoria oleae* form two-dimensional coils occurs in the female. Although the spermatozoa are deposited in the vagina and spermatheca as motile bundles, they eventually become independent and make their way up the narrow oviducts to the ovarioles (HUGHES-SCHRADER, 1946, 1948; NUR, 1962; ROBISON, 1966; ROSS and ROBISON, 1969). Before entrance into the oocyte, the spermatozoon " enters " a specialized cell, where it remains until the female gamete has completed meiosis. Within this *vestibule cell*, which was variously described and named by early morphologists, the spermatozoon coils around the nucleus four to ten times (Figs. 11 and 12). Again the spermatozoon is found in a relatively stable state of two-dimensional bending, but now, it is capable of motility and forms a coil with more revolutions. Ovaries dissected in buffered saline at this stage contain spermatozoa which are undulating, and appear to be " swimming " around the nucleus of the vestibule cell. Whether they remain active in the undissected female or are stimulated to activity by the saline could not be ascertained. Electron microscopy reveals that the spermatozoon is separated from the ground cytoplasm of the vestibule cell by a vacuolar membrane and its own plasma membrane (Figs. 12 and 13). A mated female has many vestibule cells occupied by spermatozoa simultaneously (one per mature ovariole) and some vestibule cells have more than one spermatozoon.

The coiled spermatozoa in the female, like those in the male, provide the opportunity to compare the direction of bending with the reference plane of the spermatozoon's microtublar pattern. Figs. 12 and 13 deomonstrate that the spermatozoa bend, as in the male, in a plane approximately perpendicular to the reference plane; and they bend towards the single row of microtubules. The exceptions can be explained by assuming that some spermatozoa or portions of a single spermatozoon are not aligned perfectly and that others bend back on themselves without surrounding the nucleus of the vestibule cell. The scalloped outline of spermatozoa in the female may be characteristic of spermatozoa during their motile stages, or it may be an artifact of fixation, even though all material was prepared in the same manner.

If one can assume that a flagellating spermatozoon bends in the same direction with respect to its microtubular pattern as does a coiled spermatozoon, then the above results suggest that the microtubular configurations found in coccid spermatozoa may influence the two-dimensional component of their flagella-like motion.

Microtubular basis for motility

The fact that neither doublet microtubules or any particular pattern of microtubules is necessary for flagella-like motion in coccid spermatozoa suggests that the singlet microtubule or some subunit is the basic structural unit of flagellar activity. The singlet microtubule is a common constituent of cytoplasm and it has been implicated with various cytoplasmic movements (Porter, 1966), including some undulatory activities (Grimstone and Cleveland, 1965). The demonstration of adenosine triphosphatase activity in the singlet microtubules of spermatozoa from *Steatacoccus tuberculatus* by Moses (1966) and in the flagellar fraction which contains the dissolved components of the central microtubules from a 9 + 2 motile apparatus by Gibbons (1967) indicates that singlet microtubules may have an energy-releasing system similar to that found in muscle filaments.

One might have suspected that the occurence of various patterns of microtubules could form the basis for different types of motility. However, little is known about the motile behavior of the flagella in which variants of the 9 + 2 microtubular pattern have been reported (Afzelius, 1962; Burton, 1966, 1967; Phillips, 1969; Silveira, 1969), and probably anything less than a rather gross change would be hard to evaluate considering the great variation and versitility in motile characteristics that has been reported for the 9 + 2 pattern in cilia and flagella (Fawcett, 1961; Holwill, 1966; Kinosita and Murakami, 1967; Parducz, 1967; Ringo, 1967). It is significant that coccid spermatozoa, with such unorthodox patterns of microtubules, mimic the motile characteristics of a long flagellum.

Perhaps the various microtubular patterns are merely expressions of alternate means of obtaining a basically similar type of motility. If so, and if our thesis that microtubular patterns influence motile behavior is correct, one might expect to find basic structural similarities in the various patterns of microtubules.

Most of the microtubular patterns found in coccid spermatozoa are related in that their reference plane, defined by a line which connects the two free ends of any particular pattern, divides that pattern into sectors with unequal numbers of microtubules. As pointed out by Ross and Robison (1969), some regions of coccid spermatozoa have microtubular patterns which can not be so divided. However, in *Pseudococcus obscurus* at least, these regions are near the two ends of the spermatozoon where little motility occurs.

As suggested by several investigators (SLEIGH, 1962; HOLWILL, 1966), if one assumes equal spacing (*) of the doublets of the 9 + 2 motile apparatus, the reference plane which connects the two central microtubules should divide the complex into one " half " with five and another with four doublet microtubules: Microtubule numbers one, two, three, eight and nine would constitute the major " half " (compartment) and numbers four, five, six and seven would constitute the minor " half ". The outer, coarse fibers of the 9 + 9 + 2 apparatus appear to segregate into two groups of unequal numbers also. However, the major side, or compartment, for the coarse fibers appears to be opposite the major side for the microtubules. That is, coarse fiber numbers one, two, three and nine consitute the minor side of a transected guinea pig spermatozoon and fibers four, five, six, seven and eight, the major side (FAWCETT, 1965, 1968). The proposed distribution of microtubules into major and minor compartments involves the inclusion of doublet numbers three and eight on the same side of the reference plane, whereas the major and minor compartments for the coarse fibers appear to be formed by the inclusion of fiber three on one side and number eight on the other. Opposite distribution of coarse fibers three and eight has been suggested for several species (CLELAND and ROTHSCHILD, 1959; FAWCETT, 1965; FAWCETT and ITO, 1965) and is supported by the work of GORDON and BENSCH (1968). These investigators found a distinct cortical material in the coarse fibers of guinea pig spermatozoa, which forms thickened, dense rims on some faces of the transected fibers and not on others. The dense rim on fibers three and eight always appear to face opposite sides of the 9 + 9 + 2 complex.

Therefore, it appears that all motile filaments have basic structural and functional similarities. They all exhibit two-dimensional and three-dimensional components of motility, all are composed of microtubules, and a line drawn to bisect any of their microtubular patterns in a plane perpendicular to the direction of two-dimensional bending divides the pattern into halves with unequal numbers of microtubules.

ACKNOWLEDGEMENTS. — The comments of Drs. S. W. BROWN, M. J. MOSES, and J. ROSS have been helpful in preparing this report, and Mrs. MARY WOODROW and Mrs. KAY LUCE have given technical assistance. Dr. JOHN W. BEARDSLEY has kindly collected and classified most of the insects utilized in this study.

REFERENCES

AFZELIUS B. A. (1962) – *The contractile apparatus in some invertebrate muscles and spermatozoa*. – *In* 5th International Congress for Electron Microscopy, Philadelphia. – S. S. Breese, editor. Academic Press Inc., New York, 2, M. 1.

BAWA S. R. (1964) – *Electron microscope study of spermiogenesis in a fire-brat insect,* Thermobia domestica *Pack I. Mature spermatozoon.* « J. Cell Biology », 23, 431–466.

(*) The assumption of equal spacing seems especially justified since very good superimposition of doublet images is obtained by 40° rotations using the Markham technique (see SILVEIRA, 1969).

BERLESE A. (1893) – *Le Coccіniglie italiane viventi sugli agrumi.* « Riv. Patol. Vegetale », 2, 70–109, 129–193.

BISHOP D. W. (1962) – *Sperm motility.* « Physiol. Rev. », 42, 1–59.

BURTON P. R. (1966) – *A comparative electron microscopic study of cytoplasmic microtubules and axial unit tubules in a spermatozoon and a protozoan.* « J. Morphol. », 120, 397–423.

BURTON P. R. (1967) – *Fine structure of the unique central region of the axial unit of lung-fluke spermatozoa.* « J. Ultrastructure Research », 19, 166–172.

CHAMPY C. (1913) – *Recherches sur la spermatogénèse des Batraciens, et les éléments accessoires du testicule.* « Arch. Zool. Expér. et Gén. », 52, 13–304.

CLELAND K. W. and Lord ROTHSCHILD (1959) – *The bandicoot spermatozoon: an electron microscope study of the tail.* « Proc. Roy. Soc. London », 150 B, 24–42.

DLUGOSZ J. and HARROLD J. W. (1952) – *The spermatozoon of the spider beetle* Ptinus tectus *Boieldieu as seen by light and electron microscopy.* « Proc. Roy. Soc. Edinburgh », 64 B, 353–366.

FAWCETT D. W. (1961) – *Cilia and flagella.* – *In* The cell. – Brachet J. and Mirsky A. E., editors. Academic Press, New York, 2, 217–297.

FAWCETT D. W. (1962) – *Sperm tail structure in relation to the mechanism of movement.* – *In* Spermatozoan motility. – Bishop D. W., editor. « Amer. Assoc. Adv. Sci. », Washington, D.C., 147–169.

FAWCETT D. W. (1965) – *The anatomy of the mammalian spermatozoon with particular reference to the guinea pig.* « Zeitschrift fur Zelforschung », 67, 279–296.

FAWCETT D. W. (1968) – *The topographical relationship between the plane of the central pair of flagellar fibrils and the transverse axis of the head in guinea pig spermatozoa.* « J. Cell Science », 3, 187–198.

FAWCETT D. W. and ITO S. (1965) – *The fine structure of bat spermatozoa.* « Amer. J. Anatomy », 116, 567–610.

FAWCETT D. W. and PORTER K. R. (1954) – *A study of the fine structure of ciliated epithelia.* « J. Morphol. », 94, 221–281.

GIBBONS I. R. (1961) – *The relationship between the fine structure and direction of beat in gill cilia of a lamellibranch mollusc.* « J. Biophysic. and Biochem. Cytol. », 11, 179–205.

GIBBONS I. R. (1967). – *The organization of cilia and flegella. In Molecular organization and biological function.* – Allen J. M., editor. Harper and Row, New York, 211–237.

GORDON M. and BENSCH K. G. (1968) – *Cytochemical differentiation of the guinea pig sperm flagellum with phosphotungstic acid.* « J. Ultrastructure Research », 24, 33–50.

GRIMSTONE A. V. and CLEVELAND L. R. (1965) – *The fine structure and function of the contractile axostyles of certain flagellates.* « J. Cell. Biology », 24, 387–400.

HICKMAN C. P. (1931) – *The spermiogenesis of* Succinea ovalis *Say, with special reference to the components of the sperm.* « J. Morphol. », 51, 243–289.

HOLWILL M. E. J. (1966) – *Physical aspects of flagellar movement.* – « Physiological Reviews », 46, 696–785.

HUGHES-SCHRADER S. (1946) – *A new type of spermiogenesis in iceryine coccids, with linear alignment of chromosomes in the sperm.* « J. Morphol. », 78, 43–77.

HUGHES-SCHRADER S. (1948) – *Cytology of coccids* (*Coccoidea–Homoptera*). « Adv. in Genetics », 2, 127–203.

HYMAN O. W. (1923) – *Spermic dimorphism in* Fasciolaria tulipa. « J. Morphol. », 37, 307–383.

KINOSITA H. and MURAKAMI A. (1967) – *Control of ciliary motion.* « Physiological Reviews », 47, 53–82.

MOSES M. J. (1966) – *Cytoplasmic and intra-nuclear microtubules in relation to development, chromosome morphology, and motility of an aflagellate spermatozoon.* « Science », 154, 424–425.

MOSES M. J. and COLEMAN J. R. (1964) – *Structural patterns and the functional organization of chromosomes.* – In *The role of chromosomes in development.* Locke M., editor. Academic Press, New York, 11–49.

NEBEL B. R. (1956) – *Discussion of paper by Kaufmann B. P. and McDonald M. R.*, « Cold Spring Harbor Symp. Quant. Biol. », 21, 244–246.

NEBEL B. R. (1957) – *Chromosomal and cytoplasmic microfibrillae in sperm of an iceryine coccid.* « J. Heredity », 48, 51–56.

NUR U. (1962) – *Sperms, sperm bundles and fertilization in a mealy bug,* Pseudococcus obscurus *Essig.* (*Homoptera: Coccoidea*). « J. Morphol. », 111, 173–199.

PÁRDUCZ B. (1967) – *Ciliary movement and coordination in ciliates.* International Review of Cytology, 21, 91–128.

PHILLIPS D. M. (1969) – *Exceptions to the prevailing pattern of tubules* (9+9+2) *in the sperm flagella of certain insect species.* « J. Cell Biology », 40, 28–43.

PORTER K. R. (1966) – *Cytoplasmic microtubules and their functions.* In *Principles of Biomolecular Organization.* – Wolstenhome G. E. W. and O'Connor M., editors. J. A. Churchill, Ltd., London, 308–356.

RINGO D. L. (1967) – *Flagellar motion and fine structure of the flagellar apparatus in* Chlamydomonas. « J. Cell Biology », 33, 543–571.

ROBISON W. G., Jr. (1966) – *Microtubules in relation to the motility of a sperm syncytium in an armored scale insect.* « J. Cell Biology », 29, 251–265.

ROBISON W. G., Jr. (1968 a) – *Flagellation and direction of bending in relation to unusual patterns of microtubules.* « J. Cell Biology », 39, 112 a–113 a.

ROBISON W. G., Jr. (1968 b) – *Microtubular patterns in motility of sperm and sperm bundles of coccid insects.* « J. Cell Biology », 39, 159 a.

ROBISON W. G., Jr. and MOSES M. J. (1970) – *Sperm and sperm bundles: formation, structure, and function.* – *In Biology of the Coccids.* Beardsley J. W. and Brown S. W., editors. Manuscript in preparation, copyrights reserved for Appleton–Century–Crofts, New York.

ROSS J. (1967) – *Microtubular and corkscrew structures in the motile sperm bundles of the mealybug.* « J. Cell Biology », 35, 118 a.

ROSS J. and ROBISON W. G., Jr. (1969) – *Unusual microtubular patterns and three–dimensional movement of mealybug sperm and sperm bundles.* « J. Cell Biology », 40, 426–445.

SATIR P. (1968) – *Studies on cilia:* III. *Further studies on the cilium tip and a " sliding filament " model of ciliary motility.* « J. Cell Biology », 39, 77–94.

SILVEIRA M. (1969) – *Ultrastructural studies on a " Nine plus One " flagellum* I. « J. Ultrastructure Research », 26, 274–288.

SLEIGH M. A. (1962) – *The biology of cilia and flagella.* – Macmillan Company, New York.

TARGIONI–TOZETTI A. (1867) – *Studii sulle cocciniglie.* – *Società Italiana di Scienze Naturali,* « Memorie », 3, 1–87.

TUZET O. (1930) – *Recherches sur la spermatogenèse des prosobranches* « Arch. Zool. Exp. et Gén. », 70, 95–299.

WALKER M. and MCGREGOR H. C. (1968) – *Spermatogenesis and the structure of the mature sperm in* Nucella lapillus (*L*). « J. Cell Science », 3, 95–104.

EXPLANATION OF FIGURES

Fig. 1. – Bundle of more than 80 spermatozoa from *Matsucoccus bisetosus,* showing undulations which progress from anterior (lower left) to posterior (upper right) in these filamentous cells. Looped spermatozoa (arrows) could be interpreted to demonstrate two-dimensional bending (Phase contrast, × 1,200).

Figs. 2–7. – Transected spermatozoa of various coccid insects imaged at 90,000 magnification to show variations in sperm diameter and patterns of microtubules: 2) the anterior half of the spermatozoon of *Parlatoria oleae* has 45–50 microtubules arranged in a spiral of 1 1/2 turns, around a core of chromatin; 3) the posterior half of the *Parlatoria oleae* spermatozoon has no nuclear core, but contains a moderately electron dense material; 4) the spermatozoon of *Stomacoccus plantani* has 20–30 microtubules arranged in 1 1/2 concentric rings around a very thin filament of chromatin throughout its length; 5) the spermatozoon of *Kermes sp.* has 50–60 microtubules arranged in 1 1/2–2 1/2 concentric rings around a large, often multistranded, core of chromatin which runs almost its entire length; 6) the spermatozoon of *Puto albicans* has approxomately 100 microtubules arranged in 2 1/2–3 1/2 rings around several thread-like strands of chromatin, and 7) the spermatozoon of *Matsucoccus bisetosus* has approximately 200 microtubules in 7 or more rings which form a secondary pattern of about 25 rows of whorled radii.

Fig. 8. – " Living " spermatozoa of *Parlatoria oleae* in a naturally bent state. The disc-shaped cyst contains approximately 32 filamentous spermatozoa which are grouped into two bundles. They circle within the cyst 2–4 times by bending in a single plane, toward the center of the disc (Phase contrast, ×1,700).

Fig. 9. – Transections of 5 disc-shaped cysts with naturally bent spermatozoa such as those in Figure 8, but showing only one side of each cyst. Each of the two sperm bundles of a cyst has been transected 3–4 times, once per revolution. The dense cores in the spermatozoa represent their nuclear material which runs only half their length and therefore is not seen in all transections. The plane of sectioning is perpendicular to the direction of spermatozoan bending and the centers of the cysts lie outside the figure to the lower right (×9,000).

Fig. 10. – Spiral microtublar pattern of *Parlatoria oleae* in relation to spermatozoan bending. This transection of one side of a cyst shows similarly aligned microtublar patterns for all the spermatozoa in 2 sperm bundles which have been transected 3 and 4 times each. The center of the cyst is off the micrograph, somewhat to the lower left. All the spermatozoa are aligned so that their spiral pattern of microtubules has two rows toward the periphery of the cyst and one toward the center. Therefore, the spermatozoa are bent at right angles to a reference line which would connect the two ends of their spiral microtublar patterns and divide them into two sectors with unequal numbers of microtubules (×30,000).

Fig. 11. – Spermatozoa coiled around the nucleus of a specialized cell (vestibule cell) in the female reproductive tract of *Parlatoria oleae*, where they await maturation of the oocyte (Acetocarmine squash, phase contrast, ×1,900).

Fig. 12. – Transection of a vestibule cell in the female reproductive tract of *Parlatoria oleae*, with approximately 2 spermatozoa coiled around the nucleus (×9,000).

Fig. 13. – Transection through one rim of a disc-shaped vestibule cell, showing similar orientations of the spiral microtubular pattern in several spermatozoan transections. The cell center and the direction of bending are approximately straight down (×70,000).

Discussion

AFZELIUS. – When you find small bridges at the microtubules you interpret them as something similar to FAWCETT'S satellite fibers. Would it not be more natural to conclude as does WILSON « J. Cell Biol. », 1969, 854–859 that they are the equivalent to the arms of the ciliary filaments?

ROBISON. – Your suggestion is a good one. Perhaps it would be best to make no conclusion or even to speculate on this matter until more information is available.

W. GERALD ROBISON, JR. – *Unusual arrangements of microtubules in relation to mechanisms of sperm movement.*

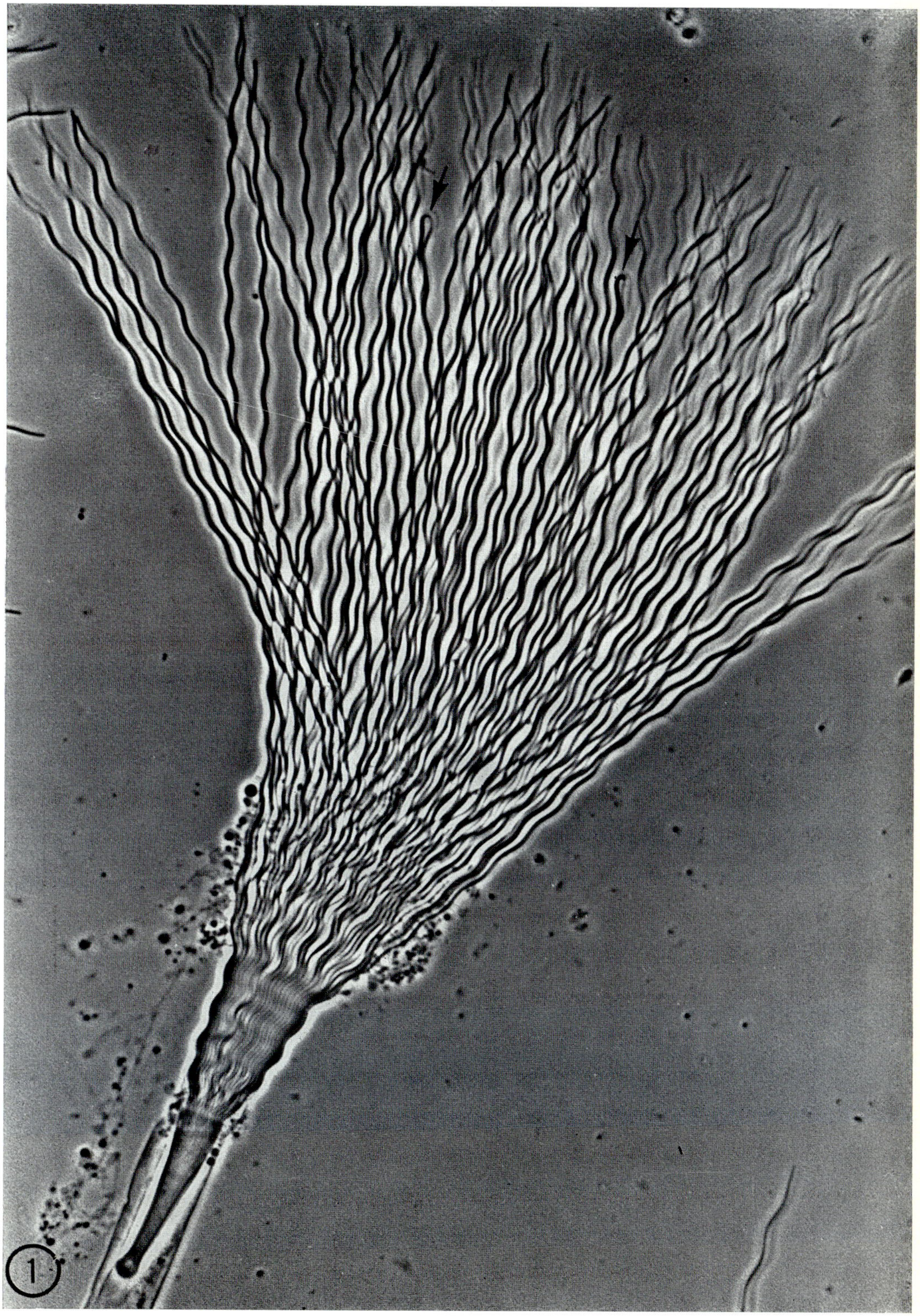

W. Gerald Robison, Jr. – *Unusual arrangements of microtubules in relation to mechanisms of sperm movement.*

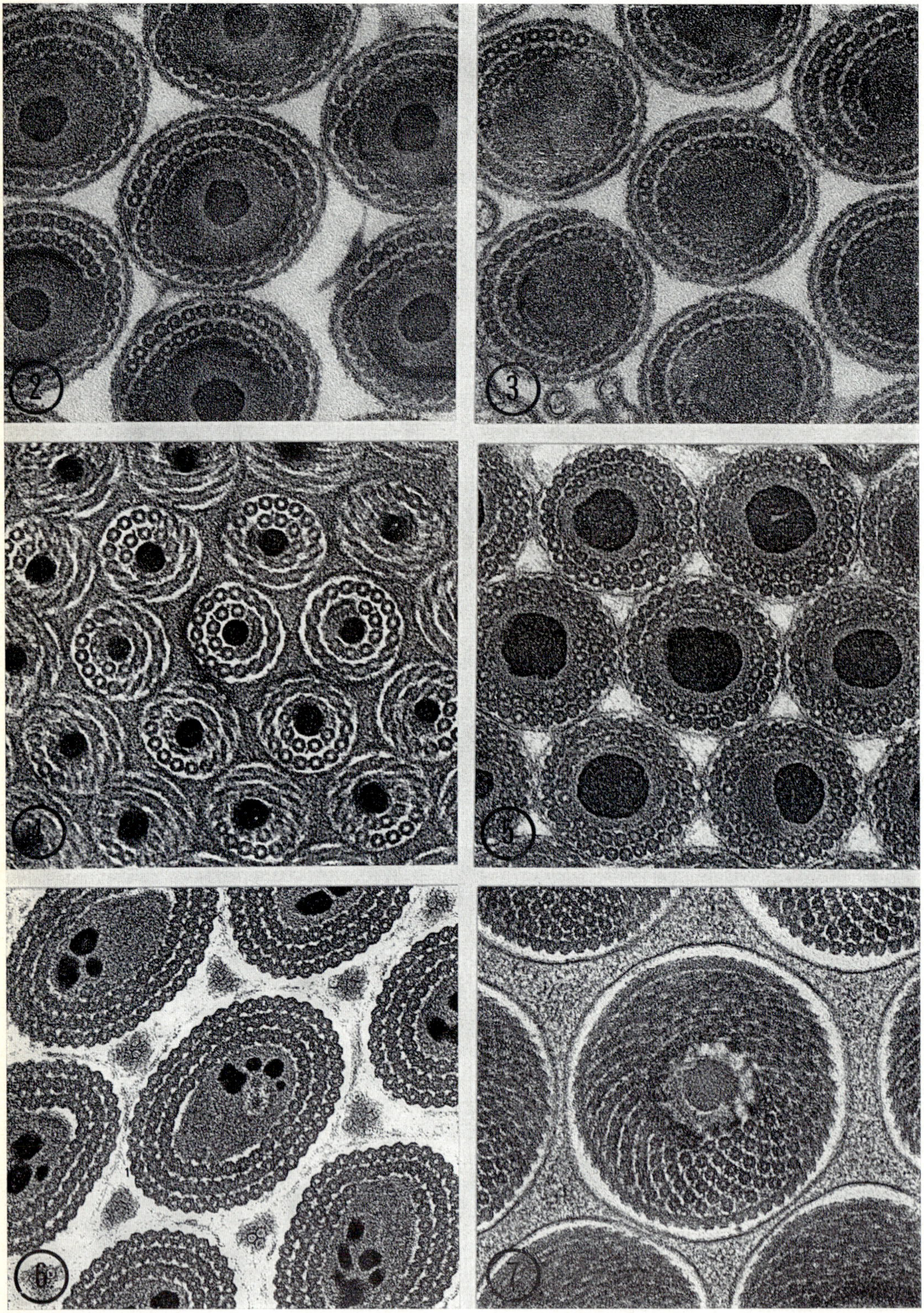

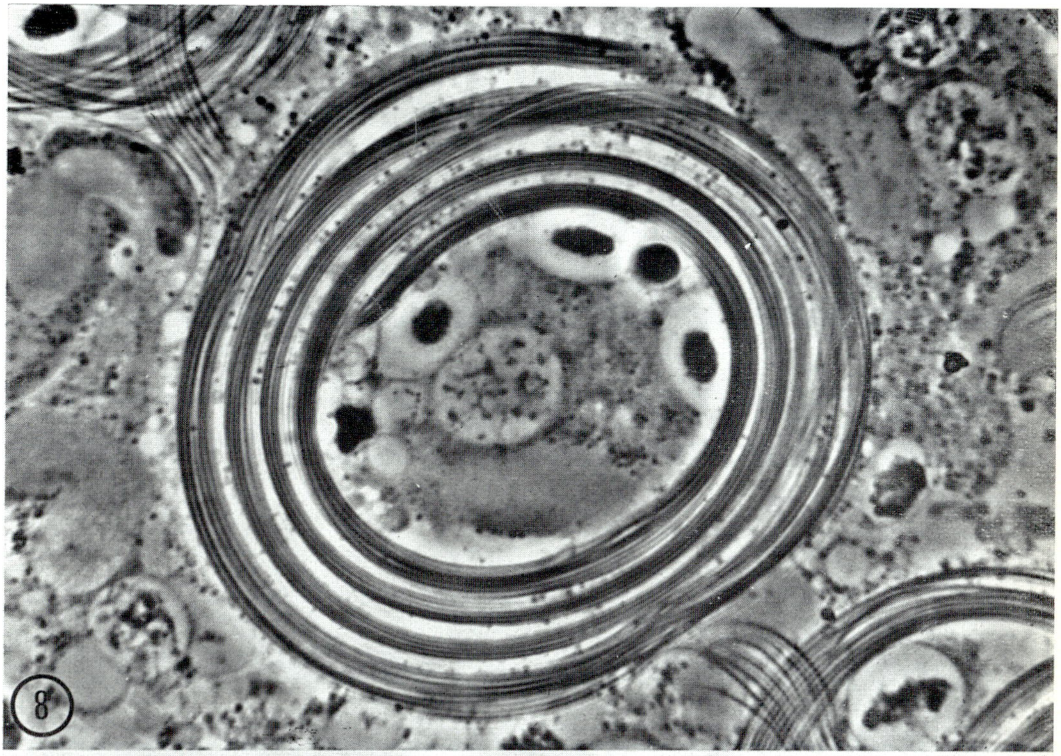
8

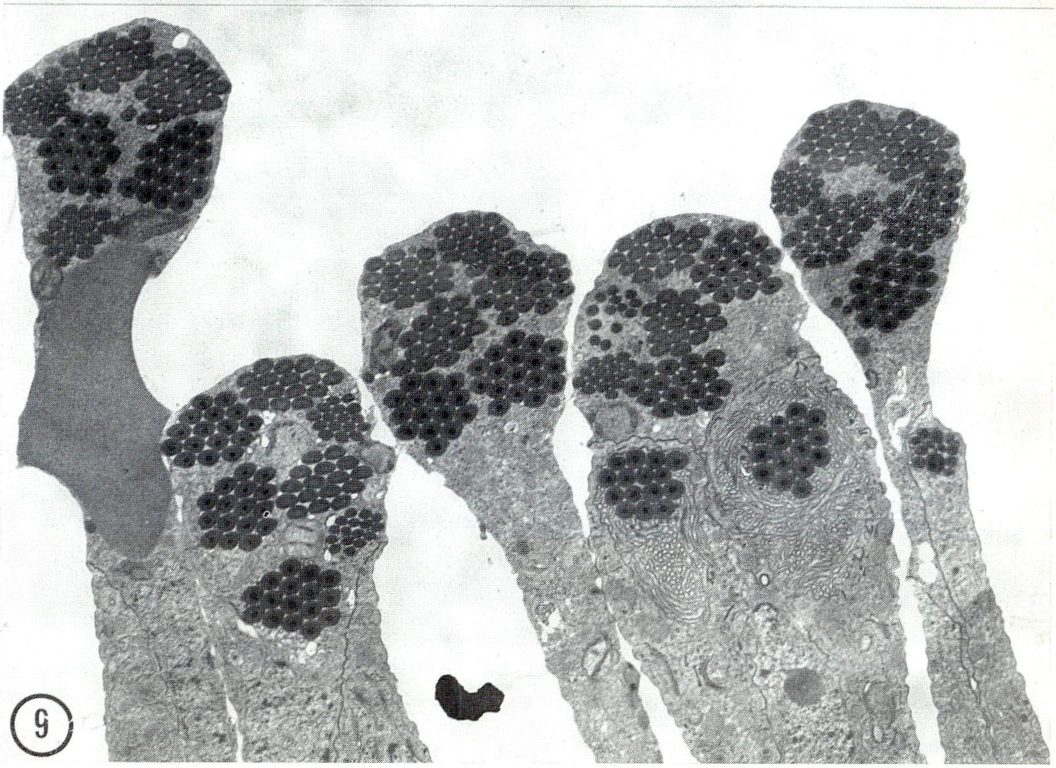
9

W. GERALD ROBISON, JR. – *Unusual arrangements of microtubules in relation to mechanism of sperm movement.*

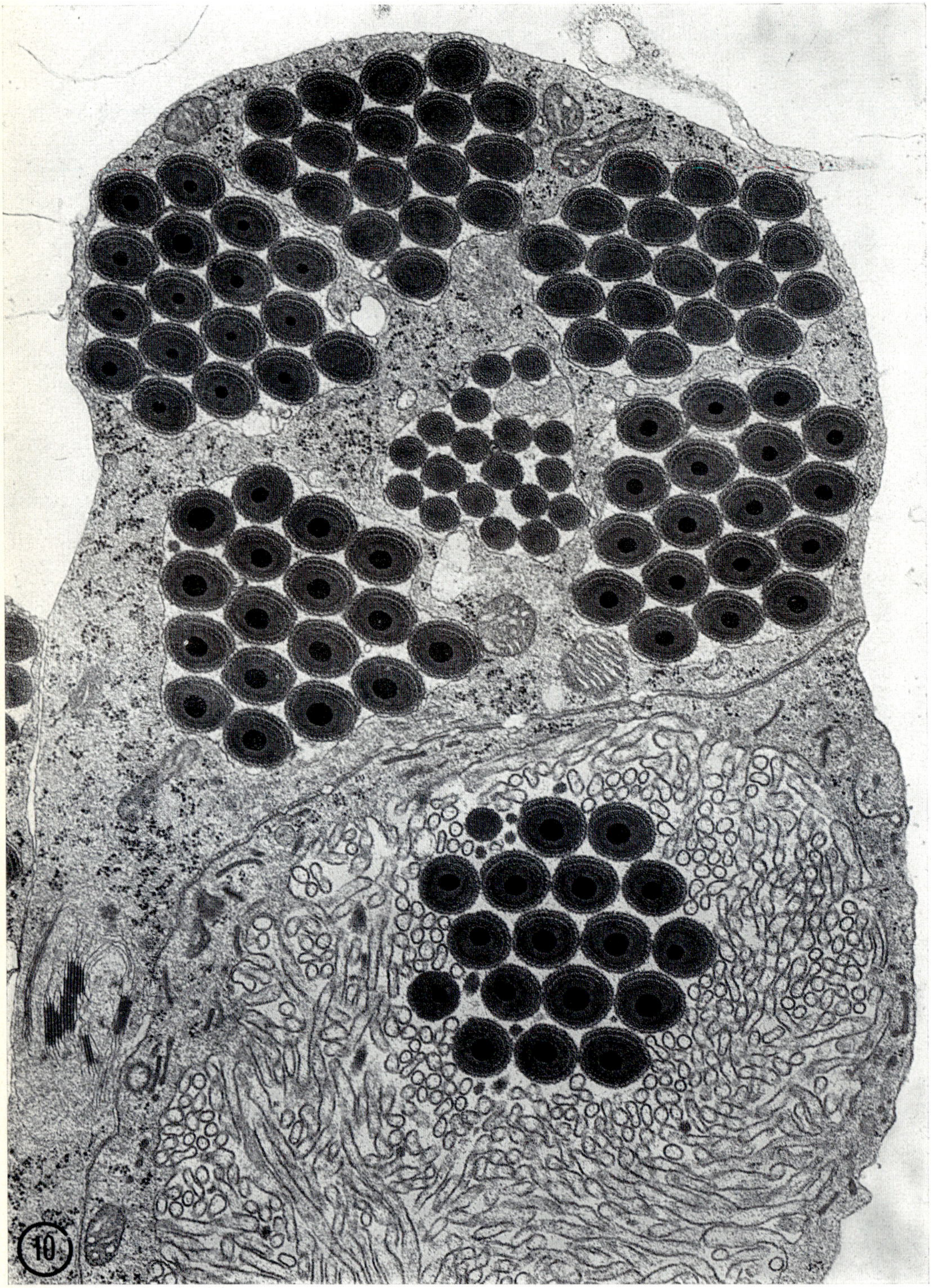

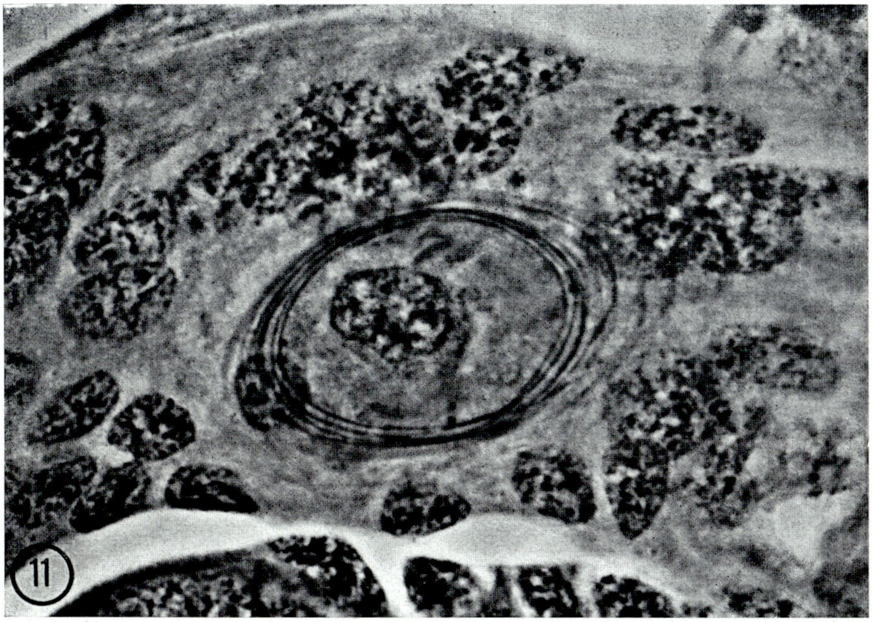

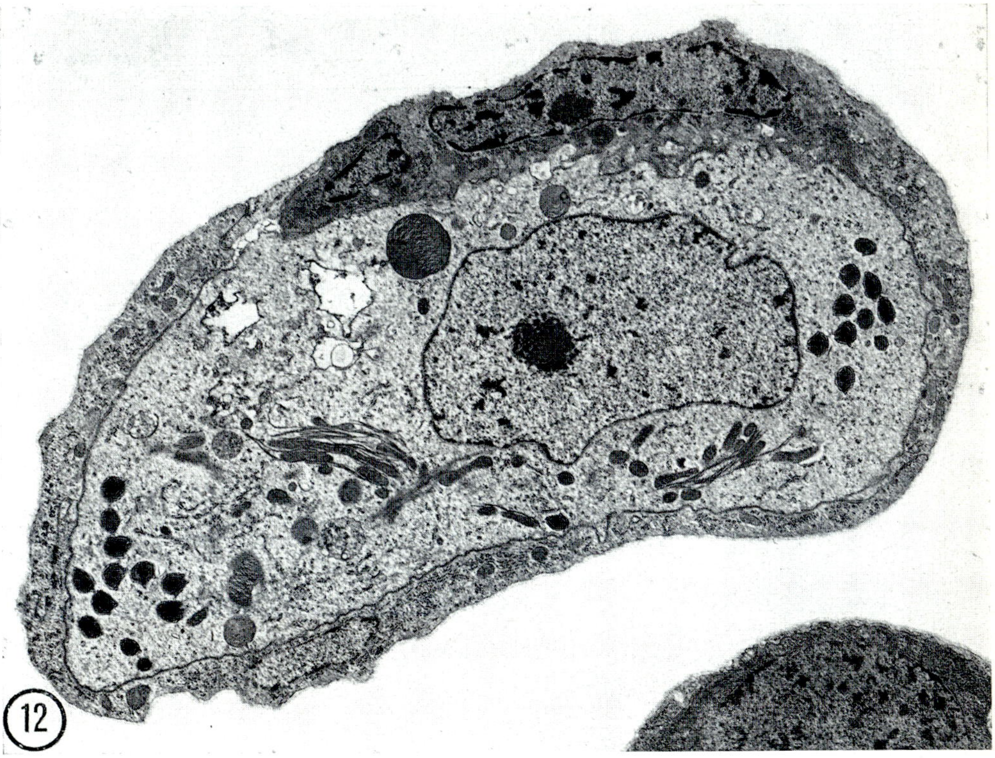

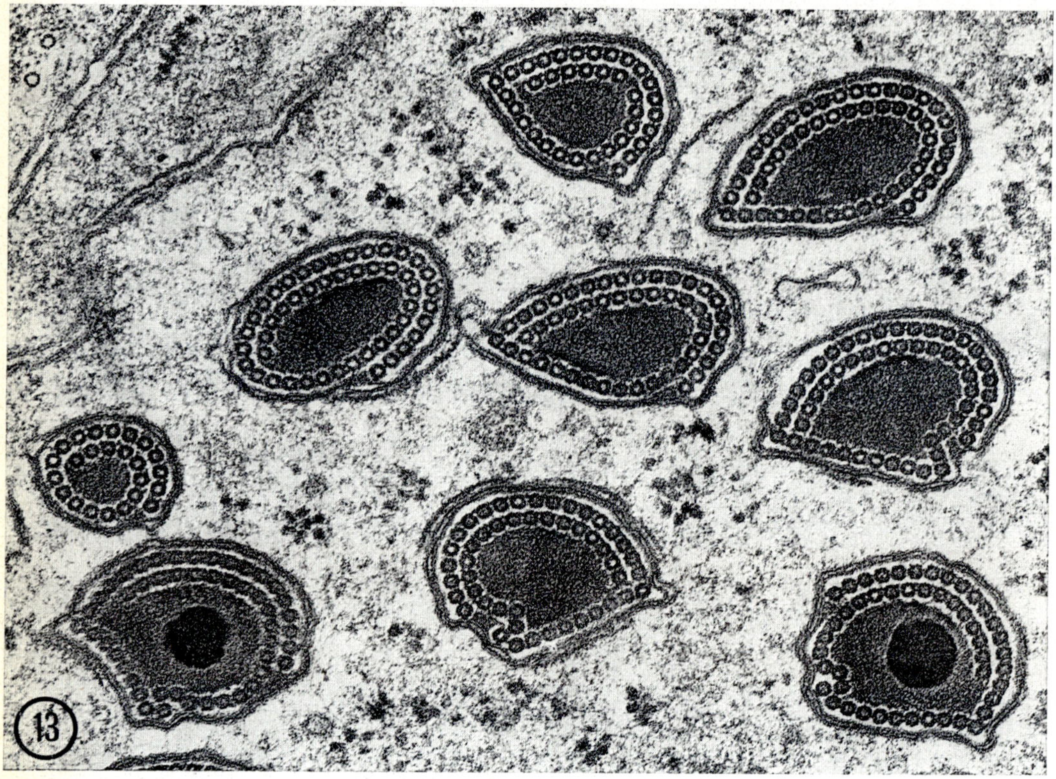
13

J. G. RIEMANN (*)

METAMORPHOSIS OF SPERM OF THE CABBAGE LOOPER, *TRICHOPLUSIA NI*, DURING PASSAGE FROM THE TESTES TO THE FEMALE SPERMATHECA (1)

SUMMARY. — Like other Lepidoptera, the cabbage looper, *Trichoplusia ni* (HÜBNER), produces both eupyrene and apyrene sperm. After lysis of the trophic cells of apyrene bundles the sperm cells separate from one another, pass through the male reproductive system, and are transferred to the female with little evidence of morphological change. However, in the case of eupyrene sperm, both the bundle as a whole and the individual sperm cells go through complex morphological changes in different parts of the reproductive system. Trophic cells of eupyrene bundles undergo lysis at about the time they leave the testes. However, a new bundle covering, together with an internal framework, is quickly rebuilt from thick strands of material possibly derived from the decayed trophic cells. The rebuilt bundle is maintained until after the sperm are transferred at mating. After degeneration of the bundle trophic cells, the individual sperm cells become surrounded by strips of amorphous material which differentiates into a thick sheath. A thin dense plate in the outer part of the sheath bears a " satellite body " which was present earlier in a somewhat different form. After the sperm are transferred to the female bursa copulatrix, there is an apparent partial rotation of the sheath around the sperm axis. The sheath of eupyrene sperm stored in the spermatheca is seen to contain a broad dense rod which runs the length of the tail. This rod is apparently formed by a concentration of intrasheath material.

RIASSUNTO. — Come altri Lepidotteri, la Nottua *Trichoplusia ni* (HÜBNER) produce tanto spermatozoi eupirenici quanto apirenici. Dopo la lisi delle cellule trofiche, nei fasci apiremici gli spermatozoi si separano l'uno dall'altro, traversano il sistema riproduttore maschile e sono trasferiti nella femmina con pochi cambiamenti morfologici. Invece, nel caso degli spermatozoi eupirenici tanto l'intero complesso degli spermatozoi quanto i singoli spermi incontrano complessi cambiamenti morfologici nelle differenti parti del sistema riproduttore. Le cellule trofiche dei fasci europirenici vanno in lisi nel momento in cui abbandonano il testicolo, e ne deriva una nuova intelaiatura e copertura per i fasci di spermatozoi, che resiste fino all'accoppiamento. I singoli spermi si trovano così avvolti da una guaina amorfa, che nella propria superficie esterna costituisce un « corpo satellite ». Dopo che gli spermatozoi si sono introdotti nella borsa copulatrice, la guaina ruota intorno all'asse dello spermio, ed al suo interno differenzia un denso bastone che corre lungo l'intera lunghezza della coda.

INTRODUCTION

The very high dosages of radiation required for sterilization of cabbage loopers, *Trichoplusia ni* (HÜBNER), may prevent sperm transfer by males during copulation (NORTH and HOLT 1968). At dosages generally permitting

(*) Metabolism and Radiation Research Laboratory, Entomology Research Division, Agr. Res. Serv., USDA, Fargo, North Dakota U.S.A.

(1) Supported in part by AEC contract no. AT (49-7) 3028.

sperm transfer, there was an increase in the quantity of anucleate (apyrene) sperm as compared to nucleate (eupyrene) sperm received by females (HOLT and NORTH, personal communication). These observations led to a study of the ultrastructure of apyrene and eupyrene *Trichoplusia* sperm in the various parts of the complex male reproductive system and in the female in an attempt to explain some of the radiation effects.

MEVES (1903) first described production of anucleate sperm as a normal process by a lepidopteran. Since then, apyrene sperm have been found in a number of lepidopteran species and are probably characteristic of the order. References and details of formation of apyrene sperm are given by FAIN-MAUREL (1966) and VIRKKI (1963).

Several investigators have studied lepidopteran testicular sperm at the ultrastructural level. ANDRÉ described the axial filament and mitochondrial derivatives of *Macroglossum* and *Pieris*, respectively (1959, 1961, 1962). Some details of *Ephestia* sperm were shown by SMITH (1968). YASUZUMI and OURA (1964 a, 1964 b, 1956 a, 1965 b) described two novel bodies, which they called the clear band and tubular structure, in spermatids of *Bombyx*. These structures occur in *Trichoplusia* sperm and have also apparently been found in all lepdopteran sperm studied thus far at the ultrastructural level. To the author's knowledge, the only electron microscope study dealing specifically with apyrene sperm has been that of *Zylberberg* (1963) on *Pieris*, although apyrene cells have been shown in the illustrations of some other papers.

The reproductive system of Lepidoptera is complex as compared to that of most insects. No detailed description or illustrations are given in the present paper, but the reproductive system of *Trichoplusia* is quite similar to those described by CALLAHAN and CHAPIN (1960) for other species of noctuid moths. Sperm are released from the testes into seminal vesicles and then pass by way of elongate vasa deferentia to the ductus ejaculatorius duplex. This paired structure (duplex) serves as a reservoir for sperm and various secretions that will be transferred to the female during copulation. During the mating period sperm from the duplex are released into the ductus ejaculatoris simplex and enclosed in a spermatophore. This latter body and its contents are deposited in the female's bursa cupulatrix from whence the sperm pass by way of the seminal duct to the spermatheca. This paper describes observations on sperm in the testes, seminal vesicles, duplex, spermatophore (within the bursa copulatrix), and the spermatheca.

MATERIALS AND METHODS

Reproductive systems of adult moths were dissected out into Belar's saline, immersed as quickly as possible in cold 2.5% glutaraldehyde in cacodylic or phosphate buffer (both *p*H 7.4), punctured with fine needles, and allowed to fix for 6 hours. They were then left overnight in buffer, postfixed 2 hours in 1% osmium tetroxide in phosphate buffer, dehydrated in ethanol and propylene oxide, and embedded in Araldite. Thin sections were mounted on either bare grids or carbon stabilized cellodin films, and stained with uranyl acetate and lead citrate (VENABLE and COGGESHALL 1965). Examination was made with an RCA EMU 3 H electron microscope.

OBSERVATIONS

1. *Testes and Seminal Vesicles.*

The axial filament of *Trichoplusia* sperm was found to be similar to that of *Macroglossum* (ANDRÉ, 1961 a). In transverse sections of bundles taken from the testes eupyrene cells were found to have a 9+2 axial filament surrounded by an outer ring of 9 dense fibers. The mitochondrial derivatives are unequal in size with the smaller one being partially embedded in the larger one (Fig. 1). Except in the area of the axial filament, cristae are inserted into the outer portions of the mitochondrial derivatives at an angle of about 45° from the sperm axis. On either side of the axial filament, there are small masses of fibrous material attached to the mitochondrial derivatives. These " fibrous rods " which extend the length of the mitochondrial derivatives have apparently not been found in other lepidopteran sperm.

Anterior to the mitochondrial derivatives, the nucleus is seen in transverse section, as a helmet–shaped structure extending along the axial filament (Fig. 2). Beyond the centriolar region the nucleus extends for a considerable distance first as a rectangular rod and then as a somewhat flattened one in association with elements of the acrosome (Fig. 3). Details of acrosome structure have not been worked out.

YASUZUMI and OURA (1965) found that the cell membrane disappeared in silkworm sperm during their development in the testes. If this occurs with *Trichoplusia*, a new membrane is formed by the time the sperm are ready for release from the testes of adult moths. No sheath is present and the enclosing membrane appears as a simple unit membrane. In the head region, the cell membrane may be widely separated from the nuclear envelope of some specimens.

An outstanding feature of *Trichoplusia* sperm, as of all other lepidopteran sperm studied at the fine structure level, is the presence of a number of regularly spaced laminate projections extending out from cells viewed in transverse (Figs. 1–2). YASUZUMI and OURA (1965) studied the formation of these projections in silkworm sperm and found that they were derived from a structure which they found to be associated at an earlier stage with the plasma membrane (1964 a, 1964 b). They called this structure the clear band and the laminate projections derived from it the clear band derivatives. In glutaraldehyde fixed *Trichoplusia* sperm, the lamellae of the clear band derivative are about 100 Å in thickess with intervening clear spaces of about 70 Å. In the tail region the lamellate projections are fairly widely separated, but in the anterior part of the nuclear area they are close enough together so as to present the appearance of a series of concentric rings.

Another outstanding feature of *Trichoplusia* sperm is the presence of a prominent body running the length of the sperm on the outside of the plasma membrane. It seems fairly definite that this structure is the same as that which was designated as the tubular structure in silkworm spermatids by YASUZUMI and OURA (1964 a, 1964 b, 1965). As the structure appears with eupyrene sperm of adult *Trichoplusia*, the term tubular structure is not descriptive and *satellite body* is used instead.

In the tail region of eupyrene sperm, the satellite body is seen as a rod attached by a series of septa to the cell membrane at a point between the axial filament and the smaller mitochondrial derivative (Fig. 1). At this position, it is immediately over one of the fibrous rods to which there are apparent connections. The satellite body is not membrane enclosed and seems to be made up of a series of very fine strands or lamellae.

In the posterior part of the sperm head, the satellite body continues in the same position relative to the axial filament as in the tail region although the connecting septa are no longer present. However, still further anterior the body moves to a position beneath the nucleus (Figs. 2–3) and assumes the form of a rather broad crescent.

Several trophic cells were found to be included in each sperm bundle. Most of these were located along the tail region, but the sperm heads appear embedded in a single *apical* cell having features somewhat different from the other trophic cells. In eupyrene bundles the cytoplasm of the trophic cells extends in between the sperm which are invested individually or in groups by extensions of the trophic cell plasma membranes. In the tail region and the posterior part of the head region, the trophic cell membrane lies directly against the clear band derivatives, but further anterior there is a fairly broad separation of the two components.

In the tail region, the origin of the membranes investing the sperm cells is obvious. However, in the head area interdigitation of membranes of the apical trophic cell with the more posterior ones made identification of the cytoplasm immediately around the sperm uncertain. It is thought, however, that projections of the posterior trophic cells form sleeves around the sperm nuclei as they extend into the apical cell.

Trichoplusia eupyrene sperm remain in bundles until after they are transferred to the female moths. However, lysis of the trophic cells occurs before or during passage of the bundles from the testes. After this a very different type of support framework is built around the sperm cells. This process of lysis and rebuilding is accompanied by formation of the sperm sheath.

Lysis of the trophic cells was found to proceed most rapidly in the tissue enclosing the individual sperm cells and this is accompanied by a degeneration of the clear band derivatives. These changes result in the formation of a granular lysate around the individual sperm cells (Fig. 4). Later the lysate becomes more homogenous and fills the space around the sperm cells. Most of this material disappears and then (open bundle stage) the interior of the bundle is apparently open to the surrounding environment (Fig. 5). However, intertwined among the sperm cells there are now numerous thick (about 50 mμ) strands which are particularly abundant around the nuclei. The appearance of the strands around the sperm cells suggest that they might be derived in some way from the trophic cell membranes, but their actual origin was not determined.

Most sperm in the open bundle stage were found in the seminal vesicles, but at least some reach this stage in the testes.

Transverse sections of eupyrene sperm in the open bundle stage are shown in Figs. 6–7. A rim of amorphous material, apparently representing remnants of the lysate formerly filling the space between the cells, is seen around each cell adhering to the plasma membrane. The appearance of the material is virtually identical from cell to cell, and, particularly in the tail region, the material is subdivided into a number of longitudinal strands so as to bring to mind the clear band derivatives of earlier stage bundles. It is not known how much the derivatives actually contribute to the new surrounding material. A heavy concentration of material under the satellite body has no earlier counterpart.

Whatever the origin of the material around the sperm after trophic cell lysis, it eventually forms the sperm sheath. An apparent early stage of sheath formation is exhibited in the cell shown in Fig. 8. A definitive sheath is present, but it is quite thin except near the tubular structure and details are not distinct. In part, this is probably due to poor fixation. However, the fact that all cells of the bundle had a generally uniform appearance suggests that the sheath was still not completely formed.

The process of bundle rebuilding was also well underway but apparently not completed in the bundle of cells shown in Fig. 8. Thick strands, such as described earlier, now formed a rather loose network over the individual sperm cells. Other strands had accumulated over the surface of the bundle as a whole to form a type of envelope. However, there were still gaps in this envelope such as were not present around some other bundles in the seminal vesicles and in duplex bundles.

During the period of trophic cell lysis and subsequent reconstruction, the satellite body retained its identity and approximate position. In the tail region it is smaller than before and the septate connections have disappeared (Fig. 6). However, it still seems to be made up of fine strands or lamellae. This is particularly evident in the nuclear region (Fig. 7). In the cells of the partially rebuilt bundle shown in Fig. 8, it can be seen that the satellite body is attached to a *dense plate* in the outer part of the sperm sheath.

According to HOLT and NORTH (in press), about 40 % of the sperm bundles in the testes of young *Trichoplusua* adults are apyrene. A transverse section of a small portion of the tail region of an apyrene bundle is shown in Fig. 9. The axial filament is similar to that of a eupyrene cell, but the two apyrene mitochondrial derivatives are equal in size and much smaller than those of eupyrene cells. Trophic cell material does not extend between the individual apyrene cells in the tail region. Also, clear band derivatives and satellite rods do not occur. A sheath is not yet present, although the enclosing membrane is rather thick.

Apyrene sperm have a short head region. In testicular bundles the individual sperm heads are, like those of eupyrene sperm, embedded in an apical trophic cell. In this area trophic cell cytoplasm lies between the individual sperm cells and the membrane seen surrounding the sperm cells shown in Fig. 10 is problably a sleeve or casing of trophic cell origin.

Two areas of electron dense material are found in the head of apyrene cells. The first of these is seen as a small cap at the anterior end. Beneath this cap is a short shaft of material of somewhat lesser density. The origin of these dense areas is not known, but the terminal cap seems to be continuous with the sheath which is at least partially formed at this stage in the head region. The dense shaft suggests a small amount of nuclear material. However, it is apparently not enclosed in a nuclear envelope and the head area of apyrene bundles is Feulgen negative.

As compared to eupyrene sperm, the changes occurring in apyrene sperm during their transit through the post–testicular organs are relatively simple. Lysis of the trophic cells of apyrene bundles is completed by the time bundles pass from the testes and henceforth the sperm cells are free from each other. In the seminal vesicle, thick strands, such as those involved in the rebuilding of eupyrene bundles, are found associated with apyrene cells (Fig. 11), but they disappear before the cells reach the duplex.

Apyrene bundle degeneration is accompanied by the formation of the sperm sheath. This seems to correspond fairly closely to the outer part of the sheath of eupyrene sperm.

2. *Ductus Ejaculatorius Duplex.*

Bundle rebuilding is probably completed by the time eupyrene bundles enter the duplex. A transverse section through the tail region of a typical duplex bundle is shown in Fig. 12. The network of thick strands around the individual cells is more extensive than it is around the cells shown in Fig. 8. Also, the enclosing envelope is now thicker with very few gaps. Around the bundle there are various types of secretory particles and some apyrene cells.

An enlargement of some of the cells from the bundle shown in Fig. 12 is given in Fig. 13. The sheath around the sperm cells is now well formed. Details of sheath structure can best be studied in sperm from the spermathecae. However, in duplex material the sheath can be seen to consist of an inner limiting portion lying against or incorporating the cell membrane and a rather thick outer limiting portion. Between there is considerable material which is present in larger quantities in the area of the satellite body than elsewhere. The satellite body itself is, as before, attached to the dense plate which is seen as an interruption of the outer limiting portion of the sheath. As far as could be determined from longitudinal sections, the appearance of the sheath and satellite body are similar in the head region to their appearance in the tail.

A few individual eupyrene cells were found in the duplex. These were always enclosed in strands similar to those of an intact bundle but usually had some obvious defect such as a break in the sheath.

Apyrene cells were found scattered throughout the duplex but were particularly abundant in the posterior portion where the eupyrene bundles were stored. A feature of apyrene sperm in the duplex, apparently not present in the seminal vesicle, was the presence of numerous fine projections extending out from around the sheath (Fig. 14). These were apparently borne on a very thin membrane which occurred over the sperm sheath. This membrane with its projections could not be detected around apyrene cells after they had left the duplex and possibly represented the result of surface interactions between the sperm cells and the surrounding secretory material.

3. *Spermatophore in the Bursa Copulatrix.*

No study has been made of sperm during most stages of movement from the male duplex to the female spermatheca. However, the contents of one spermatophore, dissected from the bursa copulatrix of a female about 20 minutes after the termination of cupulation, was studied. The eupyrene sperm were still in bundles, but the supporting network of thick strands was degenerating. With this, the bundle interior had become open to the surrounding environment so that secretory material and some apyrene sperm could be found between the eupyrene cells.

Aside from the absence of the thin outer membrane noted earlier for duplex cells, no morphological changes could be detected in the apyrene cells. However, marked differences were found in eupyrene cells as compared to their appearance in the duplex (Fig. 15). Where formerly the sheath was thickest over the smaller mitochondrial derivative and along one side of the axial filament, it was now thickest on the side opposite to the axial filament. Also, the dense plate, formerly present on one side near the axial filament, was now seen at a point opposite to the axial filament. The satellite body, as such, had disappeared but possible remnants were seen attached to the dense plates of some cells. These observations indicated that the sheath had undergone a rotation of about 120° from its previous position in regard to the internal components of the sperm.

4. *Spermatheca.*

As in other noctuid moths (CALLAHAN and CHAPIN, 1960), the spermatheca of *Trichoplusia* is divided into two lobes. The larger of these, the utriculus, was found to contain mostly eupyrene sperm. The few apyrene cells seen were located in the center of the lobe along with a mass of cellular debris. The other spermathecal lobe, the lagena, contained larger numbers of apyrene sperm along with smaller numbers of eupyrene cells.

Examination of sperm stored in the spermathecae revealed additional changes occur in eupyrene sperm beyond those already described. A striking feature was the presence of a dense rod within the sheath at a point above the dense plate and opposite to the axial filament (Fig. 16). This "intrasheath rod" runs the length of the tail and is probably formed by a concentration of the material formerly located in relatively large quantities between the inner and outer limiting portions of the sheath (Fig. 15). Generally very little of such material now remained in the tail region except near the axial filament. An interesting exception was found in a few specimens that had very small intrasheath rods. Also, much fibrous material remained within the sheath in the head region (Fig. 17).

Although the intrasheath rod is limited to the tail region, the dense plate continues along the nucleus to at least the apex of the sperm (Fig. 17). Posteriorly it has the same position as in the tail but anteriorly it is gradually displaced somewhat to one side of the nucleus. There is still not enough precise information on the position of the dense plate in the nuclear area of duplex sperm to determine whether there is a shift of the plate in the head comparable to that occuring in the tail. It will be recalled, however, that the satellite body, under which the dense plate forms, was originally beneath the anterior part of the nucleus but near the axial filament in the tail region.

Dense granules were often found attached to the dense plate in both the head and tail region. These occurred at irregular intervals along the plate and it is not known whether they represent remnants of the satellite body.

Apyrene cells in the spermatheca were probably morphologically unchanged from their earlier condition. However, the apyrene sperm in the lagena and even the few found in the utriculus were much swollen (Fig. 18). Presumably this was a fixation artifact related to the high concentration of secretory material in the spermatheca, especially in the lagena.

Conclusions

Speculation as to the functional significance of many of the complex changes in eupyrene sperm during their transit through the male and female reproductive system would be pointless without more ultrastructural and physiological research. What has been done thus far does suggest some lines of research that should be profitable. Thus, due to its close association with the dense plate, the intrasheath rod is indicated as being possibly involved in the metabolism of materials entering the sperm cell.

Of particular interest to the author was the discovery that eupyrene bundles are rebuilt and maintained until after they are transferred to the female. The key to the functional significance of this bundle rebuilding and maintenance, as well as to other unique features of lepidopteran sperm morphogenesis, may be the determination of the role of apyrene sperm. Since their discovery by Meves (1903), there has been considerable controversy as to the function of apyrene sperm and even as to whether they are transferred during mating (FAIN–MAUREL, 1966; SADO, 1963). IRIKI (1941) maintained that apyrene cells were transferred in *Bombyx* and were somehow necessary for transport of eupyrene sperm from the spermatophore to the spermatheca.

Whether or not transport of eupyrene sperm is a function of *Trichoplusia* apyrene cells, some type of interaction between the two sperm types, starting only after transfer to the female, might explain the continued maintenance of eupyrene cells in bundles until after they are deposited in the bursa copulatrix.

Containment in bundles probably also serves to shield the eupyrene cells from the several types of secretory products produced by the duplex and the accessory glands which empty into the duplex. At least some of these secretions are transferred in the spermatophore and are first found among eupyrene cells after bundle breakdown. Conceivably these products trigger the changes that seem to involve a partial rotation of the sheath axis. This rotation in itself suggests some type of activation of eupyrene cells (including a capacy for interaction with apyrene cells?).

Continued storage in the female spermatheca suggests that in *Trichoplusia* apyrene cells have a function beyond any role they may have during movement of sperm from the bursa copulatrix to the spermatheca.

REFERENCES

ANDRÉ J. (1959) – *Etude au microscope électronique de l'évolution du chondriome pendant la spermatogènese du Papillon du chou,* Pieris brassicae. « Ann. Sc. Nat. », 1, 283–305.

ANDRÉ J. (1961) – *Sur quelques détails nouvellement connus de l'ultrastructure des organites vibratiles.* « J. Ultrastruc. Res. », 5, 86–108.

ANDRÉ J. (1962) – *Contribution à la connaissance du chondriome, étude de ses modifications ultrastructurales pendant la spermatogénèse.* « J. Ultrastruc. Res. », Suppl. 3, 1–185.

CALLAHAN P. S. and CHAPIN J. B. (1960) – *Morphology of the reproductive systems and mating in two representative members of the family Noctuidae,* Pseudaletia unipuncat *and* Peridroma margaritosa, *with comparisons to* Heliothis zea. « Ann. Entomol. Soc. Amer. », 53, 763–782.

FAIN–MAUREL M. A. (1966) – *Acquisitions récentes sur les spermatogenèses atypiques.* « Ann. Biol. », 11–12, 35–564.

HOLT G. G. and NORTH D. T. – (In Press) *Spermatogenesis in the cabbage looper,* Trichoplusia ni (*Lepidoptera: Noctuidae*). « Ann. Entomol. Soc. Amer ».

IRIKI S. (1941) – *On the function of apyrene spermatozoa of the silkworm.* « Zool. Mag. », 53, 123–124. (In Japanese).

MEVES F. (1903) – *Ueber oligopyrene and apyrene Spermien und ihre Entstehung nach Beobachtungen an* Paludina *und* Pygaera. « Arch. f. Mikr. Anat. », 61, 1–84.

NORTH D. T. and HOLT G. G. (1968) – *Genetic and cytogenetic basis of radiation-induced sterility in the male cabbage looper,* Trichoplusia ni. – In: Intern. Atomic Energy Agency Symposia « Isotopes and Radiation in Entomology », Vienna, Austria, Nov. 1967, 391–403.

SADO T. (1963) – *Spermatogenesis of the silkworm and its bearing on radiation induced sterility.* II. « J. Fac. Agr. Kyushu Univ. », 12, 387–404.

SMITH D. S. (1968) – *Insect cells, their structure and function.* Oliver and Boyd, Edinburgh 372.

VENABLE J. H. and COGGESHALL R. (1965) – *A simplified lead citrate strain for use in electron microscopy.* « J. Cell Biol. », 25, 407–408.

VIRKKI N. (1963) – *Gametogenesis in the sugarcane borer moth,* Diatraea saccharallis (*F.*) *Crambidae.* « J. Agr. Univ. Puerto Rico », 47, 102–137.

YASUZUMI G. and OURA C. (1964 a) – *Differential analysis by various staining techniques of structures present in developing spermatids of the silkworm.* « Nature », 204 (5964), 1197–1198.

YASUZUMI G. (1964 b) – *Spermatogenesis in animals as revealed by electron microscopy.* XIII. *Formation of a tubular structure and two bands in the developing spermatid of the silkworm,* Bombyx mori *Linné.* « Z. Zellforsch », 64, 210–226.

YASUZUMI G. (1965 a) – *Spermatogenesis in animals as revealed by electron microscopy.* XIV. *The fine structure of the clear band and tubular structure in late stages of development of spermatids of the silkworm,* Bombyx mori *Linné.* « Z. Zellforsch. », 66, 182–196.

YASUZUMI G. (1965 b) – *Spermatogenesis in animals as revealed by electron microscopy.* XV. *The fine structure of the middle piece in the developing spermatid of the silkworm,* Bombyx mori Linné. « Z. Zellforsch. Mikrosk. Anat. », 67, 502–520.

ZYLBERBERG L. (1963) – *Remarques sur l'ultrastructure des flagelles des spermatozoïdes typiques et atypiques de* Pieris brassicae *L.* « C. R. Acad. Sci. », 256, 2702–2703.

EXPLANATION OF FIGURES

Fig. 1. – Transverse section of tail region of eupyrene sperm from intact bundle in testis. The mitochondrial derivatives (*M*) are markedly different in size. Attached to each, on either side of the axial filament (*AF*), is a fibrous rod (*FR*). Clear band derivatives (*CD*) are seen as a series of spoke-like projections around most of the cell and trophic membranes (*TM*) cover one side of the cell. The satellite body (*SB*) is attached by a series of septa to the sperm cell membrane (*CM*) over the smaller mitochondrial derivative. 55,000×.

Fig. 2. – Transverse section through the nuclear region of a cell from a eupyrene bundle in testis. The satellite body (*SB*) is seen as a crescent-shaped body near the nucleus (*N*). The projections of the clear band derivatives (*CD*) are very close together. 70,000×.

Fig. 3. – Transverse section of head of eupyrene sperm in intact bundle from testis. In this region near the apex of the sperm the clear band derivatives (*CD*) are no longer separate from each other and their lamellare are obscured. The satellite body (*SB*) is large and no longer clearly distinct from the clear band derivatives. 70,000×.

Fig. 4. – Tangential section of cells of eupyrene bundle from testis. The clear band derivatives have disappeared and a granular lysate (*GL*) has accumulated around the sperm. 40,000×.

Fig. 5. – Head region and part of tail region of eupyrene " open bundle " from seminal vesicle. A dense concentration of thick strands are found around the sperm heads with lesser numbers of strands occurring in the tail region.

Fig. 6. – Transverse section through the tail region of eupyrene sperm in open bundle stage (seminal vesicle). Masses of amorphous material (*AM*), divided by furrows into longitudinal strips, covers the cell. The material is particularly thick beneath the satellite body (*SB*). A few thick strands (*TS*) can be seen. These will eventually form a framework within the bundle. 58,000×.

Fig. 7. – Transverse section through head of eupyrene cells in open bundles stage (seminal vesicle). Amorphous material (*AM*) surrounds the entire cell but is thicker under the satellite body (*SB*). 45,000×.

Fig. 8. – Transverse section through portion of partially rebuilt eupyrene bundle from seminal vesicle. Thick strands have formed a network around the sperm cells and a rather sparse boundry over the bundle as a whole. A sheath (*S*) is present around the sperm cells but is still poorly defined. Over the smaller mitochondrial derivative the sheath is thicker than elsewhere and contains a dense plate to which the satellite body (*SB*) is attached. 31,000×.

Fig. 9. – Transverse section through tail region of portion of apyrene bundle in testis. Mitochondrial derivatives (*MD*), Axial filament (*AF*), Plasma membrane (*PM*). 40,000×.

Fig. 10. - Longitudinal section of head region of apyrene sperm bundle from testis. The head has a dense terminal cap (*DC*) back of which there is a short shaft of material of moderate density. The sheath (*S*) is at least partially formed and is covered by a thin membrane that may be of trophic cell origin. 22,000×.

Fig. 11. – Transverse section of apyrene cell in seminal vesicle. A sheath is now present. 52,000×.

Fig. 12. – Transverse section of tail region of eupyrene bundle in duplex. Thick strands have formed a more extensive network around the cells than was present in the bundle shown in Fig. 8. Also, the outer envelope is now rather thick and contains few breaks. Secretory material and a few apyrene sperm (*AS*) are seen around the bundle. 2,900×.

Fig. 13. – Enlargement of cells of bundle shown in Fig. 12. The sheath can be seen to consist of inner (*I*) and outer (O) limiting parts between which there is other dense material. The satellite body (*SB*) is attached to the dense plate (*DP*) in the outer part of the sheath. 55,000×.

Fig. 14. – Apyrene cell in duplex surrounded by secretory material. Small projections occur around the cells. These apparently arise from a thin membrane (arrow) over the sperm. 27,000×.

Fig. 15. – Transverse section of tail region of eupyrene sperm in bundle taken from a spermatophore within the bursa copulatrix. The dense plate (arrow), to which there is attached an apparent remnant of the satellite body, is now located at a point opposite to the axial filament. This indicates an approximately 120° rotation of the sperm sheath from its position as seen in Fig. 13. 55,000×.

Fig. 16. – Transverse sections of tail regions of eupyrene sperm taken from the spermatheca (utriculus). A broad dense intrasheath rod (*IS*) is present above the dense plate of the outer sheath. Granules (arrows) are attached to the dense plates of two of the cells. 55,000×.

Fig. 17. – Transverse section through head region of two eupyrene cells taken from the spermatheca (utriculus). The dense plate (arrow) is present this level, but the intrasheath rod seen in Figure 16 does not extend beyond the mitochondrial derivatives. 80,000×.

Fig. 18. – Transverse section of apyrene sperm from spermatheca (lagena). They are located in dense concentrations of secretory material and the swelling of the sperm cells may represent a fixation artifact. 47,000×.

J. G. RIEMANN – *Metamorphosis of sperm of the cabbage, looper,* Trichoplusia ni, *during passage from the testes to the female spermatheca.*

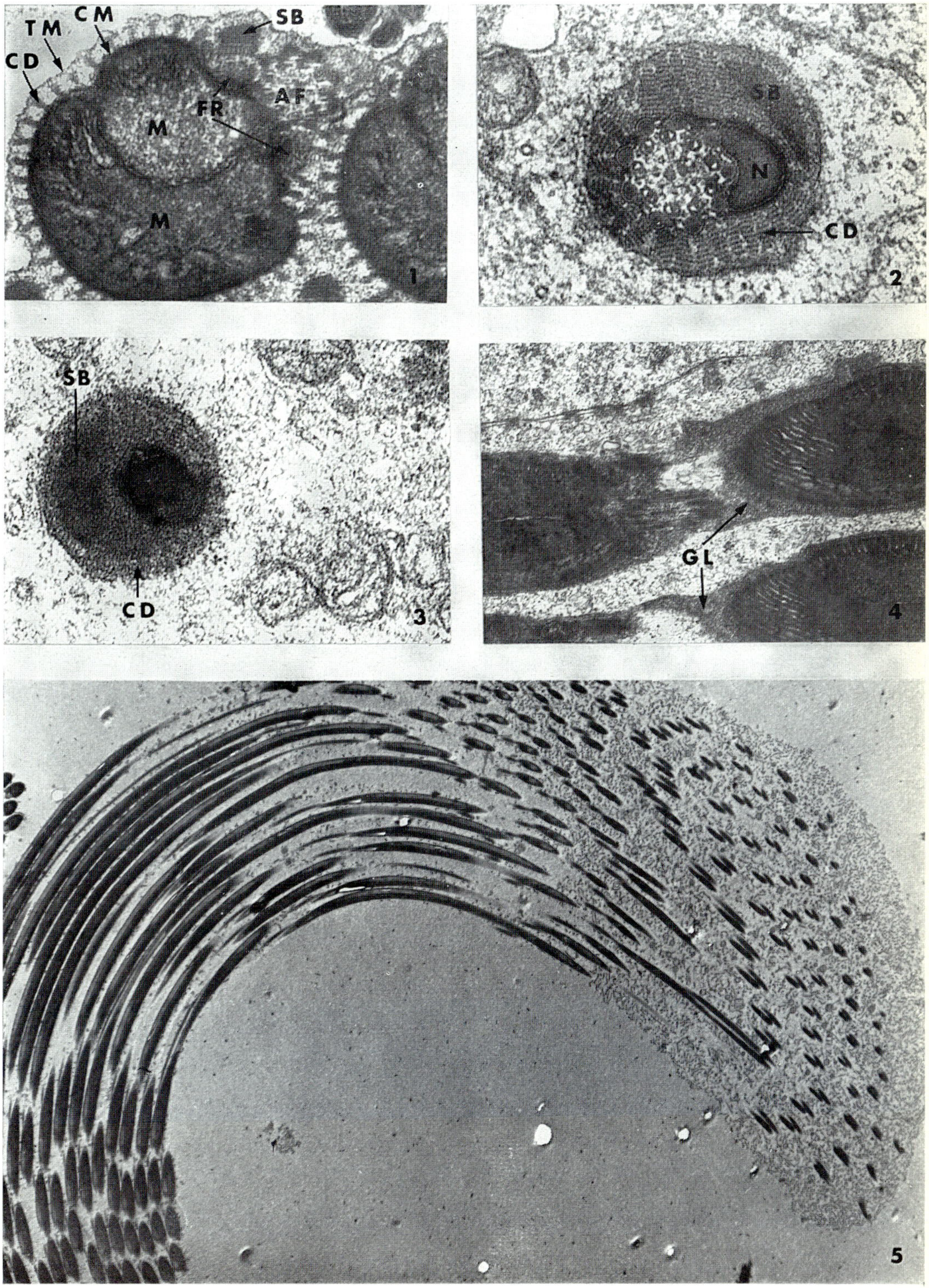

J. G. Riemann – *Metamorphosis of sperm of the cabbage looper*, Trichoplusia ni, *during passage from the testes to the female spermatheca.*

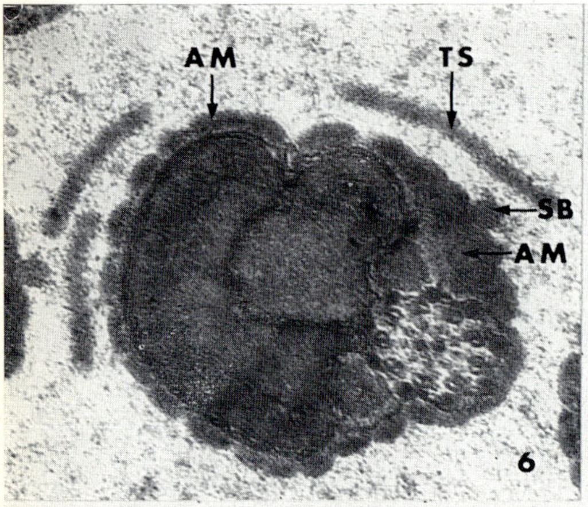

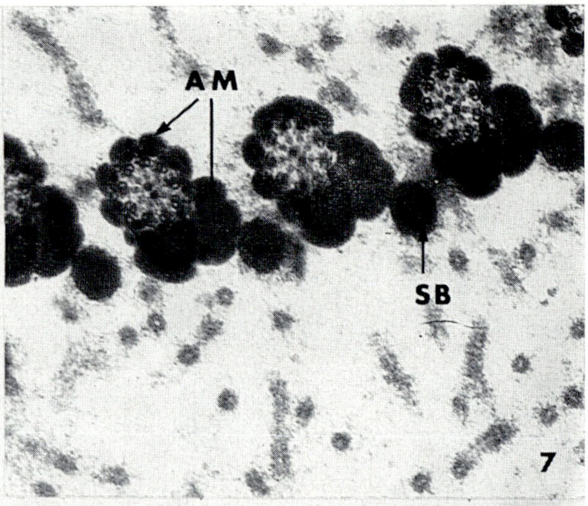

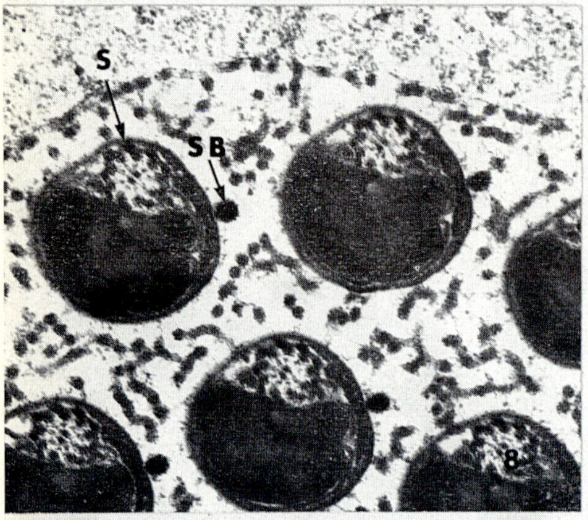

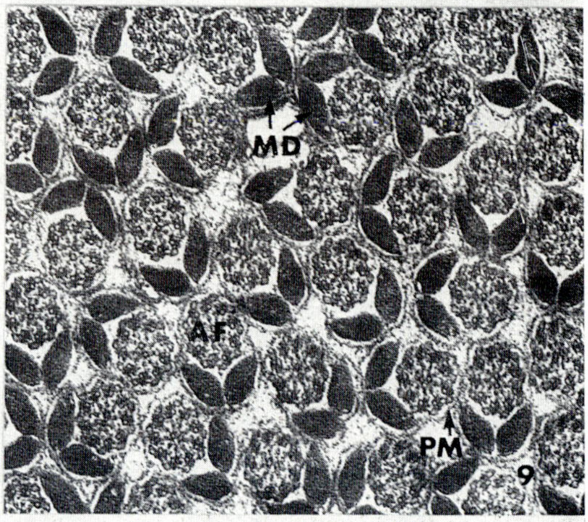

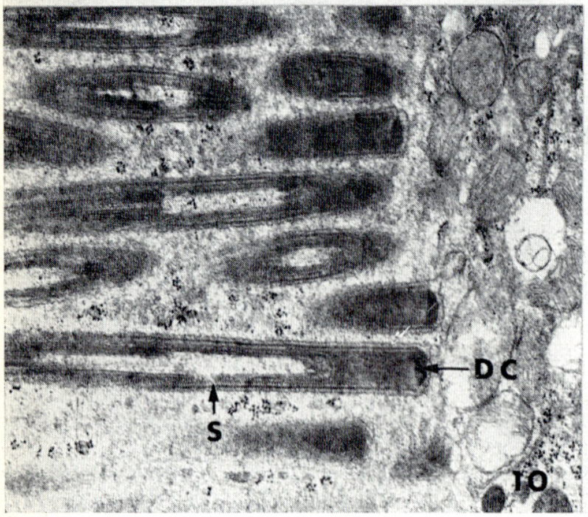

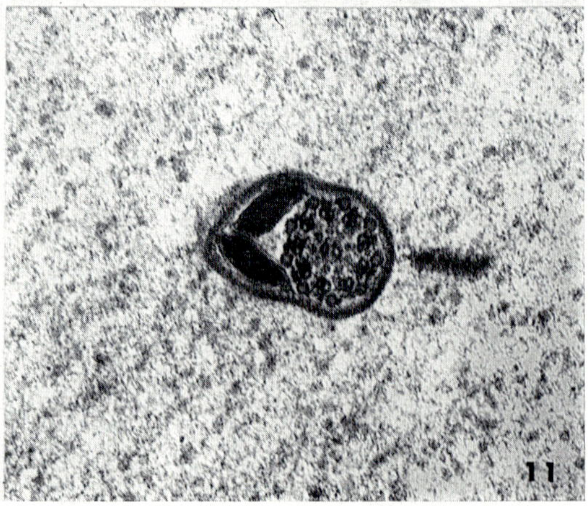

J. G. RIEMANN – *Metamorphosis of sperm of the cabbage looper,* Trichoplusia ni, *during passage from the testes to the female spermatheca.*

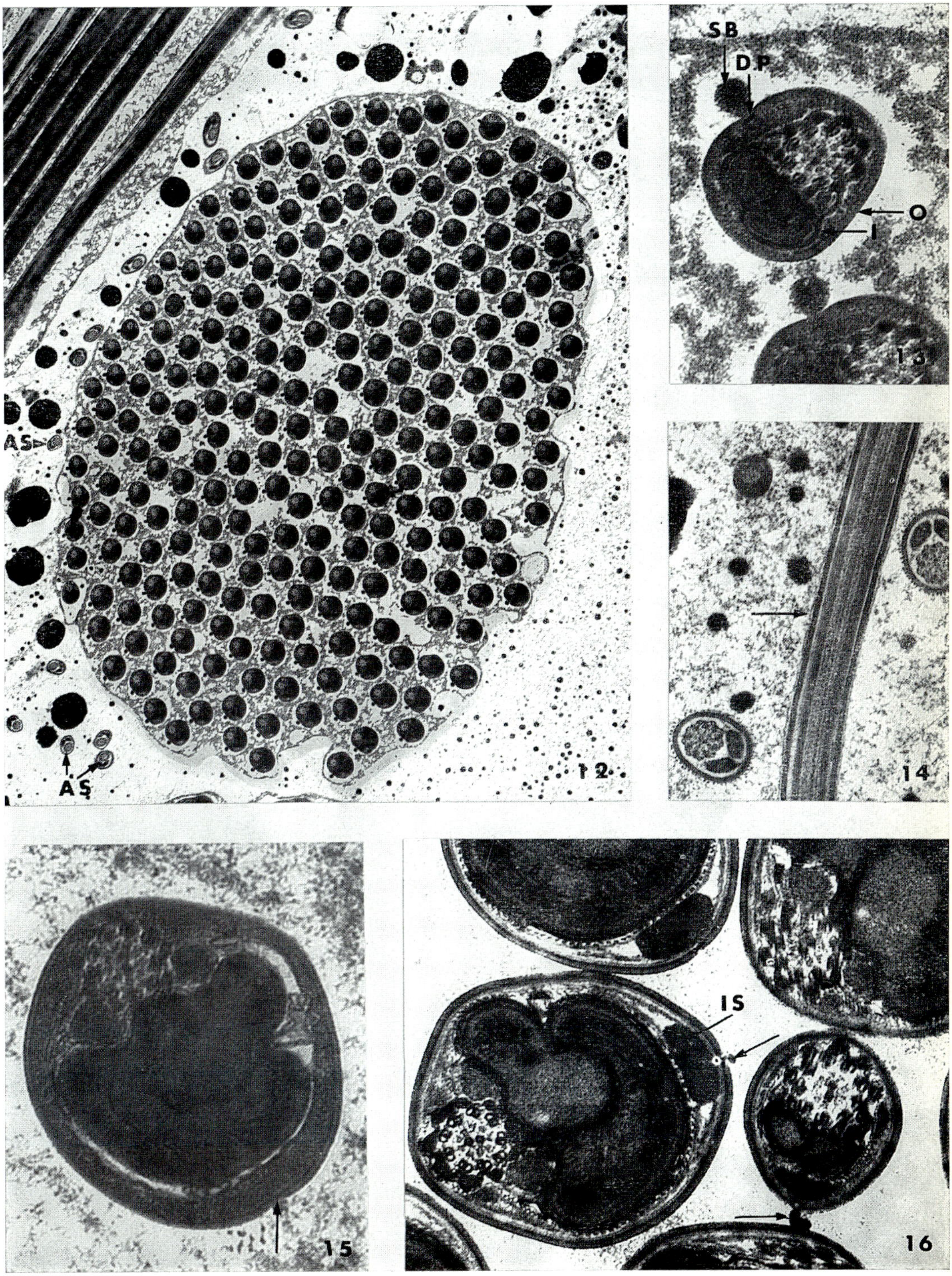

J. G. RIEMANN – *Metamorphosis of sperm of the cabbage looper*, Trichoplusia ni, *during passage from the testes to the female spermatheca.*

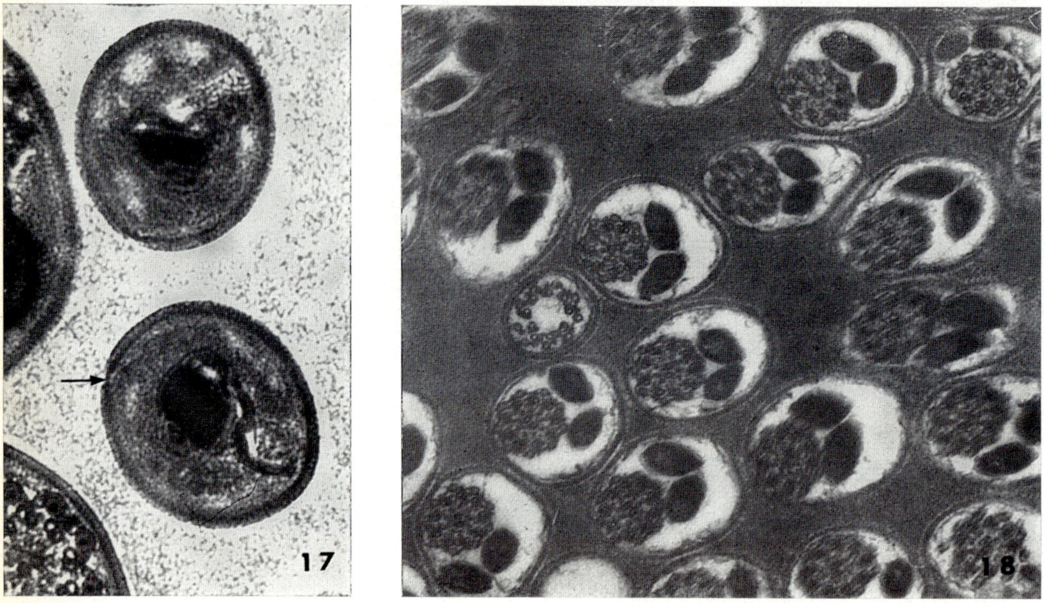

AURELIO BAIRATI (*) and M. ELISA PEROTTI (*)

SOME COMPARATIVE CONSIDERATIONS ON THE ULTRASTRUCTURE OF *DROSOPHILA MELANOGASTER* SPERMATOZOON (**)

SUMMARY. — Some details of the ultrastructure of *Drosophila melanogaster* sperm have been examined in comparison with data on spermatozoa from other species. The investigation has been carried out on ultrathin sections of embedded specimens and on negatively stained material. Serial sectioning has been employed in studying the acrosome, the neck region and the tail end piece.

The main points discussed here relate to: *i*) presence of an asymmetric plasma membrane; *ii*) presence of an acrosome with a dagger–like shape; *iii*) differentiation of a mitochondrial derivative possessing a typical paracrystalline texture; *iv*) structure of the so-called secondary fibres, which are regarded as a granular portion of a complex system of radial connections among the principal fibres; *v*) the structure of the axial filament principal fibres as revealed by the negative staining and the existence of a peculiar system of projections on the outer and the central fibres; *vi*) the organization of the tail end piece, in which a progressive tailing off of the axial filament components has been observed.

RIASSUNTO. — I risultati di indagini ultrastrutturali condotte sullo spermatozoo maturo di *Drosophila melanogaster* vengono esposti e discussi comparativamente all'ultrastruttura di spermatozoi di altre specie. Le ricerche sono state condotte sia su sezioni sottili di materiale fissato e incluso sia su sospensioni di spermi frammentati ed esaminati con la tecnica del contrasto negativo.

I risultati ottenuti possono essere così riassunti: 1) la membrana plasmatica presenta una struttura asimmetrica; 2) l'acrosoma ha una tipica forma a baionetta; 3) uno dei derivati mitocondriali possiede struttura cristallina; 4) le cosiddette « fibre secondarie » hanno struttura granulare e sono considerate come componenti di un complesso sistema di connessioni radiali esistente tra le fibre del filamento assile; 5) con la tecnica di contrasto negativo le fibre centrali e quelle periferiche appaiono fornite di tipiche proiezioni; 6) nella porzione terminale del flagello si osserva una particolare organizzazione del filamento assile, dovuta alla graduale terminazione delle diverse fibre.

Light microscopy provides very little information on the structure of *Drosophila* spermatozoon. Investigations could only evidence the head and the tail, very similar in width (0.3–0.5 μ) and distinguishable only by Feulgen positive staining of the head.

Because the sperm is so thin, nothing but merely dimensional data could be obtained. Thus, total sperm length varies, according to the techniques employed and the strains under examination, from 0.4 mm by DOBZHANSKY (1934) to 1.76 by COOPER (1950) and by others.

(*) Institute of Human Anatomy and Institute of Genetics, University of Milano, Italy.
(**) Research supported by the grant No. 115–1150–1080 from C.N.R.

Several electron microscope studies on spermatogenesis in *Drosophila* have disclosed details of spermatocytes and spermatids ultrastructure, whereas the ultrastructure of mature spermatozoa has been recently described by PEROTTI (1969) using comparative techniques of electron-microscope examination of thin sections and fragments investigated with the help of negative staining.

In this paper, latest ultrastructural features of *Drosophila melanogaster* spermatozoa are illustrated and their morphology discussed by comparison with those of other species' sperms.

The first point concerns the limiting membrane of the spermatozoon. Figs. 1, 2, clearly show the mature spermatozoon to be limited by a trilaminar plasma membrane which appears to be asymmetric; the outer, electronopaque layer is far thicker (up to 50 Å) than the other two layers. The presence of an asymmetrical plasma membrane is a relatively frequent occurrence in vertebrates tissues or in bacterial membrane, while it has been less frequently observed in insect tissues. It was found, for example, in the intestinal epithelium of Termites by NOIROT-THIMOTÉE, NOIROT and ESCAIG (1965), and in the cuticuline membrane by LOCKE (1966). No such organization of the limiting membrane, instead, has ever been demonstrated in the spermatozoa of other species. As far as the interpretation is concerned, it may be noted that the outermost layer appears thicker and more electronopaque even after fixation with OsO_4 alone, indicating that it may consist either of substances with hydrophilic groups, such as proteins, or of fatty acids, as suggested for the outermost layer of the cuticuline membrane. In any case, the basic macromolecular organization of the plasma membrane should not be modified, since the inner layer and the lipidic middle layer show the thickness typical for the unit membrane, and the outermost layer may be assumed to consist of molecules whose chemical reactivity differs from that of the most typical plasma membrane, where they are glycoproteic in nature and appear electron-clear.

The second point concerns the acrosome. Figs. 3–8 show some cross sections obtained by the serial-section method of mature spermatozoa. The acrosome exhibits a peculiar shape, and the cross sections feature different profiles as they proceed from the cephalic end towards the caudal one. While in an extreme section (Fig. 3) the acrosome appears as a thin lamina, it gradually takes a triangular shape (Figs. 4, 5) with a vertex protruding beyond the diameter of the spermatozoon head surface, until, at the level where the splicing with the nucleus is located, the acrosome section appears to be shaped like a biconvex lens (Figs. 7, 8). It is evident that the acrosome is constantly limited by a trilaminar membrane at the outermost surface of which the cell membrane is stratified. It can also be noted that the acrosome is internally formed by a material with a finely granular appearance, showing areas with a greater electronic opacity. The fact will likerwise be remarked that the material inside the acrosome may occasionally appear to be organized as in a crystal structure (Figs. 6, 7). Conclusive evidence has thus been gained of the fact that also the mature *Drosophila melanogaster* spermatozoon possesses an acrosome, as had so far been observed by SHOUP (1967) and by ANDERSON (1967) only in spermatids. The acrosome in *Drosophila* displays typical features, such as its dagger-like shape, its lateral arrangement with respect to the nucleus axis and its bayonet-like insertion. This acrosome appears simpler in organization than the acrosomes of sperms from other species, as it consists of a single compact element and no accessory structures have been observed. The only differentiation lies in zonation of the acrosome contents and was also observed in spermatids by SHOUP (1967). Zones of different densities within the acrosome have been found in the sperms of guinea pig by FAWCETT and HOLLENBERG (1963), starfish by DAN (1960), *Hydroides* and *Saccoglossus* by COLWIN and COLWIN (1961, 1963), of Crustaceans and Mollusca by several other workers. KAYE (1962) reported that in the young spermatids of crickets dense material is present in the basal half and less dense material in the apical half of the acrosomal vesicle. MORIBER (1956) in *Gerris* demonstrated that the PAS reaction is localized at the basal level of the acrosome corresponding to the zone of higher density. No cytochemical studies have been performed so far on *Drosophila melanogaster*, but a similar cytochemical difference between the two zones of the acrosome may possibly occur. Since the heterogenity observed in *Drosophila* spermatids by SHOUP (1967) persists in completely mature sperm, it is conceivable that acrosome maturation be characterized by the emergence of regional difference in density. The sharp separation of the acrosomal material into two components probably reflects certain biochemical and functional requirements for the egg penetration, as was suggested for acrosomes of compound type.

As far as the neck zone is concerned, it consists in a portion of the spermatozoon which is approximately one half micron long, and in which the base of the nucleus, a centriolar derivative, the beginnings of the mitochondrial derivatives and the granular material of the so-called " centriole adjunct " are each others interdigitated. The complicated details of this zone will be the subject of a separate paper (this Symposium, pp. 523–529).

In the tail of *Drosophila melanogaster* spermatozoon, YASUZUMI, FUJIMURA and ISHIDA (1958), MAYER (1964), BACCETTI and BAIRATI (1964), and others have demonstrated the presence of an axial complex and two mitochondrial derivatives (Fig. 9). The sperm of *Drosophila* differs from that of other Diptera in that only one of the mitochondrial derivatives becomes enormously developed, acquiring an intricate ultrastructure with a paracrystalline body, and running along the axial complex throughout its extension, while the second derivative remains as a small rod. Fig. 10 shows a cross section of the tail examined at high resolution: the principal mitochondrial derivative, irrespectively of fixation and embedding techniques, appears to consist of roundish subunits 80 Å in diameter, arranged in a hexagonal pattern. In longitudinal sections (Fig. 11), the features of the derivative appear to be quite complex, due to the arrangement of the subunits in the hexagonal lattice. A longitudinal banding is visible, caused by the alignment of cylindrical subunits. In addition, a cross banding arises from the cylindrical subunits being arranged in rows perpendicular to the derivative's long axis. Each row of subunits is separated from the next by a dense line, thus causing a periodic cross striation at 260 Å centers. A simpler pattern of the derivative cross banding is shown in Fig. 12, the 260 Å period features a marked A band and three fainter B sub-bands. All the bands are granular in appearance and the B sub-bands evidently arise from the coalescence of the grains present within the core of every cylindrical subunit being regularly aligned in transverse lines.

The difference between the appearance of mitochondrial derivatives in these two pictures, probably may be related to the phase effect caused by different focusing of electron microscope. What is the real organization is confirmed, nevertheless, by the study of negative staining specimens. In Fig. 13 the presence is clearly shown of successive rows of sub-units, separated from each other by cross bands at 260 Å. In every row the subunits appear to interconnect along the cross band, end-to-end with those belonging to the adjacent rows. The derivative features a wavy-patterned surface, depending on the subunits' longitudinal alignment being staggered, and on the cross bands protruding from the crystalline subunit plane.

The foregoing conclusively shows that the " nebenkern " of *Drosophila melanogaster* male germ cells evolves in a highly intricate pattern, originating a derivative featuring a paracrystalline organization. Such an occurrence was ascertained in the tails of other insect's and gasteropoda's spermatozoa. HEROLD and MUNZ (1967) observed in *Peregrinus maidis* a mitochondrial derivative consisting of an outer part and of an inner body. The inner body, examined in cross sections, had a paracrystalline structure made up of dots arranged in a cubic order and set 100 Å apart from each other.

PHILLIPS (1966 a) demonstrated in *Sciara copriphila* sperm a mitochondrial derivative with a crystalloid body made up of elements spaced 90 Å center to center and showing a herringbone pattern in longitudinal sections with a periodism of 450 Å. Consequently, both the inner body of *Peregrinus maidis* and the crystalloid of *Sciara coprophila* present some analogies with the mitochondrial derivative of *Drosophila melanogaster*. According to ANDRÉ'S (1962) classification based on the degree of mitochondrial differentiation, the *Drosophila melanogaster* spermatozoon should be located amongst the third type of spermatozoa. The reorganization of the original mitochondrial elements in such a complex texture raises the question of its function. The mechanical role suggested by MAYER (1964) is presumably not the most important. The intricate paracrystalline three-dimensional organization must be related to complex biochemical functions. In the absence of a specific biochemical test for this sperm, the morphological similarity with mitochondrial derivatives of other sperms (ANDRÉ, 1962; PERSONNE, 1965; ANDERSON, PERSONNE and ANDRÉ, 1968), suggests that the constituent elements of the crystalline network may be largely proteins and represent the outcome of the reorganization of the mitochondrial cristae protein occurred during spermatogenesis, and, more specifically, a peculiar state of respiratory proteins. More recently, besides, RNA synthesis has also deen demonstrated within the derivative of *Drosophila melanogaster* by CURGY and ANDERSON (1968).

Fig. 14 shows an electron microscopic picture and a diagram of the cross section of the axial filament complex of *Drosophila melanogaster* spermatozoon. This diagram had been previously suggested by BAIRATI and BACCETTI (1965) and subsequently confirmed in *Drosophila* by SHOUP (1967), KIEFER (1966), ANDERSON (1967): the same organization pattern, however, was demonstrated in the spermatozoa of many other insects by several workers. One can recognize: (*i*) the central fibres, consisting of a wall surrounding an electronopaque central core; (*ii*) the so-called secondary fibres, which in sections appear as two adjacent granules connected to the peripheral fibres; (*iii*) the doublet of the peripheral fibres; (*iv*) the outer fibres, which appear to consist of a fibre similar to the central ones surrounded by a regular mass of granular material. The outer fibres show a major axis tangential to the surface of the complex and extending into the space between peripheral fibres in a direction opposite that of fibres arms. As far as *Drosophila melanogaster* is concerned, the most original findings obtained from investigations of cross sections are those which relate to the structure of the central and outer fibres, and the presence of conspicuous granular portions at secondary fibres' level.

Certain peculiar features can be detected by supplementing observations on thin section with those on negatively-stained fragments.

The first point to be remarked is the organization of secondary fibres. Figs. 15, 16 represent a longitudinal section of a sperm. It evidences that secondary fibres, rather than being true fibres, result from the aligning of pairs of granular portions connected to the peripheral fibres and arranged at regular intervals. Moreover, the arrangement of the granular portion in one secondary fibre (Fig. 15) is slightly offset from that of adjacent ones; consequently, the lines that link the granular portions of adjacent secondary fibres form a spiral or helix. When the section plane is exactly radial with respect to the axial filament symmetry (Fig. 16) very fine connections can be seen between the so-called secondary fibres and the primary fibres of the peripheral doublets, which give rise to the two helices, left-and-right-handed, wound around the central fibres. A highly complex system of radial connections thus appears to link the different components of the axial filament.

This finding was confirmed by the subsequent examination of the negatively-stained fragments. In point of fact, a number of protruding granular expansions appear (Figs. 29, 30) closely adhering at the side of peripheral fibres, and arranged in pairs, at intervals which exactly duplicate those found in thin sections. The interference, therefore, is that, at least in *Drosophila melanogaster* sperms, secondary fibres are not true fibres, but should be regarded as granular protruding bodies connected to the main periphera fibres.

A propos of the existence of genuine secondary fibres, the data provided by the literature are discrepant. GIBBONS and GRIMSTONE (1960) and, lately, BIRGE and DOOLIN (1969), maintained that even in the cilia there exist true secondary fibres, whereas AFZELIUS (1959) and others suggest that secondary fibres should be regarded as thickenings of the radial connections between peripheral and central fibres.

As far as the spermatozoon flagellum is concerned, the most significant data supporting the existence of secondary fibres are those reported by ANDRÉ (1961), who suggested the secondary fibres of flagella may be compared with secondary myofilaments of striated muscles. As to *Drosophila*, this hypothesis must be ruled out, since the pairs of granules forming the secondary fibres are not connected with each other. From their spatial arrangement it could be inferred that they play a mechanical role in flagellum bending, acting as an anchorage for the radial strands which irradiate from them to the central fibres and peripheral doublets. Besides, the possibility that certain specific enzyme activities should occur still another interesting hypothesis to the over-all interpretation of the functions that would be performed by the individual components of the axial complex.

Another point to be debated is the one of the principal fibres' ultrastructure. From their investigations of thin sections, BAIRATI and BACCETTI (1965) had already observed that the pair of central principal fibres exhibited the same structures as the fibres included within the outer fibre, i.e. a wall consisting of globular units surrounding a central, electronopaque portion. These ultrastructual features were subsequently demonstrated by PHILLIPS (1966 b) also in the axial complex of many Insects spermatozoa. More complete and complex findings, however, were reported by PEROTTI (1969), from the study of negatively-stained tail fragments.

The points of particular interest are: (*i*) all principal fibres consist of globular sub-units, just as observed, though with different features, by several workers for the ultrastructure of flagellar fibres, cytoplasmic microtubules and bacterial flagella; (*ii*) some particular features, however, were found in *Drosophila* spermatozoa, i.e.:

(*a*) the fibres of the peripheral doublet consist of only six sub-units (Fig. 28). Such a low number of sub-filaments is quite an exceptional finding, since a similar observation on negatively stained material has been reported only by BEHNKE and FORER, who noted 3 or 4 sub-filaments in B–subfibres of rat sperm. On the other hand, in *Drosophila* the subfilaments of subfibre wall appear more widely spaced (75 Å) than the subfilaments of such cytoplasmic microtubules and flagellar fibres as have been investigated so far. In negatively stained specimens, the A subfibres appear similar in size and morphology to B subfibres unlike other components of the peripheral doublets (illustrated by ANDRÉ and THIÉRY, 1963; BEHNKE and FORER, 1967; BURTON, 1968). Moreover, the findings of this research disagree with RINGO'S hypothesis (1967) that in a doublet structure the component subfibres share some (3–4) of the subunits forming their wall. In point of fact, whenever the A– and B–subfibres appear separated, the number of their wall subfilaments is the same.

In addition to this, no features can be evidenced that may be related to the presence of such arms as are clearly visible in cross sections.

(*b*) Another peculiarity is that of the outer fibre, which exhibits a regular row of side projections at 85 Å center, which invariably protrude from the side opposite the one where the fibres are connected with the peripheral doublet (Figs. 26–27).

(*c*) Finally (Figs. 31, 32, 33), the central fibres can be seen to exhibit a row of side projections which form a spiral with a 170 Å pitch. Projections of this type from the wall of primary fibres, have been previously observed only on the A–subfibre of peripheral doublets by BEHNKE and FORER (1967) in crane-fly sperm, where they are organized in pairs spaced at 600 Å centers, and by BURTON (1968) in lung-fluke sperm, where they are visible only after KCl treatment. In both cases, the projections have been described as spokes or arms. In *Drosophila* the projections are always present on central and on outer fibres only. As to the outer fibres, no structures have been observed in thin sections of fixed, embedded sperms corresponding in either morphology or location to the lateral projections remarked in negatively-stained preparations. Since they are present only on the fibre side opposite the localization of the B–subfibres, they may be tentatively described as a kind of connection between adjacent outer fibres.

The central fibres of sperms are as resistant to preparation treatments as other axial fibres, whereas in most of the sperm previously observed (such as supported by GRIMSTONE, KLUG, 1966, and BURTON, 1968) they broke down very easily. Since every fibre of the central pair is endowed with its own helix and the two fibres do not appear to be mutually connected by the projections while, on the other hand, the only structure in the thin sections associated with the central pair is the " central sheaths ", the latter's actual structure may be assumed to consist in the helical arrangement of the central fibre projections shown by negative staining. The projections represent a component of the radial connections between the central and so-called secondary fibres; this hypothesis is substantiated by a comparison with the thin section observations of ANDRÉ (1961) on *Macroglossus* sperm axial filament, of FRIEND (1966) on *Giardia muris* flagella and of RINGO (1967) on *Clamydomonas* flagellar apparatus. Moreover, STATO and SAKODA (1967) observed in sections of lung-fluke sperm that the central unit o the sperm tail has a sheath consisting of two helical filaments with an axial pitch of 100 Å. Thus, by supplementing observations on thin sections with those performed or negatively-stained material, it has been possible to evidence in *Drosophila melanogaster* a very complex system of connections linking among the components of the axial filament. This system consists of (*i*) the double helix connecting the peripheral doublets to secondary fibres; (*ii*) the radial connections between central and secondary fibres; (*iii*) tangential connections between adjacent outer fibres. Considering that this kind of projection of flagellar fibres such as arms of peripheral fibres of cilia have been demonstrated (by GIBBONS and ROWE, 1965) to consist of a protein (dynein) possessing adenosine phosphatase activity, the possibility exists that also the three-dimensional system of connections present in *Drosophila* sperm flagellum may have something to do with the biochemical processes of axial fibre contraction.

All the ultrastructure features that have been described, therefore, show that the organization of the axial tail complex of *Drosophila melanogaster* spermatozoon is one of the most intricate reported so far. Particularly interesting appears to be the relationship existing between this remarkable ultrastructural complexity and the intricate motion patterns of this spermatozoon. In point of fact, preliminary observations performed with the help of phase-contrast microscopy have shown the *Drosophila* spermatozoon to be endowed with a fast spiralling motion around its longer axis, and with a slower undulatory motion.

The end piece of the tail is about 1 micron long and presents progressive, peculiar modifications of the axial complex organization. By resorting to the method of seriate sections, PEROTTI (1969) has been able to demonstrate how all the flagellum components are modified and how they end: to the best of our knowledge, no similar findings have been reported for other spermatozoa. Figs. 17 and 25 present a proximal-distal series of cross sections along the tail tip. In a more proximal part the principal mitochondrial derivative becomes smaller and oval with the long axis tangential to the tail surface, the paracrystalline pattern being now hardly visible. In the axial filament the Afzelius spokes and secondary fibres disappear; the peripheral doublet appears to be replaced by 9 single fibres endowed with dense cap-shaped elements. It has been ascertained that it's the A–subfibres that are lost and replaced by the dense cap-shaped elements. The nine single fibres, B–subfibres, with the cap-shaped elements are not arranged in radial symmetry, but one of them projects towards the centre giving rise to a spiral arrangement of the peripleral fibres. Gradually the tail diameter tapers, the mitochondrial derivatives disappear and the number of peripheral fibres decreases: the peripheral elements one after the other in a clockwise sequence lose their cap-shaped structure, decrease in diameter and disappear, followed by the corresponding outer fibre. Simultaneously, the remaining B–subfibres slip counter clockwise, so that the spiral decrease in number. The central fibres also decrease in size, gradually lose their sheaths and eventually separate from each other. In the end, only 4–5 peripheral fibres and the central ones are present, but they appear to be fused together so that the extreme tail tip looks dense and structureless. Along the tail end piece the sperm surface exhibits a scalloped outline, the bulges corresponding to the outer fibres.

Finally, a few considerations may be submitted.

The mature sperm of *Drosophila melanogaster* consists of two parts—a head and a tail (Diag. 1). Head and tail are connected by a very short region containing a highly modified centriole and the beginning of the mitochon-

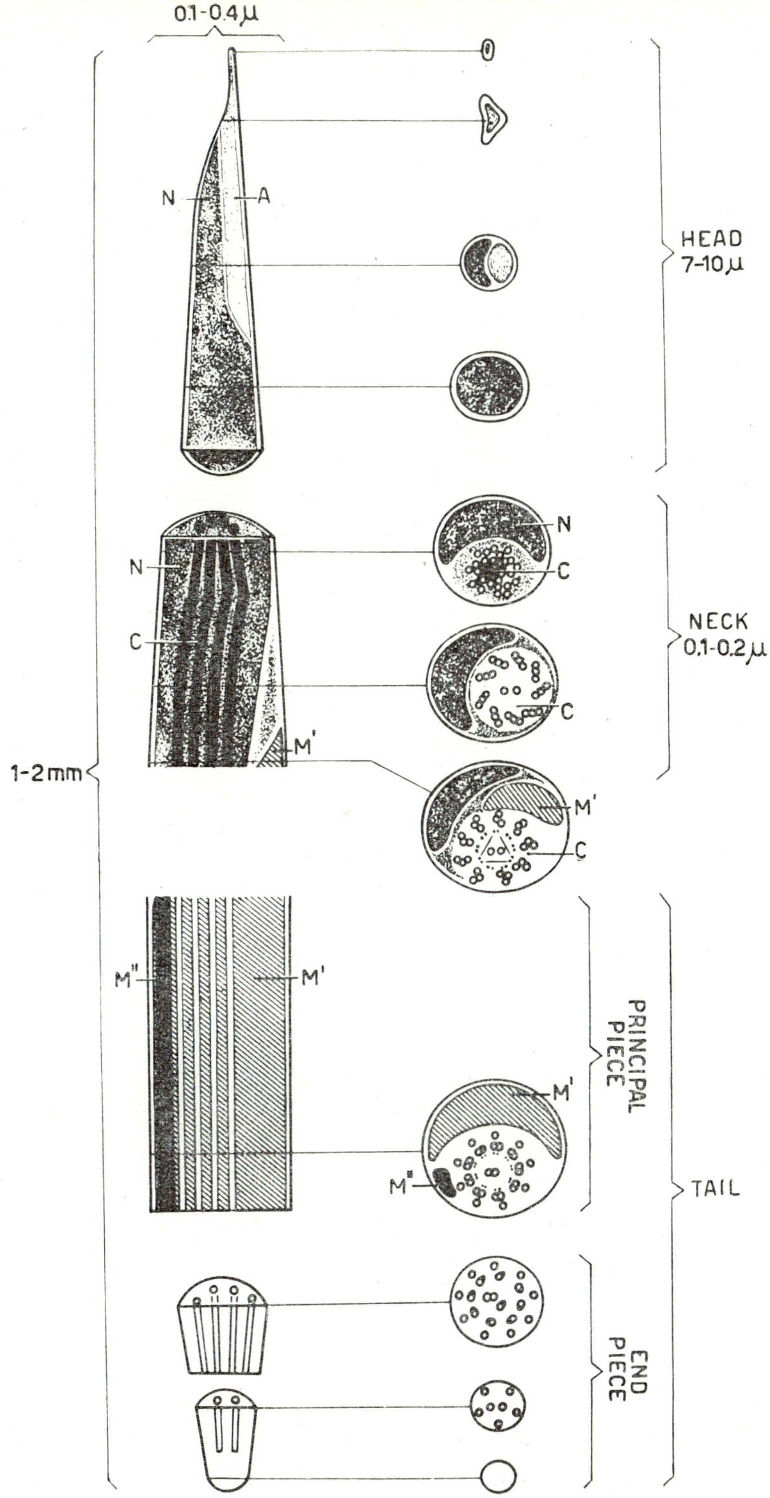

Diagram 1. – Diagram of the whole sperm illustrating the main features of the ultrastructure of its different parts.

N = nucleus; A = acrosome; C = centriole derivative; M' = principal mitochondrial derivative M'' = second mitochondrial derivative.

drial derivatives. This portion may be called a neck according to the usual terminology.

As to the tail, it is impossible to use here the classic zonation originally coined for mammal sperms, based on the presence of a " middle piece " and of a " principal piece " and " end piece " differentiated by the presence of the mitochondrial sheath along the middle piece. Since in this sperm, as in sperms of other insects, the mitochondrial derivative accompanies the axial filament through most of its length, it would be better to apply a more general terminology, as previously suggested by BACCETTI and BAIRATI (1964), based upon axial filament ultrastructure rather than on the presence of mitochondrial derivatives. Two sections can therefore be distinguished: (1) a principal piece, where the axial filament displays its most complex structure (in *Drosophila melanogaster* the mitochondrial derivatives are closely apposed to it and the secondary fibres are still present in the complex), and (2) an end piece, where the axial filament undergoes gradual changes in fibre organization showing a simpler structure. Because of the structure of its axial filament and the paracrystalline hexagonal texture of its mitochondrial derivative, the sperm of *Drosophila melanogaster* appears to be one of the most complex ever examined. It would be interesting for comparative purposes to investigate such relations as may possibly link the axial filament ultrastructure, enzyme localization, biochemical nature of the individual axial filament components, degree of specialization of the mitochondrial derivative and motion mechanism of this sperm.

REFERENCES

AFZELIUS B. A. (1959) – *Electron microscopy of the sperm tail.* « J. Biophys. Biochem. Cytol. », 5, 269–281.

ANDERSON W. A. (1967) – *Cytodifferentiation of spermatozoa in* Drosophila melanogaster: *the effect of elevated temperature on spermiogenesis.* « Mol. Gen. Genetics », 99, 257–273.

ANDERSON W. A., PERSONNE P. and ANDRÉ J. (1968) – *Chemical compartmentalization in* Helix *spermatozoa.* « J. Microscopie », 7, 367–390.

ANDRÉ J. (1961) – *Sur quelques détails nouvellement connus de l'ultrastructure des organites vibratiles.* « J. Ultrastruct. Res. », 5, 86–108.

ANDRÉ J. (1962) – *Contribution à la connaissance du condriome. Etude de ses modifications ultrastructurelles pendant la spermatogénèse.* « J. Ultrastrut. Res. », suppl. 3, 1–85.

ANDRÉ J. and THIÉRY J. (1963) – *Mise in evidence d'une sous-structure fibrillaire dans les filaments axonematiques des flagelles.* « J. Microscopie », 2, 71–80.

BACCETTI B. and BAIRATI A. (1964) – *Indagini comparative sull'ultrastruttura delle cellule germinali maschili in* Dacus oleae *Gmell ed in* Drosophila melanogaster *Meig.* « Redia », 49, 1–29.

BAIRATI A. and BACCETTI B. (1965) – *Indagini comparative sull'ultrastruttura delle cellule germinali maschili in* Dacus oleae Gmell ed in Drosophila melanogaster *Meig.* II. *Nuovi reperti ultrastrutturali sul filamento assile degli spermatozoi.* « Redia », 49, 81–85.

BEHNKE O. and FORER A. (1967) – *Evidence for four classes of microtubules in individual cells.* « J. Cell Sci. », 2, 169–192.

BIRGE W. J. and DOOLIN P. F. (1969) – *Ultrastructural organization of secondary fibers and radial links in cilia.* « J. Microscopie », 8, 167–178.

BURTON P. R. (1968) – *Effect of various treatments on microtubules and axial units of lung-fluke spermatozoa.* « Z. Zellforsch. Mikros. Anat. », 87, 226–248.

COLWIN A. L. and COLWIN L. H. (1961) – *Fine structure of the spermatozoon of* Hydroydes hexagonus (*Anellida*) *with special reference to the acrosomal region.* « J. Biophys. Biochem. Cytol. », 10, 211–230.

COLWIN A. L. and COLWIN L. H. (1963) – *Role of the gamete membranes in fertilization in* Saccoglossus kowaleskii (*Enteropneuta*). I. *The acrosome region and its changes in early stages of fertilization.* « J. Cell Biol. », 19, 477–500.

COOPER K. W. (1950) – *Normal spermatogenesis in Drosophila*: In: *Biology of Drosophila.* Ed. Demerc, Wiley and Sons, New York.

CURGY J. J. and ANDERSON W. A. (1968) – *Synthèse de* l'ARN *mitochondrial et de l'*ARN *nucleaire aux different stages de la spermatogenesis chez la Drosophile.* In: *Electron Microscopy.* IV Eur. Reg. Conf. Electron microscopy, vol. 2, 211–212. Tip. Poliglotta Vaticana. Roma.

DAN J. C. (1960) – *Studies on the acrosome.* VI. *Fine structure of the starfish acrosome.* « Exp. Cell Res. », 19, 13–28.

DOBZHANSKY T. (1934) – *Studies on hybrid sterility.* I. *Spermatogenesis in pure and hybrid* Drosophila pseudoscura. « Z. Zellforsch. Mikros. Anat. », 21, 169–233.

FAWCETT W. and HOLLENBERG R. (1963) – *Changes in the acrosome of Guinea pig spermatozoa during passage through the epididymis.* « Z. Zellforsch. Mikr. Anat. », 60, 276–292.

FRIEND D. S. (1966) – *The fine structure of* Giardia muris. « J. Cell Biol. », 29, 317–332.

GIBBONS I. R. and GRIMSTONE A. V. (1960) – *On flagellar structure in certain flagellates.* « J. Biophys. Biochem. Cytol. », 7, 697–716.

GIBBONS I. R. and ROWE A. J. (1965) – *Dynein, a protein with adenosine triphosphatasë activity from cilia.* « Science », 149, 424–426.

GRIMSTONE A. V. and KLUG A. (1966) – *Observations on the ultrastructure of flagellar fibres.* – « J. Cell Sci. », 1, 351–362.

HEROLD F. and MUNZ K. (1967) – *Ultrastructure of spermatozoa of* Peregrinus maidis (*Homoptera, Delphacidae*). « Z. Zellforsch. Mikro. Anat. », 83, 364–374.

KAYE J. S. (1962) – *Acrosome formation in the house cricket.* « J. Cell Biol. », 12, 411–431.

KIEFER N. I. (1966) – *Ultrastructural abnormalities in developing sperm of* X/O Drosophila melanogaster. « Genetics », 54, 1441–1452.

LOCKE M. (1966) – *The structure and formation of the cuticuline layer in the epicuticle of an insect,* Calpodes ethlius (*Lepidoptera, Hesperiidae*). « J. Morphol. », 118, 461–464.

MEYER G. F. (1964) – *Die parakristallinen korper in den spermienschwassen von Drosophila.* « Z. Zellforsch. Mikrosk. Anat. », 62, 762–784.

MORIBER L. G. (1956) – *A cytochemical study of Hemipteran spermatogenesis.* « J. Morphol. », 99, 271–326.

NOIROT–TIMOTHÉE C., NOIROT C. and ESCAIG J. (1965) – *Asymétrie de la membraine cellulaire dans l'intestine moyen de la reine des Termites superieurs.* « J. Microscopie », 4, 83–86.

PEROTTI M. E. (1969) – *Ultrastructure of the mature sperm of* Drosophila melanogaster *Meig.* « J. Submicr. Cytol. » 1, 171–196.

PERSONNE P. (1965) – *Etude cytochimique du dérivé mitochondrial du spermatozoide de la Testacelle: recherche des proteins et des lipides.* « J. Microscopie », 4, 627–642.

PHILLIPS D. M. (1966 a) – *Fine structure of* Sciara coprophila *sperm.* « J. Cell Biol. », 30, 499–517.

PHILLIPS D. M. (1966 b) – *Substructure of flagellar tubules.* « J. Cell Biol. », 31, 635–638.

RINGO D. L. (1967) – *The arrangement of subunits in flagellar fibres.* « J. Ultrastruct., Res. », 17, 266–277.

SHOUP J. R., (1967) – *Spermiogenesis in wild type and a male mutant of* Drosophila melanogaster. « J. Cell Biol. », 32, 663–675.

STATO M. OH M. and SAKODA K. (1967) – *Electron microscopic study of spermatogenesis in the lung-fluke* (Paragonimus miyazakii). « Z. Zellforsch. Mikroskop. Anat. », 77, 232–243.

YASUZUMI G., FUJIMURA W. and ISHIDA H. (1958) – *Spermatogenesis in animals as revealed by electron microscopy*. V. *Spermatid differentiation of* Drosophila *and grasshoper*. « Exptl. Cell Res. », 14, 258–285.

EXPLANATION OF FIGURES

Figs. 1–2. – Cross sections of mature sperm at the head (Fig. 1) and at the tail (Fig. 2) levels showing the asymmetrical structure of the plasma membrane (*Pm*). ×140,000 ×200,000.

N = nucleus; *Nm* = nuclear membrane; *Ax* = axial filament; *M'* = principal mitochondrial derivative.

Figs. 3–8. – Series of cross sections in order from proximal to distal of the head apex in a mature sperm showing the acrosome (*A*) shape at different levels and its relations with the nucleus (*N*). ×120,000.

Fig. 9. – Sperm tails cross sectioned: the principal mitochondrial derivative (*M'*) exhibits a paracrystalline structure visible also at low magnification. ×120,000.

M' = second mitochondrial derivative.

Fig. 10. – Cross section of the principal mitochondrial derivative examined at high magnification. The paracrystalline lattice consists of roundish subunits hexagonally arranged. ×500,000.

Fig. 11. – Longitudinal section of the principal mitochondrial derivative. A periodic cross striation of 260 Å is clearly visible, whereas a longitudinal banding arises from the alignement of cylindrical subunits. ×260,000.

Fig. 12. – Longitudinal section of the principal mitochondrial derivative, showing a simpler pattern of the cross period, which appears to consist of a more marked band (A band) and three fainter sub-bands (B sub-bands). ×260,000.

Fig. 13. – Principal mitochondrial derivative negatively stained with PTA; a cross period of 260 Å is present and the paracrystalline organization confirms the pattern observed in thins sections (see Fig. 11). ×260,000.

Fig. 14. – Cross section and diagram of the axial filament. ×160,000.

POF = primary outer fiber; *PPF* = primary fibers of the peripheral doublets; *PCF* = primary central fibers; *AS* = Afzelius spokes; *SF* = secondary fibers; *G* = granular material surrounding the outer fibers.

Figs. 15–16. – Longitudinal sections of sperm axial filaments showing the actual structure of the secondary fibers (*SF*) consisting of pairs of electron-opaque granules in longitudinal arrangement. In tangential sections (Fig. 15) it is possible to observe a slight stagger in the alignement of the granules of adjacent secondary fibers. In radial sections, there are thin links to be noted connecting the secondary fibers to the fibers of the peripheral doublets (*PF*) and giving rise to a double helix, right-and left-handed. ×120,000.

CF = central fiber.

Figs. 17–25. – Cross sections in order from proximal to distal of the tail end piece. The principal mitochondrial derivative shape modifies before it disappears (Fig. 17), 9 single fibers endowed with an electrondense cap-shaped structure have replaced the peripheral doublets (Figs. 17, 18) and more caudally one by one decrease in size (Fig. 19), lose their cap and disappear. The arrows point to the fiber which first undergoes modification and disappears. At the most caudal level (Fig. 24) the remaining fibers fuse together and the extreme tail tip appears dense and structureless. ×120,000.

Figs. 26–33. – Axial filament fibres isolated with ultrasounds and negatively stained with *PTA*.

Fig. 26. – Triplet of fibres consisting of an outer fibre (*OF*), the A sub-fibre (*A*) and the B-sub-fibres (*B*) of a peripheral doublet. The outer fibre is endowed with very evident side projections and in its wall 5–6 subfilaments are visible. The granular material present along the A subfibre belongs to the secondary fibres (*SF*). ×140,000.

Fig. 27. – Detail of the structure of an outer fibre. The side projections are spaced of 85 Å. ×180,000.

Fig. 28. – Detail a peripheral doublet: both the A sub-fibre (*A*) and the *B* subfibre (*B*) exhibit in their wall three beaded subfilaments. ×200,000.

SF = secondary fibre.

Figs. 29–30. – Details of the organization of secondary fibres (*SF*). Negative staining confirmed the granular structure of these fibres as observed also in thin sections (see Figs. 15, 16). The subfibres of the peripheral doublet (*PD*) are not here distinguishable from each other. ×140,000.

Figs. 31–33. – Central fibres: all over their surface there are projections to be noted spaced of 170 Å (Figs. 31, 32), which give rise to an apparent helical surface pattern (Figs. 32, 33). ×120,000. ×200,000. ×140,000.

Aurelio Bairati and M. Elisa Perotti - *Some comparative considerations on the ultrastructure of* Drosophila melanogaster *spermatozoon.*

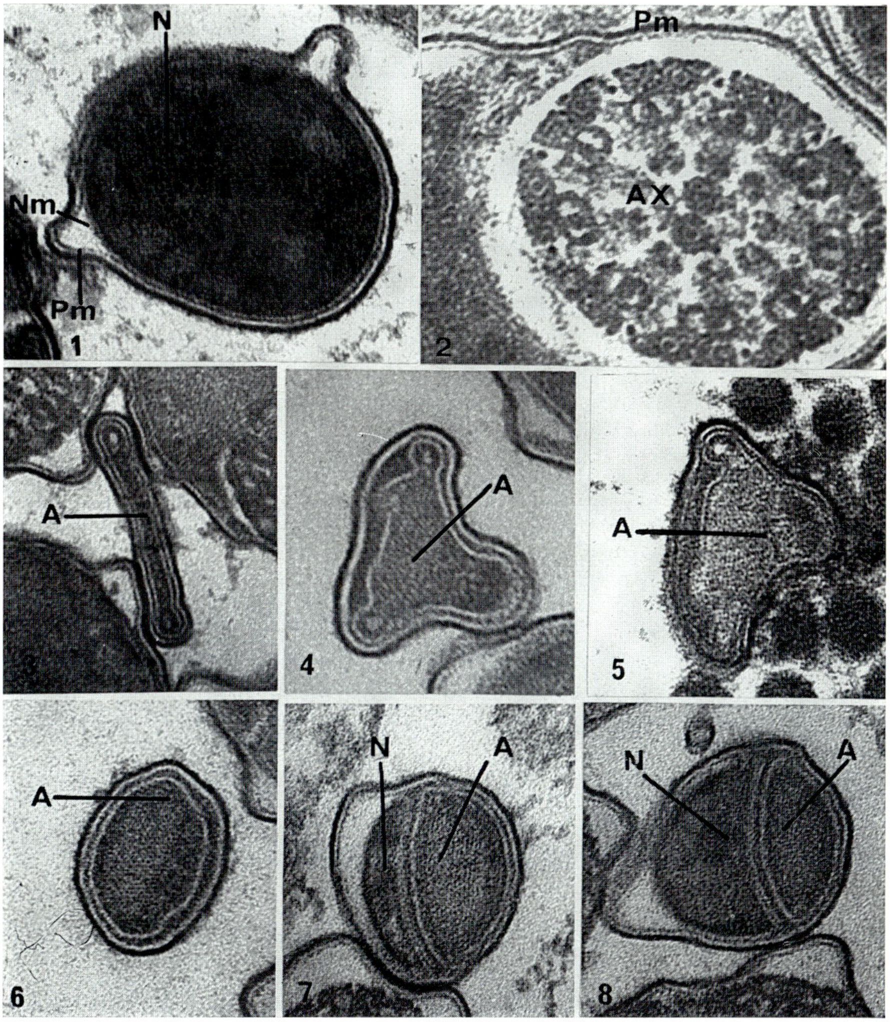

AURELIO BAIRATI and M. ELISA PEROTTI – *Some comparative considerations on the ultrastructure of* Drosophila melanogaster *spermatozoon.*

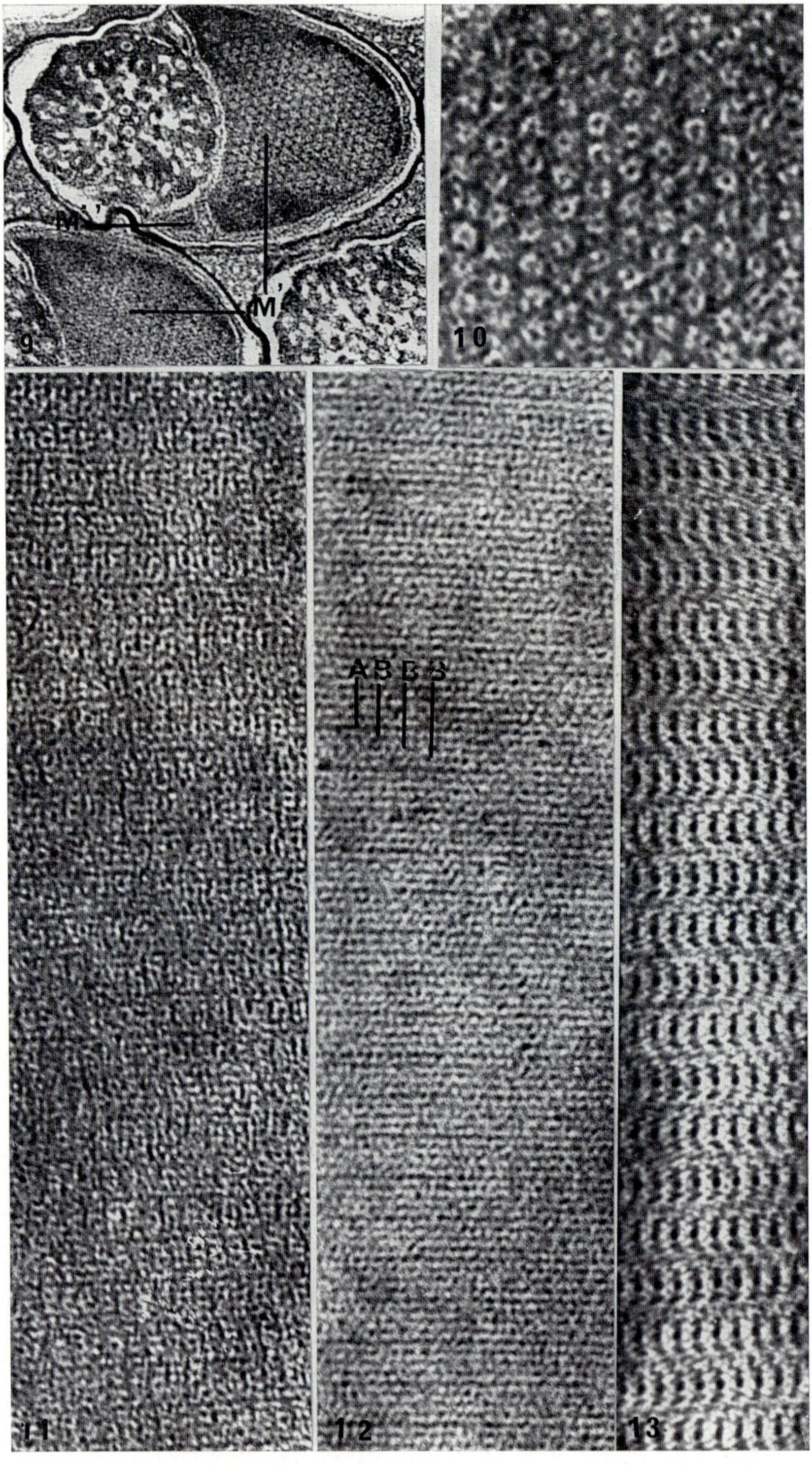

AURELIO BAIRATI and M. ELISA PEROTTI – *Some comparative considerations on the ultrastructure of* Drosophila melanogaster *spermatozoon.*

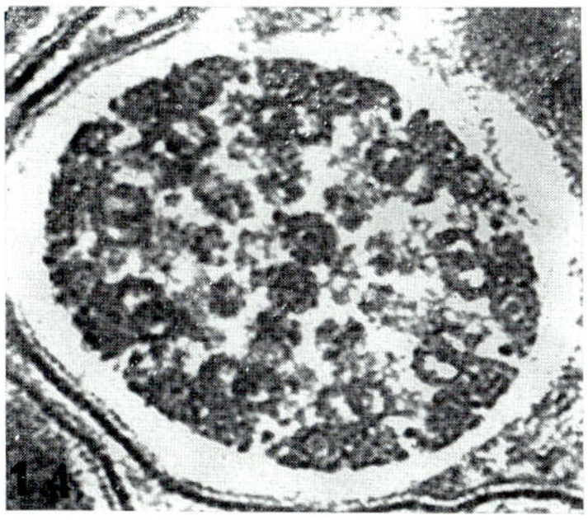

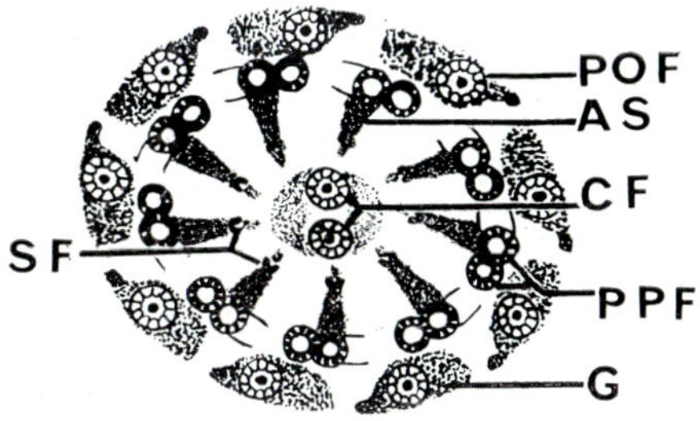

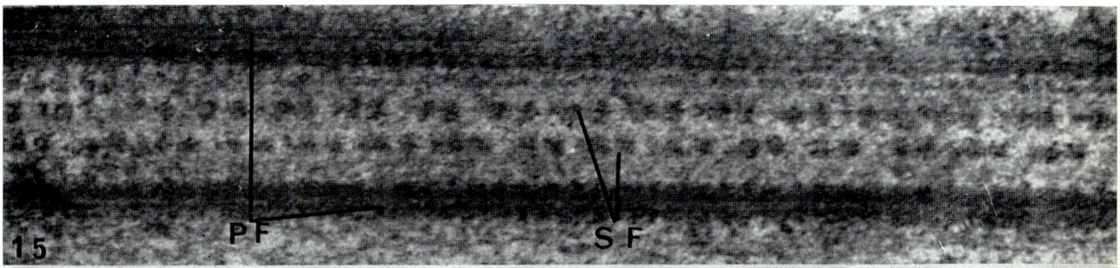

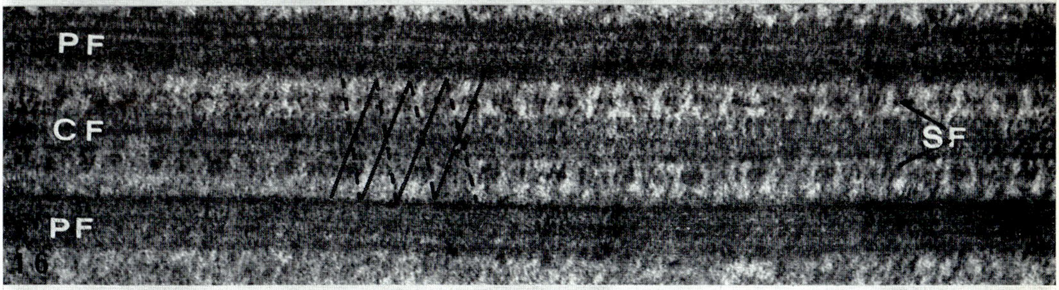

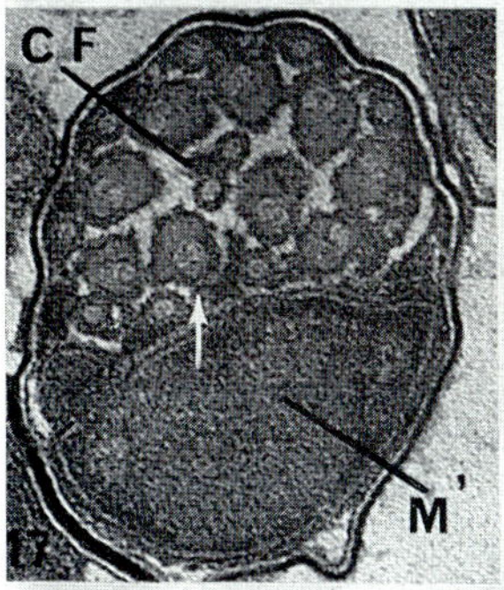

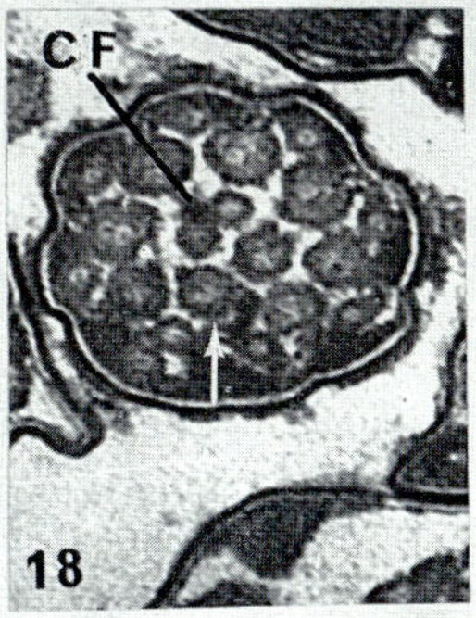

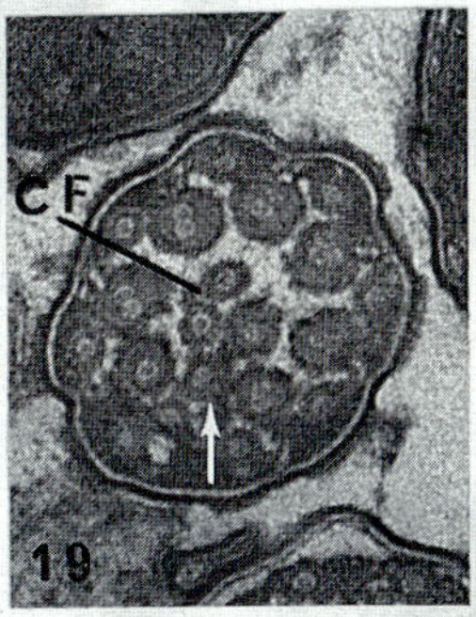

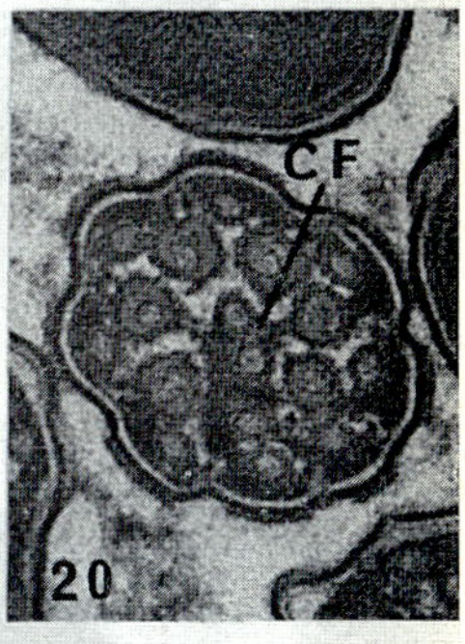

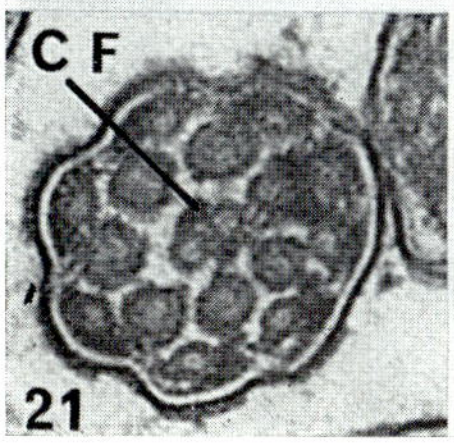

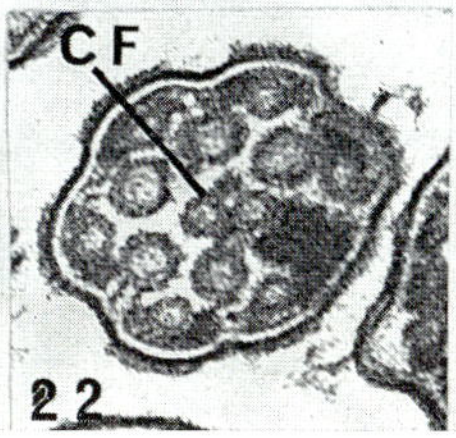

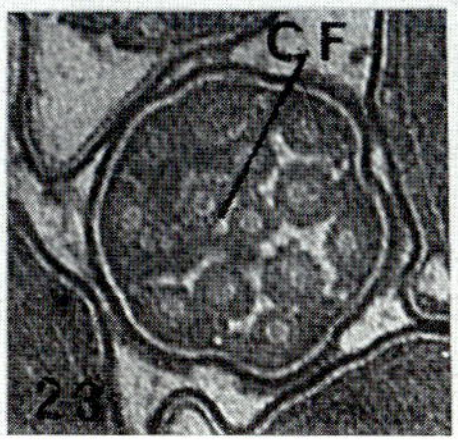

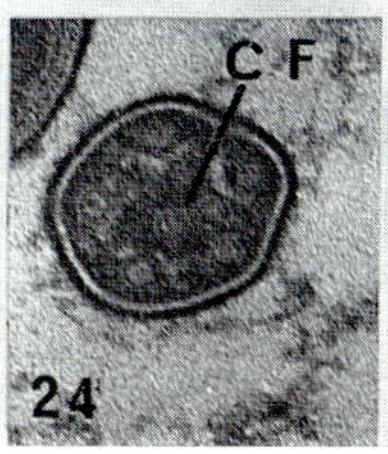

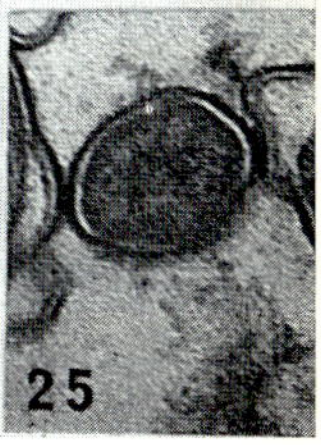

Aurelio Bairati and M. Elisa Perotti – *Some comparative considerations on the ultrastructure of* Drosophila melanogaster *spermatozoon.*

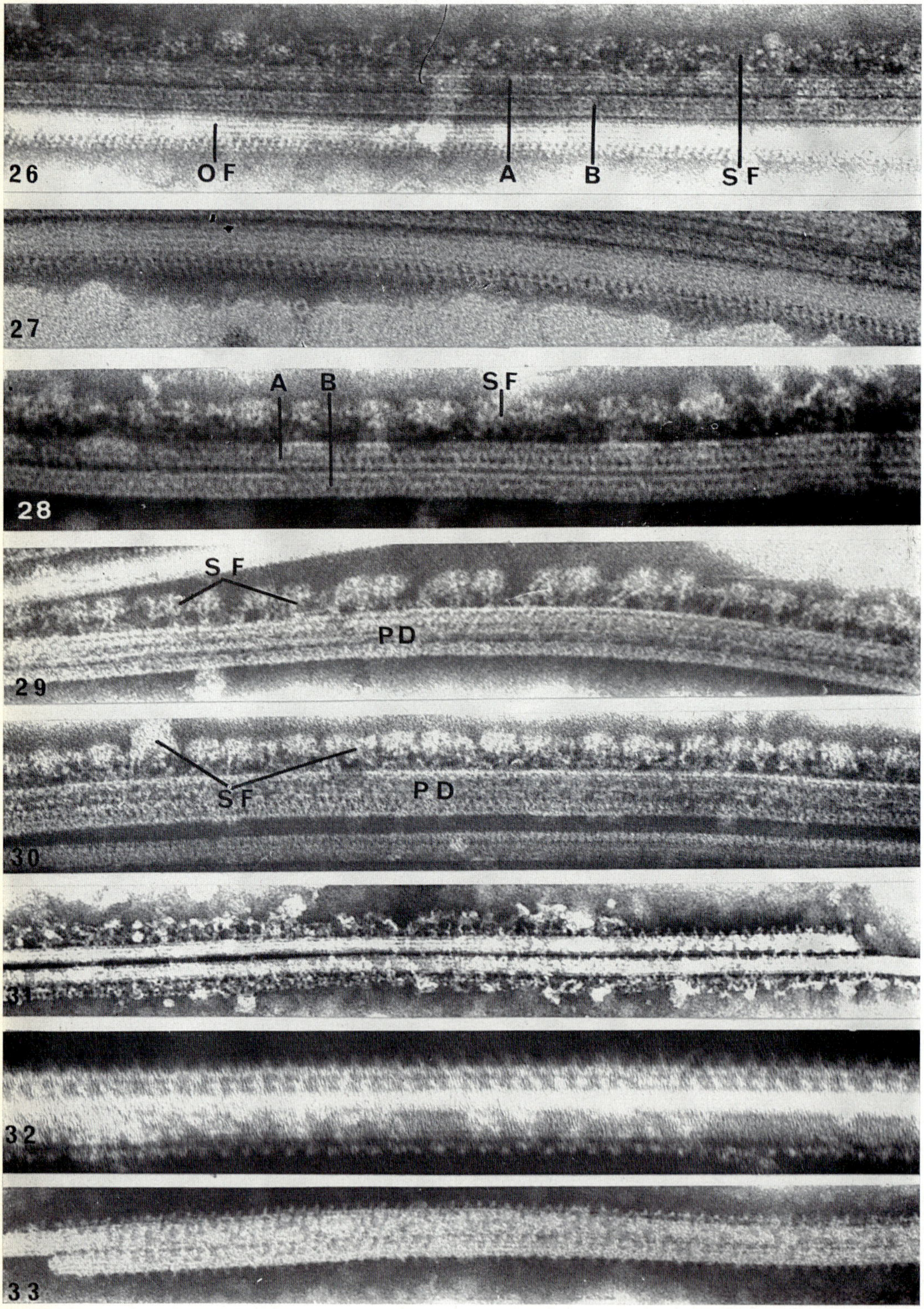

G. F. MEYER (*)

PHENOCOPIES OF Y DEFICIENCIES AND EXTRAORDINARY DIFFERENTIATION TYPES IN SPERMIOGENESIS OF *DROSOPHILA*

SUMMARY. — In *Drosophila* the spermatogenic process is under the control of genetic factors located on the Y chromosome. Partially or totally Y deficient males show many developmental aberrations in differentiating spermatids. These seem to be due to a lack of proper organization of most if not all structural sub-components that compose the spermatid organelles. Even in genetically normal males a number of aberrant gametes is observed. This number can be further increased by means of rather unspecific physical and chemical treatments which copy the differentiative defects observed in Y deficient males. The same treatments may in addition induce new types of spermatid differentiation. It seems that differentiation in cells with an inactive nucleus is especially sensitive to changes in timing and in the synthetic rates produced by environmental factors.

RIASSUNTO. — In *Drosophila* la spermatogenesi è sotto il controllo dei fattori genetici situati sul cromosoma Y. I maschi che mancano parzialmente o totalmente del cromosoma Y presentano molte aberrazioni negli spermatidi che si stanno differenziando. Queste sembrano dovute a una mancanza di organizzazione della maggior parte, se non di tutti i sub-componenti strutturali che formano gli organuli dello spermatidio. A volte, in maschi geneticamente normali, sono stati osservati gameti aberranti. Il loro numero può essere ulteriormente aumentato mediante trattamenti fisici e chimici relativamente aspecifici, che danno luogo ai difetti di differenziazione osservati nei maschi mancanti del cromosoma Y. Gli stessi trattamenti possono inoltre indurre nuovi tipi di differenziazione. Sembra che la differenziazione in cellule con nucleo inattivo sia sensibile soprattutto a cambiamenti nei tempi e nelle velocità di sintesi dovute a fattori ambientali.

INTRODUCTION

Spermiogenesis in *Drosophila* is dependent upon the presence of a complete Y chromosome (BRIDGES, 1916; STERN, 1927). Y deficient males are fully viable but sterile. It has been concluded that the (heterochromatic) Y chromosome carries a number of fertility factors indispensable for the development of normal, fertile sperm. The functional phase of these factors is characterized by the formation of giant loops at various loci on the Y chromosome (MEYER, 1963; HESS and MEYER, 1963 a; 1963 b; 1968). In partially or totally Y deficient males, many developmental aberrations in germ line cells have been observed (MEYER, 1968; HESS and MEYER, 1968)

(*) Max-Planck-Institut für Biologie, Abt. Beermann Tübingen, Germany.

which can be roughly classified into "early" and "late" effects on the process of differentiation of spermatids. This shows that different loop forming segments differ in their morphogenetic capacity and are not simply additive in function (MEYER, 1968). Electron microscopy of spermiogenesis in Y deficient males leads to the conclusion that all structural components for development of normal sperm are present but that they fail to be properly organized. Recently, it has been found that a limited number of gametes even in normal X/Y males may show identical or very similar alterations (MEYER, 1968; 1969). The number of such aberrant gametes copying the differentiative defects observed in Y deficient males (MEYER, 1969) can be further increased by means of rather unspecific physical and chemical treatments. The same treatments may in addition induce new types of spermatid differentiation.

MATERIAL AND METHODS

Light microscopical examinations of the testes of different *Drosophila* species (*D. melanogaster, D. hydei, D. virilis*) were carried out as reported previously (MEYER, 1968). For electron microscopical investigation, the testes were fixed in glutaraldehyde (GORDON *et al.*, 1963) for 30 minutes, washed in *Drosophila* Ringer (15 minutes), and postfixed for 30 minutes in a 1% OsO_4 solution (MILLONIG, 1961). The specimens were passed through a graded series of ethanol and embedded in Epon 812 (LUFT, 1961). Thin sections were made with a LKB ultratome using glass knives and mounted on formvar coated grids. Sections were stained with a saturated lead acetate solution for 10 minutes. Micrographs were made with a Siemens Elmiskop I and a Zeiss EM 9.

In order to produce developmental aberrations the following treatments were used (for details see MEYER, 1969): *Drosophila* Ringer, NaCl, KCl, $MgCl_2$, Colcemide, Cycloheximide, Actinomycin C, D_2O, elevated temperatures, X–rays, transplantation of gonads and imaginal discs according to the method developed by EPHRUSSI and BEADLE (1936), and injection of homogenates of X/O testes into X/Y larvae. In general, 3rd instar larvae (which particularly in D. hydei allow a rather exact timing) were used for the experiments. The testes of such larvae do not contain stages older than late spermatocytes. In most cases testes of adults were examined after treatment of larvae.

RESULTS

All agents used in the present experiments may result in a disturbance of the regular organizational pattern of spermatids and sperm composing a cyst as well as irregularities in the submicroscopic architecture of the sperm organelles. The majority of the effects induced in young spermatids may be observed with the light microscope whereas for the recognition of those exhibited in later developmental stages the use of the electron microscope is indispensable. The negative effects on differentiation are always restricted to a limited number of cysts and are more severe in the peripheral area. In general, increases in the dosage of chemical agents and radiation as well as in temperature cause an increase in the number of defects.

Structural aberration varies within a cyst and also between cysts, as described for Y deficiencies (MEYER, 1968). The disintegration of flagella is shown as an example (Fig. 1). Usually such severe alterations are restricted to the periphery of the cysts affected. The central region generally shows less severe defects or may even be normal. This holds true for genetically complete and fertile males, Y deficient males and phenocopies of Y deficiencies. The cyst in Fig. 1 originates from a wild type male of D. *virilis*. No normal flagellum has been formed in this area. Similar defects are observed in genetically normal testes after interspecific transplantation and subsequent fusion of gonads. Malformations in the *D. melanogaster* testis after fusion with a *D. virilis* testis shows Fig. 2. Since *D. melanogaster* normally exhibits a rather stable differentiation (MEYER, 1969), it is very likely that the disintegration of many axial fiber complexes in Fig. 1 B (arrows) results from a negative influence of the fusion process itself.

In *D. hydei* both nebenkern derivatives are transformed into material with a very regular crystalline pattern (MEYER, 1964; 1966, 1968). In contrast, in *D. melanogaster* only one nebenkern derivative is transformed while the second degenerates (Fig. 2, S_1). However, normal X/Y males of *D. melanogaster*, e.g. after ligature of the larvae or heat treatment frequently show a transformation of both nebenkern derivatives (comp. Fig. 2, S_2). It is not known whether these modified sperm later achieve motility.

Most, if not all, organizational defects at the level of the differentiating spermatid of Y deficient males can be phenocopied in males with a complete Y chromosome. All agents investigated so far, and there are certainly many more, induce alterations. This category includes specific agents such as antibiotics as well as rather unspecific (heat and X–rays). Differentiantive aberrations are not only negative, as demonstrated in Fig. 1, they may be also " positive ", or at least neutral, if instead of one nebenkern derivative both are transformed. Other, new cases of harmonic arrangement of structural subunits in spermatids are described subsequently.

Testes of males developed after injection of Ringer solution show new differentiation types in a few spermatid cysts. All spermatids of one cyst are uniformly altered (Fig. 3). In cross sections each spermatid contains a central dense body surrounded by a ring of microtubules (diameter ~ 250 Å) interconnected by a thin, diffuse band (arrows) (*). The number of the tubules surrounding the central body is in spermatid a 18, in b 19, in c 19, and in d 20. This would correspond to 9 outer doublets and 1 or 2 central ones. In addition 4 incomplete " rings " are formed. Sometimes a second body (nebenkern derivative?) is observed (Fig. 3 center, right). In the periphery of such cysts aberrant differentiation types may again occur. In other cross sections the central bodies may be elongated and dumbbell-shaped or much smaller and roundish. The ring of microtubules may be interrupted and the

(*) Further investigations of the origin of the central body within the ring of microtubules indicate that this body is a normal stage in the elongation of the nucleus. The system of nucleus, tubules and rings also shows variability possibly induced by the phenocopying treatment (see fig. 6).

number reduced to 11 or 9. Such spermatids may contain only 3 " rings " or no " ring " at all. Another new feature in these cysts is the formation of clusters of microtubules between spermatids. Further investigations on the origin of the new organelles have demonstrated that young spermatid nuclei show laterally attached double structures very similar to the incomplete " rings " in spermatid tails (Fig. 5). In later differentiation stages these rings disappear. It remains open whether or not they are transformed into lateral double structure seen in Fig. 4. The origin of the central body remains unclear, since intermediate stages have not been detected. Adjacent cysts of similar age show spermatids with growing crystals in the nebenkern derivatives. The central bodies, surrounded by microtubules do not show an outer membrane. With a few exceptions (see Fig. 3) only one body is present, whereas if indeed derived from nebenkern derivatives one would expect two.

In one case, however, spermatids have been observed with an intermediate type of organization between the normal and the new differentiation type (Fig. 6). Such spermatids contain a flagellum (*F*), a nucleus (*N*), and 4 ring-like structures. The upper spermatid in Fig. 6 shows a defective organization. Two of the four rings are translocated into a separated area of the spermatid (arrows). The same spermatid shows a flagellar fragment (*Ff*). Unfortunately the section was slightly oblique so that the fine structure of the flagellum remains unclear.

Other cysts with aberrant differentiation types are seen in Fig. 7 and 8. The cyst in Fig. 7 shows numerous microtubules in a crystalline array after preceding treatment of larvae with colcemide which does not affect flagellar fibers in *Drosophila* (comp. BEHNKE and FORER, 1967). The injection of homogenates of X/O testes into 3rd instar larvae of normal X/Y constitution may induce the formation of additional satellites (Fig. 8). Their numbers varies, being 9 or less. The differentiation of these flagella is almost completed since the central pair shows the dense mature state (comp. MEYER, 1968), despite a very defective differentiation of the cyst as a whole. No regular geometrical relation of flagella and nebenkern derivatives can be observed in such cysts.

In the foregoing section phenocopies of Y deficiencies and new differentiation types of spermatids have been described. In contrast to the cases of new differentiation or defective development of spermatids some cysts as a whole show various degrees of dedifferentiation (Fig. 9). The total contents of such cysts after a heat shock (40° C for 2 minutes) applied to larvae or pupae show no cellular organization into spermatids (Fig. 9). Several compartments of varying size and limited by membranes are developed, ribosomes (*ri*) are abundant. Other inclusions consist of homogeneous material of unknown nature. Since mitochondria are not present, the dense homogeneous inclusions may represent nebenkern derivatives. In the periphery of the cyst a few well differentiated sperm are developed consisting of flagella and crystalline nebenkern derivatives. They are connected syncytially without plasma membranes. The completely normal organization of these flagella is demonstrated in Fig. 11. Three bodies (transformed nebenkern derivatives?) are visible in the vicinity of the flagellum. An intermediate stage of cyst dedifferentiation between the cyst of Fig. 9 and normal cysts is demonstrated in Fig. 10. Nebenkern derivatives and flagella (arrows) are present. Three spermatids show a disintegration or fragmentation of nebenkern derivatives into small pieces. A single flagellum is present in each spermatid.

CONCLUSIONS

In *Drosophila* the spermatogenic process is under the control of several loci on the Y chromosome which have been called fertility factors (BRIDGES, 1916; STERN, 1927; BROSSEAU, 1960; HESS, 1968; MEYER, 1968). Y deficient males are fully viable but sterile. It appears that in partially Y deficient males most, if not all structural components of sperm organelles are present but fail to be organized into ordered complexes of typical architecture (MEYER, 1968). It is conceivable, therefore, that the Y factors control the coordination of the various synthetic and morphogenetic processes without themselves contributing structural information on the molecular level.

In primary spermatocytes the Y chromosome develops a number of giant loops at various loci whose sequence and localization have been determined by HESS (1965). Loss of a single loop pair causes sterility with the exception of the so-called pseudonucleolus (HESS, 1967; MEYER, 1968). Males deficient for this giant fused loop produce a few slightly motile sperm which may even be fertile (HESS, 1967).

It has long been known that the fertility rate in *Drosophila* wild type males (and many other organisms) depends upon age, nutrition and temperature. Elevated temperatures above 28° C cause partial or total sterility in *Drosophila* (YOUNG and PLOUGH, 1926; ANDERSON, 1967; MEYER, 1969). The investigation of such males demonstrated differentiational aberrations in a variable number of cysts. An increase in temperature increases the number of cysts with defective spermatids. Other agents (MEYER, 1969) induce similar alterations ranging from subfertility to sterility. Most aberrations in spermatids correspond to those observed in Y deficient males. Such non-hereditary copies of a known mutant phenotype have been called phenocopies by R. GOLDSCHMIDT (1935, for ref. see also 1957 *a*, *b*, and *c*). In *Drosophila*, according to GOLDSCHMIDT (1957 a), all types of morphological mutants of all organs have been copied by application of largely unspecific agents to eggs or larvae.

The process of cellular differentiation may extend over many steps until the final stage of differentiation is achieved. It seems reasonable to correlate the various aberrations in certain cysts with an effectiveness of the treatment during critical steps of differentiation. A chain of synthetic steps may be interrupted at various links always giving rise to an aberrant phenotype. Many phenocopies are produced during major morphogenetic steps, such as the formation of extremities. Others, such as those described here are expressed at the macromolecular level within single cells, or interconnected cell clusters or cell organelles (MEYER, 1969). It seems necessary that all processes of growth and differentiation must be properly integrated. This does not exclude the action of enzymes initiating certain differentiative steps or developmental reactions (GOLDSCHMIDT, 1957 a; MEYER, 1969). In male germ line cells of *Drosophila* the sequence and/or initiation of differentiative steps seems to depend on the Y chromosomal factors. The Y factors seem to control and integrate the developmental events that are characteristic for the differentiation of male germ line cells. It seems that this system is especially sensitive to changes in timing and in synthetic rates produced by environmental factors as shown by the experiments reported in this and in a previous paper (MEYER, 1969). In view of the large number of male germ line cells (including gametes) produced in all higher organisms under normal genetic and environmental conditions, a limited variation can easily be tolerated by the organism. In humans of normal fertility between 5 and 20 % of the sperm show aberrant differentiation types as determined by light microscopy (MANN, 1964). It is an open question whether these aberrant, sometimes motile sperm are fertile or not. The instability inherent in this system might require additional stabilizing mechanisms which in the case of *Drosophila* are possibly provided by the Y factors.

The molecular basis for the putative function of the Y factors still remains unclear. Some possibilities have been discussed previously (BEERMANN *et al.*, 1967; MEYER, 1968; 1969). The question arises whether chromosomes or chromosome segments which appear heterochromatic and/or genetically inert as far as structural gene content is concerned, may have some stabilizing or buffering activities in general. LINDSLEY *et al.* (1960) e.g. have shown that sex linked recessive lethals can be suppressed by the Y heterochromatin and HESS (1962) showed that the penetrance of the mutation scute^{8} is dependent upon the presence of heterochromatin. In case of variegated type position effects the Y chromosome again possesses suppressing properties (see LEWIS, 1950). The unfolding of the Y chromomeres occurring during meiotic prophase may increase such rather unspecific buffering activities proportionally to the grade of unfolding (see HESS, 1958) and the number of active loci. With decreasing number of active loci in Y deficient males buffering capacity is reduced giving raise to an increased number of malformations.

Finally, the induction of new differentiation types throws new light on the complexity and extreme variability of the process of differentiation in male germ line cells. By rather simple means all spermatids of one cyst may be uniformly altered resulting in a new harmonic arrangement of organelles. Since such modifications of spermatid fine structure are very rare, the period of sensitivity and the time of alteration of the differentiation pattern is not yet known. Some agents have been applied to spermatocytes only (3rd instar larvae) which showed after application no structural modifications at the level of the light or electron microscope. All effects were observed in testes of adults.

In general one can assume a principal hereditary pattern of cellular organization characteristic for a specific tissue and/or for a certain organism. Our experiments have shown that this fundamental pattern can be altered experimentally to a still unknown extent.

References

ANDERSON W. A. (1967) – *Cytodifferentiation of spermatozoa in* Drosophila melanogaster: *the effect of elevated temperature on spermiogenesis.* «Mol. Gen. Genetics», 99, 257–273.

BEERMANN W. HESS O. and MEYER G. F. (1967) – *Lampbrush Y chromosomes in spermiogenesis of* Drosophila, *in* E. WOLFF, *The relationship between experimental embryology and molecular biology, Gordon and Breach,* New York, 61–81.

BRIDGES C. B. (1916) – *Non-disjunction as a proof of the chromosome theory of heredity.* «Genetics», 1, 1–52.

BEHNKE O. and FORER A. (1967) – *Evidence for four classes of microtubules in individual cells.* «J. Cell Sci.», 2, 169–192.

BROSSEAU G. (1960) – *Genetic analysis of the male fertility factors on the Y chromosome of* Drosophila melanogaster. «Genetics», 45, 257–274.

EPHRUSSI B. and BEADLE G. W. (1936) – *A technique of transplantation for* Drosophila. «Am. Naturalist», 70, 218–225.

GOLDSCHMIDT R. B. (1935) – *Gen und Ausseneigenschaften,* I. «Z. indukt. Abstamm. Vererbgsl.», 69, 70–131.

GOLDSCHMIDT R. B. (1957 a) – *Problematics of the phenomenon of phenocopy.* «J. Madras Univ.», 27, 17–24.

GOLDSCHMIDT R. B. and PITERNICK L. K. (1957 b) – *The genetic background of chemically induced phenocopies in* Drosophila. «J. Exp. Zool.», 135, 127–202.

GOLDSCHMIDT R. B. and PITERNICK L. K. (1957 c) – *The genetic background of chemically induced phenocopies in* Drosophila. «J. Exp. Zool.», 136, 201–228.

GORDON G. B., MILLER L. R. and BENSCH K. G. (1963) – *Fixation of tissue culture cells for ultrastructural cytochemistry.* «Expl. Cell Res.», 31, 440–443.

HESS O. (1962) – *Die Mutation "scute-8" von* Drosophila melanogaster *als ein Letalfaktor, dessen Penetranz vom Heterochromatin abhängt.* «Verh. D. Zool. Ges. Wien.», 87–92.

HESS O. (1965) – *Strukturdifferenzierungen im Y-Chromosom von* Drosophila hydei *und ihre Beziehungen zu Gen-Aktivitäten.* III. *Sequenz und Lokalisation der Schleifen-Bildungsorte.* «Chromosoma (Berl.)», 16, 222–248.

HESS O. (1967) – *Complementation of genetic activity in translocated fragments of the Y chromosome in* Drosophila hydei. «Genetics», 56, 283–295.

HESS O. (1968) – *The function of the lampbrush loops formed by the Y chromosome of* Drosophila hydei *in spermatocyte nuclei.* «Mol. Gen. Genetics», 103, 58–71.

HESS O. and MEYER G. F. (1963 a) – *Artspezifische funktionelle Differenzierungen des Y-Heterochromatins bei* Drosophila*-Arten der* D. hydei *Subgruppe.* «Port. Acta Biol.», 7, 29–46.

HESS O. and MEYER G. F. (1963 b) – *Chromosomal differentiations of the lampbrush type formed by the Y chromosome in* Drosophila hydei *and* D. neohydei. «J. Cell Biol.», 16, 527–539.

HESS O. and MEYER G. F. (1968) – *Genetic activities of the Y chromosome in* Drosophila *during spermatogenesis.* «Advanc. Genet.», 14, 171–223.

LEWIS E. B. (1950) – *The phenomenon of the position effect.* « Advanc. Genet. », 3, 73–115.

LINDSLEY D. L., EDINGTON C. W. and VON HALLE E. S. (1960) – *Sexlinked recessive lethals in* Drosophila *whose expression is suppressed by the Y chromosome.* « Genetics », 45, 1649–1670.

LUFT I. H. (1961) – *Improvements in epoxy resin embedding methods.* « J. biophys. biochem. Cytol. », 9, 409–414.

MANN TH. (1964) – *Biochemistry of semen and of the male reproductive tract.* Methuen and Co. Ltd. London.

MEYER G. F. (1963) – *Die Funktionsstrukturen des Y–Chromosoms in den Spermatocytenkernen von* Drosophila hydei, D. neohydei, D. repleta *und einigen anderen* Drosophila – *Arten.* « Chromosoma (Berl.) », 14, 207–255.

MEYER G. F. (1964) – *Die parakristallinen Körper in den Spermienschwänzen von* Drosophila. « Z. Zellforsch. », 62, 762–784.

MEYER G. F. (1966) – *Crystalline mitochondrial derivatives in sperm.* Proc. Sixth Int. Congr. Electr. Micr. Kyoto, Vol. II, 629–630.

MEYER G. F. (1968) – *Spermiogenese in normalen und Y–defizienten Männchen von* Drosophila melanogaster *und* D. hydei, « Z. Zellforsch. », 84, 141–175.

MEYER G. F. (1969) – *Experimental studies on spermiogenesis in* Drosophila. « Genetics », 61, 79–92.

MILLONIG G. (1961) – *Advantages of a phosphate buffer for* OsO_4 *solutions in fixation.* « J. appl. Phys. », 32, 1637.

STERN C. (1927) – *Untersuchungen über Aberrationen des Y–Chromosoms von* Drosophila melanogaster. « Z. indukt. Abstamm. Vererbgsl. », 51, 253–353.

YOUNG W. C. and PLOUGH H. H. (1926) – *On the sterilization of* Drosophila *by high temperature.* « Biol. Bull. », 51, 189–198.

EXPLANATION OF FIGURES

Fig. 1. – Structural aberrations in spermatid cysts of genetically normal males of *D. virilis.* 19,000×.

Complete disintegration of the axial fiber complexes in the periphery of a cyst. Arrows, single flagellar fibers; m, crystalline nebenkern derivative

Fig. 2. – Structural aberrations in a *melanogaster–virilis* compound, *melanogaster* portion. 19,000×.

Arrows, single flagellar fibers; *F*, normal flagella; m, crystalline nebenkern derivatives; *S 1*, two normal spermatids with one transformed nebenkern derivative each; *S 2*, single spermatid with two nebenkern derivatives transformed (*D. hydei* type of transformation).

Fig. 3. – Spermatids of adult *D. hydei* exhibiting a new differentiation type, 64,000×.

18–20 microtubules interconnected by a diffuse band (arrows) are arranged around a central body. In addition each spermatid (*a–d*) contains four open ring–like structures which are thought to represent cross sections through laterally interrupted cylinders.

Fig. 4. – Spermatid nuclei showing laterally attached structures. 23,000×.

Fig. 5. – The structures laterally attached in Fig. 4 may give rise to the four ringlike structures in this figure and in Fig. 3. 23,000×.

Fig. 6. – Spermatids of adult *D. hydei* after injection of Ringer solution into 3rd instar larvae. 46,000×.

N, nucleus; *F*, flagella; *Ff*, flagellar fragment; arrows, 2 dislocated structures.

Fig. 7. – Microtubules (mt) of crystalline array after application of colcemide to 3rd instar larvae of *D. hydei*. 36,000×.

Fig. 8. – Formation of supernumerary satellites after injection of homogenates of *X/O* testes into *X/Y* larvae (3rd instar) of *D. melanogaster*. 36,000×.

Arrows, additional satellites; round bodies represent cross sectioned nebenkern derivatives.

Fig. 9. – Dedifferentiation of whole spermatid cysts of *D. hydei* following a heat shock applied to 3rd instar larvae (40° C for 2 minutes). Some flagella and transformed nebenkern derivatives are seen in the periphery of one sector of the cyst. 11,500×.

F, flagella; *ri*, ribosomes are abundant.

Fig. 10. – Slight dedifferentiation as compared with fig. 9. 5,000×.

Arrows point to cross sectioned flagella. Some spermatids show fragmented nebenkern derivatives.

Fig. 11. – Part of the cyst seen in Fig. 9, with a single cross sectioned normal flagellum many ribosomes and, possibly, three nebenkern derivatives. 46,000×.

GÜNTHER F. MEYER – *Phenocopies of Y deficiencies and extraordinary differentiation types in spermiogenesis of* Drosophila.

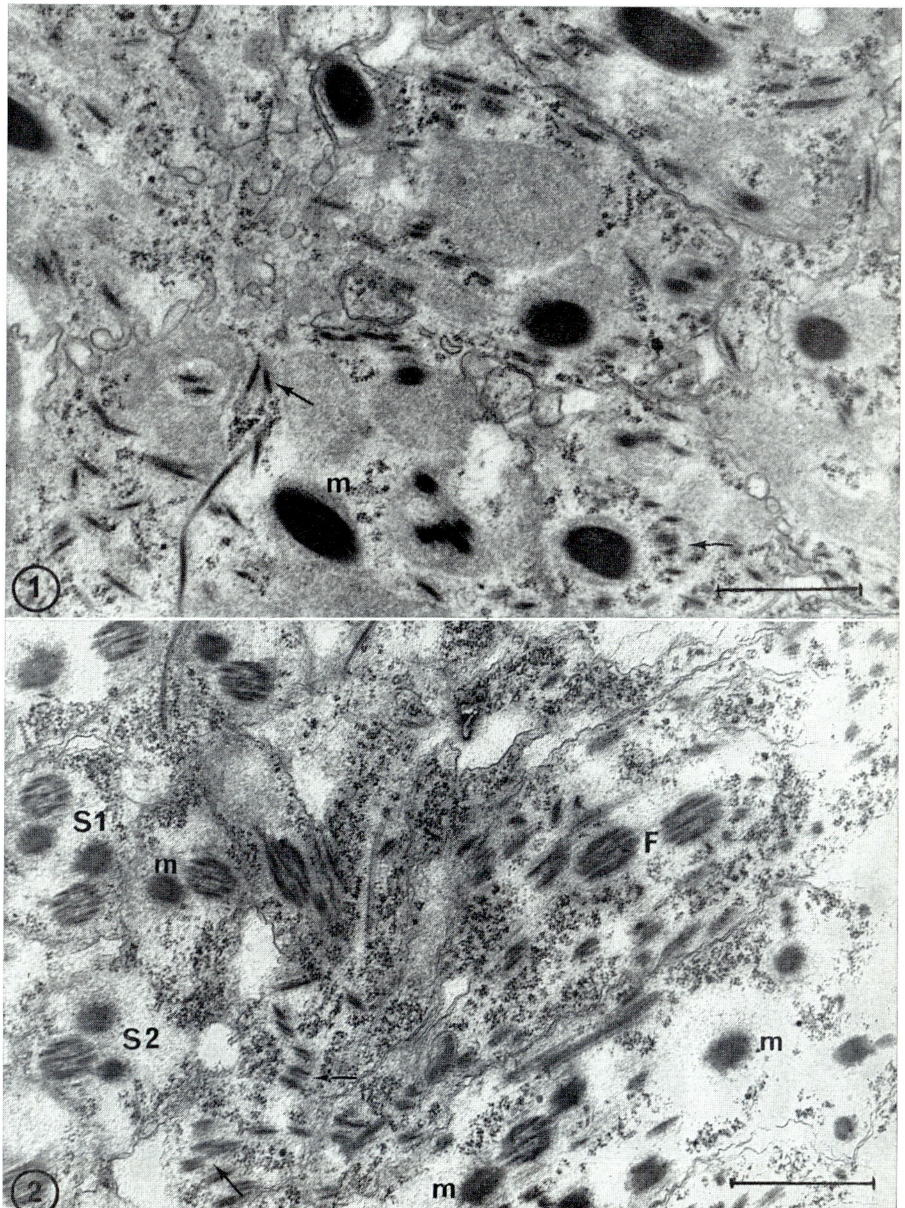

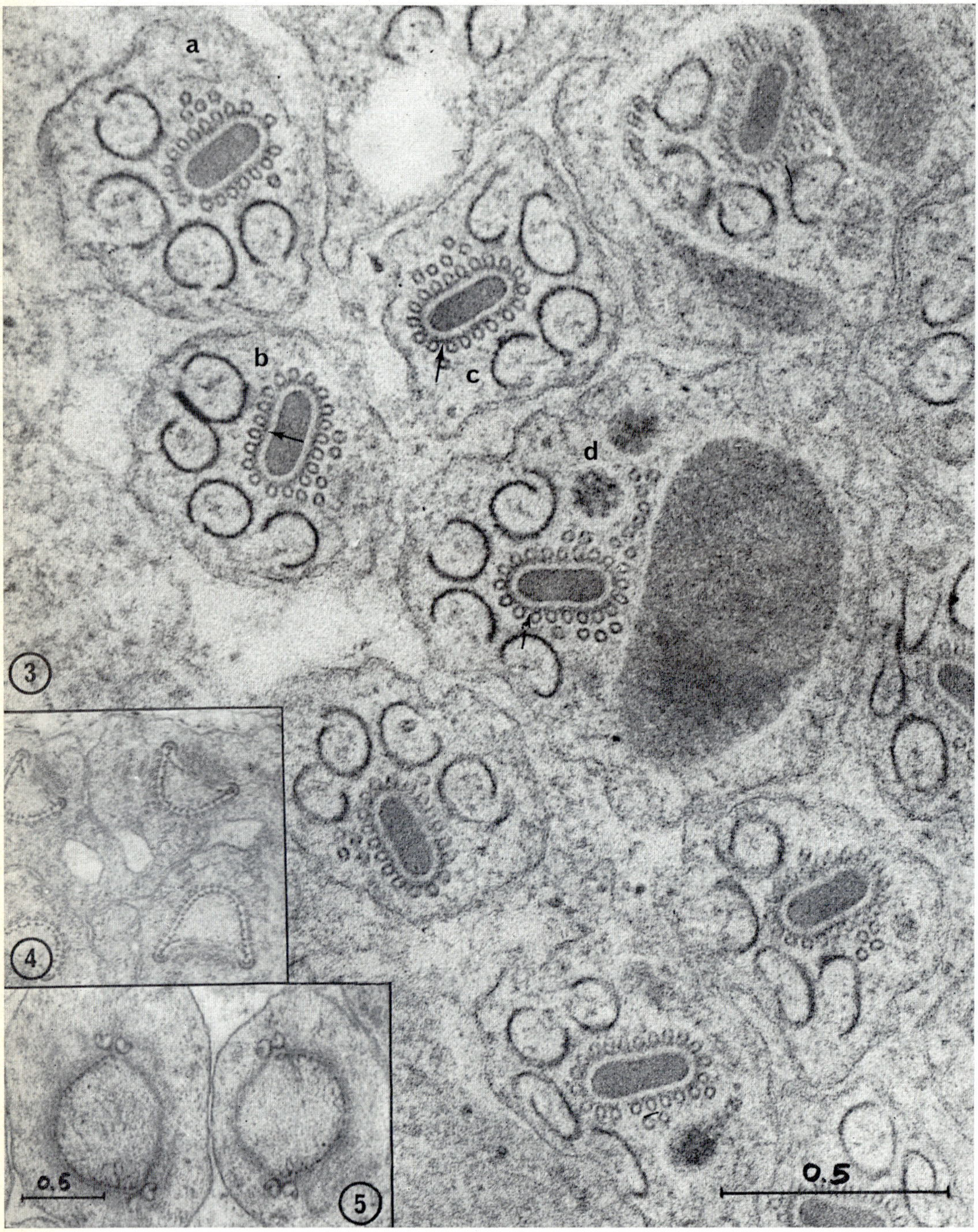
a
b
c
d
3
4
0.5
5
0.5

GÜNTHER F. MEYER – *Phenocopies of Y deficiencies and extraordinary differentiation types in spermiogenesis of* Drosophila.

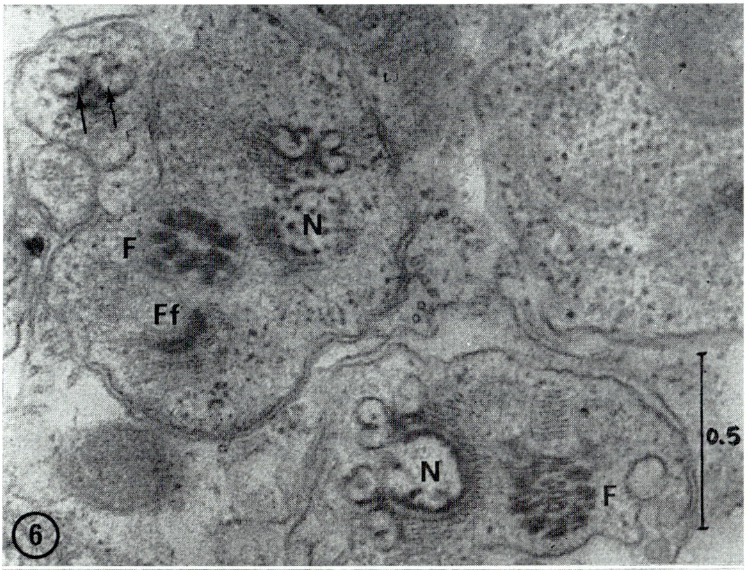

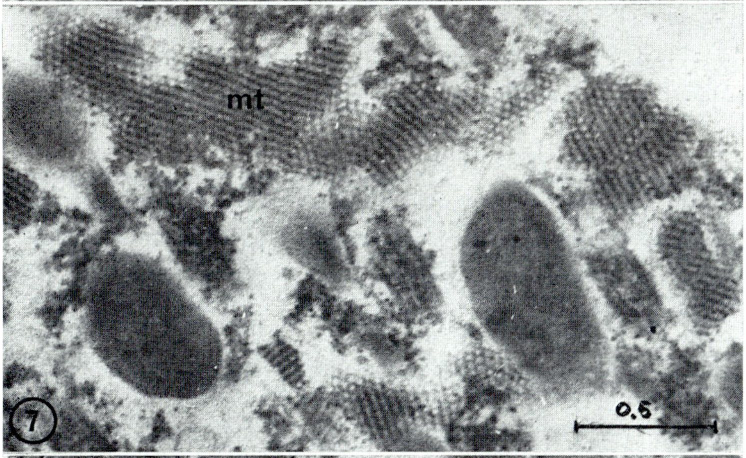

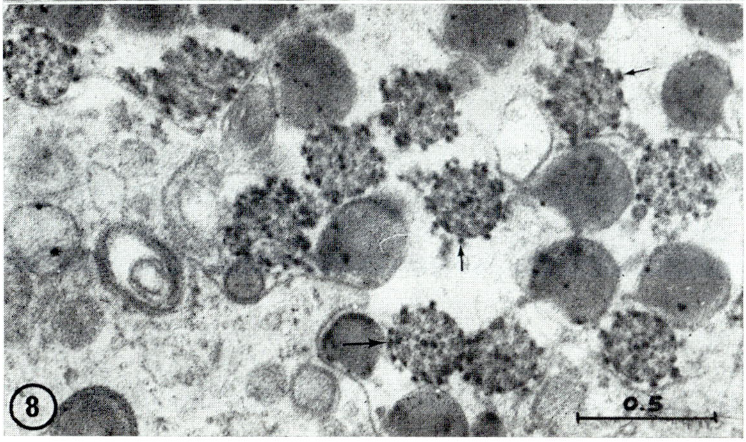

GÜNTHER F. MEYER – *Phenocopies of Y deficiencies and extraordinary differentiation types in spermiogenesis of* Drosophila.

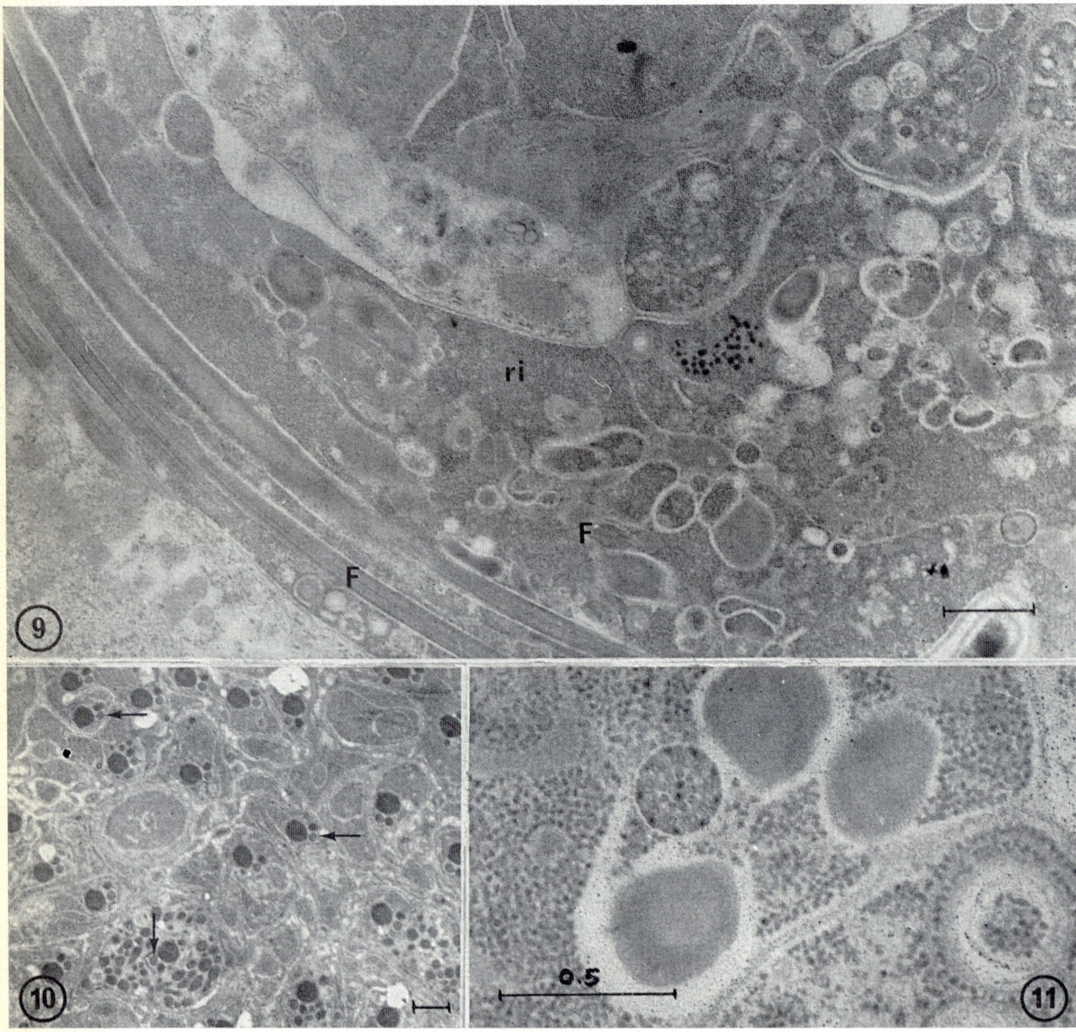

ANNA STAGNI (*) and MARIA LUISA LUCCHI (*)

ULTRASTRUCTURAL OBSERVATIONS ON THE SPERMATOGENESIS IN *HYDRA ATTENUATA*

SUMMARY. — The ultrastructural aspects of spermatogenetic process in *Hydra attenuata* has been investigated.

The spermatogonia, with large nucleolus, occur in clumps, have scattered mitochondria and few sacs of endoplasmic reticulum.

Primary spermatocytes present, within the nucleus, synaptonemal complexes at the pachytene stage and, within cytoplasm, mitochondria near the nucleus, polyribosomes, one or two Golgi apparatus.

Meiosis is quickly accomplished and secondary spermatocytes have very numerous polyribosomes, roundish or lengthened mitochondria placed around the nucleus.

Late spermatids, occurring at the tip of the spermary, show 5 or 6 large mitochondria, grouped (condriospheres) at the posterior pole and surrounding the proximal centriole.

The ripe sperm has a flattened apical region, neck with condriospheres and a long tail which, in its first tract, show a thickening of the plasma membrane. No differentiated acrosomic structure is present.

RIASSUNTO. — Gli AA. hanno studiato gli aspetti ultrastrutturali dei processi spermatogenetici e spermiogenetici in *Hydra attenuata*. Gli *spermatogoni* di questa specie si presentano riuniti in nidi, con grosso nucleolo, scarso reticolo endoplasmico; gli *spermatociti primi*, caratterizzati dai complessi sinaptinemali, hanno mitocondri che tendono a portarsi in vicinanza del nucleo e 1 o 2 apparati di Golgi. Gli *spermatociti secondi* presentano numerosi poliribosomi mentre i giovani *spermatidi* mostrano una tipica polarizzazione dei mitocondri ad un polo del nucleo. In stadi più avanzati della spermiogenesi 5 o 6 grosse condriosfere circondano il centriolo prossimale. Nello *spermio* maturo non sembrano esservi strutture acrosomiali.

Many Authors have investigated with light microscope the morphological aspects of spermatogenetic cells in Coelenterates. In extensive studies on the spermatogenesis DOWNING (1905), WILSON (1925), TUZET (1950), BRIEN and COWORKERS (1951; 1961), FRANZEN (1956) supply many accounts about the spermatogenesis of fresh–water hydras.

On the contrary very few works have been accomplished on this subject with electron microscope. BURNETT, DAVIS, HAYNES and MUMAW (1966), by studying gastrodermis regeneration, observed redifferentiation of dedifferentiated gland cells into spermatogonia, of which they briefly described the ulrastructural aspects (**).

(*) Institute of Zoology, University of Bologna, Italy.

(**) A pertinent publication of Lentz, Barrnett and Weissman has recently appeared on *Hydra littoralis* spermiogenesis (1969).

We also at a Meeting of the lower Metazoa cellular structure (Siena, October 11th–16th 1968) showed some electron micrographs of *Hydra attenuata* spermatogenesis; now we intend to demonstrate more thoroughly the whole spermatogenetic process.

Materials and methods

The hydras were reared at 18°–20° C in a 5 *l.* aquarium where aquatic plants (*Elodea* and *Myriorphyllum*) were present and fed every other day with *Daphnia*. Specimens, in different gametogenetic stages, were fixed either in 1 % solution of OsO_4 in veronal acetate buffer or in 2,5 % solution of glutaraldehyde in 0,1 M phosphate buffer, washed in 0,15 M phosphate buffer for 12 hours, and postfixed in 1 % solution of OsO_4 in 0,1 M phosphate buffer. They were dehydrated through an alcohol series, infiltrated with uranyl-acetate and embedded either in Epon or Araldite.

The sections were stained with lead salts according to MILLONIG'S method and observed with a Siemens Elmiskop I electron microscope (***).

Observations

The spermatogonia occur in clusters at the bottom of the spermary; many intercellular bridges put together these polygonal cells, showing in the scanty and dense cytoplasm several scattered mitochondria, poor endoplasmic reticulum, free ribosomes and small Golgi apparatus; their nucleus (5,3 × 2,3 μ in diameter), endowed with a large nucleolus, has a regular envelope (Fig. 1).

The primary spermatocytes, with nucleus 6,5 × 5 μ in diameter, are promptly starting meiotic prophase (Fig. 2). At high magnification, the synaptonemal complexes of the pachytene stage may be seen (Fig. 3). Perinuclear cisternae enlarge in some tracts; mitochondria occur near the nuclear membrane; the cytoplasm exhibits polyribosomes and one or two Golgi apparatus, often connected with elements of endoplasmic reticulum; lipid droplets are sometimes present.

First meiotic division is very quickly accomplished, so generating secondary spermatocytes with nuclei of 3,5 × 2,7 μ in diameter (Fig. 4). Roundish or lengthened mitochondria are now placed around the nucleus. Some small Golgi apparatus (two or three) are present. The polyribosomes are very numerous (Fig. 4).

Spermatids generally occur at the distal tip of the spermary. The early spermatids is round–shaped with a spheroidal nucleus (about 3 microns in diameter); its nucleoplasm contains small clumps of dense granules. Scanty, flattened vesicles of rough-surfaced endoplasmic reticulum occur in the cytoplasm. The small spheroidal or ellipsoidal mitochondria, formerly surrounding the nucleus, soon migrate and group at the posterior cellular pole,

(***) Preparations were carried out in the Centro di Microscopia elettronica of Bologna University.

closely applying to the nuclear membrane (Fig. 5). These mitochondria progressively become spheroidal and growth in size (0,7 μ in diameter) (Fig. 6), but their number decrease up to 5 or 6. This could lead us to suppose a fusion of the formerly small mitochondria in large ones. These large mitochondria lean against the nuclear membrane which now appears cup–like hollowed. The matrix of mitochondria becomes denser and the cristae increase in number and in length. At this stage the proximal centriole is surrounded by these large mitochondria (Fig. 8). The nucleus lengthens and its chromatin progressively condenses in the central zone (Fig. 8, 9); chromatin condensation seems to start at the apical region, where the nuclear envelope tipycally flattens (Fig. 7). Elsewhere perinuclear cisternae irregularly enlarge and some vesicles seem to be extruded into the cytoplasm (Fig. 9). At the same time some cisternae and vesicles of rough-surfaced endoplasmic reticulum are present. Two or three multivesicular bodies, different in size, occur near the Golgi region (Fig. 10); they progressively increase in diameter and their vesicles congregate arising typical lysosomes.

As differentiation continues, spermatid undergoes a loss of cytoplasm. Some cytoplasmic parts, containing elements of rough-surfaced endoplasmic reticulum, Golgi complex and large lysosome, are ejected. The plasma membrane shows an irregular outline, but in the apical region of the spermatid it adheres to the nuclear envelope, just over its flattening; therefore a truncated shape of the spermatid head results. We have never observed a differentiated acrosomial structure till now and the Golgi complex never seems to occur in close relationship to spermatid apical region. Chromatine condensation gives rise to a thick dark central body lined by a thin electron-lucent nucleoplasm layer, except at the apex of the nucleus (the flattened region) and at its base (the cup-like indented region, where are placed the mitochondria).

While the above changes are progressing, the proximal and distal centrioles and the axial filament have also appeared. The proximal centriole lies close to the nucleus, surrounded by the large mitochondria. It shows the peculiar pattern of 9 triplets encircled by a ring of satellites with thick binding arms. The distal centriole is in line with the long axis of the spermatid and from this place the tail posteriorly grows. Plasma membrane appears thickened in initial tract of the flagellum.

The ripe sperm of *Hydra attenuata* presents: *a*) the head, of about 2,8 μ in length and 1 μ in width; *b*) the neck, where 5 or 6 mitochondria are placed; *c*) the long tail (5 or 6 times longer than the head), the starting tract of which (0,3 μ) has a larger diameter and a thickened plasma membrane (Fig. 12).

The electron-lucent nucleoplasm layer is no more present. The nuclear envelope, as well as the plasma membrane surrounding the head of ripe sperm show a waved outline, except in the apical region, where they appear flattened, thickened and rather stiff. Nuclear envelope is still thickened and cup-like inflected in the basal region, where the large mitochondria seem to project into the nucleus (Fig. 12); their matrix is still denser and the cristae are numerous and crowded.

Plasma membrane of the tail seems to be rather wavy, but perhaps such outline could represent an artefact because it is frequent only after glutaraldehydic fixation.

On the whole, the ripe sperm is a very simplified one (like the first sperm type described by ANDRÉ) with flagellum, 5 or 6 chondriospheres, but lacking in a mophologically differentiated typical acrosome.

CONCLUSION

The plainly shaped ripe sperm of *Hydra attenuata* agrees with the primitive organisation of this Coelenterate.

It is of some interest to note the lack of a structurally differentiated acrosome. However we cannot exclude that the morphologically differentiated apical region of the sperm head showing a stiff and thickened flattening as a consequence of the adhesion between plasma membrane and nuclear envelope, could represent the site of some substitutive enzymatic activities.

However it is necessary to enphasize that the Golgi elements, typically involved in acrosome formation, never exhibit in *Hydra attenuata* close relationship to spermatid apical region. Golgi complex on the contrary, seems to have some activity in cytoplasmic ejection at the end of spermatogenesis.

As regards the 5 or 6 large condriospheres surrounding the proximal centriole, we suppose that a fusion of previous small mitochondria may occur, but more observations are required to clarify the way of this probable process.

REFERENCES

ANDRÉ J. (1962) – *Contribution à la connaissance du chondriome. Etude de ses modifications ultrastructurales pendant la spermatogenésè.* « J. Ultr. Res. », Suppl. 3.

BRIEN P. (1961) – *Etude d'*Hydra pirardi (*nov. spec.*). *Origine et répartition des nématocystes. Gametogénèse. Involution postgamétique. Evolution réversible des cellules interstitielles.* « Bull. Biol. », 95, 301–364.

BRIEN P. et RENIERS–DECOEN M. (1951) – *Etude d'*Hydra viridis (*Linnaeus*). (*La Blastogénèse, la Spermatogénèse, l'Ovogénèse*). « Ann. Soc. zool. Belg. », 81, 33–110.

BURNETT A. L., DAVIS L. E. and RUFFING F. E. (1966) – *A histological and ultrastructural study of germinal differentiation of interstitial cells arising from gland cells in* Hydra viridis. « J. Morph. », 120, 1–8.

DOWNING E. R. (1905) – *The spermatogenesis of* Hydra. « Zool. Jb. Anat. », 21, 379–426.

FRANZÉN Å. (1956) – *On spermiogenesis, morphology of the spermatozoon and biology of fertilization among invertebrates.* « Zool. Bidr. Uppsala », 31, 355-482.

MILLONIG G. (1961) – *A modified procedure for lead staining of thin sections.* « J. Biophysic. Biochem. Cytol. », 11, 736–739.

STAGNI A. (1968) – *Aspetti ultrastrutturali delle cellule dell'idra d'acqua dolce.* « Boll. Zool. », 35, 319.

TUZET O. (1950) – *Le spermatozoïde dans la série animale.* « Rev. Suisse Zool. », 57, 433–451.

WEISSMAN A., LENTZ T. and BARRNETT R. (1969) – *Fine structural observations on nuclear maturation during spermiogenesis in* Hydra littoralis. « J. Morph. », 128, 229–240.

WILSON E. B. (1925) – *The cell in development and heredity.* Macmillan, New York.

Explanation of figures

Fig. 1. – Spermatogonia. *Nu:* nucleolus; *m:* mitochondria; *G:* Golgi complex. 17,000×.

Fig. 2. – Primary spermatocytes. Some in meiotic prophase and others in meiotic metaphase. Uppermost some early spermatids. *ch:* chromosomes; *c:* centriole. 8,000×.

Fig. 3. – Primary spermatocytes. Synaptonemal complexes at the pachytene stage (arrows). *ch:* chromosomes. 28,000×.

Fig. 4. – Secondary spermatocytes interconnected by an intercellular bridge (arrow). *m:* mitochondria; *P:* polyribosomes. 23,000×.

Fig. 5. – Early spermatid. Small mitochondria with few cristae have grouped at the basal pole of the cell, near the nucleus. Some of these mitochondria are piled and packed. 17,000×.

Fig. 6. – Early spermatids in two different spermiogenetic stages. One of them exhibits large mitochondria (*m*) with numerous cristae and a dense matrix. *G:* Golgi complex; *mv:* multivesicular body. 14,000×.

Fig. 7. – Early spermatids with chromatin condensation at the apical region, where nuclear envelope is flattened and thickened (arrows). 23,000×.

Fig. 8. – Spermatid. The nucleus is greatly elongated and chromatin condensed in a central cone-shaped body. The flagellum is seen in association with the distal centriole (*cd*). At the right side the cross sectioned centriole presents a ring of satellites and binding arms (arrow). 29,000×.

Fig. 9. – Late spermatid. Vesicles are extruded from perinuclear cistern into the cytoplasm. The apical region is flattened. *G*: Golgi complex. 28,000×.

Fig. 10. – Spermatid. *G:* Golgi complex; *mv:* multivesicular body; *m:* mitochondria. 28,000×.

Fig. 11. – Spermatids at different spermiogenetic stages. In the middle a spermatid with a long tail and an intercellular bridge (*ib*). The other spermatids show cytoplasmic loss: two cytolysosomes (*Cy*) are seen. The apical region is flattened (arrows). Chromatin is completely condensed. 13,000×.

Fig. 12. – Ripe sperm with apical region flattened (arrow), large mitochondria. The first tail tract presents plasma membrane thickened. *cd:* distal centriole; *cp:* proximal centriole. 34,000×.

ANNA STAGNI and MARIA LUISA LUCCHI - *Ultrastructural observations on the spermatogenesis in* Hydra attenuata.

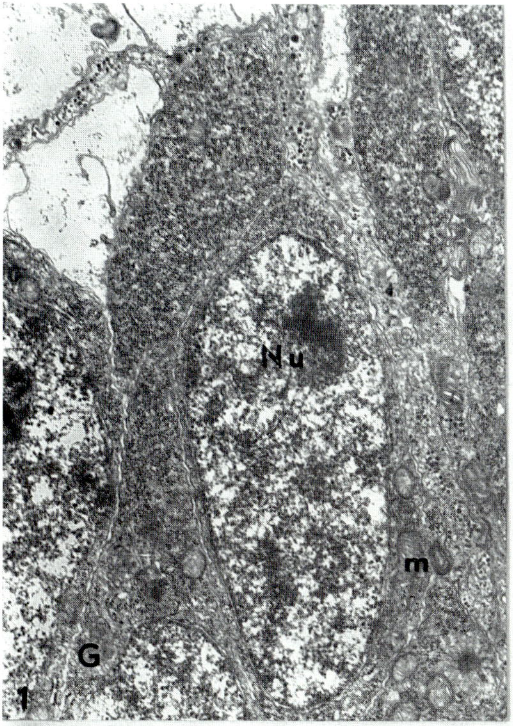

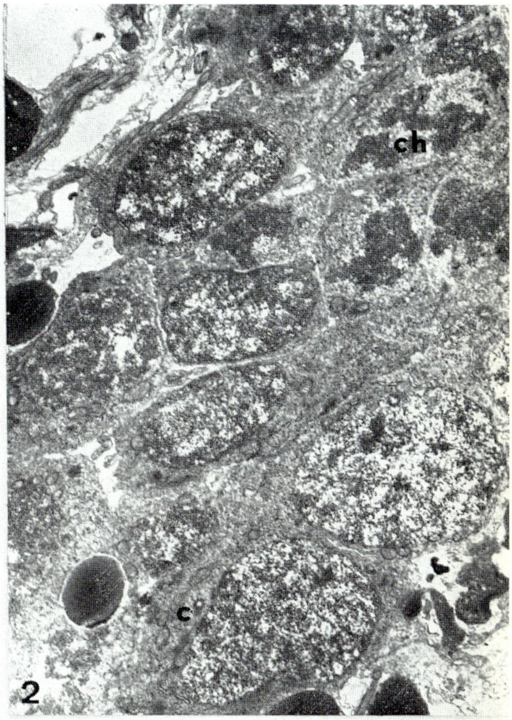

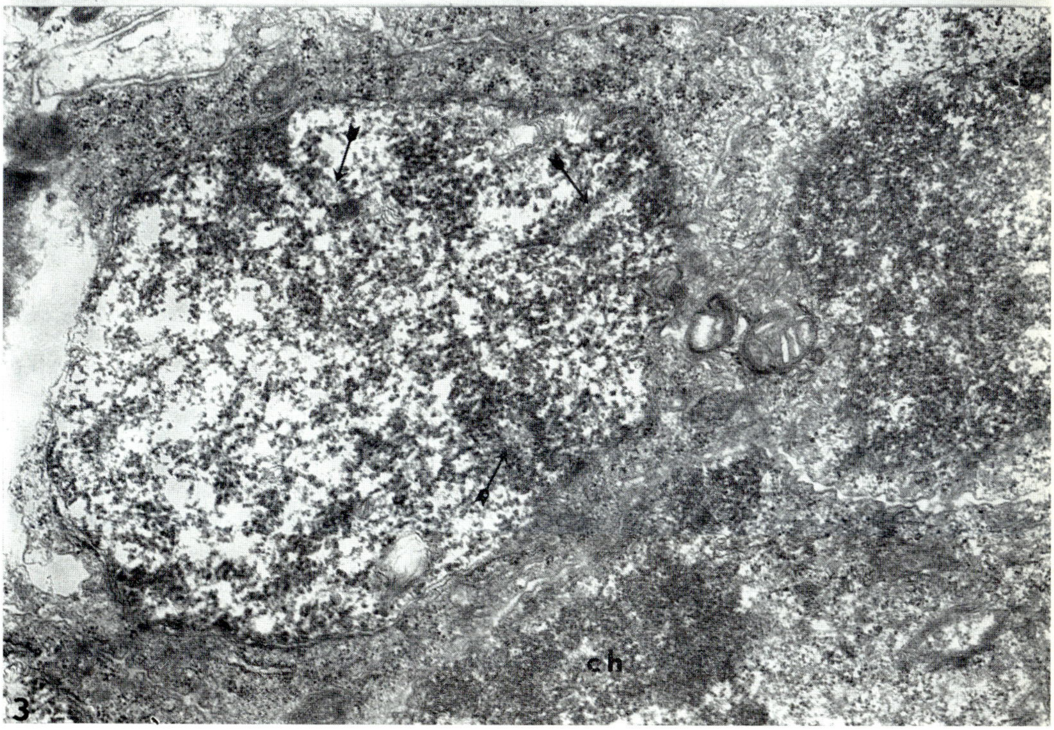

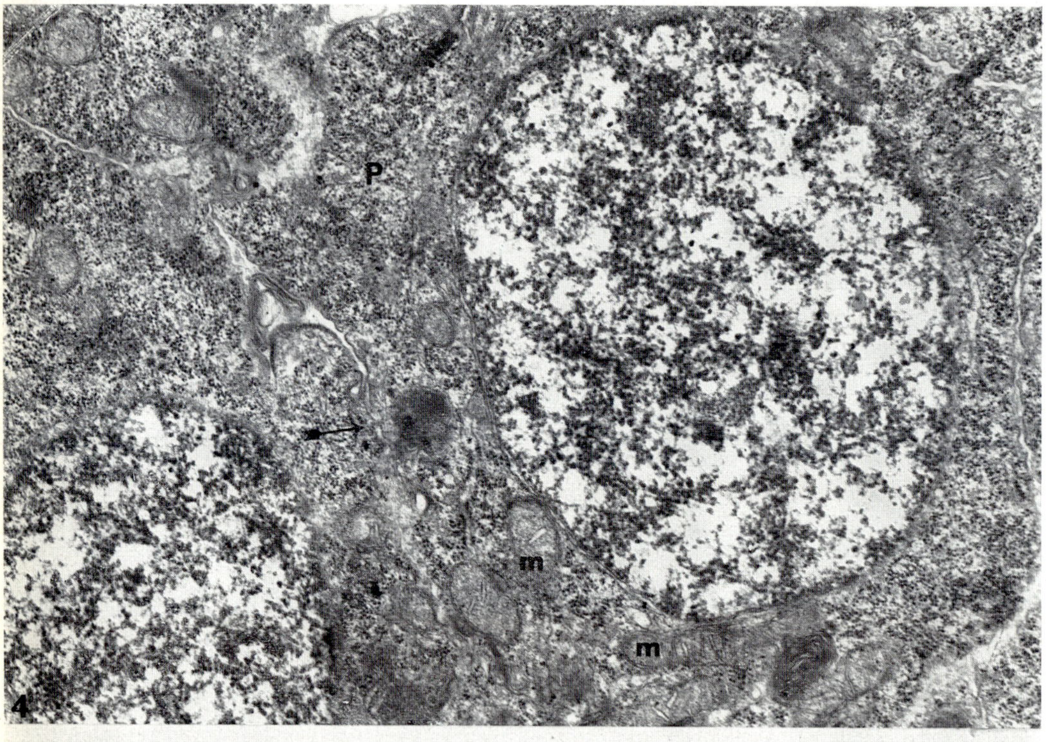
P
m
m
4

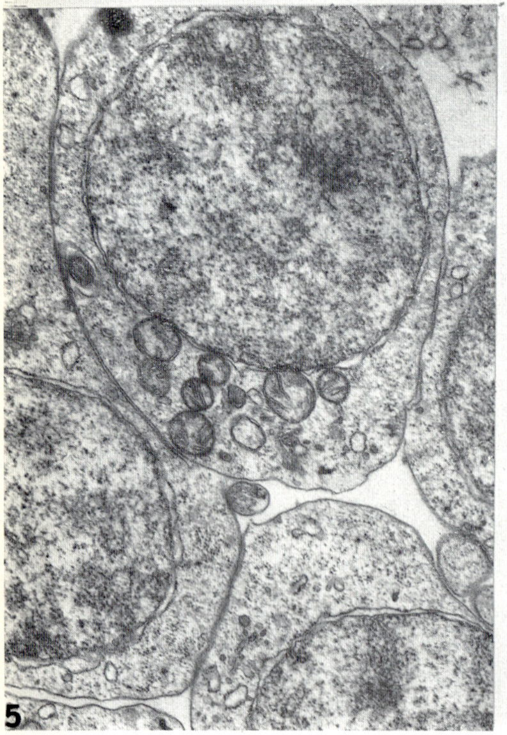
5

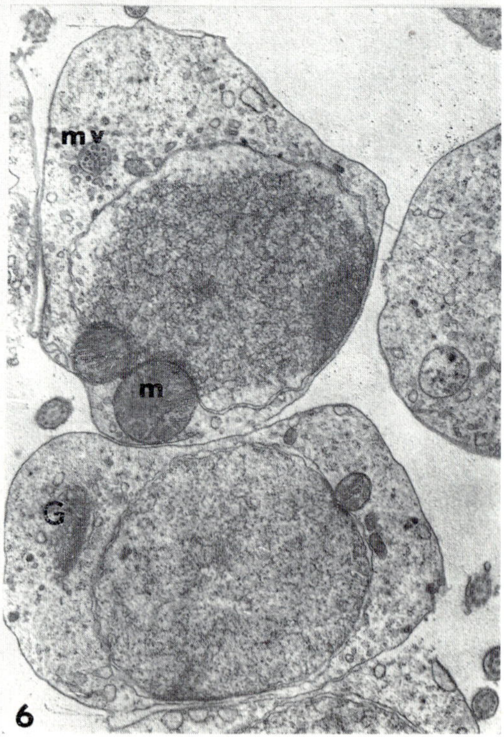
mv
m
G
6

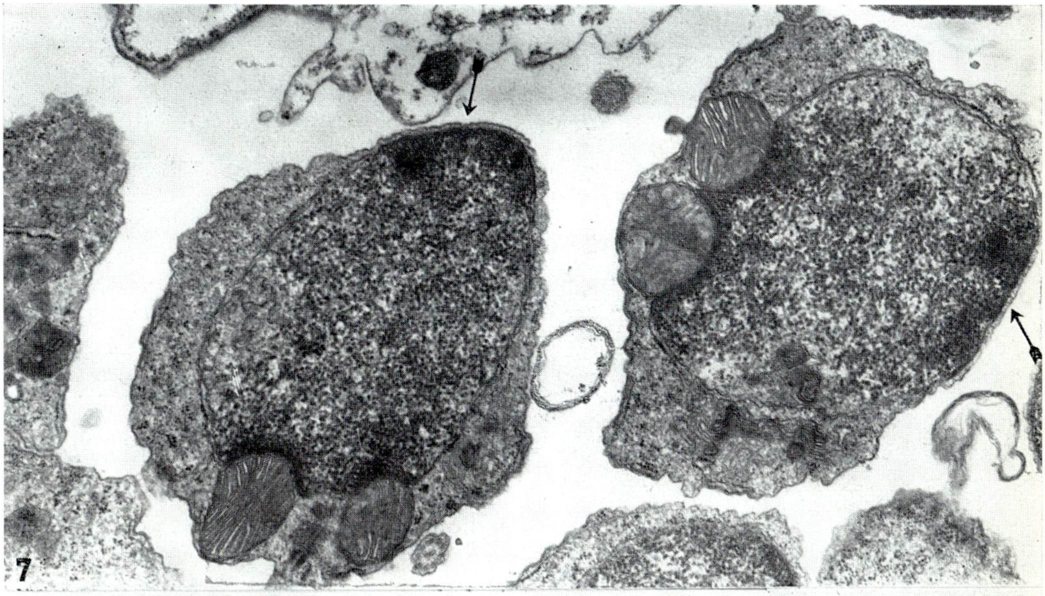

7

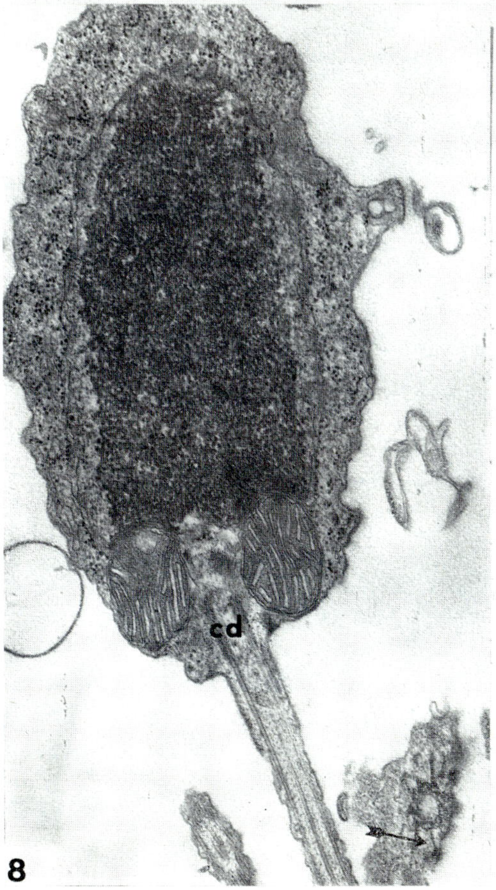

8

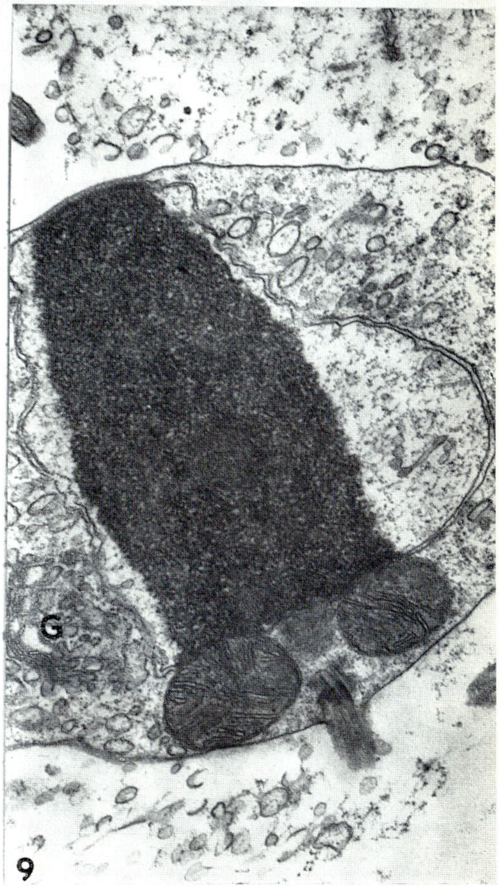

9

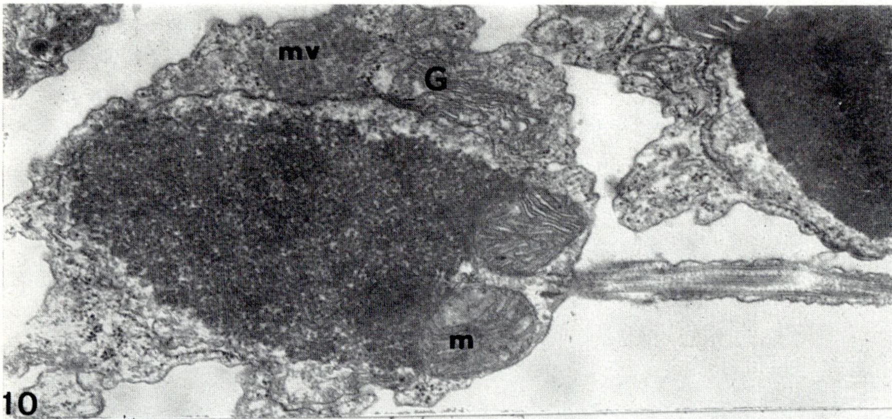
mv
G
m
10

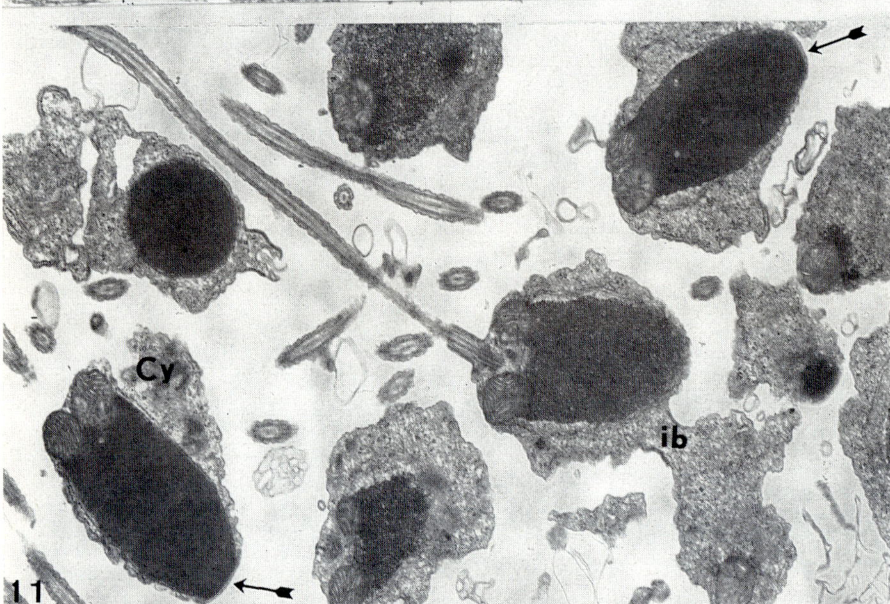
Cy
ib
11

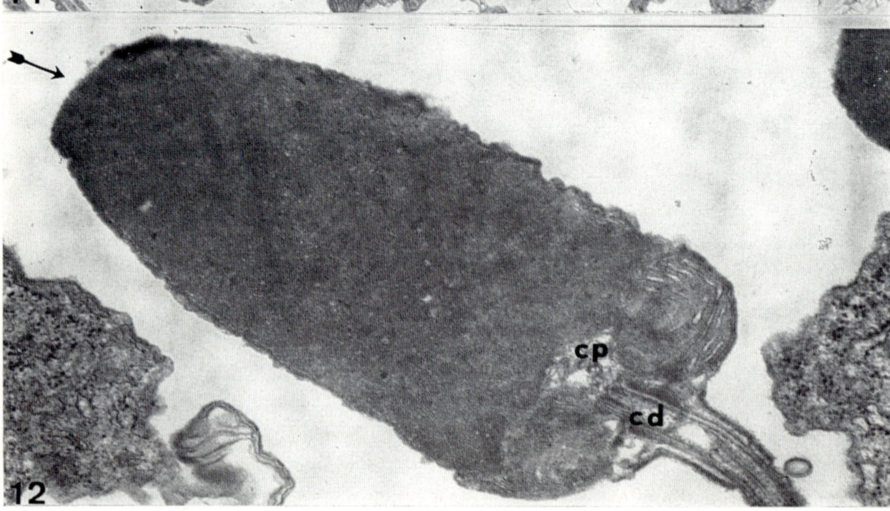
cp
cd
12

C. BEDINI (*) and F. PAPI (*)

PECULIAR PATTERNS OF MICROTUBULAR ORGANIZATION IN SPERMATOZOA OF LOWER TURBELLARIA (**)

SUMMARY. — The acoel *Convoluta psammophila* presents spermatozoa with two axial units, which show 9 + 0 fibrils for the greatest part of their length and 9+2 fibrils for a short extent at the distal end. The spermatozoa of the macrostomids *Promacrostomum gieysztori* and *Macrostomum retortum* are motile, lack axial units or flagellar-like structures but show two series of microtubules longitudinally arranged.

RIASSUNTO. — L'acelo *Convoluta psammophila* presenta spermatozoi con due filamenti assiali che mostrano organizzazione microtubulare a modello 9+0 per la maggior parte della loro lunghezza e 9+2 per un breve tratto alla estremità distale. Gli spermatozoi dei macrostomidi *Promacrostomum gieysztori* e *Macrostomum retortum* sono mobili, mancano di filamenti assiali o strutture simili a flagelli ma mostrano due serie di microtubuli ad andamento longitudinale.

In sperm flagella of all platyhelminths studied by electron microscopy (10 species of turbellarians, 6 trematodes and 4 cestodes) (AFZELIUS, 1964; BONSDORFF and TELKKÄ, 1965; CHRISTENSEN, 1961; GRESSON, 1962; GRESSON and PERRY, 1961; HENDELBERG, 1967; HERSHENOV, TULLOCH and JOHNSON, 1966; KLIMA, 1961; SHAPIRO, HERSHENOV and TULLOCH, 1961; SILVEIRA and PORTER, 1964; TULLOCH and HERSHENOV, 1967) an identical 9+1 arrangement, i.e. a single central tubule surrounded by nine peripheral doublet tubules, had been noted.

It has been observed that it is unlikely for such a character to have arisen independently in different groups of platyhelminths, and therefore it could be considered as an original character for the phylum (HENDELBERG, 1967). The report by COSTELLO *et al.* (1969) recently published by *Science* according to which an acelous turbellarian, *Childia groenlandica*, has spermatozoa with a 9+0 arrangement, is all the more interesting as acoels, which had not been studied under this point of view, are regarded by various AA. (see for references DOUGHERTY, 1963; IVANOV, 1968) as primitive forms in the evolution of all other platyhelminths.

Two arrangements of sperm microtubules, new for the platyhelminths, were observed, however, in another acoel, *Convoluta psammophila* and in two species of the close order of Macrostomida, *Macrostomum retortum* and *Promacrostomum gieysztori*.

(*) Institute of General Biology, University of Pisa, Italy.
(**) Supported by a grant from Consiglio Nazionale delle Ricerche.

Electron microscope observations were made on sections of entire animals fixed in 1% osmium tetroxide buffered with Millonig 0.2 M. or in 2.5% glutaraldeyde in cacodilate buffer and postfixed in osmium tetroxide. Embedding in Epon 812—Araldite mixture, and sections stained with uranyl acetate and lead citrate.

Convoluta has motile spermatozoa about 270 μ long, ribbon shaped and tapering somewhat abruptly to the anterior end and gradually to the posterior one.

In the sperm region, behind the nucleus, two axial units are present in the cytoplasm; they run close to the plasma membrane as far as the posterior end. Here, the tail branches into two short tips, into both of which the axial unit continues. In this two-branched region, the axial units consist of nine peripheral doublets and two central tubules, while elsewhere only nine peripheral doublets occur (Fig. 1 and 2).

Both axial units, each about 2300 Å in diameter, are separated from the other cytoplasmic organelles and inclusions by a membranous structure (Fig. 1: *M*), which runs medially along the entire length of the axial unit and side by side with it. The microtubular doublets have a diameter of about 380 Å.

In the median region of the sperm, centrally, 10 microtubules are also present. This latter have frequently organized themselves into a third atypical axial complex.

In spermatids (Figs. 3 and 4), axial units are incorporated for all their length into a cavity completely limited by a membrane (Fig. 3: *M'*). This is again surrounded by a membranous system (Fig. 3: *M''*), which appears omogeneous and strongly electron-dense on the side facing the external wall of the cell, while being elsewhere risolvable into more laminar units. 12–14 microtubules are contained between the membrane *M'* and the membranous system *M''*, in the internally facing hemicycle. The relative extension of 9+0 and 9+2 tracts is probably dependent on the spermatids stage. The 9+0 one is more distal but sometimes may be found even at the nucleus level (Fig. 3). Other longitudinally lying microtubules, in addition to those already described, are present under the plasma membrane.

Promacrostomum giesztori has thread-shaped motile spermatozoa, about 45 μ long, bearing two stiff bristles at boundary between 1st and 2nd third (Papi, 1951). *Macrostomum retortum* has identically shaped, although about 70 μ long, spermatozoa. The E. M. observations have not shown structural differences between the two species.

The spermatozoa are lacking axial units or other structures identifiable with orthodox flagella. A microtubular sheath starting from the nucleus runs up to the tail tip under the plasma membrane. This discontinues for a short way on two opposite sides (Fig. 5). The microtubules, about 250 Å in diameter, run parallel to each other and to the longitudinal axis of the sperm. In the region close to the nucleus 60–70 microtubules rather spaced from each other are counted, and at the caudal end 25–30 closely lined ones. In the middle regions transitional figures between both conditions are present.

The two bristles are thin cytoplasmic expansions with a homogeneous strongly electron-dense core (Fig. 6). In their longitudinal sections these bristles show, under the plasma membrane, a regular succession of cross-cut microtubules. This pattern can be interpreted as a close microtubular coiling around the central core.

As far as we know, the mixed 9+0 and 9+2 pattern of *Convoluta* has not been described either in turbellarians or in other animals. This pattern appears to arise from a reduction in the extension of the central tubules and this process might have led to the 9+0 pattern of *Childia*. The sperm structure of *Promacrostomum* and of *Macrostomum* recalls that of some arthropods (ROBISON, 1966). In this instance it might be derived from that of acoels as a consequence of loss of axial units and preservation, also in the mature sperm, of the other extraaxial microtubules. The present findings suggest that it is probably a hasty decision to use the structural characters of spermatozoa for phylogenetic speculations on platyhelminths at least until more species belonging to the main orders can be studied.

REFERENCES

AFZELIUS B. (1964) – *Cellen W and W-serien* 57. Wahlström and Widstrand, Stockholm.

BONSDORFF C. H. and TELKKÄ A. (1965) – *The spermatozoon flagella in* Diphyllobothrium latum (*Fish tapeworm*). « Z. Zellforsch. », 66, 643–648.

CHRISTENSEN K. (1961) – *Fine structure of an unusual spermatozoon in the flatworm* Plagiostomum. « Biol. Bull. », 121, 416.

COSTELLO P. P., HENLEY C. and AULT C. R. (1969) – *Microtubules in spermatozoa of* Childia (*Turbellaria, Acoela*) *revealed by negative staining*. « Science », 163, 678–679.

DOUGHERTY E. C. (Ed.) (1963) – *The lower metazoa*. Univ. Cal. Press, Berkeley.

GRESSON R. A. R. (1962) – *Spermatogenesis of a cestode*. « Nature », 194, 397–398.

GRESSON R. A. R. and PERRY M. M. (1961) – *Electron microscope studies of spermateleosis in* Fasciola hepatica L. « Exp. Cell Res. », 22, 1–8.

HENDELBERG J. (1967) – *On different types of spermatozoa in Polycladida, Turbellaria*. « Ark. Zoologi », 18, 267–304.

HERSHENOV B. R., TULLOCH G. S. and JOHNSON A. D. (1966) – *The fine structure of trematode* (Haematoloechus medioplexus) *sperm tails*. « Trans. Amer. Microsc. Soc. », 85, 480–483.

IVANOV A. V. (1968) – *Proiskhoždenie mnogokletočnykh životnykh*. Nauka, Leningrad.

KLIMA J. (1961) – *Elektronen mikroskopische Studien über die Feinstruktur der Tricladen* (*Turbellaria*). « Protoplasma », 54, 101–162.

PAPI F. (1951) – *Ricerche sui Turbellari Macrostomidae*. « Arch. zool. ital. », 36, 289–340.

ROBISON W. G. (1966) – *Microtubules in relation to the motility of a sperm syncytium in an armored scale insect*. « J. Cell Biol. », 29, 251–266.

SHAPIRO J. E., HERSHENOV B. R. and TULLOCH G. S. (1961) – *The fine structure of* Haematoloechus *spermatozoan tail*. « J. Biophis. Biochem. Cytol. », 9, 211–217.

SILVEIRA M. and PORTER K. R. (1964) – *The spermatozoids of flatworms and the microtubular system*. « Protoplasma », 59, 240–265.

TULLOCH G. S. and HERSHENOV B. R. (1967) – *Fine structure of platyhelminth sperm tail* (Haematoloechus medioplexus). « Nature », 213, 299–300.

Explanation of figures

Fig. 1. – Spermatozoa of *Convoluta* in cross sections, showing the two lateral axial units (1 and 1′) lacking central fibrils, the membranous structure (*M*) and the third atypical axial complex (*C*). ×24.000.

Fig. 2. – Distal part of spermatid tail of *Convoluta* showing the 9+2 pattern of the axial complex. ×65.000.

Figs. 3 and 4. – Cross sections of *Convoluta* spermatids. Note the 9+0 and 9+2 arrangement of the axial units. *M′*, *M″*: membranous structure and system. Fig. 3 ×52.000; Fig. 4 ×42.900.

Fig. 5. – Proximal and distal region of sperm tails of *Macrostomum* cross – sectioned showing microtubules. Oblique sections of bristles (*B*) are visible. ×16.000.

Fig. 6. – High magnification of a portion of bristles (*B*) showing the dense internal core and the microtubular coiling under the plasma membrane. ×48.000.

C. Bedini and F. Papi – *Peculiar patterns of microtubular organization in spermatozoa of lower turbellaria.*

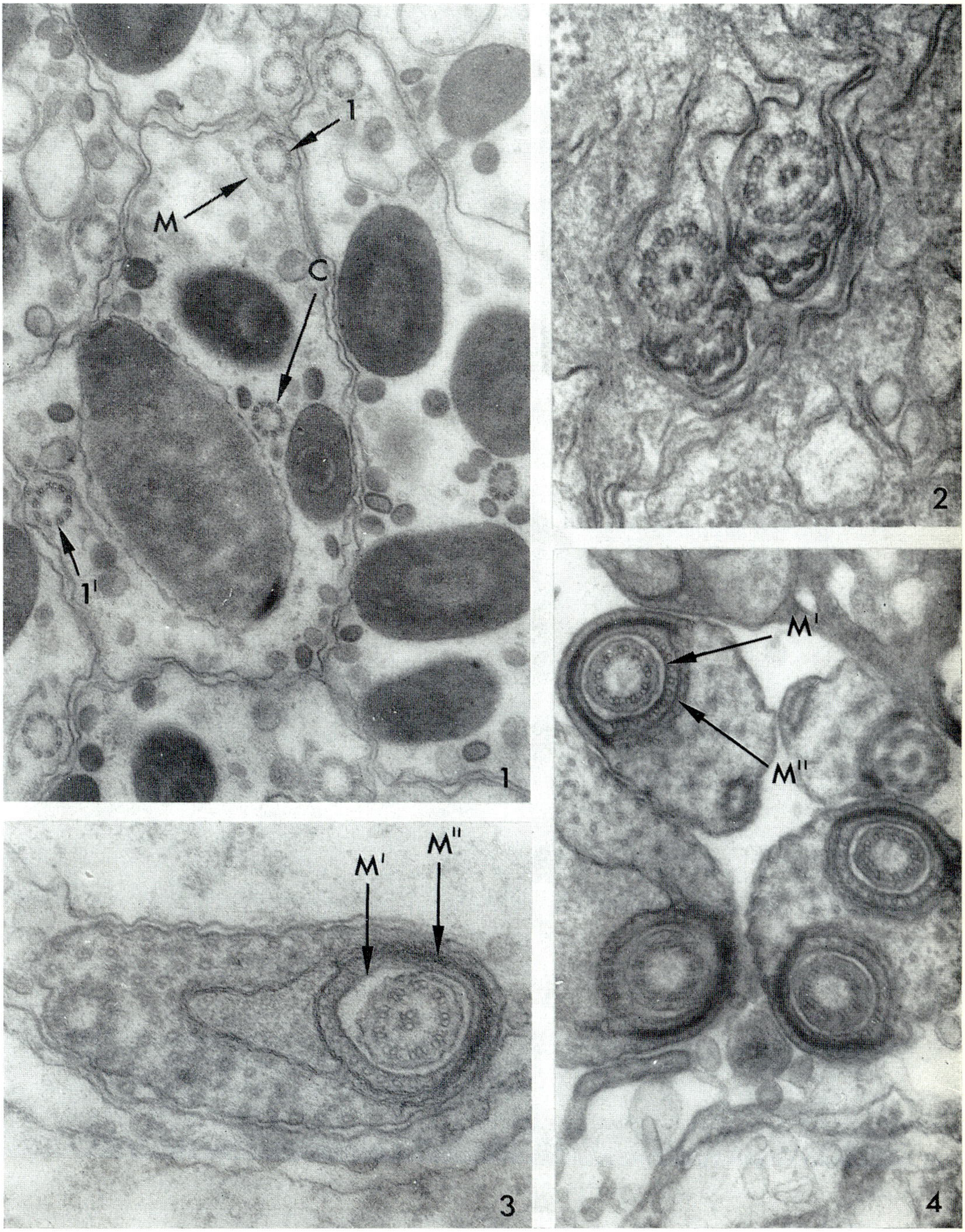

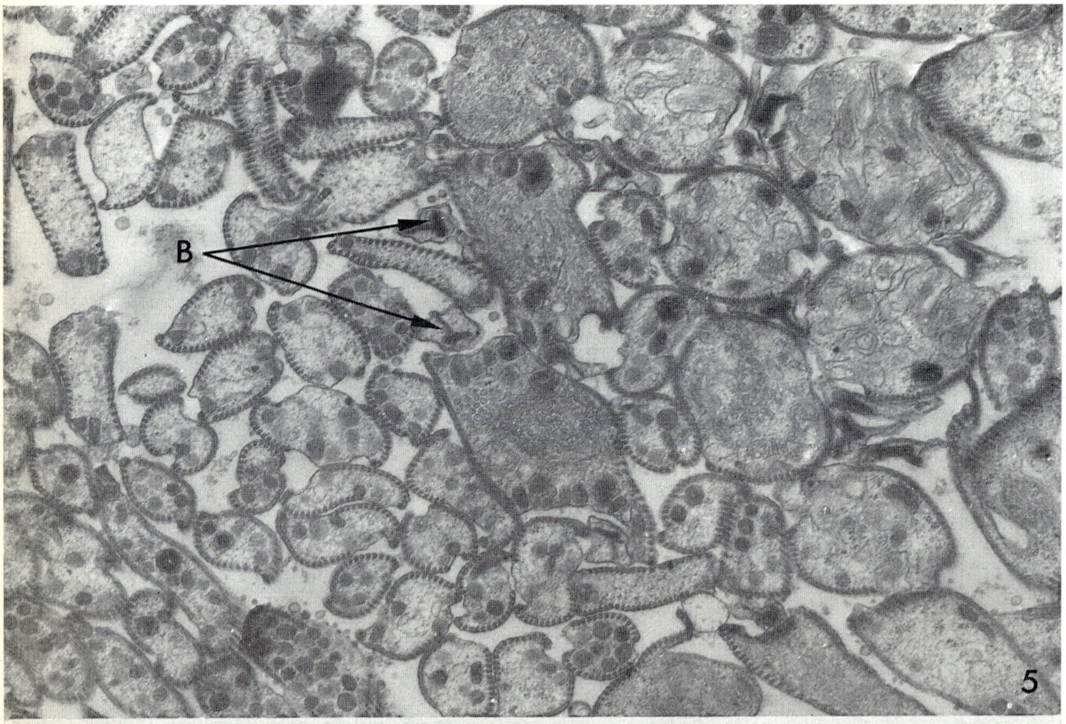
B
5

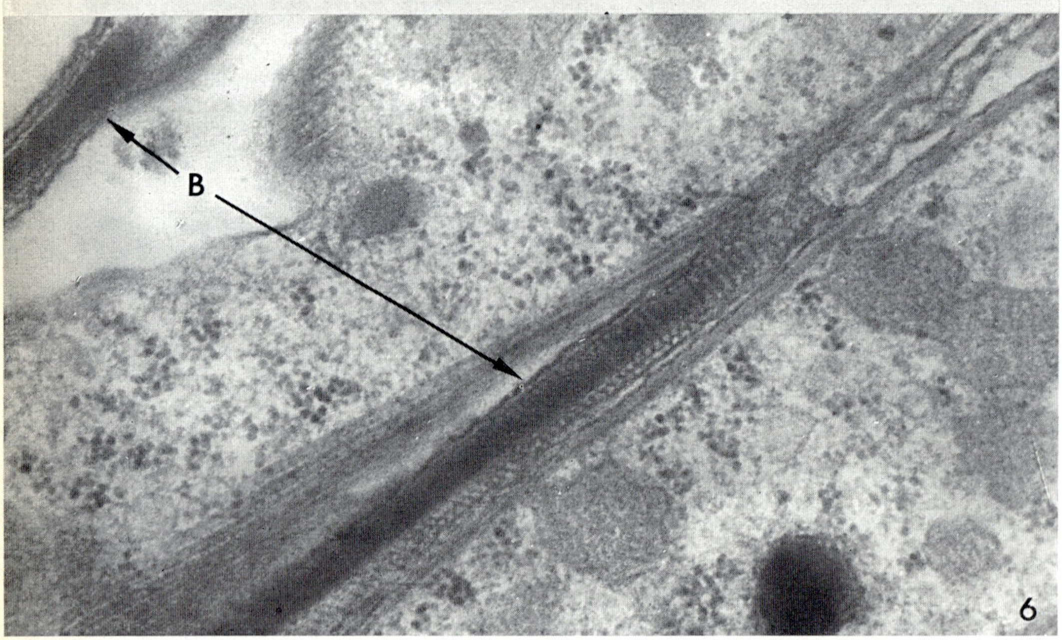
B
6

JAN HENDELBERG (*)

ON THE NUMBER AND ULTRASTRUCTURE OF THE FLAGELLA OF FLATWORM SPERMATOZOA

SUMMARY. — Two flagella have been found to grow from the young spermatids in many groups of the Platyhelminthes. This type of spermatid gives rise to many different types of spermatozoa. The widespread occurrence of two flagella, also in spermatozoa earlier regarded as monoflagellate, implies that the "Turbellarian Archetype" most probably had biflagellate spermatozoa. In some turbellarian groups the alterations during the evolution have led to a reduction in size or to complete elimination of the flagella. In the spermatozoa of the Trematoda and Cestoda the original number of flagella is two. The reported occurrence of only one flagellum in the spermatozoa of some Cestoda is explained as due to a reduction.

Contrary to the earlier known aberrant ultrastructure of the flagella in flatworm spermatozoa, the structure of the flagella in the spermatozoa of the Acoela studied by the author was found to be very reminiscent of that commonly found in cilia and flagella.

The role played by the flagella and the microtubular filaments underlying the cell membrane in the movements of the spermatozoa is dealt with briefly.

RIASSUNTO. — In molti gruppi di Platelminti dagli spermatidi hanno origine due flagelli. Questo tipo di spermatidio dà origine a molti differenti tipi di spermatozoi. La frequente presenza di due flagelli, anche negli spermatozoi prima considerati monoflagellati, implica che l'« Archetipo Turbellari » molto probabilmente abbia spermatozoi biflagellati. In alcuni gruppi di turbellari le alterazioni durante l'evoluzione hanno portato a una riduzione in misura o alla completa eliminazione del flagello. Negli spermatozoi dei Trematodi e dei Cestodi il numero originale dei flagelli è due. Il caso di un solo flagello negli spermatozoi di alcuni Cestodi viene spiegato come dovuto ad una riduzione.

Contrariamente all'ultrastruttura aberrante dei flagelli degli spermatozoi dei vermi piatti, la struttura dei flagelli degli spermatozoi degli Aceli studiati dall'autore ricorda molto quella comunemente trovata nelle ciglia e nei flagelli.

Viene trattato brevemente il ruolo giocato dai flagelli e dai filamenti microtubulari che giacciono sotto la membrana cellulare nel movimento dello spermatozoo.

The occurrence of two flagella growing from the young spermatid has been found to be a feature common to the genesis of many different types of flatworm spermatozoa. During the spermiogenesis the two flagella either become incorporated into the cell body or remain free as so-called *nebengeisseln*.

Of special interest in this respect are the *thread-shaped spermatozoa*, which occur in many different groups of the Platyhelminthes. These filiform spermatozoa with neither *nebengeisseln* nor undulating membranes were regarded

(*) Institute of Zoology, University of Uppsala, Sweden.

earlier as monoflagellate. However, my studies have revealed that many types of thread-shaped flatworm spermatozoa develop from spermatids with two flagella.

Thus, during the development of the thread-shaped, common type of spermatozoon within the Acoela (Turbellaria) two flagella first grow free, and then become incorporated (Fig. 1) into the cell body. This was found in the eight species of the Acoela with thread-shaped spermatozoa studied in this respect (HENDELBERG, 1969 a).

An incorporation of two flagella into spermatids giving rise to thread-shaped spermatozoa was found also in most of the acotylean Polycladida, in some of the Rhabdocoela (= Neorhabdocoela) (Turbellaria) and in the few Digenea (Trematoda) studied. In the spermatozoa of acotylean polyclads the two flagella were found to be very superficial—they just adhere to the outside of the cell; see Fig. 3, showing one of the two flagella (cfr. HENDELBERG, 1965). In the digenetic trematodes studied (two liver flukes) the two flagella and a median, cytoplasmic protrusion are incorporated into a common shaft during a rapid uniting process followed by a migration of the nuclear material from one end of the cell to the other (HENDELBERG, 1962). The incorporation of two flagella into trematode spermatozoa was observed by BURTON (1964) and SATO *et al.* (1967), too, and might well be the explanation of the observations reported by HERSHENOV *et al.* (1966), compare similar micrographs by GRESSON and PERRY (1961), AFZELIUS (1966, Fig. 32) and BURTON (1967; 1968) of spermatozoa from species in which an incorporation has been shown to occur.

In some Turbellaria the two flagella of the young spermatid later form the marginal filament in each of the *undulating membranes* characterizing the spermatozoon. This was found in some species of the Acoela and Polycladida studied. My results in this respect are quite in line with those arrived at by KOLTZOFF (1909) but do not agree with some other results published later (references in HENDELBERG, 1969 a). In other turbellarians two flagella may be incorporated into spermatozoa with only one undulating membrane (KOLTZOFF, 1909; HENLEY, 1968).

Two *free*, subterminally inserted flagella (*nebengeisseln*) seem to be the rule in the spermatozoa of the turbellarian groups Tricladida and Proseriata, and are found in many Polycladida and Rhabdocoela. Spermatozoa of this kind show great differences in other respects (SILVEIRA and PORTER, 1964; HENDELBERG, 1965, 1969 a). However, in all known cases the two flagella grow from the young, still approximately spherical or pear-shaped spermatids. Two (more or less?) free, terminal flagella have been reported from the spermatozoa of a few trematodes (DHINGRA, 1954; NEZ and SHORT, 1957).

The aberrant acoelan spermatozoon characterized by a *terminal bundle of filaments* has been found to develop from spermatids with two flagella in the same way as the common, thread-shaped type. The terminal filaments are a differentiation appearing in a very late phase of the spermiogenesis (HENDELBERG, 1969 a).

In the Turbellaria no spermatozoa with only one flagellum were found. The occurrence of *spermatids and spermatozoa without any flagella* was confirmed, however. Such spermatids and spermatozoa were found in some Rhabdocoela and in the Prolecithophora and Macrostomida studied (HENDELBERG, 1969 a). That the short, straight " setae " or " bristles " of the type described from the spermatozoa of many Macrostomida have an ultrastructure different from that of flagella has just been reported by BEDINI and PAPI (1969). If the more flagellum-like filaments reported earlier from some other Macrostomida are typical flagella or not remains to be investigated.

The number of flagella or axial filaments in spermatozoa of the Cestoda has been reported to be two in some species but only one in others (see e.g. GRESSON, 1962; ROSARIO, 1964; VON BONSDORFF and TELKKÄ, 1965; LUMSDEN, 1965; ŚWIDERSKI, 1968; HENDELBERG, 1969 a).

The widespread occurrence in the Turbellaria of two flagella in spermatids and spermatozoa (Schema 1) suggests that we are here concerned with a primitive feature of the group. This implies that the " Turbellarian Archetype " most probably had biflagellate spermatozoa. In some turbellarian groups the alterations during the evolution have then led to a reduction in size or to a complete elimination of the flagella (cfr. HENDELBERG, 1969 a).

The derivation of the Trematoda and the Cestoda from rhabdocoels (of dalyellioid type?) suggested by many authors (Schema 1) implies that the occurrence of two flagella in the spermatids and spermatozoa of many trematodes and of at least some cestodes ought to represent the original condition. The reported occurrence of only one flagellum or axial filament in the spermatozoa of some cestodes may then be explained as being due to a reduction.

At the beginning of the present century the theory was put forward that the occurrence of two flagella in many turbellarian spermatozoa is a primitive feature, surviving since the period before the metazoan stage. It must be stressed, however, that the occurrence of two flagella does not imply that the turbellarian spermatozoa has not evolved from the primitive, monoflagellate metazoan type. A doubling of the flagellum has been found in many other groups, too (see references in HENDELBERG, 1969 a, p. 41). Of interest are e.g. the conditions found in the Insecta by BACCETTI, DALLAI and ROSATI (1968) which in many respects seem to be analogous with those found in the Platyhelminthes. However, as far as we know, no Turbellaria have retained the primitive characteristic—one single flagellum.

The great difference between the primitive metazoan spermatozoon and the spermatozoa within the Turbellaria has been explained as depending on the strongly changed biology of propagation in the Turbellaria, which all have internal fertilization (FRANZÉN, 1956; JÄGERSTEN, 1959; AX, 1961). According to AX the " Turbellarian Archetype " had internal fertilization. My results are quite in line with these assumptions. The occurrence of a common type of spermatid within the Turbellaria, and the aberrant features in the morphology and development of this spermatid, speaks against a parallel evolution of internal fertilization in different turbellarian groups.

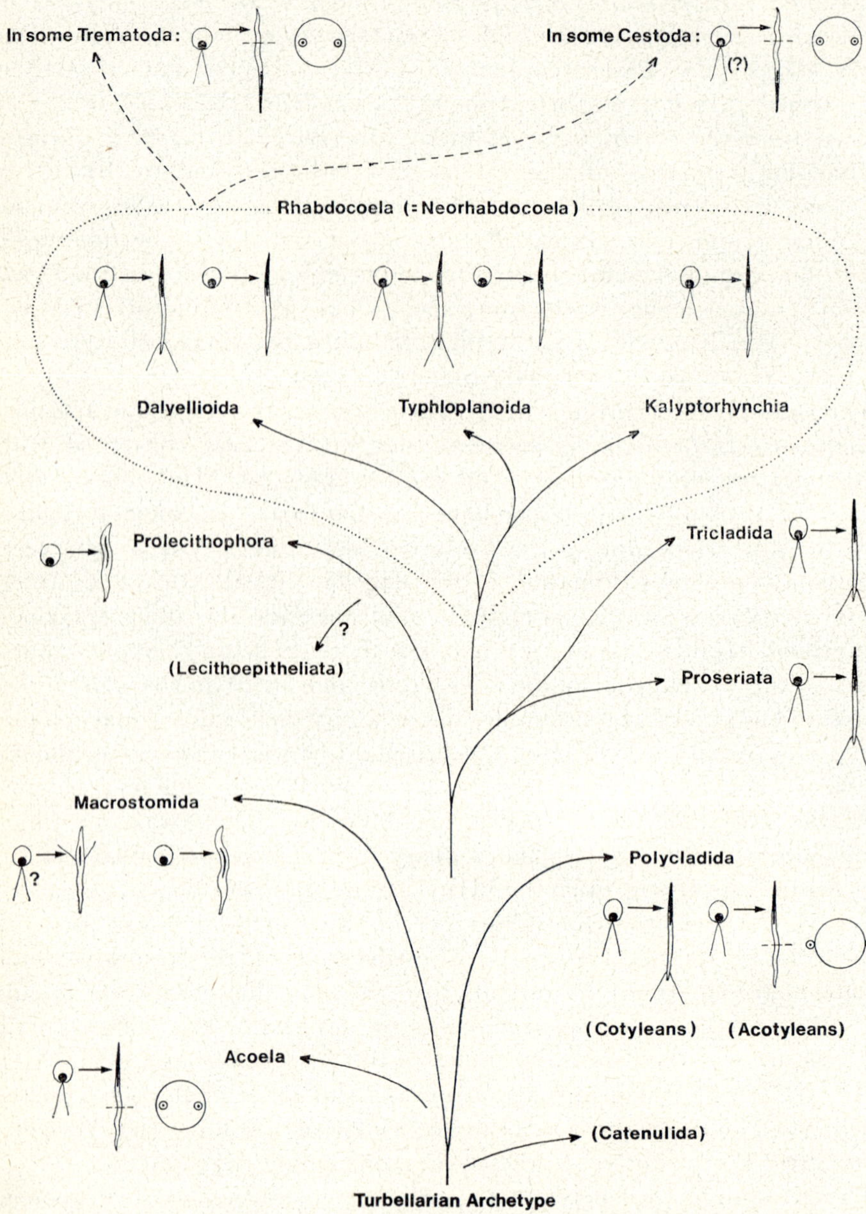

Schema I. – The results arrived at hitherto regarding the occurrence of flagella in spermatids and spermatozoa of the Turbellaria, plotted in the scheme of the evolution within the group suggested by AX (1961). The derivation of the Trematoda and the Cestoda from rhabdocoels (of dalyellioid type?) suggested by many authors is indicated in the scheme. – The development from the young spermatid to the spermatozoon is indicated by an arrow. The nuclei are marked black. The transverse sections of the spermatozoa show the position of the two incorporated flagella. (Cfr. HENDELBERG, 1969 a.)

Contrary to the earlier known (references in HENDELBERG, 1969 a, p. 41; see also SATO *et al.*, 1967; ŚWIDERSKI, 1968; SILVEIRA, 1969) aberrant ultrastructure of the flagella in flatworm spermatozoa (Fig. 3), the corresponding structure in the Acoela (Turbellaria) studied by me (Fig. 2) was found to be very reminiscent of the structure commonly found in cilia and flagella (HENDELBERG, 1969 a). Further investigations into the ultrastructure of the flagella in spermatozoa of different turbellarian groups will then be of great interest from a phylogenetic point of view.

In many flatworm spermatozoa the two flagella play an important role in the generation of the undulating movements. The role played by the microtubular filaments (*mtf* in Fig. 3) underlying the cell membrane is of interest in this connection. In e.g. the acotylean polyclads studied, the microtubular filaments occur also in that part of the spermatozoon which does not undulate. In this type of spermatozoon the flagella seem to be the direct cause of the undulations (HENDELBERG, 1965). However, other flatworm spermatozoa, having microtubular filaments but no flagella, do perform undulations (CHRISTENSEN, 1961; HENDELBERG, 1969 a, b).

REFERENCES

AFZELIUS B. (1966) – *Anatomy of the cell.* Univ. Chicago Press, Chicago and London, 127 pp.

AX P. (1961) – *Verwandtschaftsbeziehungen und Phylogenie der Turbellarien.* « Ergebn. Biol. », 24, 1–68.

BACCETTI B., DALLAI R. and ROSATI F. (1968) – *Spermatology of Rhynchotoid Insects* in Bocciarelli D. S. (*edit.*), Electron Microscopy 1968, II, Roma, 339–340.

BEDINI C. and PAPI F. (1969) – *Peculiar patterns of spermatozoa organization in lower Turbellaria.* Communication at the International Symposium on Comparative Spermatology, Roma–Siena, 1–5 July 1969.

BONSDORFF C. – H. VON and TELKKÄ A. (1965) – *The spermatozoon flagella in* Diphyllobothrium latum (*Fish tapeworm*). « Z. Zellforsch. », 66, 643–648.

BURTON P. (1964) – *Differentiation of sperm in* Haematoloechus medioplexus (*Platyhelminthes; Trematoda*). « Anat. Rec. », 148, 267.

BURTON P. (1967) – *Fine structure of the reproductive system of a frog lung fluke.* II. *Penetration of the ovum by a spermatozoon.* « J. Parasit. », 53, 994–999.

BURTON P. (1968) – *Effects of various treatments on microtubules and axial units of lung-fluke spermatozoa.* « Z. Zellforsch. », 87, 226–248.

CHRISTENSEN K. (1961) – *Fine structure of an unusual spermatozoan in the flatworm* Plagiostomum. « Biol. Bull. », Wood's Hole, 121, 416.

DHINGRA O. P. (1954) – *Gametogenesis and fertilization in* Isoparorchis eurytremum. « Res. Bull. Panjab Univ. », 44, 21–37.

FRANZÉN Å. (1956) – *On spermiogenesis, morphology of the spermatozoon, and biology of fertilization among Invertebrates.* « Zool. Bidr. Uppsala », 31, 355–482.

GRESSON R. A. R. (1962) – *Spermatogenesis of a Cestode.* « Nature », 194 (4826), 397–398.

GRESSON R. A. R. and PERRY M. M. (1961) – *Electron microscope studies of spermateleosis in* Fasciola hepatica *L.* « Exp. Cell Res. », 22, 1–8.

HENDELBERG J. (1962) – *Paired flagella and nucleus migration in the spermiogenesis of* Dicrocoelium *and* Fasciola (*Digenea, Trematoda*). « Zool. Bidr. Uppsala », 35, 569–587.

HENDELBERG J. (1965) – *On different types of spermatozoa in Polycladida, Turbellaria.* « Ark. Zool. », 18 (13), 267–304.

HENDELBERG J. (1969 a) – *On the development of different types of spermatozoa from spermatids with two flagella in the Turbellaria with remarks on the ultrastructure of the flagella.* « Zool. Bidr. Uppsala », 38, 1–50.

HENDELBERG J. (1969 b) – *Flatworm spermiogenesis and spermatozoa studied by light and electron microscope methods.* « Acta Universitatis Upsaliensis, Abstracts of Uppsala Diss. in Science », 140, 1–12.

HENLEY C. (1968) – *Refractile bodies in the developing and mature spermatozoa of* Childia groenlandica (*Turbellaria: Acoela*). « Biol. Bull. », Wood's Hole, 134, 382–397.

HERSHENOV B. R., TULLOCH G. S. and JOHNSON A. D. (1966) – *The fine structure of trematode sperm tails.* « Trans. Amer. micr. Soc. », 85, 480–483.

JÄGERSTEN G. (1959) – *Further remarks on the early phylogeny of the Metazoa.* « Zool. Bidr. Uppsala », 33, 79–108.

KOLTZOFF N. K. (1909) – *Studien über die Gestalt der Zelle.* II. *Untersuchungen über das Kopfskelett des tierischen Spermiums.* « Arch. Zellforsch. », 2, 1–65.

LUMSDEN R. D. (1965) – *Microtubules in the peripheral cytoplasm of cestode spermatozoa.* « J. Parasit. », 51, 929–931.

NEZ M. M. and SHORT R. B. (1957) – *Gametogenesis in* Schistosomatium douthitti (*Cort*) (*Schistosomatidae: Trematoda*). « J. Parasit. », 43, 167–182.

ROSARIO B. (1964) – *An electron microscope study of spermatogenesis in Cestodes.* « J. Ultrastructure Res. », 11, 412–427.

SATO M., OH M. and SAKODA K. (1967) – *Electron microscopic study of spermatogenesis in the lung fluke* (Paragonimus miyazakii). « Z. Zellforsch. », 77, 232–243.

SILVEIRA M. (1969) – *Ultrastructural studies on a " nine plus one " flagellum. 1.* « J. Ultrastructure Res. », 26, 274–288.

SILVEIRA M. and PORTER K. R. (1964) – *The spermatozoids of flatworms and their microtubular system.* « Protoplasma », 59, 240–265.

ŚWIDERSKI Z. (1968) – *The fine structure of the spermatozoon of sheep tapeworm,* Moniezia expansa (*Rud.*, 1810) (*Cyclophyllidea, Anoplocephalidae*). « Zoologica Poloniae », 18, 475–486.

EXPLANATION OF FIGURES

Fig. 1. – *Convoluta saliens* (Acoela, Turbellaria). Transverse sections of spermatozoa (in the seminal vesicle) showing among other things the incorporated flagella (*f*). Two tubular filaments are evident in the centre of each flagellum complex at all levels sectioned. ×30,000.

Fig. 2. – *C. saliens.* Transverse section of spermatozoon, showing the two tubular filaments (arrows) in the centre of each flagellum complex. ×80,000.

Fig. 3. – *Cryptocelides loveni* (Polycladida, Turbellaria). Transverse section of part of a spermatozoon showing one of the flagella (*f*) adhering to the body of the cell. The aberrant ultrastructure earlier known from the flagella of different flatworm spermatozoa is seen in the central part of the flagellum. Microtubular filaments (*mtf*) are situated under the cell membrane. ×80,000.

Figs. 1–3. – Osmium—phosphotungstic acid—epon. Siemens elmiskop I. Complementary information in Hendelberg, 1965, 1969 a.

Discussion

ANDERSON. – CHRISTENSEN described an aflagellate Platyhelminthum spermatozoon that is capable of active motility. Presumably, a subplasmalemmal system of microtubules accounts for this active motility. In species studied by you a similar microtubular system is described. Do you think it plays some role in spermatozoa motility?

HENDELBERG. – I found no evidence of this in the polyclad spermatozoa I studied in this respect. The undulations of the so-called thread-shaped polyclad spermatozoa were observed to be performed only by that part of the spermatozoon which is bordered by the two flagella. This refers to, among others, spermatozoa in which the cell membrane is underlain for the whole of the length of the spermatozoon by microtubular filaments. Thus these filaments occur also in that part of the spermatozoon which does not undulate. Also, when the two flagella were detached (by mechanical means) from the spermatozoon in the whole of their length except at the base active movements were observed in the flagella, but not in the cell body containing microtubules, from which they were detached. It is true, however, that some types of aflagellate turbellarian spermatozoa are capable of active motility. I have seen this in many *Plagiostomida*, i.e. in species related to that studied by CHRISTENSEN (1961). SILVEIRA and PORTER (1964) describe undulatory movements of the two free flagella in spermatozoa within the *Tricladida*, but also active motility of the cell body containing subplasmalemmal microtubules. However, as far as I know the role played by these microtubules in the motility has not yet been ascertained.

FRANZÉN. – It is very interesting to hear that both you Dr. HENDELBERG and Dr. BEDINI has found the ultrastructure 9 + 2 in the flagella in the Turbellarian subgroup *Acoela*. Now I would like to ask you if the different results you and Dr. AFZELIUS have obtained about the flagellum ultrastructure in a *Mecynostomum* species could be explained by the finding by Dr. BEDINI that the ultrastructure is sometimes different in different regions of the flagellum? You and AFZELIUS may have studied different regions of the flagellum?

HENDELBERG. – No, I do not think so. First I must stress that Dr. AFZELIUS and I studied different species. Secondly, the species of *Convoluta* Dr. BEDINI gave an account of evidently shows many aberrant features, e.g. the fiber sheath enveloping the flagella. Such a sheath does not occur in the species of *Convoluta* I studied. I also found the flagella to be of the 9 + 2 tubule substructure in all levels sectioned (cfr. my Fig. 1).

REGER. – Are both the 9 + 1 and the 9 + 2 tubule substructure in *Turbellaria* motile?

HENDELBERG. – Yes, they are. The motility of flagella of the so-called 9 + 1 pattern has been studied in spermatids and spermatozoa of many flatworms. The 9 + 2 pattern of flagella in flatworm spermatozoa has been demonstrated hitherto only in a few studied acoels. In these (and in other acoels with flagella of unknown ultrastructure) the part of the spermatozoon containing the two incorporated flagella has been observed to undulate. In spermatids the still unincorporated flagella often remain still, but in a few cases I have observed them to be motile.

BACCETTI. – Is it known a true 9 + 1 (not 9 + 9 + 1 or 9 + 1 of flatworms) pattern in any cilia or flagella?

AFZELIUS. – Answer to Dr. BACCETTI'S question: No, apart from the 9 + 9 + 1 flagella of the mosquitos, I know only of the *Chlamydomonas* flagellary mutants described by RANDALL and WARR. As for the problem of whether or not there are motile 9 + 0 flagella, I might say a few words, also. As I probably was the first to suggest the existance of a motile 9 + 0 flagellum I feel responsible for the idea. This suggestion was based on an examination of *Myzostomum* and presented in Philadelphia in 1962. Dr. FAWCETT suggested that the configuration was due to a dissolution of the central pair during fixation and this may well be the case. I get the same result however each summer I fix *Myzostomum*, and regardless of whether I use glutaraldehyde or osmium tetroxide. There have also been some further claims of motile 9 + 0 sperm tails or flagella: BOISSON *et al.* in Compt. rend. Acad. Sci. (Paris) 264, (1967) 2909 on the fish *Lycodontis afer* and MANTON and VON STOSCH on the diatom sperm. The ephemerid sperm described here by BACCETTI and PHILLIPS seem to be of a similar kind.

NELSON. – Variable number of central tubules or even complete absence does not necessarily influence flagellar or ciliary movement. Even in paralyzed *Chlamydomonas* mutants there are more structural deformities present than just lack of central tubules. We therefore still have no evidence of a specific role in movement for these central tubules.

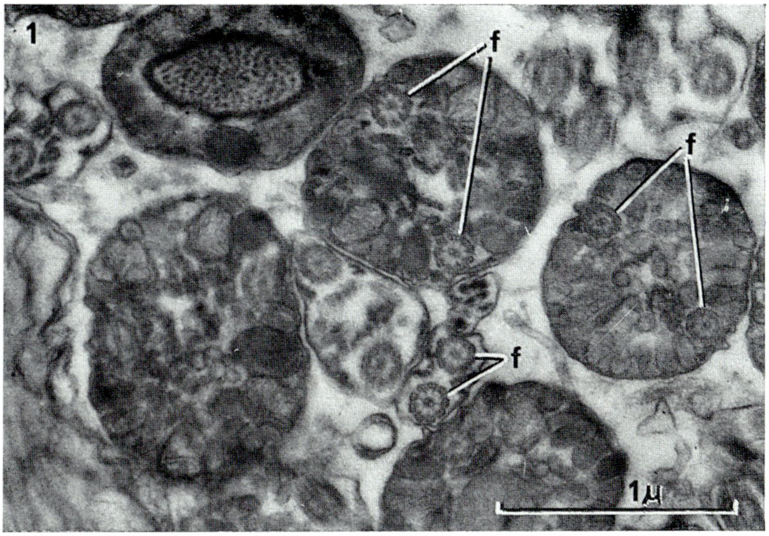
1
f
f
f
1μ

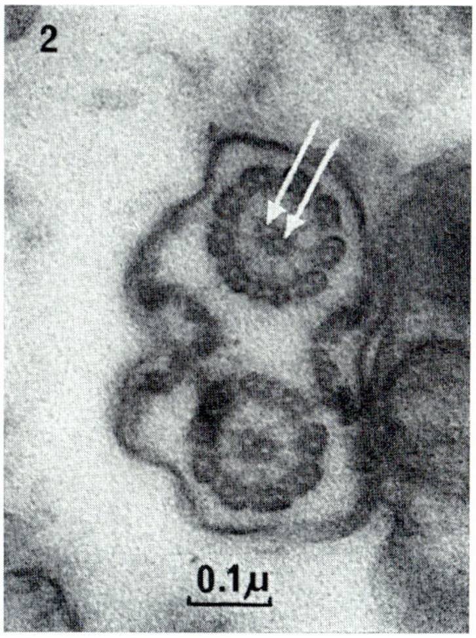
2
0.1μ

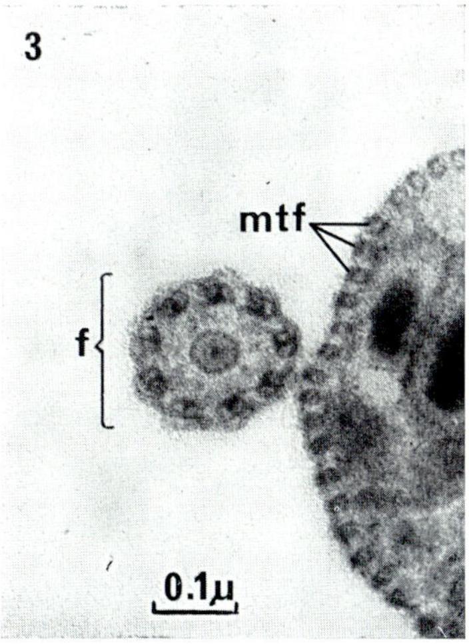
3
mtf
f
0.1μ

I. GRAEBNER (*) and H. ADAM (*)

ELECTRON MICROSCOPICAL STUDY OF SPERMATOGENESIS AND SPERM MORPHOLOGY IN GNATHOSTOMULIDS

SUMMARY. — The structural characteristics of spermatogenesis have been studied by the electron microscope in the genus *Gnathostomula*. The mature spermatozoa are aflagellate, but develop membranous protrusions the « Füsschen », which may play a role in motion of the spermatozoa. Microtubules are disposed in a single layer underneath the plasma membrane. It is suggested that they are responsible for form maintenance of the cell and probably support the motility of the spermatozoa.

RIASSUNTO. — Le caratteristiche strutturali della spermatogenesi sono state studiate con il microscopio elettronico nel genere *Gnathostomula*. Gli spermatozoi maturi sono aflagellati, ma sviluppano protrusioni membranose, i « Füsschen », che possono avere un ruolo nel moto dello spermatozoo. I microtubuli sono disposti in un unico strato al disotto della membrana plasmatica. Si ritiene che essi siano responsabili del mantenimento della forma della cellula e che probabilmente sostengano il movimento dello spermatozoo.

Rod-shaped, aflagellate spermatozoa were already observed in the genus *Gnathostomula* and *Gnathostomaria* in 1956 by Ax in the light microscope. In 1965 Ax again referred to the aberrant type of spermatozoa in *Gnathostomula paradoxa*. He stated, that the spermatozoa are of uniform structure, without a flagellum or " Nebengeissel " or any other special differentiations. KIRSTEUER (1964) first made a drawing of the shape of the spermatozoa after vital preparations of *Gnathostomula axi*.

Light and electronmicroscopical investigations of sperm-morphology and spermatogenesis have been carried out in *Gnathostomula paradoxa* and *Gnasthostomula axi*. The first species was collected from the mesopsammal of the North Sea, the latter from the mesopsammal of the North Adriatics.

Gnathostomula paradoxa.

In *Gnathostomula paradoxa* the testicular follicles are situated in the posterior region of the body forming two ventrolateral rows (Fig. 1). Each follicle is separated from the surrounding parenchyma by a membrane (Fig. 2). The epithelial (germinal) cells of the testes show a highly active Golgi apparatus. Characteristic for its activity is the large number of vesicles

(*) Zoologisches Institut der Universität Salzburg, Ferdinand Porsche-Strasse 8-5, A-5020 Salzburg, Austria.

derived from the lamellar system. In contrast to later stages the content of the vesicles is not electron dense.

Dividing spermatocytes have been found in all follicles (Fig. 3). The Golgi vesicles are arranged in a certain distance from the nucleus and come in close contact with the nucleus by means of fine bridges (Fig. 4).

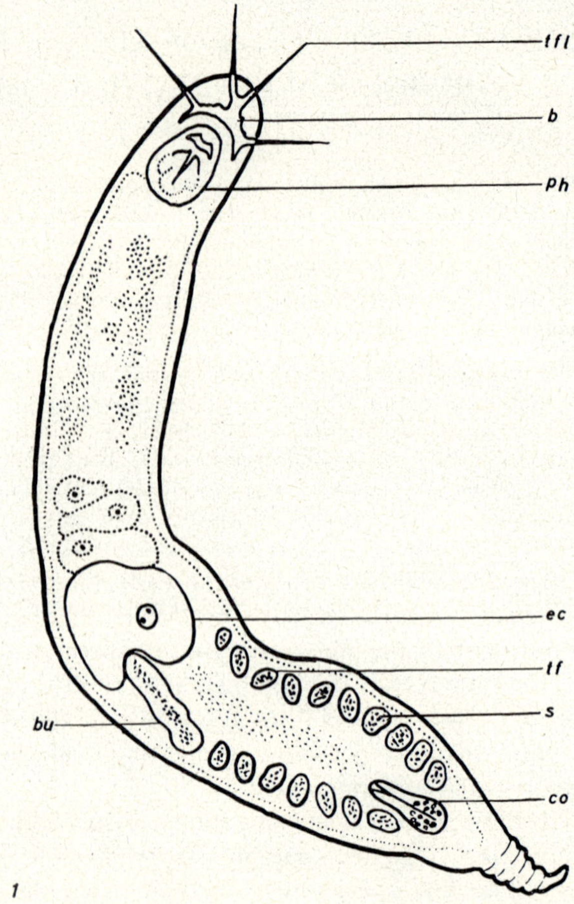

Fig. 1. – *Gnathostomula sp.*, schematic drawing, (*tfl*), tactile flagellum; (*b*), brain; (*ph*), pharynx; (*ec*), egg cell; (*tf*), testicular follicle; (*s*), spermatozoa; (*co*), copulatory organ; (*bu*), bursa. 675 : 1.

During spermatid formation two or four cells are connected by cytoplasmic bridges forming clusters of spermatids (Fig. 5) (FAWCETT, ITO and SLAUTTERBACK, 1959), a phenomenon, observed previously in some invertebrates and vertebrates (FRANZÉN, 1956; HENDELBERG, 1965; POSTWALD, 1967; ANDERSON, WEISSMAN and ELLIS, 1967). One has the impression that the Golgi vesicles migrate towards the plasma membrane and are finally located in protrusions of the limiting membrane. In these protrusions electron dense material is deposited and very often in addition membranous structures have been observed (Fig. 6, arrows).

The transformation of the free spermatid to the mature spermatozoon seems to be a very fast process. In sections through the testicular follicles of *Gnathostomula paradoxa* no intermediate stages were present or only very few cells, which can eventually be considered as intermediate stages, were found in sections of the testicular follicles of *Gnathostomula axi*. These cells are of irregular shape and inside of the cells vesicles and secretion granules are present. Partly the socalled " Füsschen " —of which I am going to talk about later on in more detail—are developed (Fig. 7).

The mature spermatozoa are about 2,5 μm long. They are embedded in the follicles in a fine granulated substance containing many granules of different size. In the mature spermatozoa one can distinguish between a more or less rounded front end and, a wider longish middle part terminating into a narrow tail end. In this stage the nucleus is oval-shaped and always placed against one plain of the cell. In that way a polarity of the cell results (Fig. 8).

Underneath the plasma membrane numerous microtubular elements forming a single layer are present. They extend longitudinally and parallel to each other along the surface of the spermatozoa. The plasma membrane itself consists of its three typical layers (1) an outer electron dense layer of about 5 nm, (2) an intermedial layer with lower electron density of about 3 nm, (3) an inner electron dense layer of about 3–4 nm thickness.

The most striking feature of the spermatozoa is the differentiation of membranous protrusion which I would like to call " Füsschen ". They are arranged in clusters at the basis of the cell and are found in single structures arround the tail end. The basal " Füsschen " are sitting on short humps of the cell into which the nucleus extends (Fig. 8). There are 4 or 5 clusters of " Füsschen " sitting medial along the main axis of the cell. The length of the " Füsschen " is 0.18 μm, the diameter 0.04 μm. The wall as well as the plasma membrane consists of three layers, however, the inner layer is 7 nm thick and therefore, twice as thick as the inner layer of the plasma membrane. In the center of every " Füsschen " membranous structures form a typical regular cross (Fig. 9). This cross extends along the longitudinal axis of the " Füsschen " up to the nucleus (Fig. 10 arrows).

The Golgi vesicles are concentrated in certain areas of the cell, in the front end, in the tail end and lateral to both sides of the nucleus. Their content is now strongly electron dense. The rest of the cytoplasm shows fine granulated material. It might be, that the vesicles among others have acrosome function, since they are derivatives of the Golgi apparatus.

The nuclei of the epithelial cells in the testicular follicles contain dense chromatin masses (Fig. 2). In the nuclei of the spermatid clusters and in the free spermatids as well chromatin-filaments of about 6 nm thickness are in irregular order. Some of them are already oriented parallel to one another (Fig. 6). In the oval nucleus of the mature spermatozoon the chromatin filaments form lamellar structures (diameter = 15 nm) which remain always clearly visible in the mature spermatozoon (Fig. 10).

In all developmental stages one or two mitochondria have been observed. They are dispersed in the cytoplasm and show neither a significant change in structure nor any special arrangement during spermatogenesis. Their shape is oval and they vary in length between 0.5 and 0.7 μm and in width between 0.1 and 0.3 μm.

The microtubular elements underneath the limiting membrane are 12–14 nm in diameter and in close contact with the membrane (Fig. 11). SILVEIRA and PORTER, 1964, report a similar contact of microtubules with the plasma membrane in spermatozoa of flat worms.

On account of vital preparation studies I was able to state motility of the spermatozoa, accompanied by a change of the form of the cell. A support of motion of the cell by means of the microtubules is suggested. In sections through the bursa spermatozoa of different bizarre forms are reckognized. In vital preparations no motility of this type of spermatozoa was observed. In the bursa the spermatozoa seem to have lost their original form and also their capacity for motion.

Gnathostomula axi.

In *Gnathostomula axi* spermatogenesis seems to take place in the same manner as in *Gnathostomula paradoxa.* Similar spermatocytes and clusters of spermatids develop (Fig. 12). In the spermatids Golgi vesicles protrude the plasma membrane in the way demonstrated in *Gnathostumula paradoxa* (Fig. 13).

The mature spermatozoon is spindle-shaped and the " Füsschen " are developed only arround the tail end (Fig. 14). The length of the spermatozoa in about 2.5 μm, and microtubules are present underneath the plasma membrane (Fig. 11). The layers of the plasma membrane and the wall of the " Füsschen " correspond with the appropriate layers in the *Gnathostomula paradoxa* spermatozoon. The " Füsschen " are in general shorter (0.12 μm) and in the interior no membranous structures are detectable. The content is electron dense and there is nevertheless a contact between the " Füsschen " and the nucleus.

The Golgi vesicles are distributed irregularely in the cytoplasm. The chromatin filaments are arranged in the mature spermatozoon to form lamellar structures. The mitochondria are inconspicuous like in *Gnathostomula paradoxa.*

Finally, I would like to mention an electron microscopical result of a new *Gnathostomula species*—that is *Gnathostomula jenneri* (RIEDL, 1969)—from North America shores (Fig. 15). In the very species the spermatids show the typical differentiation. The Golgi vesicles are located in the protruded areas and in certain places the connection with the nucleus is still visible. In the mature spermatozoon the nucleus is situated at the basis of the cell, from where 4–5 single " Füsschen " originate. They are of special length (1 μm) and their inner structure is filamentous and contacts the nucleus.

RIEDL (1969) points out a change of form of the spermatozoa in the bursa immediately after insemination of the animal.

Summarizing it can be said, that the Golgi vesicles seem to play a significant role during spermatogenesis of *Gnathostomula* and that in all three species microtubules and " Füsschen " are developed (Fig. 16). Microtubular elements have been demonstrated in flagellate and aflagellate spermatozoa of representatives of various animal groups. Microtubules, located directly underneath the limiting membrane have been observed in sperma-

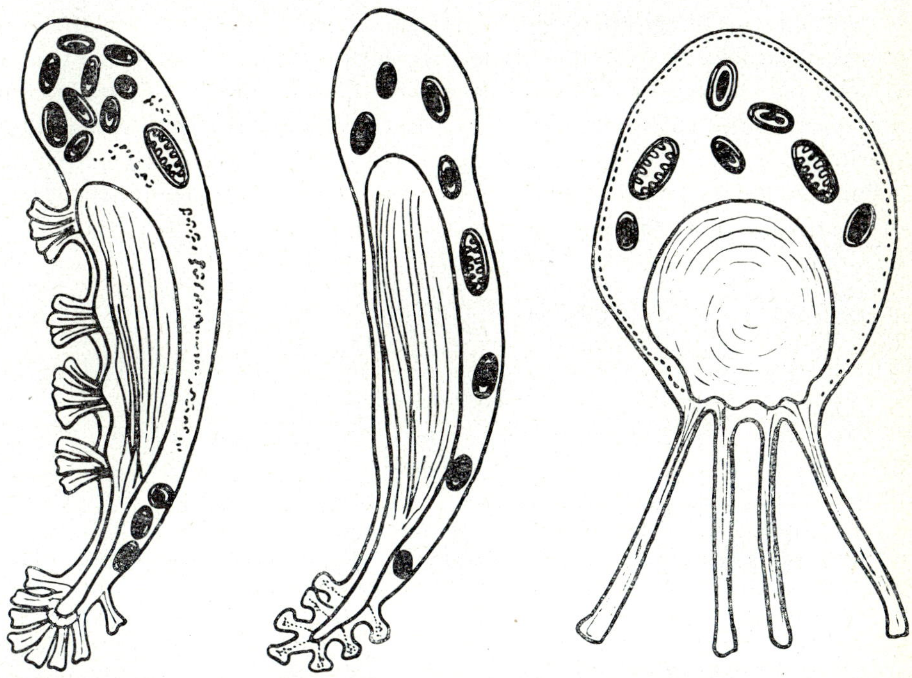

Fig. 16. – *Gnathostomula paradoxa, auxi and jenneri,* schematic drawing of the mature spermatozoa of all three mentioned species. 44.000 : 1.

tozoa of some turbellarians (CHRISTENSEN, 1961; KLIMA, 1961; SILVEIRA and PORTER, 1964; HENDELBERG, 1965) in some trematodes (SHAPIRO, MOTOW and SAKODA, 1967) and cestodes (BONSDORFF and TELKKA, 1965; ROSARIO, 1964). It is generally assumed that in spermatozoa the microtubules are responsible for maintenance of shape of the cell furthermore they are supposed to support motility. The function of microtubules as an intracellular transport system is also discussed.

The development and function of the " Füsschen " is still obscure but I would like to mention two types of peculiar motility apparatus of certain spermatids and spermatozoa, which suggest a comparison with the " Füsschen ". REGER (1961, 1962, 1963) as well as BREUCKER and HORSTMANN

(1968) recorded motile structures in spermatozoa of the tick *Amblyomma dissimili* and *Ornithodorus moubata*, covering the whole surface of the cell. In the center of these structures two fine tubuli are visible and a close relation of the structures to the endoplasmic reticulum is indicated.

ZISSLER (1969) describes " Flügelstrukturen ", i.e. wing-like structures formed by extensions of the nuclear membrane and participation of vesicles of the endoplasmic reticulum during spermatogenesis of the fresh-water ostracode *Notodromas monacha*. The " Flügelstrukturen " consist of two lamellae, each bearing numerous tubules (ZISSLER, 1969, Abb. 7).

It is most likely that the " Füsschen " are responsible for the motility of the sperm, and that the nucler membrane and in particular the Golgi vesicles play a role in the development of these organells. This presumption however, ought to be still proved. Furthermore it is interesting that the spermatozoa of the genus *Pterognathia* (STERRER, 1966) show a typical flagellum in the light microscope. An electron microscopical investigation of these spermatozoa may perhaps permit a better understanding of the development and function of the "·Füsschen ".

REFERENCES

ANDERSON W. A., WEISSMAN A. and ELLIS R. A. (1967) – *Cytodifferentiation during spermiogenesis in* Lumbricus terrestris. « J. Cell Biol. », *32*, 11–26.

AX P. (1956) – *Die Gnathostomulida, eine rätselhafte Wurmgruppe aus dem Meeressand.* « Akad. d. Wiss. u. d. Lit. Mainz. Abhandl. d. math. naturwiss. Kl. », *8*, 1–32.

AX P. (1965) – *Zur Morphologie und Systematik der Gnathostomulida.* « Z. zool. Syst. Evolutionsf. », *3*, 3–4, 259–276.

BONSDORFF C. H. v. and TELKKA A. (1965) – *The spermatozoon flagella in* Diphyllobothrium latum (*Fish tapeworm*). « Z. Zellf. », *66*, 643–648.

BREUCKER H. and HORSTMANN E. (1968) – *Die Spermatozoen der Zecke* Ornithodorus moubata (MURR). « Z. Zellf. », *88*, 1–22.

CHRISTENSEN A. K. (1961) – *Fine structure of an unusual spermatozoon in the flatworm Plagiostomum.* « Biol. Bull. », 121, 416.

FAWCETT D. W., ITO S. and SLAUTTERBACK D. B. (1959) – *The occurence of intercellular bridges in groups of cells exhibiting synchronous differentiation.* « J. Biophys. Biochem. Cytol. », *5*, 453–460.

FRANZÉN Å. (1956) – *On spermiogenesis, morphology of the spermatozoon and biology of fertilization among invertebrates.* « Zool. Bidrag (Uppsala) », *31*, 355–482.

GRAEBNER I. (1968) – *Ergebnisse einer elektronenmikroskopischen Untersuchung von Gnathostomuliden.* « Zool. Anz. », 32, Suppl. – Bd. in press.

HENDELBERG J. (1965) – *On different types of spermatozoa in Polycladida, Turbellaria.* « Arkiv f. Zoologi », *18*, 267–304.

KIRSTEUER E. (1964) – *Eine neue Gnathostomulide aus der Mangrove-Region des Archipels Los Roques, Venezuela.* « Zool. Anz. », *172*, 436–440.

KLIMA J. (1961) – *Elektronenmikroskopische Studien über die Feinstruktur der Tricladen* (*Turbellaria*). « Protoplasma », *54*, 101–162.

POSTWALD H. E. (1967) – *An electron microscope study of spermiogenesis in* Spirorbis (Laeospira) mörchi *Levinsen* (*Polychaeta*). » Z. Zellf. », *83*, 231–248.

REGER J. F. (1961) – *The fine structure of spermatids from the tick,* Amblyomma dissimili. « J. Ultrastruct. Res. », *5*, 584–599.

REGER J. F. (1962) – *A fine-structure study on spermiogenesis in the tick* Amblyomma dissimili, *with special reference to the development of motile processes.* « J. Ultrastruct. Res. », *7*, 550–565.

REGER J. F. (1963) – *Spermiogenesis in the tick,* Amblyomma dissimili, *as revealed by electron microscopy.* « J. Ultrastruct. Res. », *8*, 607–621.

RIEDL R. J. (1969) – *Gnathostomulida from America. This is the first record of the new phylum from North America.* « Science », *163* (3866), 445–452.

ROSARIO B. J. (1964) – *An electron microscope study on spermatogenesis in cestodes.* « J. Ultrastruct. Res. », *11*, 417–427.

SATO J. E., MOTOW OH and SAKODA K. (1967) – *Electron microscopic study of spermatogenesis in the lung fluke* (Paragonimus miyazakii) (*Trematoda*). « Z. Zellf. », *77*, 232–243.

SHAPIRO J. E., HERSHENOV B. R. and TULLOCH A. S. (1961) – *The fine structure of* Haematoleochus medioplexus *sperm tail.* « J. Biophys. Biochem. Cytol. », *9*, 211–217.

SILVEIRA M. and PORTER K. R. (1965) – *The spermatozoids of flatworms and their microtubular systems.* « Protoplasma », *59*, 240–265.

STERRER W. (1965) – Gnathostomula axi *Kirsteuer und Austrognathia (ein weiteres Gnathostomuldien-Genus) aus der Nord-Adria.* « Z. Morph. Ökol. Tiere », *55*, 783–795.

STERRER W. (1966) – Gnathostomula paradoxa *AX und Vertreter von Pterognathia (ein neues Gnathostomuliden-Genus) von der schwedischen Westküste.* « Ark. för Zoologi », Serie 2, *18*, 405–412.

ZISSLER D. (1969) – *Die Spermiogenese des Süsswasser-Ostracoden* Notodromas monacha O. F. MÜLLER. I. *Die ovalen und spindelförmigen Spermatiden.* « Z. Zellf. », *96*, 87–105.

ZISSLER D. (1969) – *Die Spermiohistogenese des Süsswasser-Ostracoden* Notodromas monacha O. F. MÜLLER. II. *Die spindelförmigen und schlauchförmigen Spermatiden.* « Z. Zellf. », *96*, 106–133.

EXPLANATION OF FIGURES 2–15

Fig. 2. – *Gnathostomula paradoxa,* epithelial (germinal) cells. (*GV*), Golgi vesicles; (*D*), dictyosome. 24.000 : 1.

Fig. 3. – *Gnathosomula paradoxa,* germinal cell; (*GV*). Golgi vesicles; (*D*), dictyosome. 72.000 : 1.

Fig. 4. – *Gnathostomula paradoxa,* dividing spermatocyte, (*GV*), Golgi vesicles; (*D*), dictyosome. 54.000 : 1.

Fig. 5. – *Gnathostomula paradoxa,* clusters of spermatids. 24.000 : 1.

Fig. 6. – *Gnathostomula paradoxa,* spermatids. 54.000 : 1.

Fig. 7. – *Gnathostomula axi,* developmental stage which can be considered as intermediate between the characteristic spermatid and the mature spermatozoon. (*F*), " Füsschen "; 72.000 : 1.

Fig. 8. – *Gnathostomula paradoxa,* mature spermatozoon, (*GV*), Golgi vesicles; (*F*), " Füsschen ". 74.600 : 1.

Fig. 9. – *Gnathostomula paradoxa,* transversal section of the " Füsschen ". 108.000 : 1.

Fig. 10. – *Gnathostomula paradoxa,* mature spermatozoa. The membranous cross inside the " Füsschen " is in contact with the nucleus. The chromatin material in the nucleus is arranged in lamellar formation. 72.000 : 1.

Fig. 11 a. – *Gnathostomula paradoxa*, microtubules underneath the plasma membrane, (*pm*), plasma membrane; (*mt*), microtubules. 170.000 : 1.

Fig. 11 b. – *Gnathostomula axi*, microtubules underneath the plasma membrane, (*pm*), plasma membrane; (*mt*), microtubules. 170.000 : 1.

Fig. 12. – *Gnathostomula axi*, spermatocytes, (*GV*), Golgi vesicles; 22.000 : 1.

Fig. 13. – *Gnathostomula axi*, spermatids, (*GV*), Golgi vescicles. 72.000 : 1.

Fig. 14. – *Gnathostomula axi*, spermatozoon, (*F*), " Füsschen ". 66.000 : 1.

Fig. 15. – *Gnathostomula jenneri*, spermatids and spermatozoa. 36.000 : 1.

Discussion

HORSTMANN. – Really these sperms are very unusual. You have compared the " Füsschen " with the processes on the surface of mature sperms of ticks. I do not believe that these two structures are comparable, because the processes of ticks are cristae and, as Dr. REGER has shown, are developed by a very complicate differentiation.

How do the sperms of *Gnathostomulidae* move?

GRAEBNER. – The movement of the spermatozoa in *Gnathostomula paradoxa* has an amoeboid character, no special direction in locomotion was recognizable.

I. GRAEBNER and H. ADAM – *Electron microscopical study of spermatogenesis and sperm morphology in gnathostomulids.*

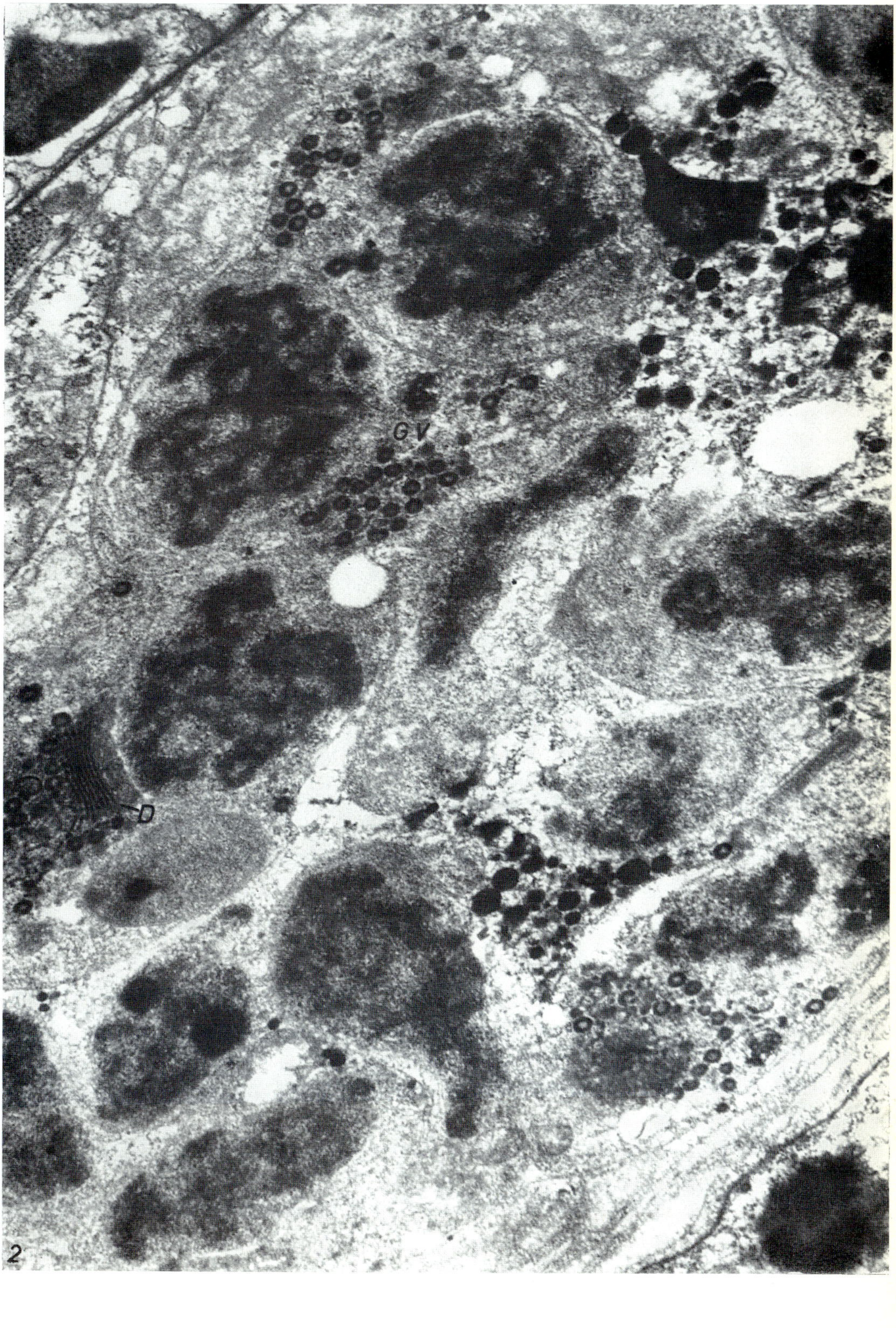

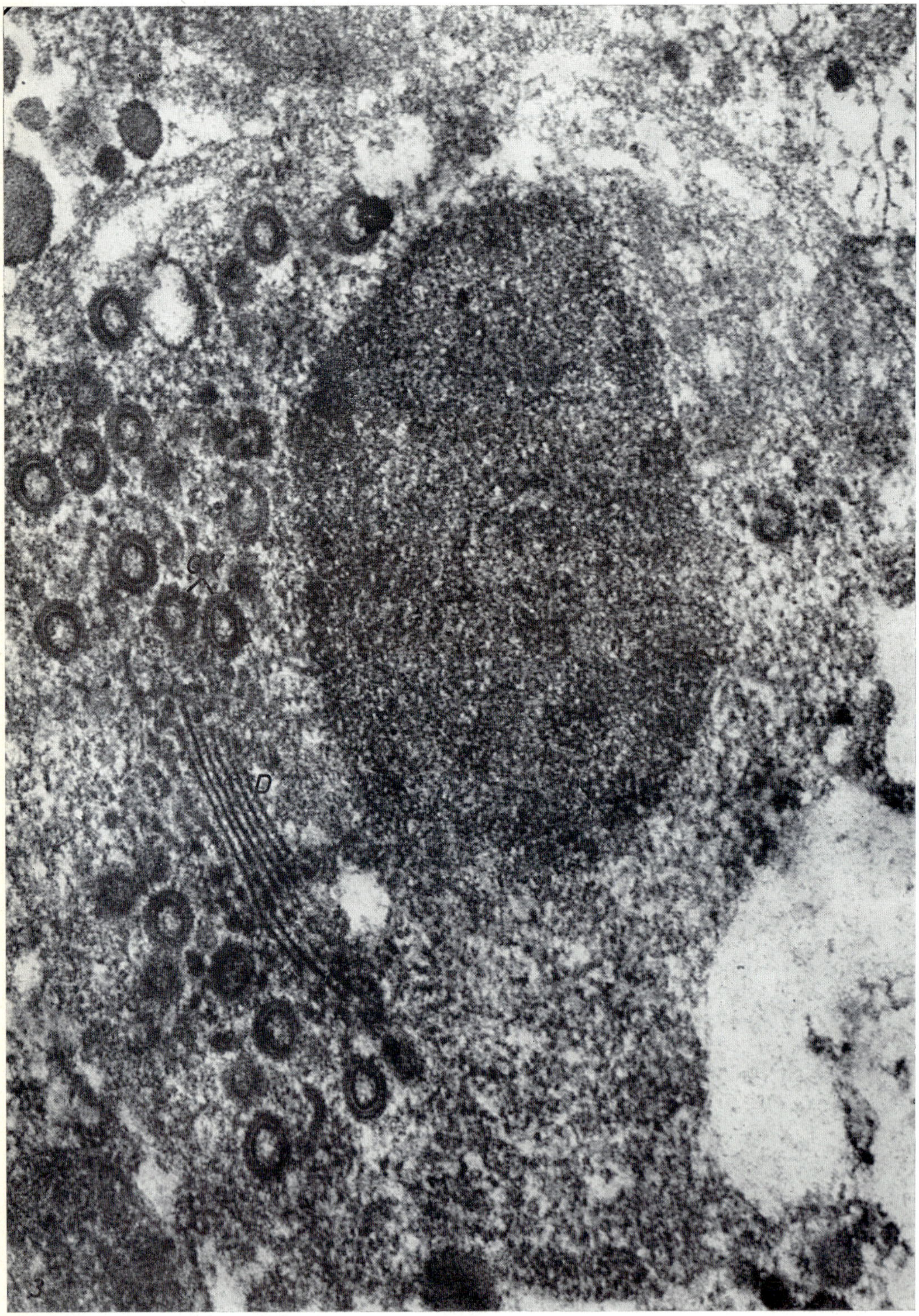
CM
D
3

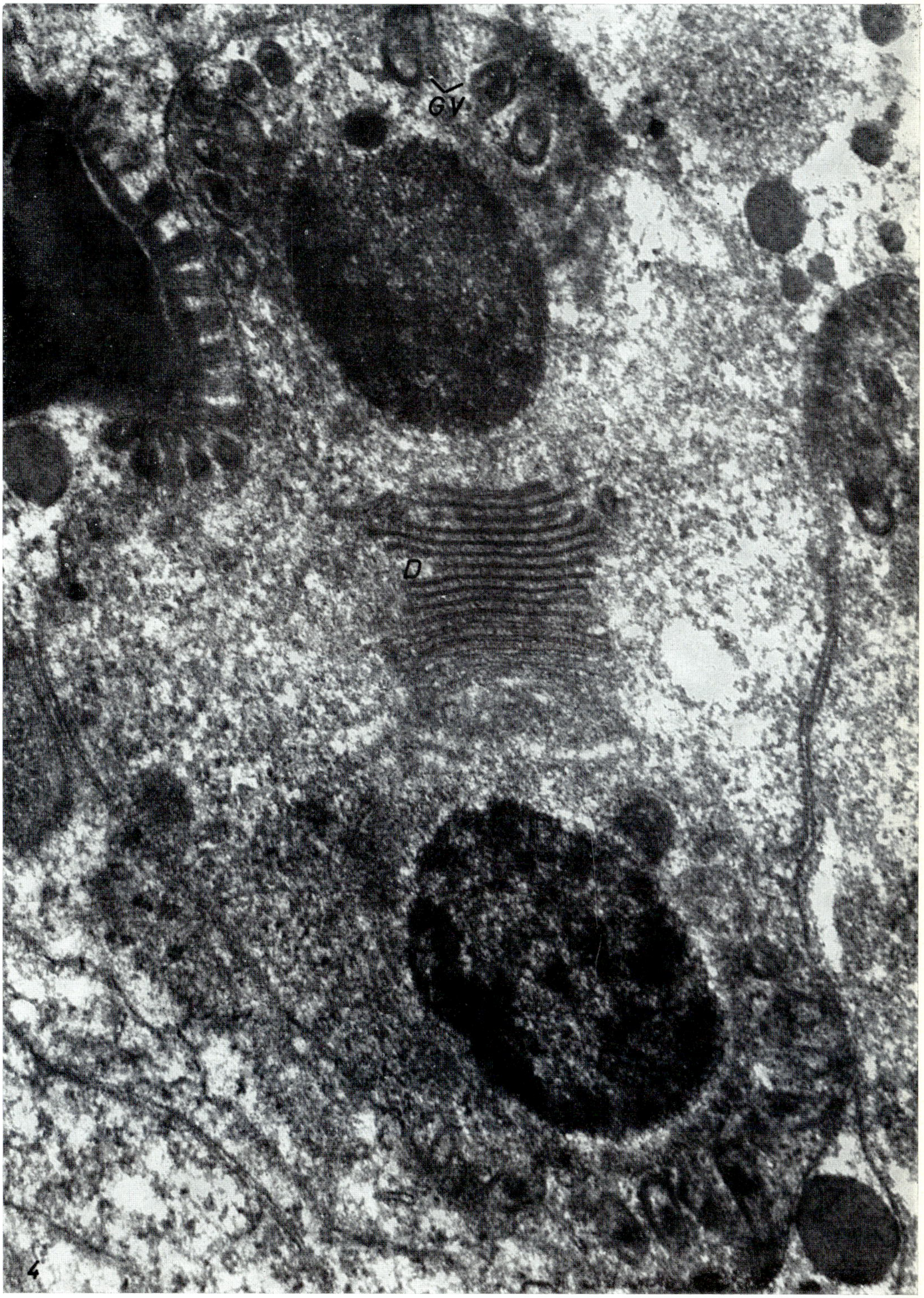
GV
D
4

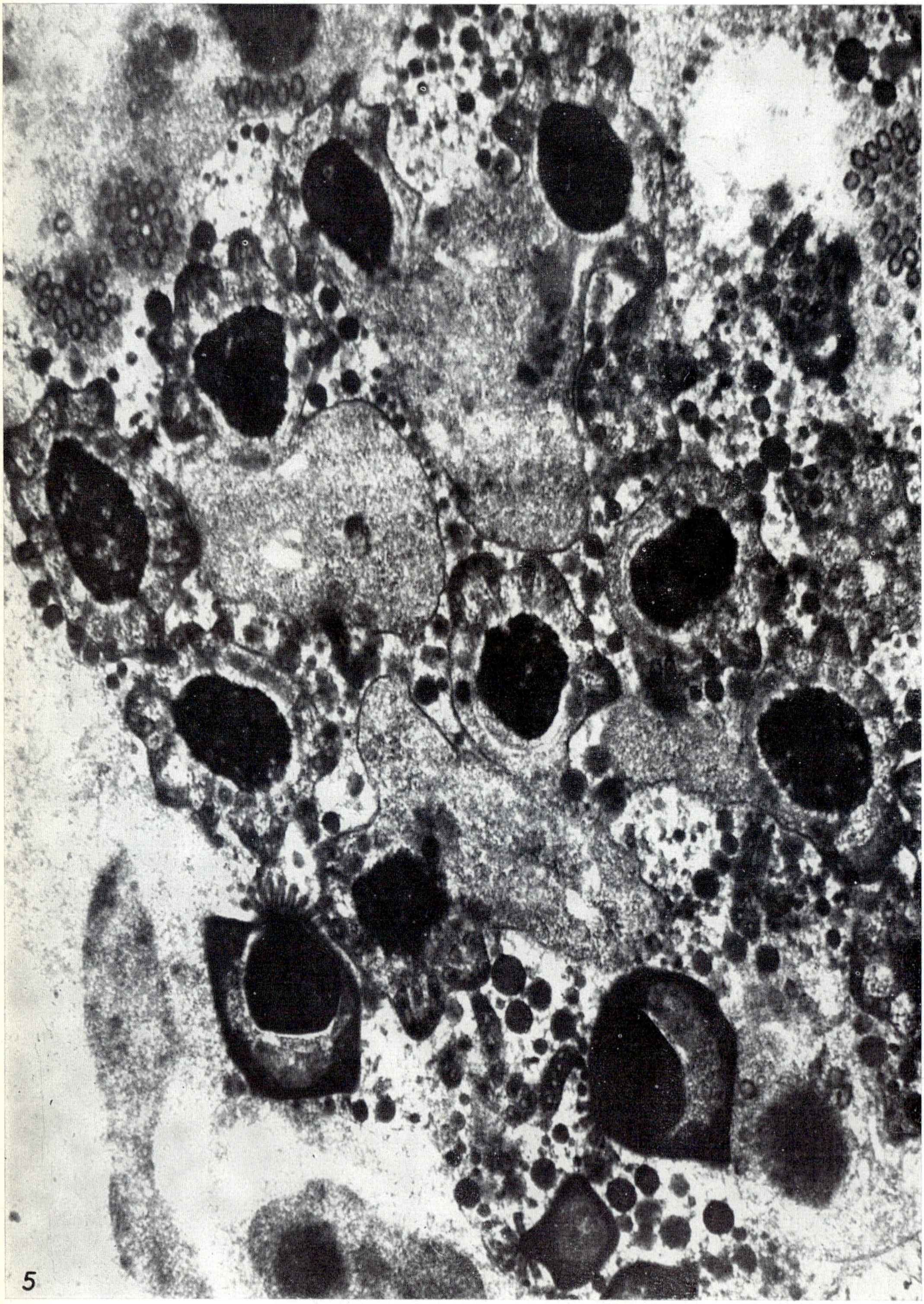

5

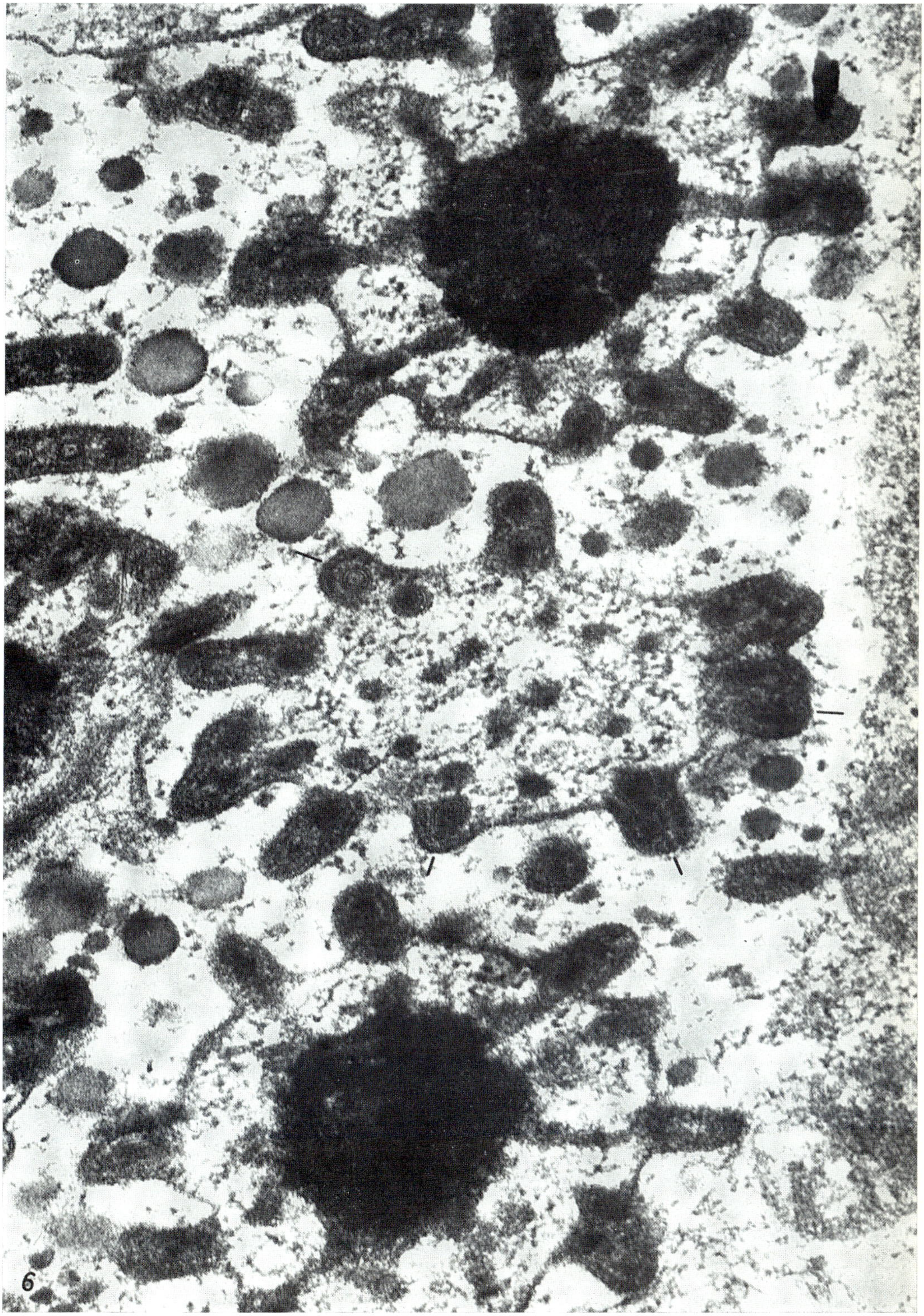
6

I. GRAEBNER and H. ADAM – *Electron microscopical study of spermatogenesis and sperm morphology in gnathostomulids.*

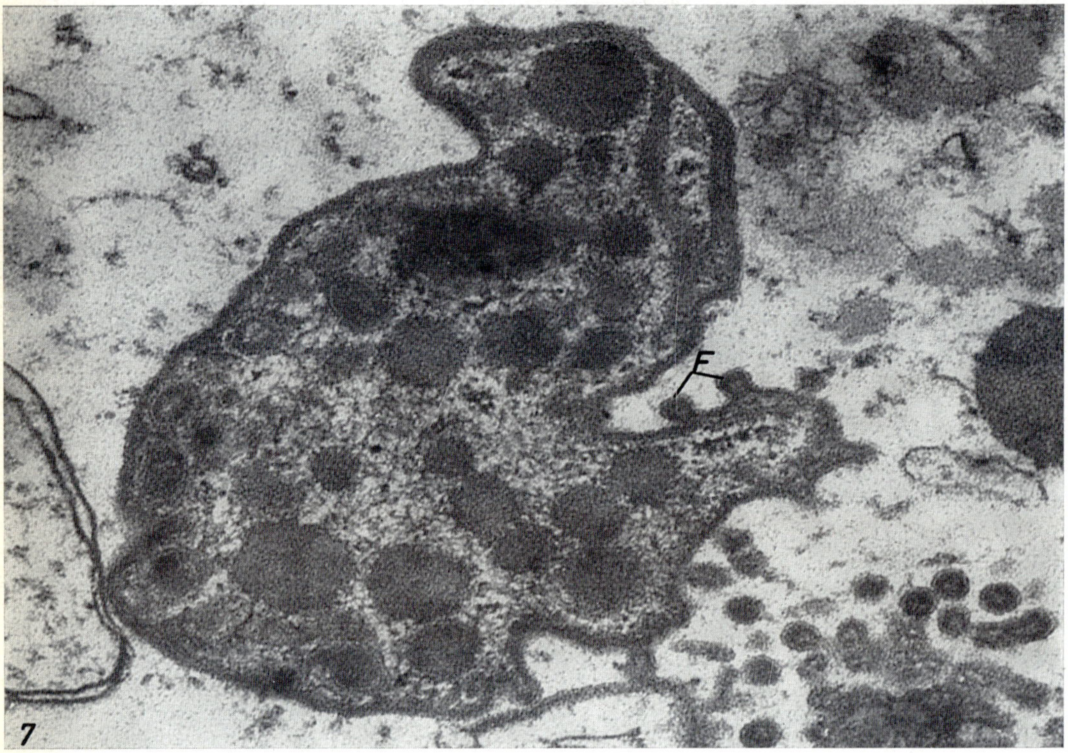

I. GRAEBNER and H. ADAM – *Electron microscopical study of spermatogenesis and sperm morphology in gnathostomulids.*

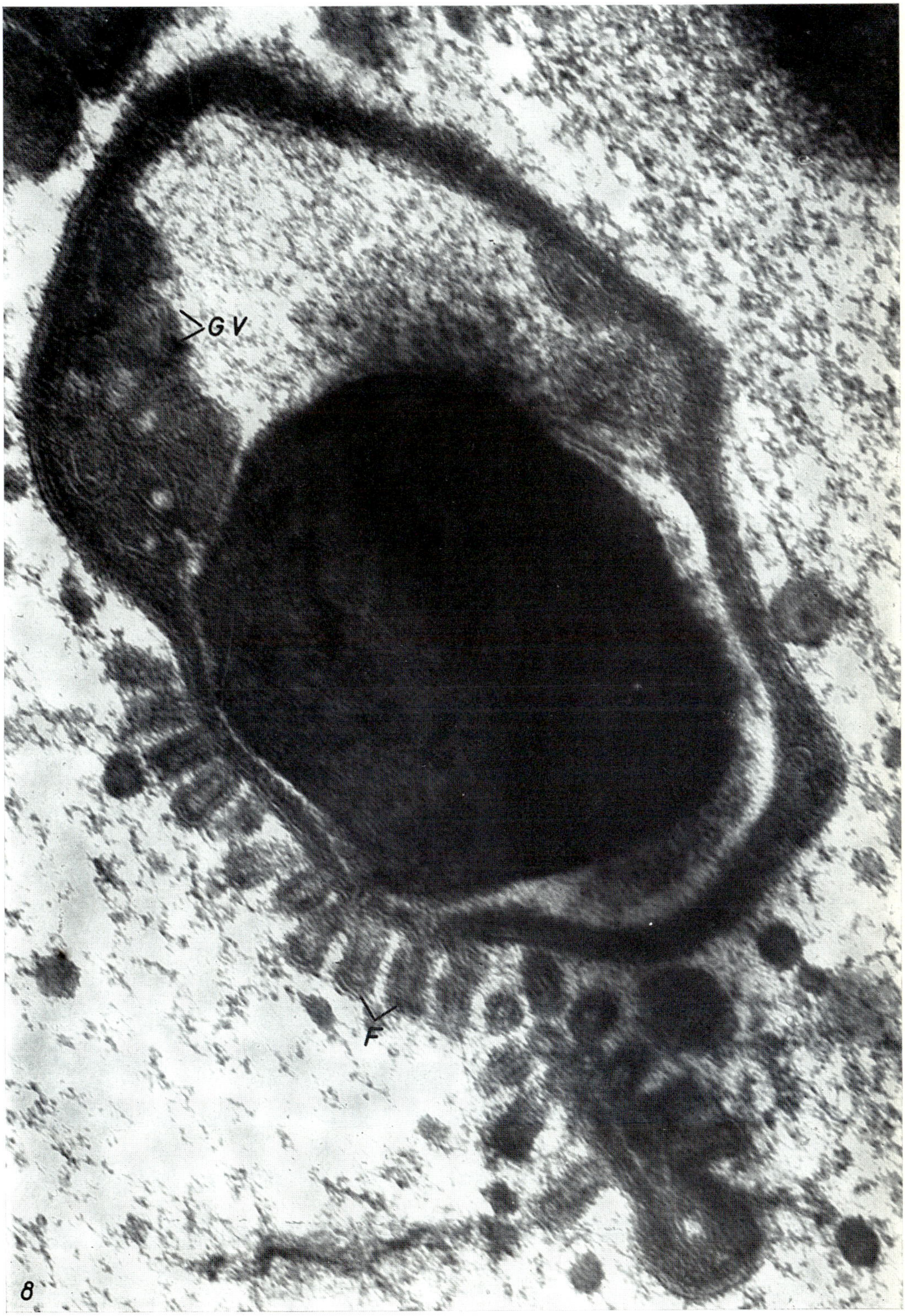

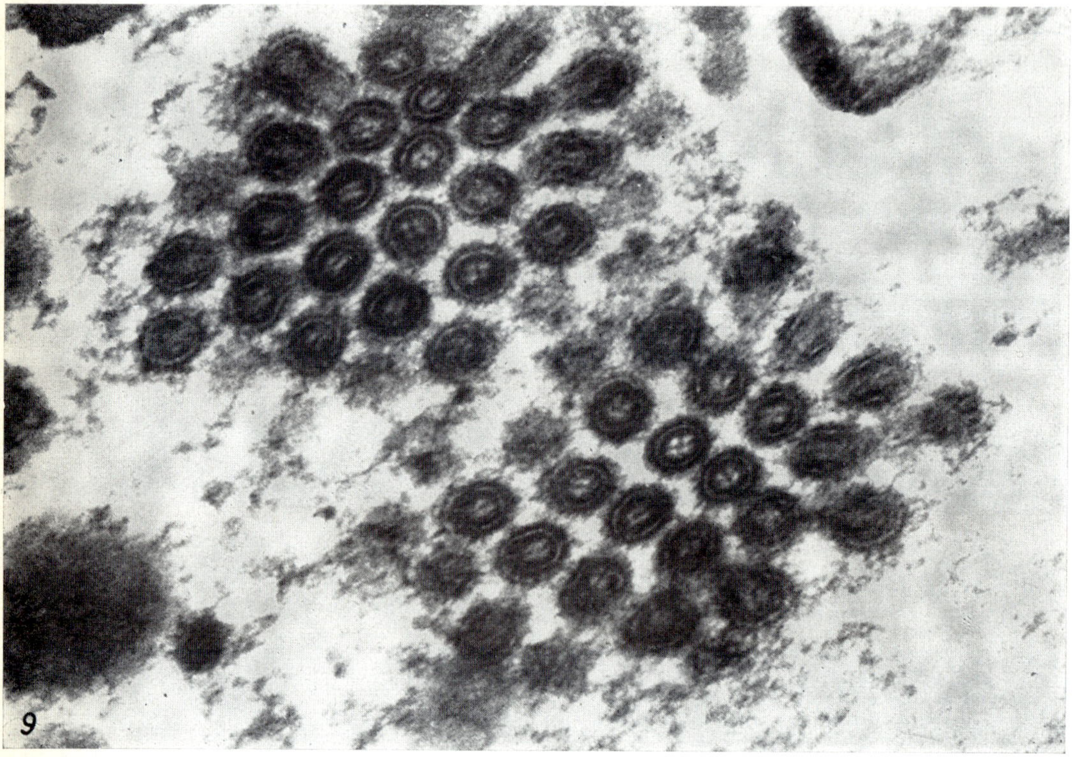
9

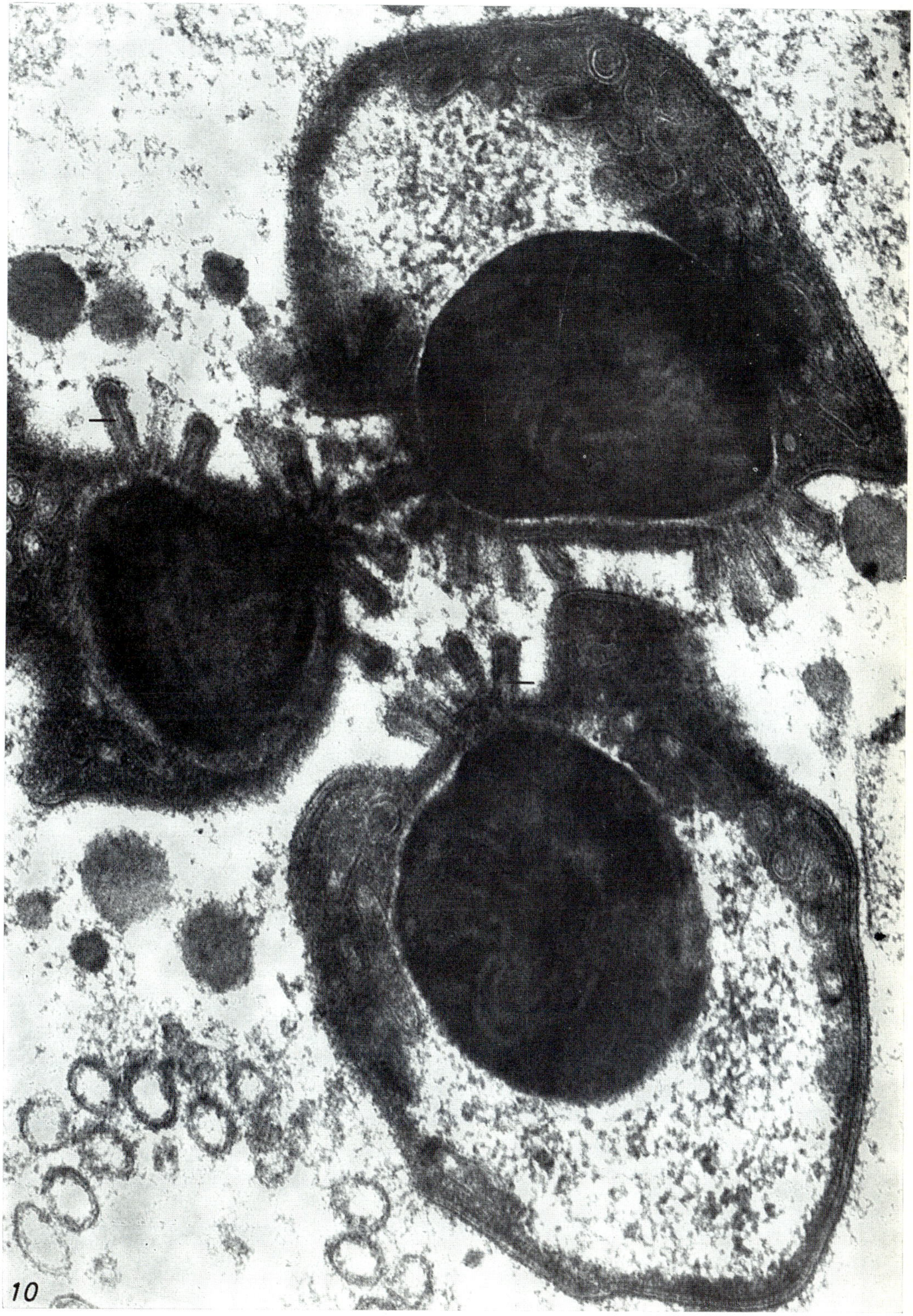

10

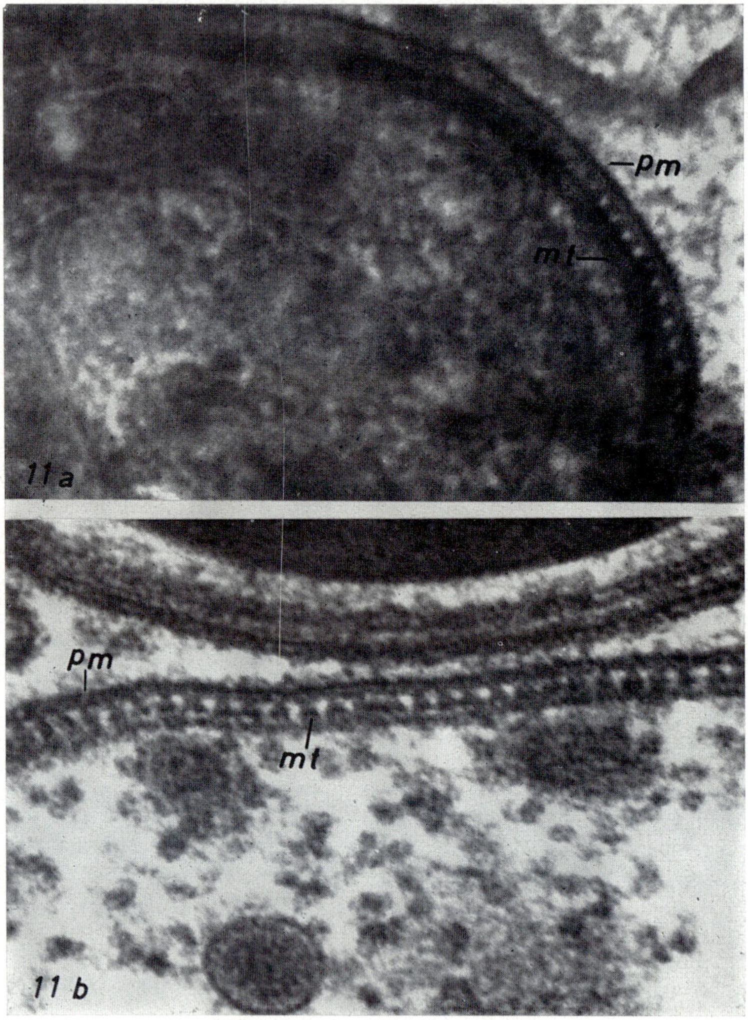
pm
mt
11a
pm
mt
11b

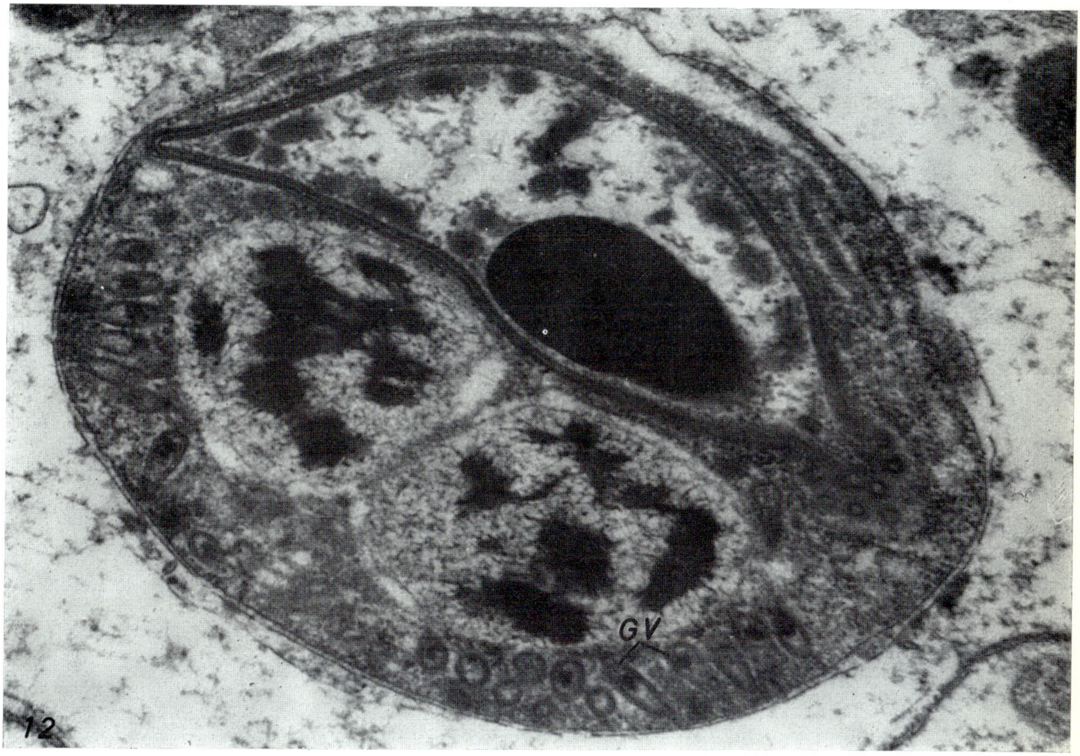
GV
12

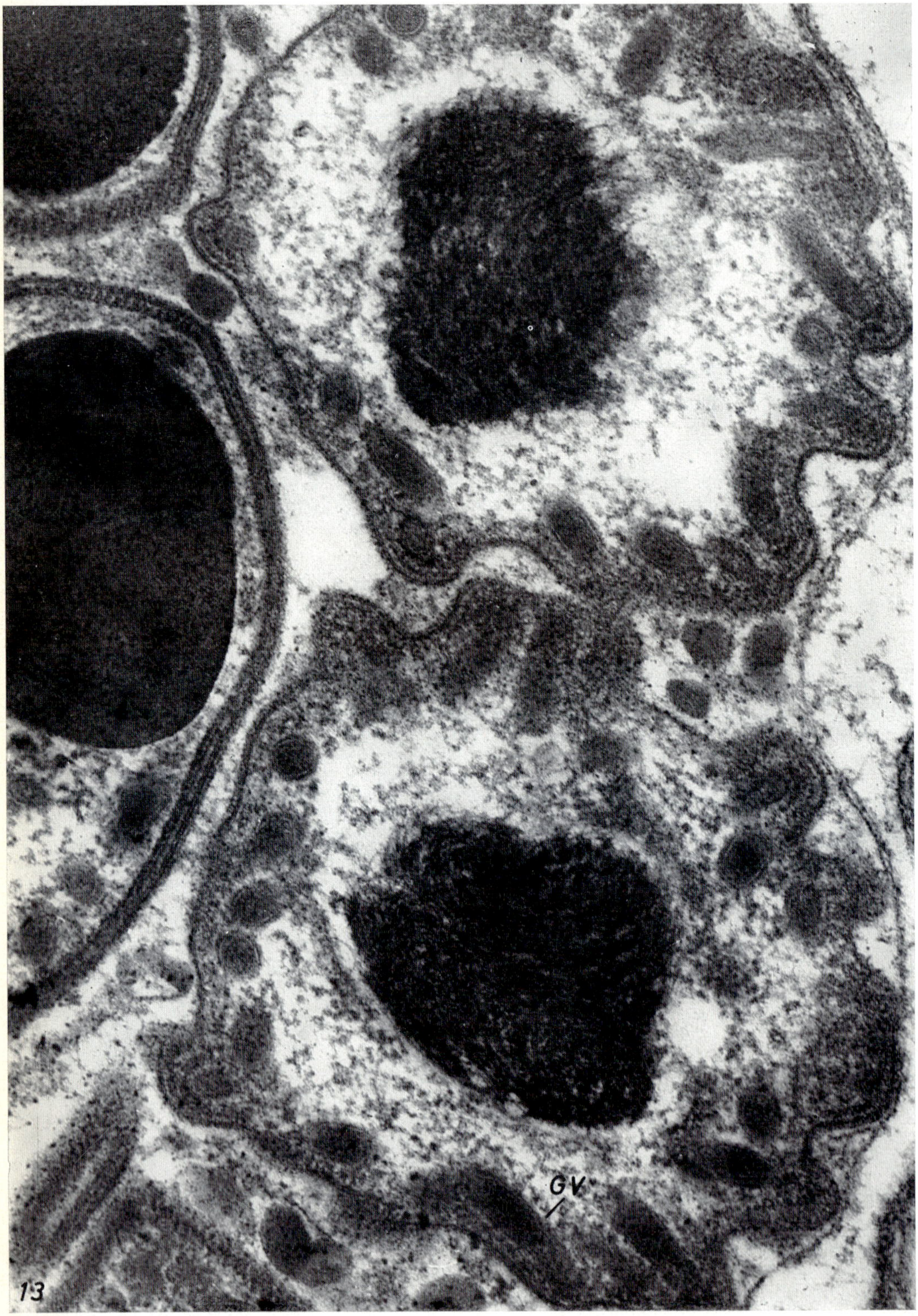
GV
13

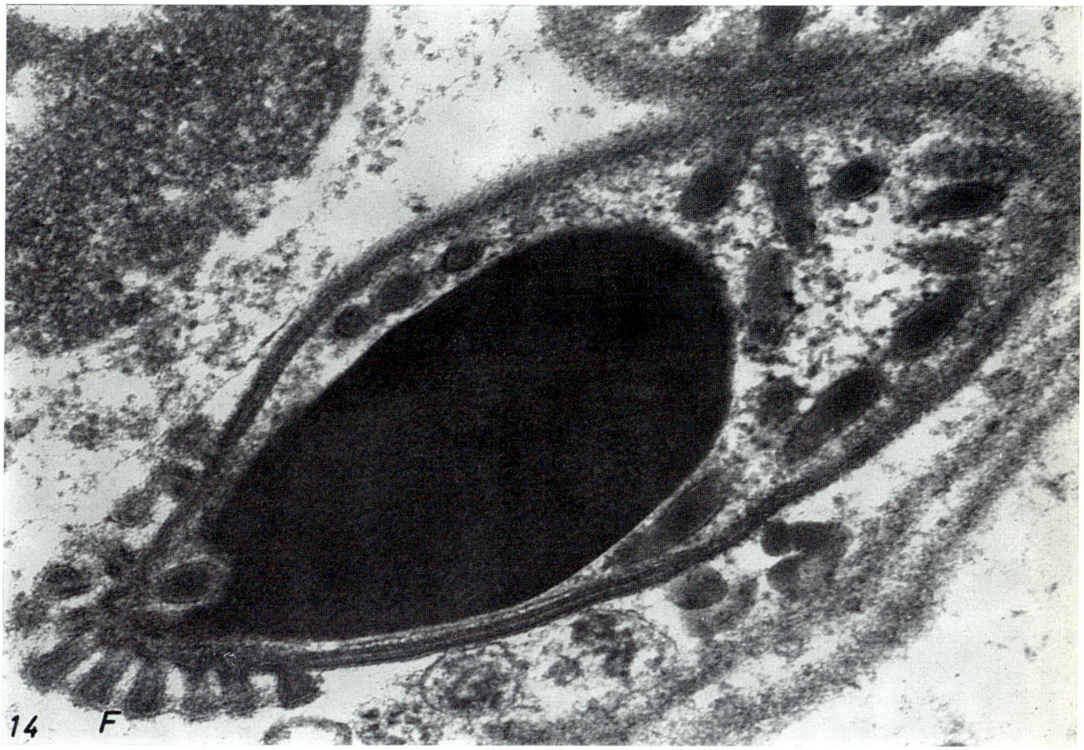
14 F

I. GRAEBNER and H. ADAM – *Electron microscopical study of spermatogenesis and sperm morphology in gnathostomulids.*

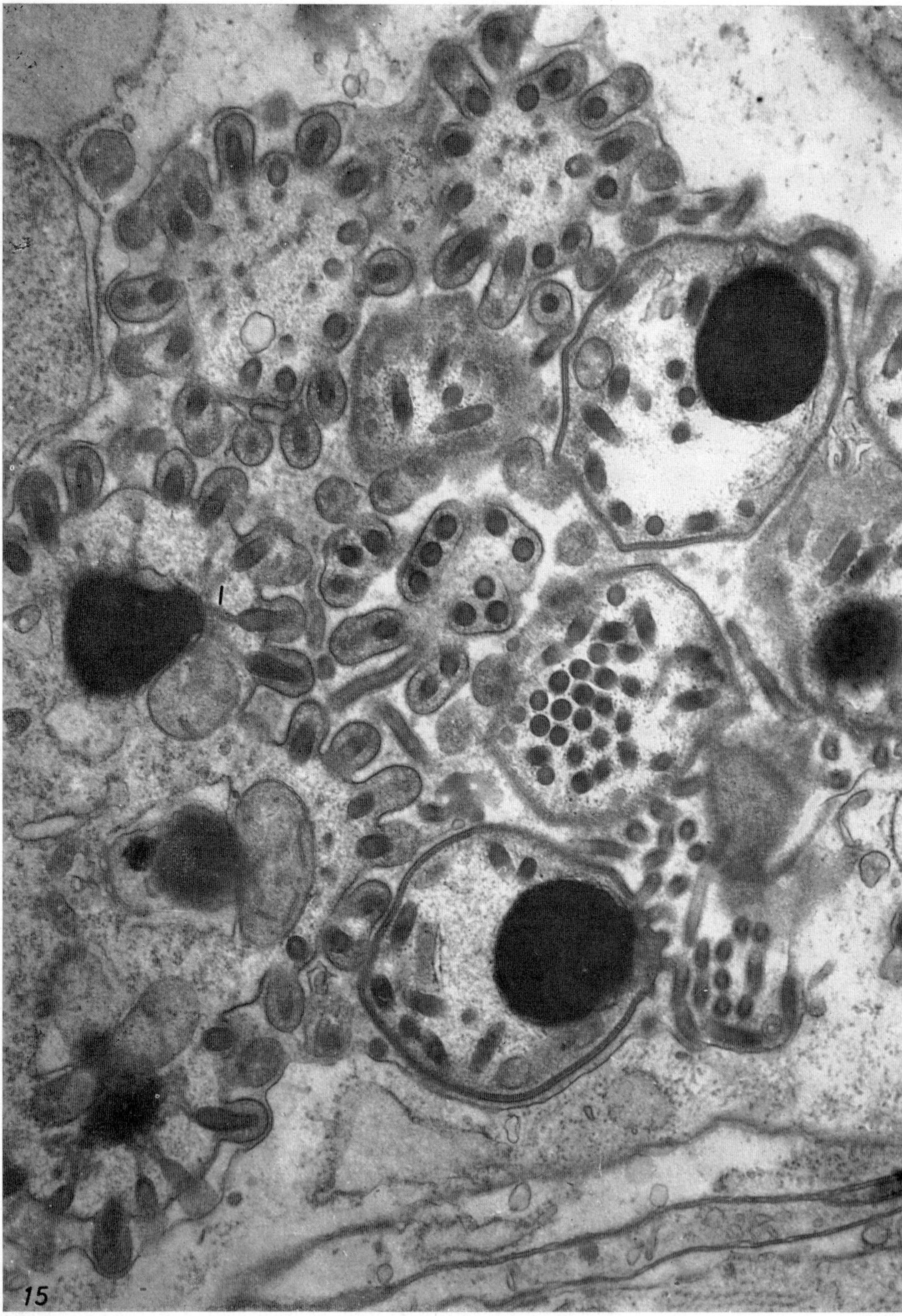

MURIEL H. WALKER (*)

SOME UNUSUAL FEATURES OF THE SPERM OF *NUCELLA LAPILLUS* (L)

SUMMARY. — The sperm of *Nucella lapillus* (L) are long and thread-like. They are about 80 μm in length and are motile throughout their length. The flagellar shaft runs the whole length of the sperm. During the early stages of spermiogenesis the nucleoprotein forms fine interlocking strands, arranged helically round the prospective long axis of the nucleus. These strands fuse to form lamellae which take up an apparent concentric array round the flagellar tube. The lamellae fuse during the final stages of elongation and the mature nucleus is homogeneous in appearance.

If the nucleus of the mature sperm is partially dispersed, the portion of the flagellar shaft which it encloses is thrown into a loose spiral and the flagellar fibers are seen to be twisted. If the nucleus is completely dispersed the flagellar shaft within the head springs back into a tight coil of 5 to 7 turns. An explanation of this coiling phenomenon is suggested.

The arrangement of the nucleoprotein within the mature sperm head has been investigated by means of experimental breakdown of the nucleus with enzymes and 8 M urea. The pattern of breakdown correlates with the pattern of nuclear condensation seen during spermiogenesis.

RIASSUNTO. — Gli spermatozoi di *Nucella lapillus* (L) sono lunghi e filamentosi. Sono lunghi circa 80 μm. La guaina flagellare corre per l'intera lunghezza dello spermio. Durante le prime fasi della spermiogenesi le nucleoproteine formano sottili corde intrecciate, disposte elicoidalmente intorno all'asse lungo del nucleo. Queste corde si uniscono a formare lamelle che assumono un'apparente disposizione concentrica intorno al tubo flagellare. Le lamelle si fondono durante le fasi finali dell'allungamento e il nucleo maturo è in apparenza omogeneo.

Se il nucleo dello spermio maturo è parzialmente disperso, la porzione della guaina flagellare che lo racchiude è modellata in un'ampia spirale e le fibre del flagello sono intrecciate. Se il nucleo è completamente disperso, la guaina flagellare nella testa discende in una stretta spirale di 5 o 7 giri. Viene suggerita una spiegazione di questo fenomeno di spiralizzazione. La disposizione delle nucleoproteine nella testa dello spermatozoo maturo è stata studiata per mezzo della rottura sperimentale del nucleo con enzimi e con urea 8 M. Il modello di rottura è confrontato con il modello di condensazione nucleare visto durante la spermiogenesi.

The sperm of the dog whelk *Nucella lapillus* (L) are long and thread like, with a pointed acrosome and a tapering tail. They are about 80 μm in length and are motile throughout their length. The nucleus is Feulgen positive and about 40 μm in length. The mid-piece is about 8 μm in length and lies immediately posterior to the nucleus. The stages of spermatogenesis are essentially similar to those seen in other species.

(*) Department of Zoology, The University, ST. ANDREWS, Fife, Scotland.

The spermatogonia are about 4 μm wide (Fig. 1). Their nuclei are large and lobed. The nuclear envelope is double and perforated by pores. The chromatin is unevenly distributed, giving the nucleus a patchy appearance. The cytoplasm contains a few mitocondria of various sizes, and numerous small granules. There are several Golgi complexes, each made up of a stack of parallel lamellae and a number of small round vesicles. Close to one of the Golgi complexes is a pair of centrioles, lying at right angles to one another In some spermatogonia four centrioles were observed. Such cells were probably about to divide mitotically.

The primary spermatocytes are 3–4 μm wide (Fig. 2). The nucleus nearly fills the cell. The chromatin is patchy and synaptinemial complexes (chromosome cores) are visible in most sections. The meiotic divisions follow in quick succession and secondary spermatocytes are rarely seen.

The early spermatids are irregularly shaped cells 3–4 μm wide. The cytoplasm of these cells contains numerous small mitochondria clustered together to one side of the nucleus. Golgi complexes are evident in some sections but have fewer associated vesicles than those of earlier stages (Fig. 3). In some sections a Golgi complex and proacrosome granulue may be seen at the opposite side of the nucleus from the mitochondrial cluster. The nuclear material is in a diffuse state and is evenly distributed throughout the nucleus.

The nucleus of the early spermatid is roughly spherical, and is about 3 μ in diameter. There is only one centriole in each spermatid. At this stage the centriole behaves in an unusual way, it bores its way through the nucleus until it comes to lie at the anterior end separated from the developing acrosome by a thin layer of nuclear material and a double layer of nuclear membrane. The spermatid nucleus is therefore penetrated by a blind ending tube lined throughout by nuclear membrane. This tube encloses part of the flagellar shaft which extends back from the centriole, and by this stage has already achieved its final length of about 80 μm (Fig. 5). The portion of the flagellar shaft enclosed by the nucleus in the early spermatid is straight.

The nucleus increases in length and is still penetrated by a straight tube (Fig. 4). The nuclear material aggregates into interwoven fibers about 100 Å in diameter, which are arranged in a loose helix around the long axis of the sperm head. The length of the flagellar tube at this stage is about 4 μm but the portion of the flagellar shaft which it encloses is much longer. As a result the flagellar shaft is thrown into a coil (Fig. 4). As condensation proceeds the strands of nucleoprotein fuse together and eventually form lamellae (Figs. 6, 7 and 8). In transverse section these lamellae are often radially arranged with respect to the flagellar tube, with one or both edges of the lamella closely applied to the nuclear membrane. The nuclear lamellae are at first widely spaced but gradually fuse as the nucleus becomes longer and narrower until between 12 and 15 apparently concentric lamellae are discernible in transverse section (Fig. 9). At this stage the periphery of the nucleus may have a fuzzy appearance and this is possibly due to the formation of microtubules. Further condensation occurs, until, in the mature sperm the nucleoprotein presents a completely homogeneous appearance (Fig. 10).

The mature sperm head consists of a cylinder of nuclear material which encloses the anterior portion of the flagellar shaft, which in the mature sperm is straight. The sperm nucleus is an elongate tube enclosed at its anterior end by a double layer of nuclear envelope. The walls of the tubular nucleus (Fig. 10) are about 100 m μm wide in the rear half of the sperm head but they narrow to about 50 m μm at the anterior end of the head. Behind the double nuclear envelope at the anterior end of the nuclear tube is the centriole showing the typical arrangement of 9 triplet elements, from which the flagellar shaft extends straight backwards. Outside the nuclear membrane, in a thin

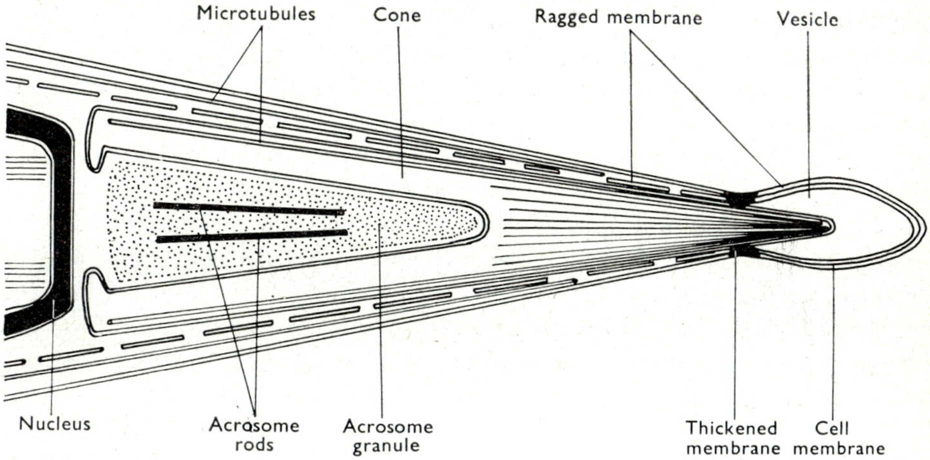

Schema 1. – Diagram of a longitudinal section through the acrosome of a mature sperm in the testis.

layer of cytoplasm which surrounds the nucleus, are microtubules which stretch backwards from the acrosome. These never surround the nucleus completely but usually appear as a row down one side of the nucleus. The microtubules lie parallel to a flat double membrane (Fig. 10) which is distinct from the nuclear membrane. This membrane is an extension of a « ragged membrane » which surrounds the acrosome.

The distinctive feature of the development of the mid-piece is the breakdown and subsequent fusion of the outer mitochondrial membranes. In the early spermatid the mitochondria that aggregate at the base of the nucleus fuse into 4 or 5 large Nebenkerne. The Nebenkerne elongate and wrap around the flagellar shaft ina spiral. The outer mitochondrial membranes of each Nebenkerne breakdown and then fuse so that the whole structure is enclosed by a common outer membrane (Fig. 11). This sack of mitochondria elongates to a final length of about 8 μm in the mature sperm (Walker and MacGregor, 1968). In the mature mid-piece the mitochondrial elements appear to be arranged in a helical fashion.

The development of the acrosome resembles that of *Acheta domestica* (KAYE, 1962; see WALKER and MACGREGOR, 1968). The acrosome of the mature sperm is terminal and pointed. It is about 1.2 μm long. Its main component is the acrosome cone which is surrounded by a bounding membrane and within which is a ring of longitudinally arranged microtubules (Schema 1; Fig. 12). These merge at their anterior ends and consequently cannot be resolved in transverse sections through the tip of the cone. At its base the cone widens slightly to form an inwardly directed lip. Within the cone, but outside the cone membrane, are five rods which appear in transverse sections as five dark patches arranged in a circle and embedded in material of a lighter shade. These rods and the matrix in which they are embedded probably corresponds to the acrosome « granule » described in *Acheta* (KAYE, 1962). In sperm taken from the testis the acrosome is separated from the cell membrane by a thin layer of cytoplasm, within which, and close to the acrosome lies a row of microtubules. Each tubule is about 200 Å in diameter. The tubules surround the acrosome and extend backwards along about 3/4 of the length of the sperm head. Between the microtubules and the acrosome cone is a discontinuous « ragged membrane ». The latter fuses with the outer cone membrane near the apex of the cone where a conspicuous thickening of the cone membrane is evident. The tip of the acrosome consists of a vesicle bounded on the inside by the outer cone membrane and on the outside by a continuation of the ragged membrane. In mature sperm taken from the testicular duct there are no microtubules in the cytoplasm surrounding the sperm nucleus (Fig. 13).

Perhaps the most unusual feature of *Nucella* sperm was first described by *Retzius* (1912) when he observed that under certain conditions the nucleus appeared to swell and the flagellar shaft enclosed within it, the « Zentralfaden » as he called it, was thrown into a loose spiral.

The living sperm of *Nucella* all look alike (Fig. 14). They are motile throughout their length, although the undulations of the head have a lower amplitude than those of the tail. For the present discussion, the flagellar shaft of *Nucella* sperm may be considered to consist of two portions: the head shaft which coils and the tail shaft which may fray but never coils (Fig. 15). Disruption of the cell and nuclear membranes without dispersal of the DNA is sufficient to allow the head shaft to start to form gentle spiral (Fig. 16). If the nucleoprotein is completely dispersed the head shaft springs back into a tight coil of 5 to 7 turns (Figs. 17 and 18). These observations and the methods involved have been described in detail by WALKER (1969).

At the electron microscope level I have looked at the coiling of the head shaft in negatively stained preparations. The spreading of mature sperm on a Langmuir trough containing sea water is sufficient to break down the cell and nuclear membranes and permit slight swelling of the nucleus. The head shaft forms a gentle spiral and negative staining with phosphotungstic acid shows the fibers if the flagellar shaft to be twisted like the wires of an electric flex. Spreading sperm on a Langmuir trough containing ×2 concentrated sea water brings about the complete dispersal of the nucleus. The head shaft forms a tight coil of 5 to 7 turns clockwise from the anterior end. The flagellar fibers of the head shaft are twisted (Fig. 19) and this twist may extend back to the anterior portion of the tail. The tail frays into its component fibers and at their posterior ends these fibers themselves fray into their subunits. The mid–piece remains intact as a tie round the ' waist ' of the sperm. Similar results can also be brought about by treatment of sperm with 50 μg/ml pronase or trypsin. The nuclear material breaks up into sheets or a meshwork of branching fibers (Figs. 20 and 21) and the head shaft forms a loose untidy coil with the flagellar fibers twisted.

On the basis of these observations I propose the following scheme to account for the coiling of the head shaft. In the very early spermatid, in which the centriole and flagellar shaft have just penetrated the nucleus, all the fibers of the flagellar shaft run straight. The length of the flagellar shaft within the nucleus increases without a corresponding increase in nuclear length, and as a result the head shaft is forced into a coil. In forming this coil the flagellar fibers become twisted and this twist remains imposed upon them. As the nuclear material condenses and the nucleus elongates to its final length of about 40 μm the head shaft is untwisted and pulled out straight. As the flagellar fibers in the sperm head are straight but are able to become twisted again when the nucleus is dispersed, they must be held under tension and torsion in the mature sperm head.

The microtubules are only present during the final stages of elongation. Their function is probably twofold. First, to assist in pulling out the nucleus to its final length, therefore extending and straightening the head shaft. Secondly, acting in a splint–like fashion, holding the nucleus straight until the nucleoprotein sets into a sufficiently rigid state to maintain its own shape in the mature sperm where the microtubules are absent. The association of microtubules with nuclei during spermiogenesis and their subsequent absence from mature sperm is a fairly common feature (KESSEL, 1966, 1967; HOAGE and KESSEL, 1968; MCINTOSH and PORTER, 1967). At what stage in spermiogenesis untwisting of the fibers of the head shaft occurs is uncertain, but after unwinding is complete the straight shaft must be locked at both ends so that it can neither shorten nor rotate. In the mature sperm the head shaft is « strait–jacketted » in a close fitting and stiff nuclear tube.

There are few reports on spread nucleoprotein from sperm (LUNG, 1968; SOLARI, 1968 a and b; GALL, 1966). From all these reports it would appear that the nucleoprotein is arranged as an unorderly meshwork of fibers, with a paucity of free ends. Observations on *Nucella* sperm with polarized light show the nucleus to be strongly birefringent indicating that the nucleoprotein is arranged predominantly parallel to the long axis of the sperm head, Treatment of *Nucella* sperm with the enzymes pronase and trypsin or with 8 M urea results inthe gradual breakdown of the nuclear materials. In the initial stages of breakdown, the nuclear material appears in the form of a sheet wrapped in a helical fashion around the long axis of the sperm head.

This sheet splits longitudinally into thinner and thinner strands, which loop out at right angles to the main axis of the sperm head (Fig. 22). Where different strands meet they appeart to fuse. Strands of varying diameter down to about 40 Å are seen and there is no evidence of free ends in the dispersed nucleoprotein.

I think it is probable that the nucleoprotein is in the mature sperm head in a supercoiled condition and that experimental treatment with enzymes and urea causes a breakdown of the supercoil allowing the nucleoprotein to unwind, hence forming loops. At this stage it is not possible to make any suggestions as to the arrangement of the chromosomes within the elongate sperm head of *Nucella*, although it is probable that the chromosomes are arranged in tandem along the length of the sperm head as suggested by TAYLOR, (1964) for the sperm of the grasshopper *Melanoplus*.

From these observations of the breakdown of the nucleus in *Nucella* it is apparent that the pattern of breakdown reflects the pattern of nuclear condensation seen during spermiogenesis. As a comparison I have begun similar investigations on sperm from the domestic fowl. During spermiogenesis in the fowl there is no evidence of sheets or lamellae in the nucleoprotein. Nuclear elongation is almost completed before condensation begins. The nucleoprotein aggregates from a fine granular state into larger granules about 350 Å in diameter. These large granules which are formed at the start of nuclear condensation increase in size and eventually fuse to give the mature nucleus which is homogeneous in appearance. The microtubular systems associated with the nucleus during spermiogenesis have been elegantly described by McINTOSH and PORTER (1967). Treatment of fowl sperm with 8 M urea results in the breakdown of the nucleus into a mass of interconnected granules about 350 Å in diameter (Fig. 24) reminiscent of isolated chromosomes (WOLFE, 1965 a) although the overall appearance of the isolated chromosomes is more fibrous. The breakdown pattern in the fowl again reflects the pattern of condensation of the maturing spermatid nucleus.

The condensation pattern seen in *Nucella* and the domestic fowl may be described " lamellar " and " granular " types respectively. There is another pattern of condensation described in the snail *Cipangopaludina* (YASUZUMI and TANAKA, 1958). Here the pattern is " fibrous ". The nuclear material aggregates into fibers in the early spermatid. These increase in diameter and fuse to give the final elongated spiral head of the mature sperm, without forming lamellae. There is also a variation of the «granular» type seen in the water beetle *Acilius*. Here, the nucleus attains its final shape prior to condensation and throughout spermiogenesis is surrounded by a complex system of microtubules. The nucleoprotein condenses in uneven patches (MACKIE, 1969).

It would be of interest to carry out similar breakdown experiments on sperm with these different condensation patterns.

References

Gall J. G. (1966) – *Chromosome fibers studied by a spreading technique.* « Chromosoma (Berl.) », 20, 221–233.

Hoage T. R. and Kessel R. G. (1968) – *An electron microscope study of the process of differentiation during spermatogenesis in the drone honey bee* (Apis mellifera (*L*)), *with special reference to centriole replication and elimination.* « J. Ultrastruct. Res. », 24, 6–32.

Kaye J. S. (1962) – *Acrosome formation in the house cricket.* « J. Cell Biol. », 12, 411–432.

Kessel R. G. (1966) – *The association between microtubules, and nuclei during spermiogenesis in the dragonfly.* « J. Ultrastruct. Res. », 16, 293–304.

Kessel R. G. (1967) – *An electron microscope study of spermiogenesis in the grasshopper with particular reference to the development of microtubular systems during differentiation.* « J. Ultrastruct. Res. », 18, 677–694.

Lung B. (1968) – *Whole mount electron microscopy of chromatin and membranes in bull and human sperm heads.* « J. Ultrastruct. Res. », 22, 485–493.

Mackie J. B. (1969) – *Personal communication.*

McIntosh J. R. and Porter K. R. (1967) – *Microtubules in the spermatids of the domestic fowl.* « J. Cell Biol. », 35, 153–173.

Retzius G. (1912) – *Ueber die Spermien der Fucacean.* « Biol. Unters. », 13.

Solari A. J. (1968 a) – *The ultrastructure of chromatin fibers.* I. *The effect of spreading conditions.* « Exp. Cell Res. », 53, 553–566.

Solari A. J. (1968 b) – *The ultrastructure of chromatin fibers.* II. *The ultrastructure of the loops from sea urchin sperm chromatin.* « Exp. Cell Res. », 53, 567–581.

Taylor J. H. (1964) – *The arrangement of chromosomes in the mature sperm of the grasshopper.* « J. Cell Biol. », 21, 286–289.

Walker M. (1969) – *Coiling of the flagellar shaft in the head region of the mature sperm of* Nucella (Purpura) lapillus (*L*). « J. Cell Sci. », 5, 211–225.

Walker M. and MacGregor H. C. (1968) – *Spermatogenesis and the structure of the mature sperm in* Nucella lapillus (*L*). « J. Cell Sci. », 3, 95–104.

Wolfe S. L. (1965) – *The fine structure of isolated metaphase chromosomes.* « Exp. Cell Res. », 37, 45–53.

Yasuzumi G. and Tanaka H. (1958) – *Spermatogenesis in animals as revealed by electron microscopy.* VI. *Researches on the spermatozoan dimorphism in a pond snail,* Cipangopaludina malleata. « J. biophys. biochem. Cytol. », 4, 621–632.

Explanation of figures

Figures reproduced by permission of the Company of Biologists Limited.

Text Fig. 1, and Figs. 1–12 from Walker and MacGregor; « J. Cell Sci. », 3, 95–104 (1968).

Fig. 1. – Spermatogonia showing the centrioles (*ce*) next to the nucleus (*n*) and Golgi material (*G*) with associated vesicles.
(*m*, mitochondria).

Fig. 2. – Primary spermatocyte. Nucleus (*n*) with chromosone cores (*cc*).
(*G*, Golgi material; *m*, mitochondria).

Fig. 3. – Early spermatid showing the flagellar shaft (*f*) penetrating the nucleus (*n*). Mitochondria (*m*) are clustered at the base of the nucleus. A conspicuous Golgi complex (*G*) lies to one side of the nucleus.

Fig. 4. – Longitudinal section of a spermatid showing the nucleus (*n*) containing the coiled portion of the flagellar shaft (*f*). The developing acrosome (*a*) lies at the anterior end of the nucleus. At the posterior end the flagellar shaft passes through the mitochondria (*m*) of the developing mid–piece.

Fig. 5. – Early spermatid in phase contrast showing the nucleus (*n*) penetrated by the flagellar shaft (*f*). The developing mid–piece (*m*) can be seen at the base of the nucleus.

Fig. 6. – Longitudinal sections of early lamellar spermatid nuclei. The nucleus (*n*) at this stage is twisted and the lamellae and flagellar shaft (*f*) follow this twist.

Fig. 7. – Transverse section of a spermatid nucleus at the stage when the nucleoprotein fibers are fusing to form lamellae.

Fig. 8. – Transverse section of a lamellar stage nucleus.

Fig. 9. – Transverse section of a late concentric lamellar–stage nucleus.

Fig. 10. – Transverse section of a mature sperm head from the testis showing one row of microtubules (arrowed).

Fig. 11. – Transverse section through the developing mid–piece showing the mitochondria (*m*) with outer membranes fused (arrowed), surrounding the flagellar shaft (*f*).

Fig. 12. – Longitudinal section through the acrosome of a sperm in the testis showing the vesicle and thickened membrane.

(*ag*, acrosome granule; *c*, cone; *cm*, cell membrane; *mt*, microtubules; *rm*, " ragged membrane "; *tm*, thickened membrane; *v*, vesicle).

Fig. 13. – Longitudinal section of part of a mature sperm head from the testicular duct. The fibers of the head shaft (*h*) run straight through the nucleus (*n*).

(*cm*, cell membrane.).

Figs. 13–18 and 20–21 from WALKER, « J. Cell Sci. », 5, 211–225. (1969).

Figs. 14–18 are phase contrast photomicrographs.

Fig. 14. – Living sperm. The head is to the top of the picture and the mid–piece is arrowed.

Fig. 15. – Sperm with fraying tail. The head is directed to the top of the picture and the mid–piece is arrowed.

Fig. 16. – Sperm with the head shaft (*h*) thrown into a gentle spiral within the swollen nucleus (*n*). The mid-piece is arrowed and the tail frayed.

Fig. 17. – Sperm with the head shaft (*h*) beginning to coil. The acrosome (*a*) is at the anterior end of the head shaft and the mid–piece arrowed.

Fig. 18. – Sperm with head shaft (*h*) in a tight coil.

Fig. 19. – Part of the head shaft of a sperm spread on a Langmuir trough containing ×2 concentrated sea water and negatively stained with phosphotungstic acid (PTA). The nuclear material is completely dispersed and the head shaft (*h*) is twisted and coiled.

Fig. 20. – Sperm head treated with 50 μ g/ml trypsin and negatively stained with PTA. The twisted head shaft (*h*) is separated from the nucleoprotein (*n*). The nucleoprotein is split into sheets. Some of the fibers of the head shaft are sharply bent (arrowed).

Fig. 21. – Sperm head treated with 50 μg/ml pronase and negatively stained with PTA. The twisted, coiled and partially disrupted head shaft (*h*) is surrounded by branching strands of nucleoprotein.

Fig. 22. – Sperm head treated with 8 M urea, dried by the critical point method and rotary shadowed at an angle of 30° with platinum/carbon. The nucleoprotein frays out into loops from the main axis of the sperm head. The narrowest fibers are about 40 Å in diameter.

Fig. 23. – Longitudinal section of spermatid nucleus from the domestic fowl. The nucleus is surrounded by microtubules (*mt*). The process of elongation of the nucleus is complete and nuclear condensation has just begun.

Fig. 24. – Sperm head from the domestic fowl treated with 8 M urea, dried by the critical point method and rotary shadowed at an angle of 30° with plantinum/carbon.

Discussion

EDDLEMAN. – Does the base of the acrosome in *Nucella* fuse to close completely as demonstrated by KAYE in *Acheta domestica*?

WALKER. – I have so far not examined the acrosome in fully mature sperm from the testicular duct. At this time therefore, it is unknown whether or not more complete fusion, as described by KAYE, occurs.

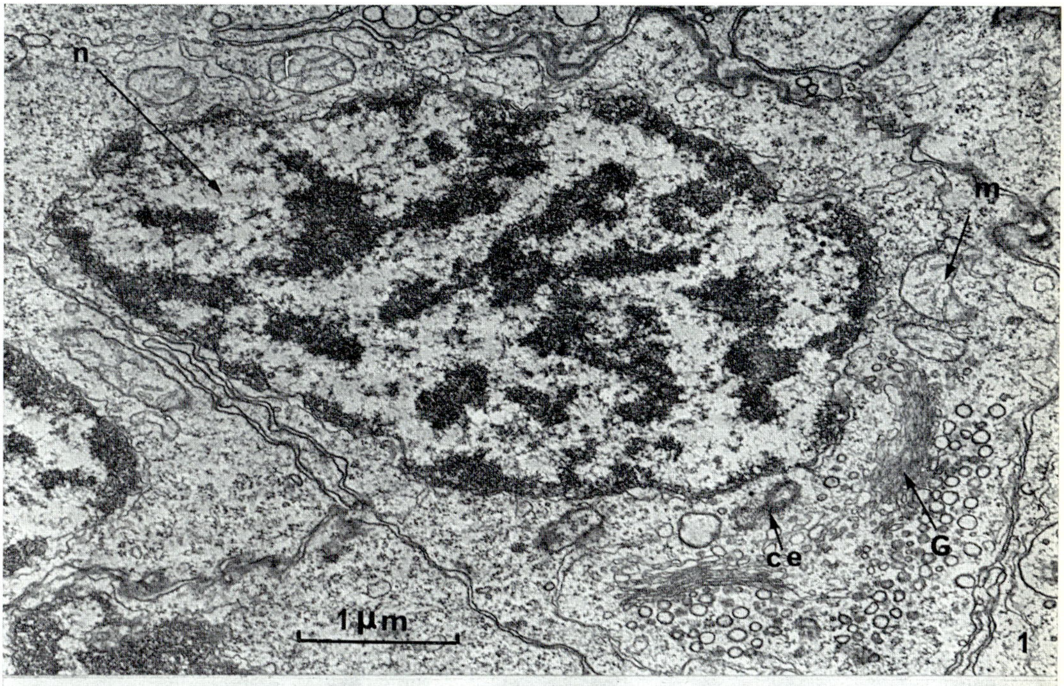
n
m
G
ce
1 µm
1

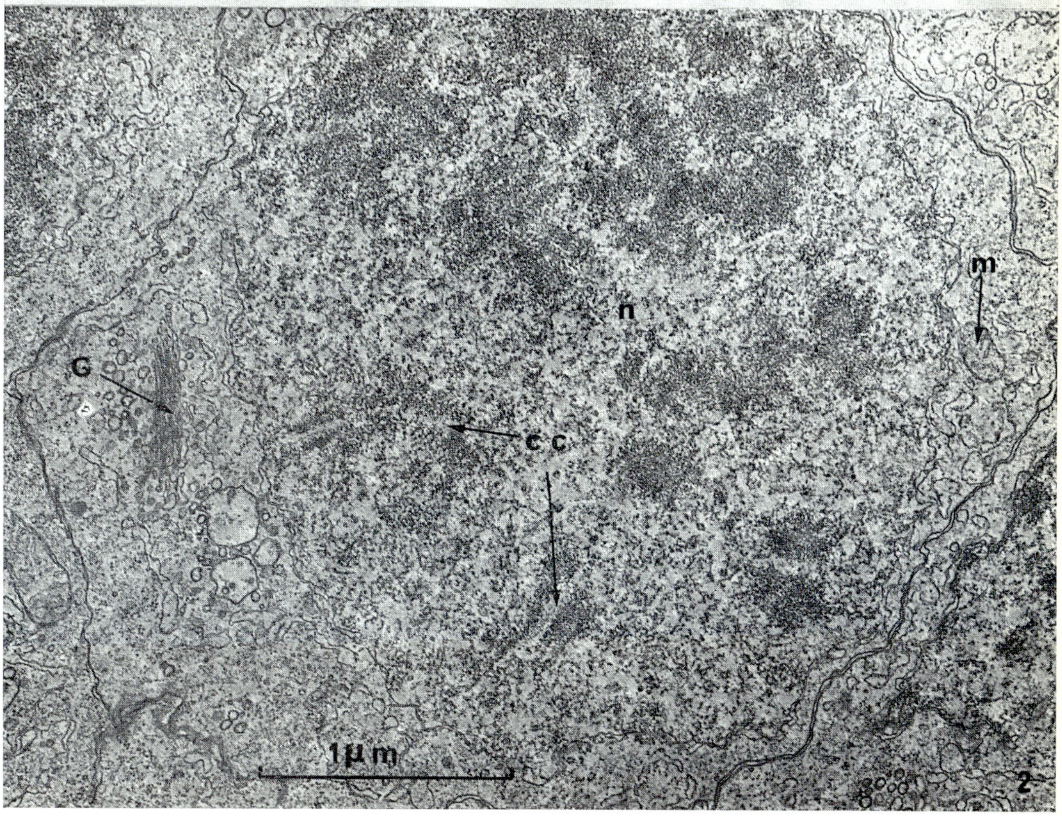
m
n
G
c c
1 µm
2

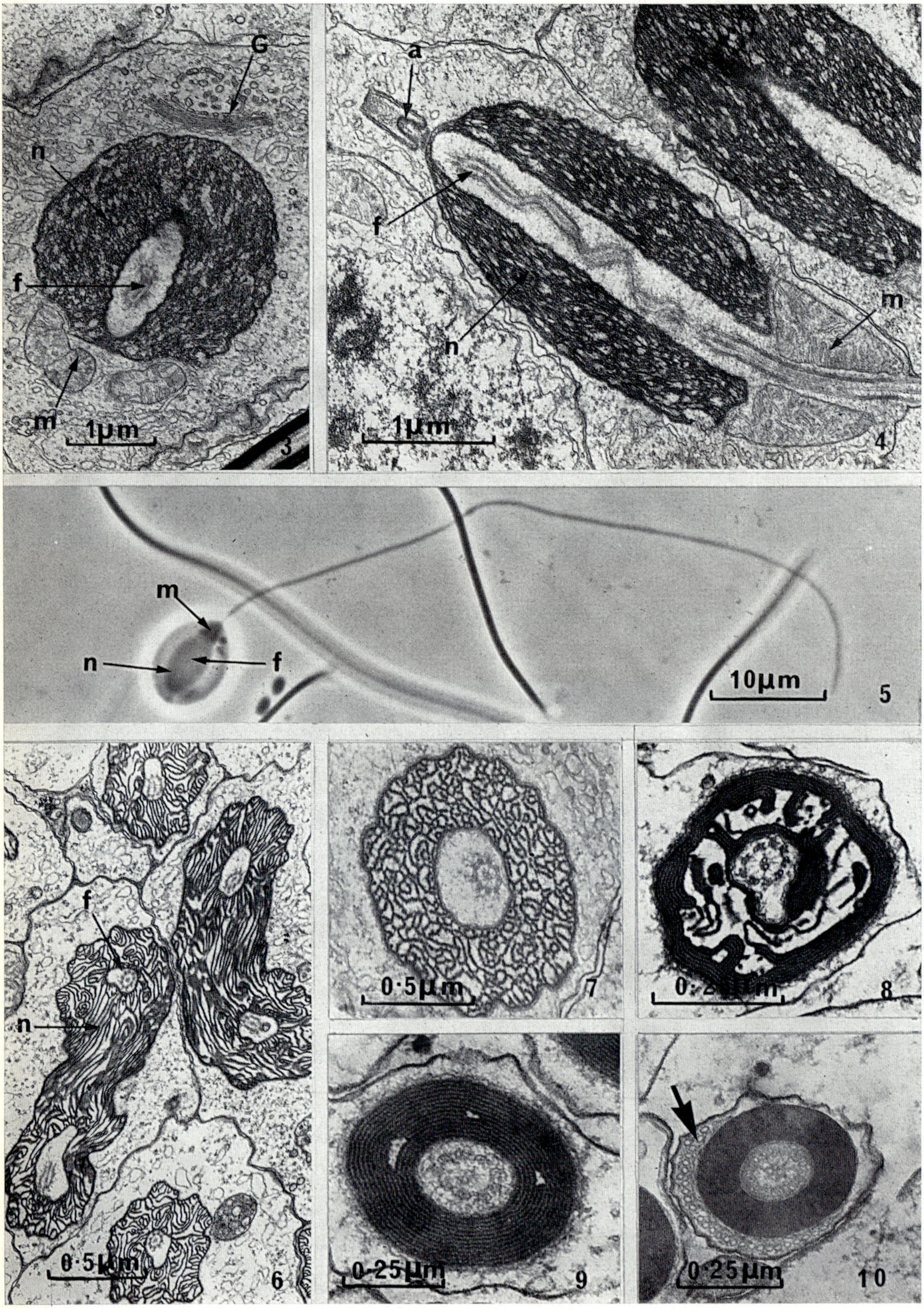
G
n
f
m
1µm
3
a
f
n
m
1µm
4
m
n
f
10µm
5
f
n
0·5µm
6
0·5µm
7
8
0·25µm
9
0·25µm
10

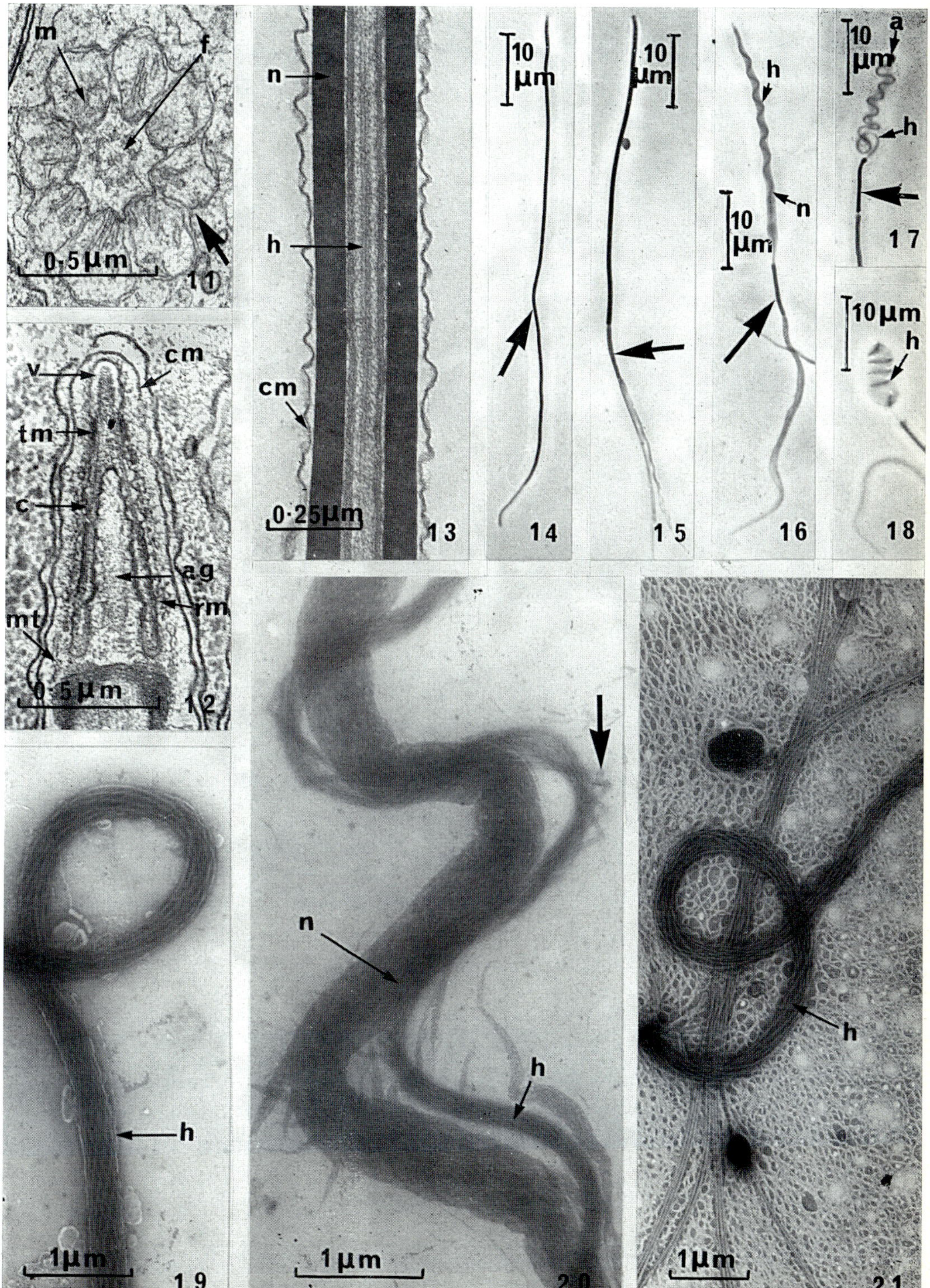
m
f
0·5 µm
11
cm
v
tm
c
ag
rm
mt
0·5 µm
12
n
h
cm
0·25µm
13
10 µm
14
10 µm
15
h
n
10 µm
16
10 µm
a
h
17
10µm
h
18
h
1µm
19
n
h
1µm
20
h
1µm
21

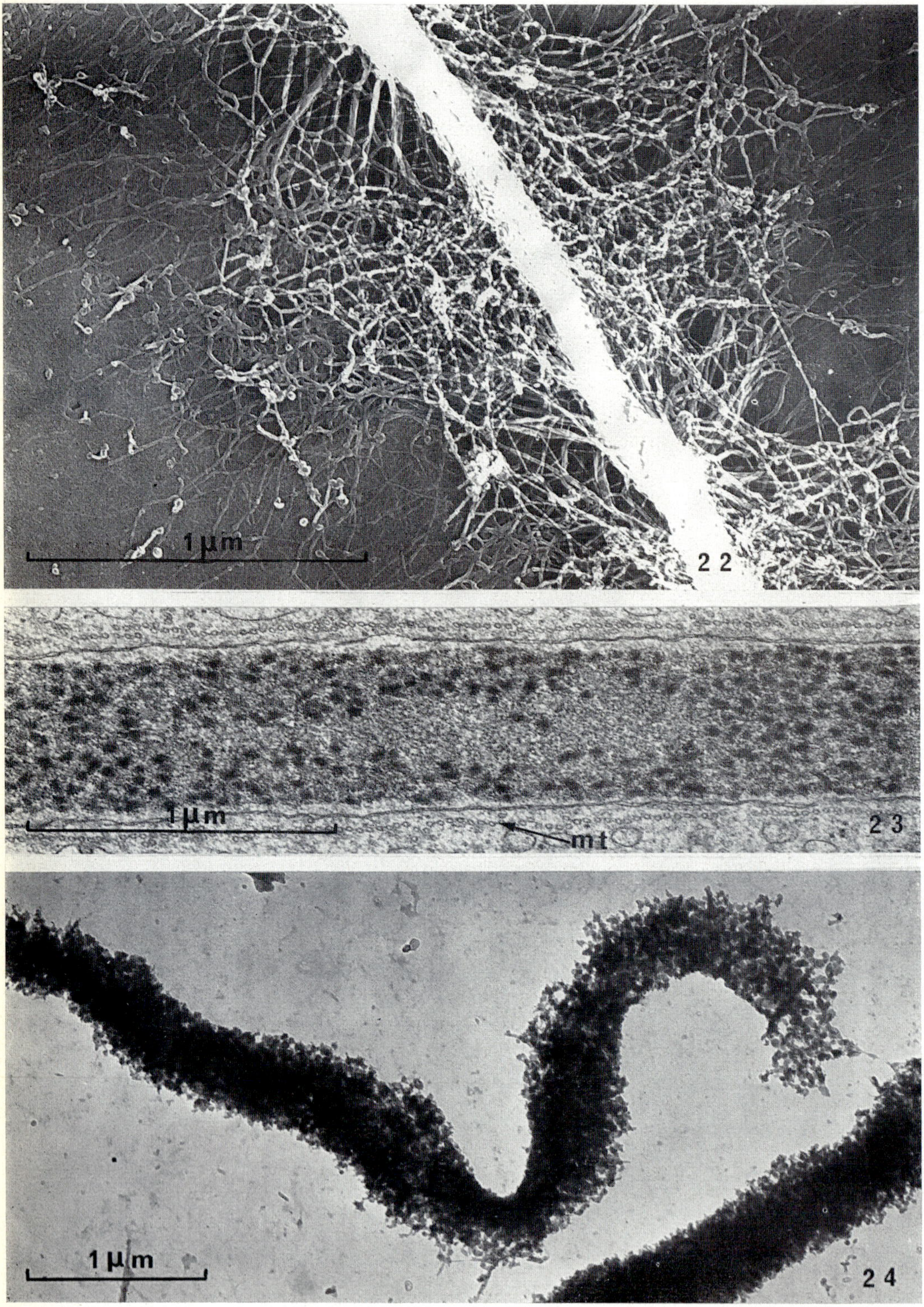
1 μm
22
1 μm
mt
23
1 μm
24

P. PERSONNE (*) et W. A. ANDERSON (**)

ÉTUDE COMPARÉE DES ÉVOLUTIONS MITOCHONDRIALES AU COURS DE LA SPERMATOGENÈSE CHEZ QUELQUES GASTÉROPODES

SUMMARY. — The study of mitochondria during spermatogenesis and in the spermatozoon allow the spermatozoons of Gastropoda to be classified in three types. One, similar to that of the Bivalva, possess a simple corona of free mitochondria at the nuclear basis. This primitive type characterizes a modality of external fertilization, and appears in some Prosobranchia. In the other Prosobranchia, in Opisthobranchia and in Pulmonata, the fertilization is internal and a middle piece is formed. The structure of the mitochondrial derivative enclosed in this middle piece and the nature of the modifications undergone by the mitochondria characterize the two other types of spermatozoons. Each of them is apparently specific of a sub-class. In Prosobranchia, i.e. Streptoneures, the cristae, always present in the mitochondrial derivative, are reorganized perpendicularly to the axis of the mitochondria that they wholly partition. In Euthyneures (Pulmonata, Opisthobranchia), the main part of the cristae disappears and a new crystalline structure fills the intermembranar space.

RIASSUNTO. — Lo studio dei mitocondri durante la spermatogenesi e negli spermatozoi permette di classificare lo spermatozoo dei Gasteropodi in 3 tipi. Uno, simile a quello dei Bivalvi, possiede una semplice corona di mitocondri liberi alla base del nucleo. Questo tipo primitivo caratterizza la fecondazione esterna, ed appare in alcuni Prosobranchi. Negli altri Prosobranchi, negli Opistobranchi e nei Polmonati, la fecondazione è interna ed è presente il « middle piece ». La struttura dei mitocondri e le modificazioni da essi subite caratterizzano gli altri 2 tipi di spermatozoi. Ciascuno di essi è apparentemente specifico di una sottoclasse. Nei Prosobranchi, p. es., Streptoneuri le creste, sempre presenti nei derivati mitocondriali, sono organizzate perpendicolarmente all'asse dei mitocondri.

Negli Eutineuri (Polmonati, Opistobranchi) scompare la maggior parte delle creste e una struttura cristallina riempie lo spazio tra le membrane.

INTRODUCTION

GRASSÉ et Coll., (1956) chez *Helix pomatia*, ANDRÉ (1962) chez *Testacella*, TAHMISIAN (1964) chez *Helix aspersa* ont montré que chez ces Gastéropodes Pulmonés les mitochondries de la spermatide fusionnent en un

(*) Laboratoire de Biologie Animale, Faculté des Sciences, 80. Amiens France, Laboratoire de Biologie Cellulaire 4, Faculté des Sciences. Orsay France. Ce travail a bénéficié de l'aide du Centre National de la Recherche Scientifique ERA 174, et de la Direction des Recherches et Moyens d'Essais (contrat 513/68).

(**) Laboratories of Human Reproduction and Reproductive Biology, Harvard Medical School, Boston, Massachusetts U.S.A.

complexe périflagellaire et subissent de profondes modifications structurales. La majeure partie des crêtes disparait et une formation nouvelle, cristalline, s'organise. KAYE (1958) a décrit chez le Prosobranche *Viviparus contectoides* une évolution différente: les mitochondries conservent leurs crêtes jusque dans le spermatozoïde. Il en est de même chez les Prosobranches *Cipangopaludina malleata* (YASUZUMI et Coll., 1958, 1959) et *Nucella lapillus* (WALKER et MACGREGOR, 1968).

Il nous a paru intéressant de rechercher si de telles différences dans l'évolution mitochondriale au cours de la spermatogenèse pouvaient avoir une valeur phylogénétique. Dans ce but, nous avons observé et comparé le comportement du chondriome pendant la spermatogenèse chez les espèces suivantes:

PROSOBRANCHES	OPISTHOBRANCHES	PULMONES
Gibbula cineraria (L.)	*Aplysia punctata* (Cuv.)	*Helix aspersa* (MÜLLER
Patella vulgata (L.)		*Helix pomatia* (L.)
Littorina obtusata (L.)		*Limnea palustris* (MÜLLER)
Littorina littorea (L.)		*Planorbis*
Purpura lapillus (L.)		*Arion aggericola* (Mab.)
Paludina fasciata (MÜLLER)		

OBSERVATIONS

I. *Les Prosobranches*:

A. *Gibbula et Patella.*

Ces Prosobranches marins ont une fécondation externe et leurs spermatozoïdes sont considérés comme primitifs dans la classification de FRANZEN (1956). Dans la jeune spermatide, les mitochondries globuleuses au nombre de 5 à 6 se groupent à la base du noyau autour des deux centrioles (Fig. 1 et 3). Au cours de la maturation de la spermatide, les crêtes mitochondriales se dilatent et la matrice se condense. Dans le spermatozoïde, les mitochondries de la couronne périflagellaire restent indépendantes. Leurs crêtes très dilatées, au contenu clair, compriment la matrice qui constitue des rubans flexueux très denses (Fig. 2). Dans ces mitochondries très peu modifiées, les structures membranaires internes conservent leur activité cytochrome oxydasique jusque dans le spermatozoïde. L'axonème de ces spermatozoïdes est dépourvu de fibres externes pleines.

B. *Paludina, Purpura, Littorina.*

La spermatogénèse se déroule de façon a peu près identique chez ces trois genres. Comme l'a montré KAYE (1958) chez *Viviparus*, les mitochondries au nombre d'une vingtaine dans le spermatocyte I fusionnent dans la jeune spermatide où il n'y a plus que 4 à 6 chondriosphéres. Celles–ci se groupent autour du flagelle à la base du noyau (Fig. 4 et 5). Les membranes externes des mitochondries adjacentes confluent, réunissant les choondriosphéres en un anneau mitochondrial périflagellaire (Fig. 5). Dans celui–ci les mitochondries gardent néanmoins leur individualité.

L'anneau mitochondrial s'allonge et s'enroule autour du flagelle (Fig. 6). Au cours de cette phase, les crêtes se réorientent et deviennent perpendiculaires à l'axe des mitochondries enroulées autour du flagelle (Figs. 7, 10 et 11). Chez le Pourpre (Fig. 7) et chez la Littorine, les crêtes sont peu nombreuses. Chez la Paludine, les crêtes très nombreuses ont une disposition périodique. Elles constituent des disques alternant régulièrement avec des disques matriciels (Figs. 10 et 11) (KAYE, 1958). Dans la gaine mitochondriale du spermatozoïde, la cytochrone oxydase reste localisée à la surface de la membrane interne (Figs. 8 et 9).

II. *Les Pulmonés.*

Chez tous les Pulmonés que nous avons étudiés, la spermatogenèse se déroule de façon semblable. Dans le jeune spermatocyte, les mitochondries, sont de courts bâtonnets aux crêtes longitudinales caractéristiques (GRASSÉ et Coll., 1956; ANDRÉ, 1962). Au cours de la croissance des spermatocytes, certaines mitochondries deviennent globuleuses et les crêtes se disposent de manière concentrique. D'autres mitochondries s'allongent; certaines de leurs crêtes se dilatent et compriment la matrice qui se condense. Le contenu clair des crêtes dilatées dénommé pseudomatrice par ANDRÉ (1962) renferme de fins filaments d'un diamètre de 70 à 90 Å (Fig. 12). Ces mitochondries allongées s'enroulent autour du flagelle (Fig. 3) puis se soudent en un seul corps mitochondrial (Fig. 14). Les filaments dans la pseudomatrice ne sont plus visibles et des amas d'un matériel finement granulaire sont apparus (Fig. 14). La fusion des mitochondries est complète, crêtes, matrices, membranes externes et membranes internes confluant. Le corps mitochondrial ainsi constitué ne comprend plus qu'un compartiment matriciel limité par ce qui subsiste de la membrane interne et entouré par la psuedomatrice volumineuse. Dans celle–ci des globules de 90 Å de diamètre apparaissent et s'organisent en bandes concentriques le long de la membrane mitochondriale externe (Fig. 15). Ces globules remplissent progressivement tout le volume pseudomatriciel, pour constituer un cristal (Fig. 16). Dans le cytoplasme résiduel, les mitochondries qui n'ont pas participé à la constitution de la pièce intermédiaire, subissent la même évolution (Fig. 17). Du point de vue des enzymes mitochondriales, la cytochrome oxydase [1] située à la surface des crêtes dans le spermatocyte (Fig. 19) se localise au niveau de la pseudomatrice dans la spermatide (Fig. 18) et au niveau du cristal dans le spermatozoïde (Fig. 20). Dans la région antérieure de la pièce intermédiaire, le cristal mitochondrial outre le compartiment matriciel est creusé d'un compartiment qui est rempli de glycogène dans le spermatozoïde mature (PERSONNE et ANDRÉ, 1964). La présence et l'agencement de ces compartiments sculptent des nervures à la surface du cristal. Chez l'Escargot, il n'existe qu'une seule nervure (Fig. 16) dans laquelle est logé un canal de glycogène. Chez la Planorbe où deux hélices contiennent du glycogène, il y a deux nervures. Chez la Limnée, deux canaux de glycogène et dans la région antérieure quatre digitations du compartiment matriciel déterminent sept nervures; dans la région médiane où le compartiment matriciel est lisse, il n'y a que deux nervures (Fig. 21). Chez la Testacelle les trois hélices correspondent l'une à un canal de glycogène et les deux autres à la matrice condensée dans deux canaux. (ANDRÉ, 1962; PERSONNE et ANDRÉ, 1964).

III. *Les Opisthobranches.*

Nous ne disposons que d'observations fragmentaires sur la spermatogénèse de ces Gastéropodes. Chez l'Aplysie, comme chez les Pulmonés, un cristal s'élaborerait dans l'espace pseudomatriciel du dérivé mitochondrial. Dans ce dérivé, les mitochondries, fusionnées en un manchon périflagellaire, resteraient individualisées.

CONCLUSIONS

Chez les Prosobranches nous avons observé, comme FRANZEN (1955), deux types de spermatozoïdes. Dans le type primitif, qui correspond à un mode de fécondation externe (FRANZEN, 1956), les mitochondries se groupent en un anneau à la base du noyau. Dans cet anneau, les mitochondries restées indépendantes ont des crêtes dilatées et une matrice condensée. Cette disposition des mitochondries se classe dans le type II A de la revue d'IDELMAN (1967). On la retrouve chez les Bivalves (GALTSOFF et PHILPOTT, 1959;

(1) Nous fondant sur le travail de SELIGMAN et Coll. (1968) nous avons utilisé la réaction DAB pour rechercher la cytochrome oxydase. Depuis BEARD et NOVIKOFF 1969 (J. Cell. Biol., 42, 501), NOVIKOFF et GOLDFISCHER 1969 (J. Histochem. Cytochem., 17, 675) ont montré que l'oxydation du DAB par les mitochondries se produisait aussi bien sur la membrane externe que sur la membrane interne. Ces résultat conduirent NOVIKOFF et Coll. à étendre à d'autres cytochromes la spécificité de la réaction DAB des mitochondries. Dans notre matériel, l'oxydation du DAB n'est donc peut-etre pas due à la seule action de la cytochrome oxydase mais à l'action de certains cytochromes. Des expériences sont en course pour tenter de préciser ce point.

PASTELLS et DE HARVEN, 1962), les Échinodermes (AFZELIUS, 1955), chez des Polychêtes (COLWIN et COLWIN, 1961) et des Poissons (BILLARD, 1969; MATTEI, 1969), dont la fécondation est aussi externe. Comme dans d'autres groupes (FRANZEN, 1956; BILLARD, 1969), une pièce intermédiaire contenant un dérivé mitochondrial plus ou moins long se constitue dans le spermatozoïde des espèces à fécondation interne. La formation de ce dérivé mitochondrial suit un schéma commun à de nombreux groupes. Les mitochondries, dont les crêtes dilatées compriment une matrice dense, s'enroulent autour du flagelle. Néanmoins, la fusion des mitochondries en un seul ensemble périflagellaire et une certaine réorganisation de l'architecture des crêtes confèrent une structure assez caractéristique au manchon mitochondrial des Prosobranches à fécondation interne. Dans ce manchon, l'abondance en crêtes est variable selon les espèces. Le nombre des espèces étudiées étant trop limité et la physiologie de ces spermatozoïdes insuffisamment connue, ce critère ne peut, pour l'instant, avoir de valeur systématique. FRANZEN (1955, 1956) a observé au contraste de phase que la pièce intermédiaire du spermatozoïde des Prosobranches était différente de celle des Pulmonés et des Opisthobranches. Nos résultats confirment ces observations et montrent que le dérivé mitochondrial des Pulmonés, et probablement celui des Opisthobranches, comprend un volumineux cristal intermembranaire. Cette structure mitochondriale nouvelle qui n'existe pas chez les Prosobranches ou Streptoneures n'a été décrite dans aucun autre groupe. Elle semble caractéristique de la pièce intermédiaire du spermatozoïde des Euthyneures: Opisthobranches, et Pulmonés. Celle–ci présenterait d'autre part des caractères propres à chacune des 2 sous–unités. Chez les Opisthobranches les mitochondries, simplement réunies comme chez les Prosobranches, par la confluence de leurs membranes externes, garderaient leur individualité. Chez les Pulmonés, les mitochondries se confondent toutes en un corps mitochondrial unifié. La surface de celui–ci est sculptée de nervures hélicoïdales qui correspondent à des canaux logés dans le cristal. Le nombre de ces nervures et la nature des canaux, différents pour chacun des genres étudiés, constituent des caractères apparemment spécifiques.

BIBLIOGRAPHIE

AFZELIUS B. A. (1955) – *The fine structure of the sea urchin spermatozoa as revealed by the electron microscope.* « Z. Zellforsch. Mikrosh. Anat. », 42, 134–148.

ANDRÉ J. (1962) – *Contribution à la connaissance du chondriome: étude de ses modifications ultrastructurales pendant la spermatogenèse.* « J. Ultrastruct. Res. », suppl. 3, 1–185.

BILLARD (1969) – *Spermiogenèse comparée de quelques Téléostéens. International Symposium on comparative spermatology.* Rome Sienne.

COLWIN A. L. et COLWIN L. H. (1961) – *Fine structure of the spermatozoon of* Hydroides hexagonous (*Annelida*) *with special references to the acrosomal region.* « J. Biochem. Biophys. Cytol. », 10, 211–230.

FRANZÉN Å. (1955) – *Comparative morphological investigation into the spermiogenesis among* Mollusca. « Zool. Bidragfran Uppsala », 30, 399–456.

FRANZÉN Å. (1956) – *On spermiogenesis, morphology of the spermatozoon, and biology of fertilization among invertebrates.* « Zool. Bidr. Uppsala », 31, 355–482.

GALTSOFF P. S. et PHILPOTT D. E. (1959) – *Electron microscope study of the sperm of* Crassostrea virginica. « Biol. Bull. », 117, 386.

GALTSOFF P. S. et PHILPOTT D. E. (1960) – *Ultrastructure of the spermatozoon of the oyster* Crassostrea virginica. « J. Ultrastr. Res. », 3, 241–253.

GRASSÉ P. P., CARASSO N. et FAVARD P. (1956) – *Les ultrastructures cellulaires au cours de la spermiogenèse de l'Escargot* Helix pomatia. *Evolution des chromosomes, du chondriome, de l'appareil de Golgi.* « Ann. Sci. Natur. Zool. », 18, 339–380.

IDELMAN S. (1967) – *Données récentes sur l'infrastructure du spermatozoïde.* « Ann. Biol. » 6, 113–190.

KAYE J. S. (1958) – *Changes in the fine structure of mitochondria during spermatogenesis.* « J. Morphol. », 102, 347–399.

MATTEI X. (1969) – *International Symposium on comparative spermatology.* Rome–Sienne.

PASTEELS J. J. et DE HARVEN E. (1962) – *Etude au microscope électronique du spermatozoïde d'un mollusque bivalve,* Barnea candida. « Arch. Biol. Belg. », 73, 445–463.

PERSONNE P. et ANDRÉ J. (1964) – *Existence de glycogène mitochondrial dans le spermatozoïde de la Testacelle.* « J. Microscopie », 3, 643–650.

SELIGMAN A. M., KARNOVSKY M. J., WASSERKRUG H. L. et HANKER J. S. (1968) – *Nondroplet ultrastructural demonstration of cytochrome oxidase activity with a polymeric osmiophilic reagent, diaminobenzidine (DAB).* « J. Cell Biol. », 38, 1–14.

TAHMISIAN T. N. (1964) – *On orderly domains of particles associated with cytomembranes during spermiogenesis in* Helix aspersa. « Z. Zellforsch. Mikrosk. Anat. », 65, 25–31.

YASUZUMI G. et TANAKA H. (1958) – *Spermatogenesis in animals as revealed by electron microscopy. Research on the spermatozoa dimorphism in a pond snail,* Cipangopaludina malleata. « J. Biophys. Biochem. Cytol. », 4, 621–632.

YASUZUMI G., TANAKA H., TEZUKA O. et NAKANOS S. (1959) – *The ultrastructure of organelles appearing in spermatids and nutritive cells of* Cipangopaludina malleata. « Z. Zellforsch. Mikrosk. Anat. », 50, 632–643.

WALKER M. et MAC GREGOR H. C. (1968) – *Spermatogenesis and the structure of the mature sperm in Nucella lapillus (L).* « J. Cell Science », 3, 95–104.

LÉGENDES DES FIGURES

Fig. 1 à 3. – Prosobranches à fécondation externe.

Fig. 1. – Gibbule. Spermatozoïde en cours de maturation. Le noyau (*N*) est surmonté d'un acrosome volumineux (*A*). A la base du noyau les 2 centrioles (*Cd* et *Cp*) sont entourés par une couronne de mitochondries globuleuses (*M*). Celles–ci ont une matrice dense (*m*) et des crêtes (*c*) peu dilatées. ×45.000.

Fig. 2. – Gibbule. Spermatozoïde mature. La condensation du matériel nucléaire est achevée. Dans les mitochondries, les crêtes (*c*) dilatées et ondulées compriment la matrice (*m*) qui constitue un réseau de lames flexueuses très denses. ×45.000.

Fig. 3. – Patelle. Spermatozoïde en cours de maturation. ×45.000.
Cd = centriole distal, *Cp* = centriole proximal, *N* = noyau, *M* = mitochondrie.

Fig. 4 à 11. – Prosobranches à fécondation interne.

Fig. 4. – Littorine. Très jeune spermatide coupée transversalement à la base du noyau (*N*). 6 mitochondries (*M*), de structure normale, sont groupées autour du flagelle (*F*) ×45.000.

Fig. 5. – Pourpre. Spermatide coupée transversalement à la base du noyau (*N*). Les mitochondries (*M*) groupées autour du flagelle se réunissent en un seul manchon, les membranes externes des mitochondries adjacentes confluant (fléches). ×45.000.

Fig. 6. – Pourpre – Coupe tangentielle d'une spermatide montrant l'allongement et l'enroulement de la gaine mitochondriale (*M*). *N* = noyau. ×45.000.

Fig. 7. – Pourpre – Spermatozoïde coupé obliquement au niveau de la pièce intermédiaire. Les mitochondries enroulées autour du flagelle sont réunies en un ensemble unique, que limite une membrane mitochondriale externe commune (*me*). Les crêtes (*c*) peu nombreuses sont disposées perpendiculairement à l'axe des mitochondries. *m* = matrice, *mi* = membrane mitochondriale interne. ×45.000.

Figs. 8–9. – Localisation de la cytochrome oxydase dans les spermatozoïdes de Pourpre. Technique de Seligman et coll. au DAB cytochrome *c* tetroxyde d'osmium.

Fig. 8. – Coupe oblique de spermatozoïde incubé dans le milieu témoin dépourvu de cytochrome *c*. ×45.000.

Fig. 9. – Coupe oblique de spermatozoïde incubé dans le milieu au DAB cytochrome *c*. Les dépôts de noir d'osmium se localisent à la surface de la membrane interne (flèches). ×45.000.

Fig. 10 et 11. – Paludine – Spermatozoïdes coupés obliquement. Dans le manchon mitochondrial périflagellaire, les mitochondries, réunies par leurs membranes externes (*me*), gardent leur individualité. Les crêtes nombreuses sont toutes issues de la face périflagellaire de la membrane interne (*mi*) (Fig. 11, flèches.). Elles constituent des disques disposés perpendiculairement au grand axe des mitochondries, séparés par des disques matriciels. ×45.000.

Fig. 12 à 21. – Pulmonés.

Fig. 12. – Escargot. Jeune spermatide dans laquelle on remarque plusieurs types de mitochondries: des mitochondries banales (M_1) semblables à celles des spermatocytes, des mitochondries allongées (M_2) qui présentent une crête centrale dilatée. Son contenu clair correspond à la pseudomatrice (*p*) et renferme des fibriles (flèches) de 70 à 90 Å de diamètre. La matrice (*m*) condensée constitue un manchon qui entoure cette crête dilatée. ×45.000.

Fig. 13. – Spermatide d'Escargot. Les mitochondries allongées (M_2) sont enroulées autour du flagelle. Le contenu de la pseudomatrice s'est modifié, les fibrilles ne sont plus visibles, mais on trouve des amas d'un matériel finament granulaire. ×25.000.

Fig. 14. – Dans cette spermatide d'Escargot plus agée, les mitochondries enroulées autour du flagelle se fusionnent. ×60.000.

me = membrane mitochondriale externe, *mi* = membrane mitochondriale interne, *c* = crête dilatée renfermant des amas d'un matériel finement granulaire, *m* = matrice.

Fig. 15 à 16. – Spermatozoïde d'Escargot en cours de maturation. Coupes transversales de la région antérieure de la pièce intermédiaire.

Fig. 15. – Au sein de la pseudomatrice 2 rangées concentriques de globules d'un diamêtre de 90 Å (flèches) se sont organisées le long de la membrane mitochondriale externe (*me*) ×45.000.

mi = membrane mitochondriale interne, *m* = matrice, *t* = microtubules.

Fig. 16. - A un stade plus évolué, les globules remplissent tout le volume pseudomatriciel et constituent un cristal. Celui–ci enserre, le flagelle, le compartiment matriciel, (*m*) limité par ce qui subsiste de la membrane mitochondriale interne (*mi*), et dans la région antérieure un compartiment rempli de glycogène dans le spermatozoïde mature. ×45.000.

Fig. 17. – Cette spermatide d'Escargot montre que des mitochondries (*M*) du cytoplasme résiduel renferment des globules (flèches) identiques à ceux du cristal de la pièce intermédiaire. (P.I.).

me = membrane mitochondriale externe, *mi* = membrane mitochondriale interne, *m* = matrice, *p* = pseudomatrice.

Fig. 18, 19, 20. – Localisation de la cytochrome oxydase au cours de la spermatogenèse de l'Escargot. Technique de Seligman et coll. au DAB cytochrome *c* tetroxyde d'osmium.

Fig. 18. – Coupe de spermatide incubé dans le milieu de Seligman. Dans la pièce intermédiaire, les dépôts se localisent au niveau du cristal (flèches). Dans les mitochondries du cytoplasme résiduel, ils se trouvent dans la pseudomatrice (*p*). ×45.000.

Fig. 19. – Mitochondrie de spermatocyte incubé dans le milieu de Seligman. Les dépôts de noir d'osmium se localisent à la surface des crêtes (flèches). ×45.000.

Fig. 20. – Spermatozoïdes incubés dans le milieu de Seligman coupés transversalement, Le cristal dans la pièce intermédiaire est, recouvert de noir d'osmium. ×45.000

Fig. 21. – Limnée. Coupes transversales de spermatozoïdes. ×30.000.

a. coupe de la région antérieure de la pièce intermédiaire montrant la surface du cristal sculptée de 7 hélices. Celles–ci correspondent aux canaux creusés dans le cristal. L'un renferme le compartiment matriciel (*m*) et présente 4 digitations; 2 autres contiennent un matériel cristallin et du glycogène (flèches).

b. coupe de la région médiane de la pièce intermédiaire, les sculptures de la surface du cristal s'estompent.

c. coupe de la région coudale remplie de glycogène périflagellaire.

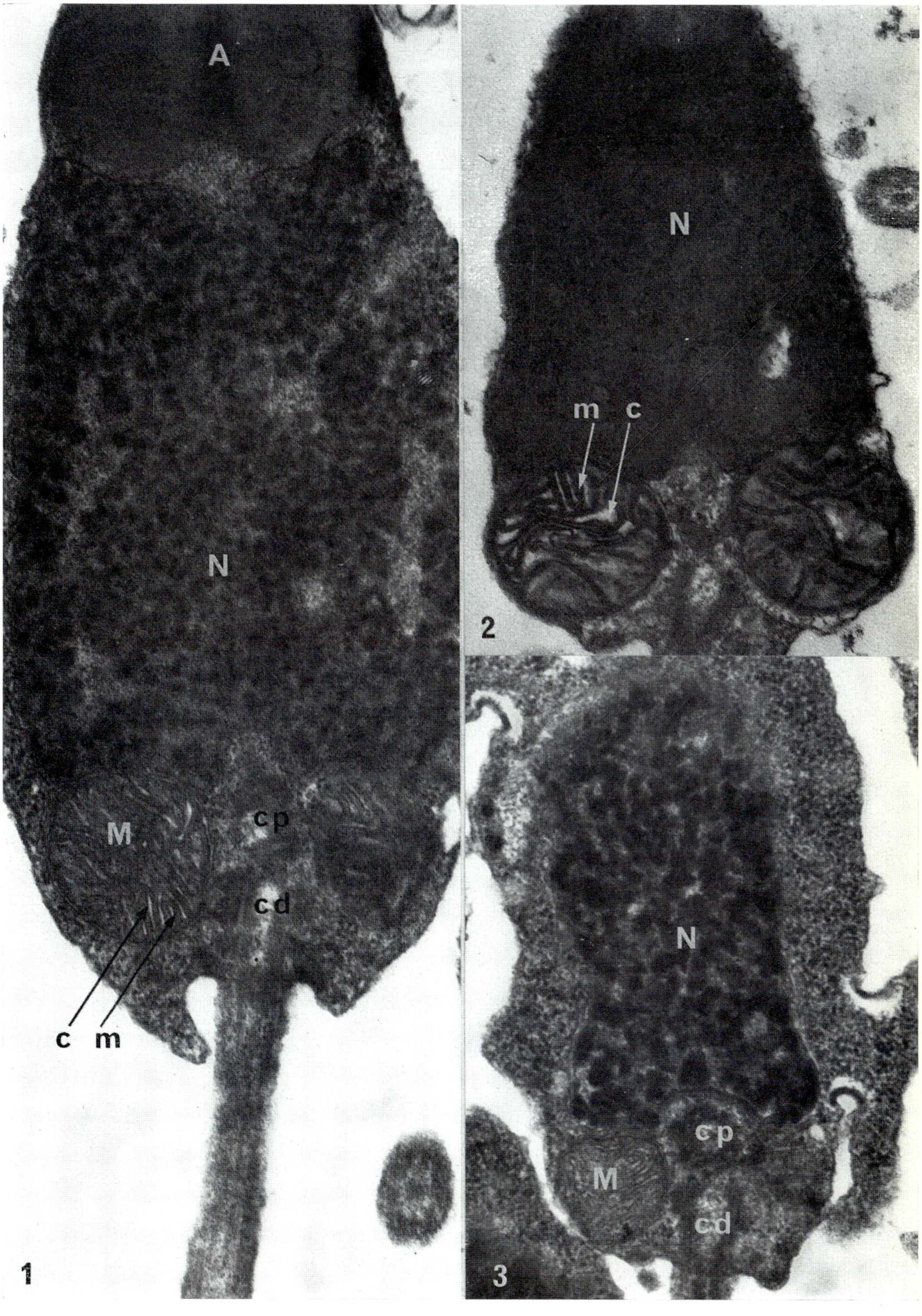
A
N
M
cp
cd
c
m
1
N
m
c
2
N
cp
M
cd
3

P. PERSONNE et W. A. ANDERSON – *Étude comparée des évolutions mitochondriales au cours de la spermatogenèse chez quelques gastéropodes.*

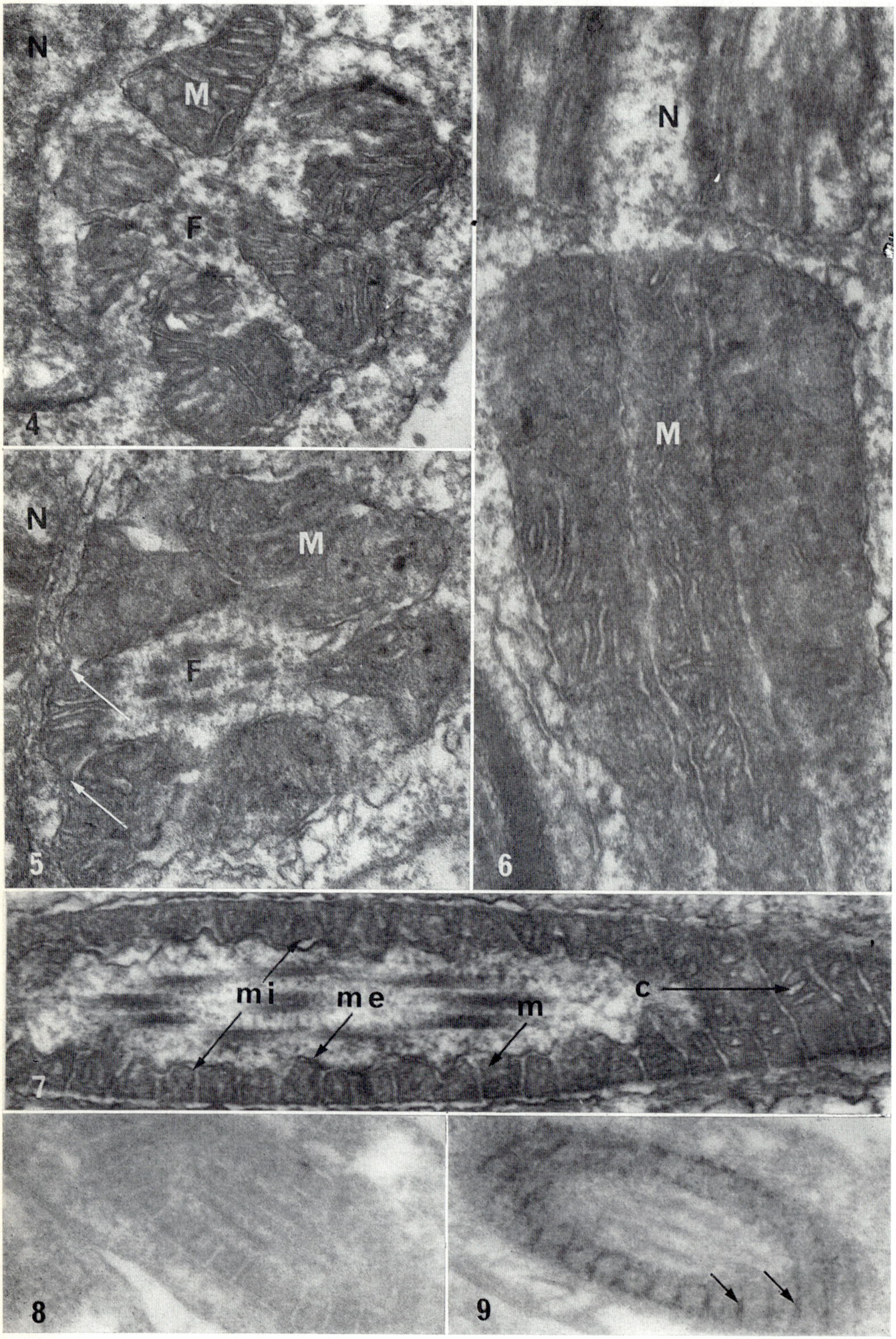

P. Personne et W. A. Anderson – *Étude comparée des évolutions mitochondriales au cours de la spermatogenèse chez quelques gastéropodes.*

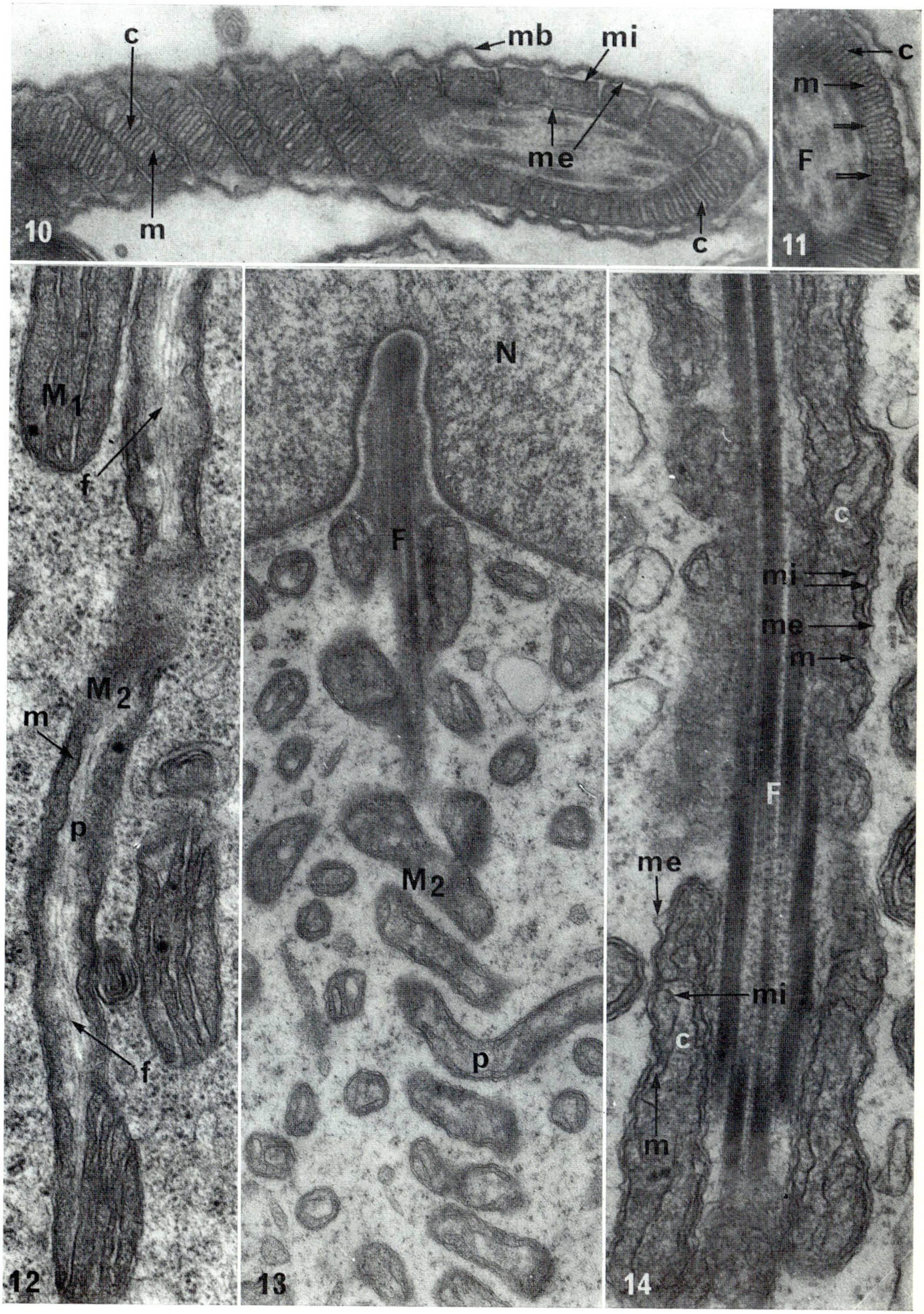

P. Personne et W. A. Anderson – *Étude comparée des évolutions mitochondriales au cous de la spermatogenèse chez quelques gastéropodes.*

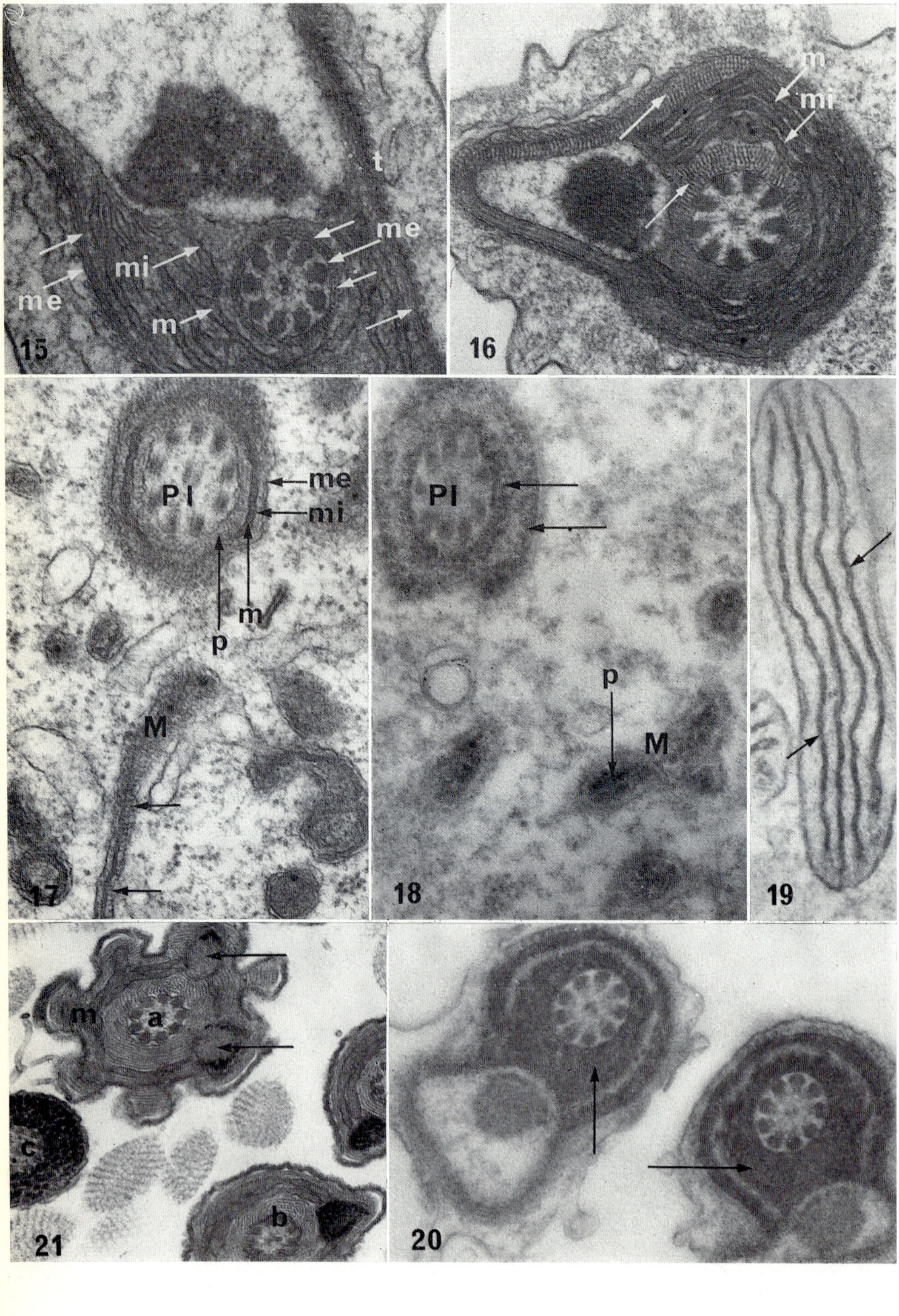

G. YASUZUMI (*), I. TSUBO (*), M. YASUDA (*), T. SUGIOKA (*), H. SAKAMOTO (*) and F. YASUZUMI (*)

ELECTRON MICROSCOPE STUDIES ON ATYPICAL SPERMATIDS OF POND SNAIL *CIPANGOPALUDINA MALLEATA* REEVE, UNDER CONSIDERATION OF CONVERSION OF DNA INTO POLYSACCHARIDE

SUMMARY. — Activities of at least five enzymes, Mg–ATPase, TPN–dependent 6DPG–dehydrogenase, UDPG–pyrophosphorylase, TPPase and acid phosphatase were observed in order to reveal the process and fine structural localization sites of glycoprotein synthesis from DNA–macromolecules in the developing atypical spermatids of the pond snail, *Cipangopaludina malleata* Reeve. These enzymes were revealed one another to be in a close relationship concerning such several metabolic processes as carbohydrate breakdown, release of DNA–macromolecules into Cytoplasm and glycoprotein synthesis occurring during the maturation of atypical spermatids. An enzyme system for the pentose-phosphate cycle was found in the smooth-surfaced endoplasmic reticulum including the nuclear envelope and in the Golgi complex on the basis of presence of TPN–dependent 6DPG–dehydrogenase and TPPase activities. It was suggested that glycogen synthesis is presumably possible in the Golgi complex through the UDPG–pyrophosphorylase activity, so far as the pond snail atypical spermatid is concerned.

RIASSUNTO. — Vengono osservate le attività di almeno cinque enzimi, Mg–ATPasi, 6–DPG deidrogenasi TPN–dipendente, UDPG–pirofosforilasi, TPPasi e fosfatasi acida per rivelare i processi e la fine localizzazione strutturale della sintesi delle glicoproteine da macromolecole di DNA negli spermatidi atipici della lumaca *Cipangopaludina malleata* Reeve. Questi enzimi sono in stretta relazione l'uno con l'altro interessando così parecchi processi metabolici come la rottura di molecole di carboidrati; il rilascio di macromolecole di DNA nel citoplasma e la sintesi di glicoproteine che avviene durante la maturazione di spermatidi atipici. Un sistema enzimatico per il ciclo del pentoso fosfato è stato trovato sulla superficie liscia del reticolo endoplasmico e nel complesso di Golgi in base alla presenza della 6DPG–deidrogenasi TPN–dipendente e della TPPasi. Si ritiene che la sintesi del glicogeno sia possibile nel complesso di Golgi attraverso la UDPG–pirofosforilasi negli spermatidi atipici della lumaca.

As the metamorphosis of atypical spermatids of the pond snail *Cipangopaludina malleata* Reeve proceeds, ribosomes free or attached to vesicular elements of the endoplasmic reticulum disappear gradually from the cytoplasmic matrix and the surfaces of the vesicles, and subsequently an amor-

(*) The Electron Microscope Research Laboratory, Department of Anatomy, Nara Medical University, Kashihara city, Nara, Japan.

phous substance makes its appearance in the smooth-surfaced vesicles. When the cytoplasm loses gradually its basophilic character showing an evidence of RNA, the contents of the vesicles are aggregated into dense granules of varying size and number, showing a Feulgen-positive reaction. As the dense granules are increased in number and size, the nucleus is gradually reduced in volume, which at last completely loses its DNA components, remaining only its basic protein. Many of chromatin granule derivatives appearing in the cytoplasm are used in the formation of the sheath of middle piece of mature atypical spermatozoa. Although the metamorphosis of atypical spermatozoa and the origin of their compositions have been made clear (YASUZUMI, 1962; 1964; YASUZUMI *et al.*, 1958, 1960, 1967) it has remained unsettled why the chromatin granule derivatives are no longer basophilic and have been converted into the periodic acid Schiff (PAS)–positive granules in the premature and mature spermatozoa.

Several authors have already reported that the middle piece sheath of atypical spermatid of several *Viviparus* is composed of polysaccharide, without making clear its origin and chemical components in detail (GALL, 1961; HANSON *et al.*, 1952; ISHIZAKI *et al.*, 1958; TOCHIMOTO, 1967). Recently, YASUZUMI *et al.* (1970) have revealed that such PAS–positive components consist of glycoprotein by means of light and electron microscopes. The existence of glycoprotein granules in the cytoplasm has been described in different tissue cells of several animals (LEBLOND *et al.*, 1957; MEYER, 1955; RAMBOURG and LEBLOND, 1967; SPIRO, 1963; THIÉRY, 1968; VAN HEYNINGEN 1965).

The present study has been cytochemically oriented towards elucidating the glycogen synthesis on the basis of the uridine diphosphate glucose (UDPG)–pyrophosphrylase activity as well as showing the presence of an enzyme system for carbohydrate breakdown, the pentose-phosphate cycle, by means of proofs of triphosphopyridine nucleotide (TPN)-dependent 6–D–phosphogluconate (6DPG) dehydrogenase and thiamine pyrophosphatase (TPPase) activities. In addition, Mg^{++} activated adenosine triphosphatase (Mg–ATPase) activity in the nuclear pore complex of the atypical spermatids and acid phosphatase activity in their nuclei have been compared with those activities in the typical spermatids. The description of these cytochemical patterns and a discussion of their functional significance form the topics of this paper.

MATERIAL AND METHODS

The materials used in the present study consisted of testis of the pond snail and liver of the mouse. Prior to observations of several enzyme activities with an electron microscope, smear preparations on glass plates or thin frozen sections of the testis or liver were incubated for 15 to 30 minutes at 37° C in several enzyme substrates either without fixation with fixative or after fixation for several minutes with several concentrations of glutaraldehyde (SABATINI, *et al.*, 1963) diluted with 0.22 M sucrose adjusted to pH 7.2 with 0.1 M sodium cacodylate buffer. After these incubated specimens were washed in buffered sucrose, they were treated with dilute ammonium sulfide and examined with a light microscope. Optimal concentrations of fixative and periods of fixation so obtained were applied for the electron microscopic observations, since several enzyme activities to be described below showed respectively different resistances against the fixation procedures.

In the acid phosphatase activity experiments, small blocks of the pond snail testis were fixed for 60 minutes at 4° C in 6.25% glutaraldehyde adjusted to pH 7.2 with 0.1 M sodium cacodylate buffer. After the fixed materials were washed for several hours in 0.22 M sucrose, their frozen sections or small slices for 15 minutes at 37° C were incubated in the Gomori medium (GOMORI, 1941) at pH 5.4 and employing sodium β–glycerophosphate as substrate, as suggested by Holt (1959). The light microscopic demonstration of acid phosphatase was performed according to Seligman–Manheimer's procedure (SELIGMAN and MANHEIMER, 1949).

Mg–ATPase activity of the pond snail testis was observed, its small blocks being fixed for 15 minutes at 4° C in 0.5% glutaraldehyde adjusted to pH 7.2 with 0.1 M sodium cacodylate buffer. After washing for 60 minutes the fixed specimens in sodium cacodylate buffer (pH 7.2) and subsequently for one minute in 0.22 M sucrose, their frozen sections were treated according to Yasuzumi–Tsubo's two step method (YASUZUMI and TSUBO, 1966) which modified an original Wachstein–Meisel procedure for ATPase activity (WACHSTEIN and MEISEL, 1957).

TPPase activity was observed in the pond snail testis fixed with a similar way as in a case of ATPase mentioned above. Frozen sections of the fixed material were incubated for 15 minutes at 37° C in a Novikoff–Goldfischer medium containing TPP (NOVIKOFF and GOLDFISCHER, 1961).

Prior to the observations of UDPG–pyrophosphrylase activity on the pond snail testis, a preliminary examination was made on the mouse liver. Although the experiments were performed in the normal mouse liver, reaction deposits showing UDPG–pyrophosphorylase activity were not found in the hepatocyte cell organelles. Thus, mice were starved for 24 hours, and subsequently fed for one hour 50% glucose per os. Small blocks of their liver were cut on a Pearse cryostat, type H in approximately 40 μ in thickness, and subsequently fixed for 10 minutes at 4° C with 0.5% glutaraldehyde adjusted to pH 7.2 with 0.1 M Na–cacodylate buffer. After the fixed materials were washed for several hours in 0.22 M sucrose, they were incubated for 20 minutes at 37° C in the following media. The medium was prepared freshly before use and had the following standard composition:

Uridine triphosphate (UTP)	0.01 M	1 ml
Glucose–1–phosphate (GIP)	0.01 M	1 ml
Magnesium chloride	2.4 mM	1 ml
Histidine buffer (pH 7.2)	0.2 M	5 ml
Lead nitrate	6.0 mM	2 ml

Three control media were also prepared as follows: medium devoid of GIP from the standard composition; medium devoid of UTP from the standard; and medium devoid of UTP and GIP from the standard.

UDPG–pyrophosphorylase activity in the atypical spermatids was observed in a similar way as in the mouse liver.

TPN–dependent 6DPG–dehydrogenase activity was examined as an enzyme of electron transfer system in the pentose–phosphate cycle in the atypical spermatids of the pond snail, by employing potassium ferricyanide as the acceptor of hydrogen. The basis of the method is that ferricyanide is reduced to ferrocyanide, and that the latter combines with copper ions to form the insoluble copper ferrocyanide. The copper ions in the medium are complexed with citrate to prevent formation of copper ferricyanide (DEVLIR *et al.*, 1956; ESTABNOOK, 1961; KARNOVSKY, 1964; KARNOVSKY *et al.*, 1964; OGAWA, *et al.*, 1968; PRESSMAN, 1955; SINGER *et al.*, 1967). The testis of pond snail was fixed for 10 minutes at 4° C in 0.5% glutaraldehyde diluted with 0.22 M sucrose adjusted to pH 7.2 with 0.1 M Na–cacodylate buffer.

After the fixed material was washed for one to two hours in 0.22 M sucrose, its frozen sections or small slices were incubated for 30 minutes at 37° C in the following medium.

TPN 1.5 mM	3.0 ml
6DPG	100.0 mg
Sodium azide	1.5 mg
Cobalt chloride	6.0 mg
Potassium ferricyanide 5 mM	2.0 ml
Cupric sulfate 30 mM	20.0 ml
Sodium citrate 0.1 M	0.6 ml
Tris-maleate buffer (pH 7.4)	15.0 ml

After all the specimens incubated in several enzyme substrates were washed in 0.22 M sucrose for several minutes, they were postfixed for 30 minutes in 1 % osmium tetroxide diluted with 0.22 M sucrose adjusted to pH 7.2 with 0.1 M Na–cacodylate buffer.

In each enzyme experiment, some material was incubated in a substrate-free medium as control.

After postfixation all the specimens were dehydrated in a series of increasing concentrations of alcohol and embedded in epoxy Epon resin (LUFT, 1961). Thin sections were cut on a Porter–Blum microtome or an LKB ultrotome with glass knives. They were mounted on Formvar–coated copper specimen grids and stained doubly with saturated aqueous uranyl acetate followed by lead citrate (REYNOLDS 1963; WATSON, 1958). These sections were examined in an electron microscope of Hitachi Co., model HU–llD–S.

RESULTS

In the early atypical spermatid the granular endoplasmic reticulum is highly developed and appears aligned in rows which are disposed parallel to one another in more or less regular intervals. The atypical spermatid at this stage is rather larger than the typical spermatid, so that the former is easily differentiated from the latter by size. The nucleus of the atypical spermatid in the early stage is also larger and more irregular in shape as compared with that of the typical spermatid. As development of the atypical spermatid proceeds, the nucleus becomes oval in shape and the cisternae of the endoplasmic reticulum invariably contain a rather electron opaque material.

At a such development stage of the atypical spermatid, dense deposits showing acid phosphatase activity are found in discrete, mostly interchromatinic foci of its nucleus (Fig. 1). Such activity has never been observed in the nuclear pore complex and on the cell surfaces. The Golgi complex is revealed to be localization site of acid phosphatase activity (Fig. 1). The development of atypical spermatids is accompanied gradually by decrease of the rough–surfaced endoplasmic reticulum in amount, and simultaneously the smooth-surfaced endoplasmic reticulum is remarkably developed in a vesicular form, containing denser material than the contents in the cisternae of the rough-surfaced endoplasmic reticulum. Final reaction deposits of acid phosphatase are visible at the interchromatinic foci of the nucleus at a such a development stage as well (Fig. 2).

In the late stage of development of atypical spermatids, the flattened navicular, and shrunken nucleus migrates to the peripheral portion of the cell, which is characterized by the low density of the nucleoplasm. Concurrently with these changes in the nuclear components and form, the cytoplasm is occupied by numerous smooth-surfaced vesicles containing dense granular components, except for the zone of the developing tail filaments. It is interesting to note that dense final reaction deposits of acid phosphatase are no longer visible in the premature nuclei, except for a part of the nuclear envelope. However, dense deposits are encountered between the tail filaments and at the proximal portion of the tail filaments (Fig. 3). Final reaction product is remarkably encountered in mature sperm tail (Fig. 4). The similar pattern of Mg–ATPase has been demonstrated in another mollusc spermatozoa by ANDERSON *et al.*, 1968). Acid phosphatase activity has never been seen in the typical spermatid nuclei through all the development stages (Fig. 5).

The electron microscopic results have been confirmed by light microscopy, employing Seligman-Manheimer's procedure (SELIGMAN *et al.*, 1949).

Non-specific staining by lead ions at the electron microscopic level reveals that any reaction product is completely absent in the atypical spermatid nuclei as well as in the tail filaments after incubation of frozen sections or small slices in a medium lacking substrate.

In the liver parenchymal cells of the mouse which was starved for 24 hours, subsequently refed for one hour 50 % glucose and incubated in the standard medium for UDPG–pyrophosphorylase, final reaction deposits occur characteristically in the endoplasmic reticulum localized in an area surrounded by mitochondria and smooth-surfaced vesicles. It is noticeable that the final reaction products are not encountered in the Golgi complex (Fig. 6). In the incubation with UTP, reaction deposits appear at random in the rough-surfaced endoplasmic reticulum and within the nuclear envelope in the similar mouse hepatocyte (Fig. 7). No reaction products have been demonstrated when the specimens are incubated either in a medium devoid of UTP or in other control media. The results concerning UDPG–pyrophosphorylase activity in hepatocytes will be described in detail elsewhere.

In the pond snail atypical spermatids incubated in the standard medium for UDPG–pyrophosphorylase, the very electron opaque deposits of irregular shape and size are found mainly between the paired membranes and seldom in the vesicles of the Golgi complex (Fig. 8). At the stage when abundant chromatin derivatives appear in the smooth-surfaced vesicles, deposits of final reaction product occur mainly in the cisternae of the Golgi complex (Fig. 9). No deposits of lead phosphate occur in the pond snail testis incubated in a medium devoid of UTP.

When the pond snail testis fixed in buffered glutaraldehyde is incubated with ATP as substrate followed by lead nitrate and postfixed in buffered osmium tetroxide, tangential sections through the atypical spermatid nuclei demonstrate finely distributed deposits of Mg–ATPase reaction product on the nuclear envelope and more dense globular deposits approximately 800 A in diameter in the nuclear pore complex (Fig. 10). Such a reaction product seems to occur remarkably at the peripheral part of the pore complex, leaving a lighter inner space. But a small deposit is found occasionally at a central point of the pore complex (Fig. 11). However, dense globular deposits showing Mg–ATPase activity within the nuclear pore complex of the developing typical spermatids are remarakably smaller in amount than those in the developing atypical spermatids. Control specimens incubated in a medium devoid of substrate have shown the negative result (Fig. 12).

Deposits of final product of TPN–dependent 6DPG–dehydrogenase are regularly confined to the smooth-surfaced endoplasmic reticulum, including smooth-surfaced vesicles, and to the inner layer of the double-layered nuclear envelope. The deposits are sometimes encountered applied to the outer surfaces of the smooth-surfaced endoplasmic reticulum (Figs. 13–15). In the flattened and shrunken nucleus of the atypical spermatid at a late stage of maturation, the inner layer of the double-layered nuclear envelope shows dense deposits in linear or in finely distributed pattern as well as in vesicular or granular appearance. No reaction product occurs in other cell organelles as well as in the cytoplasmic matrix and on the plasma membrane (Fig. 16). Any reaction product is completely absent in the specimens incubated in a medium lacking substrate (Fig. 17).

In the testis fixed in glutaraldehyde, incubated in Novikoff–Goldfischer medium containing TPP and postfixed in osmium tetroxide, dense deposits and finely distributed precipitates of final product are mainly encountered between the paired membranes of the Golgi complex. The similar pattern has been reported by MEEK and BRADBURY (1963) in *Helix aspersa*. No reaction product is observed in any other cell organelles (Fig. 18). Control experiments have not demonstrated the appearance of dense deposits.

DISCUSSION

Although STERN *et al.* (1952) have shown that acid phosphatase and ATPase are absent biochemically from the isolated nuclei, somewhat later FISCHER *et al.* (1959) and SIEBERT (1961) have demonstrated the existence of such enzymes in nuclei of normal and cancer cells. Recently, SINGH and MATHUR (1968 a, 1968 b) have reported by light microscopy that the nuclear membrane, nucleolus and chromatin material of various spermatogenetic cells of the Indian desert gerbil and the house shrew are localization sites of the acid phosphatase activity.

In the pond snail atypical spermatids observed, the acid phosphatase activity has been revealed in the Golgi complex as well as in the interchromatinic foci of the nucleus, and between the tail filaments. In the premature atypical sperm nucleus with a low density, such activity is no longer visible. The typical spermatid nucleus is completely devoid of such activity through its all the stages of the development. The role of non-specific acid phosphatase activity in the nucleus is not well known, however, the hydrolytic function of this enzyme has been well documented MUNCH–PETERSEN *et al.* 1953). So far as the atypical spermatid nucleus is concerned, the acid phosphatase activity may be related to depolymerization of DNA.

Several enzyme systems, except for acid phosphatase system, have been observed in the present materials fixed for 10 to 15 minutes at 4°C in 0.5 % glutaraldehyde diluted with 0.22 M sucrose adjusted to pH 7.2 with 0.1 M sodium cacodylate buffer, incubated in media containing several substrates, and postfixed in osmium tetroxide buffered to pH 7.2. In such preparations, several organizations of the parenchymal cells have been in general satisfactorily preserved and shown few changes that could be ascribed to the incubation procedure.

UDPG–linked pathway of glycogen synthesis can be formulated as follows (LELOIR *et al.*, 1957, 1959; MUNCH–PETERSEN *et al.*, 1953; NEUFELD *et al.*, 1957; VILLAR–PALASI *et al.*, 1960):

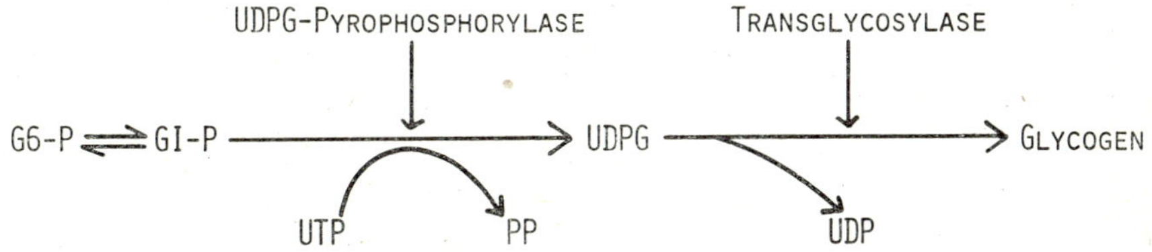

The positive results of specimens incubated in a medium containing GIP, UTP and lead ions depend upon trapping of orthophosphate as lead phosphate, which results from hydrolysis of the pyrophosphate bonds by the UDPG–pyrophosphorylase. Although the UDPG–pyrophosphorylase activity has never been demonstrated in the Golgi complex in hepatocytes of the mouse starved for 24 hours and refed for one hour 50 % glucose, such activity has been detected in the Golgi complex in the pond snail atypical spermatids. These facts have shown that there is species or cellular specificity as to localization site of enzyme. By means of PAS reaction and comparision of effects of several fixatives, it has been already assumed that the mechanism by which the DNA macromolecules are converted into polysaccharide might be attributed to function of the Golgi complex (YASUZUMI, *et al.*, 1967).

The site of reduction of the ferricyanide reflects not only the activity of the diaphorase, but is dependent on the specific substrate dehydrogenase. Therefore, it is considered that the electron transfer from substrate to ferricyanide involves at least two enzymatic steps (HESS *et al.*, 1958). The results obtained here show the localization site of enzyme, which is exhibited by dehydrogenase-diaphorase system.

By means of Nitro–BT technique, NACHLAS *et al.* (1958 a, 1958 b) have shown in the kidney and stomach of young adult white rats that whereas

DPN diaphorase has been often restricted to the mitochondria, the TPN diaphorase activity of the corresponding cells of adiacent sections has been typically distributed throughout the cytoplasm in granules too fine to be considered mitochondria.

In several stages of development of atypical spermatids, the conversion of pentose into glucose seems to occur within the smooth–surfaced endoplasmic reticulum or on its outer surfaces as well as on the inner layer of the double-layered nuclear envelope through the pentose-phosphate cycle, on the basis of the results of TPN–dependent 6DPG dehydrogenase. This assumption is supported by the certification of TPPase activity in the Golgi complex in the corresponding cells, since such enzyme is well known as an important enzyme to regulate transketolase activity in pentose-phosphate cycle DE LA HABA, *et al.*, (1955). The pentose–phosphate cycle has already revealed in cancer cell nuclei (SIEBERT, 1961, 1963) and in thymus nuclei (MCEWEN *et al.*, 1963), on the basis of glucose–6–phosphatase dehydrogenase and 6DPG dehydrogenase activities.

Several phosphatase activities such as TPPase, glucose–6–phosphatase, uridine diphosphatase and uridine triphosphatase are sometimes also revealed in the nuclear pore complex of several tissue cells of different animals (YASUZUMI, in press). So far as the nuclear envelope and its pore complex are concerned, the two step method by YASUZUMI–TSUBO (1966) reveals more numerous deposits resulting from enzyme activities than by the one step method according to a mixture of substrate and lead nitrate. However, the two step method is not available for the examination of several enzyme activities in several cell organelles, cell surfaces and intercellular space. Thus, it is assumed that the nuclear envelope and its pore complex may function as pools for orthophosphate resulting from hydrolysis of the phosphate bonds by the enzyme.

At all events, it is interesting that Mg–ATPase activity is more remarkable in the atypical spermatid than in the typical spermatid. The nuclear ATPase may be non-specific nucleoside triphosphatase, as suggested by GEORGIEV (1967), but it is assumed to be one of several permeases, since all the DNA-macromolecules of the atypical spermatid nucleus appear through the pore complex into the cytoplasm.

REFERENCES

ANDERSON W. A., PERSONNE P. and ANDRÉ J. (1968) – *Chemical compartmentalization in helix spermatozoa.* « J. Microscopie », 7, 367–390.

DE DUVE C. (1959) – *The function of intracellular hydrolases.* « Exptl. Cell Res. », Suppl. 7, 169–182.

DE LA HABA G., LEDER G. and RACKER E. (1955) – *Crystalline transketolase from Bakers' yeast: isolation and properties.* « J. Biol. Chem. », 214, 409–426.

DEVLIN T. M. and LEHNINGER A. L. (1956) – *Oxidative phosphorylation by an enzyme complex from extracts of mitochondria.* II. *The span β–hydroxybutyrate to cytochrome C.* « J. Biol. Chem. », 219, 507–518.

ESTABROOK R. W. (1961) – *Studies of oxidative phosphorylation with potassium ferricyanide as electron acceptor.* « J. Biol. Chem. », 236, 3051–3057.

FISCHER F., SIEBERT G. and ADLOFF E. (1959) – *Characterisierung von zwei Adenosintri-phosphatasen in Schweinenieren–Zellkernen.* « Biochem. Z. », 332, 131–150.

GALL J. G. (1961) – *Centriole replication. A study of spermatogenesis in the snail* Viviparus. « J. Biophys. Biochem. Cytol. », 10, 163–193.

GEORGIEV G. P. (1967) – *The nucleus.* In: *Enzyme Cytology.* (ed. ROODYN D. B.), p. 207–102. Acad. Press, London and New York.

GOMORI G. (1941) – *Distribution of acid phosphatase in the tissue under normal and under pathologic conditions.* « Arch. Pathol. », 32, 189–199.

HANSON J., RANDALL J. T. and BALEY S. T. (1952) – *The microstructure of the spermatozoa of the snail* Viviparus. « Exptl. Cell Res. », 3, 65–78.

HESS R., SCARPELLI D. G. and PEARSE A.G.E. (1958) – *The cytochemical localization of oxidative enzymes.* II. *Pyridine nucleotide-linked dehydrogenases.* « J. Biophys. Biochem. Cytol. », 4, 753–760.

HOLT S. J. (1959) – *Factors governing the validity of staining methods for enzymes, and their bearing on the Gomori acid phosphatase technique.* « Exptl. Cell Res. », Suppl. 7, 1–27.

ISHIZAKI T. and KATO K. (1958) – *The fine structure of atypical spermatozoa of the pond snail* Viviparus malleatus. « Zool. Magaz. », 67, 286–294.

KARNOVSKY M. J. (1964) – *The localization of cholinesterase activity in rat cardiac muscle by electron microscopy.* « J. Cell Biol. », 23, 217–232.

KARNOVSKY M. J. and ROOTS L. (1964) – *A « direct–coloring » technique method for cholinesterase.* « J. Histochem. Cytochem. », 12, 219–221.

LEBLOND C. P., GLEGG R. E. and EIDINGER D. (1957) – *Presence of carbohydrates with free 1,2–glycol groups in sites stained by the periodic acid–Schiff technique.* « J. Histochem. Cytochem. », 5, 445–458.

LELOIR L. F. and CARDINI C. E. (1957) – *Biosythesis of glycogen from uridine diphosphate glucose.* « J. Am. Chem. Soc. », 79, 6340–6341.

LELOIR L. F., OVAVARRIÀ J. M., GOLDENBERG S. H. and CARMINATTI H. (1959) – *Biosynthesis of glycogen from uridine diphosphate glucose.* « Arch. Biochem. Biophys. », 81, 508–520.

LUFT I. H. (1961) – *Improvements in epoxy resin embedding methods.* « J. Biophys. Biochem. Cytol. », 9, 409–414.

MCEWEN B. S., ALLFREY V. G. and MIRSKY A. E. (1963). – *Studies on energy–yielding reactions in thymus nuclei.* II. *Pathways of aerobic carbohydrate catabolism.* « J. Biol. Chem. », 238, 2571–2578.

MEEK G. A. and BRADBURY S. (1963) – *Localization of thiamine pyrophosphatase activity in the Golgi apparatus of a mollusc,* Helix aspersa. « J. Cell Biol. », 18, 73–85.

MEYER K. (1955) – *Problems of classification.* In: *Polysaccharides in Biology.* (ed. SPRINGER G. F.), p. 31–51. – Corlies, Macy and Co., New York.

MUNCH–PETERSEN A., KALCKAR H. M., CUTOLO E. and SMITH E. E. B. (1953) – *Uridyl transferases and the formation of uridine triphosphate. Enzymic production of uridine triphosphate: Uridine diphosphoglucose pyrophosphorylysis.* « Nature », 172, 1036–1037.

NACHLAS M. M., WALKER D. G. and SELIGMAN A. M. (1958 a) – *A histochemical method for the demonstration of diphosphopyridine nucleotide diaphorase.* « J. Biophys. Biochem. Cytol. », 4, 29–38.

NACHLAS M. M., WALKER D. G. and SELIGMAN A. M. (1958 b) – *The histochemical localization of triphopshopyridine nucleotide diaphorase.* « J. Biophys. Biochem. Cytol. », 4, 467–474.

NEUFELD E. F., GINSBURG V., PUTMAN E. W., FANSHIER D. and HASSID W. Z. (1957) – *Formation and interconversion of sugar nucleotides by plant extracts.* « Arch Biochem. Biophys. », 69, 602–616.

NOVIKOFF A. B. and GOLDFISCHER S. (1961) – *Nucleosidediphosphatase activity in the Golgi apparatus and its usefulness for cytological studies.* « Proc. Nat. Acad. Sci. (Wash.) », 47, 802–810.

OGAWA K., SAITO T. and MAYAHARA H. (1968) – *The site of ferricyanide reduction by reductase within mitochondria as studied by electron microscopy.* « J. Histochem. Cytochem. », 16, 49–57.

PRESSMAN B. C. (1955) – *Oxidative phosphorylation with ferricyanide as terminal electron acceptor.* « Biochem. Biophys. Acta », 17, 273–274.

RAMBOURG A. and LEBLOND C. P. (1967) – *Electron microscope observations on the carbohydrate–rich cell coat present at the surface of the cells in the rat.* « J. Cell Biol. », 32, 27–53.

REYNOLDS E. S. (1963) – *The use of lead citrate at high* pH *as an electron opaque stain in electron microscopy.* « J. Cell Biol. », 17, 208–212.

SABATINI D. D., BENSCH K. and BARRNETT R. J. (1963) – *Cytochemistry and electron microscopy.The preservation of cellular ultrastructure and enzymatic activity by aldehyde fixation.* « J. Cell Biol. », 17, 19–58.

SELIGMAN A. M. and MANHEIMER L. H. (1949) – *A new method for the histochemical demonstration of acid phosphatase.* « J. Nat. Cancer Inst. », 9, 427–434.

SIEBERT G. (1961) – *Enzyme und Substrate der Glykolyse in isolierten Zellkernen.* « Biochem. Z. », 334, 369–387.

SIEBERT G. (1963) – *Enzymes of cancer nuclei.* « Exptl. Cell Res. », Suppl. 9, 389–417.

SINGER T. P. and KEARNEY E. B. (1957) – *Determination of succinic dehydrogenase activity.* In: *Methods of Biochemical Analysis.* (ed. GLICK D.), Vol. 4, 307–333. Interscience Publishers, Inc., New York.

SINGH K. and MATHUR R. S. (1968 a) – *A comparative study on the localization of certain enzyme activities in the testes of the Indian desert gerbil and the house shrew.* « Acta Anat. », 69, 358–365.

SINGH K. and MATHUR R. S. (1968 b) – *Histochemical demonstration of certain testicular enzymes of the Indian desert gerbil* Meriones hurrianae *Jerdon and their response to unilateral cryptorchidism.* « Histochem. », 15, 204–211.

SPIRO R. G. (1963) – *Glycoproteins: Structure, metabolism and biology.* « New Eng. J. Med. », 269, 566–573 and 616–621.

STERN H., ALLFREY, V., MIRSKY A. E. and SAETREN H. (1952) – *Some enzymes of isolated nuclei.* « J. Gen. Physiol. », 35, 559–578.

THIÉRY J.–P. (1968) – *Mise en evidence de muco – et de glycoproteines dans l'appareil de Golgi.* Fourth Region. Conf. Electron Microscopy, Rome, 1968 (ed. BOCCIARELLI D. S.), Vol. 2, 59–60. Tipografia Poliglotta Vaticana, Roma.

TOCHIMOTO T. (1967) – *Comparative histochemical study on the dimorphic spermatozoa of the prosobranchia with special reference to polysaccharides.* « Sci. Rep. Tokyo Kyoiku Daigaku », Sec. B., 13, 75–109.

TSUBO L., LEE K. J., ENOMOTO Y., SAKAMOTO H., AOYAMA N., ASAI T. and YASUZUMI F. (1968) – *Electron microscope studies on ATPase activities in the nuclear pore complex of several animal tissue cells.* « J. Nara Med. Ass. », 19, 429–438.

VAN HEYNINGEN H. E. (1965) – *Correlated light and electron microscope observations on glycoprotein-containing globules in the follicular cells of the thyroid gland of the rat.* « J. Histochem. Cytochem. », 13, 286–295.

VILLAR–PALASI C. and LARNER J. (1960) – *Uridinediphosphate glucose pyrophosphrylase from skeletal muscle.* « Arch. Biochem. Biophys. », 86, 61–66.

WACHSTEIN M. and MEISEL E. (1957) – *Histochemistry of hepatic phosphatases at a physiologic* pH. « Am. J. Clin. Pathol. », 27, 13–23.

WATSON M. L. (1958) – *Staining of tissue sections for electron microscopy with heavy metals.* « J. Biophys. Biochem. Cytol. », 4, 475–478.

YASUZUMI G. (1962) – *Spermatogenesis in animals as revealed by electron microscopy.* XII. *Light and electron microscope studies on spermiogenesis of* Cipangopaludina malleata *Reeve.* J. Ultrastruct. Res. », 7, 488–503.

YASUZUMI G. (1964) – *Spermatogenesisis in animals as revealed by electron microscopy.* X. *The fine structure and function of endoplasmic reticulum and of peculiar bodies appearing in atypical maturing spermatids and nutritive cells of* Cipangopaludina malleata *Reeve.* « Am. J. Anat. », 115, 431–472.

YASUZUMI G., Unpublished data.

YASUZUMI G., LEE K. J., FUKUI H. and YOSHIDA M. (1967) – *Spermatogenesis in animals as revealed by electron microscopy.* XVII. *The fine structure of atypical spermatid cytoplasm of the pond snail with particular references to the site of hydrolytic breakdown of nucleic acids.* « Z. Zellforsch. », 80, 353–369.

YASUZUMI G. and TANAKA H. (1958) – *Spermatogenesis in animals as revealed by electron microscopy.* VI. *Researches on the spermatozoondimorphism in a pond snail,* Cipangopaludina malleata. « J. Biophys. Biochem. Cytol. », 4, 621–632.

YASUZUMI G., TANAKA H. and TEZUKA O. (1960) – *Spermatogenesis in animals as revealed by electron microscopy.* VIII. *Relation between the nutritive cells and the developing spermatids in a pond snail,* Cipangopaludina malleata *Reeve.* « J. Biophys. Biochem. Cytol. », 7, 499–504.

YASUZUMI G., NAKAI Y., TSUBO I., YASUDA M. and SUGIOKA T. (1967) – *The fine structure of nuclei as revealed by electron microscopy.* IV. *The intranuclear inclusion formation in Leydig cells of aging human testes.* « Exptl. Cell Res. », 45, 261–276.

YASUZUMI G. and TSUBO I. (1966) – *The fine structure of nuclei as revealed by electron microscopy.* III. *Adenosine triphosphatase activity in the pores of nuclear envelope of mouse choroid plexus epithelial cells.* « Exptl. Cell Res. », 43, 281–292.

YASUZUMI G., TSUBO I. and MATSUZAKI W. (1970) – *Electron microscope observations on the chemical component of the sheath of middle piece of atypical spermatozoa of the pond snail,* Cipangopaludina malleata *Reeve.* « Arch. histol. jap. » (in press).

YASUZUMI G., TSUBO I., OKADA K., TERAWAKI A. and ENOMOTO Y. (1968) – *The fine structure of nuclei as revealed by electron microscopy.* V. *Intranuclear inclusion bodies in in hepatic parenchymal cells in cases of serum hepatitis.* « J. Ultrastruct. Res. », 23, 321–332.

EXPLANATION OF FIGURES

Figs. 1–5. – Sections of the pond snail testis incubated for acid phosphatase.

Fig. 1. – Reaction product resulting from enzyme activity is found in the interchromatinic foci of the nucleus (*N*) and in the Golgi complex (*GC*) of an early atypical spermatid. ×28,000.

Fig. 2. – A more advanced atypical spermatid nucleus is reduced in its volume and amount of chromatin elements. Vesicles (*V*) contain an amorphous material of different dencities. Dense deposits showing acid phosphatase activity can be seen in the interchromatinic foci of the nucleus (*N*). ×38,000

Fig. 3. – The atypical spermatid nucleus (*FN*) of low density is flattened at a late stage of development. Fine dense deposits of acid phosphatase are no longer visible in such a flattened nucleus (*FN*), but the deposits can be seen in the developing tail filaments (*TF*). Dense deposits may bee seen at the part of the nuclear envelope and on the proximal portion of the tail filaments. Several vesicles (*V*) containing one to four dense granules appear in the cytoplasm. An early atypical spermatid appears at the upper side of the field, showing dense deposits of acid phosphatase activity in the nucleus (*N*). ×36,000.

Fig. 4. – Longitudinal section through the atypical spermatid tail. Reaction product is present between the tail filaments which are enveloped by the sheath consisting of dense bodies, each of them being surrounded by a apparently single-layered membrane. Mitochondria (*M*) are often encountered between the tail filaments. ×42,000.

Fig. 5. – No acid phosphatase activity can be seen in the typical spermatid nucleus (*N*). A part of the nebenkern (*NK*) is visible in the vicinity of the nucleus (*N*). ×54,000.

Fig. 6. – Section of a mouse liver, starved for 24 hours, subsequently refed for one hour 50% glucose, and incubated in the standard medium for UDPG–pyrophosphorylase. Reaction product is present in the endoplasmic reticulum localized in an area surrounded by mitochondria (*M*) and smooth–surfaced vesicles (*V*), but absent in the Golgi complex (*GC*). ×46,000.

Fig. 7. – Similar material as in Fig. 6, incubated in UTP as substrate. Deposits of final reaction product appear within the nuclear envelope as well as in the rough-surfaced endoplasmic reticulum at random. *N* indicates a part of the nucleus. ×50,000.

Figs. 8 and 9. – Sections from glutaraldehyde-fixed testis of the pond snail incubated in the standard medium for UDPG–pyrophosphorylase.

Fig. 8. – Two atypical spermatids demonstrate deposits of final reaction product in the lamellae and fine vesicles of the Golgi complex (*GC*). ×30,000.

Fig. 9. – Deposits of reaction product (arrows) appear mainly within the paired membranes of the Golgi complex in the more advanced atypical spermatid in which the endoplasmic reticulum is filled with a homogeneous material of intermediate density. ×46,000.

Figs. 10 and 11. – Tangential sections through the atypical spermatids incubated for Mg–ATPase activity according to Yasuzumi–Tsubo's procedure.

Fig. 10. – The nuclear envelope and especially its pore complex demonstrate the Mg–ATPase activity. ×39,000.

Fig. 11. – High power electron micrograph of the nuclear pore complex showing Mg-ATPase activity. A dense central deposit surrounded by a clear zone and numerous deposits situated peripherally are clearly differentiated in the pore complex marked by the arrow. Such differentiation is not always possible in other pore complex. ×62,000.

Fig. 12. – An atypical spermatid incubated in a control medium for Mg–ATPase. Note that the nuclear pore complex (arrow) does not demonstrate dense deposits of lead phosphate. The nucleus (*N*) contains chromatin elements in a small amount. The smooth-surfaced endoplasmic reticulum appears roughly in a parallel arrangement. ×60,000.

Figs. 13–16. – Sections of atypical spermatids of the pond snail incubated for TPN–dependent 6DPG–dehydrogenase.

Figs. 13 and 14. – Early atypical spermatid nuclei (*N*) contain a few chromatin materials. Such cells show deposits of final product on the inner layer of the double–layered nuclear envelope and within the smooth-surfaced endoplasmic reticulum or on its outer surfaces. ×46,000.

Fig. 15. – A small portion of an atypical spermatid in a more advanced stage demonstrates dense deposits within the smooth-surfaced endoplasmic reticulum running roughly in a parallel arrangement, and linear deposits on its outer surfaces. ×46,000.

Fig. 16. – Several patterns of deposits of final product, linear (*L*) or finely distributed (*FD*) or irregularly shaped precipitates (*P*), appear within the nuclear envelope or closely related to its inner layer of the navicular nucleus (*N*) in a late maturation stage. Developing tail filaments (*TF*) appear attached closely to the nucleus (*N*). ×44,000.

Fig. 17. – Section of an atypical spermatid incubated in a control medium for TPN–dependent 6DPG–dehydrogenase shows a shrunken nucleus (*N*), mitochondria (*M*), vesicles (*V*) containing one to four dense granules, and developing tail filaments (*TF*), but no reaction product can be seen in any parts. ×23,000.

Fig. 18. – The Golgi complex in an atypical spermatid incubated for TPPase activity. Remarkably dense deposits (large arrow) and finely distributed deposits (small arrows) of lead phosphate are found in the cisternae of the Golgi complex. ×56,000.

Discussion

NELSON. – Have you done any biochemical analyses to substantiate the beautiful histochemical studies?

YASUZUMI. – Isolated nuclei were biochemically analyzed by ion exchangecolumn chromatography to confirm the histochemical results.

PALLINI. – Is it possible to detect histochemically a hydrolytic enzyme acting on DNA?

YASUZUMI. – It is possible to detect histochemically alkaline DNAase, but it was not possible in the atypical spermatid nuclei of the present material. However, it was found in the nutritive cell nuclei of the similar material.

PALLINI. – Which is the fate of the purine and pyrimidine bases, which are only slightly soluble in water?

YASUZUMI. – It is impossible histochemically to detect the fate of free purine and pyrimidine bases in the presente technique.

G. Yasuzumi et al. – *Electron microscope studies on atypical spermatids of Pond Snail* Cipangopaludina malleata *Reeve, under consideration of conversion of* DNA *into polysaccharide.*

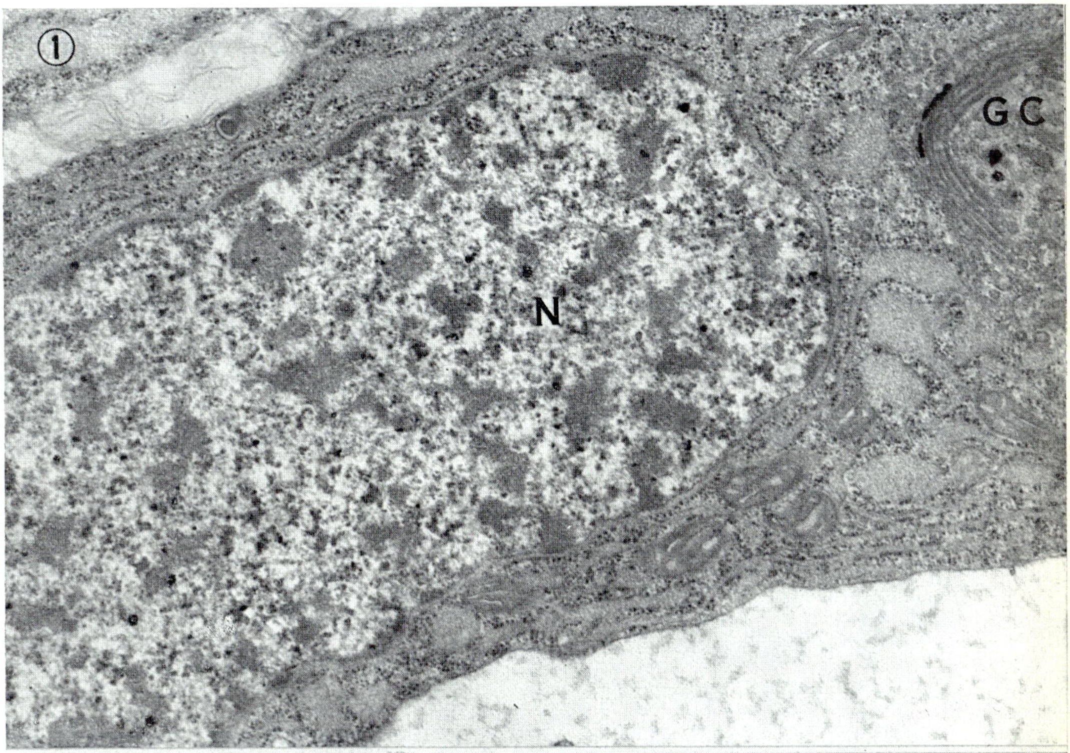

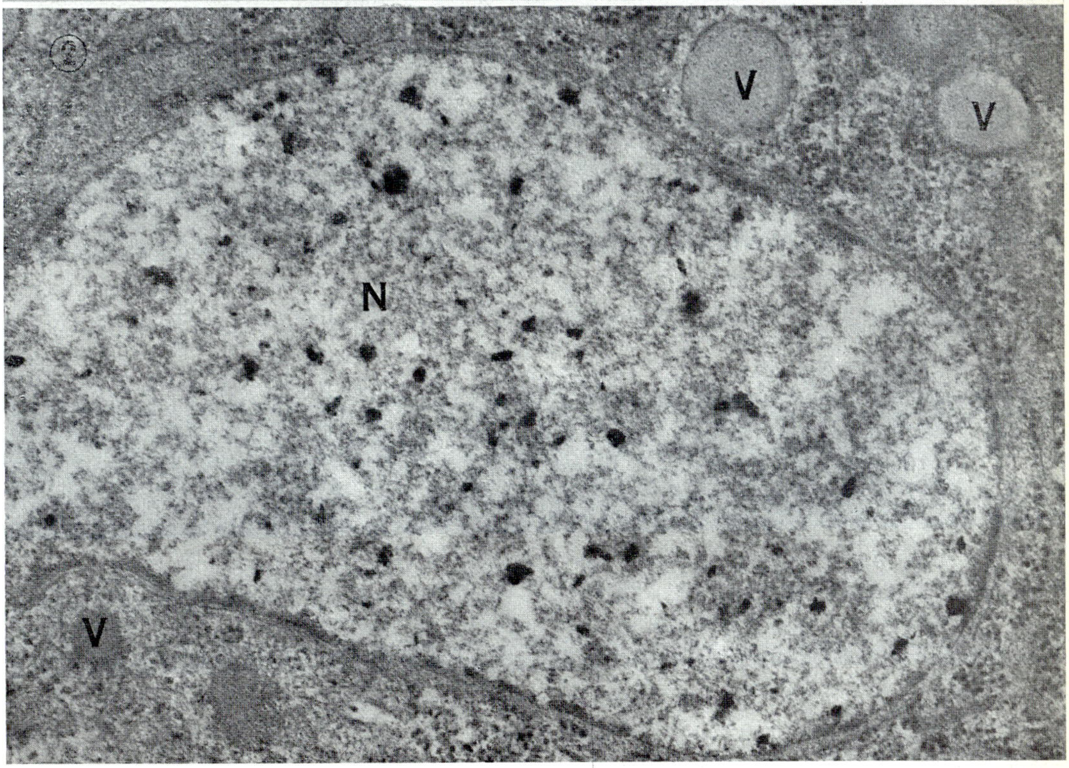

G. Yasuzumi et al. – *Electron microscope studies on atypical spermatids of Pond Snail* Cipangopaludina malleata *Reeve, under consideration of conversion of* DNA *into polysaccharide.*

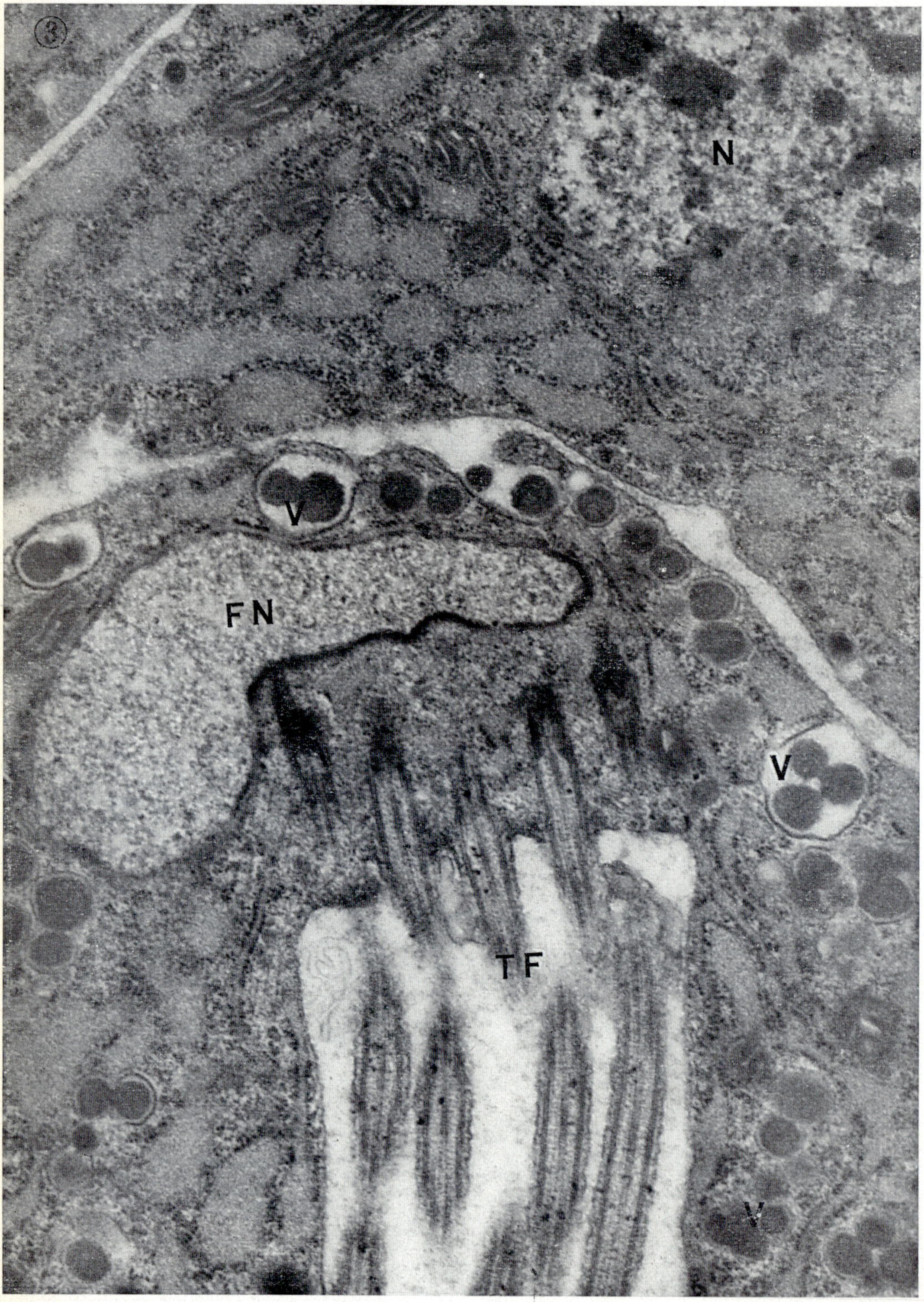

G. YASUZUMI et AL. – *Electron microscope studies on atypical spermatids of Pond Snail* Cipangopaludina malleata *Reeve, under consideration of conversion of* DNA *into polysaccharide.*

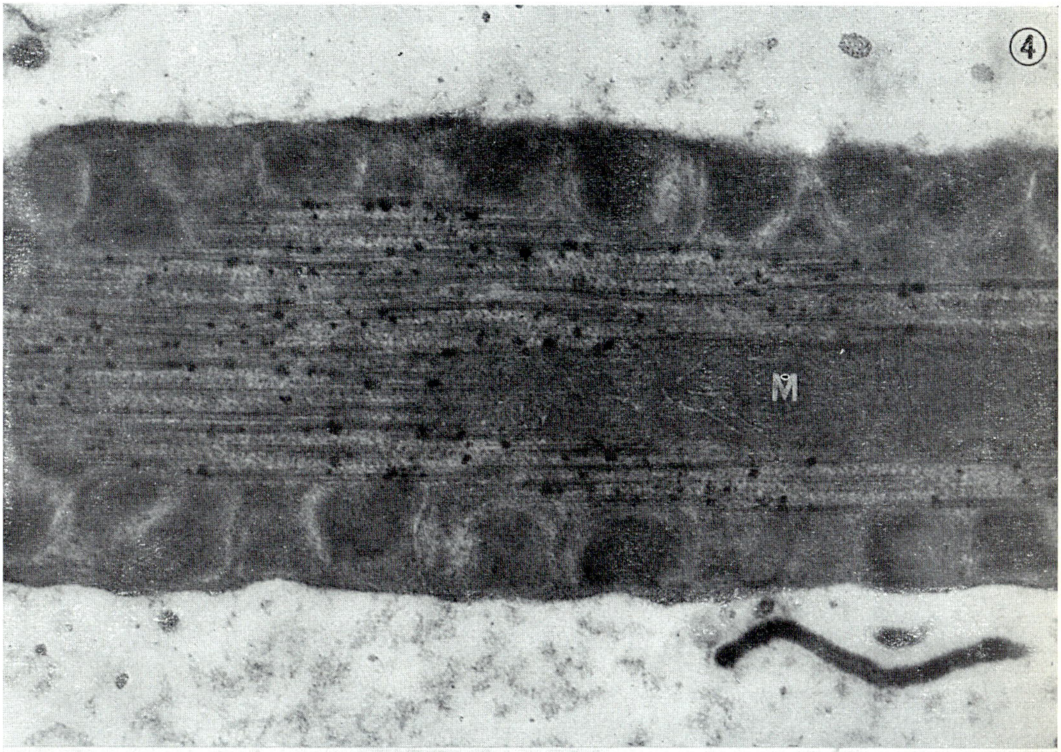

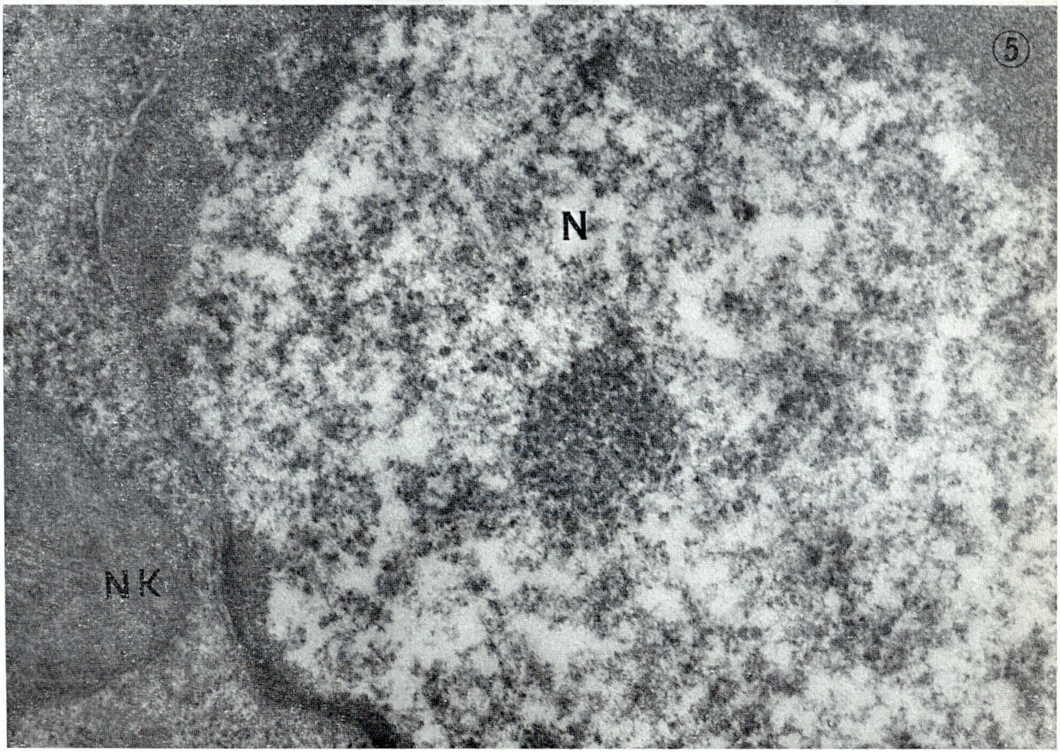

G. YASUZUMI et AL. – *Electron microscope studies on atypical spermatids of Pond Snail* Cipangopaludina malleata *Reeve, under consideration of conversion of* DNA *into polysaccharide.*

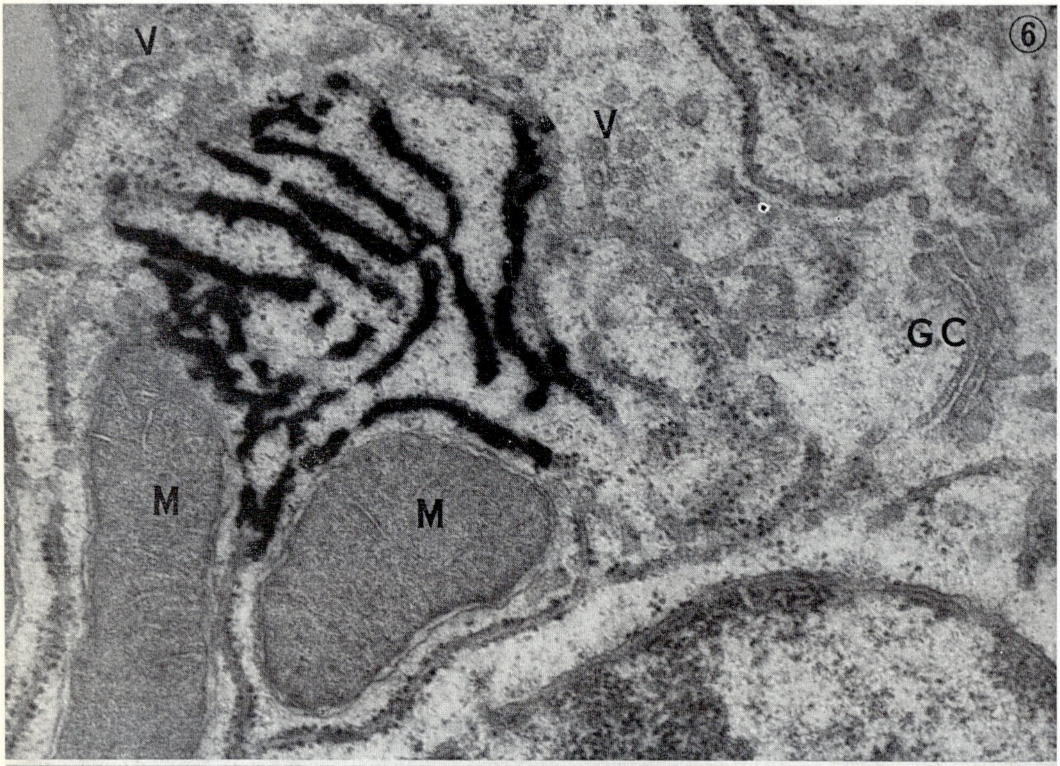

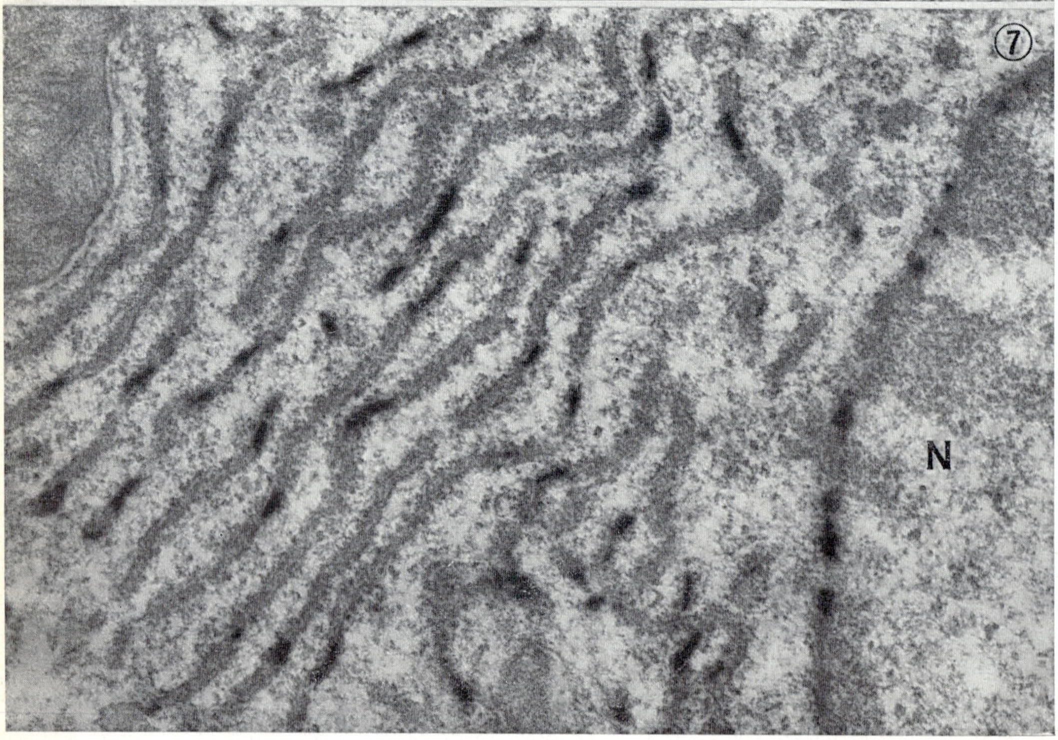

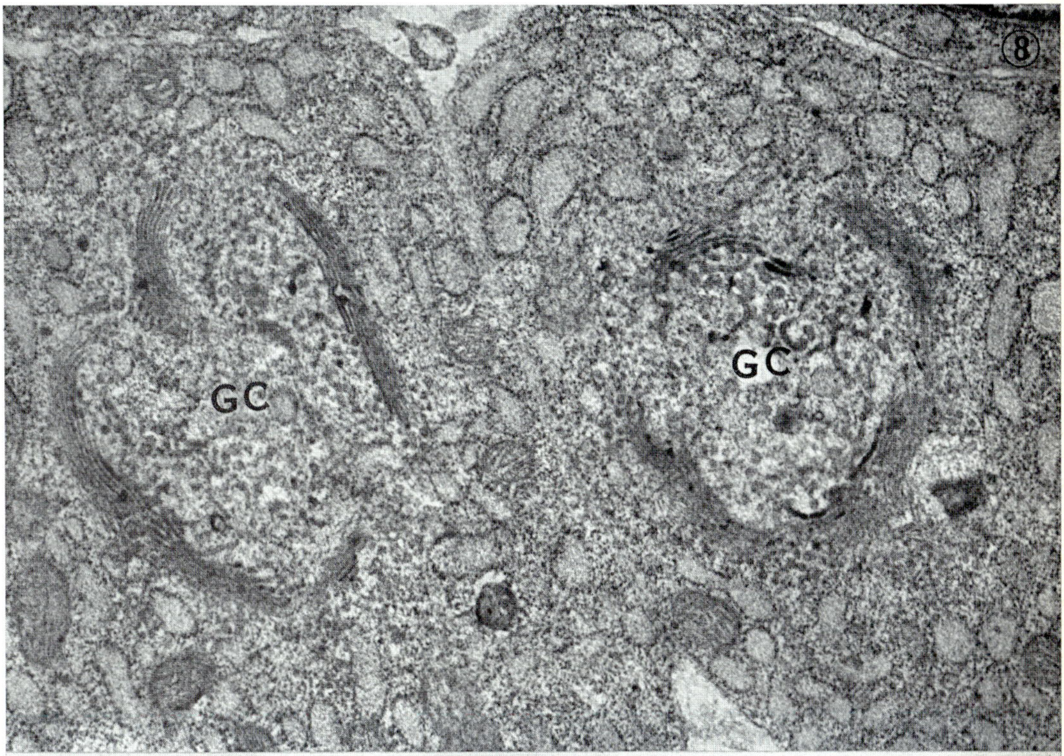
8
GC
GC

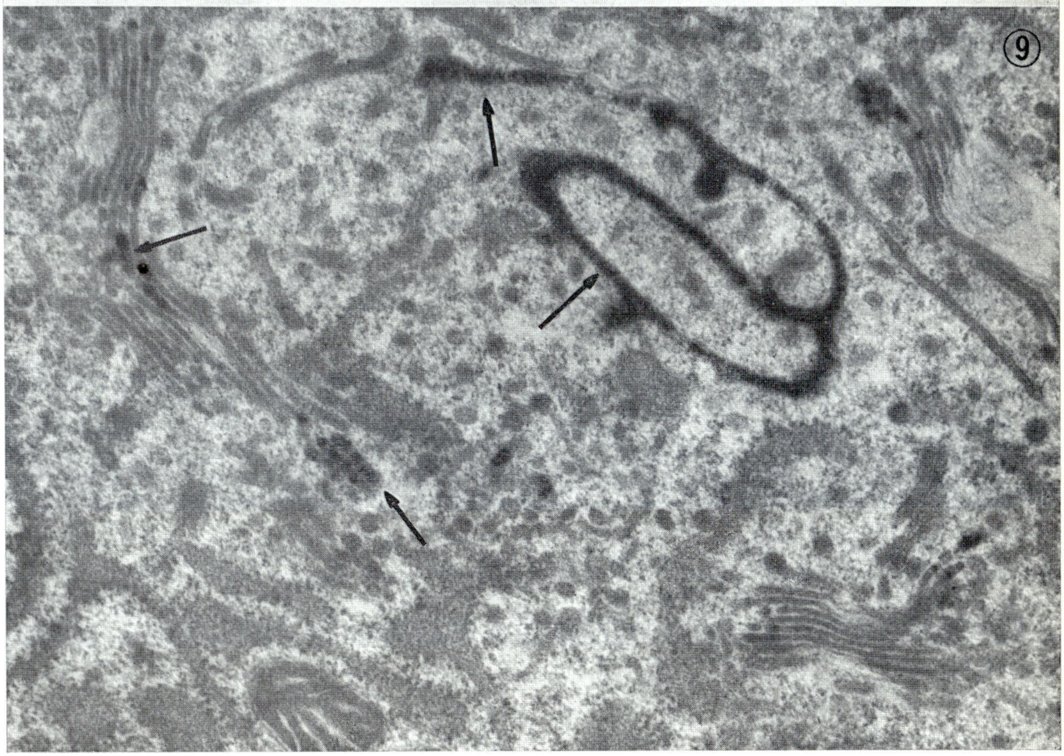
9

G. Yasuzumi et al. – *Electron microscope studies on atypical spermatids of Pond Snail* Cipangopaludina malleata *Reeve, under consideration of conversion of* DNA *into polysaccharide.*

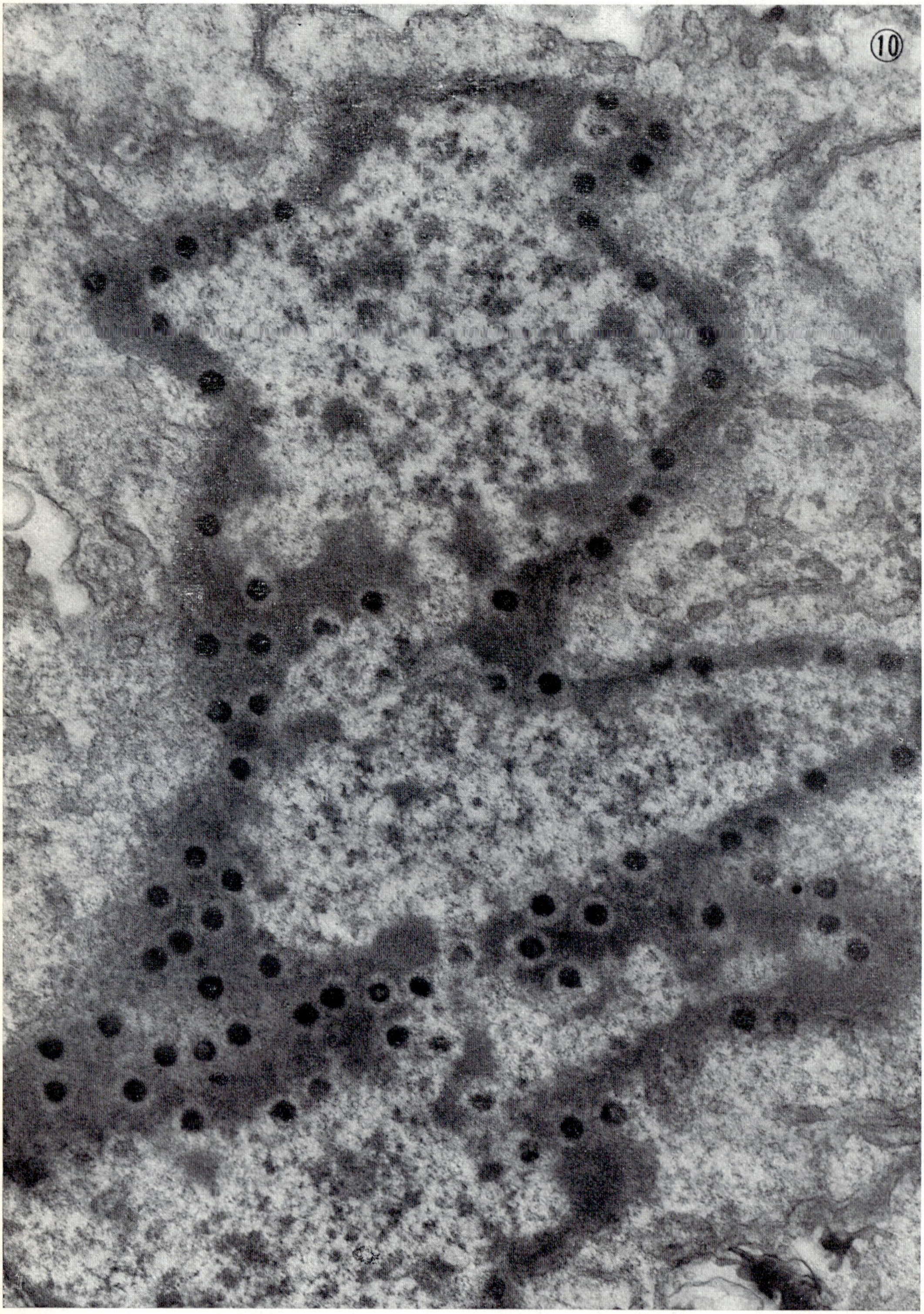

G. Yasuzumi et al. – *Electron microscope studies on atypical spermatids of Pond Snail* Cipangopaludina malleata *Reeve, under consideration of conversion of* DNA *into polysaccharide.*

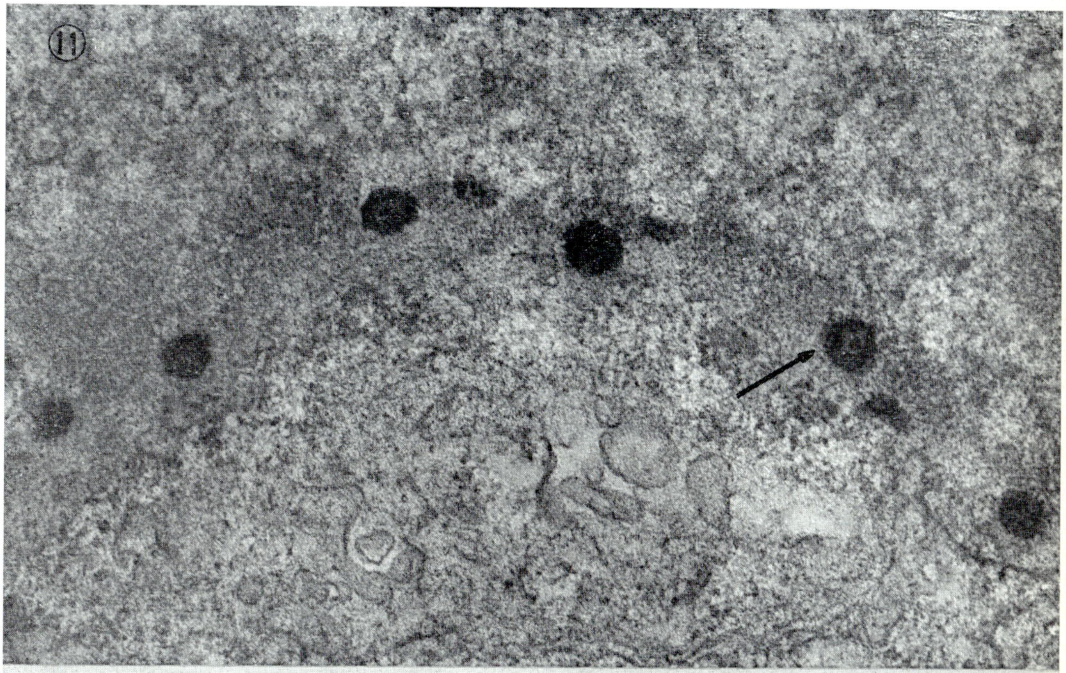

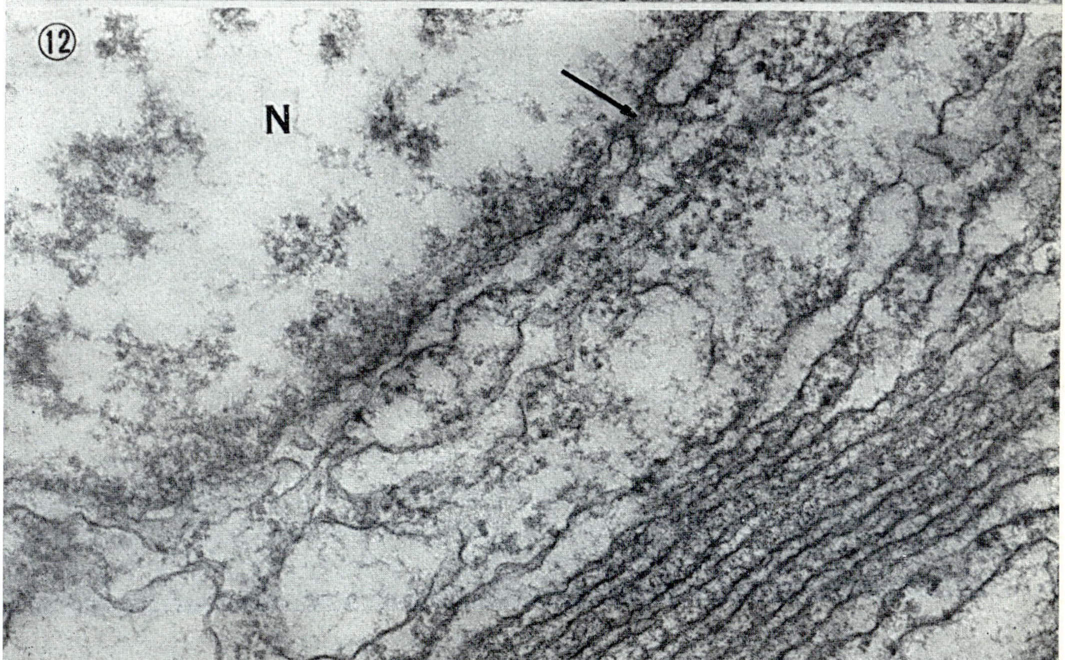

G. Yasuzumi et al. – *Electron microscope studies on atypical spermatids of Pond Snail* Cipangopaludina malleata *Reeve, under consideration of conversion of* DNA *into polysaccharide.*

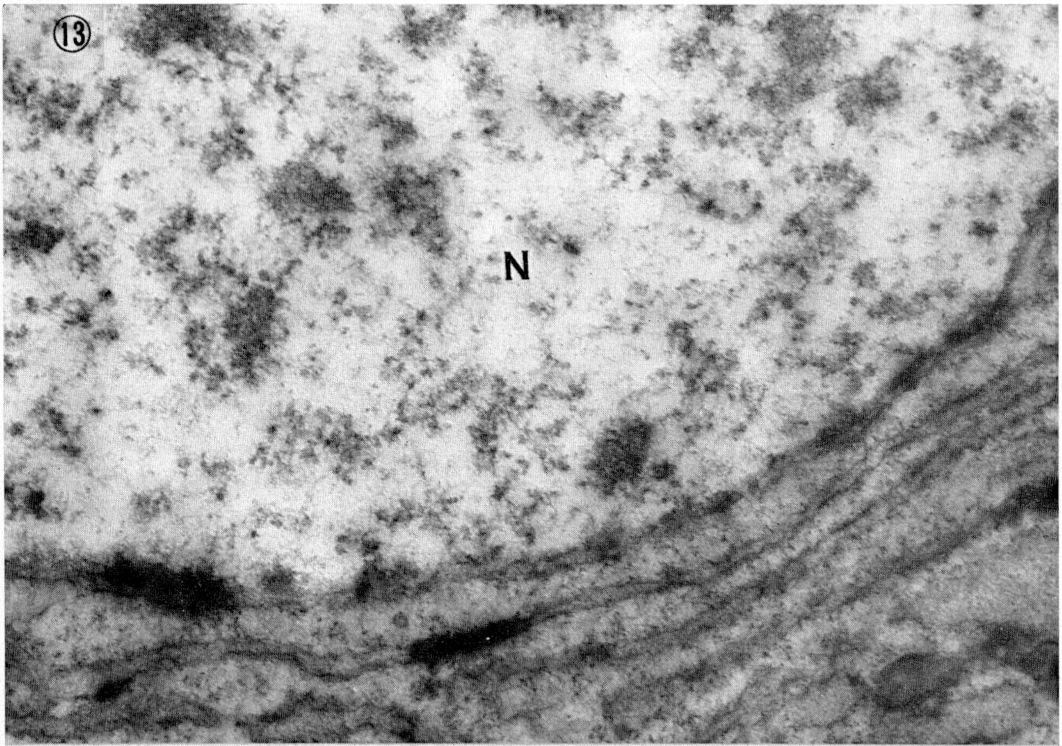

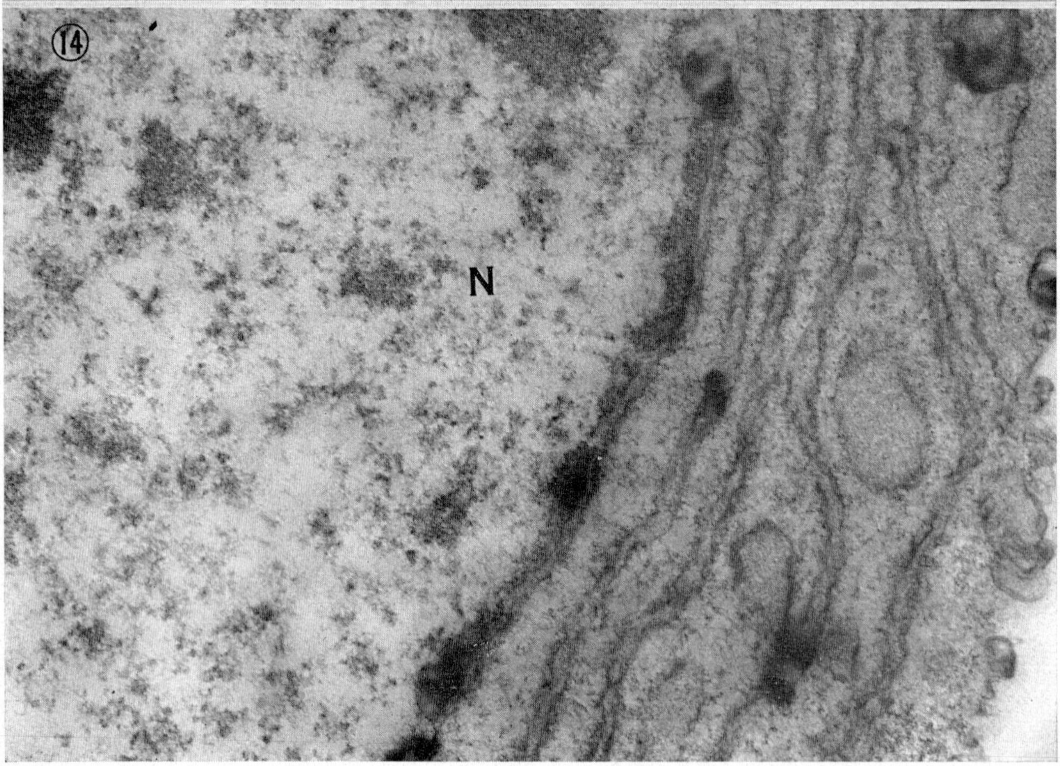

G. Yasuzumi et al. - *Electron microscope studies on atypical spermatids of Pond Snail* Cipangopaludina malleata *Reeve, under consideration of conversion of* DNA *into polysaccharide.*

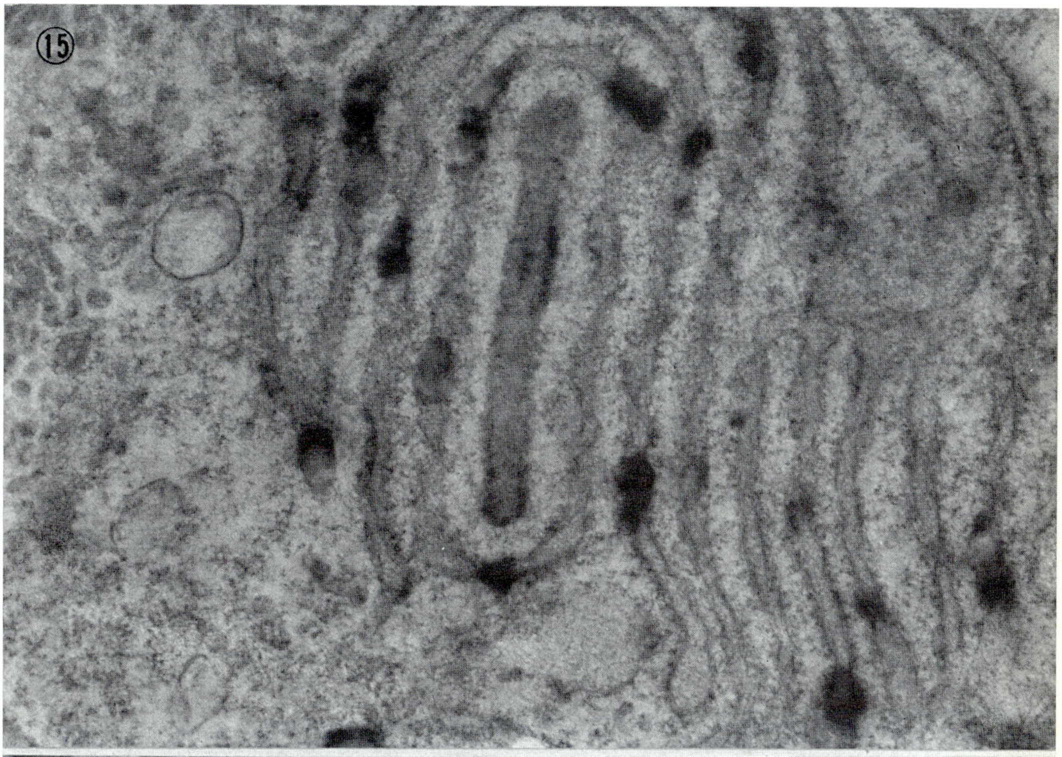

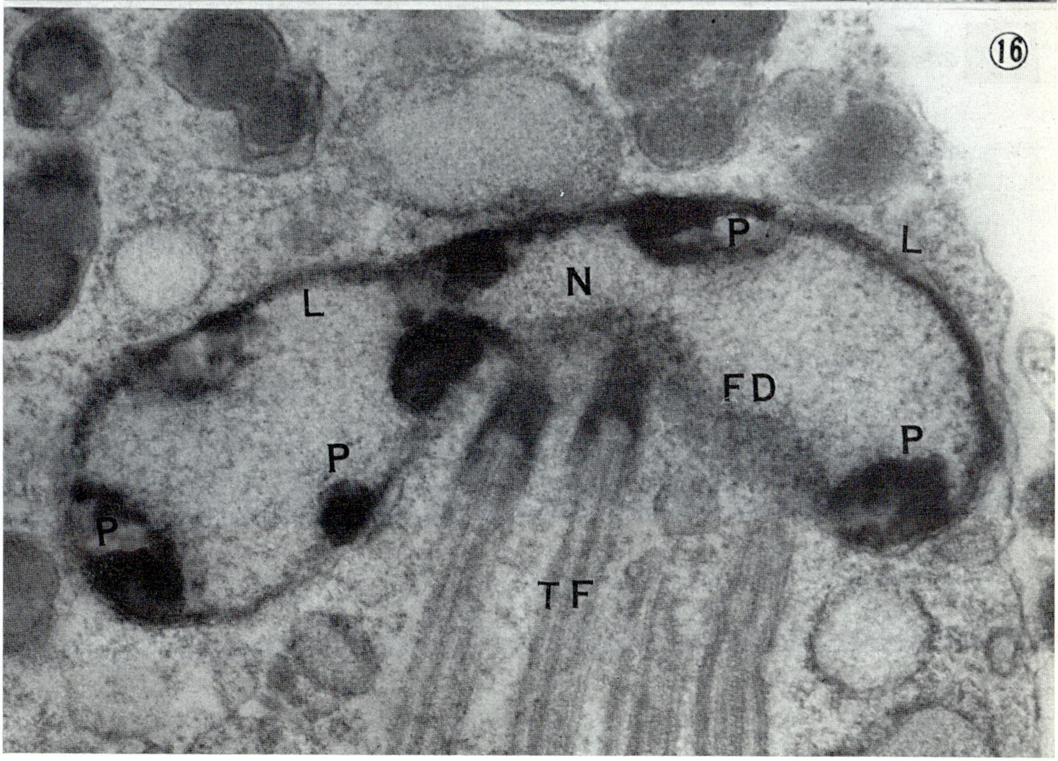

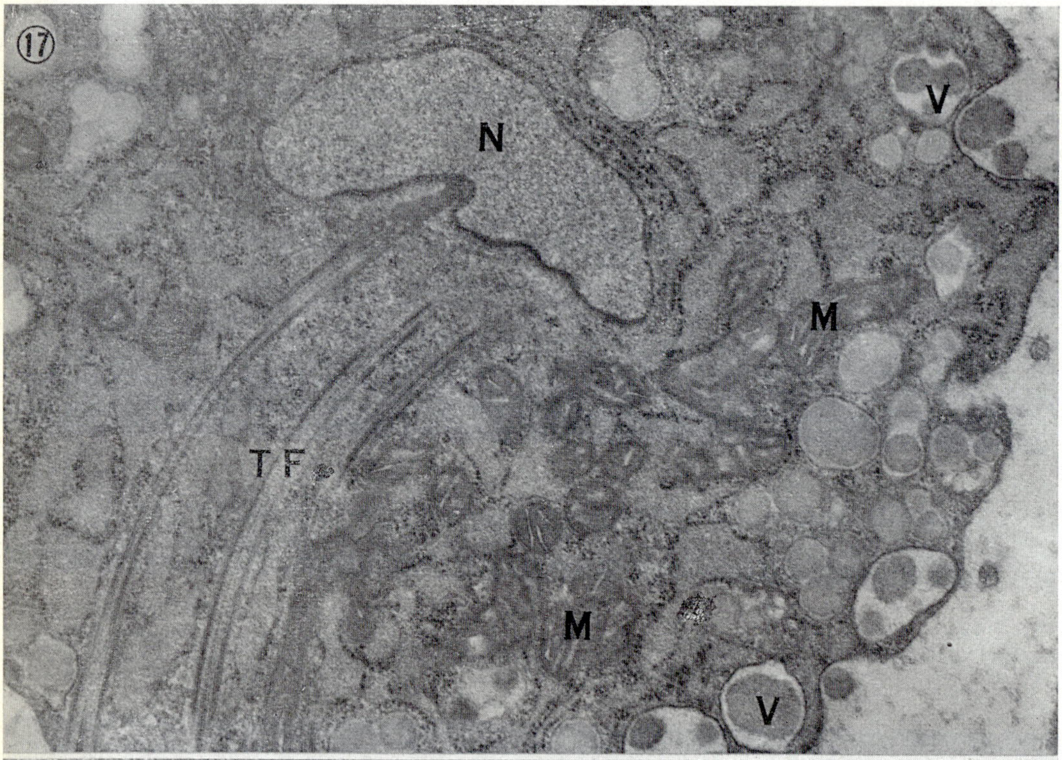
17
N
V
M
TF
M
V

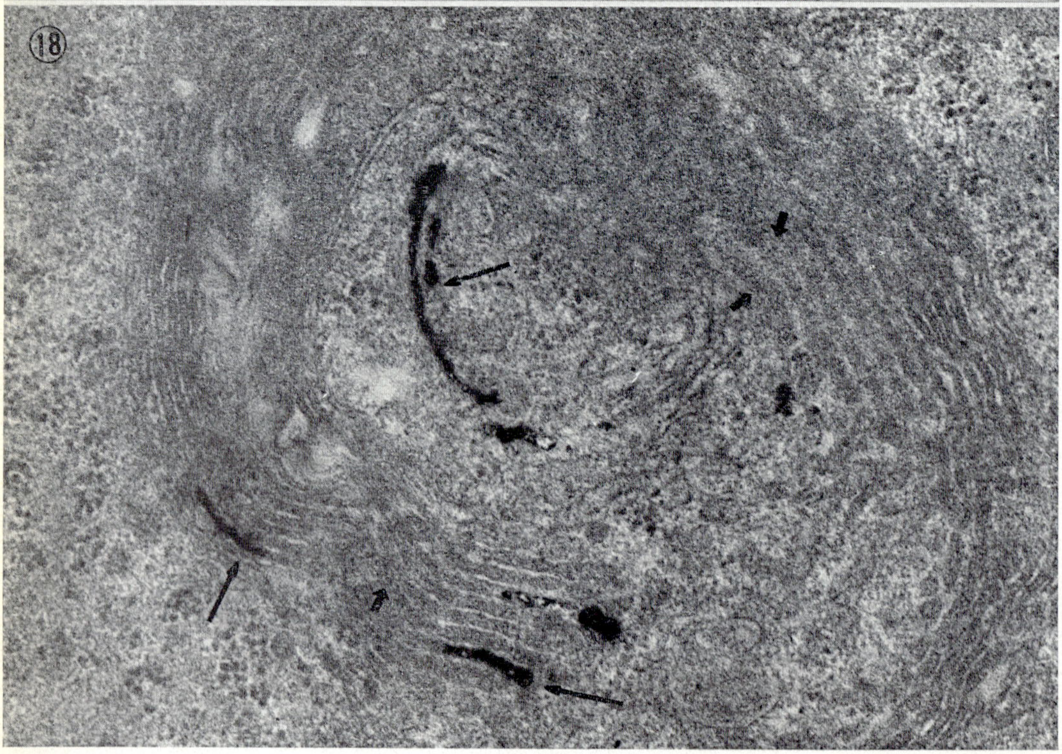
18

Pierre Favard (*) and Jean André (**)

THE MITOCHONDRIA OF SPERMATOZOA

SUMMARY. — The repartition and fine structure of the mitochondria in sperm cells are reviewed. A few groups of animals have aflagellate sperm with the mitochondria dispersed at random in the cytoplasm, or flagellate sperm with the mitochondria located in the nuclear area. In most of the animal groups, the mitochondria are clumped behind the nucleus, localized in the so called middle piece. In this case, the mitochondria may have simply gathered in this region with no structural modification, or have fused and spiralized with more or less extensive modifications. The climax in this remodelling is reached by Insects and Gastropods.

As a whole, the characteristics of sperm mitochondria are less an image of the Systematics than that of the fertilization procedures. Sperm are very highly specialized cells for which survival in the medium, where they are released or stored, and potency to reach the egg have played the main role in their modelling during evolution.

RIASSUNTO. — Viene studiata la ripartizione e la fine struttura dei mitocondri nelle cellule spermatiche. Pochi gruppi di animali hanno spermi aflagellati con i mitocondri dispersi irregolarmente nel citoplasma, o spermi flagellati con i mitocondri situati nell'area nucleare. Nella maggior parte dei gruppi animali, i mitocondri sono raggruppati dietro il nucleo, localizzati nel così detto « middle piece ». In questo caso, i mitocondri possono essere semplicemente riuniti in questa regione senza nessuna modificazione strutturale, o essere fusi e spiralizzati con modificazioni più o meno estensive. Il culmine di questo rimaneggiamento è raggiunto dagli Insetti e dai Gasteropodi.

Nell'insieme, le caratteristiche dei mitocondri spermatici sono più importanti per i processi di fecondazione che non per la sistematica. Gli spermatozoi sono cellule altamente specializzate per cui la sopravvivenza nel mezzo in cui essi sono rilasciati o conservati, e la potenza per raggiungere l'uovo hanno giocato il ruolo più importante nel loro modellamento durante l'evoluzione.

With the exception of the Cestodes, Trematodes, Coccids and primitive Decapods (Bonsdorff and Telkka, 1965; Rosario, 1964; Hendelberg 1962; Gresson and Perry, 1961; Robison, 1966; Brown and Metz, 1967) all animal spermatozoa contain mitochondria. From a morphological point of view, comparative spermatology shows a great number of variations in mitochondria among the different phyla and even at the level of different species. From a physiological point of view, another variability exists, which comes from the different origin and nature of the oxidizable substrates that

(*) Laboratoire de Biologie Cellulaire P.C.E.M., Faculté des Sciences, Paris, France.
(**) Laboratoire de Biologie Cellulaire, Faculté des Sciences, Orsay, France.

the spermatozoa can utilize. Finally, from an evolutionary point of view, certain tendencies can be drawn from these variations in structure and physiology. Our purpose here is to summarize the main lines in the morphology, the physiology and the evolution of the sperm cell mitochondria.

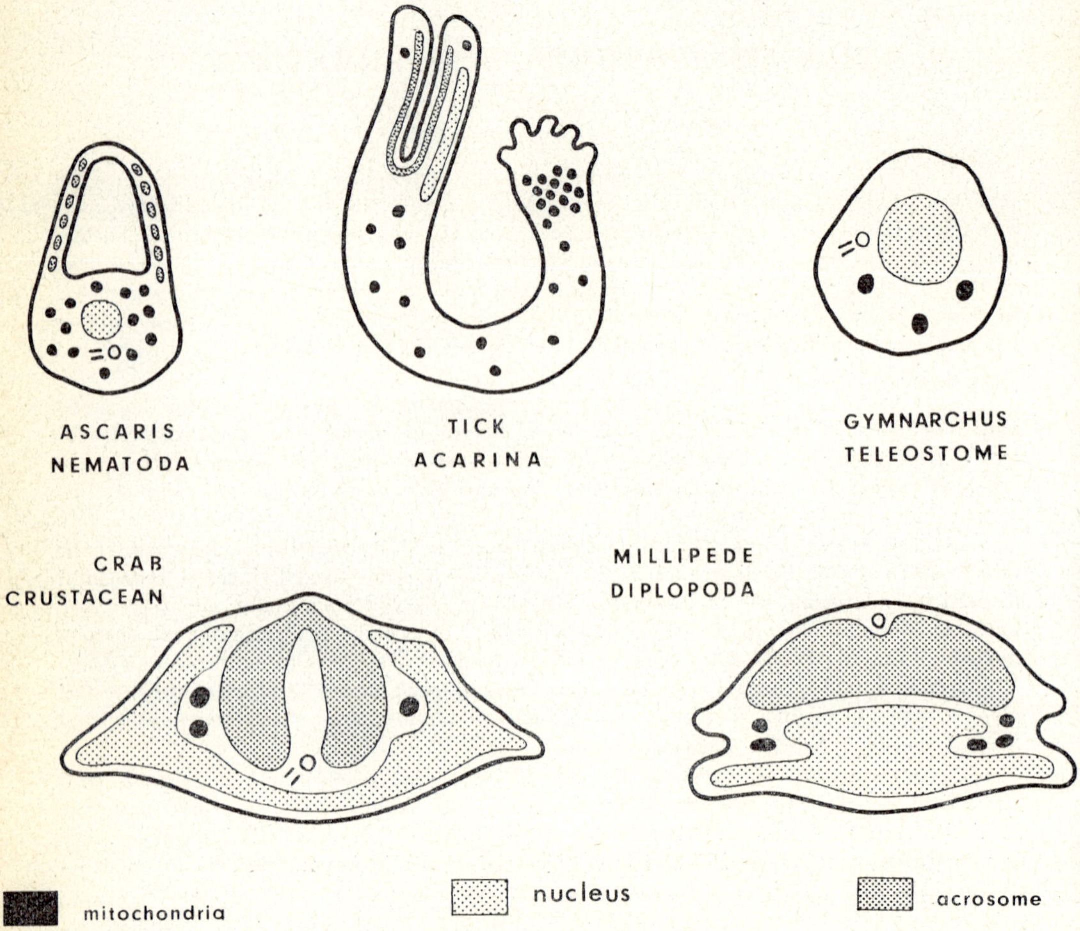

Diagram 1. – Sperm cells with mitochondria dispersed at random in the cytoplasm. *Ascaris* after Favard (1961); Tick after Reger (1963); *Gymnarchus* after Mattei (1969); Crab after Pochon–Masson (1968); Millipede after Grassé *et al.* (1956 b).

I. Morphology

If we examine the ultrastructure of their mitochondria, the various spermatozoa of the animal kingdom can be separated into two classes: first, those in which the general architecture of the normal mitochondrion persists intact or with only minor modifications; second, those in which the mitochondria have been transformed into a mitochondrial derivative by the way of a long and complicated metamorphosis.

A. *Sperm cells with normal mitochondria (diagrams 1–4).*

In this first class the basic mitochondrial structure is either not changed at all or only slightly altered during the course of spermatogenesis. In every case, the mitochondrial envelope, the matrix and the intermembrane spaces are easily recognizable. Only the location of the mitochondria in the cell is variable and allows us to distinguish the three following situations:

1. In the first, the mitochondria are dispersed at random in the cytoplasm (diagram 1). This is the case in aflagellate sperm. When the cytoplasm remains relatively abundant at the end of the maturation of the sperm, mito-

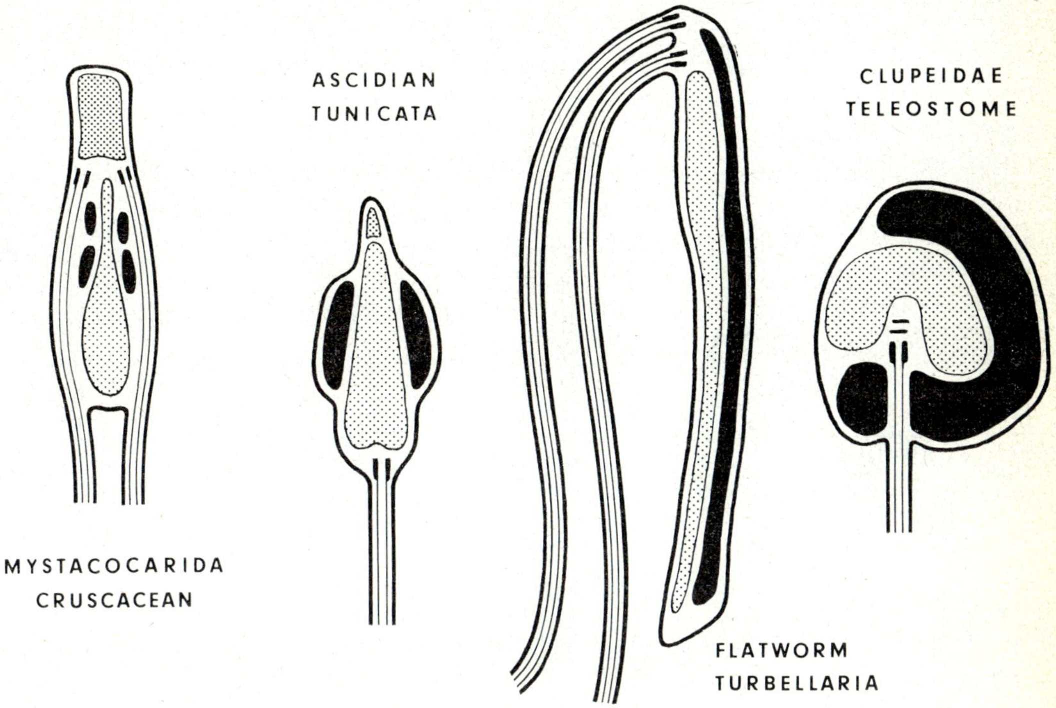

Diagram 2. – Sperm cells with mitochondria located in the nuclear area. *Mystacocarida* after Brown and Metz (1967); Ascidian after Ezell (1963); Flatworm after Silveira and Porter (1964); Clupeidae after Mattei (1969).

chondria can be found everywhere in the cell. This situation is found in *Ascaris*, in ticks and, astonishingly enough, in a Vertebrate, the teleost *Gymnarchus* (Mattei *et al.*, 1967; Mattei, 1969). Conversely, if the cytoplasmic background is scarce, the mitochondria are forcedly restricted to these cytoplasmic areas; for example, in crabs and in the millipede *Spirostreptus*, they are located between the acrosome and the nucleus.

2. In the second, the mitochondria are located in the nuclear area (diagram 2). In this case, the mitochondria can remain independent from each other. This is rare, however, being known only in a primitive Crus-

tacean group, the *Mystacocarida* (BROWN and METZ, 1967). More often, the mitochondria fuse during the process of spermatogenesis and form a single mitochondrial structure which corresponds to a typical Nebenkern. This situation has been described for the Prochordates and for the Planerian *Bdelloura* (SILVEIRA and PORTER, 1964). Finally, a disposition of the Nebenkern which is a compromise between a position lateral to the nucleus and one encircling the flagellum has been observed among certain Clupeid teleosts (MATTEI, 1969). In fact, the posterior portion of the mitochondrial structure in these fishes partially surrounds the flagellum.

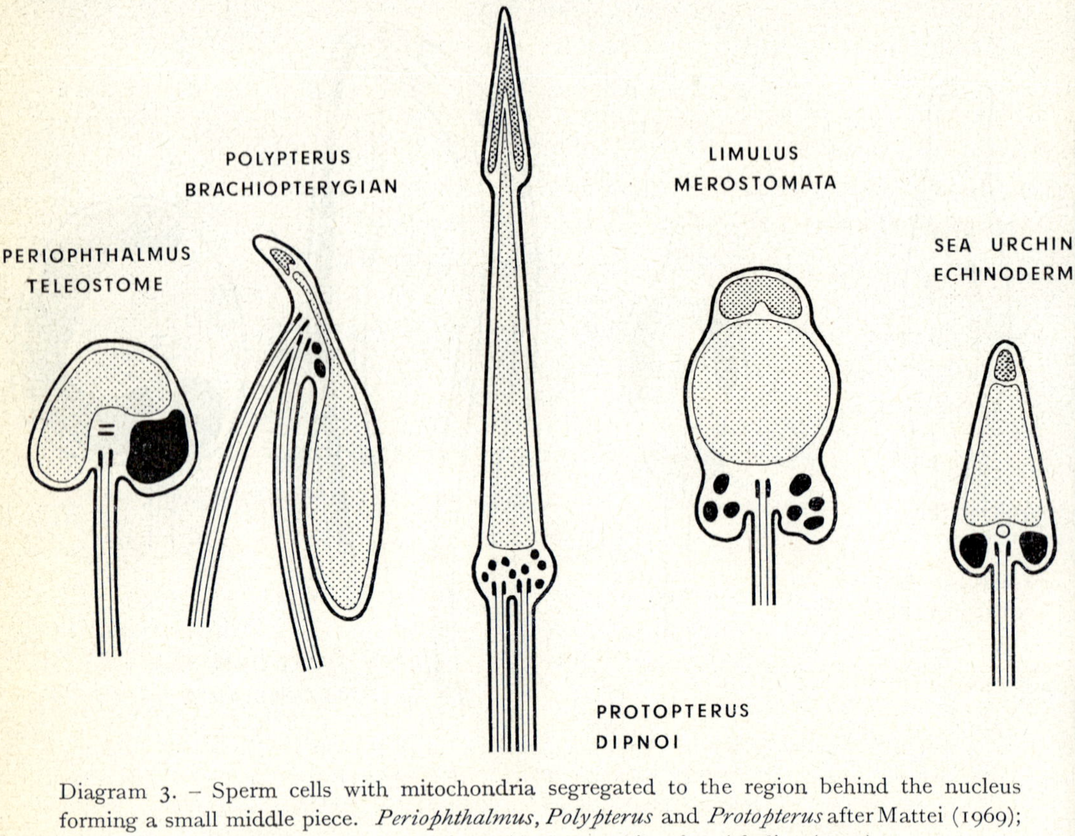

Diagram 3. – Sperm cells with mitochondria segregated to the region behind the nucleus forming a small middle piece. *Periophthalmus*, *Polypterus* and *Protopterus* after Mattei (1969); *Limulus* after André (1965 b); Sea urchin after Afzelius (1955).

3. In the third situation, the mitochondria are segregated to the region behind the nucleus. In these cases, the mitochondria participate in the formation of the middle piece, a very common occurrence, which can be developed to a greater or lesser extent according to the species, as RETZIUS pointed out long ago.

When the sperm is endowed with a small middle piece only (diagram 3), the mitochondria may be located either to one side of the centriolar apparatus – this is the case of the fishes, *Periophthalmus* and *Polypterus* – or, more commonly, around the centriolar apparatus as seen in *Protopterus*, in the horse-shoe crab *Limulus*, in sea urchins and in the Lamellibranchs. Sometimes, the mitochondria conserve their individuality (as in *Polypterus*, *Protopterus* and *Limulus*) or they may fuse during spermatogenesis to form a single mitochondrial body (as in certain sea urchins and teleosts).

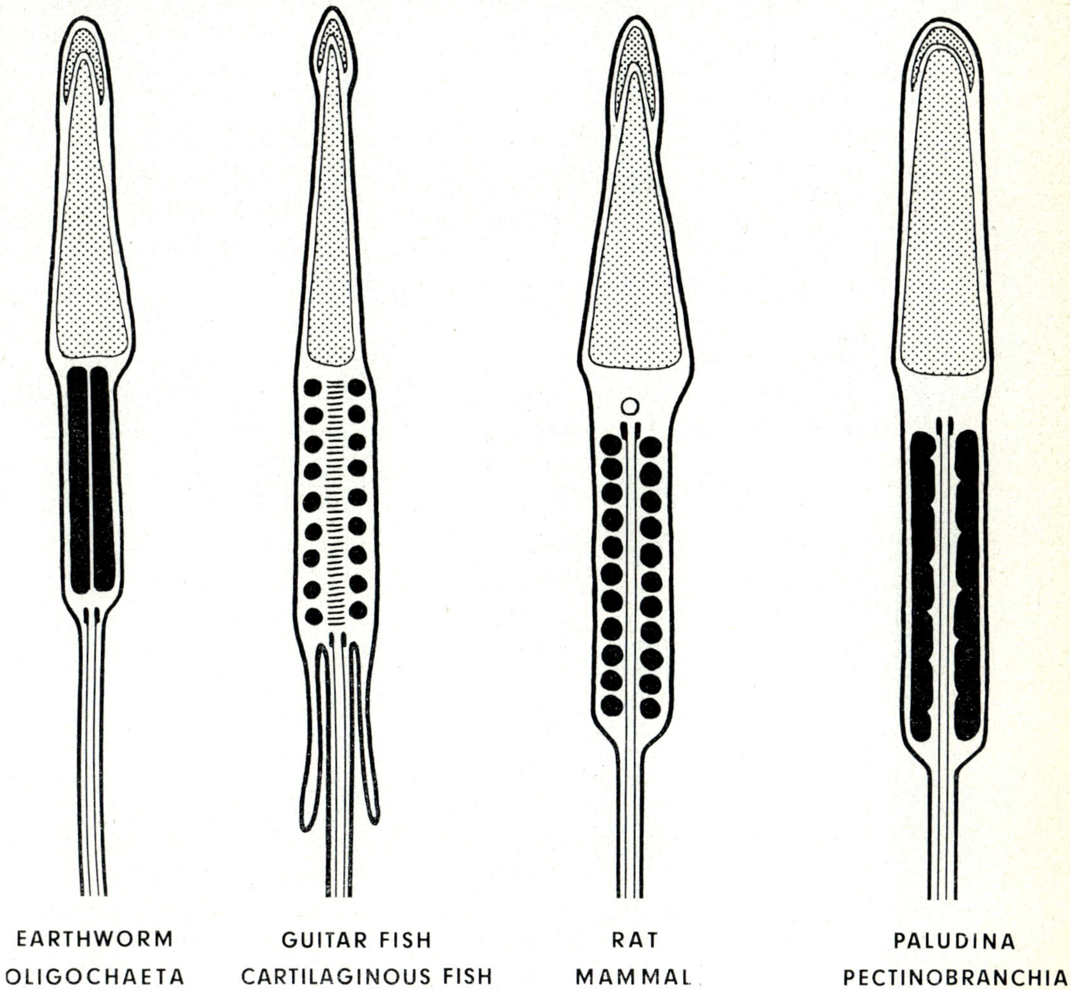

Diagram 4. – Sperm cells with mitochondria segregated to the region behind the nucleus forming a large middle piece. Earthworm after Anderson *et al.* (1967;) Guitar fish after Mattei (1969); Rat after Fawcett (1958); *Paludina* after Kaye (1958).

Conversely, when the sperm is endowed with a well developed middle piece (diagram 4) two variations can be described: one in which the mitochondria are placed between the centriolar apparatus and the nucleus; the other in which the mitochondria form a sheath around the flagellum. Examples of the first variation can be found in the Oligochaetes and the Hirudinea, where the mitochondria are assembled in a bundle anterior to the centriole, and in the

Chondrichthyes, where the mitochondria are disposed around a periodic axis situated anterior to the centriole. In the second variation, where the mitochondria form a sheath around the flagellum, they are generally arranged in a helical pattern and can remain separate, as in the mammals, or they can fuse together as in the Pectinibranch Gastropods. In this latter case, however, the cristae are extensively modified and finally become stacked in periodic arrays where some grooves may represent the point of fusion of the original mitochondria (KAYE, 1958).

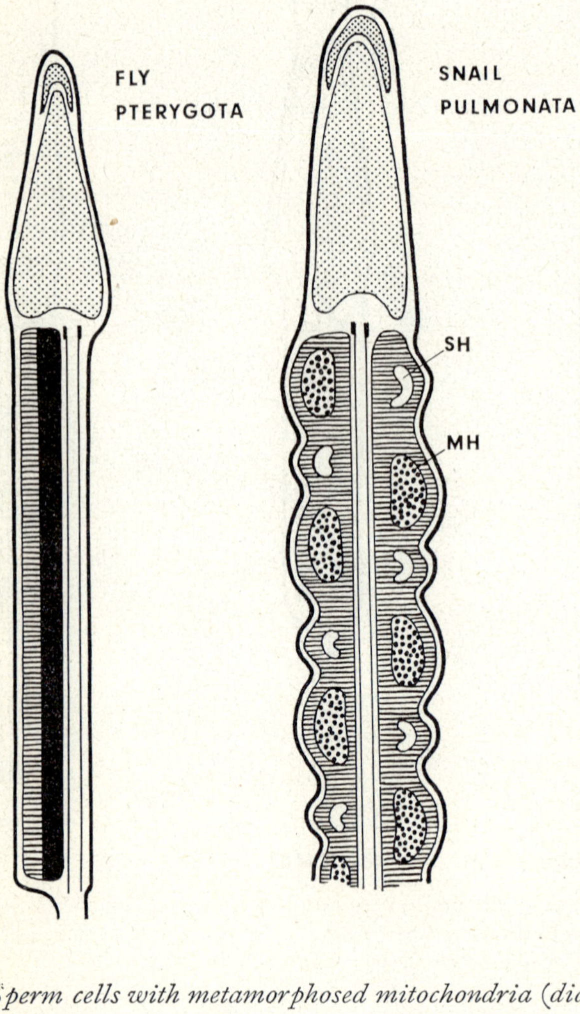

Diagram 5. – Sperm cells with metamorphosed mitochondria. Fly after Meyer (1664); Snail after André (1962). MH: major helix; SH: minor helix.

B. *Sperm cells with metamorphosed mitochondria (diagram 5).*

In this class, one or two elongated structures may be observed, either alongside of the nucleus or posterior to it. The study of spermatogenesis in these animals reveals that the structures result from a fusion of mitochondria, followed by a metamorphosis, in which the typical mitochondrial morphology becomes completely lost. This is encountered in the Insects and in the Pulmonate Gastropods.

In the Insects, the mitochondria of the young spermatid gather and clump together to form an enormous sphere, bigger than the nucleus – the famous Nebenkern, as discovered and named by v. LA VALLETTE ST. GEORGE in 1867 (bibliography in ANDRÉ, 1962). As PRATT (1968) has beautifully demonstrated, the Nebenkern divides precisely into two mitochondrial derivatives which elongate enormously along the axoneme. Meanwhile, the mitochondrial structure undergoes a metamorphosis, giving rise to completely transformed bodies, a variety of which have been described by PHILLIPS (1966 a and b, and this Symposium). One of the main riddles concerning these bodies is the general presence of some crystallized material, probably proteinacious in nature.

The Pulmonate Gastropods probably represent the climax in mitochondrial remodelling. As we have already shown several years ago (GRASSÉ *et al.*, 1956 a; ANDRÉ, 1962), the mitochondria of the young spermatid gather at the back of the nucleus, around the growing flagellum. Thereafter, they fuse in a continuous sheath around the axoneme, and elongate extensively (diagram 6). At the same time, a metamorphosis also occurs here. Most of the

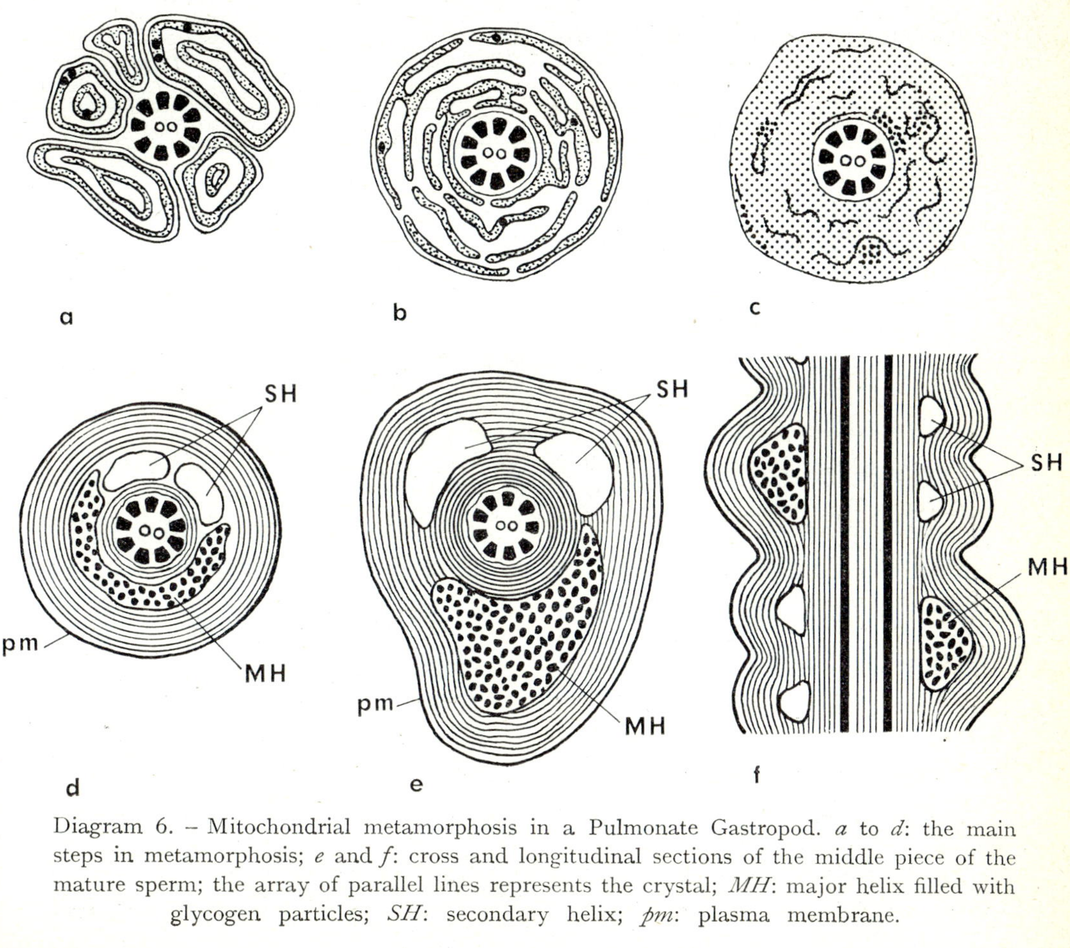

Diagram 6. – Mitochondrial metamorphosis in a Pulmonate Gastropod. *a* to *d*: the main steps in metamorphosis; *e* and *f*: cross and longitudinal sections of the middle piece of the mature sperm; the array of parallel lines represents the crystal; *MH*: major helix filled with glycogen particles; *SH*: secondary helix; *pm*: plasma membrane.

volume of the emerging mitochondrial derivative is made of a proteinacious crystal whose basic element is a globule or hollow rodlet, 90 Å in diameter. This crystal is traversed by two or more helically–coiled canals of two different kinds. One of them, which we have named the major helix, is filled with a large quantity of glycogen, as cytochemically demonstrated by PERSONNE and ANDRÉ (1964). The other or secondary helix, is derived from the matrix areas of the original mitochondria (figure 1).

II. PHYSIOLOGY

It is evident that the presence of mitochondria in spermatozoa is closely linked to the aerobic metabolism of these cells. The APT produced by oxidative phosphorylation is transformed into mechanical energy which permits fertilization to occur. Depending on the species, the sperm are released into a medium which may or may not contain an oxidizable substrate.

A. *Medium containing oxidizable metabolites.*

In the case of internal fertilization, the metabolites can be taken up from the extracellular medium according to the needs of the sperm. The most well known example is that of the Mammals where the seminal fluid contains fructose (MANN, 1964). The sperm themselves do not contain any metabolic reserves.

B. *Medium lacking oxidizable metabolites.*

In those animals where fertilization is external, the spermatozoa are released into fresh or salt water and their survival depends on their own metabolic reserves. It has been established that these materials can be either phospholipids or glycogen.

The degradation of phospholipids has been demonstrated in the sperm of sea urchins. As shown by AFZELIUS and MOHRI (1966), the ageing process of motile sperm is accompanied by a gradual disappearance of the mitochondrial cristae.

Certain spermatozoa contain a reserve of glycogen whose location may be either peri- or intra-mitochondrial (ANDERSON and PERSONNE, 1970). Peri-mitochondrial glycogen has been found in a variety of species. Intramitochondrial glycogen has been found in the sea urchin *Arbacia* (ANDERSON, 1968), and most strikingly in the Pulmonate Gastropods (LANZA, 1965; PERSONNE and ANDRÉ, 1964; ANDRÉ, 1965 a; LANZA and QUATTRINI, 1964). In this latter case, a phosphorylase activity can be demostrated. It should be emphasized here that this activity does not exist in other mitochondria and therefore is an enzymatic expression of mitochondrial specialization (PERSONNE and ANDERSON, 1970).

The situation encountered in the Pulmonate Gastropods is unique and deserves special consideration. These sperm have been the subject of numerous cytochemical studies that ANDERSON and PERSONNE will develop during this Symposium. To summarize, it has been shown that the mitochondrial metamorphosis consists of a redistribution of the chemical constituents. Cytochromes are present in the crystal (RITTER and ANDRÉ, in preparation;

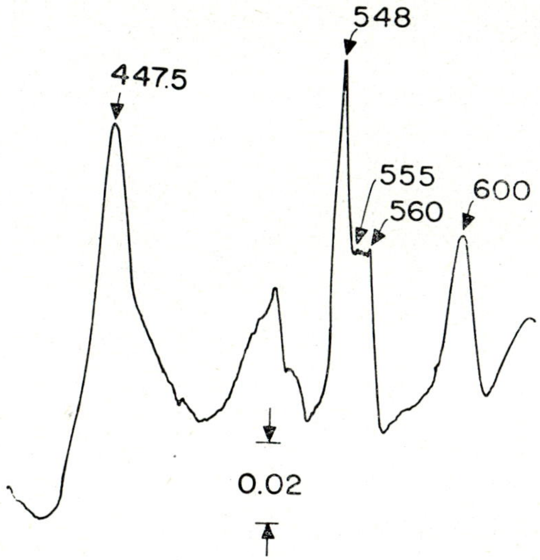

Diagram 7. – Difference spectrum of a suspension of fresh snail sperm. Absorption peaks show the presence of cytochromes $a+a_3$, *b*, and *c* in high concentration. Courtesy of C. RITTER.

diagram 7 and fig. 2), whereas the Krebs cycle enzymes are confined to the secondary helices (ANDERSON *et al.*, 1968; PERSONNE and ANDERSON, 1969; fig. 3). The third entity, the major helix, contains a large quantity of glycogen together with a phosphorylase activity (figs. 4 and 5).

III. EVOLUTION VERSUS SPECIALIZATION

It has been shown by BACCETTI and his collaborators (BACCETTI, 1967; BACCETTI *et al.*, 1969 a and b; BACCETTI, this Symposium). that for the Insects, the ultrastructural details of the axoneme follow the systematics of the class and therefore, can bring new data or can indicate new trends in the phylogenetic parenthood between species or families.

Contrarily, while being highly pleomorphic, the chondriome of spermatozoa does not show any clear evolutionary tendencies, at least when we consider the animal kingdom as a whole. For example, on the one hand, unmodified mitochondria are encountered in groups as far apart as the Nematodes, the Arthropods and the Vertebrates. On the other hand, highly metamorphosed mitochondria are characteristic mainly of Insects and Gastropods. It is only in the case of some narrow divisions of the systematics that the characters of the mitochondria have an evolutionary significance, as we have pointed out several years ago for the Scorpions where the Chactidae family is well separated from the Buthidae family (ANDRÉ, 1963). The same is true for the Blenniidae, a family of teleosts; however, if we consider the whole group of teleosts, we must conclude that a large diversity of variations are realized (MATTEI, 1969).

Therefore, when considered at the level of the animal kingdom, we arrive at the conclusion that the variations observed in sperm mitochondria have but little evolutionary significance. It is only if we consider the degree of specialization, that is the adaptive features, that some trends can be disclosed. It has been estimated by COWDRY (1924) that the sperm cell is the utmost in specialization achieved by the living world. This is very true for the Vertebrates and the Insects, for example. It is not true for those species whose sperm are amoeboid. In this case precisely, the mitochondria are unmodified and most probably function as any other somatic mitochondria during fertilization. The sperm are deposited very close to the egg; the need for energy is scant.

In the flagellate sperm, diverse degrees of specialization are present. The most striking characteristic of this specialization is the concentration of the energetic machinery in a given segment of the sperm, the so-called middle piece, in close proximity to the centriolar apparatus and the axoneme. When the sperm are released externally, in a watery medium, the middle piece is short – said to be primitive – and the sperm is short lived. The chances for fertilization are low, but they are augmented by the enormous number of sperm released. On the contrary, when fertilization is performed internally, and thus in a much more viscous medium, the middle piece becomes elongated. So appears a second characteristic of the specialization: an increase in the ratio of the volume of the chondriome to the volume of the rest of the cell. This is consistent with the fact that the biogenesis of mitochondria is so extensive in the spermatocytes of Vertebrates.

At the same time, the mitochondrial material condenses, becomes less hydrated, and may acquire new morphologic and physiologic features which however, are still efficient in the transformation of energy. This is well realized in the two main evolutionary summits: Mammals and Insects. Curiously enough, the climax is reached by a far less successful group, the Pulmonate Gastropods. Here the chondriome represents about 95 % of the volume of the cell – by far much larger than the nucleus. Moreover, the energetic machinery acquires unique features: the electron transport intermediates are highly concentrated in a crystal, while the Krebs cycle enzymes are compartmentalized in a confined space. Still further, another compartment is present which contains a large stock of glucoside reserves along with the necessary enzymes for their metabolism and entrance into the oxidative process. Owing to these adaptative features, the snail sperm can withstand a very long storage in the female tract. The mitochondrial specialization appears here at its maximum to carry out the sperm function, that is to transport intact the genetic message.

REFERENCES

AFZELIUS B. A. (1955) – *The fine structure of the sea urchin spermatozoa as revealed by the electron microscope.* « Z. Zellforsch », 42, 134–148.

AFZELIUS B. A. and MOHRI H. (1966) – *Mitochondria respiring without exogenous substrate. A study of aged sea urchin spermatozoa.* « Exp. Cell Res. », 42, 10–17.

ANDERSON W. A. (1968) – *Cytochemistry of sea urchin gametes.* I. *Intramitochondrial localization of glycogen, glucose–6–phosphatase and adenosine triphosphatase activity in spermatozoa of* Paracentrotus lividus. « J. Ultrastructure Res. », 24, 398–411.

ANDERSON W. A. and PERSONNE P. (1970) – *The localization of glycogen in the spermatozoa of various invertebrate and vertebrate species.* « J. Cell. Biol. », 44, 29–51.

ANDERSON W. A., PERSONNE P. and ANDRÉ J. (1968) – *Chemical compartmentalization in* Helix *spermatozoa.* « J. Microscopie », 7, 367–390.

ANDERSON W. A., WEISSMAN A. and ELLIS R. A. (1967). – *Cytodifferentiation during spermiogenesis in* Lumbricus terrestris. « J. Cell Biol. », 32, 11–26.

ANDRÉ J. (1962) – *Contribution à la connaissance du chondriome. Etude de ses modifications ultrastructurales pendant la spermatogenèse.* « J. Ultrastructure Res. », suppl. 3, 1–185.

ANDRÉ J. (1963) – *Some aspects of specialization in sperm.* in D. Mazia and A. Tyler: General Physiology of cell specialization. McGraw–Hill Book Co., New York, 91–115.

ANDRÉ J. (1965 a) – *Quelques données récentes sur la structure et la physiologie des mitochondries: glycogène, particules élémentaires, acides nucléiques.* « Arch. Biol. », 76, 277–304.

ANDRÉ J. (1965 b) – *A propos d'une leçon sur la Limule.* « Ann. Fac. Sci. », Clermont–Ferrand, 26, 27–38.

BACCETTI B. (1967) – *Spermatologia comparata degli Artropodi.* « Atti VII Congr. Naz. Ital. Ent., Atti Accad. Naz. Ital. Ent. », 15, 32–61.

BACCETTI B. (1969) – This Symposium.

BACCETTI B., DALLAI R. and ROSATI F. (1969 a) – *The spermatozoon of Arthropoda.* III. *The lowest holometabolic insects.* « J. Microscopie », 8, 233–248.

BACCETTI B., DALLAI R. and ROSATI F. (1969 b). – *The spermatozoon of Arthropoda.* IV. *Corrodentia, Mallophaga and Thysanoptera.* « J. Microscopie », 8, 249–262.

BONSDORFF C. H. von and TELKKA A. (1965) – *The spermatozoon flagella of* Diphyllobothrium latum (fish tapeworm). « Z. Zellforsch. », 66, 643–648.

BROWN G. C. and METZ C. B. (1967) – *Ultrastructural studies on the spermatozoa of two primitive crustaceans* Hutchinsoniella macrocantha *and* Derocheilocaris typicus. « Z. Zellforsch. », 80, 78–92.

COWDRY E. V. (1924) – *General Cytology.* The University of Chicago Press, Chicago.

EZELL S. D. (1963) – *The lateral body of* Ciona intestinalis *spermatozoa.* « Exp. Cell Res. », 30, 615–617.

FAVARD P. (1961) – *Evolution des ultrastructures cellulaires au cours de la spermatogenèse de l'Ascaris.* « Ann. Sci. Nat., Zool. », 12e série, 3, 53–152.

FAWCETT D. W. (1958) – *The structure of the mammalian spermatozoon.* « Intern. Rev. Cytol. », 7, 195–234.

GRASSÉ P. P., CARASSO N. and FAVARD P. (1956 a) – *Les ultrastructures cellulaires au cours de la spermiogenèse de l'Escargot* (Helix pomatia *L.*): *évolution des chromosomes, du chondriome, de l'appareil de Golgi, etc.* « Ann. Sci. Nat., Zool. », 11e série, 339–380.

GRASSÉ P. P., TUZET O. and CARASSO N. (1965 b) – *Ultrastructure d'un spermatozoïde aberrant d'un Iule,* Spirostreptus castaneus *Attems* (*Myriapode, Diplopode*) *avec des remarques sur les chromosomes.* « C. R. Acad. Sc. », 243, 337–343.

GRESSON R.A.R. and PERRY M. M. (1961) – *Electron microscope studies of spermateleosis in* Fasciola hepatica *L.* « Exp. Cell Res. », 22, 1–8.

HENDELBERG J. (1962) – *Paired flagella and nucleus migration in the spermiogenesis of* Dicrocoelium *and* Fasciola (Digena, Trematoda). « Zool. Bidr. Uppsala », 35, 569–589.

KAYE J. S. (1958) – *Changes in the fine structure of mitochondria during spermatogenesis.* « J. Morphol. », 102, 347–399.

LANZA B. (1965) – *Note su gli spermatidi e gli spermi di alcuni Gasteropodi: glicogeno intramitocondriale e cariolinfoteca.* « Boll. Zool. », 32, 1080–1086.

LANZA B. and QUATTRINI D. (1964) – *Observazioni sul contenuto in glicogeno degli spermi e degli epiteli della gonade e delle vie sessuali ermafrodite di* Vaginulus borellianus (Colosi) (Mollusca Gastropoda Soleolifera). « Boll. Soc. Ital. Biol. Sper. », 40, 1154–1155.

LA VALLETTE St. GEORGE von (1867) – *Über die genese der Samenkörper.* II. « Archiv. Mikroskop. Anat. », 3, 263–273.

MANN T. (1964) – *Biochemistry of semen and the male reproductive tract.* – Methuen and Co., Inc., London.

MATTEI X. (1969) – *Contribution à l'étude de la spermiogenèse et des spermatozoïdes de Poissons par les méthodes de la microscopie électronique.* Thèse, Faculté des Sciences, Université de Montpellier, 1–148.

MATTEI X., BOISSON C., MATTEI C. and REIZER C. (1967) – *Spermatozoïdes aflagellés chez un Poisson:* Gymnarchus niloticus (*Téléostéen,* Gymnarchidae). « C. R. Acad. Sc. », 265, 2010–2012.

MEYER G. (1964) – *Die parakristallinen Körper in den Spermienschwanzen von* Drosophila. « Z. Zellforsch. », 62, 762–784.

PERSONNE P. and ANDERSON W. A. (1969) – *Compartimentage des activités enzymatiques dans le spermatozoïde de certains mollusques.* I. *Localization des déshydrogénases.* « J. Cell Sci. », 4, 693–707.

PERSONNE P. and ANDERSON W. A. (1970) – *Localisation mitochondriale d'enzymes liées au métabolisme du glycogène dans le spermatozoïde de l'escargot.* « J. Cell Biol. », 44, 20–28.

PERSONNE P. and ANDRÉ J. (1964) – *Existence de glycogène mitochondrial dans le spermatozoïde de la Testacelle.* « J. Microscopie », 3, 643–650.

PHILLIPS D. M. (1966 a) – *Observations on spermiogenesis in the fungus gnat* Sciara coprophila. « J. Cell Biol. », 30, 477–497.

PHILLIPS D. M. (1966 b) – *Fine structure of* Sciara coprophila *sperm.* « J. Cell Biol. », 30, 499–517.

PHILLIPS D. M. (1969) – This symposium.

POCHON-MASSON J. (1968) – *L'ultrastructure des spermatozoïdes vésiculaires chez les Crustacés décapodes avant et au cours de leur dévagination expérimentale.* I. *Brachyoures et Anomoures.* II. *Macroures. Discussion et conclusions.* « Ann. Sci. Nat. », 12e série, 10, 1–99 et 367–454.

PRATT S. A. (1968) – *An electron microscope study of Nebenkern formation and differentiation in spermatids of* Murgantia histrionica (*Hemiptera, Pentatomidae*). « J. Morphol. », 126, 31–66.

REGER J. F. (1963) – *Spermiogenesis in the tick* Amblyomma dissimili. « J. Ultrastructure Res. », 8, 607–621.

RITTER C. and ANDRÉ J. – *Cytochromes in sperm of* Helix aspersa, in preparation.

ROBISON G. W. (1966) – *Microtubules in relation to the mobility of a sperm syncytium in an armored scale insect.* « J. Cell Biol. », 29, 251–265.

ROSARIO B. (1964) – *An electron microscope study on spermatogenesis in Cestodes.* « J. Ultrastructure Res. », 11, 412–427.

SELIGMAN A. M., KARNOVSKY M. J., WASSERKRUG H. L. and HANKER J. S. (1968) – *Nondroplet ultrastructural demonstration of cytochrome oxidase activity with a polymerizing osmiophilic reagent, diaminobenzidine* (*DAB*). « J. Cell Biol. », 38, 1–14.

SELIGMAN A. M., UENO H., MORIZONO Y., WASSERKRUG H. L., KATZOFF L. and HANKER J. S. (1967) – *Electron microscopic demonstration of dehydrogenase activity with a new osmiophilic ditetrazolium salt* (*TC-NBT*). « J. Histochem. Cytochem. », 15, 1–14.

SILVEIRA M. and PORTER K. R. (1964) – *The spermatozoïdes of flatworms and their microtubular systems.* « Protoplasma », 59, 240–265.

THIÉRY J. – P. (1967) – *Mise en évidence des polysaccharides sur coupes fines en microscopie électronique.* « J. Microscopie », 6, 987–1018.

EXPLANATION OF FIGURES

Fig. 1. – Transverse section through the mitochondrial derivative of the middle piece of a snail sperm showing the cytochemical compartmentalization. The cytochromes are localized in the crystal, the Krebs cycle enzymatic activities in the secondary helix, and the glycogen and phosphorylase activity (PRase) in the major helix. Courtesy of W. Anderson and P. Personne × 160,000.

Figs. 2 and 3. – Cytochemical reactions for cytochromes (Fig. 2) and succinic dehydrogenase activity (Fig. 3). The black deposits are obtained by the methods of SELIGMAN *et al.* (1967; 1968). Courtesy of W. ANDERSON and P. PERSONNE. × 45,000.

Figs. 4 and 5. – Presence of glycogen in the major helix in snail sperm. Glycogen particles in typical α clusters stained by the conventional uranyl-lead technique (Fig. 4); glycogen in β particles stained by the THIÉRY method (1967) (Fig. 5). ×60,000.

Discussion

AFZELIUS. – You believe that the crystalline mitochondrial derivatives represent the most effective form of arrangement of the mitochondrial enzymes in order to produce ATP. I believe on the opposite that it represents the least effective form, in other words that they are incapable of ATP-production. My reasons for this belief are these:

1) If this was an effective arrangement I believe it would appear more often, and not only in spermatozoa which swim for a short while.

2) The crystalline arrangement, although it looks beautiful in the micrographs represents a low degree of order. You may think of the usual mitochondrial membranes as 2–dimensional arrangement of mitochondrial enzymes, but here the enzymes do not see each other; it is so to say not even a 1–dimensional arrangment of the enzymes. And when they do not come together they will have difficulties to cooperate effectively. It is probably more realistic to look upon the crystal as a degenerated product or a storage substance. The oxidative phosphorylation seems to require something more organized; enzyme arrays surrounded on both sides by lipid layers.

3) Spermatozoa with simple mitochondria seem more active as a rule. The sea urchin sperm swims actively for at least an hour. Many of these big spermatozoa with an enormous crystal do hardly move at all. The *Notonecta* sperm has feeble movements, in spite of its gigantic mitochondrial crystal, the *Discoglossus* sperm swims for just a few seconds, etc.

My question is: is there any proof of these crystals being capable of manufacturing ATP?

ANDRÉ. – We may have used a poor expression, but we never meant that the crystal represents the *most effective* distribution of mitochondrial enzymes. What we meant is that this sperm is *still effective* in transforming energy, even if, obviously enough, the enzymes are no longer distributed in a two dimensional array. We do not know if it is still the same pathway which is working (I mean dehydrogenase activity, electron transport and coupled phosphorylation). What we know at present is:

1) The complete set of cytochromes is still there, as has been shown during the presentation, from spectrophotometric data obtained with Carl Ritter in Britton Chance's lab.

2) We have not measured the rate of phosphorylation, if present, but we know that oxidizable substrates are used oxidatively: in aerated medium, the suppression of the endogenous glycogen by amylase causes the cytochromes to remain in the oxidized state; if we then add succinate, or another oxidizable substrate, the cytochromes become reduced, which is a proof that the electron transport chain is still functional.

3) Snail sperm can be artificially activated by trypsin (which probably removes some enzymatic inhibition). A thick suspension of snail sperm to which you add trypsin becomes fantastically active within 10 minutes. The sperm move in groups so that the suspension is no longer homogeneous, when observed with the naked eye. Usually, the sperm climb up the walls of the beaker and escape on the bench. After 30 minutes this activity decreases, but some sperm are still moving after 5 hours. Obviously, snail sperm are metabolically much more active than those you are referring to, which move only a few seconds. Moreover, a variety of enzymatic activities can be detected cytochemically, as will be shown by Winston Anderson and Paul Personne, in their presentation.

I agree with you, Björn, when you say that most often, biological crystals, particularly proteinacious crystals, are storage stages of molecules transitorily left aside by metabolism. But this is not always the case. Muscles, for example, are complex repetitive arrangements of molecules, the ATP-ase activity of which is greatly enhanced by their repetitivity. The same is probably true for the retina rodlets, in which piles of saccules are very efficient in transforming light energy into electrical impulses, and for the trichocysts of *Paramecium* in which a tridimensional array of molecules is the seat of an explosive production of mechanical energy. We do not know yet if the crystal of the snail sperm is endowed with such unusual properties; what I think is that we must keep an open mind until more is known about it.

NELSON. – This was a beautiful presentation. When sperm of mammals are inseminated in female reproductive tract, they usually leave the seminal plasma at the cervical barrier, and have only been exposed to the female accessory secretions for a very brief period of time. Unless the sperm can utilize the secretory products of the female tract, e.g. lactate, they have to rely on their own ATP-regenerating mechanism, because as you have shown there are no intracellular reserves in mammalian sperms.

ANDRÉ. – Thank you Dr. Nelson, for this information.

BACCETTI. – I ask more details on the sperms in which mitochondria disappear during the sperm maturation.

ANDRÉ. – Obviously, this is not an easy problem, and very few data are available to answer this question. A first remark is that these unusual sperm are very different from each other according to the species and probably they do not all utilize the same metabolic pathway. Second, most of them are nonmotile or creep very slowly, that is to say do not require much energy for movement. Third, orthodox respiration is not the only source of ATP; glycolysis is certainly utilized by several species; we can even hypothesize that some unusual metabolic pathways such as the glyoxylic cycle, or primitive respiratory mechanisms known to occur in peroxisomes for example are in use.

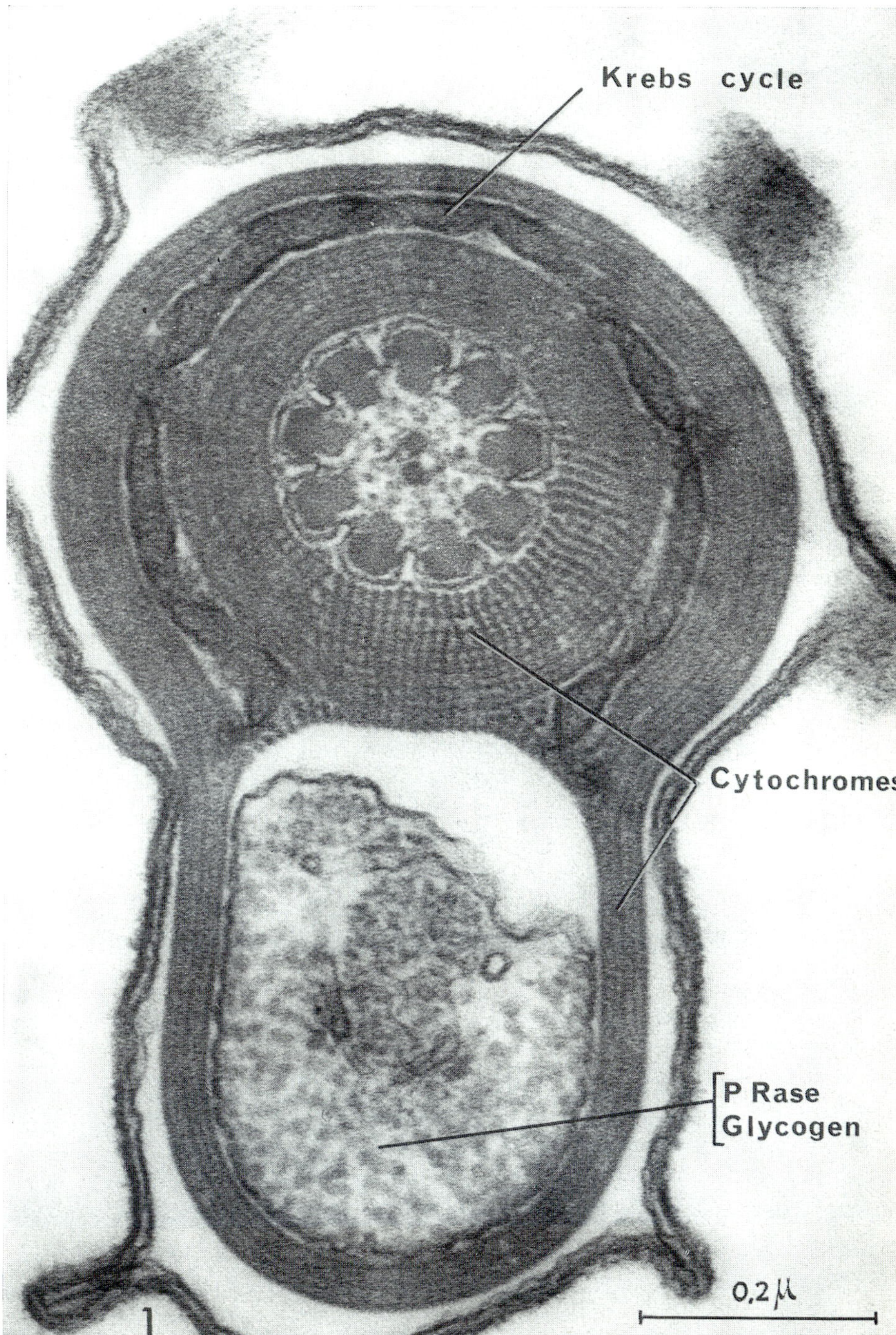
Krebs cycle
Cytochromes
P Rase
Glycogen
0,2 μ
1

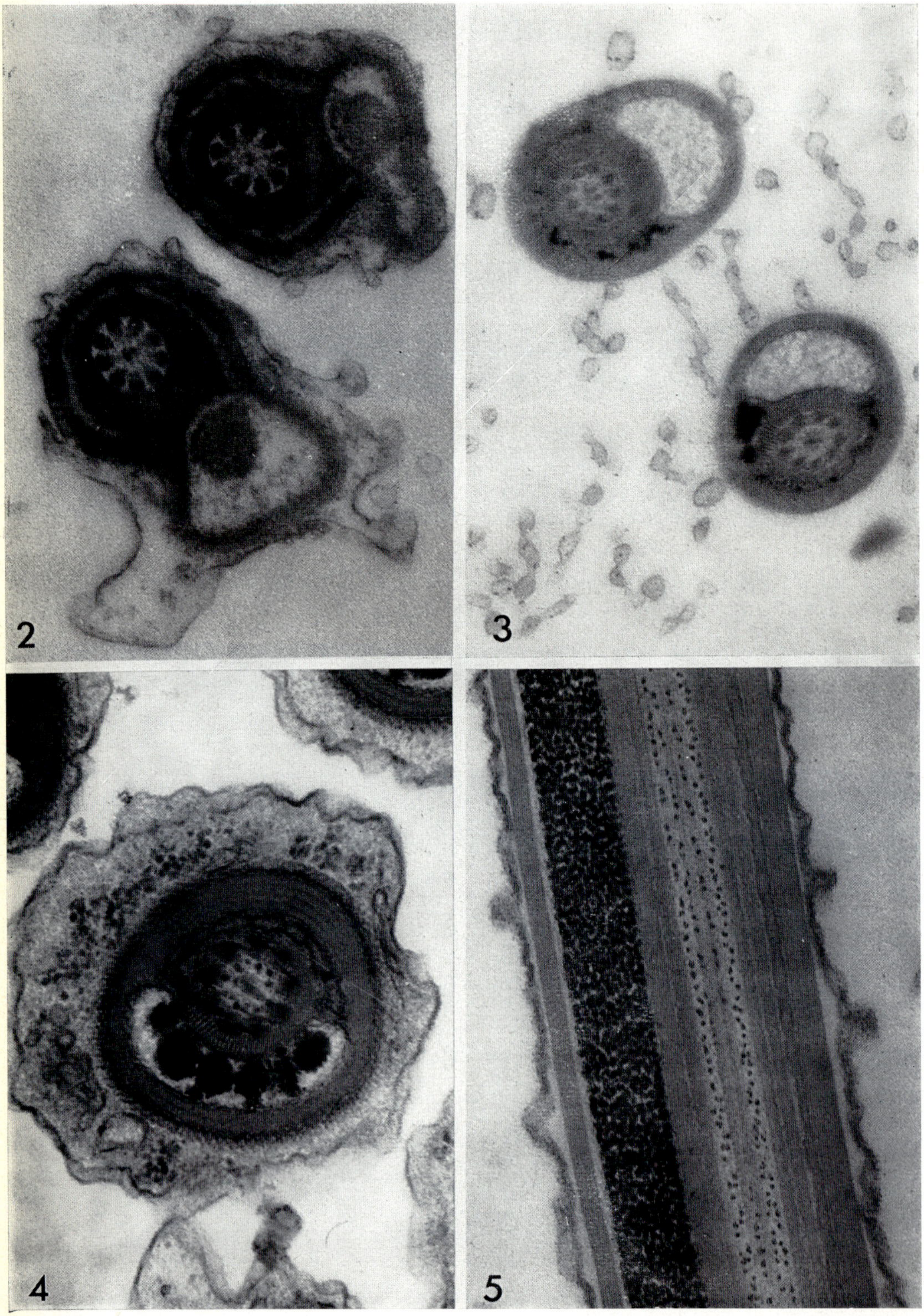
2
3
4
5

WINSTON A. ANDERSON (*) and PAUL PERSONNE (*)

RECENT CYTOCHEMICAL STUDIES ON SPERMATOZOA OF SOME INVERTEBRATE AND VERTEBRATE SPECIES (**)

SUMMARY. — The contributions of cytochemistry to the study of spermatozoan metabolism and function are considered in this report.

By means of electron microscope cytochemistry evidence is presented for the existence of significant amounts of glycogen in mature spermatozoa of some invertebrate and vertebrate species. Evidence is also presented that glycogen synthetic and glycolytic enzyme systems occupy the glycogen compartment within the mitochondrial derivative of sperm of pulmonate gastropods.

Sites of activity of some oxidative and respiratory chain enzymes are localized in membranous and in paracrystalline mitochondrial derivatives of some invertebrate spermatozoa. Hypotheses on the mechanism of energy conversion during spermatozoan metabolism are discussed.

The relationship of the sites of ATPase activity and their possible implications in spermatozoan motility are also considered.

RIASSUNTO. — In questo lavoro vengono considerati i contributi della citochimica allo studio del metabolismo e della funzione degli spermatozoi.

Per mezzo della citochimica al microscopio elettronico è stata dimostrata l'esistenza di significativi ammassi di glicogeno negli spermatozoi maturi di alcune specie di invertebrati e vertebrati. Vengono anche presentate prove che la sintesi del glicogeno e gli enzimi glicolitici occupano il compartimento del glicogeno nei derivati mitocondriali degli spermatozoi di gasteropodi polmonati.

L'attività di alcuni enzimi ossidativi e di enzimi della catena respiratoria è localizzata sulle membrane e nei derivati mitocondriali paracristallini degli spermatozoi di alcuni invertebrati. Sono discusse ipotesi sul meccanismo di conversione dell'energia durante il metabolismo dello spermatozoo.

Vengono anche considerate le relazioni tra i siti di attività ATPasica e le loro possibili implicazioni nella motilità dello spermatozoo.

In the course of evolution, a number of variations have developed in the pattern of spermatozoan development, physiology and function, and in the mechanism of fertilization. However, a marked correlation is observed

(*) (Laboratories of Human Reproduction and Reproductive Biology and the Department of Anatomy, Harvard Medical School, Boston, Mass., USA; Laboratoire de Biologie Cellulaire 4, Faculté des Sciences, Orsay, France; and, Laboratoire de Biologie Animale, Faculté des Sciences, Université d'Amiens, 80-Amiens, France).

(**) Supported in part by grant No. HD-02344 from the Institute of General Medical Sciences, National Institutes of Health, United States Public Health Service, and in part by grant 513/68 from the Direction des Recherches et Moyens d'Essais, France.

between spermatozoan morphology and function, and the physiological demands of the environment (FRANZEN, 1956). Spermatozoa are therefore somewhat adapted to survive under overcrowded conditions and low oxygen tension in male and female storage organs, to resist the unusual physiological conditions of the immediate prefertilization environment, and to transport male genetic material to complementary ova. The male gamete is thus endowed with the structural and chemical capacity to ensure, in part, the success of fertilization and karyogamy.

The mature spermatozoon is a product of complex cytomorphogenetic processes, which include the conservation of nuclear, mitochondrial and axonemal components and the elimination of excess nucleoplasm and cytoplasm (FAWCETT, 1958; ANDRÉ, 1962; ANDERSON *et al.*, 1967). Equally extensive chemical changes underlie these morphogenetic processes (TICE and BARRNETT, 1963; ANDERSON *et al.*, 1968). The resultant spermatozoon usually is devoid of active DNA and RNA templates and cytoplasm, and is thus endowed with limited biosynthetic ability. However, it possesses the physiological capacity for maintaining the energetic demands for its metabolism and motility for some time. Endogenous substrates, enzyme systems, cofactors etc. essential to spermatozoan metabolism are primarily located in their mitochondrial and axonemal compartments. In this report an attempt is made to localize endogenous metabolites and enzyme pathways related to sperm metabolism, and to correlate spermatozoan submicroscopic morphology and chemistry. Attention is mainly directed to the demonstration of intracellular polysaccharide reserves in some invertebrate and vertebrate spermatozoa, and to the relationship of glycolytic, oxidative, and respiratory enzyme systems in energy production and motility. No attempt is made to survey all the available data on spermatozoan metabolism, since this subject is already adequately considered (ROTHSCHILD, 1951; BISHOP, 1961; GONSE, 1962; SALISBURY and LODGE, 1962; MANN, 1964; NELSON, 1967). Thus, only the contributions of cytochemistry in the study of sperm metabolism and function are considered here.

The Demonstration of Intracellular Polysaccharide Reserves in Spermatozoa.

Spermatozoa of most vertebrate and invertebrate species have the ability to respire (ROTHSCHILD, 1951; SALISBURY and LODGE, 1962; MANN, 1964). Moreover, sperm of mammals and of some other species can utilize either respiratory or glycolytic processes in energy production. Although intracellular phospholipids are oxidized aerobically in the absence of extracellular metabolites, under normal conditions a wide range of glycolyzable substances, and some oxidizable fatty acids and polyols present in the semen provide the main source of energy for the metabolism of mammalian spermatozoa (MANN, 1964; 1967).

Spermatozoa of some invertebrate and vertebrate species are released into an aqueous prefertilization environment from which metabolizable nutrients are absent. According to some studies, energy-production in sperm of sea urchins for example, is exclusively derived from the aerobic oxidation of intracellular phospholipids (AFZELIUS and MOHRI, 1966). Presumably these sperm are endowed with little ability to utilize glycolytic processes. Other studies indicate however, that when oxidative processes are inhibited sperm of some marine invertebrate species are capable of metabolizing added carbohydrates (HUMPHREY, 1950). It is also reported that sperm of some marine molluscs and ascidians contain significant amounts of glycogen, while sperm of echinoderms contain lesser amounts (SPIKES, 1949; ROTHSCHILD and MANN, 1950; RESTIVO and REVERBERI, 1957). In recent morphological and cytochemical studies, large amounts of intracellular glycogen stores have been demonstrated in sperm of some gastropod molluscs, annelids, and echinoderms (LANZA and QUATTRINI, 1964; PERSONNE and ANDRÉ, 1964; ANDRÉ, 1965; ANDERSON *et al.*, 1967; ANDERSON, 1968). The phenomenon of glycogen storage by invertebrate and vertebrate spermatozoa may be of important physiological significance in spermatozoan metabolism. How widespread this phenomenon is, will be demonstrated in this electron microscope cytochemical survey, in which the periodic acid—thiosemicarbazide—silver proteinate (PA–TSC–SP) procedure for demonstrating polysaccharides in thin sections (THIERY, 1967) was used. Correlated enzymatic extraction and biochemical isolation procedures substantiate the existence of polysaccharide stores in spermatozoa.

Spermatozoa of lamellibranch molluscs (*Pecten*, *Mytilus*, *Spisula*, *Ostrea*) and the gastropods (*Gibbula*, *Patella*, *Diadora*) are classified as " primitive " according to FRANZEN (1956). Their middle piece is composed of relatively unmodified mitochondria located at the base of the nucleus. When tissues are prepared for electron microscopy and stained with uranyl acetate and lead citrate no unusual structures appear in the middle piece. However, when thin sections are treated with the PA–TSC–SP procedure according to THIERY (1967) significant amounts of polysaccharide become apparent in their middle piece. The intensely stained granules which disappear after treatment with α–amylase solutions or saliva are considered to be glycogen. In these " primitive " spermatozoa, β–glycogen particles (nomenclature according to DROCHMANS, 1962) consistently appear in the matrix between adjacent mitochondria and surrounding the basal body (Figs. 1 and 2). Glycogen also appears in the lumen of centrioles and in indentations of the nucleus.

Spermatozoa of the amphibians (*Rana*, *Bufo*) and of the fish (*Opsanus*, *Lebistes*) possess noticeable amounts of cytoplasm in their middle piece. In mature sperm of these species, β–glycogen particles are randomly scattered in the cytoplasm between the mitochondria (Fig. 3). Rosettes of α–particles are also present in the middle piece of sperm of *Lebistes*. Similarly, α–particles also are present in the matrix surrounding the nucleus and mitochondria of mature sperm of *Ciona* and *Molgula*.

Flagellate spermatozoa of the annelids (*Lumbricus*, *Hirudo*) and of the molluscs (*Littorina*, *Purpura*) possess a cylindrical middle piece that lies immediately behind their elongate nucleus. Their mitochondria are markedly more modified than those of the "primitive" spermatozoa. Sperm of these species lack noticeable amounts of residual cytoplasm. Glycogen granules are totally absent from their middle piece, instead they are consistently present in sperm tails of these species (ANDERSON and PERSONNE, 1970; ANDERSON *et al.*, 1967). The glycogen granules are moderately stained with REYNOLD's (1963) lead citrate solutions, but they are intensely contrasted after treatment with the PA–TSC–SP procedure. The granules are tightly packed in the matrix between the flagellar membrane and the outer doublets of the axoneme (Figs. 4, 6, and 7). They are however separated from the doublets by a pepsin extractable, proteinaceous material. The glycogen granules are extracted after treatment with α–amylase solution (Fig. 5).

Spermatozoa of cirriped crustaceans are flagellate and are capable of motility. These sperm contain large amounts of glycogen. In sperm of *Lepas* for example, the glycogen particles are disposed as a thick ridge on one side of the axoneme and as a single row on the opposite side (Fig. 8).

Spermatozoa of fresh-water pulmonate gastropods (*Planorbis*, *Lymnaea*, *Helisoma*) and filliform sperm of the prosobranch gastropods (*Pomacea*, *Viviparus*) possess a highly differentiated mitochondrial derivative and an enormous tail piece. Particles with staining properties similar to glycogen occupy the matrix between the central tubules and outer doublets of the axoneme (Figs. 9, 11 and 12; PERSONNE and ANDERSON, in preparation. Glycogen storage seems to be a widespread characteristic in sperm of fresh-water and terrestrial pulmonate gastropods, since mature sperm of all species studied so far contain glycogen reserves within their middle piece. These sperm possess a highly modified mitochondrial derivative that is composed in part of a paracrystalline compartment (ANDRÉ, 1962; PERSONNE, 1965). Depending upon the species, the glycogen reserves are located in one or more compartments that course low-pitched helices within the paracrystalline compartment of sperm of *Testacella*, *Vaginalis* and *Helix* (LANZA and QUATTRINI, 1964; PERSONNE and ANDRÉ, 1964; ANDRÉ, 1965). The glycogen reserves occupy membrane-bounded compartments, and as such are set apart from the paracrystalline derivative (Figs. 9–11). Similarly, in relatively unmodified mitochondria that form the middle piece of sperm of of *Paracentrotus* the glycogen reserves occupy membrane-limited compartments (ANDERSON, 1968). Glycogen granules form a thick mantle around the axoneme in the tail piece of sperm of fresh-water pulmonate gastropods (Fig. 12).

Based on morphological findings, glycogen-like granules have been detected in sperm of the Plathyhelminthes and Chilopoda (SILVERIA and PORTER, 1964; VON BONSDORFF and TELKKA, 1965; HORSTMAN, 1968). The outer fibers of the axoneme of sperm of some insects contain an active polysaccharide with properties similar to glycogen (BACCETTI *et al.*, 1969 a; 1969 b). So far however, typical glycogen granules have not been observed in mature sperm of mammals, birds, and insects that have been studied by us (ANDERSON and PERSONNE, 1970).

According to these cytochemical findings, glycogen granules are detected in centrioles and basal bodies, in the matrix between the axonemal doublets and the flagellar membrane, at the level of the secondary fibers between the central tubules and the outer doublets, in the packing cytoplasm between mitochondria of the middle piece, and in membrane-limited compartments in unmodified and in highly modified mitochondrial derivatives of sperm of some invertebrate and vertebrate species. A more detailed study on glycogen storage in spermatozoa is presented in another report (ANDERSON and PERSONNE, 1970). Glycogen storage in spermatozoa seems to be a relatively widespread phenomenon. The intracellular glycogen accumulation commences subsequent to the completion of spermatozoan maturation, since developing spermatids and immature spermatozoa lacked recognizable glycogen deposits. It is speculated that this polysaccharide is an intracellular constituent of considerable importance in the economy of the cell. Endogenous glycogen stores in these spermatozoa are believed to represent an important source of glycolyzable material for the production of energy.

The Localization of Enzymes Related to the Metabolism of Glycogen.

Demonstration of Amylophosphorylase Activity.

The presence of intracellular glycogen stores implies the existence of functional pathways for glycogen metabolism in spermatozoa. It is well established that regulation of glycogen metabolism is carried out mainly through the activities of phosphorylase and glycogen synthetase (CORI *et al.*, 1938; KREBS and FISCHER, 1962; LELOIR, 1967). These two enzymes catalyze respectively the *in vivo* degradation and synthesis of glycogen. When appropriately stimulated, phosphorylase can catalyze the *in vitro* synthesis of glycogen (MORDOCH *et al.*, 1965; WANSON and DROCHMANS, 1968). Thus by simultaneously activating phosphorylase *b*–kinase with either 5–AMP, cyclic 3,5–AMP, or ATP and Mg^{++} ions, and by inactivating phosphorylase phosphatase by NaF, the conversion of nonactivated phosphorylase *b* to activated phosphorylase *a* is effected (TAKEUCHI and KURIAKI, 1955; GUHA and WEGMANN, 1959; 1961). In the presence of glucose–1–phosphate, ATP, Mg^{++} ions and NaF, phosphorylase *a* catalyzes the *in vivo* synthesis of glycogen (PERSONNE and ANDERSON, 1970). The newly-formed glycogen molecules appear on the surface of preformed glycogen particles that occupy the mitochondrial derivative of sperm of pulmonate gastropods (Figs. 14 and 15). Newly-formed glycogen molecules are absent from specimens incubated in medium lacking glucose–1–phosphate (Fig. 13). The neoformed granules disappear after treatment with α–amylase solution. However, they persist after treatment with β–amylase suggesting the branched nature of the polysaccharide molecules and the participation of the branching enzyme in their synthesis. Our findings therefore concur with those of WANSON and

DROCHMANS (1968) that the locus of amylophosphorylase activity is the surface of preformed glycogen granules. These findings further indicate that an active phosphorylase and other enzymes participating in glycogen synthesis are located in the mitochondrial derivative of glycogen-containing spermatozoa. It must be pointed out however, that although under appropriate conditions phosphorylase catalyzes the synthesis of glycogen, under normal physiological conditions this enzyme functions in glycogen degradation. Attempts to localize phosphorylase activity in sperm that lack glycogen stores (eg. mammalian spermatozoa) have so far been unsuccessful.

Demonstration of Glucose–6–phosphatase Activity.

Glucose–6–phosphate occupies a key position in glycogen metabolism since it is a common intermediate in glycogenesis, glycogenolysis, and glycolysis (KREBS and FISCHER, 1962). Consequently, activity of glucose–6–phosphatase directly influences the disposition of this substrate and is thus of great importance in the regulation of glycogen metabolism. Glucose–6–phosphatase is generally considered a microsomal enzyme (BEAUFAY and DE DUVE, 1957), that is cytochemically localized in the lumen of the endoplasmic reticulum (GOLDFISCHER *et al.*, 1964). It is highly unusual then to consistently localize this enzyme within the middle piece of sperm of pulmonate gastropods (ANDERSON *et al.*, 1968). In sperm of *Helix*, enzyme reaction product for this enzyme is mainly localized in the matrix between the fibers of the axoneme and on the membrane that limits the matrical compartment of this mitochondrion (Fig. 16). Control specimens show no activity for glucose–6–phosphatase (Fig. 17). Even in relatively unmodified mitochondria of the sea urchin spermatozoa, glucose–6–phosphatase activity appears on the matrical side of the internal membranes (Fig. 18), while control specimens are unreactive for this enzyme (Fig. 19). The significance of glucose–6–phosphatase activity in the axonemal and mitochondrial compartments of spermatozoa is unresolved at this time, however it is speculated that this enzyme may play an important role in glycogen metabolism in these spermatozoa (ANDERSON, 1968; ANDERSON *et al.*, 1968). Extreme caution must however be exercised in the interpretation of these findings, for other phosphatases or a polyphosphatase with broad substrate specificity could also be responsible for the hydrolysis of glucose–6–phosphate.

The Demonstration of Glycolytic Dehydrogenases in Spermatozoa.

Numerous studies have established that ATP is the main source of energy for spermatozoan motility and metabolism (LARDY and PHILLIPS, 1945; MANN, 1945; 1964; ROTHSCHILD and MANN, 1950). The ATP level is maintained by either glycolytic or oxidative phosphorylation, or by both processes in some cases. It is speculated that intracellular glycogen reserves may serve as an important source of glycolyzable material in sperm that store this polysaccharide. Acetyl radicals provided by glycolysis may also be utilized oxidatively by sperm of some species.

Numerous technical difficulties interfere with the cytochemical demonstration of enzymes of the Embden–Meyerhof pathway. These enzymes are soluble in aqueous medium and attempts to localize them in unfixed and frozen tissues results in their diffusion from intracellular sites. Prefixation in glutaraldehyde normally inhibits enzymatic activity. However, prefixation in formaldehyde solution according to FAHIMI and KARNOVSKY (1966) for no longer than 10–20 mins preserves enzyme activity and prevents extracellular diffusion. Moreover, to detect maximal activity for the glycolytic dehydrogenases it is essential to include small amounts of phenazine methosulfate (PMS) in the incubation medium. PMS largely transfers electron from reduced NAD directly to the tetrazolium salts, significantly bypassing the associated $NADH_2$–tetrazolium reductases (FARBER *et al.*, 1964). Using PMS and tetra nitro blue tetrazolium salts (T–NBT) FAHIMI and KARNOVSKY (1966) demonstrated activity for glyceraldehyde–3–phosphate dehydrogenase (GAPD) and lactate dehydrogenase (LDH) in the lumen of the sarcoplasmic reticulum and in mitochondria of striated muscle. Enzyme reaction product in mitochondria is thought to represent either $NADH_2$–tetrazolium reductase activity due to the incomplete bypassing by PMS or the existence of an active intramitochondrial isozyme.

Spermatozoa with intracellular glycogen stores (*Helix*, *Helisoma*, *Otala*) are intensely reactive for both GAPD and LDH. When the incubation medium contained PMS so that the staining system was largely independent of the tissue diaphorase system, NAD–linked enzyme activity for these dehydrogenases appears in the glycogen compartment and in the matrix compartment of these mitochondrial derivatives (Fig. 20). In the absence of PMS, reaction product indicating activity for the $NADH_2$–tetrazolium reductases associated with GAPD and LDH is relegated to the matrix compartment (Fig. 21). It appears then that PMS not only suppresses activity for the $NADH_2$–tetrazolium reductases, but augments activity for the glycolytic dehydrogenases. In tissues incubated in medium lacking substrate, but containing T–NBT or thiocarbamyl–NBT (TC–NBT) and PMS, intracellular formazan deposits were absent. Moreover, the complete inhibition of GAPD and LDH activity respectively with iodoacetate and iodine indicates the enzymatic nature of these reactions. These findings demonstrate therefore that the dehydrogenases that catalyze the oxidation-reduction reactions of the glycolytic pathway are localized mainly in the glycogen compartment, but are present in the matrix compartment as well. These findings further support the suggestion that the glycolytic enzymes are located in close proximity to the glycogen reserves within the mitochondrial derivatives of sperm of pulmonate gastropods.

Spermatozoa of some species that lack intracellular glycogen reserves are known to contain the complete system of enzymes of the Embden-Meyerhof pathway. Moreover, when extracellular metabolites are available, sperm of mammals utilize glycolysis preferentially even in the presence of oxygen. By means of light microscope cytochemical procedures, enzyme systems associated with the glycolytic dehydrogenases have been localized in the middle piece of these spermatozoa (BALOGH and COHEN, 1964). At the light microscope level the opaque formazan deposits completely fill the middle piece; it thus obscures the underlying components and limits resolution of the interfaces responsible for enzyme activity.

However, electron microscope cytochemical findings indicate that in the absence of PMS, the $NADH_2$–tetrazolium system associated with LDH activity is primarily localized in the matrix of mitochondria that compose their middle piece. However, in the presence of PMS enzyme activity in the mitochondria deminishes, and formazan deposits now appear in the axonemal compartment. Specifically, formazan deposits appear at the interface of adjacent coarse fibers. Based on these findings, it is suggested that two distinct species of LDH exist within the middle piece of the rat spermatozoon. These findings are supported by data obtained from electrophoretic analyses of homogenates of washed epididymal spermatozoa, in which at least 2 slow-moving LDH isozymes are most prominent. The slow-moving LDH isozymes are known to function in glycolytically active tissues, by catalyzing the anaerobic production of lactate with the simultaneous oxidation of $NADH_2$–NAD. (KAPLAN, 1965). LDH may therefore play a significant role in the metabolism of these spermatozoa by regulating the balance of $NADH_2$–NAD under conditions of low oxygen tension.

The Demonstration of Sorbitol Dehydrogenase Activity in Spermatozoa.

Polyols (glycerol and sorbitol) which are normally present in the semen are metabolized by spermatozoa of mammals (MANN, 1964). Sorbitol for example, is oxidized to fructose–1–6–diphosphate which is subsequently metabolised via glycolysis. Polyols could therefore serve as an important source of energy in spermatozoan metabolism. Sorbitol dehydrogenase catalyzes the oxidation of sorbitol and could significantly regulate the glycolytic metabolism of these spermatozoa. Enzyme activity indicating the $NADH_2$–tetrazolium reductase system associated with sorbitol dehydrogenase activity is consistently localized in the middle piece of mammalian spermatozoa (BISHOP, 1967). In sperm of pulmonate gastropods, the $NADH_2$–tetrazolium reductase system allied to sorbitol dehydrogenase is relegated to the matrix compartment of the mitochondrial derivative (ANDERSON and PERSONNE, 1969 b).

The Localization of Oxidative and Respiratory Enzymes in Spermatozoa.

Actively motile spermatozoa generally possess a distinct mitochondrial derivative that is closely associated with their kinetic apparatus. However, the degree of structural modification and juxtaposition to the axoneme varies extensively with the species. Thus for example, primitive sperm of marine invertebrates usually possess relatively unmodified mitochondria, whereas sperm of some molluscs and insects possess complex crystalline derivatives. Still, in motile sperm of some species (eg. coccids) a recognizable mitochondrial derivative is absent (ROBISON, 1966). Indeed, the degree of structural modification may represent physiological adaptation for survival in the milieu in which they are stored and released. Thus sperm of mammals are known to utilize glycolysis preferentially even in the presence of oxygen, and are thus equipped to survive in the carbohydrate-rich seminal fluid. However even the extensively modified mitochondria appear to possess the the enzyme systems and chemical intermediates that maintain the metabolic and energetic demands for motile activity. Chemical similarity to typical mitochondria of somatic cells is indicated by biochemical studies on mitochondria isolated from vertebrate and invertebrate spermatozoa (MOHRI *et al.*, 1964).

Cytochemical data at the light and electron microscope levels concur with data from biochemistry that succinate dehydrogenase (SDH) activity is relegated to the mitochondrial middle piece of sperm of mammals (NELSON, 1958; 1959; 1962; NACHLAS *et al.*, 1958; BIRNS and MASEK, 1961; EDWARDS and VALENTINE, 1963) and of some invertebrates (ANDRÉ, 1962; GUPTA, 1962). BALOGH and COHEN (1964) further localized diaphorase activity associated with malate and isocitrate dehydrogenase and SDH activity in the middle piece of air-dried spermatozoa. These findings do not permit the precise localization of the diaphorase or SDH tetrazolium reductase activity since formazan deposits obscure the underlying components responsible for enzyme activity. Using techniques that offer better resolution, an extramitochondrial SDH tetrazolium reductase is demonstrated in the coarse fibers of sperm tails of mammals (NELSON, 1959). More recent studies using TC–NBT (according to SELIGMAN *et al.*, 1967) localize SDH–tetrazolium reductase activity specifically on or in the internal membranes of mitochondria of the guinea pig sperm. Even when PMS is added to the incubation medium the coarse fibers remain unreactive for SDH–tetrazolium reductase. As in mitochondria of somatic cells, SDH activity resides on or in the internal membranes of mitochondria from mammalian spermatozoa.

Spermatozoa of pulmonate gastropods possess an enormous mitochondrial derivative that is composed in part of a proteinaceous, paracrystalline compartment (ANDRÉ, 1962; PERSONNE, 1965). The crystal encases a membrane-limited matrix compartment named the secondary helix by ANDRÉ (1962). Using T–NBT or TC–NBT and appropriate substrates and cofactors, SDH–tetrazolium reductase and $NADH_2$–tetrazolium reductases associated with the Kreb's cycle dehydrogenases are localized within the matrix compartment of these mitochondrial derivatives (PERSONNE and ANDERSON, 1969 a). Opaque formazan deposits indicating SDH–tetrazolium reductase activity are shown in the secondary helix of sperm of *Helisoma* (Fig. 22). This is a highly unusual finding that differs significantly from observations of unmodified mitochondria in which SDH activity appears on or in the internal membranes (SELIGMAN *et al.*, 1967). Studies using the copper ferricyanide technique for demonstrating SDH activity (KERPEL–FRONIUS and HAJOS, 1968), support the observation that the Kreb's tricarboxylic acid cycle enzymes occupy the matrix compartment (secondary helix) of these mitochondrial derivatives.

Whereas the Kreb's cycle enzymes occupy the matrix compartment, recent cytochemical findings indicate that activity for cytochrome oxidase appears in the paracrystalline compartment of these mitochondrial derivatives. Spectrophotometric data further indicate that these spermatozoa contain all the enzymes of the respiratory chain (RITTER and ANDRÉ, unpublished). It seems apparent that in these unusual mitochondria the Kreb's cycle and respiratory enzymes are spatially separated in juxtaposed compartments.

Mitochondrial metamorphosis during spermiogenesis of prosobranch gastropods is extensive (KAYE, 1959). In these species typical mitochondria aggregate and coalesce to form two ovoid derivatives located at the base of the nucleus. Subsequent mitochondrial metamorphosis involves the condensation of the matrix and the formation of a highly laminated system of internal membranes. The helical mitochondrial derivative completely ensheathes a portion of the axoneme. Using improved techniques according to SELIGMAN and coworkers (1968) cytochrome oxidase activity is demonstrated in metamorphosing mitochondria during spermiogenesis of *Viviparus* and *Pomacea.* In typical mitochondria and in the ovoid mitochondrial complex, cytochrome oxidase activity is restricted to the outer surface of the internal membranes (Fig. 23). During the phase of mitochondrial elongation the cristae lose their regularity and continuity, and portions of the cristal material are randomly scattered in the matrix. Isolated clumps of matrix material also stain positively for cytochrome oxidase activity. By mechanisms that are still undetermined the internal membranes become organized into a continuous, regularly-repeating system of laminae that encase portions of the opaque matrix and which delimit the clear intracristal compartments. In these mitochondrial derivatives, cytochrome oxidase activity appears only on the outer surface of the internal membranes (Fig. 24). In over-reacted specimen, opaque deposits for cytochrome oxidase activity completely fill the intracristal space. Therefore, the sites of cytochrome oxidase activity and SDH–tetrazolium reductase activity are identical in these mitochondria. These findings support the view that the locus for both parts of the respiratory chain may be located in or on the outer surface of the internal membranes of membranous mitochondria (SELIGMAN *et al.*, 1968).

Comparative studies on the highly compartmentalized mitochondrial derivatives of spermatozoa might yield information on the loci of oxidative and respiratory enzymes and on their relationship to each other within mitochondrial compartments. Data from cytochemistry indicate that in the membranous mitochondrial derivatives of sperm of mammals and of prosobranch gastropods, the respiratory chain from flavoprotein to cytochrome *c* appear in or on the outer surface of the internal membranes that delimit the intracristal space. Thus sites for SDH–cytochrome *b* to cytochrome *c* are closely related or identical. In this way they resemble typical mitochondria from somatic cells (SELIGMAN *et al.*, 1968). A highly contrasting situation is demonstrated by the paracrystalline mitochondrial derivative of sperm of pulmonate gastropods, in which SDH activity occupies a matrix compartment while cytochrome oxidase activity is relegated to the crystalline compartment. As ANDRÉ (1965) suggested the subunits of the crystal bear some resemblance to the elementary particles described by FERNANDEZ–MORAN *et al.*, (1964). It is further speculated that these subunits which contain the respiratory chain enzymes are arranged in repetitive array. These mitochondria exhibit therefore the complete spatial segregation of systems of enzymes of the Kreb's cycle and of the respiratory pathways. Dehydrogenases located in the matrix compartment probably discharge the reducing equivalents to the respiratory chain components of the crystalline compartment. The complete elucidation of the oxidative phosphorylation processes occurring in these mitochondrial derivatives must await further biochemical and cytochemical studies. Indeed, the extreme structural and chemical compartmentation exhibited by these mitochondria may be related to the efficiency of the oxidative and phosphorylation processes and to the translocation of high-energy intermediates to the kinetic apparatus.

The Demonstration of ATPase Activity in Spermatozoa.

The uniformity of the dimension and arrangement of the longitudinal fibers of sperm tails of mammals and some invertebrates is well-established by electron microscopy (AFZELIUS, 1959; ANDRÉ, 1961; FAWCETT, 1965). Their constant presence in the motile apparatus of spermatozoa strongly suggests that intrinsic mechanochemical changes in their structure may produce the forces of contraction. However, although this subject has been extensively studied with a variety of cytochemical, cytoimmunochemical and biochemical procedures, there is still no clear evidence that contractility of the longitudinal fibers is involved in spermatozoan motility.

In addition to microtubules that form the axoneme, accessory coarse fibers are present in sperm tails of mammals, birds, some insects and molluscs. The degree of development of the coarse fibers varies with the species (CLELAND and ROTSCHILD, 1959; FAWCETT, 1962; 1965; FAWCETT and ITO, 1965). In sperm of some species the coarse fibers and outer doublets are juxtaposed (ANDERSON and PERSONNE, 1967), whereas in others they are located at great distances from the peripheral doublets (CLELAND and ROTHSCHILD, 1959). They are directly continuous with the segmented columns forming the neck of sperm of pulmonate gastropods, while in most mammals they are separate and distinct elements attached to the columns of the connecting piece (FAWCETT, 1965). Coarse fibers are generally present in sperm possessing a large middle piece and in those that effect internal fertilization. Although contractility of the coarse fibers is yet to be proven, these structures are thought to function in collaboration with the axoneme in bending the middle piece. Their shape and arrangement are consistent with their presumed role in concentrating the contractile thrust in one major plane (FAWCETT, 1968; FAWCETT and ITO, 1965). Satellite fibers occupying the matrix between the coarse fibers (Fig. 27), the thin filaments (spokes and secondary fibers surrounding the central tubules, and the projections (arms) on subfiber A of the outer doublets are considered to represent the structural components that perform essential functions of spermatozoan motility (ANDRÉ, 1961; GIBBONS, 1965; FAWCETT, 1968). These structural components within the axoneme may well represent contractile proteins as well as sites of glycolytic and hydrolytic enzymes, while the seemingly structureless matrix may represent the pathway for the transfer of soluble substances (eg. ATP, ADP, ions, et.) to and from the mitochondrial and axonemal compartments.

Correlated biochemical and anatomical studies of glycerinated models of spermatozoa (BISHOP, 1962; BISHOP and HOFFMANN–BERLING, 1959) and of extractions of flagella (ENGELHARDT, 1945; ENGELHARDT and BURNASHEVA, 1957; BURNASHEVA, 1958; TIBBS, 1962; GIBBONS, 1965; 1968) indicate that the energy for spermatozoan motility is provided by the dephosphorylation of ATP. The specificity for ATP is high, as other nucleoside triphosphates support little or no motility of flagella (Brokaw, 1961). The requirement for Mg^{++} and Ca^{++} ions is also high, although cytochemical and biochemical evidence concur on the existence of both Mg^{++} and Ca^{++} stimulated ATPases in sperm tails (GIBBONS, 1965; GORDON and BARRNETT, 1967). At *p*H 7.0, M_9^{++} stimulated ATPase predominates; ATPase activity appears in the mitochondria and in the axoneme (NAGANO, 1965; ANDERSON and PERSONNE, 1969 a; ANDERSON *et al.*, 1968). At pH 9.0, Ca^{++} stimulated ATPase predominates (NELSON, 1958), but its activity also appears at *p*H 7.0 (GORDON and BARRNETT, 1967). Indeed, the presence of several ATPases in sperm tails is not surprising in view of the variety of metabolic pathways in these cell that require the dephosphorylation of ATP.

Based on extraction and reconstitution studies (GIBBONS, 1965; GIBBONS and ROWE, 1965) strong evidence is provided that the arms on subfiber A of the outer doublets of fish and sea urchin sperm tails are largely composed of a contractile protein called " dynein ". Dynein bears some similarity to muscle myosin, but these proteins differ somewhat in their enzymatic properties and molecular dimensions. Dynein possesses high ATPase activity. It is speculated that interaction between the arms and subfiber B of the adjacent doublet may provide the forces essential to motility (GIBBONS, 1965). However, based on cytochemical studies, activity for Mg^{++} stimulated ATPase is not restricted to the arms on the outer tubules. Enzyme-reaction product is localized at the interface between adjacent coarse fibers and doublets, and on the surface of the central tubules (Fig. 25, see also NAGANO, 1965; GORDON and BARRNETT, 1967; ANDERSON *et al.*, 1968; ANDERSON and PERSONNE, 1969 a). In over-reacted specimens, enzyme-reaction product occupies the matrix between the coarse fibers and between the outer and central tubules (Figs. 26 and 28). Underlying satellite fibers and thin filaments may account for the hydrolysis of ATP within the axoneme of sperm tails.

References

Afzelius B. (1959) – *Electron microscopy of the sperm tail: results obtained with a new fixative.* « J. Biophys. Biochem. Cytol. », 5, 269–278.

Afzelius B. and Mohri H. (1966) – *Mitochondria respiring without exogenous substrate. A study of aged sea urchin spermatozoa.* « Exp. Cell Res. », 42, 10.

Anderson W. A. (1968) – *Cytochemistry of sea urchin gametes.* I. *Intramitochondrial localization of glycogen, glucose–6–phosphatase and adenosine triphosphatase activity in spermatozoa of* Paracentrotus lividus. « J. Ultrastruct. Res. », 24, 398–411.

Anderson W. A. and Personne P. (1967) – *The fine structure of the neck region of spermatozoa of* Helix aspersa. « J. Microscopie », 6, 1033–1042.

Anderson W. A. and Personne P. (1969 a) – *Structure and histochemistry of the basal body derivative, neck and axoneme of spermatozoa of* Helix aspersa. « J. Microscopie », 8, 87–96.

Anderson W. A. and Personne P. (1969 b) – *The cytochemical localization of sorbitol dehydrogenase activity in spermatozoa of* Helix aspersa. « J. Microscopie », 8, 97–102.

Anderson W. A. and Personne P. (1970) – *The localization of glycogen in the spermatozoa of various invertebrate and vertebrate species.* (In preparation).

Anderson W. A., Personne P. and André J. (1968) – *Chemical compartmentalization in* Helix *spermatozoa.* « J. Microscopie », 7, 367–390.

Anderson W. A., Weissman A. and Ellis R. A. (1967) – *Cytodifferentiation during spermiogenesis in* Lumbricus terrestris. « J. Cell Biol. », 32, 11–26.

André J. (1961) – *Sur quelques détails nouvellement connus de l'ultrastructure des organites vibratiles.* « J. Ultrastruct. Res. », 5, 86–108.

André J. (1962) – *Contribution à la connaissance du chondriome: étude de ses modifications ultrastructurales pendant la spermatogenèse.* « J. Ultrastruct. Res. », suppl. 3, 1–185.

André J. (1965) – *Quelques données récentes sur la structure et la physiologie des mitochondries: Glycogène, particules élémentaires, acides nucléiques.* « Arch. Biol., Liege. », 76, 277–304.

Baccetti B., Dallai R. and Rosati F. (1969 a) – *The spermatozoon of Arthropoda.* III. *The lowest holometabolic insects.* « J. Microscopie », 8, 233–248.

Baccetti B., Bigliardi E., Dallai R. and Rosati F. (1969 b) – *The outer coarse fibers the axial filament complex of insect spermatozoa.* « J. Microscopie », 8, 32 a.

Balogh K. and Cohen R. B. (1964) – *A cytochemical technic for studying oxidative enzyme systems in mammalian spermatozoa in semen smears.* « Fertility Sterility », 15, 35–39.

Beaufay H. and de Duve C. (1957) – *Altération précoce des lysosomes au cours de la nécrose massive d'un lobe hépatique.* « Arch. Inter. Physiol. Biochem. », 65, 156–157.

Birns M. and Masek B. (1961) – *Localization of enzyme activities in frozen-substituted-fixed cells.* « J. Histochem. Cytochem. », 9, 204–206.

Bishop D. W. (1961) – *Biology of spermatozoa.* – In Sex and Internal Secretions. Young, W. C. ed. Williams and Wilkins, Baltimore, Md. 2, 707–796.

Bishop D. W. (1962) – *Reactivation of sperm cell models in relation to the mechanism of motility. In* Spermatozoan Motility. Bishop, D. W. ed. Am. Assoc. Advanc. Sci. Press., Washington, D. C. pp. 251–268.

Bishop D. W. (1967) – *Significance of testicular sorbitol dehydrogenase (SDH).* « J. Gen. Physiol. », 50, 2504.

Bishop D. W. and Hoffmann–Berling H. (1959) – *Extracted mammalian sperm models.* I. *Preparation and reactivation with adenosine triphosphate.* « J. Cellular Comp. Physiol. », 53, 445–466.

von Bonsdorff C–H. and Telkka A. (1965) – *The spermatozoon flagella of* Diphyllobothrium latum (*fish tapeworm*). « Z. Zellforsch. », 66, 543.

Brokaw C. J. (1961) – *Movement and nucleoside polyphosphatase activity of isolated flagella from* Polytoma uvella. « Exp. Cell Res. », 22, 151–162.

BURNASHEVA S. A. (1958) – *Properties of spermosin, a contractile protein in sperm cells.* « Biokhimia », 23, 558–563.

CLELAND K. W. and LORD ROTHSCHILD (1959) – *The bandicoot spermatozoon: an electron microscope study of the tail.* « Proc. Royal. Soc. », Series B, 50, 24–42.

CORI G. T., COLOWICK S. P. and CORI C. F. (1938) – *The action of nucleotides in the disruptive phosphorylation of glycogen.* « J. Biol. Chem. », 123, 381–389.

DROCHMANS P. (1962) – *Morphologie du glycogene. Etude au microscope electronique de colorations negatives du glycogene particulaire.* « J. Ultrastruct. Res. », 6, 141–1.

EDWARDS R. G. and VALENTINE R. C. (1963) – *Cytochemical demonstration of succinic dehydrogenase in intact rabbit spermatozoa.* « Exp. Cell Res. », 31, 508–516.

ENGELDARDT V. A. (1945) – *Phosphoric acids and cell functions.* « Bull. Acad. Sci. USSR », Biol. Series 2, 182–195.

ENGELDARDT V. A. and BURNASHEVA S. A. (1957) – *Localization of the protein spermosin in sperm cells.* « Biochemistry », 22, 513–518.

FAHIMI H. D. and KARNOVSKY M. J. (1966) – *Cytochemical localization of two glycolytic dehydrogenases in wite skeletal muscle.* « J. Cell Biol. », 29, 113–128.

FARBER E., STERNBERG W. H. and DUNLAP C. E. (1954) – *Histochemical localization of specific oxidative enzymes.* I. *Tetrazolium stains for diphosphopyridine nucleotide diaphorase and triphosphopyridine nucleotide diaphorase.* « J. Histochem. Cytochem. », 4, 254–265.

FAWCETT D. W. (1958) – *The structure of the mammalian spermatozoon.* « Int. Rev. Cytol. », 7, 195–235.

FAWCETT D. W. (1962) – *Sperm tail structure in relation to the mechanism of movement.* In « Spermatozoan Motility » Bishop, D. W. ed. Am. Assoc. Advanc. Sci. Press, Washington, D. C. pp. 147–169.

FAWCETT D. W. (1965) – *The anatomy of the mammalian spermatozoon with particular reference to the guinea pig.* « Z. Zellforsch. », 67, 279–296.

FAWCETT D. W. (1968) – *The topographical relationship between the plane of the central pair of flagellar fibrils and the transverse axis of the head in guinea-pig spermatozoa.* « J. Cell Sci. », 3, 187–198.

FAWCETT D. W. and ITO S. (1965) – *The fine structure of bat spermatozoa.* « Am. J. Anat. », 116, 567–610.

FERNANDEZ-MORAN H., ODA T., BLAIR P. V. and GREEN D. E. (1964) – *A macromolecular repeating unit of mitochondrial structure and function.* « J. Cell Biol. », 22, 63–100.

FRANZEN A. (1956) – *On spermiogenesis, morphiology of the spermatozoon, and biology of fertilization among invertebrates.* « Zool. Bidr. Uppsala », 31, 355–482.

GIBBONS I. R. (1965) – *Chemical dissection of cilia.* « Arch. Biol., Liege », 76, 317–352.

GIBBONS I. R. (1968) – The *biochemistry of motility.* « Ann. Rev. of Biochem. », 37, 521–546.

GIBBONS I. R. and ROWE A. J. (1965) – *Dynein: a protein with adenosine triphosphatase activity from cilia.* « Science », 149, 424–426.

GOLDFISCHER S., ESSNER E. and NOVIKOFF A. B. (1964) – *The localization of phosphatase activities at the level of ultrastructure.* « J. Histochem. Cytochem. », 12, 72–95.

GONSE P. H. (1962) – *Respiration and oxidative phosphorylation in relation to sperm motility.* In « Spermatozoan Motility », Bishop, D. W. ed. Am. Assoc. Advanc. Sci. Press, Washington, D. C. 99–132.

GORDON M. and BARRNETT R. J. (1967) – *Fine structural cytochemical localizations of phosphatase activities of rat and guineapig spermatozoa.* « Exp. Cell Res. », 48, 395–411.

GUHA S. and WEGMANN R. (1959) – *Etudes sur l'activité phosphorylasique.* I. *Une nouvelle méthode de mise en évidence de la phosphorylase.* « Ann. Histochem. », 4, 103–114.

GUHA S. and WEGMANN R. (1961) – *Phosphorylase in chick-embryo liver.* « J. Histochem. Cytochem. » 9, 454–455.

GUPTA B. L. (1962) – *Histochemical localization of succinic dehydrogenase activity in the mitochondria of some invertebrate spermatozoa.* « Nature », 193, 788.

HORSTMANN E. (1968) – *Die spermatozoen von* Geophilus Tinearis *Koch* (*cliopada*). « Z. Zellforsch. », 89, 410–429.

HUMPHREY G. F. (1950) – *The metabolism of oyster spermatozoa.* « Aust. J. Exp. Biol. Med. Sci. », 28, 1.

KAPLAN N. O. (1965) – *Evolution of dehydrogenases.* In « Evolving Genes and Proteins, Bryson V. and Vogel H. J., eds. Academic Press Inc., New York and London, 243–277.

KAYE J. S. (1958) – *Changes in the fine structure of mitochondria during spermatogenesis.* « J. Morphol. », 102, 347–3.

KERPEL–FRONIUS S. and HAJOS F. (1968) – *The use of ferricyanide for the light and electron microscope demonstration of succinic dehydrogenase activity.* « Histochemie », 14, 343–351.

KREBS E. G. and FISHER E. H. (1962) – *Molecular properties and transformations of glycogen phosphorylase in animal tissues.* « Advances in Enzymology », 24, 263–290.

LANZA B. and QUATTRINI D. (1964) – *Observazioni sul contenuto in glicogeno degli spermi epiteli della ganade e delle vie sessuali ermafrodite di* Vaginalus borellianus (*Colosi*) (*Mollusca, Gastropoda, Soleolifera*). « Boll. Società Italiana Biol. Spermentale », 40, 1154–1155.

LARDY H. A. and PHILLIPS P. H. (1945) – *Studies of fat and carbohydrate oxidation in mammalian spermatozoa.* « Arch. Biochem. », 6, 53–61.

LELOIR L. F. (1967) – *Regulation of glycogen metabolism.* In. « International Symposium Enzymatic Aspects of Metabolic Regulation » National Cancer Instit. Monograph. U. S. Dept. of Health Education and Welfare, No. 27, 3–18.

MANN T. (1945) – *Metabolism of semen.* I. *General aspects. Occurrence and distribution of cytochrome, certain enzymes and coenzymes.* « Biochem. J. », 39, 451–458.

MANN T. (1964) – *Biochemistry of Senem.* «Methuen and Co Ltd. », London.

MANN T. (1967) – *Sperm metabolism.* In « Fertilization », Metz. C.B. and Monroy, A. eds. Academic Press Inc., New York and London, 1, 99–116.

MOHRI H., MOHRI T. and ERNSTER L. (1964) – *Biochemical properties of bull–sperm mitochondria.* « Biochem. J. », 92, 38 P.

MORDOH J., LELOIR L. F. and KRISMAN C. R. (1965) – In vitro *synthesis of particulate glycogen.* « Proc. Natl. Acad. Sci. », 53, 86–91.

NACHLAS M. M., TSOU K. C., DE SOUZA E., CHENG C. S. and SELIGMAN A. M. (1957) – *Cytochemical demonstration of succinic dehydrogenase by the use of a new p-nitrophenyl substituted ditetrazole.* « J. Histochem. Cytochem. », 5, 420–436.

NAGANO T. (1965) – *Localization of adenosine triphosphatase activity in the rat sperm tail as revealed by electron microscopy.* « J. Cell Biol. », 25, 101–112.

NELSON L. (1958) – *Cytochemical studies with the electron microscope.* I. *Adenosinetriphosphatase in rat spermatozoa.* « Biochem. Biophys. Acta », 27, 634–641.

NELSON L. (1959) – *Cytochemical studies with the electron microscope.* II. *Succinic dehydrogenase in rat spermatozoa.* « Exp. Cell Res. », 16, 403–410.

NELSON L. (1962) – *Cytochemical aspects of spermatozoan motility.* In « Spermatozoan Motility », Bishop D. W., ed. Am. Assoc. Advanc. Sci. Press, Washington, D. C. pp. 171–187.

NELSON L. (1967) – *Sperm motility.* In Fertilization, Metz, C. B. and Monroy, A., eds. Academic Press Inc., New York and London, 1, 27–97.

PERSONNE P. (1965) – *Etude cytochemique du dérivé mitochondrial du spermatozoide de la Testacelle: recherche des protéines et des lipides.* « J. Microscopie », 4, 627–641.

PERSONNE P. and ANDERSON W. A. (1969 a) – *Compartimentage des activités enzymatiques dans le spermatoide de certains Mollusques Gastéropodes.* I. *Localisation des dehydrogenases.* « J. Cell Sci. », 4, 693–707.

PERSONNE P. and ANDERSON W. A. (1970) – *Localisation mitochondriale d'enzymes liées au métabolisme du glycogène dans le spermatozoide de l'escargot.* « J. Cell Biol. », 44, 20–28.

PERSONNE P. and ANDERSON W. A. – *Existence de glycogène intraflagellaire dans le spermatozoïde des Gastéropodes Pulmonés* (in preparation).

PERSONNE P. and ANDRÉ J. (1964) – *Existence de glycogène mitochondrial dans le spermatozoïde de la Testacelle.* « J. Microscopie », 3, 643–650.

RESTIVO F. and REVERBERI G. (1957) – *Ricerche sugli spermi di* Ciona *e di* Patella. *Localizzazione della citocromo-ossidasi della succino-deidrogenasi e del glicogeno.* « Acta Embryol. Morphol. Exp. », 1, 164–170.

REYNOLDS E. S. (1963) – *The use of lead citrate at high pH as an electron opaque stain in electron microscopy.* « J. Cell Biol. », 17, 208–212.

RITTER C. and ANDRÉ J. *Cytochromes and hemoglobin in sperm of* Helix aspersa (*Muller*) (unpublished results).

ROBISON W. B. (1966) – *Microtubules in relation to the motility of asperm syncytium in an armored scale insect.* « J. Cell Biol. », 29, 251–266.

ROTHSCHILD LORD (1951) – *Sea-urchin spermatozoa.* « Biol. Revs. », 26, 1–27.

ROTHSCHILD LORD and MANN T. (1950) – *Carbohydrate and adenosine-triphosphate in sea-urchin semen.* « Nature », 166, 781–782.

SALISBURY G. W. and LODGE J. R. (1962) – *Metabolism of spermatozoa.* « Advanc. Enzymol. », 24, 35–104.

SELIGMAN A. M., UENO H., MORIZONO Y., WASSERKRUG H. L., KATZOFF L. and HANKER J. S. (1967) – *Electron microscopic demonstration of dehydrogenase activity with a new osmiophilic ditetrazolium salt (TC–NBT).* « J. Histochem. Cytochem. », 15, 1–13.

SELIGMAN A. M., KARNOVSKY M. J., WASSERKRUG H. L. and HANKER J. S. (1968) – *Non-droplet ultrastructural demonstration of cytochrome oxidase activity with a polymerizing osmiophilic reagent, diaminobenzidine (DAB).* « J. Cell Biol. », 38, 1–14,

SILVEIRA M. and PORTER K. (1964) – *The spermatozoids of flatworms and their microtubular system.* « Protoplasma », 49, 240–265.

SPIKES J. D. (1949) – *Metabolism of sea urchin sperm.* « Am. Natural. », 83, 285–298.

TAKEUCHI T. and KURIAKI H. (1955) – *Histochemical demonstration of phosphorylase in animal tissues.* « J. Histochem. Cytochem. », 3, 153–160.

THIÉRY J. P. (1967) – *Mise en évidence des polysaccharides sur coupes fines en microscopie électronique.* « J. Microscopie », 6, 987–1018.

TIBBS J. (1962) – *Adenosine triphosphatase and acetylcholinesterase in relation to sperm motility.* In « Spermatozoan Motility », Bishop, D. W. ed. Am. Assoc. Advanc. Sci. Press, Washington, D. C. 233–250.

TICE L. W. and BARRNETT R. J. (1962) – *Fine structural localization of adenosine triphosphatase activity in heart muscle myofibrils.* « J. Cell Biol. », 15, 401–416.

WANSON J. C. and DROCHMANS P. (1968) – *Detection of phosphorylase with the electron microscope.* In Control of Glucogen Metabolism, Universitets forlaget, Oslo. 169–177.

EXPLANATION OF FIGURES

The micrographs shown in Figs. 1–4 and 6–12 are taken from sections treated by the periodic acid – thiosemicarbazide – silver proteinate procedure for the demonstration of polysaccharides.

Figs. 1 and 2. – Longitudinal sections through the middle piece of *Pecten* (Fig. 1) and of Mytilus (Fig. 2) are shown here. Glycogen granules occupy the matrix (arrow, Fig. 1) between mitochondria (*M*) and the nucleus (*N*), and around the proximal centriole (*C*) and basal body. Glycogen granules are present in the lumen (arrow, Fig. 2) of the proximal centriole. ×30,000.

Fig. 3. – In a longitudinal section through portions of the nucleus (*N*) and middle piece of a spermatozoon of *Opsanus tau*, appear to be randomly scattered (arrow) in the packing cytoplasm between mitochondria (*M*). ×30,000.

Fig. 4. – Transverse section of sperm tails of *Hirudo* are illustrated here. Glycogen granules occupy the matrix (arrow) between the outer doublets of the axoneme (*A*) and the flagellar membrane. ×40,000.

Fig. 5. – When thin sections are treated with 0.5% α–amylase solution, glycogen granules completely disappear from the region (arrow) around the axoneme (*A*) of sperm tails of *Hirudo*. ×40,000.

Fig. 6. – In this micrograph, transverse sections through sperm tails of *Littorina* are shown. Beta glycogen particles form a thick mantle around the axoneme (*A*). ×50,000.

Fig. 7. – A longitudinal section through a portion of the middle piece and tail of sperm of *Nucella lapillus* is shown in this micrograph. Glycogen granules surround the axoneme (*A*) in the tail but are absent from the middle piece. ×110,000.

Fig. 8. – In this micrograph, glycogen granules are shown in the region surrounding the the axoneme (*A*) in the tail of sperm of *Lepas*. ×110,000.

Fig. 9. – A longitudinal section through the middle piece (*M*) of sperm of the slug, *Arion*, is shown here. Glycogen granules (large arrows) are regularly arranged within the axoneme (*A*). Beta glycogen particles completely fill the membrane-bounded compartment within the mitochondrial derivative (small arrows). ×70,000.

Figs. 10 and 11. – These micrographs show transverse sections through the middle piece of of sperm of *Lymnaea* (Fig. 10) and *Planorbis* (Fig. 11) Beta glycogen granules occupy the membrane-bounded compartments (Fig. 10, arrow) within the mitochondrial derivative. Glycogen granules also occupy the matrix (arrow, Fig. 11) between the central tubules and the outer doublets of the axoneme (*A*). ×70,000.

Fig. 12. – A transverse section through the tail piece of *Lymnaea* is illustrated here. These beta glycogen granules form a thick mantle around the axoneme (*A*), while single particles (arrow) are located between the peripheral doublets and the central tubules. ×70,000.

The micrographs shown in Figs. 13–15 are taken from experiments indicating the involvement of an active amylophosphorylase in glycogen synthesis within the middle piece of sperm of *Helix*.

Fig. 13. – A control specimen incubated in medium containing ATP, Mg^{++} ions, and NaF, but lacking glucose–1–phosphate is shown here. After treatment with the PA–TSC–SP procedure individual beta glycogen particles (arrow) are apparent. (*F*), axoneme. ×60,000.

Figs. 14 and 15. – In sections incubated in complete medium containing glucose–1–phosphate finely-granular glycogen particles now completely fills the compartment within the mitochondrial derivative (*M*). The newly-formed particles (approximately 30–40 A in diameter) appear on the surface and prevent visualization of the preformed β–particles. ×60,000.

Fig. 16. – Enzyme-reaction product indicating glucose–6–phosphatase activity appears in the axoneme (*F*) and on the membranes surrounding the matrical compartment (*SH*). ×75,000.

Fig. 17. – Glucose–6–phosphatase activity is absent from the matrical compartment (*SH*) and axoneme (*F*) in the middle piece of control specimens incubated in complete medium lacking glucose–6–phosphate. ×75,000.

Fig. 18. – A portion of the nucleus (*N*) and middle piece (*M*) of a spermatozoon of *Paracentrotus lividus* is illustrated here. Enzyme–end product for glucose–6–phosphathase activity appears on the matrical surface of negatively-stained cristae (arrow) in this tissue that was postfixed in glutaraldehyde. ×90,000.

Fig. 19. – A control specimen that was fixed in osmium tetroxide shows no enzyme-reaction product for glucose-6-phosphatase activity. (*N*), nucleus; (*M*), mitochondria. ×110,000.

Fig. 20. – This micrograph illustrates lactate dehydrogenase activity in the middle piece of a spermatozoon of *Otala*. In a specimen incubated in complete medium containing phenazine methosulphate, formazan deposits appear in the matrix compartment (*SH*) and in the glycogen compartment (arrows) of the mitochondrial derivative. ×70,000.

Fig. 21. – In samples incubated in complete medium lacking PMS, formazan deposits appear in the matrix compartment (*SH*), but are absent from the glycogen compartment (arrow). ×80,000.

Fig. 22. – Enzyme-reaction product indicating succinate dehydrogenase activity completely fills the matrix compartment (*SH*) of the mitochondrial derivative of sperm of *Helisoma*. The glycogen compartment (arrow) lacks formazan deposits. ×90,000.

Fig. 23. – The mitochondrial complex (*M*) at the base of the nucleus (*N*) of a spermatid of *Viviparus* is shown in this micrographs. Cytochrome oxidase activity appears mainly on the outer surface of the cristate membranes (large arrow). Opaque material in the matrix is also positive for cytochrome oxidase activity (small arrow). ×45,000.

Fig. 24. – A longitudinal section through the middle piece of a mature spermatozoon of *Viviparus* is shown here. Deposits of osmium black, indicating cytochrome oxidase activity, are relegated to the outer surface of the internal membranes that border the intercristae space (arrow). (*M*), mitochondrion; (*N*), nucleus. ×40,000.

Fig. 25. – In a transverse section through the mitochondrial derivative of sperm of *Helix*, lead phosphate deposits indicating Mg^{++} stimulated ATPase activity appear at the interface (arrows) of adjacent coarse fibers (*cf*) and on the surface of the central tubules of the axoneme. (*M*), mitochondrial derivative. ×80,000.

Fig. 26. – In a longitudinal section, ATPase activity appears only within the axoneme (arrow) that is surrounded by the paracrystalline mitochondrial derivative (*M*). ×50,000.

Fig. 27. – A transverse section through the middle piece of a spermatozoon of the ground squirrel, *Citellus*, is shown here. Following *en bloc* alcoholic-PTA staining, the satellite fibers (*S*) are apparent between the coarse fibers (*cf*). ×40,000.

Fig. 28. – A transverse section trough the tail piece of a spermatozoon of *Citellus* is illustrated here. Lead phosphate deposits indicating ATPase activity (arrow) appear in the matrix between the coarse fibers (*cf*) and around the central tubules (*A*). ×30,000.

Discussion

NELSON. – Succinic dehydrogenase is present in outer coarse longitudinal fibers of rat sperm by tetrazolium, tellurite reduction and also malonate. Otherwise a very impressive paper, but I'm not sure that indiscriminate extrapolation from one species to another is feasible.

BROKAW. – Has it been possible to demonstrate the disappearance of glycogen granules from sea urchin spermatozoa after periods of either aerobic or anaerobic motility?

ANDERSON. – Our results so far have been inconsistent. After incubation in sea water either under aerobic or anaerobic conditions, glycogen disappears from mitochondria of some sperm, but remains in others.

PALLINI. – Have you any result about the effect of cyclic AMP and hormones on the glycogen content of sperm cells?

ANDERSON. – It appears that in the presence of glucose–1–phosphate and NaF, either cyclic AMP or glucagon may stimulate synthesis of glycogen in sperm of *Helix*. Phosphorylase *a* may be involved in glycogen synthesis.

ANDRÉ. – After this superb piece of cytochemical work, I would like to emphasize two points:

1) This evoluted sperm appears to contain a large variety of enzymatic activities which can be classified in 3 families: phosphorus transferases, dehydrogenases, electron transport intermediates; all 3 families are involved in energy metabolism; therefore, this sperm must be considered as metabolically very active, as I already indicated this morning after BJORN AFZELIUS suggestion that crystallisation could be a sign of decline in activity;

2) Unexpectedly enough, the secondary fibers contain a polysaccharide which reacts cytochemically like glycogen; this is a new and important data which probably invalidates my former suggestion on the possible role of the secondary fiber, which Dr. BAIRATI recalled yesterday; another hypothesis has to be looked for.

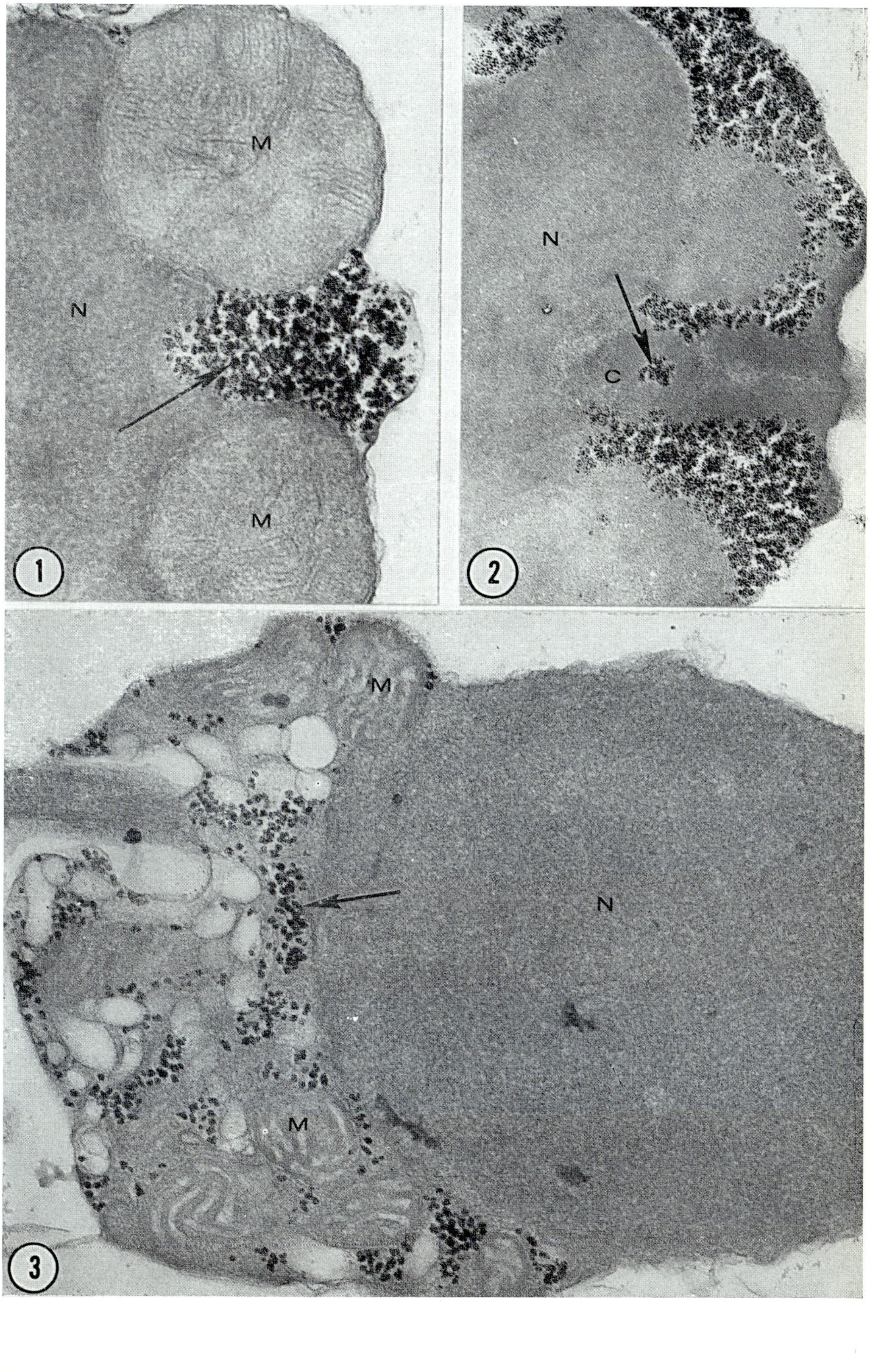
M
N
M
1
N
C
2
M
N
M
3

W. A. ANDERSON and P. PERSONNE – *Recent cytochemical studies on spermatozoa of some invertebrate and vertebrate species.*

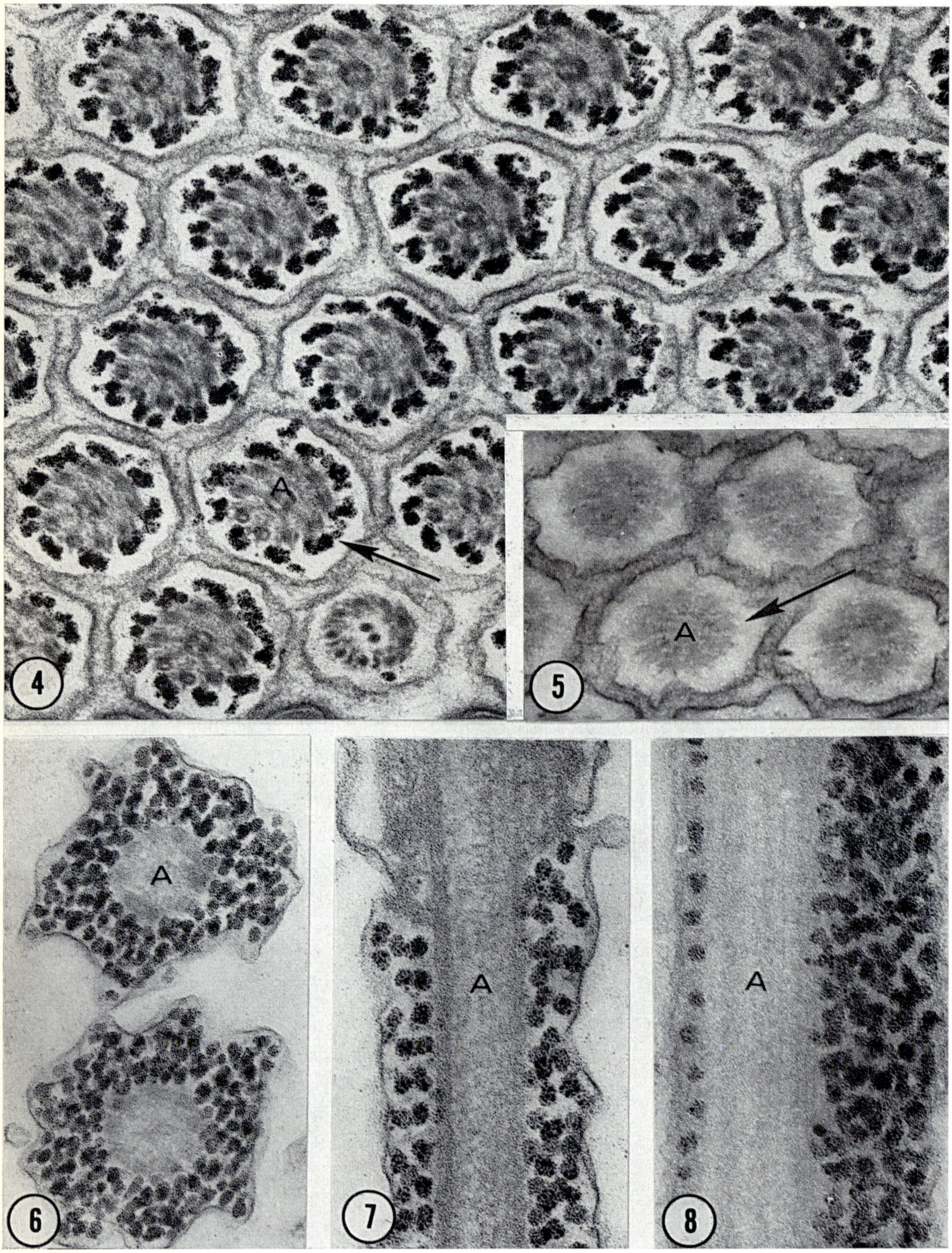

W. A. Anderson and P. Personne – *Recent cytochemical studies on spermatozoa of some invertebrate and vertebrate species.*

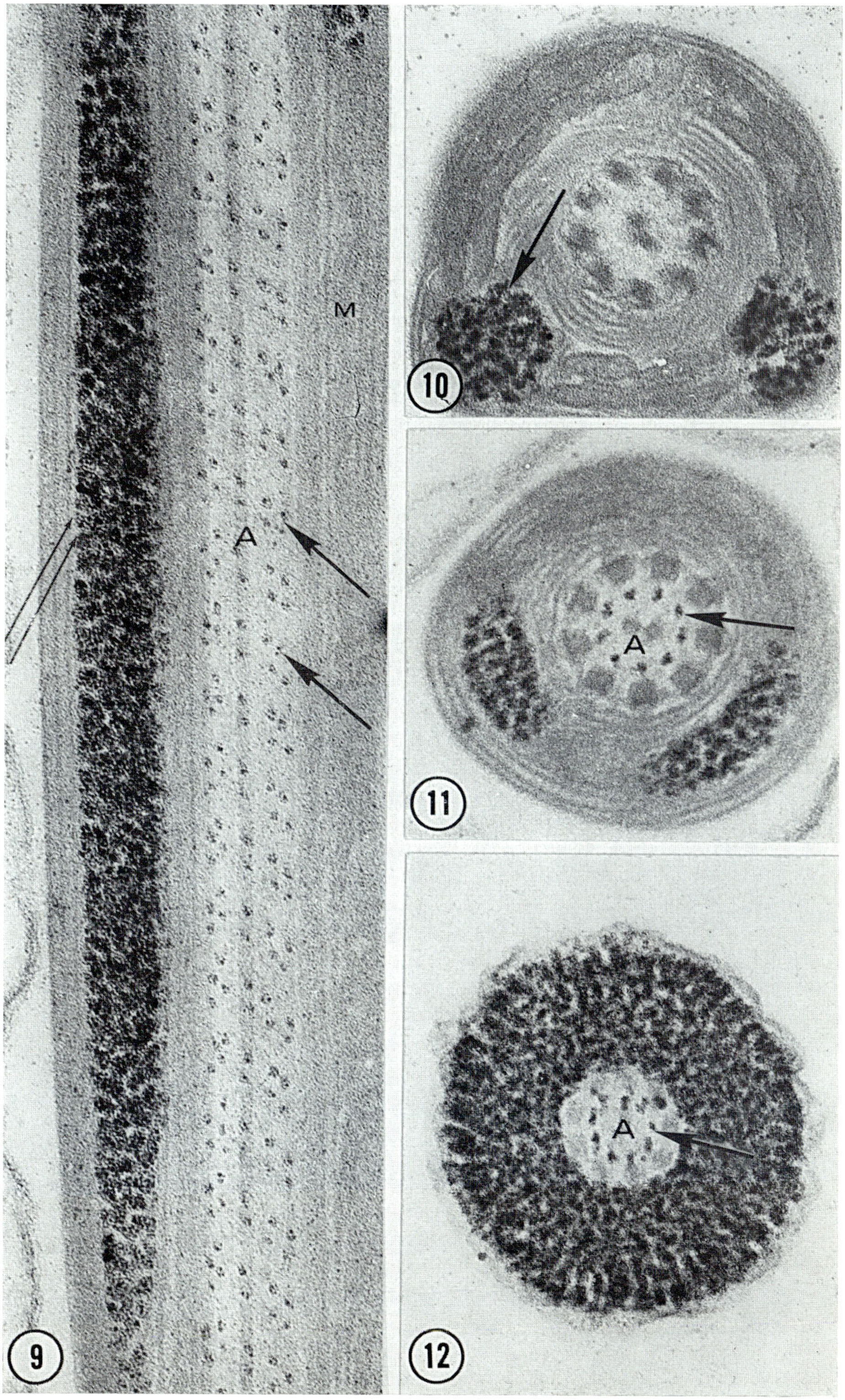

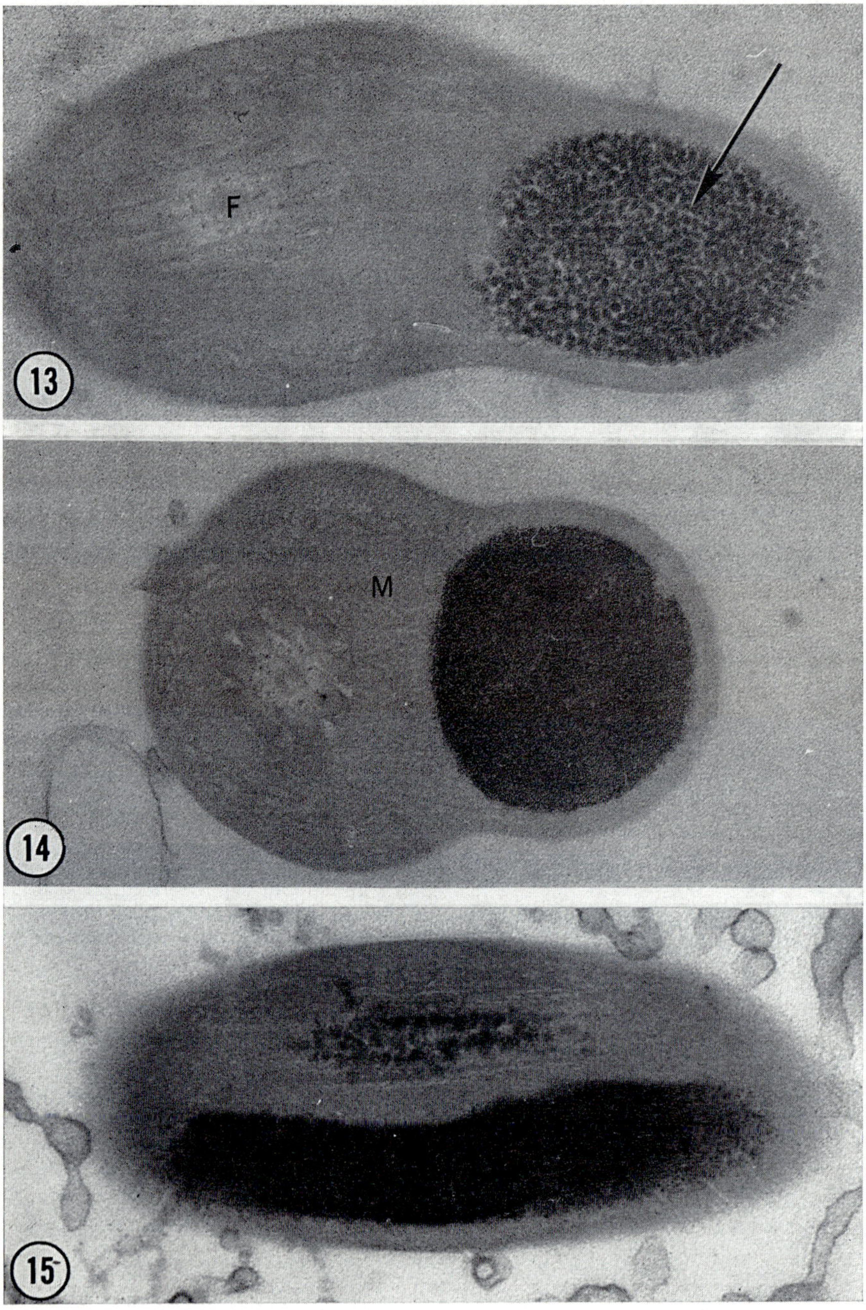
F
13
M
14
15

W. A. ANDERSON and P. PERSONNE – *Recent cytochemical studies on spermatozoa of some invertebrate and vertebrate species.*

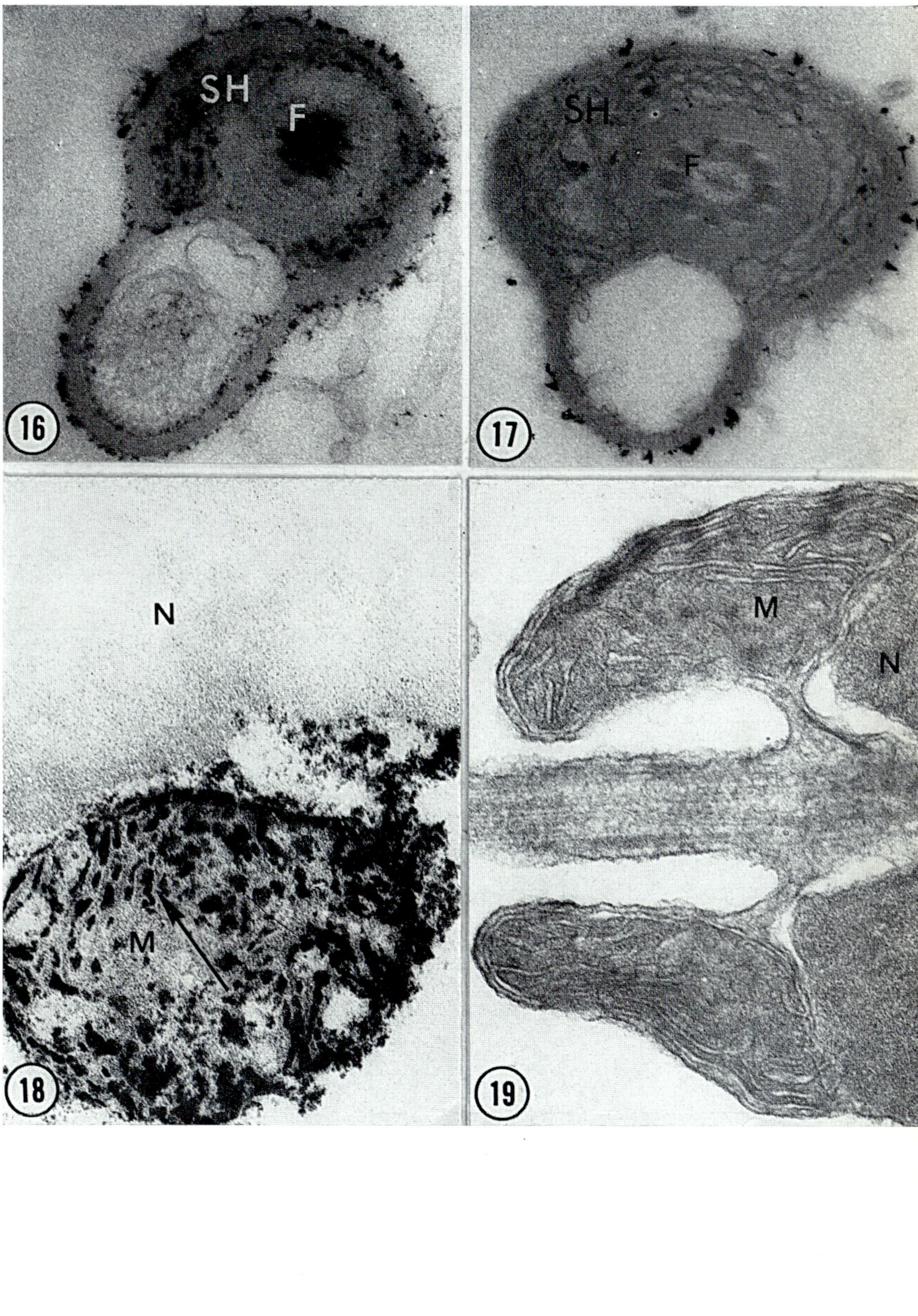

W. A. ANDERSON and P. PERSONNE – *Recent cytochemical studies on spermatozoa of some invertebrate and vertebrate species.*

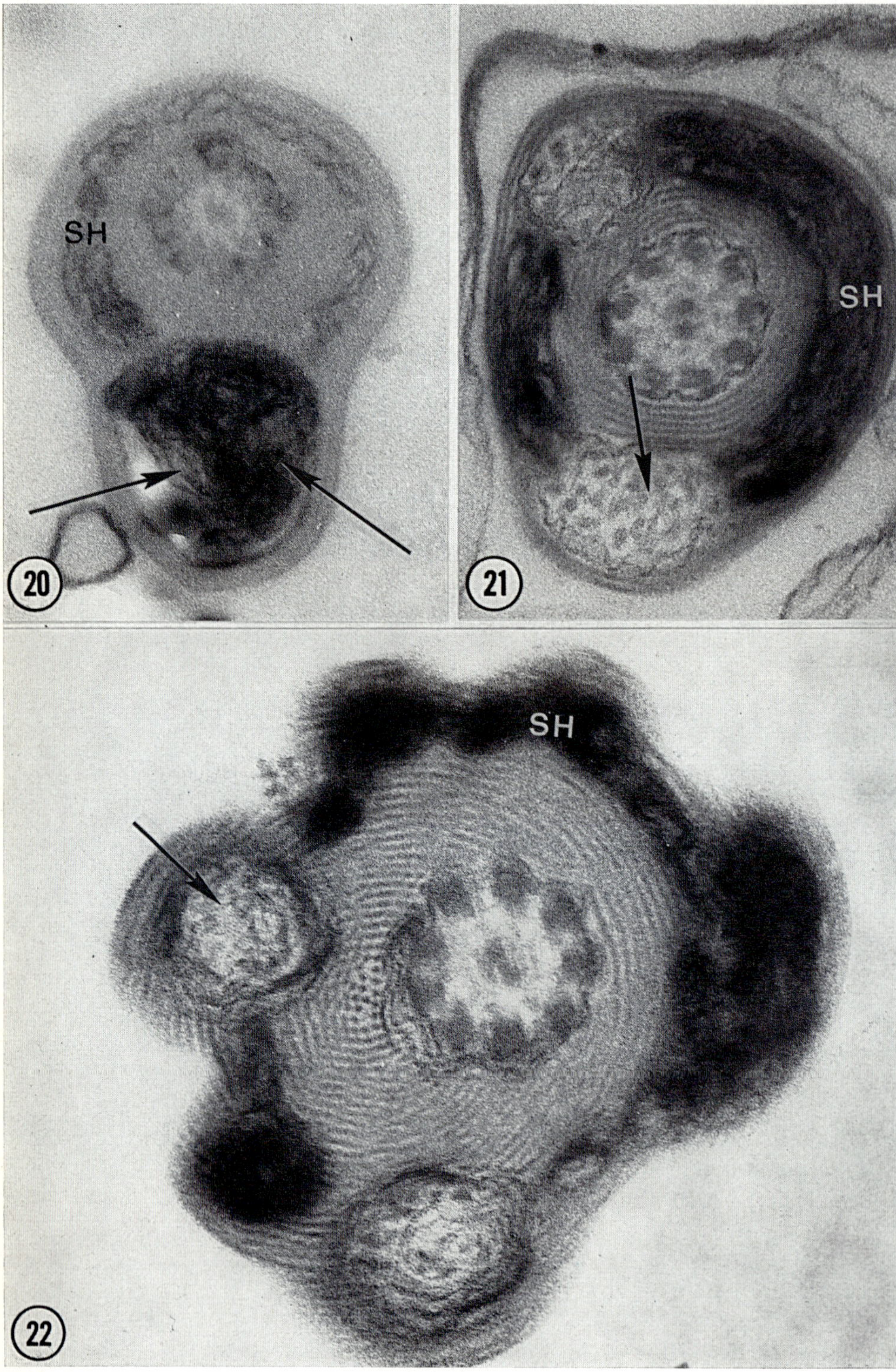

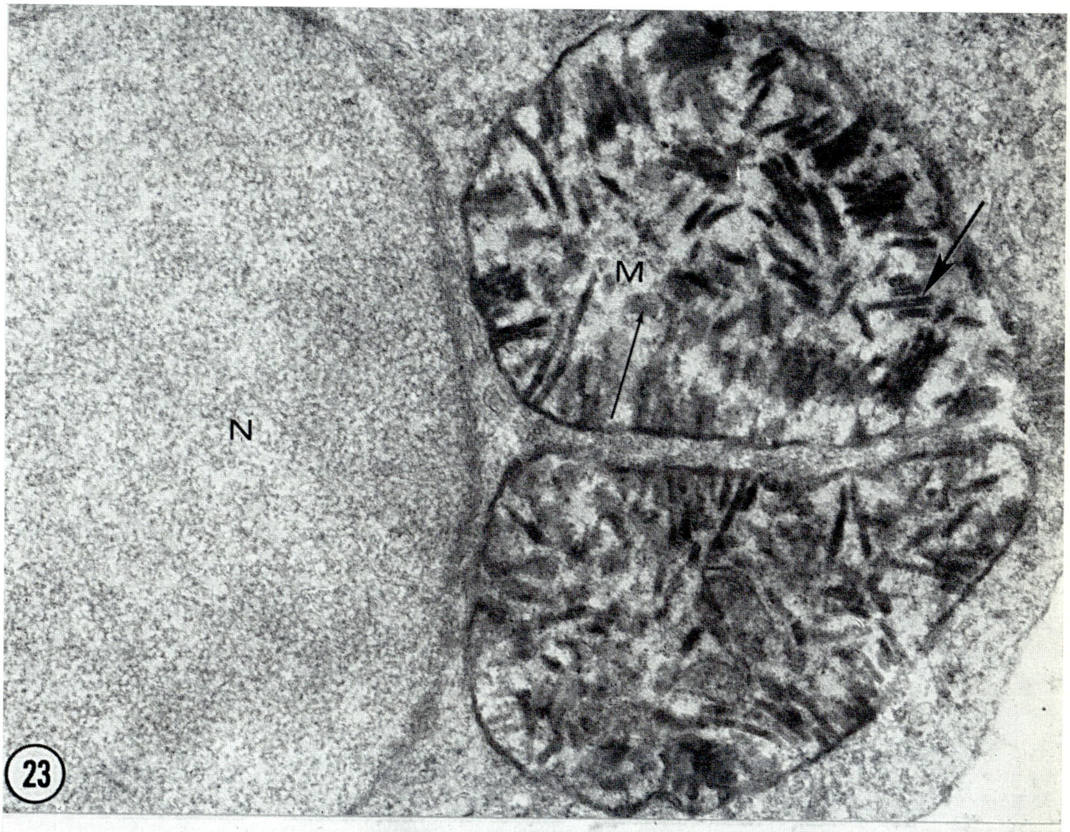
M
N
23

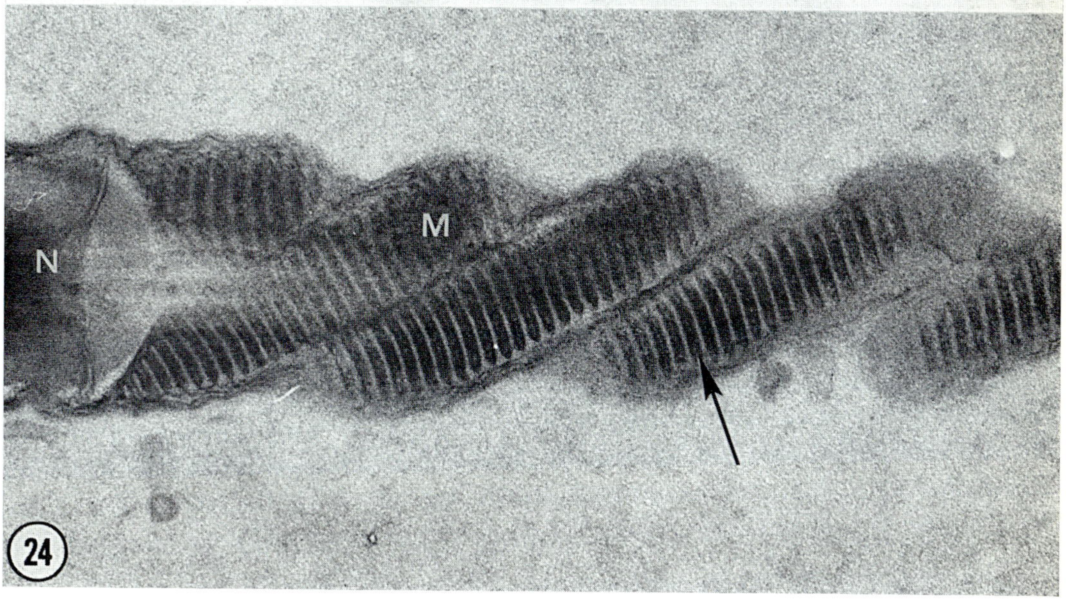
M
N
24

W. A. ANDERSON and P. PERSONNE – *Recent cytochemical studies on spermatozoa of some invertebrate and vertebrate species.*

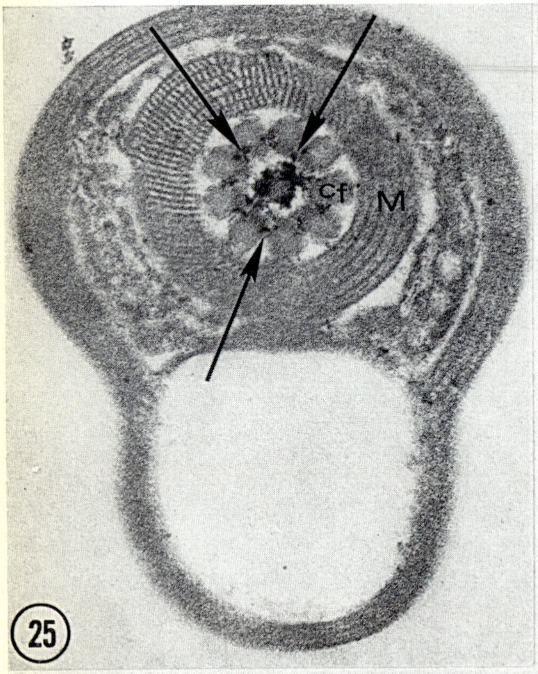

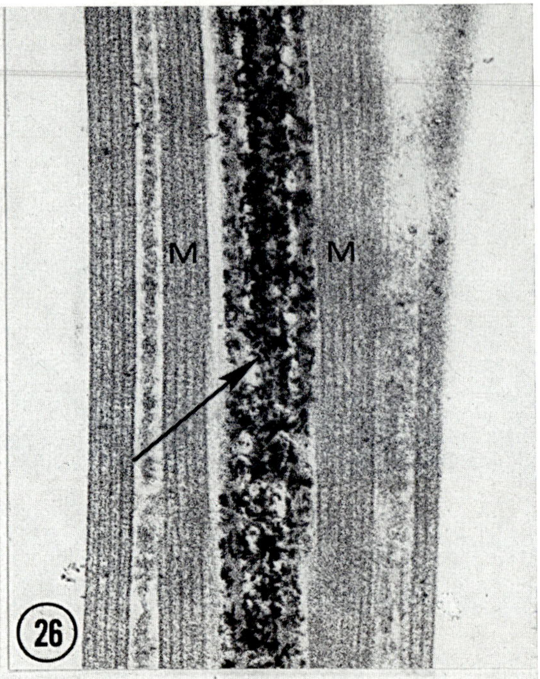

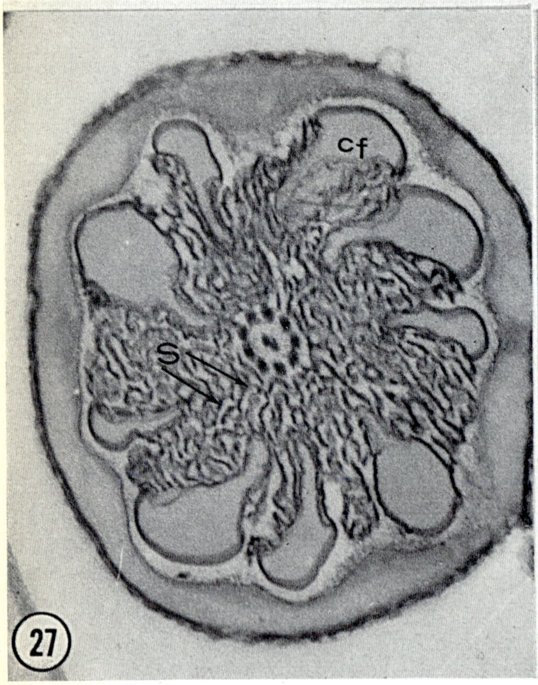

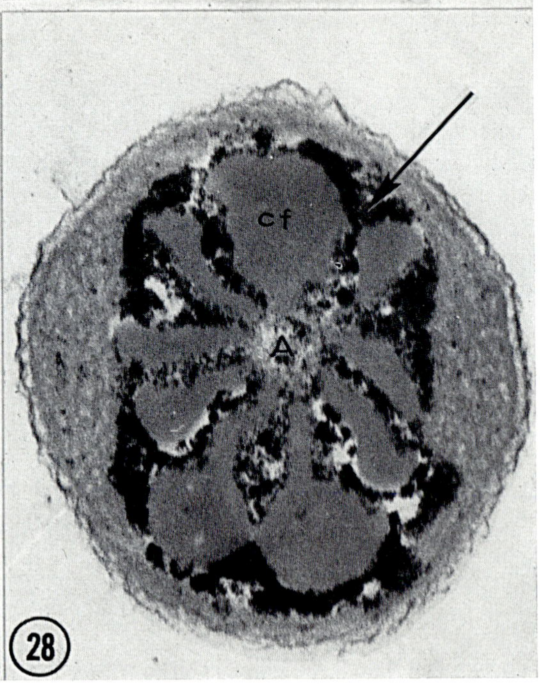

E. BIGLIARDI (*), B. BACCETTI (*), A. G. BURRINI (*) and V. PALLINI (*)

THE SPERMATOZOON OF ARTHROPODA. XII. THE DISTRIBUTION OF SOME ENZYMES IN THE INSECT SPERM TAIL (**)

SUMMARY. — In the *Bacillus* and *Ceratitis* sperms studied by us, only UTPase and, in *Ceratitis*, cytochrome-oxidase are abundant in mitochondria, while the other enzymes are almost exclusively localized in the axial filament complex, both in the accessory outer (succinic-dehydrogenase, cytochrome-oxidase), in the double (glucose-6-phosphate phosphatase) and in the secondary (cytochrome-oxidase) fibers.

Acid phosphatase, UTPase, and ATPase are found in the interspaces among these fibers. The last kind of distribution is found also for glucose-6-phosphate phosphatase in *Ceratitis*. The cytochrome oxidase activity is localized around the mitochondrial crystalline derivatives in *Ceratitis* sperms, while the mitochondrial derivatives of *Bacillus* sperms are absent.

RIASSUNTO. — Negli spermatozoi di *Bacillus* e *Ceratitis*, soltanto l'UTP–asi e, in *Ceratitis*, la citocromo–ossidasi sono abbondanti nei mitocondri, mentre gli altri enzimi sono quasi esclusivamente localizzati nel filamento assile, sia nelle fibre accessorie (succinico-deidrogenasi e citocromo ossidasi), che nei doppietti (glucoso–6–fosfato fosfatasi) e nelle fibre secondarie (citocromo–ossidasi).

Fosfatasi acida, UTP–asi, e ATP–asi sono localizzate negli interspazi tra queste fibre. Negli spermi di *Ceratitis* è così distribuita anche la glucoso–6–fosfato fosfatasi.

La citocromo–ossidasi è localizzata intorno ai derivati mitocondriali negli spermatozoi di *Ceratitis*, mentre i derivati mitocondriali degli spermi di *Bacillus* sono assenti.

An important way to clarify the role played by the different elements of the tail during sperm movement is the study of the submicroscopic localization of enzymes or other metabolic substances. Several observations have been carried out on Mammalian sperms (NELSON, 1955, 1958; 1959, 1967; NAGANO, 1964, 1965), or on the sperms of various invertebrates, as Molluscs (ANDERSON and PERSONNE, 1967, 1969; ANDERSON, PERSONNE and ANDRÉ, 1968; PERSONNE and ANDERSON, 1969), Echinoderms (ANDERSON, 1968 a, b and c) and marine crustacea (YASUZUMI and LEE, 1966). Only two brief observations have been made, to our knowledge, on the Insect sperm tail: ATP-ase in *Drosophila* axial filament (DAEMS, PERSIJN and TATES, 1963) and respiratory proteins in mitochondria (MEYER, 1964 and ANDRÉ, 1962). The problem in Insects is, nevertheless, very important, because this sperm

(*) Institute of Zoology and Institute of Biochemistry, University of Siena. Italy.
(**) Research performed under C.N.R. contract.

has attained a particular structure (9 microtubular accessory fibers, crystalline mitochondrial derivatives) in relation to the definitely established internal fertilization.

Materials and methods

Histochemical and electron microscope techniques.

Acid phosphatase activity. Small pieces of testes and seminal vescicles were fixed at 0° C for 10′–20′ in 2,5 % cacodylate buffered glutaraldehyde containing 7 % sucrose at pH 7,2. After fixation the tissues, rinsed in cold cacodylate buffer for 10′–15′, were incubated at 37° C for 30′–60′ in GOMORI's acid phosphatase medium (1952). Control samples were incubated in a substrate-free medium. After incubation the specimens were rinsed for 10′–15′ in 0,1 M sodium cacodylate buffer (pH 7,2) and postfixed for 15′ in OsO_4 solution.

Alkaline phosphatase activity. Glutaraldehyde fixed spermatozoa, rinsed in sodium cacodylate buffer at pH 7,2, were incubated for 1 h in an alkaline phosphatase medium containing β–glycerophosphate, lead nitrate, Tris-maleate buffer (0,2 M, pH 9), and distilled water. Control specimens were incubated in a medium without substrate. Incubated pieces, rinsed in cacodylate buffer for 10′–15′, were postfixed in 1 % OsO_4 solution.

Nucleoside phosphate phosphatase activity. Unfixed and glutaraldehyde-fixed (10′–15′) spermatozoa, washed in cacodylate buffer at pH 7,2, were incubated for 45′–60′ at 37° C in a medium containing ATP, magnesium sulfate, lead nitrate and Tris-maleate buffer at pH 7,2 (WACHSTEIN and MEISEL, 1957), and rinsed in sodium cacodylate buffer. In control experiments, the specimens were incubated in a medium lacking ATP. Subsequently, the unfixed spermatozoa were fixed in 2,5 % cacodylate-buffered-glutaraldehyde for 45′ an washed in cacodylate buffer. All the samples were then postfixed in 1 % OsO_4 solution for 15′.

Other experiments were carried out using UTP as substrate, in the same medium of incubation.

Glucose-6-phosphatase activity. Unfixed and glutaraldehyde-fixed spermatozoa (10′–15′) were used to demonstrate glucose-6-phosphatase activity.

The specimens were rinsed in cacodylate buffer at pH 7,2 for 10′, and then incubated at 37° C for 45′–60′ in medium of CHIQUOINE (1953) containing glucose-6-phosphate, lead nitrate and Tris-maleate buffer at pH 6,7. Glucose-6-phosphate was omitted from the incubation medium in control experiments. After incubation, all the specimens were washed in cacodylate buffer for 10′. Subsequently, glutaraldehyde-fixed spermatozoa were postfixed in 1 % OsO_4; unfixed spermatozoa were fixed in 2,5 % cacodylate-buffered glutaraldehyde for 45′, rinsed in cacodylate buffer and postfixed in 1 % OsO_4 for 15′.

Succinic-dehydrogenase activity. Unfixed spermatozoa and spermatozoa fixed for 10–15′ in 2,5 % cacodylate-buffered glutaraldehyde were rinsed in cacodylate buffer and incubated at 37° C for 1 h in medium containing sodium succinate, Nitro-BT and phosphate buffer at pH 7,6 (NACHLAS *et al.*, 1957) and again washed in cacodylate buffer. Unfixed spermatozoa were then fixed in 2,5 % cacodylate-buffered glutaraldehyde and rinsed in cacodylate buffer. All the specimens were postfixed for 15′ in 1 % OsO_4 solution.

Cytochrome c *oxidase activity.* Unfixed spermatozoa were incubated at 37° C for 45′ in a modified medium of SELIGMAN consisting of a solution of cytochrome c and 3–3′–diaminobenzidine tetra HCl in phosphate buffer. In the control the cytochrome c was absent. After incubation the specimens were rinsed in 0,1 M phosphate buffer for 15′. Subsequently the spermatozoa were fixed in gluteraldehyde for 15′ and postfixed in 1 % OsO_4 for 15′.

Electron microscope techniques. After fixation in glutaraldehyde and OsO_4 solution, the specimens were dehydrated in a graded series of ethylic alcohols and embedded in Epon 812. The sections, obtained by the ultramicrotome LKB III, mounted on grids and stained with uranyl acetate, were observed and photographed with Siemens Elmiskop I electron microscope.

The presence of glycogen and polysaccharides was demonstrated by THIÉRY's method (1967) on thin sections.

Other sections were oxidized for 7′ in 12 V H_2O_2, rinsed in distilled water and then incubated for 45′ at 37° C in 0,1 % α-amylase solution in 0,1 M phosphate buffer at pH 6,9.

For the demonstration of proteins, thin sections were oxidized for 7′ in 12 V H_2O_2, thoroughly rinsed in distilled water and treated with 0,1 % pepsin solution in 0,1 M Mc Ilvaine buffer at pH 2,2 for 15′ at 37° C.

Biochemical experiments.

a) *Sperm.* It is possible to obtain pure and abundant preparations of sperm cells from *Bacillus* by squeezing the seminal vesicles and testes. Sperms were usually collected in 15% Glycerol, a medium in which stability of enzyme activities was observed, upon storage at 4° C.

The sperm suspension was centrifuged at 105000×g for 1 h. The sperm pellet was resuspended in the same medium. Enzyme and protein determinations were carried out both on the sperm cells and the supernatant fluid.

b) *Materials.* pNO_2 Phenylphosphate, AMP, ADP, ATP, UTP, and CTP were Na salts and Sigma products. GTP (Li salt) and G–6–P (Na salt) were Boehringer products. Cytochrome C, type III, from horse heart was Sigma product.

c) *Methods.* Totale proteins were determined with the micromethod of LOWRY *et al.*

Acid and alkaline phosphatase were determined in a 0,05 M Acetate buffer pH 4,6 or in a 0,05 Glycine buffer pH 10,5 with a substrate concentration of 1 mg/ml, in the final volume of 1 ml. At the end of incubation, 0,2 ml of 2 M Na OH were added, and p. Nitrophenol determined at 410 mμ.

The hydrolysis of various nucleotides was followed in 0,1 M TRIS–HCI buffer pH 7,5, in the presence of mM $MgCl_2$, with a 5 mM substrate concentration. The final volume of the reaction mixtures was 0,120 ml. After incubation at 37° C, 0,030 ml of 30% Trichloroacetic acid were added, the precipitated protein removed by centrifugation and 0,1 ml of the supernatant fluid were used for inorganic phosphate determination after a micro-modification of the LOWRY method. Suitable blanks were run in each determination.

Glucose-6-Phosphate phosphatase was determined with a similar procedure, using 0,05 M Citrate or Imidazole–HCl buffers of pH 6.

Succinate-oxidase was detected after GREEN *et al.*

Cytochrome-oxidase was detected using COOPERSTEIN and LAZAROW method.

OBSERVATIONS

a) *Morphological and chemical aspects of the general construction of* Ceratitis *and* Bacillus *sperm tail.*

Both *Bacillus* (a Phasmid) and *Ceratitis* (a fruit fly) have a 9+9+2 sperm tail with two crystalline bodies of different origin extending through the whole length of the tail. In transverse sections the fibrils appear to be similar in the two species, with the exception of the inner 2 and outer 9 single tubules provided with an osmiophilic axis in *Ceratitis* (Fig. 4), moderately and homogeneously opaque in *Bacillus* (Fig. 1). The mitochondrial derivatives appear cylindrical, with a crystalline core and brief peripheral cristae in the former, absent, and substituted by two S shaped in cross section, bodies and totally crystalline in the latter. These bodies are probably originated from the Golgi complex.

By treating this material with some simple histochemical tests, we can observe that in *Ceratitis* the 2 central and the 9 accessory tubules are 150 Å in diameter, and contain very small amounts of polysaccharides (Fig. 5), stained by Thiéry's method for glycogen and removed by α-amylase treatment (Fig. 6).

Pepsin digestion reveals a diffuse content of proteins within these tubules (Fig. 7). Small granular deposits of glycogen appear on the secondary fibrils.

The peripheral doublets seem to be entirely proteinaceous and, treated by pepsin, disappear short time after the single tubules.

In *Bacillus* the situation is somewhat different. The peripheral singlets reach 200 Å in diameter and, like the two central units, contain a very small amount of diffuse proteins and concentrated polysaccharides stored in the form of globular units (Fig. 2). This polysaccharide seems to be more abundant in the spermatids (Fig. 3), and decreases during the maturation of the sperm.

The secondary fibrils appear devoid of glycogen; the peripheral doublets, as in *Ceratitis*, proteinaceous.

b) *Acid phosphatase*. In *Bacillus* sperm the reaction becomes highly positive only after 1 h incubation. In sectioned material large deposits of granules can be observed throughout the entire length of the tail, close to the single microtubules, both of the outer accessory units and of the inner two central units. The spaces between these elements, i.e. the peripheral doublets, the secondary fibrils and the intervals, are always completely negative at all. The most caudal levels of the tail show a quite similar enzyme distribution. The elements of the tail other than the axial filament complex, as S–shaped bodies, plasma membrane etc., are always devoid of reaction products (Figs. 11–12).

In *Ceratitis* the situation is slightly different, essentially because of the more intense reactivity of the enzyme, which seems to be more abundant. After 30′ incubation the reaction appears strongly positive in the interspaces between the fibrillar components of the axial filament complex, without any particular order. After 1 h incubation the reaction appears to be particularly positive around the outer and central single tubules, and on the plasma membrane surrounding mitochondria and fibrils. After 1 h 30′ incubation, the positivity is very intense at all the levels of the filament complex, but negative in fibrils and in mitochondria (Figs. 8–9–10).

The results of the biochemical estimation of this enzyme showed its presence both in the sperm cells and in the supernatant fluid (Diag. 1).

The hydrolysis of p NO_2 phenyl-phosphate is a linear function both of the time and of the protein concentration.

It was observed that the optimum pH of the reaction is the same both with sperm cells and with supernatant fluid (Diag. 2). This fact suggests the presence of a same enzyme in the two fractions. This conclusion is further substantiated by the observation that the acid phosphatase activity may be almost completely removed from the sperms by repeated washings with glycerol or isotonic NaCl.

Therefore, acid phosphatase appears to be an enzyme not strictly linked with the sperm organelles, but somewhat diffused in its cytoplasm. These observations confirm the histochemically demonstrated distribution.

Versene, Mg Cl_2 or Ca Cl_2 have no effect on the activity up to a 0,01 M concentration.

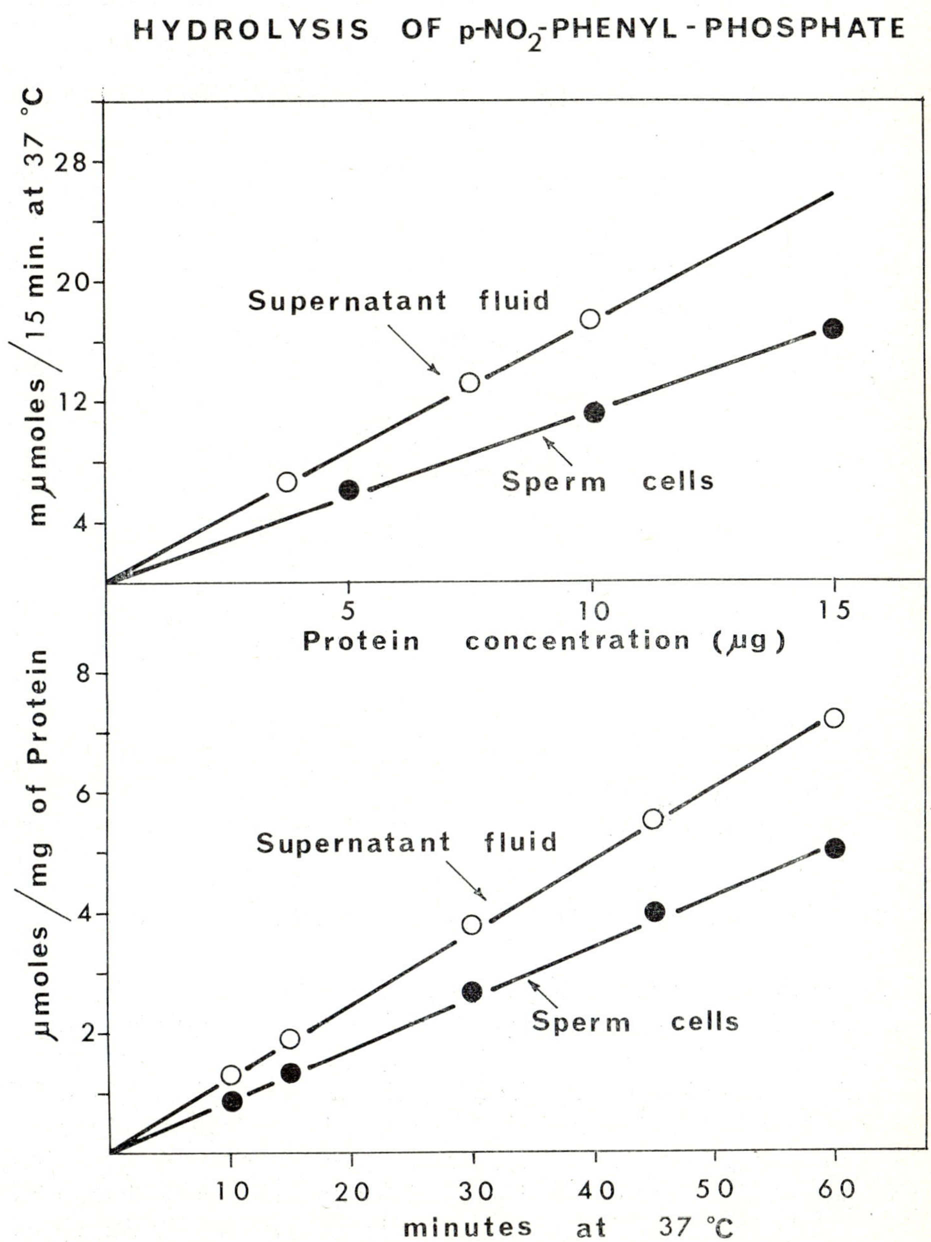

Diagram 1. – Acid phosphatase activity in *Bacillus* sperms and supernatant fluid.

c) *Alkaline phosphatase.* All the histochemical reactions carried out by us both on *Bacillus* and *Ceratitis* sperms have always given negative results.

The rate of hydrolysis of p NO_2 phenyl phosphate measured in the sperm cells with biochemical methods at pH 10,5 and 7,5 is about 0,03 μ moles hydrolysed per hour per mg of sperm protein, i.e., about 100 times slower than at pH 4,6. Alkaline phosphatase activity was not detectable in the supernatant fluid.

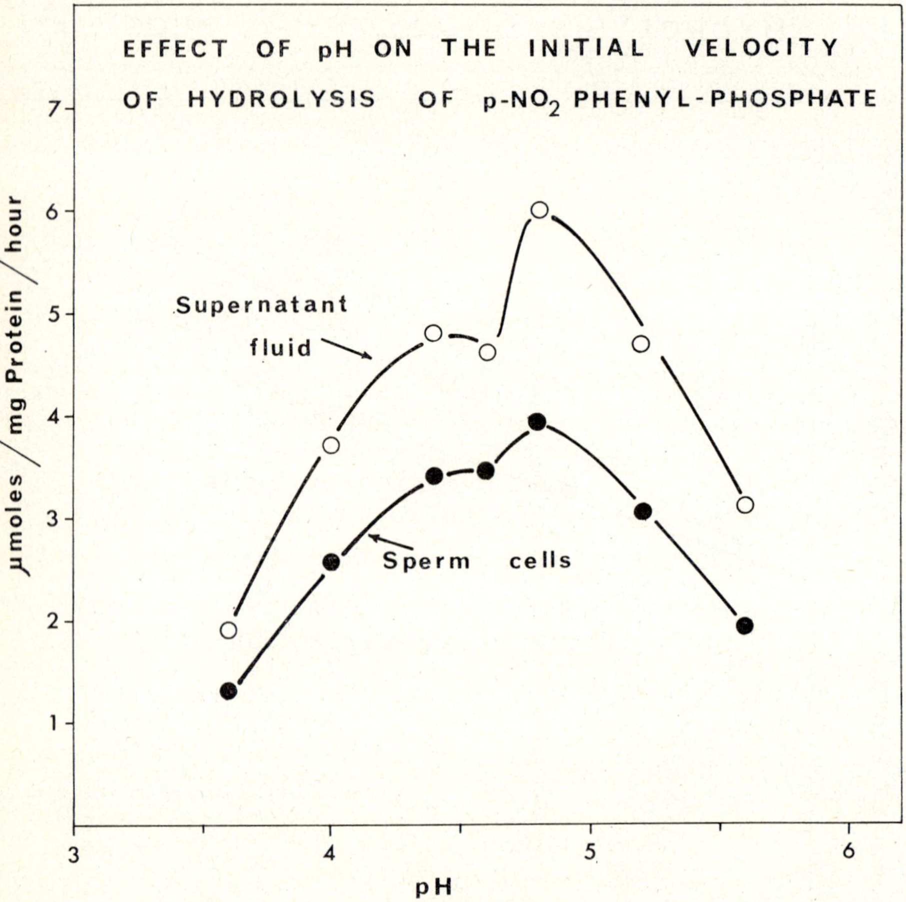

Diagram 2. – Optimum pH of the acid phosphatase activity in *Bacillus* sperms.

d) *Nucleoside phosphato-phosphatases.* The submicroscopic distribution of this class of enzymes in *Bacillus* and in *Ceratitis* sperm tails is vast.

After 45′–1 h incubation, on moderately glutaraldehyde fixed material (postosmicated after incubation), the inorganic phosphate released from ATP appears strictly localized around the outer and inner single tubules of the axial filament complex, and in the interspaces between the peripheral doublets.

In unfixed *Bacillus* material incubated for 45′ and postfixed the distribution of ATP–ase seems the same, whereas in *Ceratitis* the reaction appears much more intense, and the products completely occupy the space of the axial filament complex, avoiding only the 9+9+2 fibrillar elements. In this material the enzyme is also localized around the crystalline masses of the mitochondrial derivatives (Figs. 13–14–16–17).

A quantitative determination with biochemical methods revealed in *Bacillus* sperms the presence of an ATP splitting activity in the range of 0,2 moles of inorganic phosphate released per mg of sperm protein per hour of incubation at 37° C.

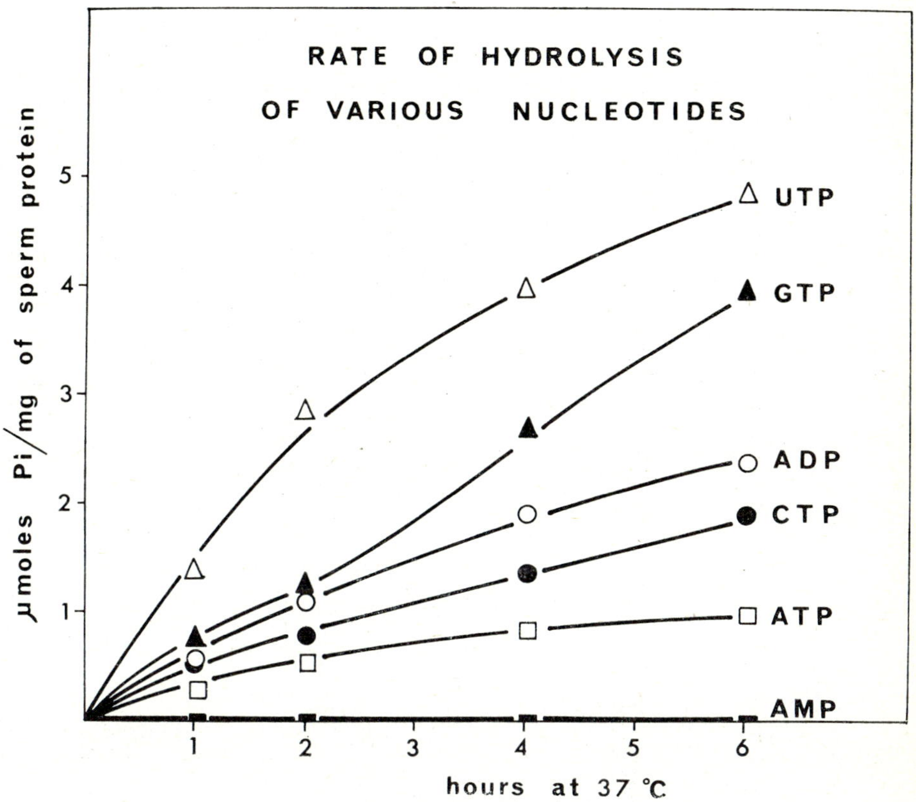

Diagram 3. – Nucleoside phosphatase activity in *Bacillus* sperms.

Using other nucleoside-phosphates as substrates (Figs. 15, 18), we found that UTP is hydrolysed at the hyghest rate: about five times faster than ATP. This result is consistent with histochemical determinations.

The relative rates of hydrolysis of these substrates are shown in the figure (Diag. 3).

It is interesting to note that 5'–AMP apparently is not attacked at all. This fact suggests the presence of an enzyme (or enzymes) specific for the pyrophosphate bond. This is also consistent with the negligible rate of hydrolysis of pNO_2 phenyl phosphate at neutral pH.

The nucleoside phosphate hydrolysing activity is apparently bound to the sperm organelles, since it is not detectable in the supernatant fluid.

We do not yet know whether UTP and the other nucleoside-triphosphates are hydrolysed by an enzyme endowed with low specificity or whether several specific enzymes are present. Very preliminary results have shown that the UTP–splitting activity is more sensitive to activation by Mg^{++} ions.

e) *Glucose–6–phosphato–phosphatase.* In histochemically examined mature *Bacillus* spermatozoa this enzyme seems to be absent, but in immature stages of spermiogenesis the reaction gives an interesting result, being highly

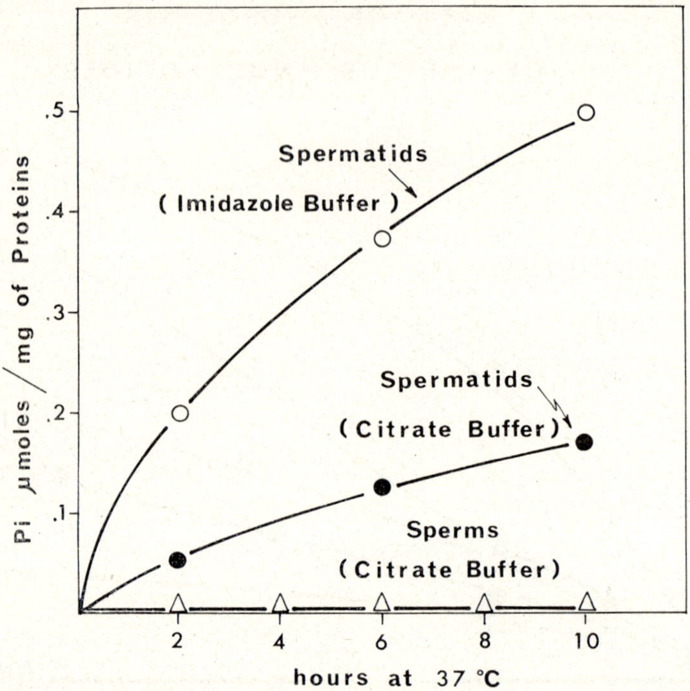

Diagram 4. – Hydrolysis of glucose-6-phosphate in different male germe cells of *Bacillus*.

positive inside the B subfiber of the 9 peripheral doublets. Only exceptionally we have observed a positive reaction inside one central singlet (Figs. 21, 22).

In *Ceratitis* the situation is very different. Mature spermatozoa react positively at the level of the axial filament complex, showing a distribution of the glucose–6–phosphatase between the outer 9 single tubules and around the central two, like the enzymes previously examined (Figs. 19, 20).

Attempts to detect glucose–6–phosphate phosphatase in mature *Bacillus* sperm cells using pH 6 citrate buffer gave negative results, even using 0,1 % deoxycholate as an unmasking agent.

On the contrary, according to the histochemical data, the activity was found in spermatids (Diag. 4).

The use of imidazole instead of citrate buffer gave an higher activity.

f) *Succinic-dehydrogenase and cytochrome-c-oxidase.* The distribution of the succinic-dehydrogenase histochemically detected both in *Bacillus* and in *Ceratitis* sperm seems to be the same.

It is important to note that only in a few cases we have been able to obtain positive results for reasons that are still unclear.

In any case only the 9 outer accessory fibers react positively, becoming uniformly electrondense. In *Bacillus* a positive reaction can be given also by the 2 central tubules (Figs. 23, 24).

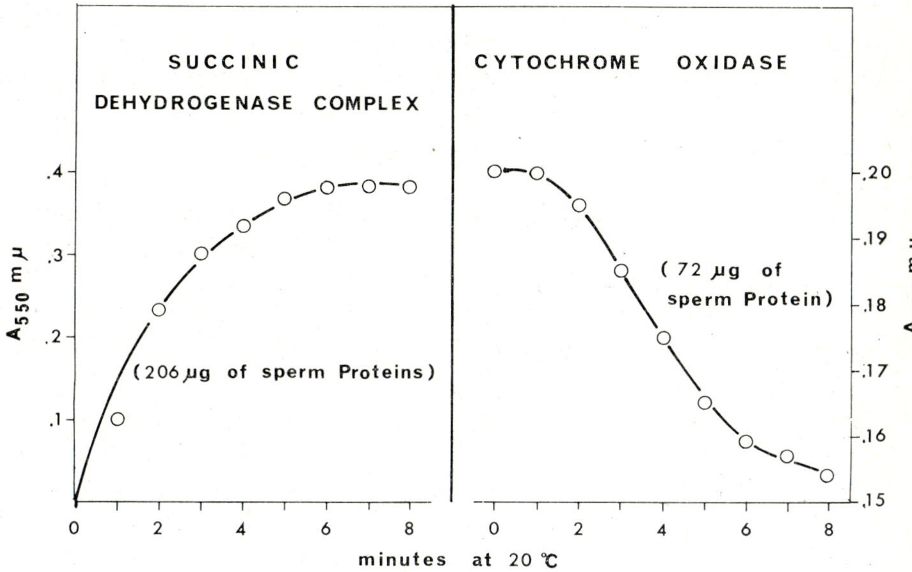

Diagram 5. – Respiratory activities in *Bacillus* sperm cells.

The cytochrome-c-oxidase is in both species localized in the outer accessory fibers as the succinic-dehydrogenase. In *Ceratitis* the crown of secondary fibrils too reacts positively. The mitochondria don't present a high cytochrome oxidase content: in *Ceratitis* only the brief peripheral cristae give a positive reaction. In *Bacillus*, where the mitochondrial derivatives are absent, the S–shaped bodies appear negative. In any case the crystalline masses appear devoid of enzyme (Figs. 25, 26, 27, 28).

In a biochemical assay system, we found that cytochrome c is promptly reduced in the presence of succinate by *Bacillus* sperm suspensions. Even in the absence of succinate we observed a low but noticeable " endogenous " reduction by sperm cells suspended in glycerol (Diag. 5).

Reduced cytochrome c may be in turn oxidized by sperm cells. A quantitative estimation of these activities was not attempted, since they decrease quickly, during storage of the sperm suspension.

CONCLUSIONS

On the basis of our data it is reasonable to think that insect sperms are endowed with a complete electron transporting system, at least starting from succinate, which may be involved with the production of high energy compounds.

We do not yet have data about the glycolytic activity of insect sperms.

These cells also possess an active acid phosphatase. Other phosphatases are present which hydrolyse nucleoside triphosphates and diphosphates at neutral pH.

As far as the hystochemical localization of these enzymes is concerned, comparing our data on insect sperm tails with the data available in the literature about the sperms of other phyla, it is possible to point out the following differences.

In the species examined so far (Gastropods, Echinoderms and Mammals), succinic-dehydrogenase, cytochrome oxidase, sorbitol dehydrogenase, glucose-6-phosphate phosphatase and acetylcholinesterase are essentially localized in mitochondria (NELSON, 1966; ANDERSON and PERSONNE, 1967, 1968; ANDRÉ, 1962; and MEYER, 1964, 1968), where glycogen is also sometimes present (ANDRÉ and PERSONNE, 1964; ANDERSON and PERSONNE, 1967 b). Only acid phosphatase and sometimes ATP-ase and glucose-6-phosphate phosphatase are localized around the fibers of the axial filament complex in molluscans (ANDERSON, PERSONNE and ANDRÉ, 1968; ANDERSON and PERSONNE, 1969) whereas in mammals the outer coarse fibers contain succinic dehydrogenase, ATP-ase and inorganic pyrophosphatase (NELSON, 1959, 1967).

In the insect sperms studied by us, only UTP–ase and, in *Ceratitis*, cytochrome–c–oxidase are abundant in mitochondria, while the other enzymes are almost exclusively localized in the axial filament complex, both in the outer (succinic-dehydrogenase, cytochrome–c–oxidase), in the double (glucose–6–phosphate phosphatase) and in secondary (cytochrome–c–oxidase) fibers. Acid phosphatase, UTP–ase and ATP–ase are found in the interspaces among these fibers. The last kind of distribution is found also for glucose–6–phosphate phosphatase in *Ceratitis*.

These enzymes seem to be strictly bound to the structure, while acid phosphatase may be easily removed.

The localization of so many enzyme activities in the axial filament complex, typical of the insect sperms studied by us, may be connected with the evolution in these cells of mitochondria into peculiar crystalline proteinaceous masses and with the localization of a glycogen-like polysaccharide at the level of the outer fibers and of the *Ceratitis* secondary fibrils.

References

ANDERSON W. A. (1968) – *Cytochemistry of Sea Urchin Gametes* I. *Intramitochondrial localization of glycogen, glucose-6-phosphatase and* ATP–*ase activity in spermatozoa of Paracentrotus lividus.* « J. Ultrastr. Research. », 24, 398–411.

ANDERSON W. A. (1968) – *Cytochemistry of Sea Urchin Gametes.* II. *Ruthenium Red Staining of Gamete Membranes of Sea Urchins.* « J. Ultrastr. Research. », 24, 322–333.

ANDERSON W. A. (1968) – *Cytochemistry of Sea Urchin Gametes.* III. *Acid and alkaline phosphatase activity of spermatozoa and fertilization.* « J. Ultrastr. Research. », 25, 1–14.

ANDERSON W. A. and PERSONNE P. (1969) – *Structure and histochemistry of the basal body derivative, neck and axoneme of spermatozoa of Helix aspersa.* « J. Microscopie », 8, 87–96.

ANDERSON W. A. and PERSONNE P. (1969) – *The cytochemical localization of sorbitol dehydrogenase activity in spermatozoa of Helix aspersa.* « J. Microscopie », 8, 97–102.

ANDERSON W. A., PERSONNE P. and ANDRÉ J. (1968) – *Chemical compartmentalization in Helix spermatozoa.* « J. Microscopie », 7, 367.

ANDRÉ J. (1962) – *Contribution à la connaissance du chondriome, étude de ses modifications ultrastructurales pendant la spermatogénèse.* « J. Ultrastr. Res. », Suppl. 3, 185 pp.

CHIQUOINE A. D. (1953) – *The distribution of glucose-6-phosphatase in the liver and kidney of the mouse.* « J. Histochem. Cytochem. », 1, 429–435.

COOPERSTEIN S. J. and LAZAROW A. (1951) – *A microspectrophotometric method for the determination of cytochrome oxidase.* « J. Biol. Chem. », 189, 665–670.

DAEMS W. T., PERSIJN J. P. and TATES A. D. (1963) – *Fine structural localization of* ATP–*ase activity in mature sperm of Drosophila melanogaster.* « Exp. Cell Res. », 32, 163–167.

GOMORI G. (1952) – *Microscopic Histochem.*, Univ. Chicago Press, Chicago, Illinois.

GREEN D. E., MII S. and KOHOUT P. M. (1955) – *Studies on the terminal electron transport system. I. Succinic dehydrogenase.* « J. Biol. Chem. », 217, 551–567.

LOWRY O. H. and LOPEZ J. A. (1946) – *The determination of inorganic phosphate in the presence of labile phosphate esters.* « J. Biol. Chem.» , 162, 421–428.

LOWRY O. H., ROSEBROUGH N. J., FARR A. L. and RAUDALL R. J. (1951) – *Protein measurement with the Folin phenol reagent.* « J. Biol. Chem. », 193, 265–275.

MEYER G. F. (1964) – *Die parakristallinen korper in der spermienschwanzen von Drosophila.* «Zeit. Zellforsch. », 62, 762–784.

NACHLAS M. M., TSOU K. C., DE SOUZA E., CHENG C. S. and SELIGMAN A. M. (1957) – *Cytochemical demonstration of succinic dehydrogenase by the use of a new p–nitrophenyl substituted ditetrazole.* « J. Histochem. Cytochem. » 5, 420, 436.

NAGANO T. (1964) – *Electron microscopic observations on the rat sperm tail with special reference to the localization of phosphatase activities.* « Symp. Cell Chem. », 14, 251–260.

NAGANO T. (1965) – *Localization of adenosine triphosphatase activity in the rat sperm tail as revealed by electron microscopy.* « J. Cell Biol. », 25, 101–112.

NELSON L. (1955) – *Adenosine triphosphatase of Mytilus spermatozoa.* I. *Effects of* pH, *calcium and magnesium, and concentration of enzyme and substrate.* « Biol. Bull. », 109, 295–305.

NELSON L. (1958) – *Cytochemical studies with the electron microscope.* I: *Adenosine triphosphatase in rat spermatozoa.* « Bioch. Bioph. Acta », 27, 634–641.

NELSON L. (1959) – *Cytochemical studies with the electron microscope.* II: *succinic dehydrogenase in rat spermatozoa.* « Exp. Cell Res. », 16, 403–410.

NELSON L. (1967) – *Sperm motility.* In « *Fertilization* ». Vol. I, Acad. Press, New York and London.

PERSONNE P. and ANDERSON W. A. (1967) – *Recherche de déshydrogenases par cytochemie ultrastructurale.* « J. Microscopie », 6, 35 a.

PERSONNE P. and ANDERSON W. A. (1969) – *Compartimentage des activités enzymatiques dans le spermatozoide de certains mollusques gastéropodes.* I: *Localization des déshydrogénases.* « J. Cell Sci. », 4, 693.

SELIGMAN A. M., PLAPINGER R. E., WASSERKRUG H. L., DEB C. and HANKER J. S. (1967) – *Ultrastructural demonstration of cytochrome oxidase activity by the NADI reaction with osmiophilic reagents.* « J. Cell Biol. », 34, 787–800.

THIÉRY J. P. (1967) – *Mise en evidence des polysaccharides sur coupes fines en microscopie électronique.* « J. Microscopie », 6, 987–1018.

WACHSTEIN M. and MEISEL E. (1957) – « Am. J. Clin. Pathol. », 27, 13.

YASUZUMI G. and LEE K. J. (1966) – *Spermatogenesis in animals as revealed by electron microscopy.* VI. *The microtubular structure and sites of thiamine pyrophosphatase activity in premature sperm of the japanese Crayfish.* « Zeit. Zellforsch. », 73, 384–404.

EXPLANATION OF FIGURES

Fig. 1. – Cross section of *Bacillus rossius* sperm tail. 90,000×.

Fig. 2. – Cross section of *Bacillus rossius* sperm tails treated by Thiéry's method for glycogen. 75,000×.

Fig. 3. – Spermatids of *Bacillus* after treatment by α–amylase solution. 24,000×.

Fig. 4. – Cross section of *Ceratitis capitata* sperm tails. 90,000×

Fig. 5. – Sperm cells of *Ceratitis capitata* treated by Thiéry's method for glycogen. 60,000×.

Fig. 6. – Cross section of spermatids of *Ceratitis* after treatment by α-amylase solution. 60,000×.

Fig. 7. – Pepsin digestion of sperm tails of *Ceratitis capitata.* 60,000×.

Figs. 8–9–10. – Acid phosphatase activity in *Ceratitis* sperms. Control (8), 1 h incubation (9), 1 h, 30′ incubation (10).

Figs. 11–12. – Acid phosphatase activity in *Bacillus* sperms: control (11), reaction (12).

Figs. 13–14–15. – Nucleoside phosphate phosphatase activity in *Ceratitis* sperms: control (13), ATPase (14), UTPase (15).

Figs. 16–17–18. – Nucleoside phosphate phosphatase activity in *Bacillus* sperms: control (16), ATPase (17), UTPase (18).

Figs. 19–20. – Glucose-6-phosphate phosphatase activity in *Ceratitis* sperms: control (19), reaction (20).

Figs. 21–22. – Glucose-6-phosphate phosphatase activity in *Bacillus* sperms: control (21), reaction (22).

Figs. 23–24. – Succinic dehydrogenase activity in *Bacillus* sperms: control (23), reaction (24).

Figs. 25–26. – Cytochrome-c-oxidase activity in *Ceratitis* sperms: control (25), reaction (26).

Figs. 27–28. – Cytochrome-c-oxidase activity in *Bacillus* sperms: control (27), reaction (28).

Discussion

ANDRÉ. – You did succeed in obtaining a very good reaction for several nucleotide triphosphatases. An ATP–ase activity is quite satisfactory in view of energy metabolism for the production of flagellar movement. But you obtained a very strong reaction for UTP–ase activity. Have you an explanation for such a strong reaction in the general context of flagellar metabolism?

BIGLIARDI. – I cannot propose an explanation for this point, for which I am astonished as you.

NELSON. – This beautiful demonstration of the morphological distribution of key enzymes should help clarify their role in the production of the insect sperm flagellar wave.

BROKAW. – (Comment after NELSON): In a protozoan flagellum, adenylate kinase activity appears to be about 100 times greater than ATP–ase activity, if it is measured directly. The ATP-ase activity of the sea urchin sperm flagellum also varies greatly depending on the treatment. Apparently the ATP–ase activity can be either transformed or "uncoupled" from other components, thus increasing its activity.

E. BIGLIARDI et AL. – *The spermatozoon of Arthropoda.* XII. *The distribution of some enzymes in the insect sperm tail.*

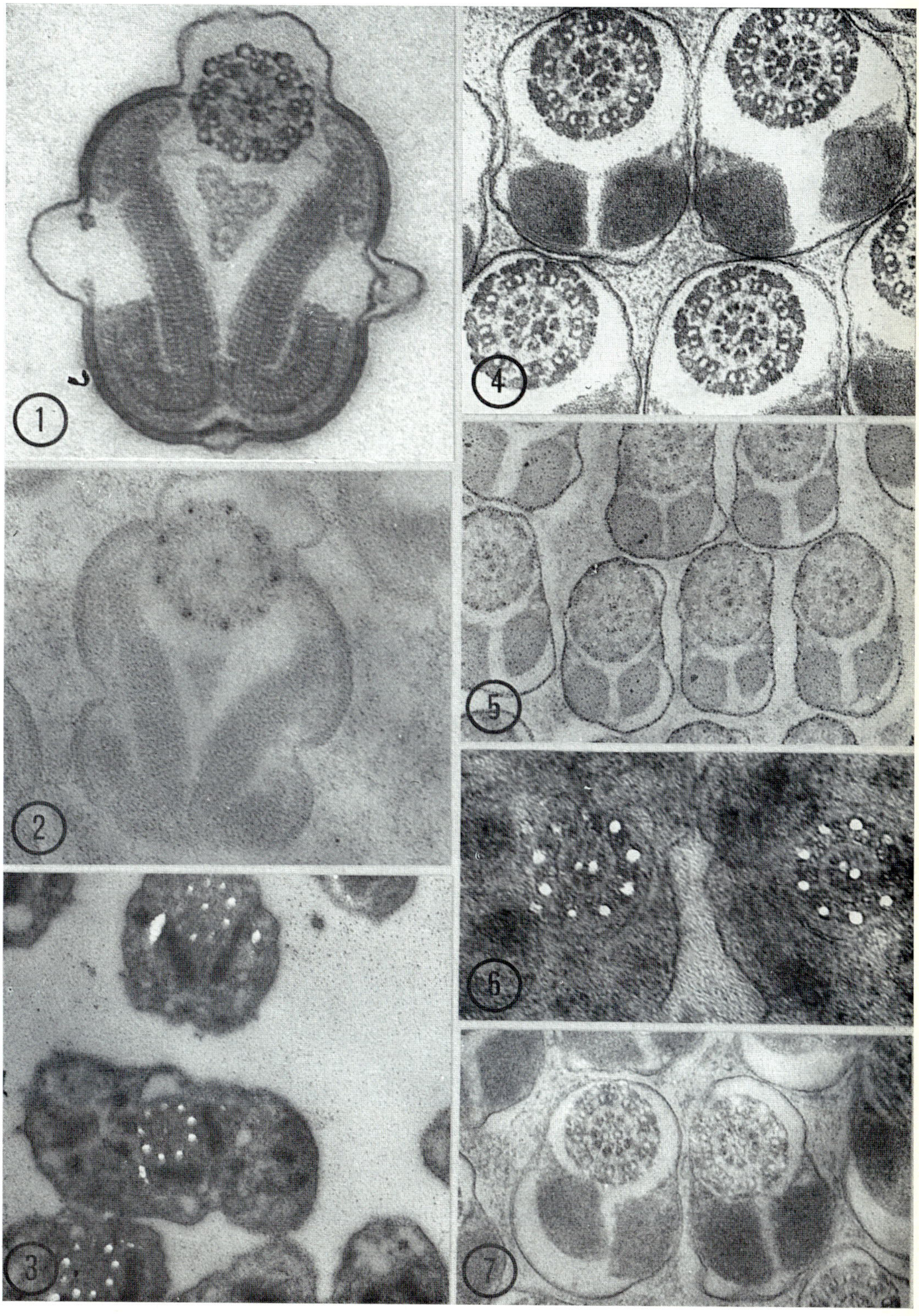

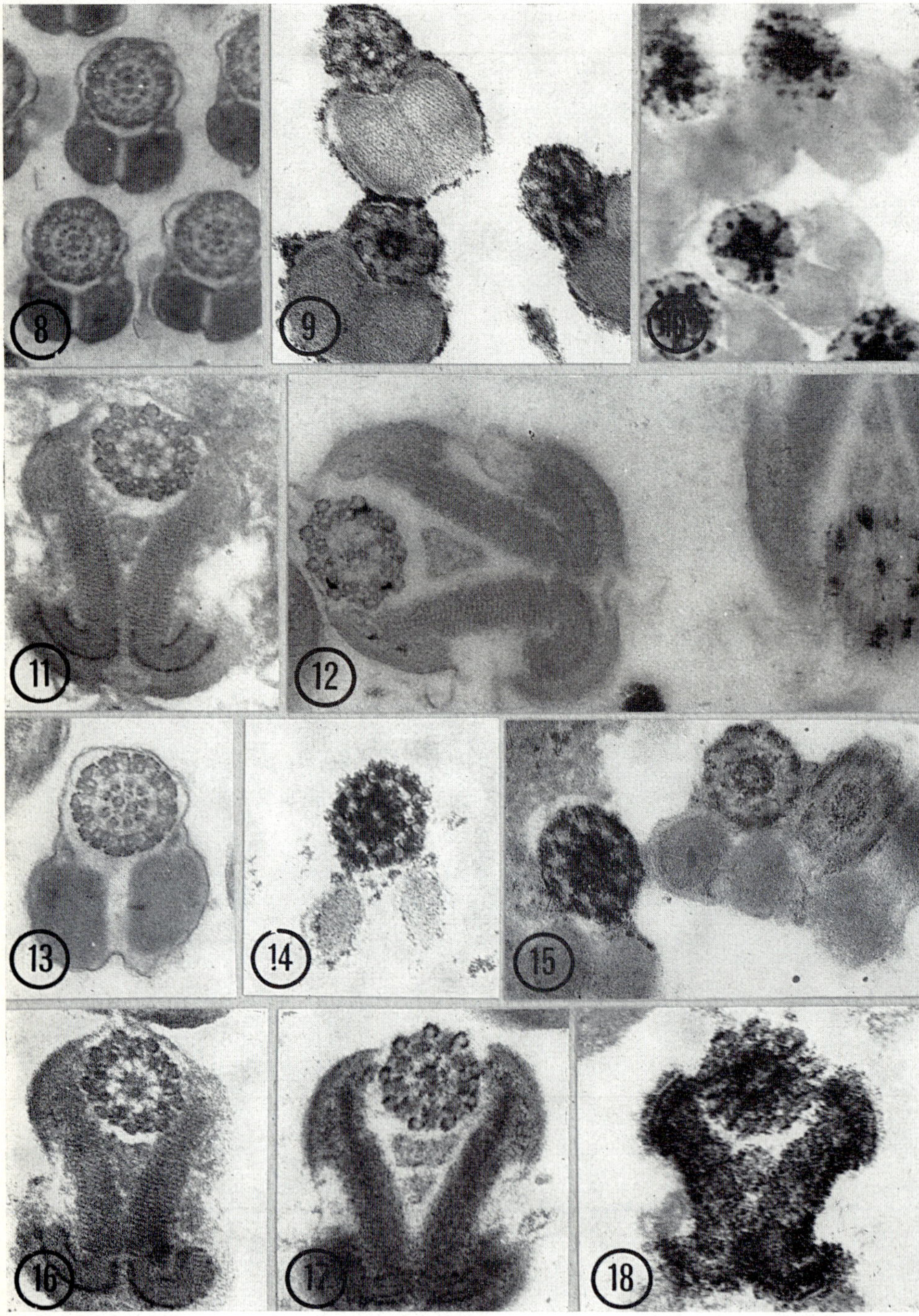
8
9
10
11
12
13
14
15
16
17
18

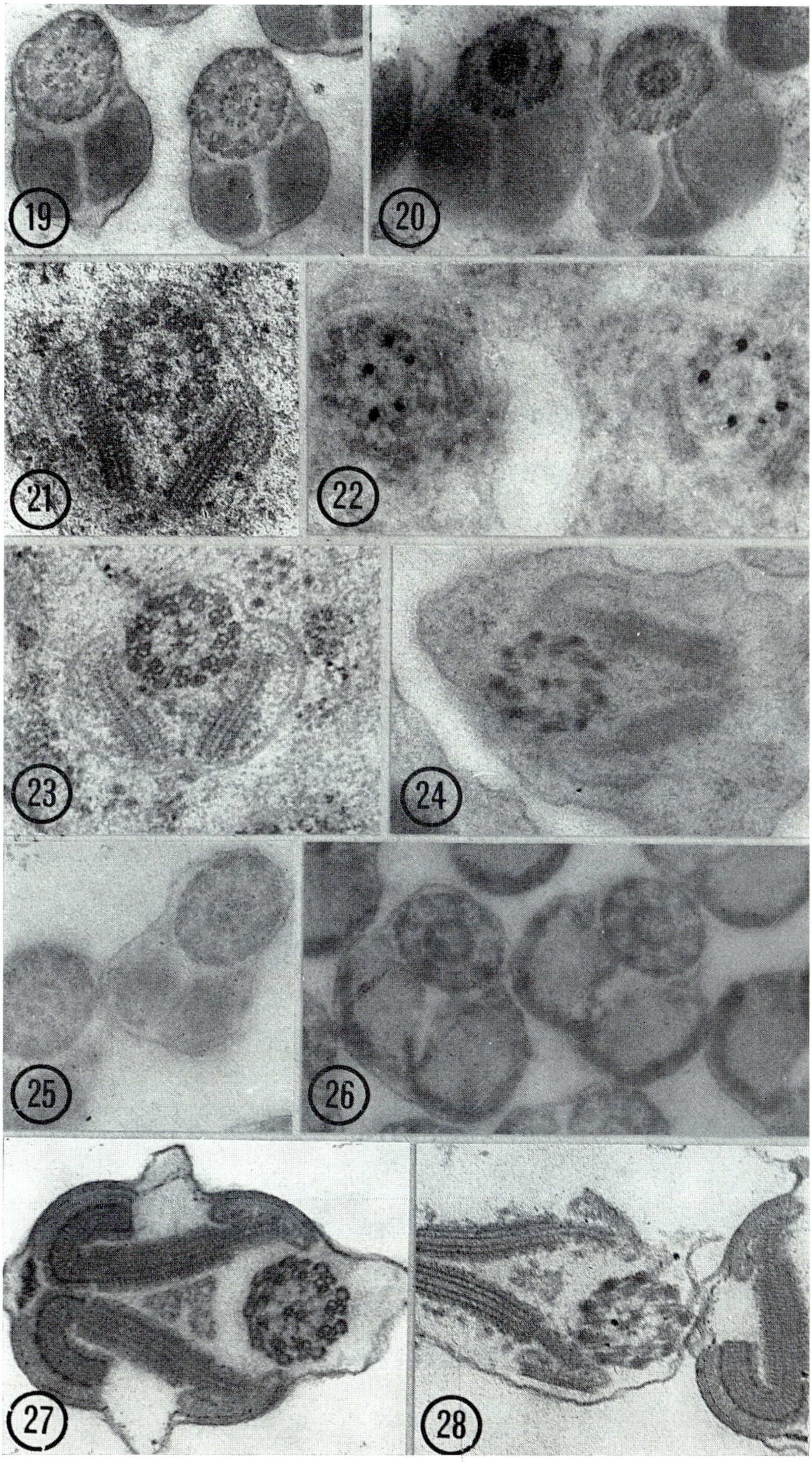
19
20
21
22
23
24
25
26
27
28

L. NELSON (*), A. V. MC GRADY (*) and M. E. FANGBONER (*)

CONTROL OF FLAGELLAR MOVEMENT (**)

SUMMARY. — Coordination and propagation of the flagellar wave are essential conditions for effective sperm cell propulsion. Glycerinated " models " of mammalian spermatozoa may be reactivated by adenosine triphosphate, but although they twitch repetitively at isolated segments along the flagellum, they cannot make progressive movements. Since glycerination causes some morphological alterations, and also the loss of some substrates and enzymes, but not others, the matter was investigated at both biochemical and cytochemical levels.

One of the lesions, loss of integrity of the cell membrane may be directly or indirectly responsible for interruption of the conductile system. Acetylcholinesterase, which is usually associated with rhythmic activity, impulse transmission and propagation of membrane depolarization in excitable systems is highly active in rat, bull and mussel sperm flagella. Eserine competitively inhibits the flagellar enzyme. Electron microscopic examination reveals that this enzyme, true specific acetylcholinesterase is localized on the mitochondrial surfaces in the midpiece, and on the fibrous sheath of the tail in bull sperm. However, the proximal centriole appears to exhibit no positive cytochemical reactivity for this enzyme.

RIASSUNTO. — Il coordinamento e la propagazione dell'onda flagellare sono condizioni essenziali per la propulsione dello spermatozoo. «Modelli» glicerinati di spermatozoi di mammiferi possono essere riattivati con ATP, ma sebbene segmenti isolati lungo il flagello si contraggano ripetutamente, essi non possono compiere movimenti progressivi. Poiché il trattamento con glicerina provoca alterazioni morfologiche ed anche la perdita di alcuni substrati ed enzimi, il problema viene investigato sia a livello biochimico che citochimico.

Una delle lesioni, la perdita dell'integrità della membrana cellulare può essere direttamente o indirettamente responsabile dell'interruzione del sistema di conduzione. L'acetilcolinesterasi, che è di solito associata con l'attività ritmica e provoca la trasmissione e la propagazione della depolarizzazione della membrana nei sistemi eccitabili, è molto attiva nei flagelli degli spermatozoi di ratto, toro e mitilo. L'eserina inibisce competitivamente l'enzima flagellare. L'esame submicroscopico rivela che questo enzima, una vera acetilcolinesterasi specifica, è localizzato sulla superficie mitocondriale nella regione intermedia, e sulla guaina fibrosa della coda negli spermi di toro. Tuttavia, il centriolo prossimale non presenta nessuna reazione positiva per questo enzima.

Flagella isolated from seminal ejaculates containing naturally decapitated bull spermatozoa (NELSON, 1966) and from specially prepared samples of the alga *Polytoma* (BROKAW, 1961) under appropriate conditions, carry on seemingly normal motile activity. Normal motile activity, for the purposes of this discussion, signifies effective forward propulsion in which the flagella

(*) Department of Physiology Medical College of Ohio at Toledo, Toledo, Ohio.
(**) Supported by USPHS Research Grant 5RO1 HD 03266-02.

are driven by waves, the amplitude and frequency of which may fall within the range of the natural biological condition. The sperm head in the one case, and the cell body in the second may therefore be eliminated from consideration as the seat of control of the flagellar undulatory process. The control of flagellar activity is apparently intrinsic in some of the various physical and chemical attributes of the flagellum or in their interaction with its environment.

Glycerinated models prepared from bull (BISHOP and HOFFMANN–BERLING, 1959) and from *Strongylocentrotus* (BROKAW, 1963) spermatozoa exhibit vigorous repetitive vibratile activity on reactivation by ATP, but with the loss of wave propagation have also lost their capacity for progressive movement. Reactivated models of the sperm of the sea urchins *Hemicentrotus* (KINOSHITA, 1959), *Arbacia* (CLAYBROOK and NELSON, 1968) and *Lytechinus* and of the tunicate *Ciona* and the annelid *Chaetopterus* (BROKAW, 1964), on the other hand, can simulate forward swimming activity. In the case of the *Hemicentrotus* sperm a motility inducing factor, subsequently identified as the MARSH–BENDALL relaxing factor, myokinase, was found to be an essential ingredient of the reactivation medium along with ATP and Mg^{++}; but when this sperm cell has been "thoroughly" extracted additional sarcoplasmic components were needed (KINOSHITA, 1959). The possibility that a tropomyosinlike protein, extractable from sperm constitutes part of this system is being examined at present. On the other hand, the MARSH–BENDALL factor prevented restoration of the bull sperm models unless this relaxing factor was inactivated by calcium ions (BISHOP and HOFFMANN–BERLING, 1959). Even though calcium is not otherwise essential, its presence in the reactivating medium "definitely improves the quality of flagellation" leading BISHOP and HOFFMANN–BERLING (1959) to conclude that its effect may be on a relaxing system in the sperm. Other relaxing factors (usually ATP–regenerating systems) such as creatine–ATP–phosphokinase and phospho–enol–pyruvate kinase as well as plasticizing agents including inorganic pyrophosphate and ATP itself have been nominated for roles in regulating the contraction-relaxation cycles of muscle as well as sperm (NELSON, 1959).

One concomitant of the preparative procedures in the above studies, in which ATP reactivation of the glycerol-extracted model fails to restore propulsive motion, held in common with more drastic measures for the separation of flagella from sperm heads, e.g., homogenization or ultrasonically-induced dismemberment, along with a greater or lesser degree of morphological disruption, is the loss of chemical integrity.

These observations serve to substantiate the conclusion that contractile elements distributed along its entire length underly the alternating processes leading to translatory motion of the flagellum. These repetitive cycles provide the necessary, but demonstrably not the sufficient, conditions for effective propulsion. Coordination required to propagate the waves of active bending must be superimposed upon the periodic contraction-relaxation cycles enabling the flagellum to achieve normal motile activity.

One of the lesions induced by glycerination, loss of physiological integrity of the cell membrane, as well as extraction of particular substrates and enzymes and structural protein sub-units may contribute to the interruption of a critical conductile mechanism.

The acetylcholine-acetylcholinesterase interaction which is frequently associated with rhythmic biological activity, impulse transmission and propagation of depolarization of excitable membranes and thereby ion flux regulation, is highly active in boar (SEKINE, 1951), ram (MANN, 1954), mussel (APPLEGATE and NELSON, 1962), and bull (NELSON, 1964, 66) spermatozoa. Eserine competitively inhibits this enzyme which, in general, possesses the characteristics ascribed to " true ", specific acetylcholinesterase (NELSON, 1966).

An analysis of the spatial distribution of this enzyme among the structural components of the sperm flagellum should provide some useful insights into its possible role as a mediator (coordination, conduction) between mechanochemical transduction (ATP–ATPase/plasticizer, ATP–regenerator; contraction/relaxation cycles) and effective flagellar movement (wave-propagation, propulsion). We have therefore undertaken an electron microscopic cytochemical study and we are beginning an examination of some of the electrophysiological parameters of spermatozoan movement.

MATERIALS AND METHODS

The cytochemistry has been applied to semen obtained from a Guernsey bull whose ejaculates contain only decapitated sperm (NELSON, 1964), that is, sperm heads and motile and non-motile flagella in about equal proportions; and also to the spermatozoa flushed from bull epididymides obtained at a local abattoir. The electrophysiological studies are being conducted on " raw " bull semen provided through the courtesy of the Northern Ohio Breeders Association.

Crevier and Bélanger's Thiolacetic acid method (CREVIER and BELANGER, 1955; KOELLE and HORN, 1968) was applied to the " decapitated " semen, a droplet of which had been rapidly frozen in liquid propane at —175° C and dried *in vacuo* at —40° C (GERSH. *et al.*, 1957). After coming to room temperature, the dried specimen was transferred directly to the incubation medium which consisted of 0.12 M thiolacetic acid buffered at pH 7.2 in veronal acetate containing 0.001 M lead acetate.

The specimens were incubated at room temperature for thirty minutes, rinsed in buffer and then in dilute (0.01 M) yellow ammonium sulfide for five minutes. After rinsing in buffer again, the specimen was dehydrated in ethanol and imbedded in methacrylate (Figs. 1, 3). Thiolacetic acid was omitted from the control preparatiosn (Fig. 2).

The epididymal sperm were suspended and washed in 0.9% NaCl and then treated for five minutes in 1% Triton X–100 before fixing in ice-cold 3.5% glutaraldehyde, 0.2 M sucrose buffered to pH 7.0 with 0.05 M sodium cacodylate. After fixation for one hour the specimens were washed for two hours in buffered sucrose. Incubation took one hour in 0.12 M Thiolacetic acid in the presence of 10^{-3} M lead acetate in cacodylate buffer pH 7.0 (Fig. 4). Thiolacetic acid was omitted from the control specimens (Fig. 5). The preparations were rinsed in buffered lead acetate and then in buffer and dehydrated to 95% ethyl alcohol. Bulk staining was performed in 5% platinum tetrabomide in 95% alcohol for an hour. After several fifteen-minute rinses in 95% and absolute alcohol, the specimens were transferred through two fifteen-minute changes of propylene oxide, agitated in a 50 : 50 mixture of propylene oxide and epoxy resin for two hours. After increasing the resin to a 2 : 1 mixture with overnight agitation the specimens were embedded in epoxy and polymerized at 35° C, 45° C and 60° C for twenty-four hours each. (In one set, experimental and control, Fig. 6, pretreatment with Triton X–100 was omitted).

The methacrylate blocks were sectioned with glass knives using a Huxley microtome and examined in a Siemens Elmiskop I electron microscope. The epoxy embedded material was sectioned on an LBK Ultratome I with glass knives and examined in a Philips electron microscope Model EM 300.

RESULTS

Biochemical analysis of the distribution of acetylcholinesterase in the subcellular components of bull spermatozoa has revealed interesting variations, some of which may be technologically-based, such as cross-contamination of the fractions in the mechanically disrupted specimens while others may be related to enzyme stability or to steric problems such as accessibility of reagents to the enzymatic sites. For not only did epididymal sperm tails exhibit quite considerably lower specific activity than did the naturally-decapitated flagella, but of the latter, the non-motile flagella were twice as active as the motile flagella with respect to acetylcholinesterase. Table I summarizes data assembled from previous experiences in the author's laboratory.

The first systematic difference occurs in the appearance of both acetylcholinesterase and adenosine triphosphatase-adenylate kinase in the head fraction of the mechanically-disrupted sperm and the absence of these enzymes from the naturally-decapitated heads. This can be ascribed, with a high degree of assurance to the difficulty of completely removing minute tail fragment residues from the " heads " (verified microscopically). The enzyme content of the tail or flagellar fractions appeared consistently greatest in both mechanically and naturally disrupted specimens. Apparently, however, ultrasonic disintegration had a considerably less deleterious effect than did glass-homogenization of partially frozen sperm suspensions.

Finally, and perhaps most striking, are differences in enzyme activity between the motile and non-motile flagella separated by differential centrifugation from the naturally-decapitated ejaculates. Electron micrographs (unpublished observations) revealed that vigorous motile activity was associated with those flagella which retained intact plasma membranes, while the non-motile flagella could readily be distinguished by partial or complete destruction of their plasmalemma. Adenosine triphosphatase is reportedly a relatively unstable enzyme, and adenylate kinase (or myokinase) while comparatively indestructible, is however quite soluble in solutions of low ionic strength, and so could be easily washed out from the damaged flagella during the course of preparation. These factors could readily account for the depression of the phosphohydrolase activity of the non-motile flagella.

On the other hand, acetylcholinesterase is allegedly a comparatively stable enzyme, while its substrate, acetylcholine, a highly polar molecule would encounter resistance in penetrating the intact cell. Therefore, since the enzyme has greater accessibility in the more or less denuded non-motile flagellum, its activity there would be predictably higher than in the intact motile flagellum.

TABLE I.

ENZYME (Source and Condition)	SPECIFIC ENZYME ACTIVITY			
	μg reactant hydrolyzed or product liberated		mg protein	hour
	Heads	Midpieces	Tails	" whole "
AChEase . . . . Epididymal Sonicated	17	20	76	32
ATPase-Ad-Kinase . . . . Epididymal Sonicated	10	72	252	—
ATPase-Ad-Kinase . . . . Ejaculate Frozen-Homogenized	5	43	150	48
	Heads	Motile Flagella	Non Motile Flagella	
AChEase . . . . Ejaculate Nat.–Decapitated	0	168	323	
ATPase–Ad–Kinase . . . . Ejaculate Nat.–Decapitated	0	315	114	

Some of these biochemical observations are nicely supported by the cytochemical evidence. Illustrations 1, 2 and 3 are of frozen-dried, naturally-decapitated bull sperm cells. Figure 1 includes longitudinal, transverse and tangential sections of sperm tails and midpieces after incubation in thiolacetic acid and lead nitrate. Hydrolysis of thiolacetic acid by acetylcholinesterase liberated hydrogen sulfide which precipitates as finely granular and highly insoluble lead sulfide at the presumed site of the enzyme action. Here this appears to occur just below the plasmalemma on the fibrous sheath of the tail (*T*) and on or near the mitochondrial surfaces in the midpiece (*M*).

Since these specimens were neither post-fixed in osmic acid nor counter-stained, while it may be somewhat difficult to distinguish the longitudinal filaments or other non-reactive flagellar constituents, we have a clear and unimpeded view of the enzymatically active sites. Figure 2 is a control specimen of the same preparation, from which only the thiolacetic acid has been omitted. Again, while the flagellar fine structure exhibits no enhanced electron opacity, and there are a few random deposits of lead salt scattered throughout both the longitudinal and transverse sections, we have here a satisfactory demonstration of the cytochemical dependence on the enzymatic hydrolysis of the appropriate substrate. What Figure 3 may lack in esthetic appeal it more than makes up in its confirmation that the site of the lead sulfide deposit most likely corresponds to the actual site of acetylcholinesterase activity. This fortuitous section through a kinoplasmic (cytoplasmic) droplet shows that diffusion and secondary deposition of the reaction product does not occur under these experimental conditions. For here there is no non-selective adsorption of the granular deposits at the cell-seminal plasma interface, rather the lead sulfide appears specifically on the fibrous sheath.

If one resorts to chemical fixation and contrast-staining it becomes possible to resolve the fine details of spermatozoan ultrastructure, but unfortunately at the cost of a considerable loss of intensity of the cytochemical reaction. Embedding in epoxy literally demands bulk-staining to preclude loss of the specimen in the polymerized block. Nevertheless, it is possible to salvage some of the cytochemical information. Figures 4 and 5 represent respectively experimental and control specimens of Triton X–100–treated, glutaraldehyde-fixed epididymal bull sperm prepared for acetylcholinesterase localization. The longitudinal section of the midpiece in Fig. 4 clearly shows the close association of the cytochemically-reactive material with the mitochondrial surface. The cross-section of the tail (*T*) shows not only enhanced electron opacity of the fibrous sheath, but also perhaps some involvement of the doublets and the central filament pair. In contrast, the latter structures are apparently absent in the control section in Fig. 5. Since both experimental and control preparations were stained in bulk with alcoholic 5 % platinum tetrabromide, the coarse outer longitudinal filaments show up quite clearly while in the midpiece cross sections (*M*) the nine doublets and central pair are also quite distinguishable.

In Fig. 6, the specimens have not been pretreated with the detergent Triton X–100, but both the experimental (6 *A*) and the control (6 *B*) specimens were prefixed in glutaraldehyde and bulk–stained in platinum tetrabromide after the cytochemical processing.

As previously stated the presence of intact plasma membranes may impose fairly severe limitations on the penetrability of the reactants. Some increased contrast may be detected in the mitochondrial surface in Fig. 6 A compared to those in 6 B. But in these micrographs of the neck region, the proximal centriole appears quite unreactive by usual cytochemical standards.

Conclusion

The biochemical and cytochemical evidence for flagellar localization of acetylcholinesterase in bull spermatozoa complement each other. Moreover, in none of the electron microscopic preparations do any of the fine structural elements of the sperm head betray any positive reaction for the enzyme. This is certainly consistent with the ability of morphologically intact naturally-decapitated motile flagella to propel themselves so vigorously as to exhibit en masse synchronous movement, referred to as " wave-formation " when observed at low magnification. Propulsive movement is also encountered when the isolated glycerinated sperm flagella of some species of invertebrates are reactivated with ATP. Evidently the head contributes very little if anything positive to the propulsive activity of the otherwise intact flagellum. And so we may confidently look elsewhere for the regulatory seat of flagellar power, the coordinating system essential for wave initiation and propagation. Of some possible significance is the fact of the apparent complete cytochemical non-reactivity of the centriole (see Fig. 6. The frozen-dried centrioles were also cytochemically negative. This evidence in itself may not be entirely conclusive. RIKMENSPOEL and VAN HERPEN (1969), on the basis of X–irradiation and proton bombardment damage to sperm motility invoke target theory to zero in on an organelle with a diameter of 160 mμ and volume of 0.75×10^{-15} cm^3 and nominate the " centriole " as the control center of sperm motility. Mathematically this may be a valid conclusion. However, a comparable amount of disruption of the plasma membrane or other structure could equally well adversely affect bull sperm motility. For instance, GOLDSTEIN and BROKAW (1968) showed by means of a 2 μ diameter laser beam that in some marine invertebrates' sperm, the portion of the flagellum anterior to the beam's damage continued to beat, only if that portion was longer than the normal length of one flagellar bend, namely, 10–12 μ. This supports other evidence that initiation of wave movement is centered at the anterior end of the flagellum, and it also suggests that destructive damage is not necessarily limited to the 160 mμ bulls-eye of the sensitive target. Moreover while the control center need not possess acetylcholinesterase activity (and our evidence clearly indicates that the centriole lacks this particular enzyme and the several others so far assayed cytochemically), if conduction is essential to wave propagation, some mechanism providing impulse transmission from the center to the conductile apparatus could be expected.

BRADFIELD (1955) assumed that the nine fiber doublets were capable of propagating contractions and that the central pair are specialized for more rapid conduction; he also thought that impulses producing contraction arise rhythmically at a point in the " basal corpuscle ", directly beneath one of the nine doublets and each impulse travels around the other eight fibers and then dies out. On the basis of the observations of GRIGG and HODGE (1949) on the morphology of rooster spermatozoa, who suggested that the central fibers may perform an excitatory function, BRADFIELD likened these to the giant nerve fibers of an earthworm causing contraction almost simultaneously along the entire length of the outer fibers on one side of the flagellum. Such a mechanism could perhaps subserve two-dimensional ciliary beat, but sequential firing, conduction and propagation would more nearly meet the demands of the three-dimensional flagellar wave.

A priori judgments based exclusively on strictly morphological studies can lead us to speculate that an intracellular conductile system should initiate its activities in the region of the centriole and by extrapolation we are further led to implicate either the central pair of axial filaments or some more superficially disposed structure at or near the plasma membrane. Frequently, in the frozen-dried preparations, deposits of lead sulfide appeared along the central axial region of the flagellum, but these were neither so vivid nor so consistent as those in the subplasmalemmar regions on or near the mitochondrial surfaces and seemingly permeating the fibrous sheath of the principal piece of the tail.

At this stage we can only tentatively conclude that a highly stable, true specific acetylcholinesterase is " advantageously " arrayed in close morphological approximation to the outer coarse longitudinal contractile fibers of the mammalian sperm flagellum. Here it may, by propagated depolarization of the overlying plasma membrane, govern the coordination of the flagellar wave. We cannot at present account for a presumed conductile function of the central fiber pair, although this could possibly be a heritage from the invertebrates' sperms and cilia which lack both outer coarse fibers and fibrous sheaths.

Preliminary measurements ol bioelectric potentials with microelectrodes, one inserted in the bull sperm head, and one placed externally in the medium, fairly consistently exhibit a potential difference of about ten millivolts. Bull sperm flagella average about ten beats per second (GRAY, 1958; LORD ROTHSCHILD, 1953), and if each of the nine fibers is firing in sequence about 11 % out of phase this would require a spacing of about one pulse every 10–12 milliseconds. We are planning to examine the correlation between impulse production and acetylcholinesterase activity and their mutual response to the influence of sympathomimetic agents. It is not immediately apparent whether either the cytochemical or electrophysiological approach can establish an involvement of the centriole in the regulation of flagellar moment. In fact, we may have to conclude that it may be nothing more than a romantic quest to seek in the centriole any other than its primary, if not sole, function as the synthetic center for flagellar *fiber* generation, as the induction organelle or template for initiation of the *self-assembly* of microtubular proteins. If that were all, it would be enough!

References

Applegate A. and Nelson L. (1962) – *Acetylcholinesterase in Mytilus Spermatozoa.* « Biol. Bull. », 123, 475.

Bishop D. W. and Hoffmann–Berling H. (1959) – *Extracted Mammalian Sperm Models. I. Preparation and Reactivation with Adenosine-triphosphate.* « J. Cell Comp. Physiol. », 53, 445–466.

Bradfield J. R. G. (1955) – *Fibre Patterns in Animal Flagella and Cilia.* « Symp. Soc. Exp. Biol. », 9, 306–334.

Brokaw C. J. (1961) – *Movement and Nucleoside Polyphosphatase Activity of Isolated Flagella from* Polytoma uvella. « Exp. Cell Res. », 22, 151–162.

Brokaw C. J. (1963) – *Movement of the Flagella of* Polytoma uvella. « J. Exp. Biol. », 40, 149–156.

Brokaw C. J. (1964) – *Thiourea-Induced Alterations of Flagellar Wave Forms.* « J. Cell Biol. », 23, 15 A.

Claybrook J. R. and Nelson L. (1968) – *Flagellar Adenosine Triphosphatase from Sea Urchin Sperm: Properties and Relation to Motility.* « Science », 162, 1134–1136.

Crevier M. and Belanger L. F. (1955) – *Simple Method for Histochemical Detection of Esterase Activity.* « Science », 122, 556.

Gersh I., Isenberg I., Stephenson J. and Bondareff W. (1957) – *Submicroscopic Structure of Frozen-Dried Liver Specifically Stained for Electron Microscopy.* Part. I. *Technical.* « Anat. Rec. », 128, 91–108.

Goldstein S. F. and Brokaw C. J. (1968) – *Laser Microbeam Irradiation Studies in the Control of Flagellar Bending.* « Biophys. J. », 8, A–122.

Gray J. (1958) – *The Movement of the Spermatozoa of the Bull.* « J. Exp. Biol. », 35, 96–108.

Grigg G. W. and Hodge A. J. (1949) – *Electron Microscopic Studies of Spermatozoa. I. The Morphology of the Spermatozoon of the Common Domestic Fowl* (Gallus Domesticus). « Austral. J. Sci. Res. », Ser. B. 2, 271–286.

Kinoshita S. (1959) – *On the Identity of the Motility-Inducing Factor of Flagellum and the Relaxing Factor of Muscle.* « J. Fac. Sci., Univ. of Tokyo », Section IV, 8, 427–437.

Koelle G. B. and Horn R. S. (1968) – *Acetyl Disulfide,* $(CH_3COS)_2$, *a Major Active Component in the Thiolacetic Acid Histochemical Method for Acetylcholinesterase.* « J. Histochem. Cytochem. », 16, 743–753.

Mann T. (1954) – *The Biochemistry of Semen,* p. 174. Methuen and Co., Ltd, London.

Nelson L. (1959) – *Adenosinetriphosphatase of Mytilus Spermatozoa. II. Effects of Sulfhydryl Reagents, Temperature and Inorganic Pyrophosphate.* « Biol. Bull. », 117, 327–339.

Nelson L. (1964) – *Acetylcholinesterase in Bull Spermatozoa.* « J. Reprod. Fertil. », 7, 65–71.

Nelson L. (1966) – *Enzyme Distribution in « Naturally–Decapitated » Bull Spermatozoa: Acetylcholinesterase, Adenylpyrophosphatase and Adenosine triphosphatase.* « J. Cell Physiol. », 68, 113–116.

Rikmenspoel R. and Van Herpen G. (1969) – *Radiation Damage to Bull Sperm Motility. I. X–Ray Effects and Target Theory.* « Biophys. J. », 9, 822–832.

Rikmenspoel R. and Van Herpen G. (1969) – *Radiation Damage to Bull Sperm Motility. II. Proton Irradiation and Respiration Measurements.* « Biophys. J. », 9, 833–844.

Rothschild Lord (1953) – *The Movements of Spermatozoa,* in *Mammalian Germ Cells.* 122–133, Ciba Fdn. Symp. London.

Sekine T. (1951) – *Cholinesterase in Pig Spermatozoa.* « J. Biochem., Tokyo », 38, 171–179.

EXPLANATION OF FIGURES

Fig. 1. – Frozen-dried, naturally-decapitated, ejaculated bull sperm, incubated in 0.12 M thioacetic acid, 0.001 M lead acetate for 30 minutes at room temperature embedded in methacrylate. Longitudinal and transverse sections of midpiece (*M*) and tail (*T*). Lead sulfide deposit at mitochondrial surfaces and in fibrous tail sheath mark sites of acetylcholinesterase activity.

Fig. 2. – Frozen-dried, naturally-decapitated ejaculated bull sperm, control specimens—thiolacetic acid omitted from incubation medium. Longitudinal, transverse and tangential sections of midpiece and tail. Random small deposits of lead salt due to incomplete removal of lead at washing and precipitated during treatment with dilute ammonium sulfide.

Fig. 3. – Cross-section through frozen-dried specimen at level of the knoplasmic droplet. Treatment by Belanger method shows lead sulfide deposit at mitochondrial membrane surface, but none at cytoplasm-seminal plasma interface. This precludes possible secondary deposition due to resolubilization and diffusion to a non-specific adsorbing surface.

Fig. 4. – Glutaraldehyde-fixed epididymal bull sperm, treated with Triton X–100, incubated one hour in the Belanger medium and counterstained with alcoholic platinumtetrabromide. Cross-section of tail shows enhanced electron—opacity of fibrous sheath and central pair of axial filaments as well as of the nine doublets. Longitudinal, tangential and transverse section of a segment of the midpiece shows particulate deposits exclusively on the mitochondrial membrane surface. (All glutaraldehyde-fixed specimens embedded in epoxy).

Fig. 5. – Glutaraldehyde-fixed control specimens (thiolacetic acid omitted from incubation medium). Very little electron-scattering in tail (*T*) and midpiece (*M*) cross-sections. Central pair of fibers not visible in tail but discernible in midpiece. Neck region (*N*) is not particularly striking.

Fig. 6. – Glutaraldehyde-fixed, epididymal bull sperm, not treated with Triton X–100, but stained with platinum tetrabomide:

A. Incubated in complete Belanger medium. Major increased contrast on mitochondrial surfaces. Proximal Centriole (*PC*) remarkable only for lack of reactivity.

B. Control specimens—no thiolacetic acid in incubation medium. Quite similar in appearance to Figure 6 A, except that there are no deposits at the mitochondrial surfaces.

Discussion

NICANDER. – TEICHMANN has recently shown acid phosphatase activity in membranes of rabbit spermatozoa. Have you studied this enzyme?

NELSON. – No, we have not yet conducted any biochemical or cytochemical studies on acid phosphatase, but showed several years ago that alkaline phosphatase was localized at the plasma membrane in the rat sperm tail.

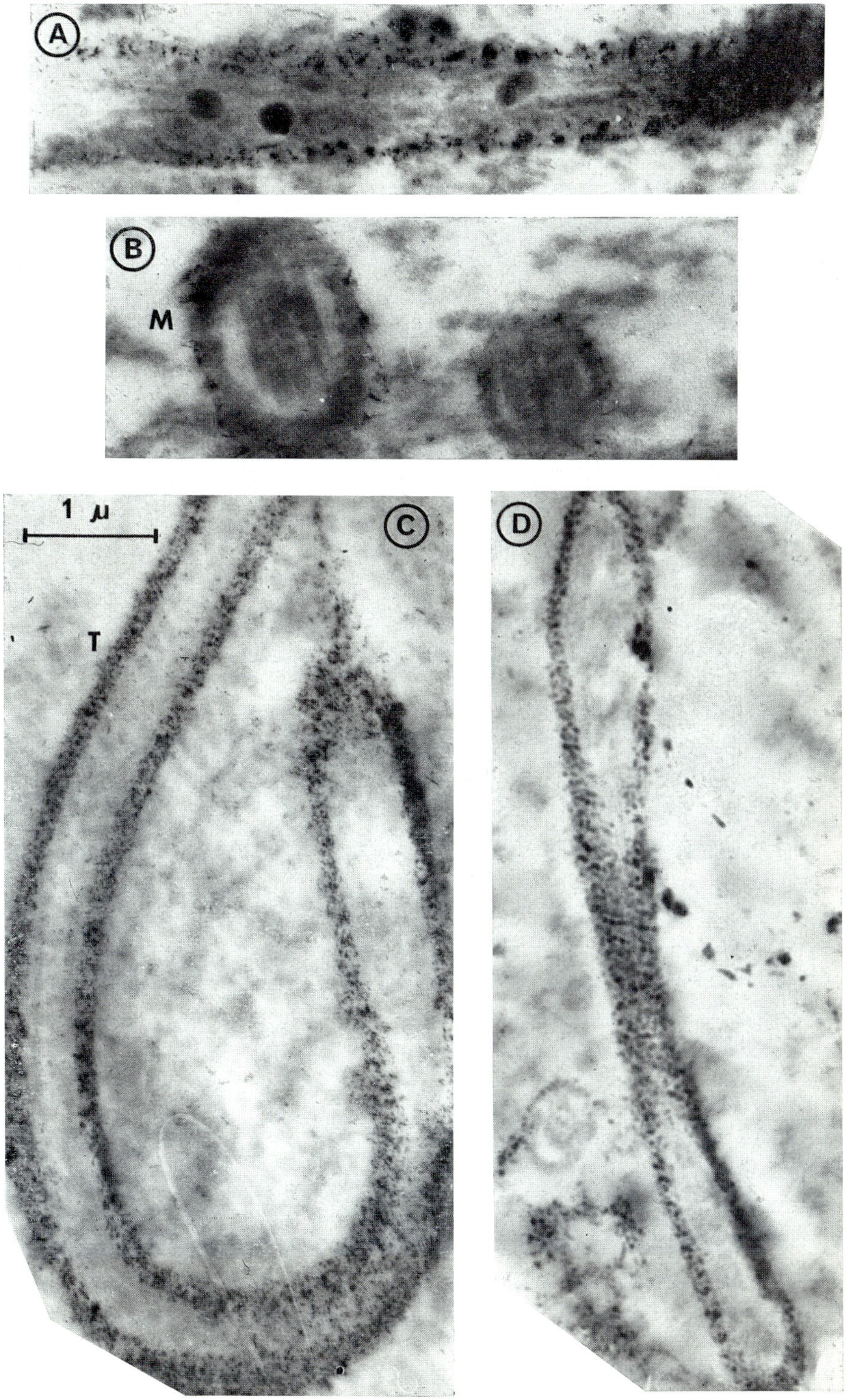

Fig. 1.

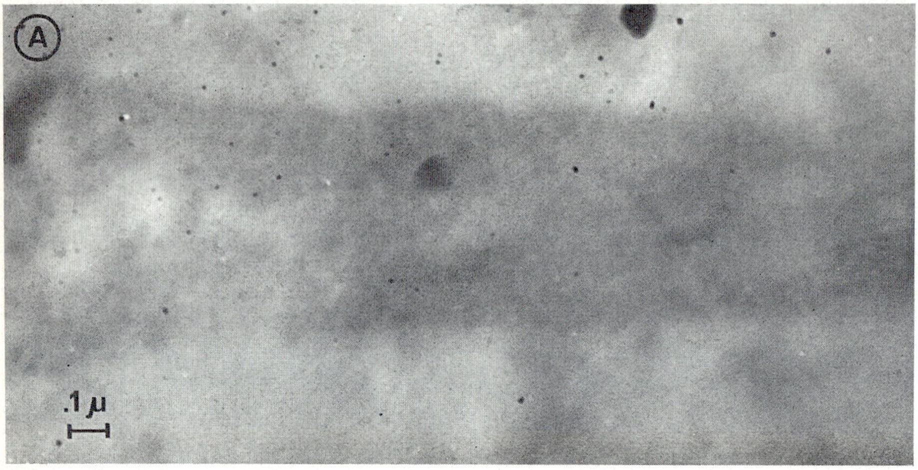

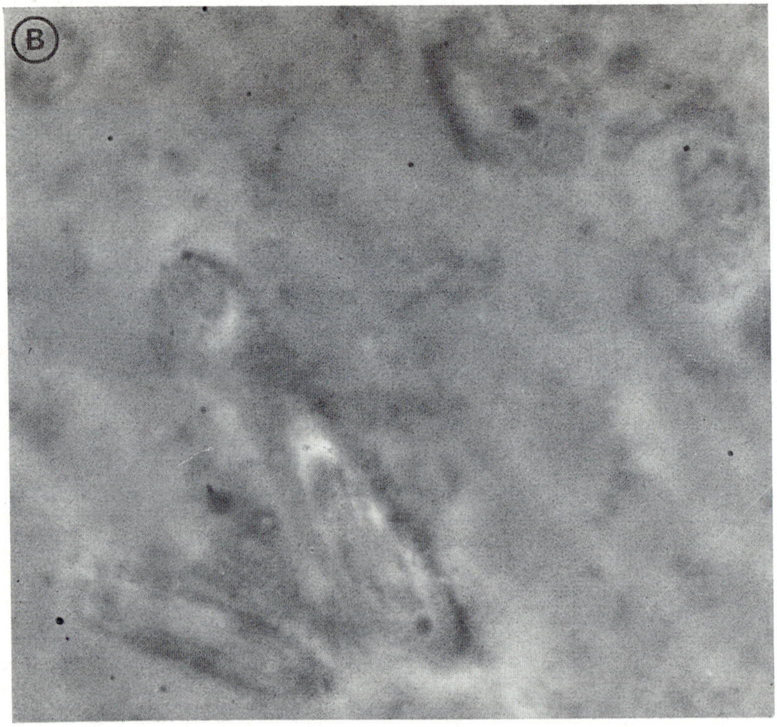

Fig. 2.

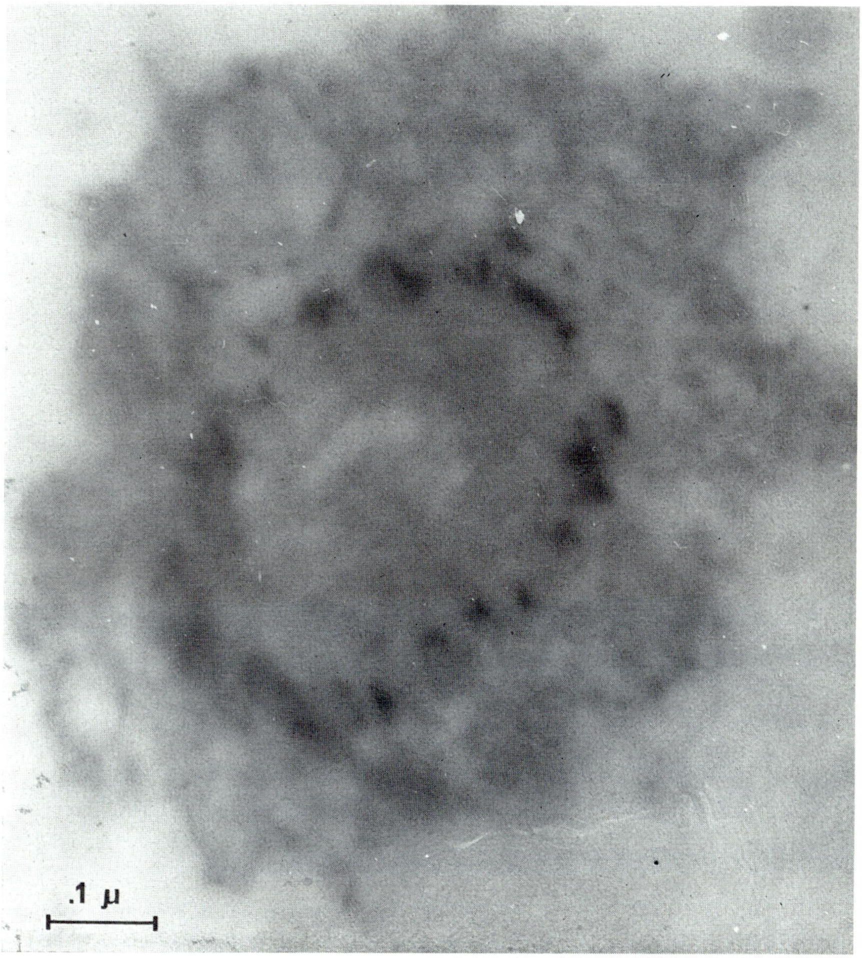

Fig. 3.

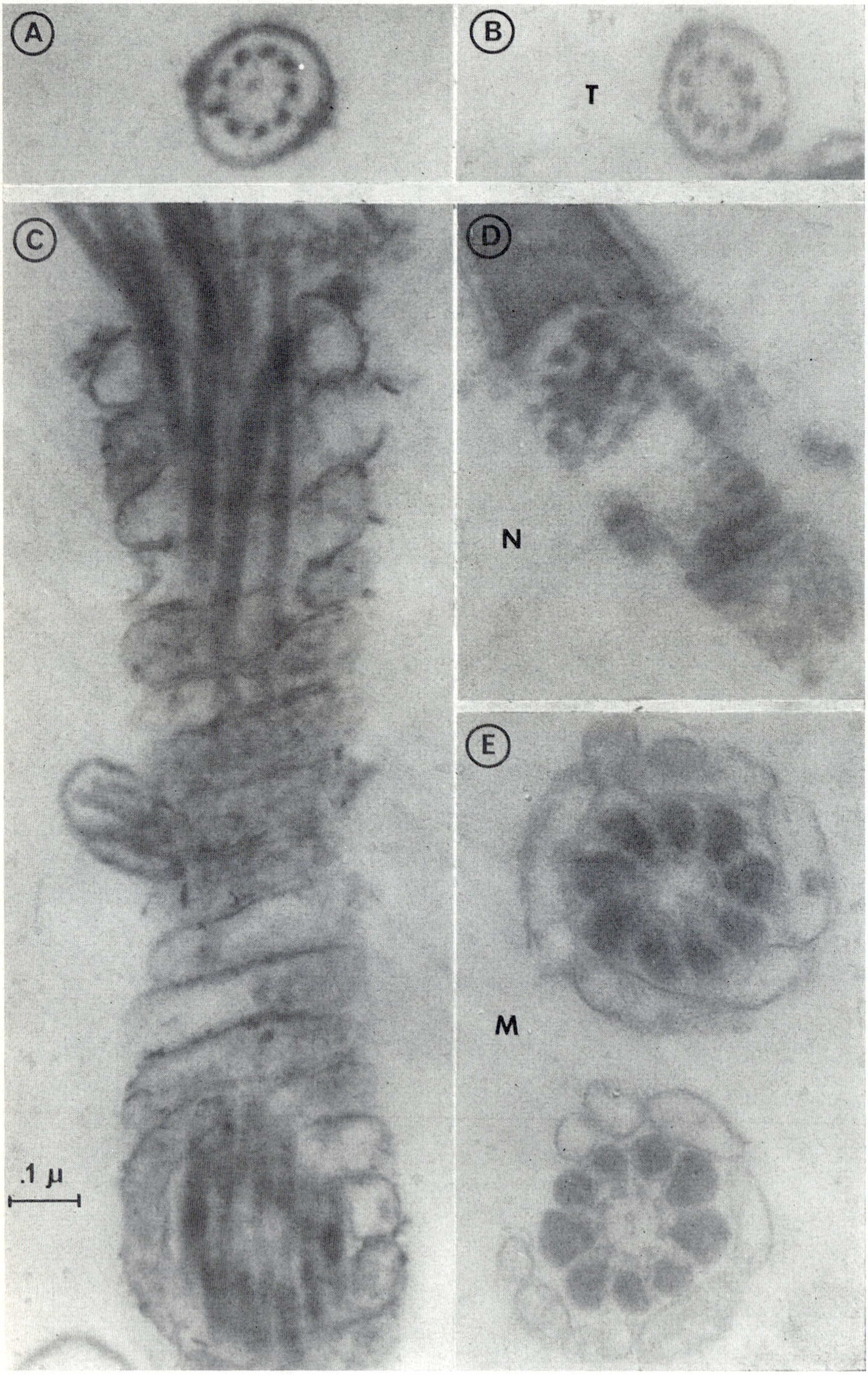

Fig. 4.

Fig. 5.

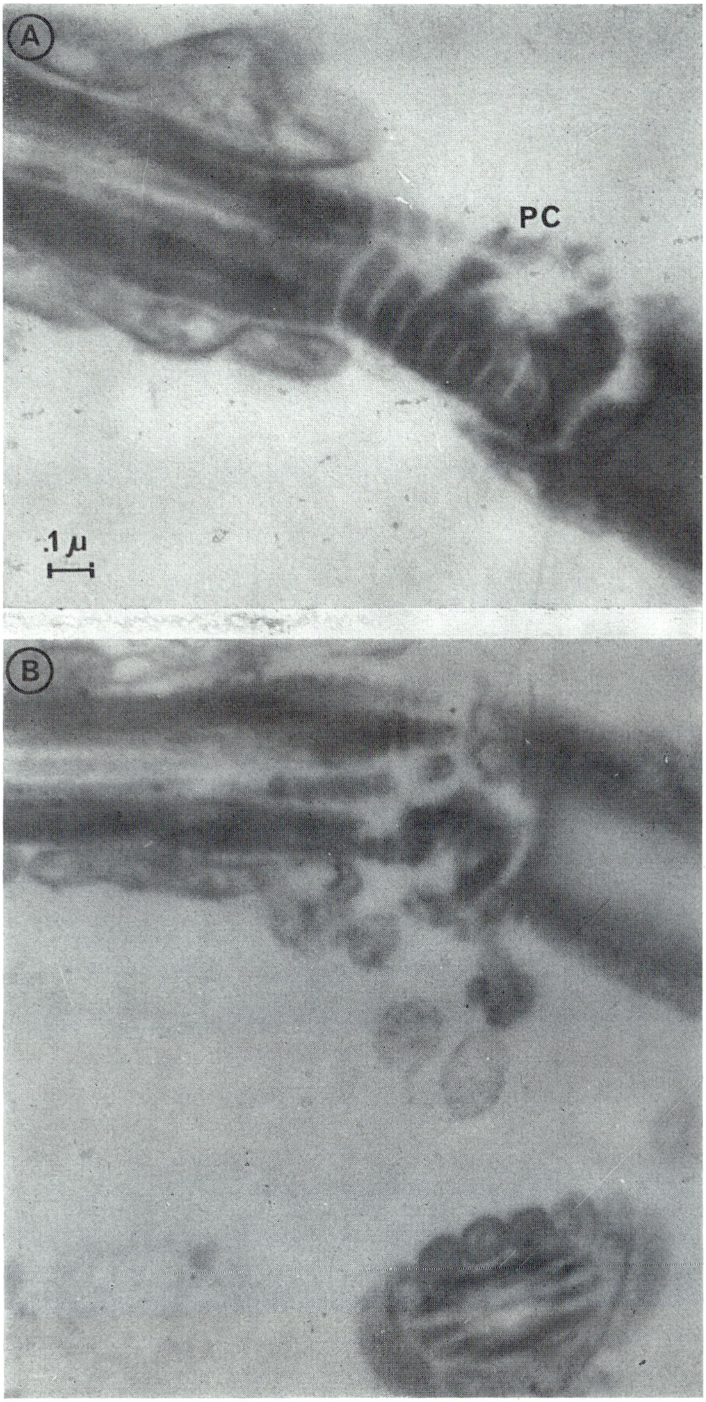

Fig. 6.

C. J. BROKAW, S. F. GOLDSTEIN (*) and R. L. MILLER (**)

RECENT STUDIES ON THE MOTILITY OF SPERMATOZOA FROM SOME MARINE INVERTEBRATES (***)

SUMMARY. — We have attempted to show briefly that techniques are now available which can yield, with a minimum of effort and expense, complete and precise information about the movement of the flagellum of « simple » spermatozoa such as those of sea urchins and some other readily available marine invertebrates. Although only a limited amount of work has so far been done with these techniques, they have already revealed significant differences between the behavior of spermatozoa from different animals; differences which have not yet been correlated with evidence from comparative studies with the electron microscope or with biochemical techniques. We suggest that the information available in this way is an important, if not essential, basis for studying the mechanisms of sperm motility, and that spermatozoa on which this information can be obtained should be a principal focus of research on comparative spermatology to the extent that it seeks to understand the mechanisms of sperm motility.

RIASSUNTO. — Esistono ora tecniche che possono dare, con minimo sforzo e spesa, un'informazione completa e precisa sul movimento del flagello di « semplici » spermatozoi come quelli del riccio di mare e di altri invertebrati marini. Sebbene ci siano per ora pochi lavori fatti con queste tecniche, questi hanno già rivelato differenze significative nel funzionamento di spermatozoi di differenti animali; differenze che non sono state ancora correlate con prove mediante studi comparativi col microscopio elettronico o con tecniche biochimiche.

Noi pensiamo che le informazioni ottenibili in questa maniera siano una importante, se non essenziale, base per lo studio del meccanismo del movimento dello spermatozoo, e che gli spermatozoi su cui queste informazioni possono essere ottenute dovrebbero essere il centro principale di ricerca di spermatologia comparata al fine di capire il meccanismo del moto dello spermatozoo.

Sea urchin spermatozoa were the subjects of the first detailed study, based on photographic evidence, of the movement of the sperm flagellum (GRAY, 1955). These spermatozoa, and spermatozoa with similar morphology and properties from some other marine invertebrates, continue to be particularly suitable subjects for experimental studies. Their flagella contain the classic " nine-plus-two " pattern of microtubules, and very little in the

(*) Present address: Department of Physiology–Anatomy, University of California, Berkeley, California, 94720.

(**) Present address: Department of Biology, Temple University, Philadelphia, Pennsylvania, 19122.

(***) From the Division of Biology, California Institute of Technology, Pasadena, California. This work has been supported in part by a grant from the United States Public Health Service (GM–14613).

way of other visible structures. They appear to be uniform in size and construction throughout their length, except for modifications at the distal end and, possibly, near the base. The sperm flagellum retains its ability to swim by generating bending waves for at least a short time after removal of the head and midpiece (BROKAW, 1965). In these respects, they can be considered to be relatively simple spermatozoa, in which the basic mechanisms of ciliary and flagellar motility can be studied with a minimum of confusion.

Because some of these spermatozoa can be obtained in reasonable quantities, with uniform properties, they are also suitable for physiological and biochemical studies such as biochemical characterization of the components of isolated tails (STEVENS, RENAUD and GIBBONS, 1967; YANIGASAWA, HASEGAWA and MOHRI, 1968; CLAYBROOK and NELSON, 1968) or measurements of parameters such as oxygen consumption, where suspensions of uniformly motile spermatozoa are required (BROKAW and BENEDICT, 1968 b).

Their movements, also, are made easier to study by the fact that the bending of the sperm flagellum takes place predominantly in a single plane (GRAY, 1955). This feature, plus the tendency of these spermatozoa to accumulate near interfaces with the plane of beat parallel to the interface as they swim, makes it possible to obtain photomicrographs of good resolution in which the entire flagellum is in focus, and which therefore contain all the important information about the shape of the flagellum at any instant. A series of such photographs will therefore completely describe the movement of the flagellum.

In the following pages, we will review some of the experimental work from this laboratory, based on photographic study of the movement of the sperm flagellum, and consider a few of the questions which remain to be answered about the mechanisms of movement of these spermatozoa. The photographic techniques which we have used have been described in various previous publications, but the flash illuminator used in earlier work has now been made obsolete by the availability of a more efficient flash illuminator, which is commercially available from the Chadwick-Helmuth Company, Monrovia, California, USA (Model 135 N). Fig. 2 is an example of a photograph made with this new illuminator.

The pattern of bending.

The photographs of moving sea urchin spermatozoa studied by GRAY (1955) suggested that the flagellum was bent in the form of a sinusoidal wave. Mathematical treatments based on this conclusion were developed by GRAY and HANCOCK (1955) to compare theoretical and observed swimming velocities, by CARLSON (1959) and others to find the energy expenditure during movement, and by MACHIN (1958) to analyze a suggested mechanism for wave propagation. Higher resolution photographs of flagella obtained by BROKAW and WRIGHT (1963) and BROKAW (1965) indicated that the bending pattern was not a sinusoidal wave, but could, instead, be matched more closely by a waveform consisting of circular arcs connected by straight lines. This subject is not yet closed, however, for recently Mr. TAKAO SARASHINA, of Hokkaido University, has demonstrated that the bending waves of the sea urchin sperm flagellum in the photographs of BROKAW (1965) can also be accurately matched by a function known as a sine-generated curve (SARASHINA, personal communication). Although the differences between these curves are small, they have very different implications for the mechanism of bending.

The bending of the flagellum can perhaps most usefully be described by a curve showing its curvature, $d\theta/ds$, as a function of distance, s, measured along the flagellum; where θ is an angle between a line tangent to the flagellum at the point s and a convenient reference line. Curves of this type, which can be referred to as wave generating functions, for some possible bending patterns are illustrated in Fig. 1. Such curves will also illustrate the curvature, or amount of bend, at any point on the flagellum as a function of time, if the bending is propagating uniformly along the flagellum. Similarly, a curve showing the second derivative, $d^2\theta/ds^2$, will indicate the rate of change of curvature, or the actual amount of bending, occurring at a particular point on the flagellum, as a function of time. This is the information which is important to obtain from flagellar photographs, in order to describe the bending of the flagellum in terms which can be directly related to its internal bending mechanisms.

A sinusoidal bending wave, generated by curve 5 in Fig. 1, differs from the other curves in being defined in terms of distance along the axis of symmetry of the wave, rather than the distance s; consequently the curves of θ or its derivatives as functions of s are mathematically more complicated than a sinusoidal function. For this reason alone, a sinusoidal wave might be considered to be an unikely waveform to be produced by a system of biologically generated bending, unless the similarities of the system to the passive bending wave propagation by an elastic rod completely dominate the biological mechanism. In any event, the photographs provide evidence against a sinusoidal wave or a " triangle generated " wave (number 4 in Fig. 1), or any wave in which the curvature of the wave ($d\theta/ds$) changes rapidly near the crests of the waves, because the bends on such waves could not be closely fitted by segments of a circle.

The first three bending patterns defined in Fig. 1 all involve a fairly constant curvature of the flagellum near the crests of the bending waves, and therefore all will produce bending waves in which the bent regions can be matched reasonably well by a segment of a circle. It may prove to be impossible to distinguish between these possibilities by analysis of photographs of flagella.

The sine-generated wave produced by pattern 3 in Fig. 1 has been applied to description of the form of river meanders, and is also the curve of minimum energy of bending for an elastic filament subject to certain constraints (LEOPOLD and LANGBEIN, 1966 a, b). If the curvature of points on the flagellum is determined by biological control mechanisms, the sine-generated wave would appear to be unnecessarily complex; however, if elastic forces are predominant in shaping the wave it may be a more reasonable choice.

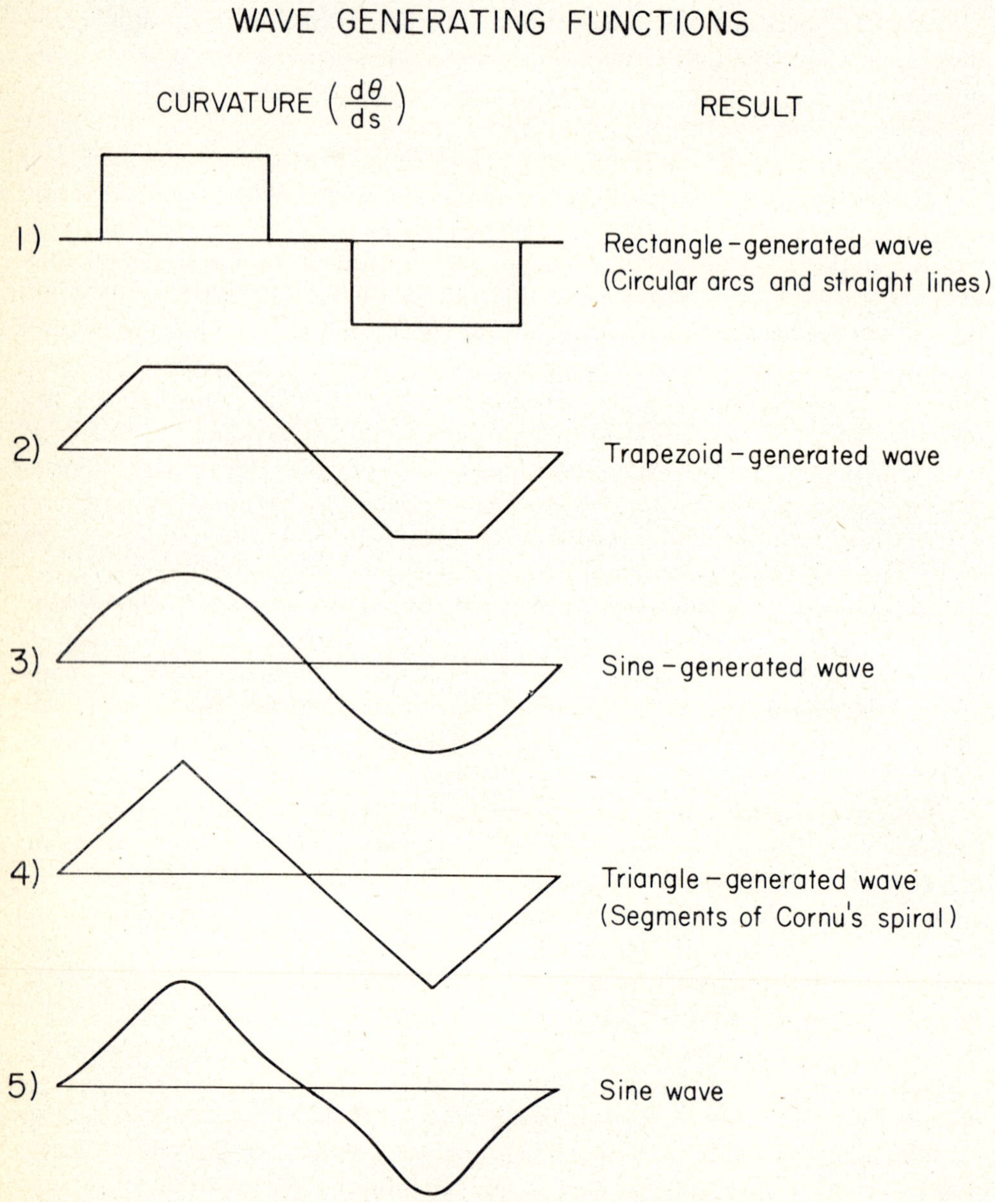

Fig. 1. – Generating functions for some possible flagellar wave patterns. Each curve shows the curvature of the flagellum as a function of distance measured along the flagellum, for one full bending wave. The amplitudes of these curves have been adjusted to produce bending patterns having equal total angles of bend.

Pattern 1, which generates a wave containing circular arcs and straight regions, and pattern 2, which also generates a wave containing circular arcs, would appear to be particularly simple forms to be generated by a biological control mechanism, since each point on the flagellum can be controlled by signals which simply instruct it to switch to an alternate state, when the signal is received. A " switching " mechanism of this type appears particularly attractive in the light of results from measurements of the amount of ATP used during flagellar bending (BROKAW and BENEDICT, 1968 a, b), which demonstrate that on the average, the number of ATP molecules used by a flagellum each time a bend is propagated along it is approximately equal to the number of molecules of the ATP–dephosphorylating enzyme, dynein, which the flagellum contains. This result raises the intriguing possibility that at the molecular level, the passage of a bend along the flagellum may correspond to the use of just one ATP molecule by each molecule of dynein. Such a mechanism might be expected to generate waves according to patterns 1 or 2 of Fig. 1. A preference for pattern 1 over pattern 2 might be based on indications that flagella do in fact have a neutral straight state; for instance, the laser microbeam irradiation experiments described below provide some support for this concept.

Bending Moments.

A sea urchin spermatozoon swimming in sea water is operating under hydrodynamic conditions corresponding to a very low Reynold's number, where the resistance offered by the surrounding medium can be described entirely in terms of viscous forces. For movement restricted to a plane, any element of flagellar length, *ds*, is subject to a viscous resisting force with normal (F_N) and tangential (F_L) components defined by

$$F_N = -C_N V_N \, ds \qquad \text{and} \qquad F_L = -C_L V_L \, ds \, .$$

V_N and V_L are the normal and tangential components of the velocity of the element *ds*, and C_N and C_L are normal and tangential drag coefficients. A hydrodynamically unsophisticated treatment of these forces, which assumes that the drag coefficients are independent of velocity and independent of the movement of neighboring regions of the flagellum, has been utilized by GRAY and HANCOCK (1955) and BROKAW (1965) to correctly predict the swimming velocity from the parameters of the bending waves.

This approach can be extended to calculate the bending moment, M_v, which will be produced at any point *s* on the flagellum as the result of all the F_N and F_L forces acting on the flagellum as it moves through the viscous medium. The movement of the flagellum must result from active bending moments (M_a) generated by mechanochemical processes within the flagellum. At any point at which the flagellum is bending in opposition to M_v, M_a must be greater in magnitude than M_v and in the opposite direction. There is also likely to be an elastic resistance to bending, represented by a moment M_e, which must be overcome by the active bending moment, so that the magnitude of M_a must be greater than $M_v + M_e$. At an unbending point, M_e may assist M_a in overcoming M_v.

Equations giving M_v for the very special, and rather unrealistic, case of an infinitely long flagellum propagating symmetrical bending waves have been published (BROKAW, 1965). These equations, or similarly based equations used by other workers, indicate that the viscous forces which the flagellum must overcome as it moves will account for a sizeable fraction of the energy available from metabolism or ATP dephosphorylation (cf. BROKAW and BENEDICT, 1968 b). The viscous forces acting on the flagellum, as represented by the values of M_v at the points where the flagellum is bending or unbending, must at least set some limits on the bending behavior of the flagellum, and may play a more significant role in determining the rate and distribution of bending.

Significant information about the mechanisms of flagellar bending might be obtained by comparing the bending behavior of points on the flagellum with the values of M_v at those points. The published equations for M_v are not adequate for a thorough analysis. We are currently working on the development of methods for calculation of M_v for flagella of finite length and having any pattern of bending, including asymmetrical patterns. Sufficient progress has been made on these methods to suggest that it will soon become possible to take much fuller advantage of the information contained in photographs of moving sperm flagella, by using this information, and computer calculation of M_v, to efficiently examine a variety of questions about the mechanisms of flagellar bending, including the following:

1) Is a flagellum able to generate an active bending moment (M_a) during both bending and unbending, in contrast to muscle, which can generate tension only during contraction? If a flagellum can generate M_a only during bending, then presumably an elastic moment is responsible for overcoming M_v during unbending. Previous indications have suggested that it is unlikely that elastic moments can be totally responsible for unbending (BROKAW, 1968), but a more rigorous analysis of this point is needed.

2) What is the relation between active bending moment and the concentration of ATP? The effect of ATP concentration on the rate of bend propagation along ATP-reactivated, glycerinated sea urchin spermatozoa does not match the ATP–binding characteristics of the flagellar ATPase, dynein, obtained from measurements of the rate of ATP dephosphorylation as a function of ATP concentration. This observation might possibly be rationalized if M_a is determined by the degree of ATP binding by dynein, and if the propagation velocity is then secondarily determined by interaction between M_a and M_v. We have been collecting data on the effects of ATP concentration on the movement of glycerinated sea urchin spermatozoa which appear to support this explanation, but the completion of this work is awaiting a more thorough analysis of the viscous bending moments.

3) Does the active bending moment vary with the amount of curvature of the flagellum or the rate of bend propagation? Does the propagation velocity of a bend depend on the local values of M_v which must be overcome as it moves along the flagellum? Does a bend propagate as an integrated unit, or is it merely the result of the independent propagation of a bending point and an unbending point? These questions can be investigated by analyzing data obtained from photographs which compare the movements of the flagella of spermatozoa beating with their heads attached to the microscope slide with the movements of freely swimming spermatozoa (BROKAW, 1965), from photographs of spermatozoa with flagella of different lengths, (BROKAW, 1965), and from photographs of spermatozoa swimming in solutions containing methyl cellulose to alter the viscosity (BROKAW, 1966).

The viscosity data are particularly interesting because they reveal some interesting differences between the behavior of spermatozoa of different species. At increased viscosities, sea urchin spermatozoa, and spermatozoa of the tunicate, *Ciona*, maintain a constant degree of curvature in the bent regions of the flagellum, while the beat frequency, wavelength, and amplitude of the bending patterns decrease. The estimated values of M_v at the points of bending and unbending also appear to remain constant as the viscosity increases. On the other hand, a very different result was obtained with spermatozoa of the annelid worm, *Chaetopterus*. The degree of curvature of the bent regions of the flagellum increases with increasing viscosity, and the estimated values of M_v also increase, more or less in proportion to the degree of curvature. This behavior does not appear to be unique to *Chaetopterus* spermatozoa, however, since similar behavior was obtained with sea urchin spermatozoa, but not with *Ciona* spermatozoa, when their movements were slowed down by an inhibitor, thiourea. Although these results can be more fully interpreted when a more complete analysis of M_v is available, they already point out the value of comparative studies on different species, to prevent us from forming too hurried conclusions about universal mechanisms of spermatozoan movement.

Non-uniform bending patterns.

The discussion up to this point has focussed on the bending patterns of normal flagella, which may have relatively simple geometry. Important additional information about the mechanisms of flagellar bending may also be obtained from examples of movement which do not conform to an ideal bending pattern. The commonest such deviation is perhaps the generation of asymmetrical bending waves. This and other types of deviations have been discussed in previous papers (BROKAW, 1965; 1968) but no systematic study of the implications of these deviations has yet been carried out. A particularly interesting type of experimentally produced alteration in the normal bending behaviour of a sperm flagellum has been described by GOLDSTEIN (1969). Goldstein's experiments involved the use of a laser microbeam to damage a small part of the sperm flagellum. An example of the type of result obtained in these experiments is shown in Fig. 3.

The laser experiments utilized a pulsed ruby laser, with a pulse duration of a few hundred microseconds, which made it possible to hit a small spot on the sperm flagellum while the flagellum was actively beating. The laser beam was sent backwards down through the microscope, and focussed by the objective lens into a spot of approximately 2 microns diameter. A spermatozoon was selected which was beating with its head fastened to the microscope slide, and stroboscopic light flashing at the same frequency as the sperm tail was used to observe the spermatozoon during focussing and alignment of a desired part of the bending pattern on the sperm tail with the cross hairs which located the target area of the laser beam. The laser beam was then fired in sychrony with the stroboscopic illuminator, in order to ensure that the flagellum would be at the target spot at the time of the laser pulse. Photographs of the sperm flagellum were taken with higher intensity flashes, at the same time as the laser pulse, and at intervals after the laser pulse. Fig. 3 is a multiple exposure made with three photographic flashes.

In most cases, the laser pulse produced a visible break in the sperm flagellum at the target spot, and apparently welded the tail to the microscope slide at that spot. The most important result, illustrated by Fig. 3, is the demonstration that a bend which has already passed the point of laser irradiation is able to continue independently to end of the flagellum, but that the flagellum is unable to generate any new bends beyond the point of irradiation. This result implies that there is a part of the tail near its base which has special properties required for bend initiation; this result has also been implied by other observations (VAN HERPEN and RIKMERSPOEL, 1968). Several considerations suggest that the inability of the flagellum to initiate new bends beyond the point of irradiation is not due to exhaustion of the supply of ATP which it normally receives from the midpiece of the spermatozoon. The most direct evidence is provided by similar results obtained in experiments using glycerinated spermatozoa activated by an external source of ATP.

When the target for the laser pulse was within a bent region, rather than between bent regions as illustrated in Fig. 3, the most usual result was complete disappearance, that is, failure to propagate, of the target bend. Although several alternative explanations of this result are possible, it seems to suggest that a bent region, or bend, on the flagellum, is in some sense a unit of bending, which is distinct from the preceding and following bends, but which is more than just the summation of local bending activity within a particular region. This result may suggest that bending waves are generated according to curve 1 in Fig. 1. Other implications are discussed in BROKAW (1968) and GOLDSTEIN (1969).

In many cases, the bends which continued to propagate beyond a region of laser irradiation showed a variety of changes in rate of propagation or the form of the bent region. These changes have not yet been exhaustively analyzed, in part because it has not been possible to isolate the effects which might be produced by the altered distribution of viscous bending moments which will exist on the flagellum as it moves after irradiation. This analysis may be possible in the near future, as further experimental data from laser irradiation experiments becomes available. The laser irradiation technique appears to be an especially valuable technique to use with sperm flagella, because of its ability to damage the sperm flagellum within a very short time period.

Changes in flagellar bending during chemotactic responses.

Attraction of spermatozoa to eggs by chemotaxis has been well established in lower plants for many years, particularly since the classic study by Pfeffer on the chemotaxis of fern spermatozoids (PFEFFER, 1884). Despite much debate over the years, a through demonstration of sperm chemotaxis in animals has only recently been presented, and even now it appears that this is not a common method for assisting fertilization in animals.

Animal sperm chemotaxis occurs in the hydroids *Campanularia flexuosa* and *C. calceolifera* (MIILLER, 1966 a), *Tubularia crocea* and *Gonothyrea loveni* (MILLER, 1966 b), *Tubularia marina* and *T. larynx* (MILLER, unpublished observations). In all of these species, the eggs are enclosed in gonangia which the spermatozoa must enter by swimming through a narrow opening. This situation resembles the attraction of fern spermatozoids to eggs contained within archegonia, except that many of the attracting substances involved in hydroid sperm chemotaxis appear to act species-specifically (MILLER, 1966 b). None of the attracting substances involved in hydroid sperm chemotaxis has yet been chemically identified.

Analysis of the tracks of *Campanularia* spermatozoa obtained by frame by frame plotting of data from 16 mm motion pictures has demonstrated the chemotactic response of the spermatozoa to either female gonangia or capillary tubes containing extracts of female gonangia (MILLER, 1966 a). The records demonstrate that the chemotactic aggregation is the result of directed turning movements made by the spermatozoa, which make them swim towards the source of the chemical stimulus. Similar evidence has been accumulated for the chemotactic response of the spermatozoids of the bracken fern (ROTHSCHILD, 1952; BROKAW, 1958).

Although the chemotactic response of bracken fern spermatozoids can be defined precisely in terms of change in the direction of the axis of the helical path of the spermatozoid in response to a chemical or electrical gradient (BROKAW, 1958; 1959), there appears to be little hope of establishing the role of their flagella in causing changes in direction, since they have about 50 flagella arranged in a very complex array. Hydroid spermatozoa, on the other hand, present a much more favorable situation for analyzing the role of the flagellum in chemotactic response, since they are morphologically no more complex than, say, a sea urchin spermatozoon. We have, therefore, been attempting to take pictures which show the behavior of the flagellum of a hydroid spermatozoon while it is changing its direction of swimming in response to a chemotactic stimulus. Fig. 4 is an example of the progress we have made so far in this direction. We have photographed a considerable number of "turns" made by spermatozoa in the vicinity of the tips of pipettes filled with extracts of female gonangia. These consistently show altered patterns of flagellar beating of the type illustrated in Fig. 4, and it seems reasonable to conclude that this illustrates a change in flagellar bending pattern which is responsible for the change in the swimming direction of a spermatozoon when it responds to a chemotactic stimulus.

What we have not yet been able to establish is any quantitative relationship between the response of the flagellum and the stimulus to which it is exposed, nor are we able to state how the response of the sperm flagellum is controlled so as to ensure that the change in swimming direction of a spermatozoon will cause it to swim towards the source of chemical stimulation. Hopefully, further study will make it possible.

References

BROKAW C. J. (1958) – *Chemotaxis of bracken spermatozoids. Implications of electrochemical orientation.* « J. Exptl. Biol. », 35, 197–212.

BROKAW C. J. (1959) – *Random and oriented movements of bracken spermatozoids.* « J. Cell. Comp. Physiol. », 54, 95–101.

BROKAW C. J. (1965) – *Non-sinusoidal bending waves of sperm flagella.* « J. Exptl. Biol. », 43, 155–169.

BROKAW C. J. (1966) – *Effects of increased viscosity on the movements of some invertebrate spermatozoa.* « J. Exptl. Biol. », 45, 113–139.

BROKAW C. J. (1968) – *Mechanisms of sperm movement.* « Symp. Soc. Exptl. Biol. », 22, 101–116.

BROKAW C. J. and BENEDICT B. (1968 a) – *Mechanochemical coupling in flagella.* I *Movement dependent dephosphorylation of ATP by glycerinated spermatozoa.* « Arch. Biochem. Biophys. », 125, 770–778.

BROKAW C. J. and BENEDICT B. (1968 b) – *Mechanochemical coupling in flagella.* II. *Effects of viscosity and thiourea on metabolism and motility of* Ciona *spermatozoa.* « J. Gen. Physiol. », 52, 283–299.

BROKAW C. J. and WRIGHT L. (1963) – *Bending waves of the posterior flagellum of* Ceratium. « Science », 142, 1169–1170.

CARLSON F. D. (1959) – *The motile power of a swimming spermatozoon.* Proc. First Natl. Biophysics. Conf. (Quastler, H. and Morowitz, H. J., eds, Yale University Press) 443–449.

CLAYBROOK J. R. and NELSON L. (1968) – *Flagellar adenosine triphosphatase from sea urchin sperm: properties and relation to motility.* « Science », 162, 1134–1136.

GOLDSTEIN S. F. (1969) – *Irradiation of sperm tails by laser microbeam.* « J. Exptl. Biol. », 51, 431–441.

GRAY J. (1955) – *The movement of sea-urchin spermatozoa.* « J. Exptl. Biol. », 32, 775–801.

GRAY J. and HANCOCK G. J. (1955) – *The propulsion of sea urchin spermatozoa.* « J. Exptl. Biol. », 32, 802–814.

LEOPOLD L. B. and LANGBEIN W. B. (1966 a) – *River Meanders.* « Scientific American », 214, (6), 60–70.

LEOPOLD L. B. and LANGBEIN W. B. (1966 b) – *River meanders – Theory of minimum variance.* Geological Survey Professional Paper 422–H, U.S. Govt. Printing Office, Washington, D.C. 1–15.

MACHIN K. E. (1958) – *Wave propagation along flagella.* « J. Exptl. Biol. », 796–806.

MILLER R. L. (1966 a) – *Chemotaxis during fertilization in the hydroid* Campanularia. « J. Exptl. Zool. », 162, 23–44.

MILLER R. L. (1966 b) – *Chemotaxis during fertilization in the hydroids* Tubularia *and* Gonothyrea. « Amer. Zool. », 6, 509.

PFEFFER W. (1884) – *Locomotorische Richtungsbewegungen durch chemische Reize.* « Untersuch. Botanische. Inst. Tübingen », 1, 363–481.

ROTHSCHILD LORD (1952) – *The behavior of spermatozoa in the neighborhood of eggs.* « Internat. Rev. Cytol. », 1, 257–263.

STEVENS R. E., RENAUD F. L. and GIBBONS I. R. (1967) – *Guanine nucleotide associated with the outer fibers of flagella and cilia.* « Science », 156, 1606–1608.

VAN HERPEN G. and RIKMENSPOEL R. (1968) – *Search for a control center for sperm motility.* « Biophys. J. », 8, A 121.

YANAGISAWA T., HASEGAWA S. and MOHRI H. (1968) – *The bound nucleotides of the isolated microtubules of sea-urchin sperm flagella and their possible role in flagellar movement.* « Exptl. Cell Research », 52, 86–100.

EXPLANATION OF FIGURES 2–4

Fig. 2. – Multiple flash photomicrograph of a spermatozoon from the sea urchin, *Strongylocentrotus purpuratus.* The flash frequency was slightly greater than half the flagellar beat frequency, so that the photograph illustrates successive stages in propagation of bends along the flagellum, but in reversed sequence.
This photographs was obtained with a Zeiss 40× apochromat objective with iris diaphragm giving a total magnification of 190× on Kodak Tri–X film. The white scale bar is 25 microns in length. The flash illuminator was operating at about 1 watt-second per flash with a flash duration less than 50 microseconds, according to the manufacturers specifications.

Fig. 3. – Multiple flash photomicrograph of a laser irradiated sea urchin spermatozoon. The arrow points to the irradiated spot. The first flash occurred just before irradiation; subsequent flashes were at 20 msec intervals. (from GOLDSTEIN, 1969).

Fig. 4. – Multiple flash photomicrograph of a spermatozoon of the hydroid, *Campanularia calceolifera,* in the vicinity of a source of female gonangial extract (lower right corner). The flash frequency was approximately half of the flagellar beat frequency.

Discussion

BROWN. – Are there other cases of sperm attraction in the animal kingdom?

BROKAW. – There have been suggestions that chemotaxis may occur in other phyla, but as far as I know, conclusive evidence for animal sperm chemotaxis is only available for the hydroids.

KOEHLER. – Have you seen a chemotactic response with headless hydroid sperm?

BROKAW. – We have not tried to do this yet: it would be a very interesting experiment, but not an easy one.

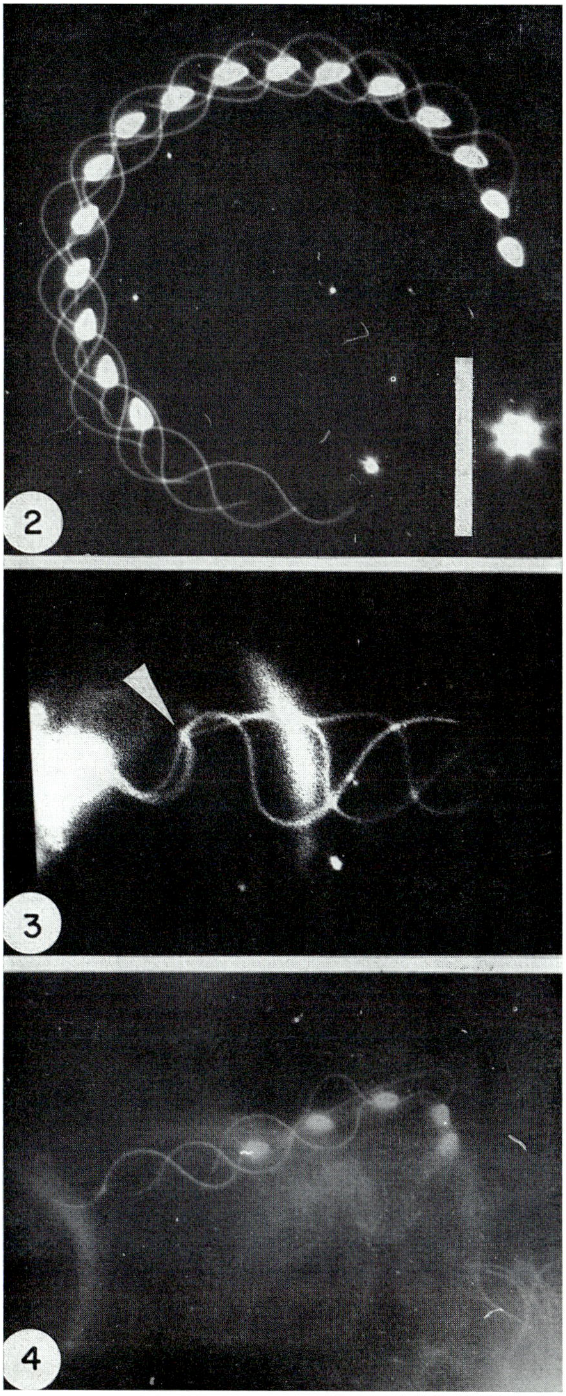
2
3
4

JEAN C. DAN (*)

THE ACROSOMAL PROCESS MEMBRANE

SUMMARY. — The often extensive synthesis of new membrane that occurs during the formation of the acrosomal process in some spermatozoa is the basis for the assumption that the intact mature acrosome must include a stock of membrane precursor substances. In echinoderm acrosomes, a conspicuous complex of stratified materials is interpreted as representing such precursors; in the *Mytilus* acrosome, the corresponding component is a portion of the acrosomal membrane which, however, appears somewhat thicker and more osmiophilic than the adjacent plasma membrane.

An investigation of acrosome formation in *Mytilus* and two starfishes (*Asterias, Asterina*) shows that in both cases one side of the proacrosome is distinguished by the gradual deposition of a layer of osmiophilic material. This differentiation begins early in spermatid development, while Golgi material is still being added to the proacrosome, and its location is apparently determined by the position of the Golgi cisternae.

In the starfishes, this material is incorporated into the process membrane precursor complex. In *Mytilus*, some of it appears to be utilized during the synthesis of new membrane to form the tubular invagination of the acrosomal vesicle. It is suggested that the osmiophilia characterizing the posterior part of the *Mytilus* acrosomal membrane may be due to lipid deposited here for use in further membrane synthesis when the acrosome reacts.

RIASSUNTO. — La sintesi di nuove membrane che avviene durante la formazione del processo acrosomiale in alcuni spermatozoi fa ritenere che l'acrosoma maturo includa una quantità di materiali precursori delle membrane. Nell'acrosoma degli echinodermi un cospicuo complesso di materiale stratificato viene interpretato come rappresentante di tali precursori; nell'acrosoma di *Mytilus*, il componente corrispondente è una porzione della membrana acrosomiale che, tuttavia, appare talvolta più spessa e più osmiofila della membrana plasmatica.

Un'indagine sulla formazione dell'acrosoma in *Mytilus* e in due stelle di mare (*Asterias, Asterina*) dimostra che in entrambi i casi da un lato del pro–acrosoma si deposita uno strato di materiale osmiofilo. Questa differenziazione comincia presto durante lo sviluppo degli spermatidi, mentre il complesso di Golgi è ancora aggiunto al proacrosoma, e la sua localizzazione è apparentemente determinata dalla posizione delle cisterne del Golgi.

Nelle stelle di mare, questo materiale è incorporato nel complesso precursore della membrana. In *Mytilus* un poco di questo materiale è utilizzato durante la sintesi di nuove membrane per formare l'invaginazione tubulare della vescicola acrosomiale. Si pensa che l'osmiofilia che caratterizza la parte posteriore della membrana acrosomiale del *Mytilus* sia dovuta a un deposito di lipidi che possono essere usati in ulteriori sintesi di membrane quando l'acrosoma reagisce.

The importance of the acrosomal process membrane is fully attested to by the observations of the COLWINS (1961 a, b, c; 1963 a, b; 1967), who have demonstrated that it is this part of the spermatozoon which unites with

(*) Department of Biology, Ochanomizu University, Tokyo and Department of Biology, Illinois Institute of Technology, Chicago U.S.A.

the egg plasma membrane. The confirmation of this finding by several investigators working with pelecypod molluscs (PASTEELS, 1965; NIIJIMA, 1963), sea urchins (FRANKLIN, 1965) and an echiuroid (TYLER, 1965) establishes the generality of such membrane fusion as the essential event in sperm entry, and emphasizes the necessity to know more about the conditions underlying it.

So far as can be learned from the observations cited above on the species in which the fine structure of the intact acrosome and its changes has been thoroughly investigated, the membrane forming the surface component of acrosomal processes is derived from the adnuclear part of the vesicle which is a prominent part of the acrosomal complex in *Hydroides*, *Saccoglossus*, *Barnea*, *Mytilus* and *Urechis*. The situation in the sea urchin and starfish is a partial exception to this rule in that a constant arrangement of stratified substances, with appearance and dimensions different from those of usual membranes, plays a comparable role in the spermatozoa of these animals.

The observation that such components give rise, during the acrosome reaction, to the membrane of the acrosomal proces, has led to the concept of « acrosomal process membrane precursors ». In view of the fact that acrosomal process formation in the species with a membrane-bounded acrosomal vesicle also involves a considerable increase in membrane area to cover the elongated process, it has seemed a valid exercise to regard the process-membrane-forming part of the acrosomal vesicle in the same way, and attempt to find in it special properties connected with its unusual capacity for expansion.

No high resolution studies have yet been performed to elucidate the fine structure of the membrane constituting the acrosomal vesicle. Since fusion takes place between the egg plasmalemma and the acrosomal process membrane, one is encouraged to assume, on the basis of the still unproved assumption that identity of structure is a prerequisite for membrane fusion, that the latter is a trilamellate membrane around 100 A in thickness. That only the tip of the process consists of such a membrane, if indeed it does, is suggested by published electron micrographs showing early stages of gamete fusion (e.g., FRANKLIN, 1965), in which the more basal part of the process membrane appears to be thicker than the adjacent egg plasmalemma. In any case, the possibility exists that at least the process membrane-forming portion of the acrosomal vesicle in the mature spermatozoon incorporates a supply of membrane precursor substances and to this extent departs from the ordinary concept of « cytomembrane ».

An effort has been started in our group to resolve the fine structure of the *Mytilus edulis* acrosomal membrane, in order to obtain direct evidence on this point. In the meantime, investigations of acrosome formation during spermiogenesis in *Mytilus* and two starfishes, *Asterias amurensis* and *Asterina pectinifera*, have added several new observations which are related to this problem.

Although the acrosomal processes formed by the spermatozoa of these two animal groups are basically similar, the changes leading to their formation are very different, as would be anticipated from the structural differences between the intact acrosomes. One of these differences depends on the fact that in *Mytilus* (Fig. 1 A), the process membrane precursor part of the acrosomal vesicle projects anteriorly, for about 1.5 μ, in the direction of future elongation, as a characteristically shaped invagination of the posterior side of the vesicle. In the starfish (Fig. 1 B), the comparable component is primarily a bowl-shaped complex of denser and less dense materials, with the further possibility that the central components also take part in forming part of the process membrane (DAN and HAGIWARA, 1967).

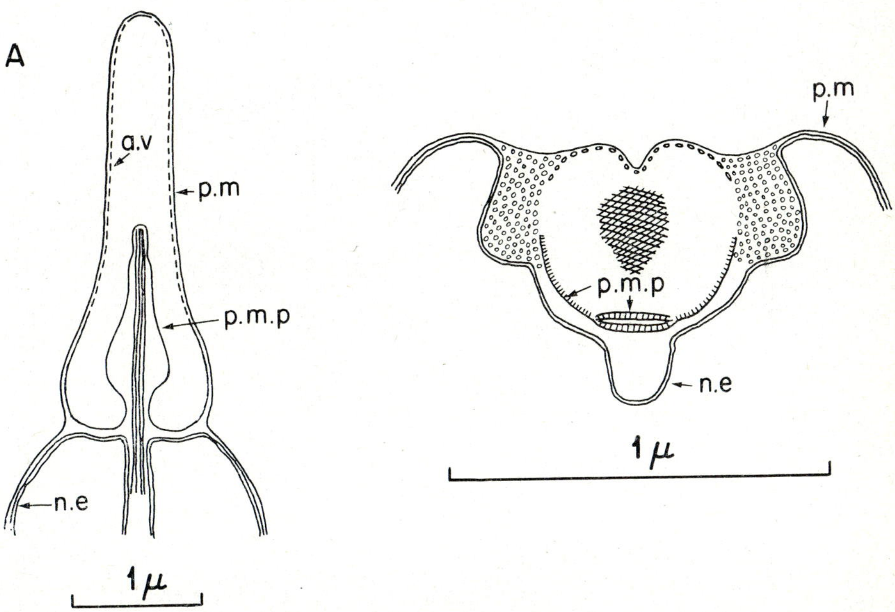

Fig. 1. – Diagrammatic representation of two types of acrosomal process membrane precursors. Axial sections of acrosomal region; some components not directly concerned with process membrane formation have been omitted.

A. *Mytilus edulis*. Broken line indicates portion of acrosomal vesicle which is removed during acrosome reaction. B. *Asterias amurensis*. a.v.: acrosomal vesicle membrane. n.e.: nuclear envelope. p.m.: plasma membrane. p.m.p.: process membrane precursor.

When the *Mytilus* spermatozoon reaches the egg covering, its acrosome reacts very rapidly (Fig. 2 A-E); the changes leading to the formation of the acrosomal process and the fusion of its membrane with the egg plasmalemma are completed within 2–3 seconds (NIIJIMA, 1963; NIIJIMA and DAN, 1965). These changes consist essentially in a local rupture of the plasma and acrosomal membranes at the tip of the acrosome and their fusion to each other (Fig. 2 A).

This membrane complex is immediately turned backward (Fig. 2, B, C), exposing the invaginated part of the acrosomal vesicle, which elongates, together with its axial rod, as the acrosomal process (Fig. 2 D). In fertilization, these changes take place close to the egg surface, so that an increase in length of only 1 to 2 μ is sufficient to bring the tip of the acrosomal process into contact with the egg plasma membrane (Fig. 2 E). When suspended spermatozoa are exposed to an excess of Ca'', however, the acrosome reaction is induced and the process formed in this case may be as long as 14 μ (Fig. 2 F).

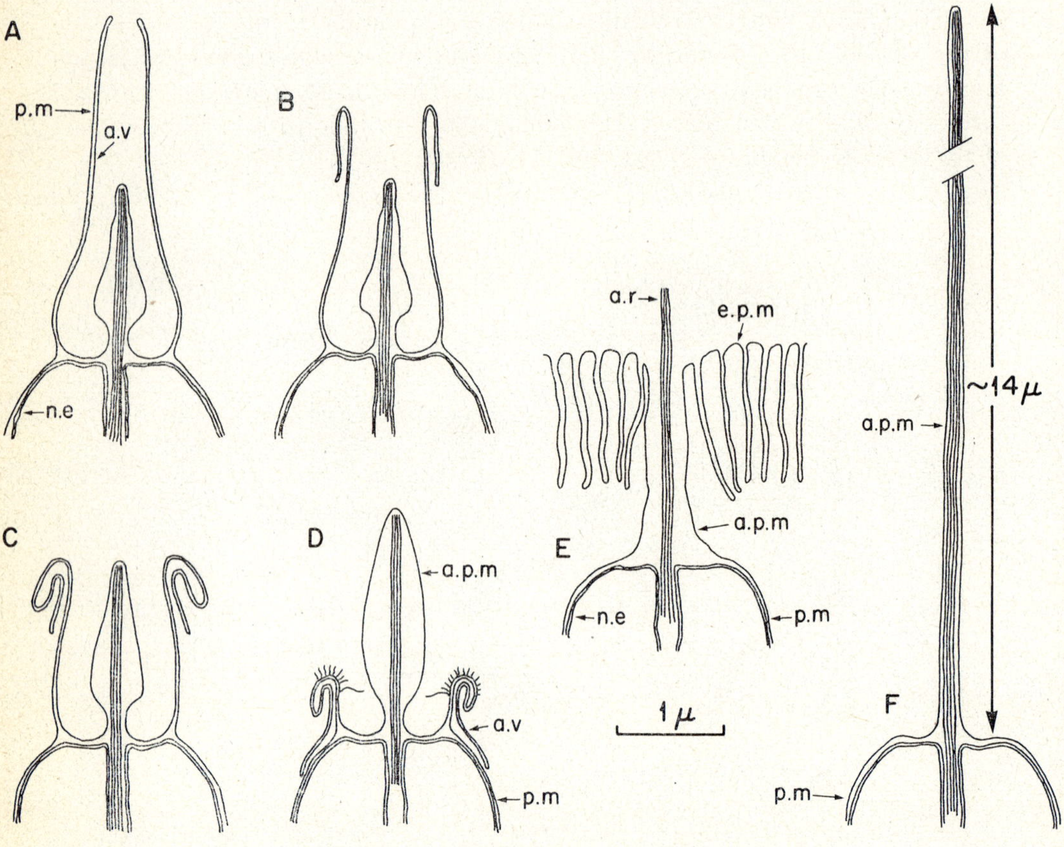

Fig. 2. – Course of acrosome reaction in *Mytilus edulis*.

A. Acrosomal and plasma membranes rupture and fuse at sperm apex. *B, C*. Successive stages in reflection of fused membranes; invaginated tubule exposed during first second of reaction. *D*. Beginning of acrosomal process elongation. *E*. After 2–3 seconds, acrosomal process membrane fused with egg plasma membrane. *F*. Long process formed by suspended spermatozoon treated with excess Ca''. *a.p.m.*: acrosomal process membrane. *a.r.*: axial rod. *a.v.*: acrosomal vesicle membrane. *e.p.m.*: egg plasma membrane. *n.e.*: nuclear envelope. *p.m.*: plasma membrane (of sperm).

The more complicated acrosomal reaction of starfish spermatozoa (DAN and HAGIWARA, 1967) can be induced by treating them with dissolved jelly-coat mucopolysaccharide. In samples fixed at 1 second (Fig. 3 A-C), it is found that the acrosome opens and the material at its center flows out over the anterior rim of the nucleus, exposing the bowl-shaped process membrane precursor complex (m1', m2'). The flat base of the bowl (m1') gives rise to the membrane of a slender blind tubule (m1), which elongates at least to the length shown in Figure 3 C within 1 second. What is interpreted as an extent of new membrane is deposited at the interface between the outflowing central material and the structures underlying it (Fig. 3 C); residual debris of this membrane formation can be seen for a few seconds before it disperses completely (Fig. 3 C, D, E).

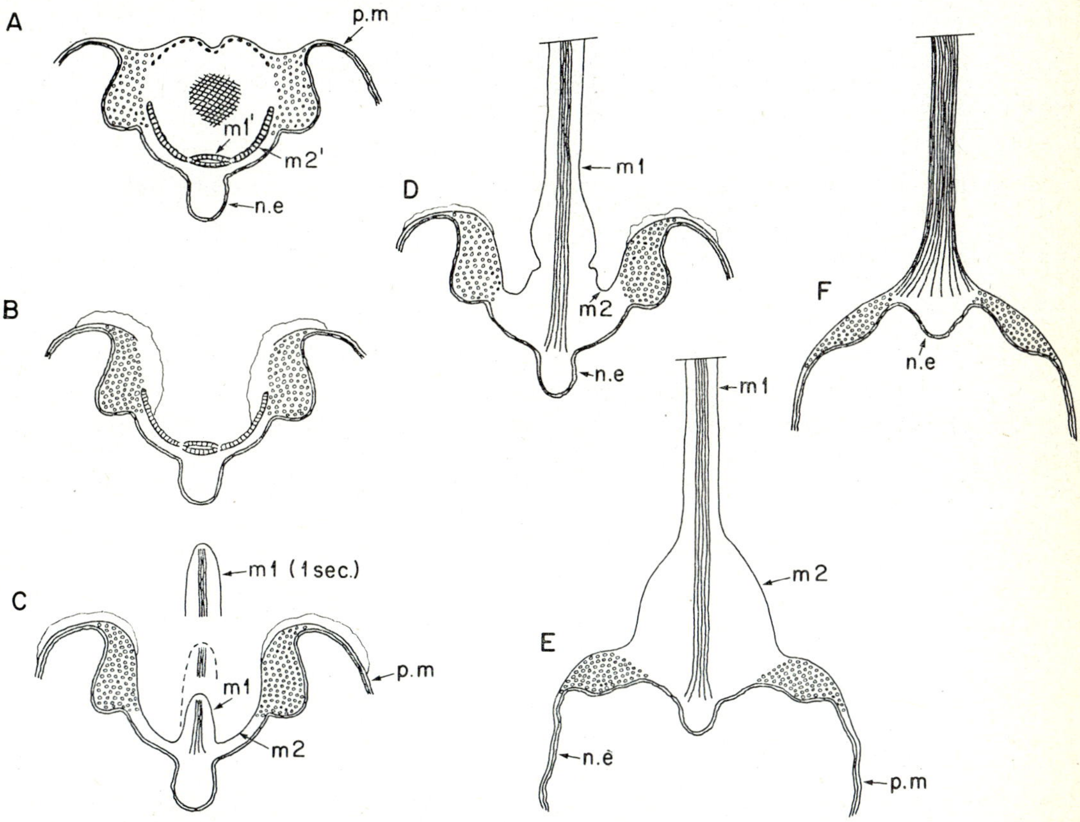

Fig. 3. – Course of acrosome reaction in *Asterias amurensis*.

A. Intact acrosome. *B*. Immediately after treatment with egg-jelly solution. Central component of acrosome flows out of acrosomal depression, exposing process membrane precursors (m1', m2'). *C*. Precursors give rise to process membrane (m1, m2). Blind tubule of early process ca. 1 μ long at 1 second. *D*. (4 sec.). m2 membrane drawn out of acrosomal depression. E. (ca. 6 sec.). Nucleus rounds up, obliterating acrosomal depression. *F*. (30–60 sec.). Base of fully formed acrosomal process. m1', m2': precursors of acrosomal process membrane. m1, m2: distal, proximal portions of process membrane. *n.e.*: nuclear envelope. *p.m.* plasma membrane.

By 4 seconds the process tubule is probably longer than 10 μ (Fig. 3 D, m1). Up to this time the adjoining component (m2) has remained in place, although it also has changed into a membrane similar to the tubule membrane with which it is continuous. After about 4 seconds (Fig. 3 D, m2), this component is drawn outwards to form part of the process membrane. The process continues to elongate; the time required for it to acquire its full length of ca. 25 μ is difficult to measure accurately, but the early observations of JUST (1929) and CHAMBERS (1930), that the fertilizing spermatozoon is connected (through the 20–25 μ-thick jelly coat) with the egg surface by 5 to 15 seconds after insemination, afford evidence that elongation proceeds steadily and rapidly to completion.

After this second membrane precursor component is drawn out of the acrosomal depression, the latter is obliterated by the rounding-up of the nucleus (Fig. 3 E, F). A certain amount of fluid included in the basal part of the process (Fig. 3 E) gradually diminishes, and by ca. 30 seconds after the beginning of these changes (Fig. 3 F), the process membrane closely invests a slender rod which forms in the axis of the tubule as it elongates, and connects laterally with the original plasma membrane. Such a comparison of the changes through which similar acrosomal processes are formed by two quite different types of acrosomes suggests that the diversity characterizing the acrosomes of various animals should be regarded as adaptive to the conditions set by the very different properties of the protective layers covering their respective eggs. If these two examples can for the moment be taken as representative of acrosomes which form a process as a preliminary to membrane fusion and transfer of the sperm nucleus into the egg, one observes a trend toward conformity in the structure of acrosomal processes, possibly reflecting the uniformity of egg plasmalemmas.

At the other end of this "life-history" of the acrosome, the studies which have been made of acrosome formation during spermiogenesis consistently show that the earliest stages in acrosomal development, from lower invertebrates to mammals, are so alike as to be virtually indistinguishable. A generalized account of the successive changes occurring in invertebrate acrosomes from their Golgi origin to their final role in fertilization thus presents a picture of a common starting point, followed by differentiation into widely diverse organelles in the mature spermatozoa of various animal groups. These different acrosomes in turn react to produce an acrosomal process, or processes, that may be long or short, with or without a rigid axial component, but is always covered by a membrane capable of uniting with the egg plasmalemma.

Even the most detailed studies of acrosomal process formation in animals representing several invertebrate phyla (Annelida: COLWIN and COLWIN, 1961 a, b, c; Enteropneusta: COLWIN and COLWIN, 1963 a, b; Mollusca: NIIJIMA and DAN, 1965 a, b; Echinodermata: DAN et al., 1964; DAN and HAGIWARA, 1967) have failed to afford much illumination as to the precise nature of the changes which occur in and between the acrosomal components to produce these structures. The rapidity of the changes and the fact that they occur in the absence of synthesizing organelles and even of cytoplasmic sap, however, strongly suggest the existence of precursor components within the acrosomal complex. In an effort to obtain some information as to the manner in which the various components are laid down in the developing acrosome, the course of spermiogenesis has been followed in *Mytilus edulis* and in two starfishes, *Asterias amurensis* and *Asterina pectinifera*. The following account will deal principally with those aspects of acrosome differentiation which concern the process membrane precursor components.

In osmium-fixed testes of *Mytilus edulis*, the proacrosomal material first appears in the early spermatid as numerous minute vesicles containing a product of Golgi synthetic activity (Fig. 4). These vesicles unite to form a single membrane-bounded mass of uniformly dense substance between 1 and 2 μ in diameter. Differentiation of this proacrosome begins with the appearance of a layer of osmiophilic material lining the inner surface of its membrane, at the side farthest from the Golgi cisternae (Fig. 5). This represents the earliest detectable stage in the development of the acrosomal process membrane precursor.

The diameter of the proacrosomal vesicle increases markedly in the next stage, and its contents segregate into a dense central, and a disperse peripheral, phase (Fig. 6). The proacrosome rotates, if necessary, as it approaches the nucleus, so that the extent of its membrane which is lined with the gradually thickening osmiophilic layer faces the nuclear envelope (Fig. 7). The apposing surfaces of both nucleus and acrosome flatten; a small accumulation of additional osmiophilic material (Fig. 8) marks the midpoint of the process membrane precursor. The dense mass near the center of the vesicle shifts away from its adnuclear side (Fig. 7), and the acrosome begins to elongate along the axis thus established (Fig. 9). As this occurs, strictly localized membrane-synthetic activity at the center of the process membrane precursor gives rise to a slender tubule of uniform diameter, which forms an invagination into the elongating vesicle. The layer of osmiophilic material covers the outer surface of this tubule, becoming less conspicuous as the tubule lengthens (Figs. 9, 10).

As the spermatid continues to differentiate, the tubule extends into the posterior part of the apically located mass of dense material, some of which apparently flows backwards along the wall of the tubule to fill the ring-shaped basal portion of the vesicle (Fig. 11). In the nearly mature spermatid (Fig. 12), the osmiophilic lining layer is no longer detectable, although the conspicuous appearance of the membrane constituting the invaginated tubule and the basal part of the acrosomal vesicle suggests that it may have incorporated some of this osmiophilic material. Its thickness and ultrastructure have not yet been precisely determined.

The first precursors of the starfish acrosome also appear as numerous small vesicles in the general neighborhood of the conspicuous Golgi complex (Figs. 13, 14). These unite to form a single mass of proacrosomal material (Fig. 15), which appears not to be completely membrane-bounded, since Golgi-derived vesicles enter it with their membranes intect (Fig. 16).

As this mass grows larger, it becomes increasingly lens-shaped (Figs. 15–17) and one of its faces acquires an inner layer of osmiophilic material. As in the *Mytilus* spermatid, this material accumulates at the side opposite to that from which the Golgi-derived vesicles join the acrosomal mass, and marks the side of the proacrosome which will face the nucleus and form the bowl-shaped complex of acrosome process membrane precursors.

Soon after polarization is established, several additional layers of osmiophilic material accumulate at the center of the membrane precursor complex to produce the flat base of the bowl which, as was described above, gives rise to the first-formed part of the acrosomal process membrane (Fig. 17). While this differentiation is taking place at the surface, the bulk of the proacrosomal substance segregates into peripheral and central components with mutually different texture and degree of osmiophily. In both genera, the central component is at first sparse and only moderately osmiophilic (Figs. 15, 17), but as soon as the proacrosome begins to condense, a strongly osmiophilic substance accumulates centrally in *Asterias* (Fig. 18), whereas in *Asterina* it remains dispersed even at a very late stage in spermiogenesis (Fig. 19).

As the acrosome becomes embedded in the nucleus (Figs. 18–20), its contents condense, its size diminishes and its general shape changes to hemispherical. A moderately dense material, which gives rise to the rigid supporting components of the acrosomal process at the time of reaction (DAN and HAGIWARA, 1967), is gradually deposited in a conspicuous zone between the nuclear envelope and membrane precursor complex (Figs. 18–21).

This comparison of the series of changes followed by the developing acrosome in two types of spermatids brings to light what seems to be an important aspect of this process; i.e., the leading role played by the part of the proacrosomal complex that is destined to form the acrosomal process membrane. In both *Mytilus* and the starfishes, there is sufficient evidence to show that this role is not determined by the spatial relation of the proacrosome to the nucleus; as described above, the available micrographs consistently show that the side the proacrosome farthest from the Golgi cisternae acquires this character. The osmiophilic material characteristic of this particular part of the proacrosome accumulates gradually during early spermiogenesis. In *Mytilus* it becomes apparent very early, even before the proacrosomal granule reaches its largest size, and while its contents otherwise form a uniform mixture. While the major components of the proacrosomal contents are undergoing various changes, the amount of this osmiophilic material slowly increases, to reach a maximum just before the formation of the tubular invagination. It is no longer detectable as a discrete layer in the mature acrosome, but the membrane forming the base of the acrosomal versicle appears thick and osmiophilic to an unusual degree. The available evidence supports the interpretation that this osmiophilic material represents a lipid, presumably a phospholipid, part of which is used to synthesize the new membrane making up the invaginated tubule, while the remainder is stored in or adjacent to the vesicle membrane around the base of the tubule. The presence of this stock of excess lipid would then constitute the chief detectable peculiarity of such a " membrane precursor ". Obviously, appropriate protein constituents must also be present, but the nature of these is unknown and their location cannot be determined by simple electron microscopy.

The situation observed in the starfish acrosome differs from this scheme in that no actual formation of new membrane comparable to the invaginated tubule of the *Mytilus* acrosome takes place during spermiogenesis. The various components of the mature starfish acrosome which are found to give rise to the distal, proximal and basal parts of the acrosomal process membrane are believed to represent fairly constant amounts of protein and lipid, stored in a metastable condition, which is maintained as long as the acrosome remains intact. On this basis, the changes leading to the formation of the acrosomal process, which begin within the first second after the plasma membrane is broken, would constitute the final steps in membrane synthesis resulting from the sudden availability of water and salt ions to react with, or catalyze reactions among, the precursor substances.

The considerable degree of condensation observed in the later stages of acrosomal development suggests that these precursor substances may be a condition to react vigorously with water. Whatever the nature of these changes is, any real understanding of them must be preceded by more specific information regarding the protein constituents of cellular membranes and the mechanisms controlling membrane synthesis in general.

REFERENCES

The electron micrographs shown as Figs. 4, 10 and 12 were made by F. SUZUKI; Figs. 5, 6, 7, 8, 9 and 11, by S. TUNA; and Figs. 13–21, by A. SIRAKAMI, of the Department of Biology, Ochanomizu University, Tokyo. This work was supported by grants in aid of research from the Japanese Ministry of Education.

CHAMBERS R. (1930) – *The manner of sperm entry in the starfish egg.* « Biol. Bull. », *58*, 344–369.

COLWIN A. L. and COLWIN L. H. (1961 a) – *Fine structure of the spermatozoon of* Hydroides hexagonus (*Annelida*), *with special reference to the acrosomal region.* « J. Biophys. Biochem. Cytol. », *10*, 211–230.

COLWIN L. H. and COLWIN A. L. (1961 b) – *Changes in the spermatozoon during fertilization in* Hydroides hexagonus (*Annelida*). I. *Passage of the acrosomal region through the vitelline membrane.* « J. Biophys. Biochem. Cytol. », *10*, 231–254.

COLWIN A. L. and COLWIN L. H. (1961 c) – *Changes in the spermatozoon during fertilization in* Hydroides hexagonus (*Annelida*). II. *Incorporation with the egg.* « J. Biophys. Biochem. Cytol. », *10*, 255–274.

COLWIN A. L. and COLWIN L. H. (1963 a) – *Role of the gamete membranes in fertilization in* Saccoglossus kowalevskii (*Enteropneusta*). I. *The acrosomal region and its changes in early stages of fertilization.* « J. Cell Biol. », *19*, 477–500.

COLWIN L. H. and COLWIN A. L. (1963 b) – *Role of the gamete membranes in fertilization in* Saccoglossus kowalevskii (*Enteropneusta*). II. *Zygote formation by membrane fusion.* « J. Cell Biol. », *19*, 501–518.

COLWIN A. L. and COLWIN L. H. (1967) – *Behavior of the spermatozoon during sperm-blastomere fusion and its significance for fertilization* (Saccoglossus kowalevskii: *Hemichordata*). « Ztschr. Zellforsch. », *78*, 208–220.

DAN J. and HAGIWARA Y. (1967) – *Studies on the acrosome.* IX. *Course of acrosome reaction in the starfish.* « J. Ultrastruct. Res. », *18*, 562–579.

DAN J., OHORI Y. and KUSHIDA K. (1964) – *Studies on the acrosome.* VII. *Formation of the acrosomal process in sea urchin spermatozoa.* « J. Ultrastruct. Res. », *11*, 508–524.

FRANKLIN L. E. (1965) – *Morphology of gamete membrane fusion and of sperm entry into oocytes of the sea urchin.* « J. Cell Biol. », No. 2 Pt. 2, 81–100.

JUST E. E. (1929) – *The production of filaments by echinoderm ova as a response to insemination, with special reference to the phenomenon as exhibited by ova of the genus Asterias.* « Biol. Bull. », *57*, 311–325.

NIIJIMA L. (1963) – *Acrosome reaction and sperm entry in* Mytilus edulis. « Bull. Marine Biol. Station Asamushi », *11*, 217–221.

NIIJIMA L. and DAN J. (1965) – *The acrosome reaction in* Mytilus edulis. II. *Stages in the reaction, observed in supernumerary and calcium-treated spermatozoa.* « J. Cell Biol. », *25*, 249–259.

PASTEELS J. J. (1965) – *Aspects structuraux de la fécondation vus au microscope électronique.* « Arch. Biol. (Liège) », *76*, 463–509.

TYLER A. (1965) – *The biology and chemistry of fertilization.* « Amer. Nat. », *99*, 309–334.

EXPLANATION OF FIGURES 4–21

Fig. 4. – Golgi regions of 2 early *Mytilus* spermatids, showing dark proacrosomal granule and small Golgi-derived vesicles in lower cell, Golgi cisternae and vesicles in upper cell. ×15,000.

Fig. 5. – Early *Mytilus* spermatid; proacrosome with layer of osmiophilic material lining side farthest from Golgi cisternae. ×30,000.

Fig. 6. – *Mytilus* spermatid; contents of proacrosome segregating into dense and sparse phases as it approaches nucleus. ×30,000.

Fig. 7. – Dense material has moved to apical side of acrosomal vesicle, which is now close to nuclear membrane. ×32,000.

Fig. 8. – Detail of Mytilus acrosomal process membrane precursor. ×50,000.

Fig. 9. – Beginning of acrosomal elongation and formation of invaginated tubule. ×30,000.

Fig. 10. – Tubular invagination becomes longer; substances within vesicle segregating. Osmiophilic material lines adnuclear side of acrosome and outer wall of tubule. ×45,000.

Fig. 11. – Diagonal section through somewhat more mature acrosome; some of apical dense material moving to basal ring. ×20,000.

Fig. 12. – Acrosome of nearly mature *Mytilus* spermatozoon. Osmiophilic lining layer no longer detectable; conspicuous osmiophilia associated with part of acrosomal membrane. ×30,000.

Fig. 13. – Golgi complex of early *Asterina* spermatid, including fairly large and very small vesicles containing proacrosomal material. ×30,000.

Fig. 14. – Golgi region of 2 *Asterias* spermatids; proacrosomal material in vesicles. ×30,000.

Fig. 15. – *Asterina* spermatid. Larger Golgi vesicles fused to form one proacrosomal mass more than 1 μ in diameter. Small Golgi vesicles joining mass; first appearance of osmiophilic layer at side farthest from Golgi cisternae. ×30,000.

Fig. 16. – *Asterias* spermatid at same stage as above. Note small membrane-bounded vesicles within proacrosomal mass. ×30,000.

Fig. 17. – *Asterias* spermatid. Proacrosome lens-shaped, bounded on one face by an increasingly conspicuous osmiophilic layer, with differentiation of process membrane precursor at its center; further segregation of central constituents. ×30,000.

Fig. 18. – *Asterias* spermatid. Acrosome becoming embedded in nucleus. Osmiophilic material accumulating at center, very small vesicles prominent at apical side. Material of moderate density being deposited at outer side of process membrane precursor. ×30,000.

Fig. 19. – Late *Asterina* spermatid. Note that osmiophilic constituent of central component is still associated with peripheral material. ×30,000.

Fig. 20. – Late *Asterias* spermatid. Osmiophilic material increasingly accumulated in center and in process membrane precursors. ×30,000.

Fig. 21. – Very late *Asterias* spermatid. Note especially deposition of osmiophilic material in process membrane precursor complex, and large amount of rigid component precursor material adjacent to nuclear envelope. ×50,000.

Discussion

NELSON. – Does the calcium content of the sea water affect the acrosome reaction? It appears that the formation of the acrosome filament membrane does not require any simultaneous protein synthesis. Instead this may be an almost instantaneous physical reorientation of Ca-protein-phospholipid molecules at the acrosome-sea water interface resembling the famous, historical " surface precipitation reaction ". The necessary protein synthetic reactions probably have occurred during the differentiation of the acrosomal process.

DAN. – Devising an adequate way of testing this point is difficult because no acrosome reaction occurs in the absence of calcium. Offhand, I would expect the " famous surface precipitation reaction " to require the presence of a certain amount of " cytoplasm " – i.e., cell sap containing the necessary components to combine with calcium from the sea water. Since there is no such cytoplasm in the vicinity of the acrosomes we have studied, we have resorted to the idea of appropriately located " precursor materials ", which may very well pick up calcium ion in the course of becoming reoriented to form the process membrane.

NICANDER. – Studies just made by DR. BEDFORD and me have shown changes in the fine structure of the acrosome membrane during spermiogenesis in mammals, and an asymmetry in the fine structure of this membrane in mature spermatozoa. A passerine bird, *Cashanatis taeniopupge*, has an acrosome membrane much thicker than the plasma membrane.

BACCETTI. – I would ask you to summarize the actual knowledge on the enzymes demonstrated in the different parts of the acrosome.

DAN. – In mammalian spermatozoa, the acrosomal vesicle is known to contain hyaluronidase.

In the case of invertebrates, the Colwins believe that the lytic substance which they extracted from *Hydroides* spermatozoa, and which has properties appropriate for an enzyme, is located in the central part of the acrosomal vesicle.

In *Mytilus edulis*, the work of Wada et al. (1956) and of Niijima & Dan (1965) indicates that material located apically and in a ring at the base of the acrosome represents the enzymatic vitelline coat lysin which is recovered from the supernatant of sperm suspensions after induced acrosome reaction.

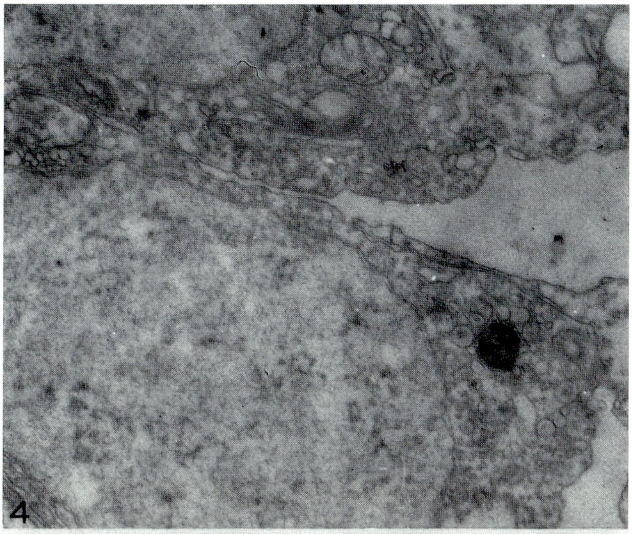

4

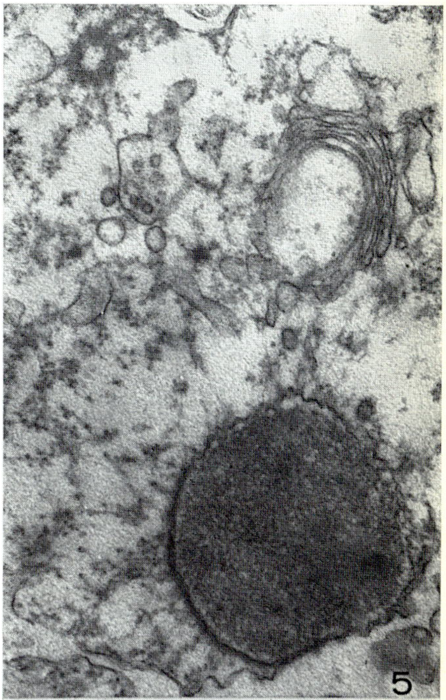

5

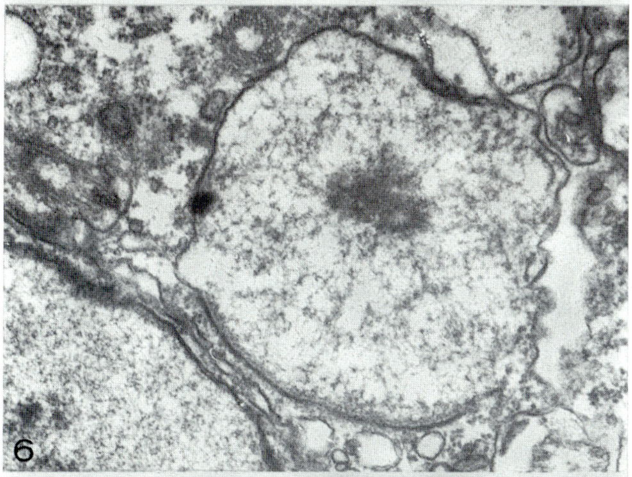

6

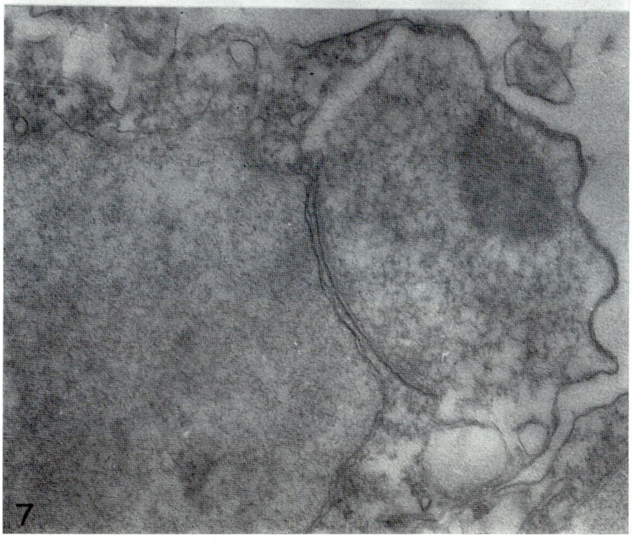

7

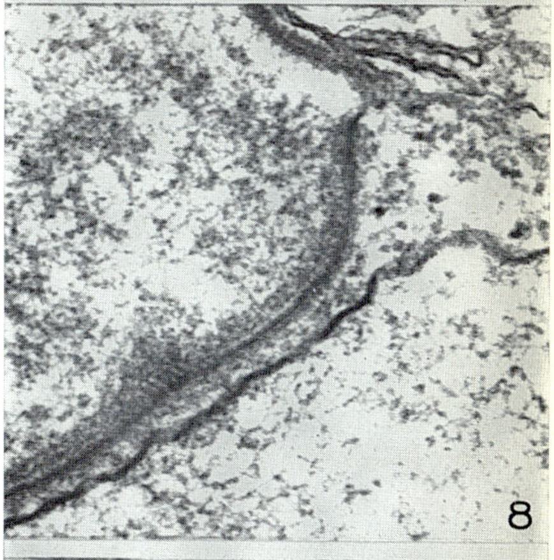

8

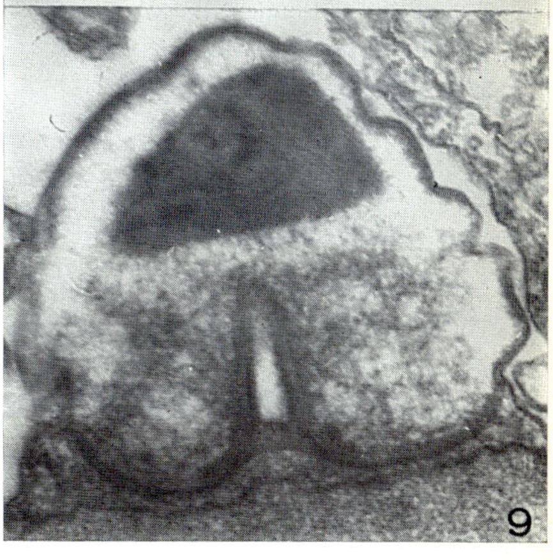

9

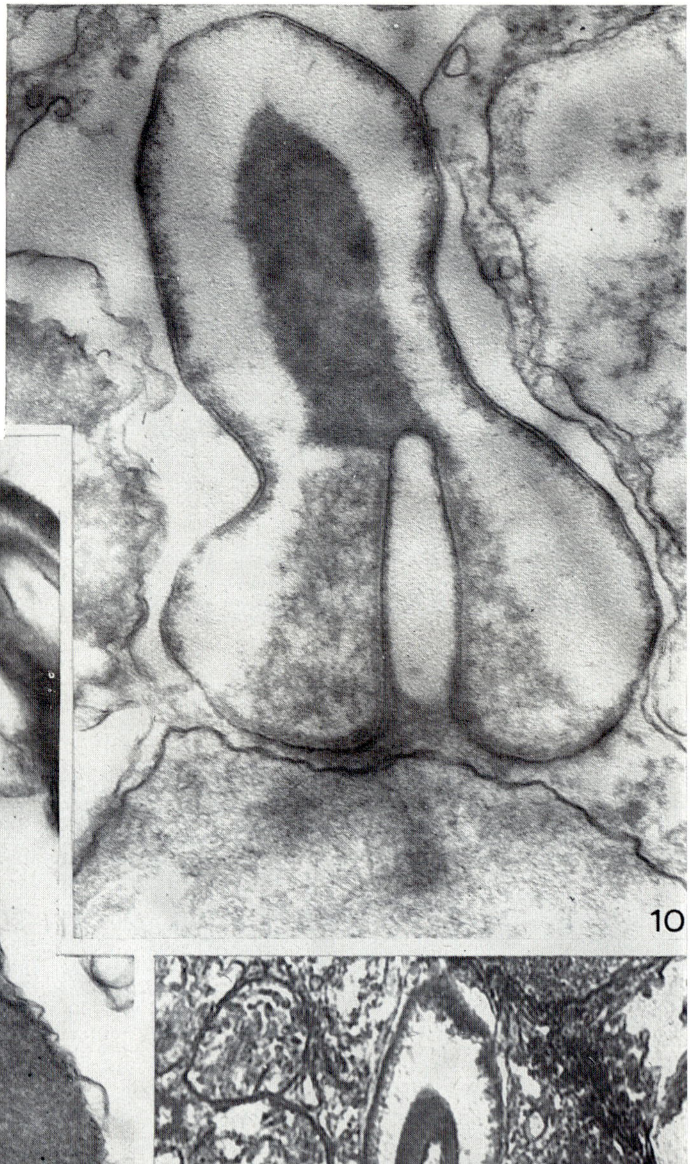

10

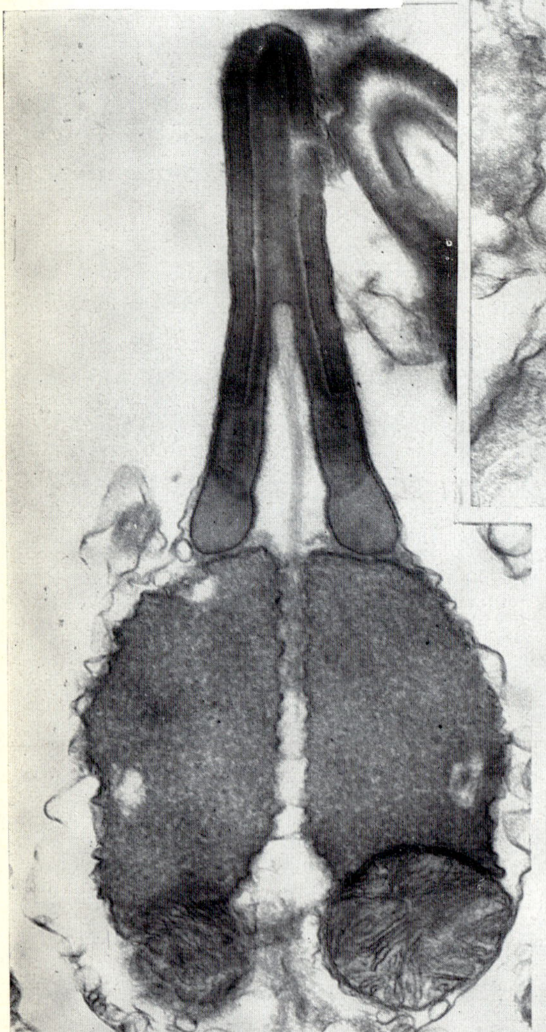

12

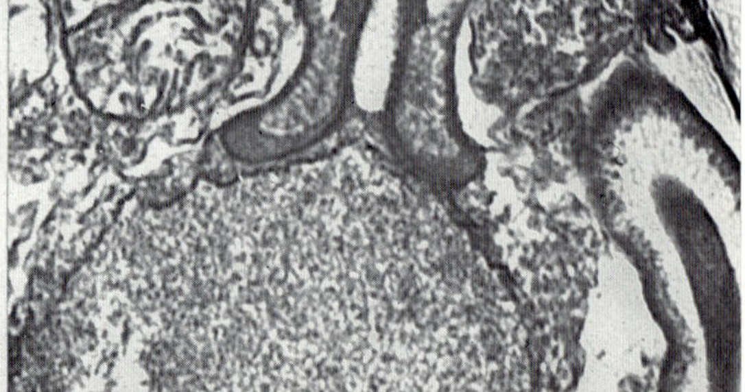

11

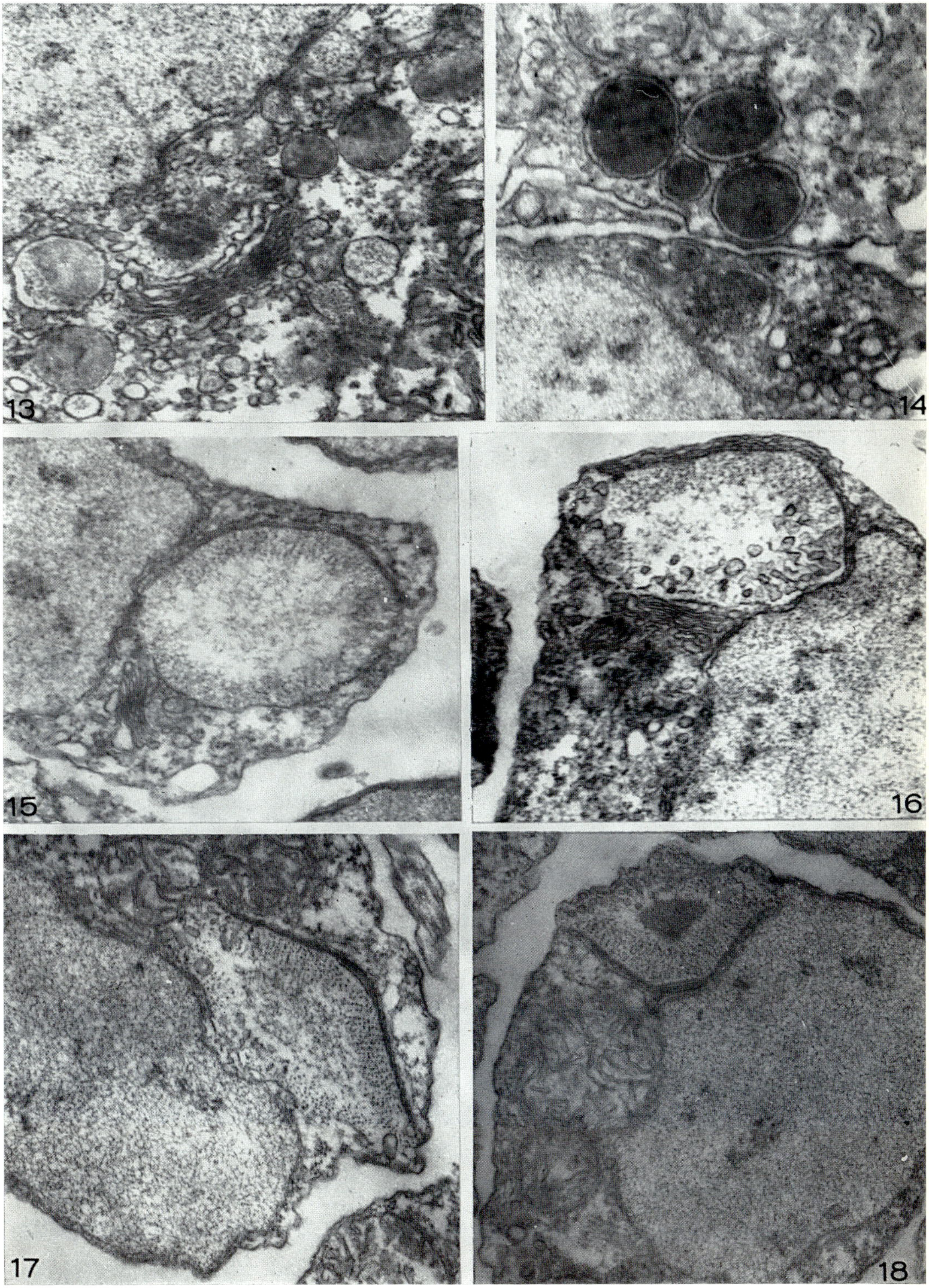
13
14
15
16
17
18

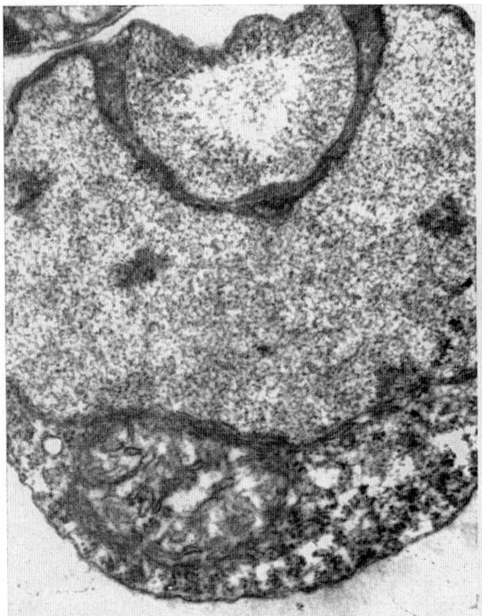

19

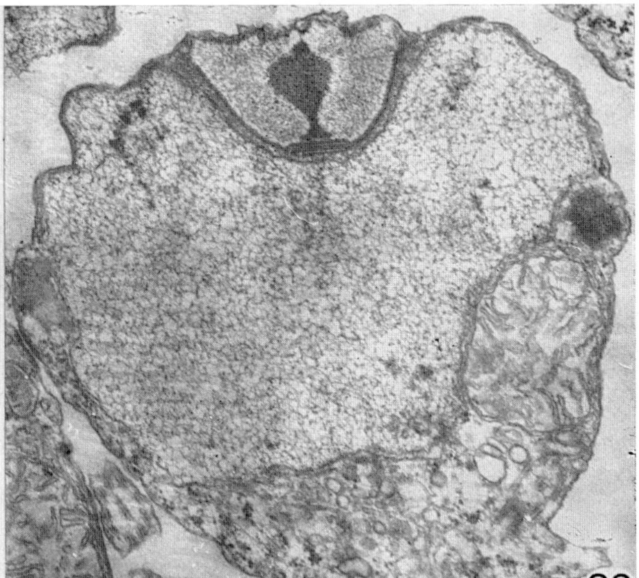

20

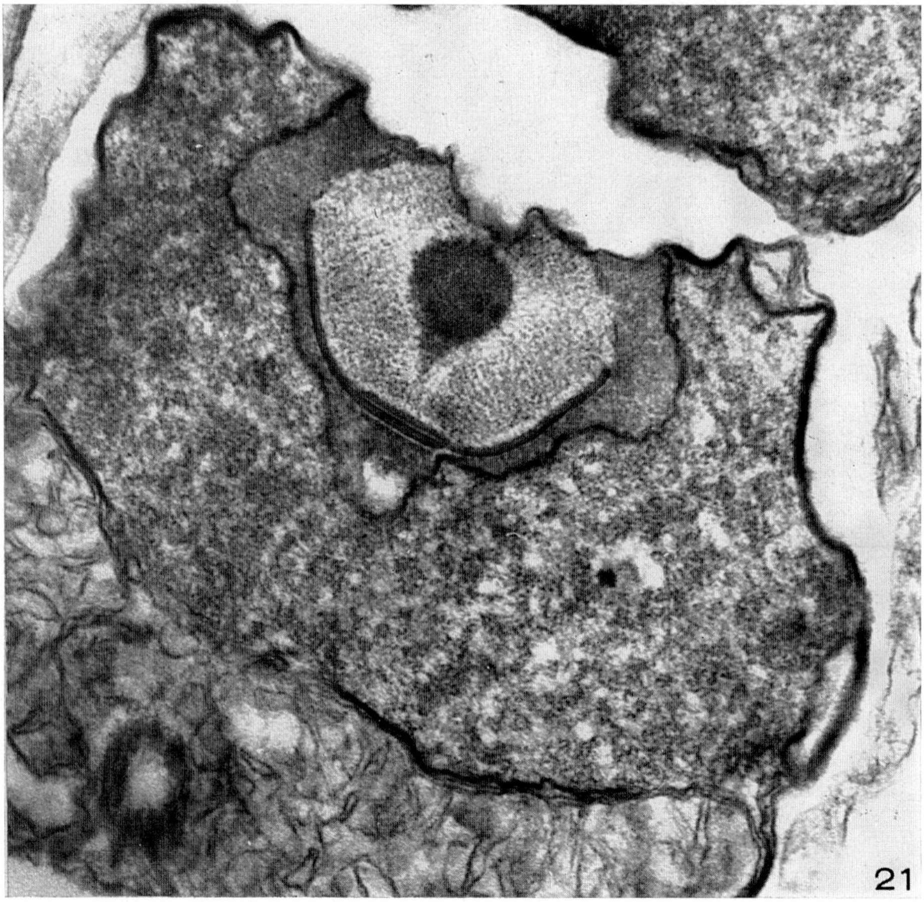

21

P. Chevaillier (*)

LE NOYAU DU SPERMATOZOÏDE ET SON ÉVOLUTION AU COURS DE LA SPERMIOGENÈSE

Summary. — A brief review concerning structural, chemical, physical and molecular aspects of mature sperm nucleus organization is presented. Some of the properties of these highly specialized cells appearing during spermiogenesis are discussed. Anomalous characters of sperm nuclei in some species are quoted. Numerous problems remain unsolved and need re-investigation.

Riassunto. — Viene presentata una breve indagine sugli aspetti strutturali, fisici, chimici e molecolari dell'organizzazione nucleare dello spermatozoo maturo. Sono discusse alcune proprietà di questa cellula altamente specializzata che compaiono durante la spermiogenesi. Vengono citati caratteri anomali dei nuclei degli spermatozoi in alcune specie. Numerosi problemi rimangono insoluti e necessitano di un'ulteriore indagine.

Les communications présentées au cours des séances qui ont précédé celle-ci nous ont appris que le spermatozoïde mûr était une cellule hautement spécialisée dans laquelle les différents organites cytoplasmiques - appareil de Golgi, mitochondries, centrioles - sont différenciés en systèmes parfois complexes et toujours originaux. Ces particularités structurales et leur acquisition ont donné lieu à de nombreux travaux et les plus récents nous ont été présentés ces jours-ci. Par contre, l'étude du noyau du spermatozoïde paraît actuellement susciter moins de travaux, sans doute en raison de son apparente homogénéité de structure et de la répétition au cours de la spermiogenèse, dans la majorité des espèces étudiées, de phénomènes similaires. Nous pensons néanmoins que le noyau du spermatozoïde pose en raison de sa structure particulière et de son inertie métabolique de nombreux problèmes qui sont loin d'être résolus.

Nous essaierons de dégager dans cette brève revue l'originalité de structure et de composition chimique du noyau du spermatozoïde, de noter au passage des exemples qui s'écartent du schéma-type, et d'évoquer les phénomènes affectant le noyau lors de la spermiogenèse.

Caractères généraux

Le noyau du spermatozoïde apparaît généralement comme une masse dense, de forme régulière, allongée ou compacte, située en arrière de l'acrosome et en avant de la pièce intermédiaire. Il renferme un génôme haploïde,

(*) Laboratoire de Biologie Cellulaire, Faculté des Sciences, Rennes, France.

c'est-à-dire l'équivalent de *n* chromosomes. Il est classique d'ajouter que le patrimoine génétique de l'espèce est protégé par des protéines plus basiques que celles qui existent dans les noyaux somatiques.

En fait, chacun des caractères que nous venons de définir souffre de nombreuses exceptions dont nous verrons des exemples au cours de cet exposé: anomalies de forme, de structure, de position, et anomalies de composition chimique tant du point de vue qualitatif que du point de vue quantitatif.

Dans la majorité des espèces, il n'existe qu'un seul type nucléaire caractéristique de l'espèce. En fait, il n'en est pas toujours ainsi. Par exemple, chez un Hyménoptère du genre *Dahlbominus*, il existe des têtes nucléaires à enroulement hélicoïdal dextre, d'autres à enroulement sénestre [LEE et WILKES (1965); WILKES et LEE (1965)].

Dans d'autres cas, le dimorphisme nucléaire peut être beaucoup plus accusé et puisque nous parlons du noyau du spermatozoïde, disons quelques mots de ceux qui n'en ont pas ou en ont peu. C'est le cas chez certains Mollusques. Par exemple, dans le genre *Conus*, il existe une lignée de spermatozoïdes dont le noyau subit une évolution normale avec condensation et élongation du noyau; il en existe une seconde, dite atypique, dont le noyau se vacuolise et dont la chromatine finit par disparaître laissant une vésicule vide: cette seconde lignée donne naissance aux spermatozoïdes apyrènes. Dans une autre espèce, chez *Cerithium*, il existe également une double spermatogenèse, l'une normale qui aboutit à la formation de spermatozoïdes eupyrènes à noyau ovoïde, l'autre, atypique, qui donne naissance à des spermatozoïdes oligopyrènes à noyau punctiforme (TUZET, 1930).

CARACTÈRES PHYSIQUES

Ils ont été définis aussi bien par les méthodes de la biophysique que par les méthodes microscopiques.

WILKINS *et coll.* (1953, 1956) en obtenant des diagrammes de diffraction aux rayons X démontrent que le matériel intra-nucléaire a un agencement tridimensionnel périodique caractéristique d'une structure cristalline. Les diagrammes obtenus à partir des tête entières de certains spermatozoïdes (*Sepia*, *Loligo*) peuvent être rapprochés de ceux obtenus avec des fibres de DNA. Pour WILKINS, ces diagrammes peuvent êtres interprètés de la façon suivante: le matériel intra-nucléaire est constitué de molécules de DNA en double hélice orientées de façon presque – mais pas exactement – parallèles entre elles. Ce type d'organisation n'est cependant pas général. Par exemple, chez la Truite, les diagrammes obtenus ressemblent aux précédents, mais chaque arc est devenu un anneau complet; pour WILKINS, ceci correspond à une orientation au hasard des chaînes nucléoprotéiques. Dans tous ces cas, les protéines associées au DNA sont des protéines simples mais très basiques, les protamines, et WILKINS les situe dans la petite gorge du DNA. Dans d'autres cas, chez l'Oursin par exemple, les diagrammes obtenus sont bien différents des précédents et sont identiques à ceux des nucléoprotéines somatiques.

Les méthodes physiques d'étude de la cellule à l'aide du microscope ont permis de compléter ces données et d'obtenir des renseignements précieux sur l'organisation du matériel intra-nucléaire dans le spermatozoïde.

En premier lieu, il faut signaler la très grande densité du matériel intranucléaire dont la masse sèche, évaluée par microinterférométrie, a été estimée (MELLORS *et coll.*, 1954, 1955) à 440 mg/ml, concentration comparable à celle qui existe dans les chromosomes mitotiques.

Une autre propriété liée à l'organisation du matériel intra-nucléaire et qui peut être étudiée au microscope est la biréfringence. Chez certaines espèces, l'observation au microscope à lumière polarisée permet de démontrer l'anisotropie du noyau. Dans ces cas, cette anisotropie n'est acquise que progressivement au cours de la spermiogenèse: les premiers stades ont des noyaux isotropes alors que le spermatozoïde montre une biréfringence très marquée. A l'aide d'un microscope polarisant très perfectionné, INOUÉ et SATO (1962, 1966) ont pu étudier de façon précise la distribution de la biréfringence le long du noyau du spermatozoïde. Ils mettent ainsi en évidence un arrangement hélicoïdal des régions biréfringentes, qui se répartissent en microdomaines dans lesquels les axes cristallins ne sont pas parallèles à l'axe longitudinal mais inclinés par rapport à lui. L'arrangement cristallin ainsi observé est détruit par une irradiation par les UV polarisés à 45° par rapport à l'axe nucléaire. De toutes ces données, INOUÉ et SATO ont proposé une série de modèles dont celui-ci a leur préférence: le matériel intra-nucléaire se trouve organisé en 2 super-hélices de 8000 Å de diamètre, chacune résultant de l'enroulement hélicoïdal d'une hélice de 1500 Å de diamètre, elle-même formée par des faisceaux de molécules de DNA de 200 Å de diamètre.

Ceci n'est pas sans rappeler le schéma de ZUBAY (1964) relatif à la structure des nucléohistones, et à la constitution de super-hélices imposées aux molécules de DNA par des ponts d'histones.

Il faut noter cependant que MC INNES et URETZ (1968), analysant chez 8 espèces d'Orthoptères – parmi lesquelles celle étudiée par INOUÉ et SATO – la polarisation de la fluorescence émise par des noyaux de spermatozoïdes traités par l'orangé d'acridine, arrivent à des conclusions totalement différentes: d'après leurs résultats, le DNA est disposé parallèlement au grand axe du spermatozoïde et, contrairement aux observations de INOUÉ et SATO, ne forme pas de super-hélices.

Les observations de INOUÉ et SATO suggèrent néanmoins la présence de ruptures tout le long de la super-hélice qui pourraient correspondre à des extrémités de chromosomes qui seraient disposés bout à bout. Un tel arrangement en tandem des chromosomes dans le noyau, au moins chez certaines espèces, repose sur un petit nombre de données. HUGHES-SCHRADER (1946, 1955) suit l'évolution nucléaire chez certains Coccides dont le nombre haploïde est 2. Dans la jeune spermatide apparaît une petite papille nucléaire qui repousse le cytoplasme puis la membrane cellulaire. Ce diverticule s'allonge et les 2 chromosomes y pénètrent successivement dans un ordre constant.

Un autre exemple d'arrangement en tandem nous est fourni dans le travail de DOUGLAS (1965); dans les noyaux de spermatides âgées de Hamster traités par une solution hypotonique renfermant de l'EDTA, on révèle des éléments chromosomiques disposés les uns à la suite des autres et le plus souvent en nombre correspondant au nombre haploïde de l'espèce.

Citons également les observations de TAYLOR (1964), sur un Orthoptère *Romalea microptera*, qui a utilisé la thymidine comme marqueur de la chromatine. Le marquage se fait selon 3 modalités: 1/. les spermatozoïdes sont marqués sur toute leur longueur; 2/. il existe une zone non marquée alors que tout le reste du noyau l'est; 3/. une 3e catégorie est constituée de spermatozoïdes marqués seulement sur un court segment. Ce segment à comportement particulier correspond probablement au chromosome X dont la réplication est décalée dans le temps par rapport à celle des autosomes. Ces résultats suggèrent que le chromosome X et probablement tous les autres chromosomes sont disposés bout à bout en une file tout au long du noyau.

Un autre exemple d'arrangement linéaire des chromosomes a été signalé dans le règne végétal chez une Hépatique du genre *Shaerocarpus* (REITBERGER, 1964).

Il est bien évident qu'une telle organisation nucléaire ne peut se concevoir que pour des espèces ayant un noyau fortement allongé et à anisotropie marquée. Dans les autres cas, les chromosomes doivent être, ou bien repliés sur eux–mêmes, ou bien disposés côte à côte. Dans les noyaux isotropes, l'orientation du matériel intra–nucléaire est quelconque.

CARACTÈRES STRUCTURAUX

En microscopie électronique, le noyau apparaît généralement très dense aux électrons, finement ou grossièrement fibrillaire ou granulaire ou encore totalement homogène. De nombreux exemples de ces types structuraux existent dans la littérature. Nous n'y reviendrons pas.

L'évolution structurale de la chromatine au cours de la spermiogenèse a été suivie chez de nombreuses espèces. Nous prendrons comme référence l'évolution nucléaire de *Philaenus spumarius* (Fig. 1–7). La spermatide jeune a un noyau homogène peu dense, finement fibrillaire; la distinction entre régions eu – et hétérochromatiques a disparu. Alors que le noyau continue son élongation, le noyau devient plus hétérogène; le matériel intra–nucléaire se condense en fibres moins nombreuses de diamètre plus important. La condensation commence ou bien à la périphérie ou bien au centre du noyau. De plus, dans certains cas, la condensation ne se fait pas de façon régulière pour l'ensemble du noyau, certaines régions semblant en avance dans leur condensation sur d'autres et ne suivant pas les mêmes étapes au cours de leur évolution. L'orientation des fibres de chromatine est longitudinale. Les fibres dont le diamètre continue à augmenter forment des lames par rapprochement de fibres qui perdent ensuite leur individualité. Les lamelles d'abord isolées confluent pour former un réseau de plus en plus serré où le nucléoplasme devient de plus en plus réduit. Finalement, le noyau est dense et homogène.

Les aspects observés varient suivant les espèces. Chez certaines espèces, des figures très régulières s'observent au cours de la spermiogenèse et une disposition en nid d'abeille est parfois obtenue (YASUZUMI et ISHIDA, 1957). RIS (1962) a signalé la formation dans la spermatide âgée de fibres de nucléoprotamines de 40 Å à partir des fibres de nucléohistones de 100 Å de la jeune spermatide.

En fait, même dans le cas où le noyau parait homogène, cette uniformité de structure n'est qu'apparente et l'on peut démontrer qu'en réalité il n'en est pas ainsi. Par exemple, KOEHLER (1966), par la technique du « freeze-etching », a révélé l'existence dans le noyau du spermatozoïde de taureau de structures lamellaires empilées, à peu près parallèles entre elles et à orientation longitudinale. D'autre part, en rompant les membranes entourant le noyau et en étalant le matériel ainsi dispersé, LUNG (1968) observe des fibrilles de 140 à 200 Å de diamètre formant un réseau qui doit être très dense dans le noyau intact.

Il existe des exceptions à l'uniformité de structure du noyau. Par exemple, chez un Chilopode du genre *Geophilus*, HORSTMANN (1968) note une dualité de structure du noyau, dont la partie centrale est fibrillaire alors que la partie périphérique disposée en hélice par rapport à la précédente est granulaire. Cette partie centrale est constituée de fibres parallèles entre elles à orientation longitudinale. Une structure nucléaire particulièrement hétérogène a été également signalée chez certains Homoptères du groupe des Psylles (LE MENN, 1966) où la chromatine caractérisée par le DNA qu'elle contient s'individualise du reste du noyau.

La persistence de structures lamellaires à orientation longitudinale s'observe dans les spermatozoïdes mûrs de Thysanoures où ces lamelles sont organisées de façon régulière (BAWA, 1964). Des systèmes lamellaires subsistent également dans le noyau de Tiques, comme l'ont montré BREUCKER et HORSTMANN (1968). Dans ce cas, les lamelles sont réparties de façon irrégulière dans la chromatine.

Chez certains Urodèles, il existe parallèlement au noyau proprement dit une côte nucléaire longitudinale à structure alvéolaire, alors que la zone chromatinienne est dense et homogène (PICHERAL, 1966, 1967). Nous aurons l'occasion de revenir sur sa structure et sa composition.

Les profondes modifications de structure du matériel intra-nucléaire s'accompagnent également de remaniements au niveau de la membrane nucléaire. Dans certains cas, par exemple chez les Annélides (ANDERSON et coll., 1967; POTSWALD, 1967), chez certains Insectes (BACCETTI et coll., 1969; WERNER, 1965) et chez certains Mammifères (ANDRÉ, 1963; FRANKLIN, 1968), on observe la formation au cours de la spermiogenèse de vastes poches limitées par la membrane nucléaire; selon les cas, ces extrusions sont apparemment vides de tout matériel nucléaire ou au contraire renferment un matériel finement granulaire toujours peu dense. Le devenir de ces évaginations de la membrane nucléaire et de leur contenu ne semble pas avoir été suivi, sauf par WERNER qui leur attribue un rôle dans la formation de l'annexe centriolaire.

Les pores nucléaires voient généralement leur nombre diminuer au cours de la spermiogenèse. C'est dans la région postérieure du noyau qu'ils se maintiennent le plus longtemps. En général, la membrane nucléaire du spermatozoïde mûr est totalement dépourvue de pores nucléaires. Elle présente d'autre part des régions densifiées le long du feuillet interne au niveau de l'acrosome et, dans certains cas, au niveau du pôle postérieur du noyau (CLARK, 1967).

Le caractère dense du noyau du spermatozoïde mûr souffre des exceptions. Ces exceptions s'observent chez des Platodes (VON BONSDORFF et TELKKÄ, 1965) dont le noyau apparaît hétérogène, finement fibrillaire et peu dense aux électrons. On observe également des formes à noyau très hétérogène chez les Turbellariés où la structure du noyau ayant terminé sa maturation est double: une partie fibrillaire chromatinienne est enveloppée par du matériel moins dense finement granulaire individualisé du reste de la chromatine mais demeurant intra-nucléaire (SILVEIRA et PORTER, 1964).

Dans d'autres spermatozoïdes mûrs, le noyau ressemble à un noyau interphasique et comprend de l'hétérochromatine condensée le long de la membrane nucléaire et des régions euchromatiques centrale et périphériques à texture beaucoup plus lâche. De tels aspects se retrouvent dans les noyaux de spermatozoïdes d'un Téléostéen du genre *Gymnarchus* (MATTEI et coll., 1967), des Cestodes décrits par ROSARIO (1964) et chez certains Myriapodes, où régions hétérochromatiques et euchromatiques alternent (Fig. 8). Dans ce dernier cas, la membrane nucléaire ne semble pas nettement définie sur toute sa longueur. Elle peut avoir complètement disparu, au moins sur toute une face du noyau, chez d'autres Myriapodes (Fig. 9). Elle est totalement absente du côté de la vésicule acrosomienne, qui paraît ici relativement simple et constituée d'une zone centrale à structure fibrillaire et d'une calotte périphérique très dense aux électrons. Cette situation se retrouve chez les Crustacés Décapodes que nous avons plus particulièrement étudiés (Fig. 10). La membrane nucléaire persiste le long de ce que l'on peut appeler la région postérieure du spermatozoïde et les parties latérales du noyau mais a disparu dans la région qui est en contact avec la capsule cytoplasmique. On doit noter la structure particulière du noyau, sa faible densité comparée à l'aspect uniformément dense de la capsule.

CARACTÉRISTIQUES CHIMIQUES

L'analyse cytochimique ou biochimique révèle que le noyau du spermatozoïde mûr est constitué essentiellement d'une certaine quantité de DNA auquel sont associées des protéines dont une partie au moins est représentée par des protéines basiques. La recherche du RNA est négative. L'analyse qualitative et quantitative du DNA peut être réalisée facilement par les méthodes cytochimiques, cytophotométriques ou biochimiques. Il peut être également mis en évidence après extraction, déprotéinisation par le phénol, étalement puis ombrage comme cela a été fait par SOLARI (1965–1968) pour le DNA du spermatozoïde d'Oursin. Le DNA apparaît alors en très longues molécules apparemment linéaires.

La teneur en DNA, très variable selon les espèces, équivaut généralement à la quantité correspondant à la valeur haploïde de l'espèce. En fait, certaines lignées atypiques de spermatozoïdes comme celles que nous avons signalées ci-dessus ne renferment qu'un faible pourcentage de DNA ou en sont totalement dépourvues. Dans d'autres cas, au contraire, on peut observer une valeur supérieure à la valeur haploïde normale, comme c'est le cas chez la Patelle où certains spermatozoïdes ont en DNA l'équivalent de 2 *n* (INDELICATO et STREIFF, 1969). Des spermatozoïdes polyploïdes ont également été décrits (BOUIX, 1963). L'observation de teneurs aberrantes en DNA a été mise en relation chez le Taureau avec le pouvoir fécondant, les animaux stériles ayant une teneur moindre en DNA; notons également une plus forte teneur en protéines nucléaires déduite de la recherche de l'arginine et du fait que, les masses sèches des animaux fertiles et stériles sont voisines, les rapports DNA/arginine et DNA/protéines nucléaires sont plus faibles chez les animaux stériles (LEUCHTENBERGER et coll., 1956).

Les protéines basiques associées au DNA les mieux connues sont les protamines que l'on trouve dans les noyaux des spermatozoïdes de certains Poissons, de certains Oiseaux et de certaines espèces de Mollusques. Ce sont chez les Poissons que ces protamines ont été le mieux étudiées. (FELIX, 1956, 1960; MAZEN, 1962; VENDRELY et VENDRELY, 1966). Elles ont été classées parfois selon le nombre d'acides aminés basiques qu'elles renferment en mono –, di – ou triprotamines. Ces protamines sont très basiques comme en témoigne leur point isoélectrique élevé et qui est d'autant plus élevé que la teneur en arginine est importante. Les protamines, et les monoprotamines en particulier, sont des polypeptides simples renfermant un petit nombre d'acides aminés parmi lesquels les acides aminés basiques (arginine, lysine, histidine) dominent très nettement. Dans les monoprotamines, l'arginine peut représenter jusqu'à 90 % des acides aminés. La proline est l'acide aminé N-terminal le plus souvent représenté, alors que l'arginine se rencontre en position C-terminale. Le poids moléculaire se situe généralement aux environs de 5000 et varie entre 4000 et 8000.

En fait, il semble bien qu'il n'existerait pas qu'une seule espèce moléculaire de protamine par noyau, mais plutôt une famille plus ou moins importante de protamines de composition voisine. La seule analyse séquentielle complète publiée à ce jour a été réalisée pour la clupéine d'un Hareng *Clupea pallasii* par l'école japonaise d'ANDO (ANDO et SUZUKI, 1966). Il a réussi à séparer par chromatographie 3 polypeptides Y I, Y II et Z dont il a réalisé l'analyse complète. Chaque chaîne comprend 30 ou 31 acides aminés, parmi lesquels on retrouve la proline et l'alanine en position N–terminale et l'arginine en position C–terminale.

Néanmoins, il ne faudrait pas croire que toutes les protéines basiques associées au DNA dans le noyau du spermatozoïde sont des protamines. En fait, il existe tous les intermédiaires entre les histones somatiques et les protamines (BLOCH, 1966; VENDRELY et VENDRELY, 1966). Pour simplifier, on a distingué des espèces dont le DNA est associé à des histones typiques, d'autres à des histones enrichies en arginine et d'autres enfin à des protamines. Ces 3 cas se retrouvent chez les Poissons où la Truite par exemple renferme une protamine, la Carpe une histone typique et où le Brochet présente une situation intermédiaire. Il peut être intéressant de rapprocher ces particularités biochimiques, le degré d'évolution morphologique de chacun de ces spermatozoïdes comme l'a défini BILLARD (ce symposium) et également l'aspect du noyau au microscope électronique, dont la densité et l'homogénéité augmentent de la Carpe à la Truite.

Signalons un autre exemple permettant de relier structure et composition. Chez la Drosophile, le noyau de spermatozoïde mûr est homogène et dense; le DNA est associé à des histones riches en arginine. Chez un mutant stérile (SHOUP, 1967), le noyau ne se condense pas, demeure fibrillaire et la transition histones somatiques→histones enrichies en arginine ne se produit pas.

Les protéines nucléaires caractéristiques des spermatozoïdes de certaines espèces (histones enrichies en arginine ou protamines) succèdent au cours de la spermiogenèse aux protéines de type histones qui existent dans les noyaux des stades précédents (ALFERT, 1956; BLOCH, 1960, 1966; DAS et coll., 1964; LISON, 1955). Les modalités de cette transition sont encore très mal connues. La synthèse de ces nouvelles protéines pourrait se faire dans le cytoplasme (BLOCH et BRACK, 1964; INGLES et coll., 1966) à partir de RNA–messagers synthétisés avant la méiose ou au début de la spermiogenèse (CLAYPOOL et BLOCH, 1967; MONESI, 1964, 1968). Le problème même du site de synthèse de ces protéines est loin d'être résolu.

Il est banal de dire qu'au cours de la spermiogenèse le RNA disparaît du noyau (DALED, 1951); il est beaucoup plus difficile de suivre cette évolution. Dans la spermatide d'un Homoptère du genre *Philaenus* et seulement dans la spermatide, jamais à un stade antérieur, MAILLET et GOURANTON ont observé des travées de granules reliées au noyau et semblant s'échapper par les pores nucléaires (Fig. 11). En microscopie photonique, ils ont détecté du RNA associé à cette formation transitoire qui est éliminée avec le reliquat cytoplasmique. C'est le seul cas à notre connaissance d'une démonstration aussi nette de la disparition des ribonucléoprotéines nucléaires au cours de la spermiogenèse.

Certains spermatozoïdes ont un noyau dont la structure et la composition sont aberrantes. Lorsque l'on cherche à détecter les protéines du spermatozoïde de certains Crustacés Décapodes, le Pagure par exemple, qu'il s'agisse de la recherche des protéines totales ou des protéines basiques, on obtient toujours les mêmes résultats: seule la vésicule cytoplasmique homologuée par certains auteurs à un acrosome réagit de façon positive. Le noyau est toujours invisible. Nous avons montré (1965–1968) que cette capsule renferme des protéines dont une partie plus ou moins importante suivant les espèces, est représentée par des protéines basiques libres non associées à un acide nucléique, DNA ou RNA. Le noyau a en microscopie électronique une structure qui s'apparente à celle du DNA de Procaryote ou du DNA cytoplasmique. Le matériel qu'il renferme réagit aux conditions de fixation comme le DNA bactérien. Par exemple, il est conservé de façon correcte en fibres de diamètre uniforme de 30–40 Å dans les fixateurs renfermant des cations, Ca^{++} ou spermine, alors que le test au versène de RYTER et KELLENBERGER coagule à nouveau le DNA (Figs. 12 et 13). Le matériel intranucléaire résiste aux digestions par les protéases (Figs. 14 et 15) alors que les protéines capsulaires sont facilement extraites. La ribonucléase (Fig. 16) ne provoque aucune extraction mais se recombine aux fibres en leur conférant un plus grand contraste. La désoxyribonucléase (Fig. 17) attaque rapidement ces fibres en les faisant disparaître complètement pour des temps variant de 1 à 3 heures. Les différentes données cytochimiques et structurales permettent de conclure que le DNA des Anomoures, des Brachyoures et de certains Macroures est comme le DNA bactérien dépourvu d'histones et aucune protéine nucléaire n'est cytochimiquement décelable.

Les protéines nucléaires quittent le noyau tout au long de la spermatogenèse à partir du stade spermatocytes primaires. Elles se localisent tout d'abord en lames osmiophiles dans l'espace périnucléaire qui apparait considérablement dilaté (Figs. 21 et 22); elles constituent ensuite des grains à structure parfois très régulière (Fig. 21) qui s'individualisent et passent dans le cytoplasme. Il s'agit comme permettent de le dire les méthodes cytochimiques de protéines non–histones. La nature protéique de ces grains peut également être vérifiée au microscope électronique par des extractions par les protéases (Figs 18 et 20). Ces grains riches en protéines non–histones confluent et forment dans le cytoplasme une volumineuse vésicule à laquelle viennent s'associer dans une dernière phase les protéines basiques du noyau formant la capsule définitive (Fig. 10).

La structure apparemment voisine du spermatozoïde de certains Myriapodes du groupe des Diplopodes nous a amené à entreprendre l'étude de la volumineuse vésicule cytoplasmique plus ou moins enchâssée dans le noyau (Fig. 9) considérée comme un acrosome. Aucun acide nucléique n'a pu y être détecté, pas plus que des protéines basiques libres. Cette région est néanmoins très riche en protéines non–histones qui renferment de la cystéine et une quantité importante d'arginine. La cystine ne se trouve que dans la partie centrale paracristalline. Chez l'espèce que nous avons étudiée, aucun polysaccharide neutre ou acide n'a été mis en évidence. Nous rapprochons l'extrême richesse en protéines non-histones de cette vésicule, l'absence de membrane nucléaire et les observations de HORSTMANN (ce symposium) sur un autre Diplopode du genre *Spirostreptus* suggèrant un passage de matériel nucléaire en direction de la vésicule acrosomienne. Le Tableau I résume nos observations cytochimiques.

TABLEAU I.

Analyse cytochimique du spermatozoïde de Iulus *sp.*

	Noyau	Vésicule cytoplasmique (= acrosome)
Acides nucléiques:		
DNA	+	—
RNA	—	—
Protéines:		
Protéines totales	+	+
Protéines basiques libres	—	—
Protéines basiques liées au DNA . .	+	—
arginine.	+	+
tryptophane	—	—
cystéine	+	+
cystine	+	+ (*)
Polysaccharides:	—	—

(*) La présence de cystine est limitée à la partie axiale paracristalline.

Nous avons également entrepris l'analyse cytochimique du noyau, de la côte nucléaire et du cou du spermatozoïde de Pleurodèle (Figs. 23–28). Les méthodes cytochimiques en microscopie photonique ont permis de dresser ce premier inventaire des substances présentes dans chacune de ces trois régions (Tableau II).

De ce tableau, il découle que la côte nucléaire renferme des protéines non–histones riches en ponts disulfures; que le noyau proprement dit contient du DNA normalement associé à des protéines basiques et enfin que le cou, région extra – mais juxta – nucléaire, contient des protéines basiques libres riches en arginine. Les méthodes cytochimiques ultrastructurales (Figs. 23–28) permettent de confirmer ces données; les protéines de la zone chromatinienne et du cou sont facilement extraites par la trypsine ou la pronase; les protéines du cou, libres de toute association, étant extraites les premières. Par contre, les protéines de la côte nucléaire, que nous avons montré comme étant riches en cystine, nécessitent des temps d'extraction beaucoup plus longs. Nous assistons donc ici à une ségrégation à l'intérieur du noyau de protéines non-histones par rapport à la chromatine constituée de DNA et d'histones. D'autre part, l'existence de protéines basiques libres et l'observation d'images suggèrant des relations entre le noyau d'une part et le cou en formation d'autre part, nous font penser à un autre exemple de ségrégation de matériel nucléaire, ici des protéines basiques, qui migreraient dans le cytoplasme.

TABLEAU II.

Analyse cytochimique des constituants de la tête du spermatozoïde de Pleurodeles Waltlii.

	Noyau	Côte nucléaire	Cou
Acides nucléiques:			
DNA	+	—	—
RNA	—	—	—
Protéines:			
Protéines totales	+	+	+
Protéines basiques libres	—	—	+
Protéines basiques liées au DNA . .	—	—	—
Acides aminés:			
arginine.	+	—	+
tryptophane	—	—	—
cystéine	—	—	—
cystine	—	+	—
Polysaccharides:	—	—	—

De telles protéines basiques localisées dans le cytoplasme où elles sont associées à du RNA ont été décrites dans le cytoplasme des spermatides de Rat dans la « sphère chromatophile » étudiée par VAUGHN (VAUGHN, 1966). Ces protéines basiques riches en lysine sont éliminées avec le reliquat cytoplasmique. Dans d'autres cas (Diplopodes, Décapodes, Pleurodèle), des protéines primitivement nucléaires se ségrègeraient de la chromatine en restant intranucléaires (cas de la côte nucléaire du spermatozoïde de Pleurodèle) ou en donnant naissance à des formations cytoplasmiques (capsule des spermatozoïdes de Décapodes et de Diplopodes; cou du spermatozoïde de Pleurodèle).

Remerciements. – Je tiens à remercier Messieurs FOLLIOT et GOURANTON qui m'ont communiqué les clichés qui composent les planches I et IV, et Messieurs B. PICHERAL et J.-P. PRIGENT qui m'ont fourni les données ultrastructurales relatives aux spermatozoïdes et à la spermiogenèse des Urodèles d'une part, et des Myriapodes d'autre part. Les résultats d'ordre cytochimique concernant le spermatozoïde de Pleurodèle et ceux de *Glomeris* et de *Iulus* ont été obtenus avec leur collaboration. Je remercie également très vivement toutes les personnes qui m'ont aidé dans la préparation de ce travail et dans l'obtention des résultats qu'il contient, en particulier Madame BASSEZ et Monsieur MORILLE.

BIBLIOGRAPHIE

Cet index qui n'a nullement la prétention d'être complet groupe seulement les travaux dont il a été fait référence dans le texte.

ALFERT M. (1956) – *Chemical differentiation of nuclear proteins during spermatogenesis in the Salmon.* « J. Biophys. Biochem. Cytol. », 2, 109–114.

ANDERSON W. A., WEISSMAN A. et ELLIS R. A. (1967) – *Cytodifferentiation during spermiogenesis in* Lumbricus terrestris. « J. Cell Biol. », 32, 11–26.

ANDO T. et HASHIMOTO C. (1958) – *Studies on protamines.* IV. *The basic proteins of the testis cell nuclei of adult and immature rainbow-trout in breeding season.* « J. Biochem. », 45, 453–460.

ANDO T. et SUZUKI K. (1967) – *The amino-acid sequence of the third component of clupeine.* « Biochim. Biophys. Acta », 140, 375–377.

ANDRÉ J. (1963) – *Some aspects of specialization in sperm.* In: *General physiology of cell specialization*, Mazia D. and Tyler A. édit., Mc Graw-Hill Book Co., New York., 91–115.

BACCETTI B., DALLAI R. et ROSATI F. (1969) – *The spermatozoon of Arthropoda.* III. *The lowest holometabolic insects.* « J. Microscopie », 8, 233–248.

BAWA S. R. (1964) – *Electron microscope study of spermiogenesis in a firebrat insect,* Thermobia domestica *Pack.* I. *Mature spermatozoon.* « J. Cell Biol. », 23, 431–446.

BERNSTEIN M. H. et MAZIA D. (1953) – *The desoxyribonucleoprotein of sea urchin sperm.* I. *Isolation and analysis.* « Biochim. Biophys. Acta », 10, 600–606.

BERNSTEIN M. H. et MAZIA D. (1953) – *The desoxyribonucleoprotein of sea urchin sperm.* II. *Properties.* « Biochim. Biophys. Acta », 11, 59–68.

BERRY R. E. et MAYER D. T. (1960) – *The histone-like basic protein of bovine spermatozoa.* « Exper. Cell Res. », 20, 116–126.

BLOCH D. P. (1966) – *Cytochemistry of the histones.* « Protoplasmatologia », 5, 1–56.

BLOCH D. P. et BRACK S. D. (1964) – *Evidence for the cytoplasmic synthesis of nuclear histone during spermiogenesis in the grasshopper* Chortophaga viridifasciata (*De Geer*). « J. Cell Biol. », 22, 327–340.

BLOCH D. P. et HEW H. Y. C. (1960) – *Schedule of spermatogenesis in the Pulmonate snail* Helix aspersa, *with special reference to histone transition.* « J. Biophys. Biochem. Cytol. », 7, 515–532.

BONSDORFF C. H. VON et TELKKÄ A. (1965) – *The spermatozoon flagella in* Diphyllobothrium latum (*fish tapeworm*). « Z. Zellforsch. Mikr. Anat. », 66, 643–648.

BOUIX G. (1963) – *Sur la spermatogenèse des Carabes* (*Col. Car.*)*: modalité et fréquence de la spermiogenèse atypique.* « C. R. Acad. Sci. », 256, 2698–2701.

BREUCKER H. et HORSTMANN E. (1968) – *Die Spermatozoen der Zecke* Ornithodorus moubata (*Murr.*). « Z. Zellforsch. Mikr. Anat. », 88, 1–22.

BRIL-PETERSEN E. et WESTENBRINIK H. G. K. (1963) – *A structural basic protein as a counterpart of deoxyribonucleic acid in mammalian spermatozoa.* « Biochim. Biophys. Acta », 76, 152–154.

CHEVAILLIER P. (1966) – *Contribution à l'étude du complexe ADN–histone dans le spermatozoïde du Pagure* Eupagurus bernhardus *L.* « J. Microscopie », 5, 739–758.

CHEVAILLIER P. (1966) – *Structure et constitution cytochimique de la capsule des Crustacés Décapodes.* « C. R. Acad. Sci. », 262, 1546–1549.

CHEVAILLIER P. (1967) – *Mise en évidence et étude cytochimique d'une protéine basique extranucléaire dans les spermatozoïdes des Crustacés Décapodes.* « J. Cell Biol. », 32, 547–556.

CHEVAILLIER P. (1967) – *Relations* DNA–*histones au cours de la spermatogenèse des Crustacés Décapodes.* « C. R. Soc. Biol. », 161, 435–436.

CHEVAILLIER P. (1967) – *Nouvelles observations sur la structure des fibres intra-nucléaires du spermatozoïde du Pagure* Eupagurus bernhardus (*Crustacé Décapode*). « J. Microscopie », 6, 853–856.

CHEVAILLIER P. (1968) – *Etude cytochimique ultrastructurale des nucléoprotéines dans le spermatozoïde du Pagure* Eupagurus bernhardus *L.* « J. Microscopie », 7, 107–114.

CHEVAILLIER P. et MAILLET P. L. (1965) – *Structure fine et constitution cytochimique du spermatozoïde de la Langoustine* Nephrops norvegicus *L.* (*Crustacé Décapode*). « J. Microscopie », 4, 679–700.

CHEVAILLIER P. et PICHERAL B. – *Constitution cytochimique et structure du noyau du spermatozoïde d'un Urodèle,* Pleurodeles Waltlii *Michah.* Manuscrit en préparation.

CHEVAILLIER P. et PRIGENT J. – P. – *Structure et analyse cytochimique du spermatozoïde de* Iulus londinensis (*Myriapode Diplopode*). Manuscrit en préparation.

CHEVAILLIER P. et PRIGENT J. P. – *Analyse ultrastructurale et cytochimique des constituants du spermatozoïde d'un Myriapode,* Glomeris marginata. Manuscrit en préparation.

CLARK A. W. (1967) – *Some aspects of spermiogenesis in a lizard.* « Am. J. Anat. », 121, 369–400.

CLAYPOOL C. J. et BLOCH D. P. (1967) – *Synthesis of ribonucleic acid and histone change during spermatogenesis in the grasshopper* Chortophaga viridifasciata. « Nature », 215, 966–967.

DALED H. J. (1951) – *Etude cytochimique sur l'évolution de l'acide ribonucléique dans la spermatogenèse du rat.* « Archiv. Anat. Micr. Morphol. Expér. », 40, 183–194.

DAS C. C., KAUFMANN B. P. et GAY H. (1964) – *Autoradiographic evidence of synthesis of an arginin-rich histone during spermiogenesis in* Drosophila melanogaster. « Nature », 204, 1008–1009.

DAS C. C., KAUFMANN B. P. et GAY H. (1964) – *Histone-protein transition in* Drosophila melanogaster. I. *Changes during spermatogenesis.* « Exper. Cell Res. », 35, 507–514.

DOUGLAS L. T. (1965) – *Evidence for tandem arrangement of chromosomal elements in spermatid nuclei of the chinese hamster.* « Genetica », 36, 59–64.

FELIX K., FISCHER H. et KREKELS A. (1956) – *Protamines and nucleoprotamines.* « Progress in Biophysics and Biophysical Chemistry », 6, 2–23.

FELIX K. (1960) – *Protamines.* « Advances in Protein Chemistry », 15, 1–56.

FRANKLIN L. E. (1968) – *Formation of the redundant nuclear envelope in Monkey spermatids.* « Anat. Rec. », 161, 149–161.

HORSTMANN E. (1968) – *Die Spermatozoen von* Geophilus linearis *Koch* (*Chilopoda*). « Z. Zellforsch. Mikr. Anat. », 89, 410–429.

HUGHES-SCHRADER S. (1946) – *A new type of spermiogenesis in Iceryine Coccids with linear alignement of chromosomes in the sperm.* « J. Morphol. », 78, 43–84.

HUGHES-SCHRADER S. (1955) – *The chromosomes of the giant scale* Aspidoproctus maximus *Louns.* (*Coccoïdea–Margarodidae*) *with special reference to asynapsis and sperm formation.* « Chromosoma », 7, 420–438.

INDELICATO I. et STREIFF W. (1969). – *Etude statistique et cytophotométrique de la dimégalie des spermatozoïdes chez* Patella coerulea *L., Mollusques, Gastéropodes, Prosobranches.* « C. R. Acad. Sc. », 268, 2091–2094.

INGLES C. J. TREVITHICK J. R., SMITH M. et DIXON G. H. (1966) – *Biosynthesis of protamine during spermatogenesis in Salmonoid fish.* « Biochem. Biophys. Res. Commun. », 22, 627–634.

INOUE S. et SATO H. (1962) – *Arrangement of* DNA *in living sperm: a biophysical analysis.* « Science », 136, 1122–1124.

INOUE S. et SATO H. (1966) – *Deoxyribonucleic acid arrangement in living sperm.* In *Molecular architecture in cell physiology*, Hayashi et Szent–Györgyi édit., 209–248.

KOEHLER J. K. (1966) – *Fine structure observations in frozen-etched bovine spermatozoa.* « J. Ultr. Res. », 16, 359–375.

LEE E. et WILKES A. (1965) – *Polymorphic spermatozoa in the Hymenopterous wasp* Dahlbominus. « Science », 147, 1445–1446.

LEUCHTENBERGER C., MURMANIS I., MURMANIS L., ITO S. et WEIR D. R. (1956) – *Interferometric dry mass and microscopectrophotometric arginine determination on bull sperm nuclei with normal and abnormal* DNA *content.* « Chromosoma », 8, 73–86.

LE MENN R. (1966) – *Observations sur la spermiogenèse et le spermatozoïde des Psyllides* (*Homoptera, Psylloïdea*). « C. R. Acad. Sc. », 262, 1731–1733.

LISON L. (1955) – *Variation de la basophilie pendant la maturation du spermatozoïde chez le Rat et sa signification histochimique.* « Acta Histochem. », 2, 47–67.

LUNG B. (1968) – *Whole–mount electron microscopy of chromatin and membranes in bull and human sperm heads.* « J. Ultr. Res. », 22, 485–493.

MACINNES J. W. et URETZ R. B. (1968) – DNA *organization in the mature sperm of several Orthoptera by the method of polarized fluorescence microscopy.* « J. Cell Biol. », 38, 426–436.

MAILLET P. L. et GOURANTON J. (1965) – *Sur l'expulsion de l'acide ribonucléique nucléaire par les spermatides de* Philaenus spumarius *L.* (*Homoptera, Cercopidae*). « C. R. Acad. Sc. », 261, 1417–1419.

MATTEI X., BOISSON C., MATTEI C. et REIZER C. (1967) – *Spermatozoïdes aflagellés chez un Poisson:* Gymnarchus niloticus (*Téléostéen, Gymnarchidae*). « C. R. Acad. Sc. », 265, 2010–2012.

MAZEN A. (1962) – *Contribution à l'étude biochimique des nucléohistones et nucléoprotamines du noyau cellulaire.* « Bull. Biol. Fr. Belg. », 96, 305–361.

MELLORS R. C. et HLINKA J. (1955) – *Quantitative cytology and cytopathology* IV. *Interferometric measurement of the anhydrous organic mass* (*dry weight*) *of genetic material in sperm nuclei of the mouse, the rat and guinea pig.* « Exper. Cell Res. », 9, 128–134.

MONESI V. (1964) – *Autoradiographic evidence of a nuclear histone synthesis during mouse spermiogenesis in the absence of detectable quantities of nuclear ribonucleic acid.* « Exper. Cell Res. », 36, 683–688.

MONESI V. (1968) – *Ribonucleic acid and protein synthesis during differentiation of male germ cells in the mouse.* « Archiv. Anat. Micr. Morphol. Expér. », 56, 61–74.

PICHERAL B. (1967) – *Structure et organisation du spermatozoïde de* Pleurodeles Waltlii *Michah.* (*Amphibien Urodèle*). « Arch. Biol. », 78, 193–221.

PICHERAL B., FOLLIOT R. et MAILLET P. L. (1966) – *Sur la structure du noyau du spermatozoïde de* Pleurodeles waltlii *Michah.* (*Amphibien Urodèle*). « C. R. Acad. Sc. », 262, 1579–1582.

POTSWALD H. E. (1967) – *An electron microscope study of spermiogenesis in* Spirobis (Laeospira) mörchi *Levinsen* (*Polychaeta*). « Z. Zellforsch Mikr. Anat. », 83, 231–248.

REITBERGER A. (1964) – *Lineare Anordnung der Chromosomen in Kern des Spermatozoen des Lebermoses* Sphaerocarpus donnellii. « Naturwiss. », 16, 395–396.

RIS H. (1962) – *Interpretation of ultrastructure in the cell nucleus.* In: *The interpretation of ultrastructure,* « Symp. Internat. Soc. Cell. Biol. », Harris édit., 69–88.

ROSARIO B. (1964) – *An electron microscope study on spermatogenesis in Cestodes.* « J. Ultr. Res. », II, 412–427.

SHOUP J. R. (1967) – *Spermiogenesis in wild type and in a male sterility mutant of* Drosophila melanogaster. « J. Cell Biol. », 32, 662–675.

SILVEIRA M. et PORTER K. R. (1964) – *The spermatozoids of flatworms and their microtubular systems.* « Protoplasma », 59, 240–265.

SOLARI A. J. (1965) – *Electron microscopy of native DNA in sea urchin cells.* « J. Ultr. Res. », 17, 421–438.

SOLARI A. J. (1965) – *Structure of the chromatin in sea urchin sperm.* « Proc. Nat. Acad. Sci. », 53, 503–510.

SOLARI A. J. (1968) – *The ultrastructure of chromatin fibers.* I. *The effect of spreading conditions.* « Exper. Cell Res. », 53, 553–566.

SOLARI A. J. (1968) – *The ultrastructure of chromatin fibers.* II. *The ultrastructure of the loops from sea urchin sperm chromatin.* « Exper. Cell Res. », 53, 567–581.

TAYLOR J. H. (1964) – *The arrangement of chromosomes in the mature sperm of the grasshopper.* « J. Cell Biol. », 21, 286–289.

VAUGHN J. C. (1966) – *The relationship of the « sphère chromatophile » to the fate of displaced histones following histone transition in rat spermiogenesis.* « J. Cell Biol. », 31, 257–278.

VENDRELY R. et VENDRELY C. (1966) – *Biochemistry of histones and protamines.* – « Protoplasmatologia », 5, 1–88.

WERNER G. (1965) – *Untersuchungen über die Spermiogenese beim Sandläufer,* Cicindela campestris *L.* « Z. Zellforsch. Mikr. Anat. », 66, 255–275.

WILKES A. et LEE P. E. (1965) – *The ultrastructure of dimorphic spermatozoa in the Hymenopteron* Dahlbonimus fuscipennis (*Zett.*) (*Eulophidae*). « Canad. J. Genet. Cytol. », 7, 609–619.

WILKINS M. H. F. (1956) – *Physical studies of the molecular structure of deoxyribose nucleic acid and nucleoprotein.* « Cold Spring Harbor Symposia on Quantitative Biology », 21, 278–293.

WILKINS M. H. F. et RANDALL J. T. (1953) – *Crystallinity in sperm heads: molecular structure of nucleoprotein in vivo.* « Biochim. Biophys. Acta », 10, 192.

YASUZUMI G. et ISHIDA H. (1957) – *Spermatogenesis in animals as revealed by electron microscopy.* II. *Submicroscopic structure of developing spermatid nuclei of grasshopper.* « J. Biophys. Biochem. Cytol. », 3, 663–668.

ZUBAY G. (1964) – *Nucleohistone structure and function.* In *The nucleohistones*, Bonner et Ts'o édit., Holden-Day, San Francisco, 95–107.

LÉGENDES DES FIGURES

Figs. 1–7. – Evolution de la chromatine au cours de la spermiogenèse de *Philaenus spumarius* (Homoptère). (*Clichés R. Folliot*).

Fig. 1: ×20.000. Fig. 3,4: ×40.000.
Fig. 2: ×25.000. Fig. 5,6,7: ×50.000.
(*mc*: membrane cellulaire; *mN*: membrane nucléaire; *mt*: microtubules).

Fig. 8. – Spermatozoïde mûr de *Glomeris marginata*; noter l'aspect interphasique du noyau présentant des régions euchromatiques et hétérochromatiques. La membrane nucléaire ne semble pas toujours bien définie; ×20.000.

Fig. 9. – Spermatozoïde de *Iulus londinensis*. Noter la structure de la chromatine, l'absence de membrane nucléaire séparant le noyau et la vésicule acrosomienne et la double structure de cette vésicule avec sa partie axiale d'aspect paracristallin et sa région périphérique très dense; ×33.000.

(*C*: vésicule acrosomienne; *fa*: formation axiale; *Gl*: glycogène; *m*: mitochondries; *mN*: membrane nucléaire; *N*: noyau).

Fig. 10. – Spermatozoïde mûr du Pagure *Eupagurus bernhardus* (Crustacé Décapode). Noter le noyau peu dense et hétérogène et la capsule de structure uniforme et très dense; ×16.500.

(*C*: capsule; *c*: centriole; *fa*: filament axial; *ga*: granule apical; *m*: mitochondries; *mc*: membrane cellulaire; *N*: noyau; *t*: microtubules).

Fig. 11. – Echanges nucléo–cytoplasmiques dans la spermatide de *Philaenus spumarius* (Homoptère). Des granules de nature ribonucléoprotéique sont éliminés du noyau par les pores nucléaires; ×22.000 (*cliché J. Gouranton*).

(*A.*: acrosome; *F.*: flagelle; *G.*: dictyosome; *N.*: noyau; *Ne.*: nebenkern mitochondrial).

Figs. 12–20. – Etude cytochimique ultrastructurale du contenu nucléaire du spermatozoïde du Pagure *Eupagurus bernhardus* (Crustacé Décapode).

Fig. 12: matériel fixé selon la méthode de Ryter et Kellenberger à l'osmium-calcium et post–fixation par l'acétate d'uranyle; ×75.000.

Fig. 13: matériel fixé par l'osmium–calcium et post-traitement par le versène. Le DNA apparait coagulé comme le DNA bactérien après ce traitement; ×75.000.

Fig. 14: extraction par la trypsine; ×50.000.

Fig. 15: extraction par la pronase; ×50.000.

Fig. 16: traitement par la ribonucléase après inclusion dans le glycol-méthacrylate; ×50.000.

Fig. 17: même inclusion; extraction par la désoxyribonucléase; ×50.000.

Fig. 18: grain protéique non traité; ×50.000.

Fig. 10: extraction par la pronase; ×50.000.

Fig. 20: extraction par la pepsine; ×50.000.

Fig. 21–22. – Echanges nucléo–cytoplasmiques dans les spermatides d'*Eupagurus bernhardus* (Crustacé Décapode): formation de lames denses dans l'espace périnucléaire qui donnent naissance à des grains protéiques qui s'individualisent et migrent dans le cytoplasme. Ce sont ces grains qui, en fusionnant, forment la première ébauche de la capsule.

Fig. 21: ×16.500. Fig. 22: ×46.000.

(*f.e.*: feuillet externe; *f.i.*: feuillet interne; *g.p.*: grain protéique; *m.n.*: membrane nucléaire; *N.*: noyau).

Figs. 23–28. – Etude cytochimique ultrastructurale de la côte nucléaire et du cou du spermatozoïde du Pleurodèle (*Pleurodeles Waltlii*).

Fig. 23: observation au microscope optique de la région antérieure du spermatozoïde; ×1.800.

Fig. 24: coupe transversale non traitée montrant la structure dense de la chromatine et la structure alvéolaire de la côte nucléaire; ×46.000.

Fig. 25: extraction par la trypsine; ×46.000.

Fig. 26: extraction par la pronase; ×46.000.

Fig. 27: coupe transversale non traitée de la région postérieure de la tête du spermatozoïde montrant le cou entouré d'un anneau de chromatine; ×46.000.

Fig. 28: extraction par la pronase; ×46.000.

(*A.*: acrosome; *AX.*: filament axial; *CN.*: côte nucléaire; *Co.*: cou; *mN.*: membrane nucléaire; *N.*: noyau; *ZC*: zone chromatinienne).

Discussion

POCHON–MASSON. – Pouvez–vous préciser les corrélations entre la présence centriolaire, ou centriolaire et flagellaire, et l'évolution nucléaire au cours de la spermiogenèse?

CHEVAILLIER. – Il ne semble pas qu'il y ait de corrélation directe entre la présence des centrioles ou du flagelle et l'évolution du noyau au cours de la spermiogenèse, ni du point de vue morphologique, ni du point de vue – et encore moins – de sa constitution.

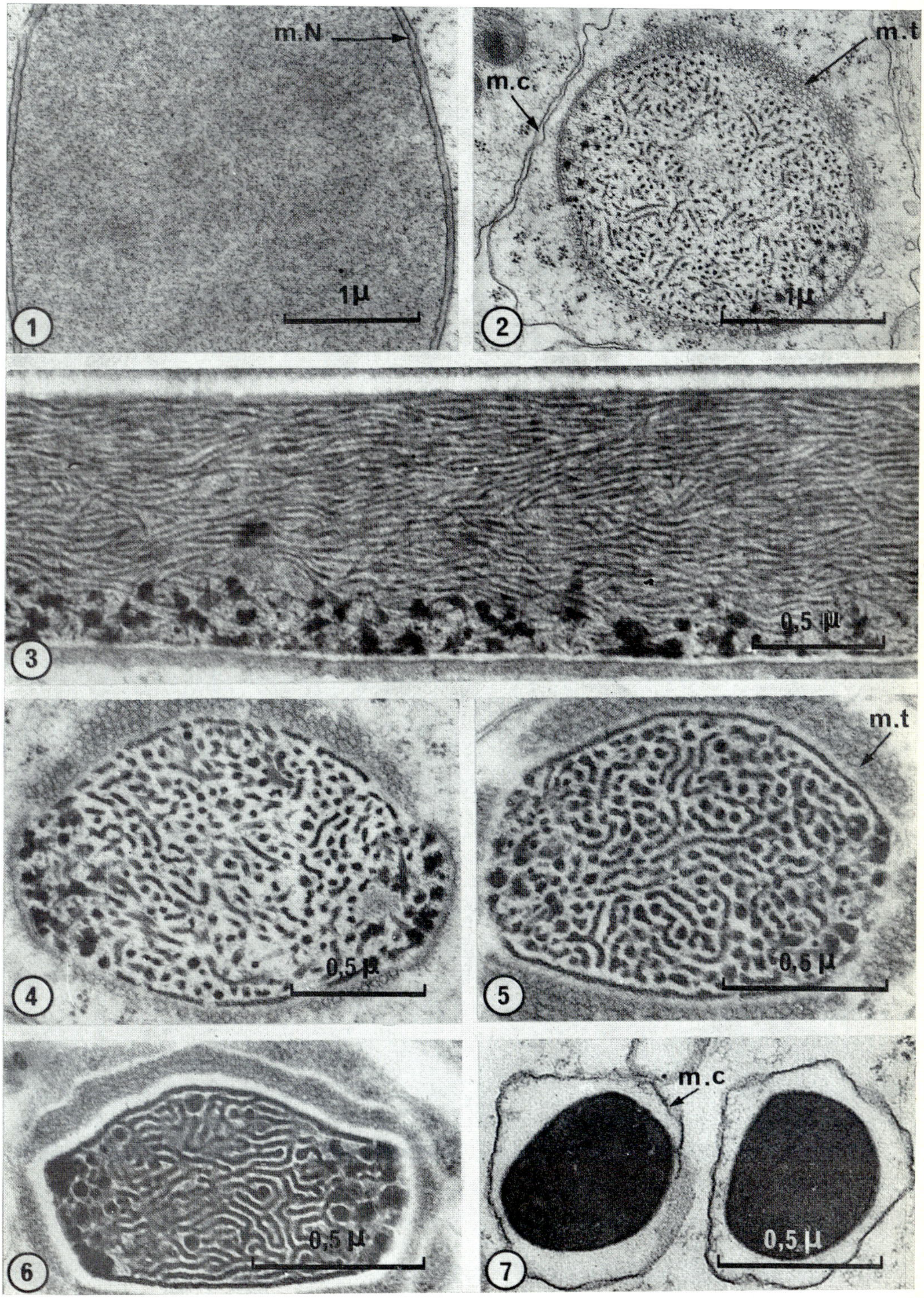
m.N
1µ
1
m.c
m.t
1µ
2
0,5 µ
3
0,5 µ
4
m.t
0,5 µ
5
0,5 µ
6
m.c
0,5 µ
7

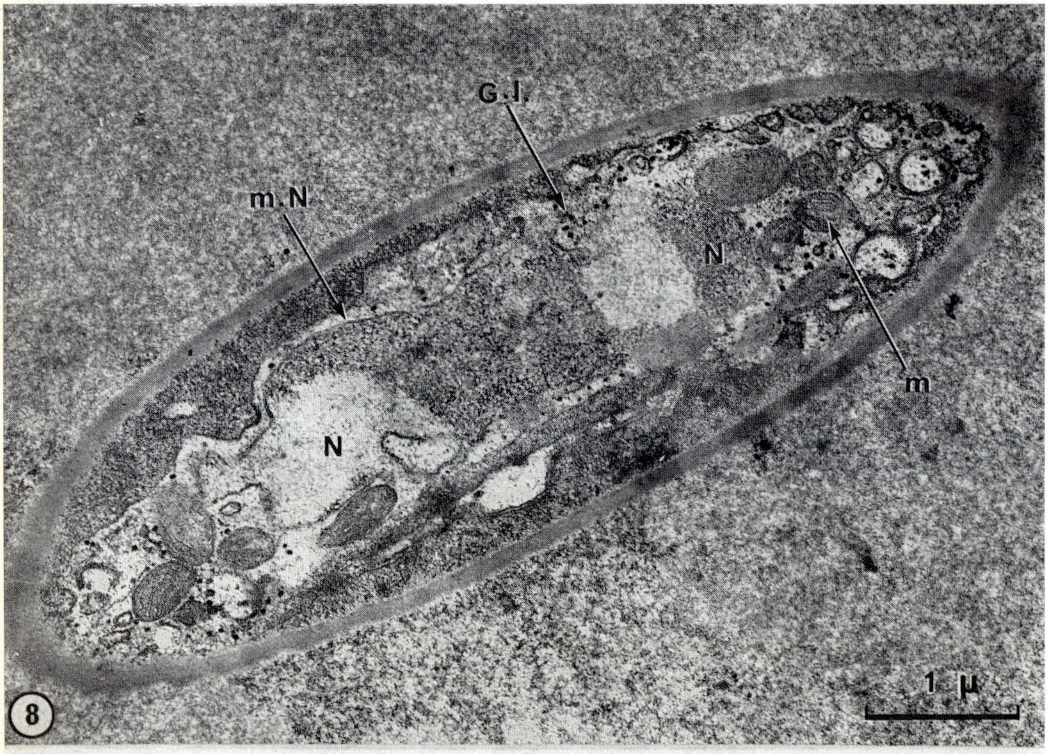
G.I.
m.N
N
N
m
1 µ
8

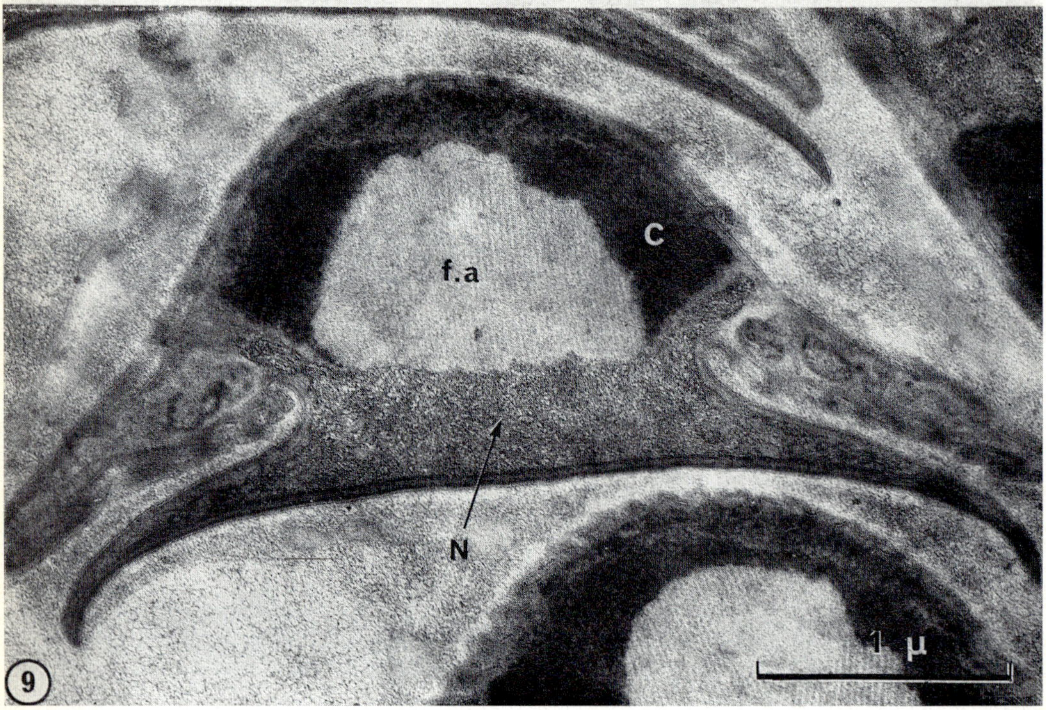
C
f.a
N
1 µ
9

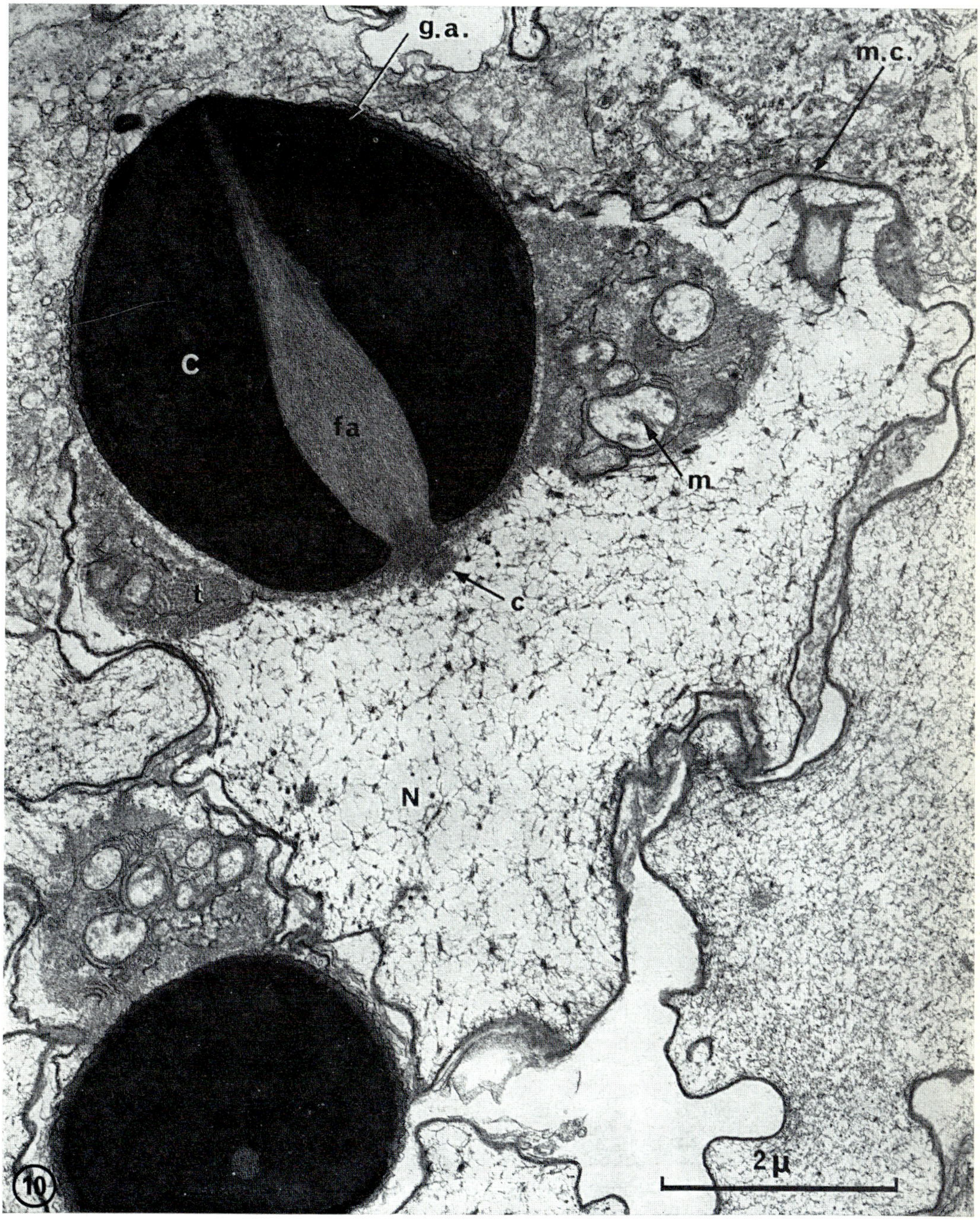
g.a.
m.c.
C
fa
m
t
c
N
2μ
10

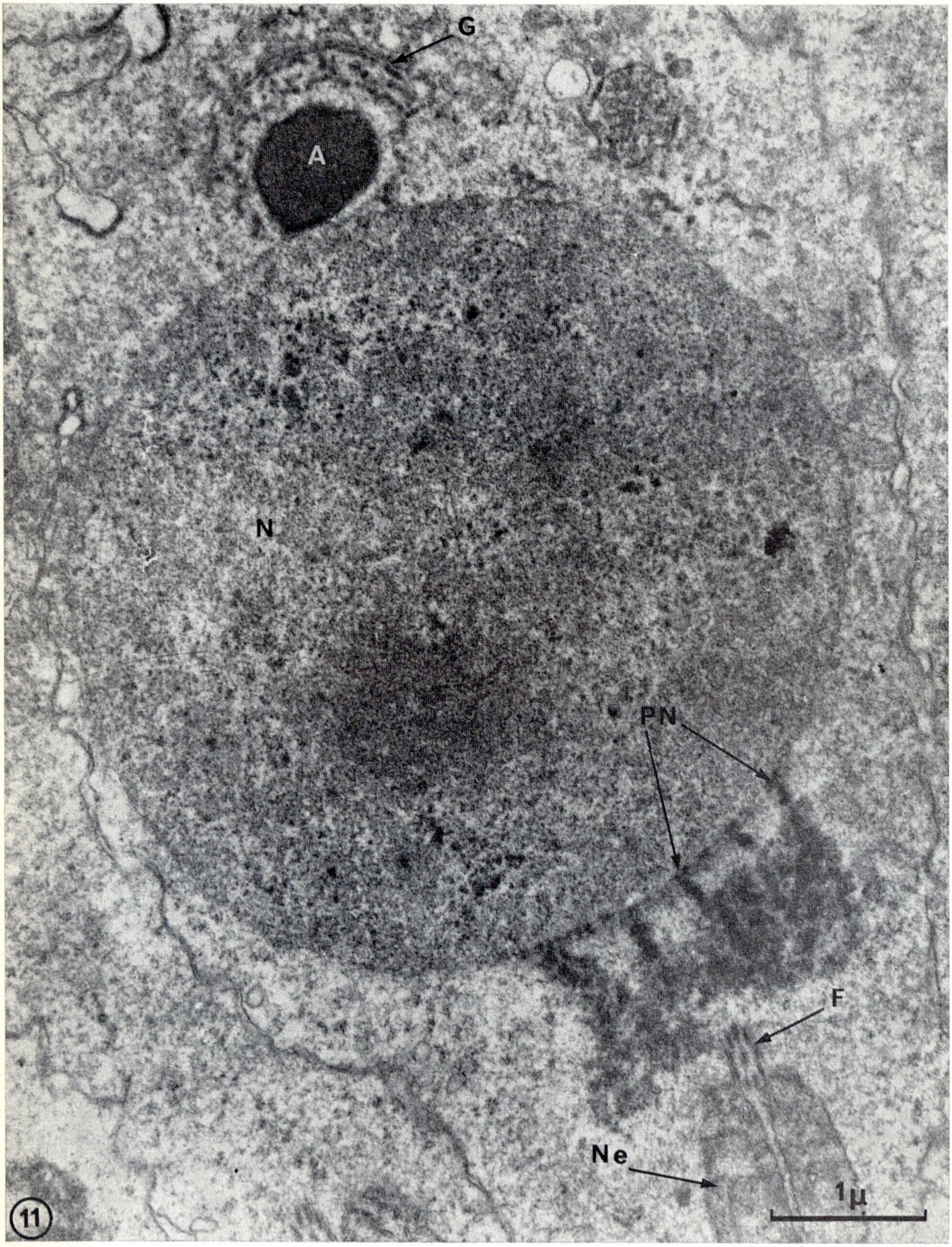
G
A
N
PN
F
Ne
1µ
11

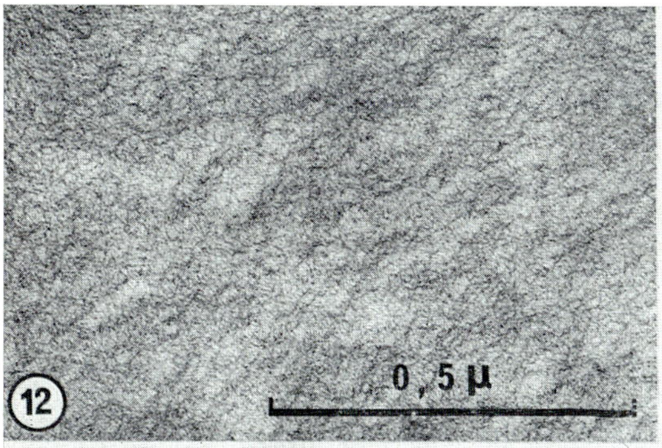
12
0,5 µ

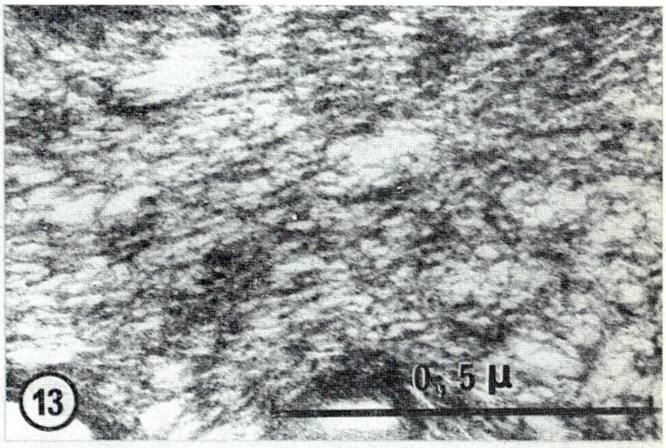
13
0,5 µ

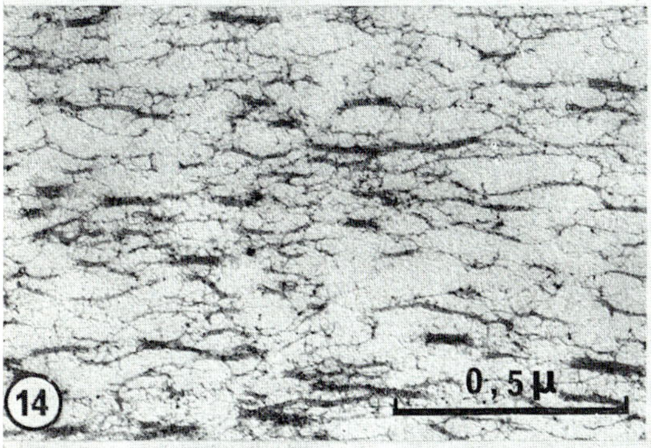
14
0,5 µ

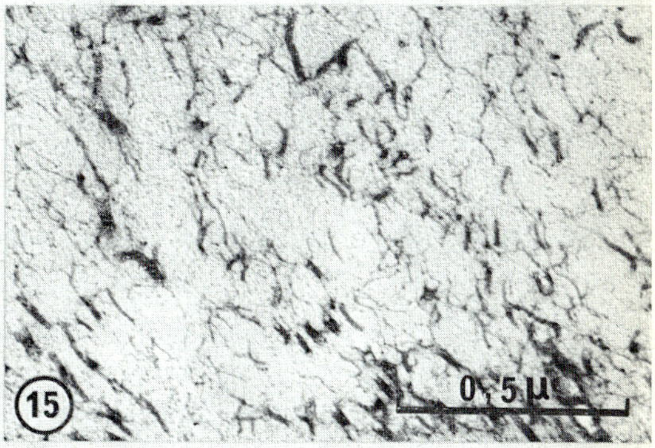
15
0,5 µ

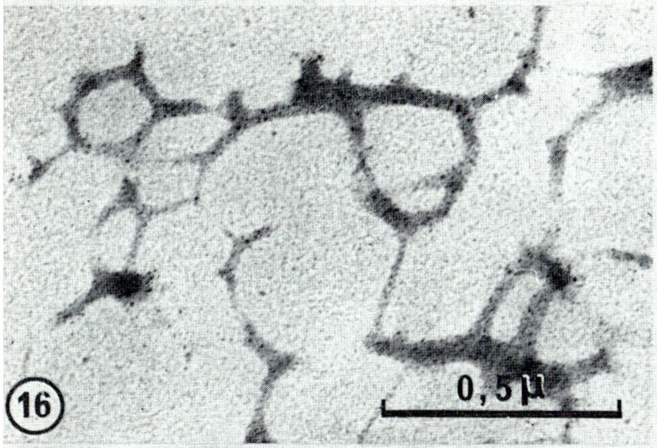
16
0,5 µ

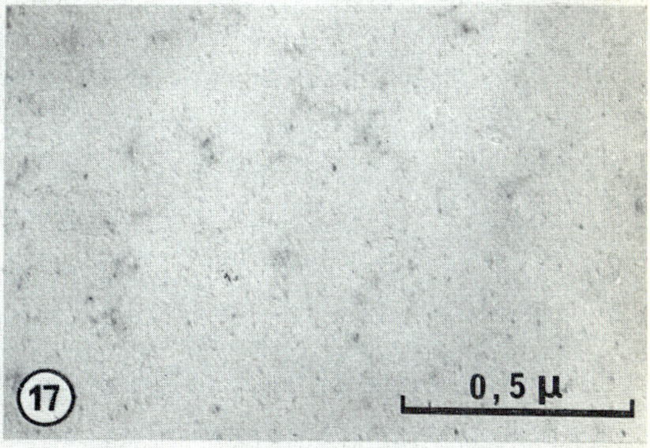
17
0,5 µ

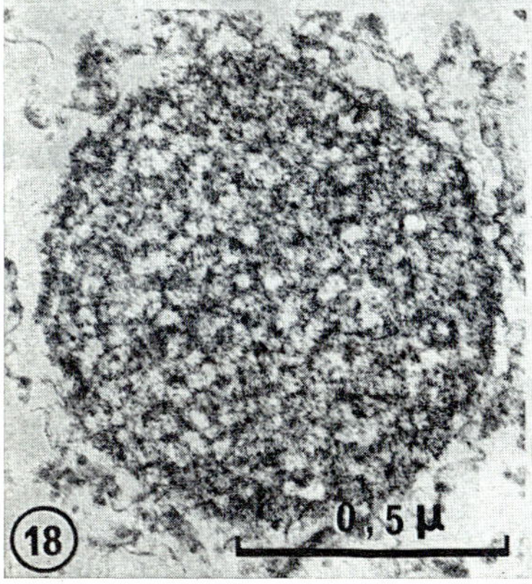
18
0,5 µ

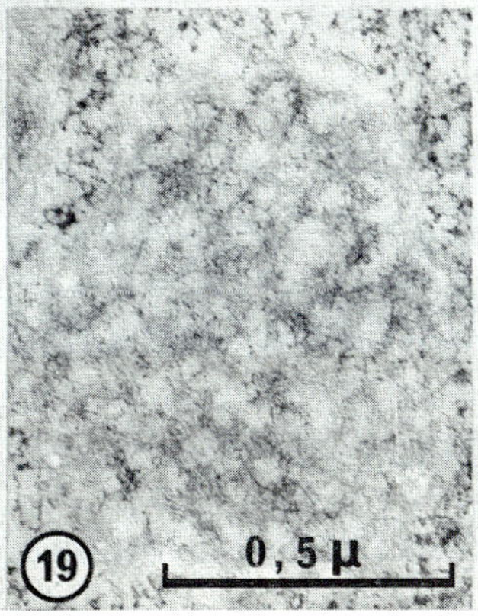
19
0,5 µ

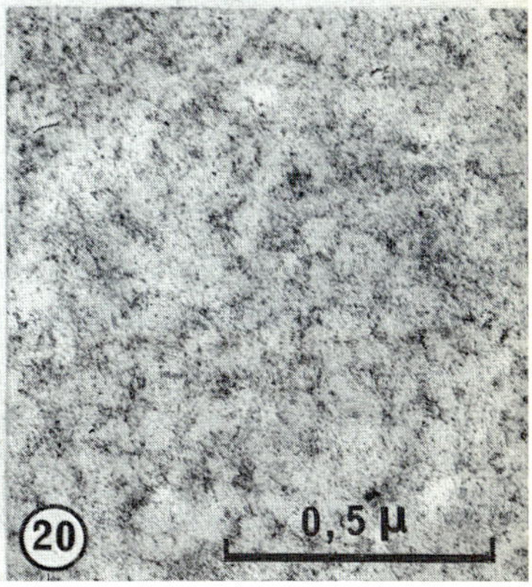
20
0,5 µ

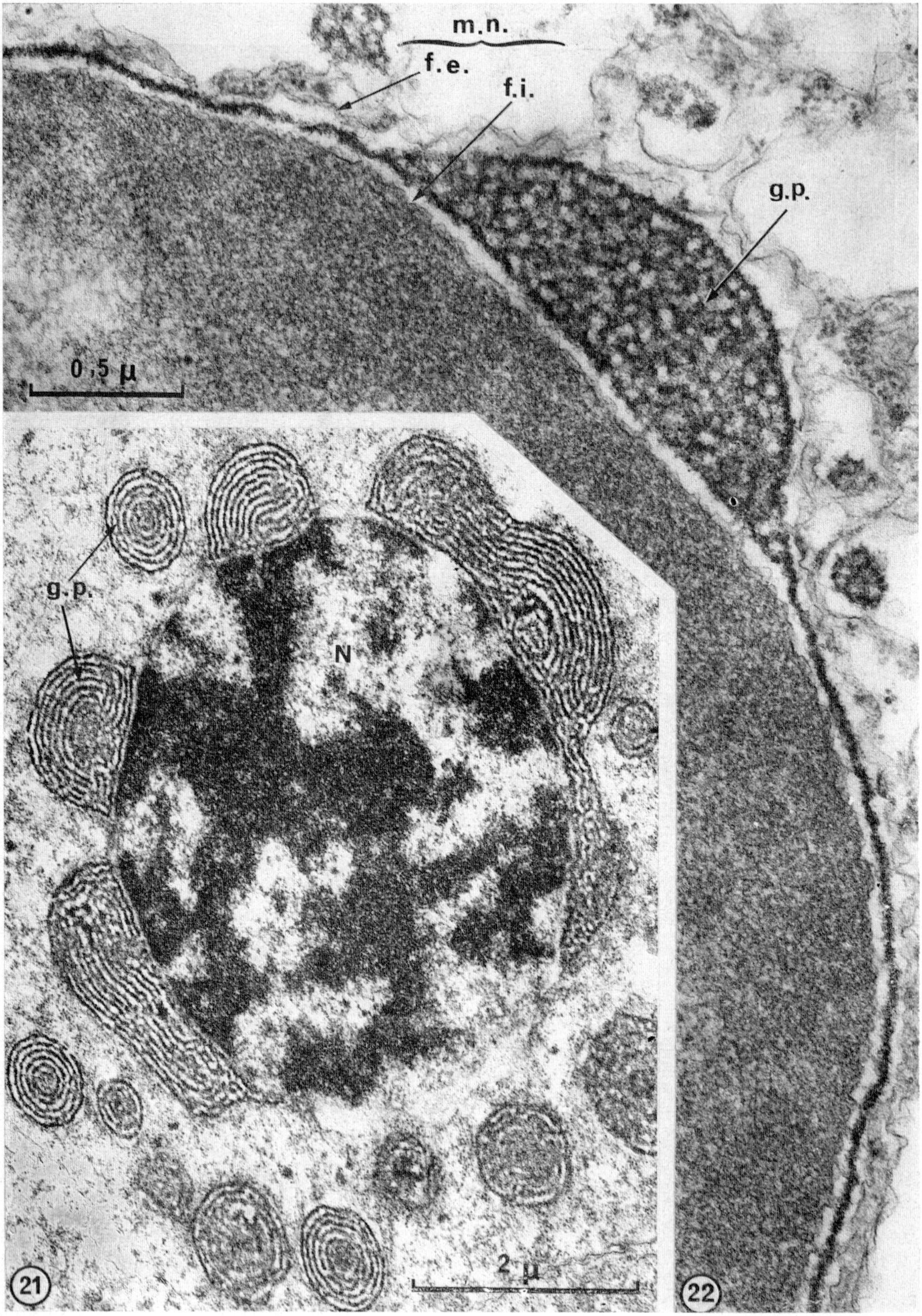
m.n.
f.e.
f.i.
g.p.
0,5 μ
g.p.
N
2 μ
21
22

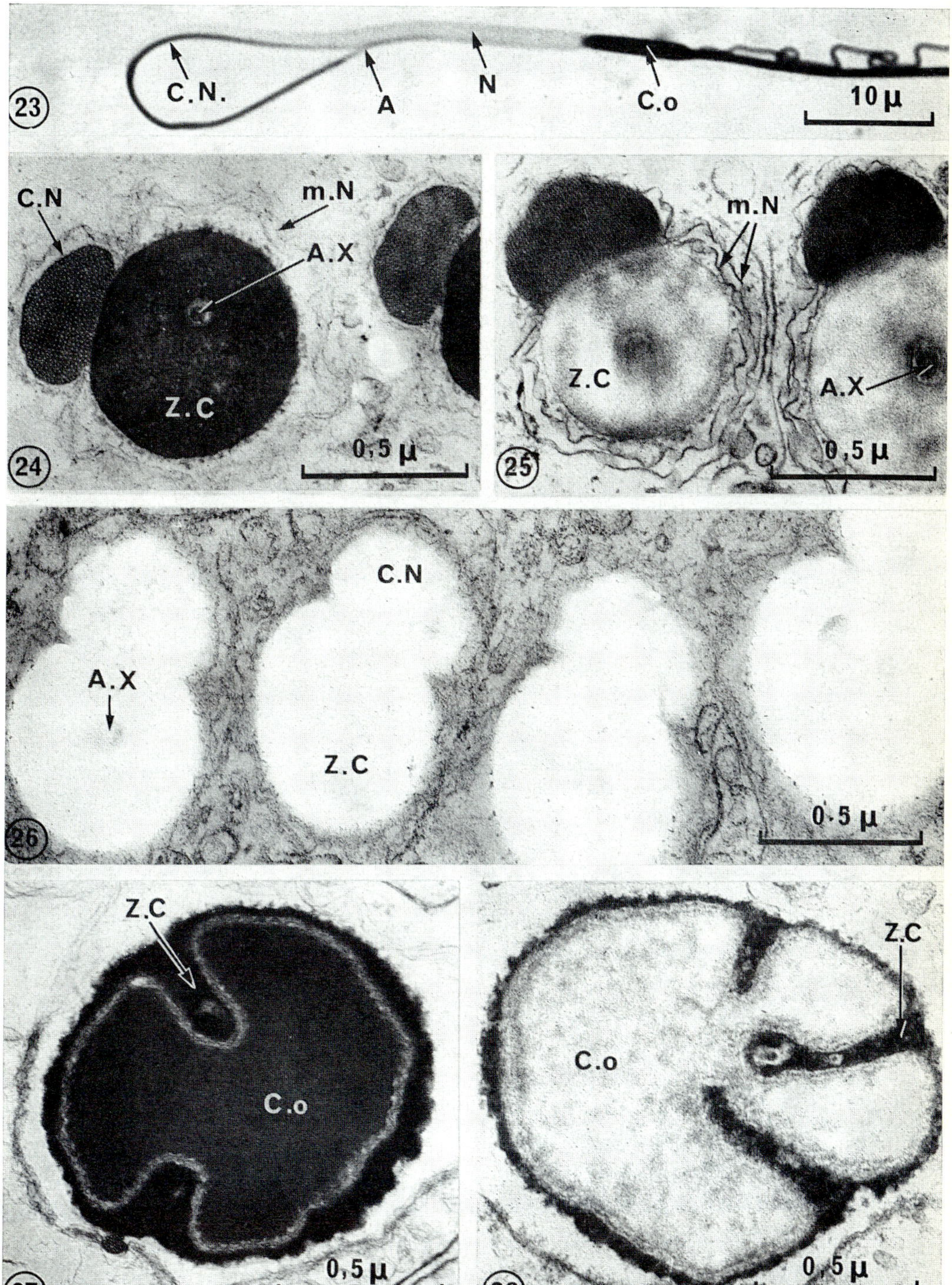
23
C.N.
A
N
C.o
10 µ
24
C.N
m.N
A.X
Z.C
0,5 µ
25
m.N
Z.C
A.X
0,5 µ
26
C.N
A.X
Z.C
0.5 µ
27
Z.C
C.o
0,5 µ
28
Z.C
C.o
0,5 µ

J. K. KOEHLER (*)

FREEZE-ETCHING STUDIES ON SPERMATOZOA WITH PARTICULAR REFERENCE TO NUCLEAR AND POST-NUCLEAR CAP STRUCTURE (**)

SUMMARY. — Ejaculated spermatozoa of the rabbit, human and rainbow trout have been subjected to fine structural analysis using the freeze-etching technique. Views of the " post-nuclear cap " in mammalian sperm show a complex arrangement of several components including cords or stria of material associated with the implantation fossa. The trout sperm have no similar specialization in this region. The arrangement of nucleoprotein in the case of the mammalian species is observed to be in the form of layers of lamellae giving rise to a strong orientational dependence on birefringence. The trout sperm do not exhibit the lamellar arrangement and show no particular orientational dependence with the polarization microscope.

RIASSUNTO. — Spermatozoi eiaculati di coniglio, uomo e trota sono stati sottoposti ad una analisi strutturale usanto la tecnica del « freeze-etching ». Immagini della « calotta postnucleare » degli spermatozoi di mammiferi mostrano una complessa disposizione di numerose componenti includendo le corde o strie di materiale associato con la cavità di impianto. Lo spermio di trota non presenta una simile specializzazione in questa regione. Le nucleoproteine, nel caso dei mammiferi, sono disposte a formare strati di lamelle che danno origine ad una forte birifrangenza. Lo spermatozoo di trota non presenta disposizione lamellare e non mostra nessuna particolare birifrangenza con il microscopio polarizzatore.

INTRODUCTION

This report concerns two aspects of spermatozoan head structure. One of these deals with the so-called " post-nuclear cap " first studied intensively in mammalian sperm by GATENBY and his associates in the 1920's and 1930's (GATENBY and WIGODER, 1929). Early observations were to a great extent dependent on silver impregnation methods which appeared to reveal a uniform material covering the posterior portion of the nucleus. Over the years, the " post-nuclear cap " has come under frequent criticism and has periodically been interpreted as an artifact. NATH (1965) briefly summarizes some of these historical details and also quotes studies by DHILLON and DUIJN indicating that a differentiated, posteriorly located region can be observed in living mammalian spermatozoa of several species under phase contrast. Several workers in the fine structure field have commented on the presence of dense,

(*) Department of Biological Structure University of Washington Seattle, Washington.

(**) Supported by research grants from the National Science Foundation (GB 8165) and USPHS (GM 16598) from the National Institutes of Health.

membrane associated material in the post-nuclear region. FAWCETT and ITO (1965) have demonstrated an organized cytoplasmic component in the area of the " post-nuclear cap " of bat spermatozoa. Furthermore, FAWCETT (1965) has suggested that the term " post-nuclear cap " is not descriptive of the actual structure present in mammalian sperm and should be discarded. The problem is further complicated by the fact that we have no obvious functional role for this structural entity.

The second and to some extent independent aspect of sperm head structure to be discussed is the conformation of the nuclear material. Electron microscopic studies of chemically fixed, mature spermatozoa have revealed little, if any, structural pattern of detail in the nuclear region. This area is typically occupied by a very dense, almost amorphous mass of material. This appearance is modified in only very minor ways by different chemical fixations including aldehydes, potassium permanganate and osmium tetroxide. Occasionally, rounded clumps or a variety of finely filamentous material can be discerned, but no indication of paracrystalline order is to be detected. In contrast to the lack of discernible fine structure in mature sperm nuclei, there is considerable evidence showing a variety of structural modes in developing spermatid nuclei. These include plate-like lamellae in grasshopper spermatids (DASS and RIS, 1958), similar structures in locust spermatids (GIBBONS and BRADFIELD, 1956), and many other modifications too numerous to detail here. The usual line of thought suggests that the phenomenon of compactation and " crystallization " of the nuclear material obscures structural patterns that might otherwise be revealed by fine structural analysis. It is difficult to explain why just at a stage when the electron microscope fails to reveal structural detail of a periodic nature, the birefringence of sperm nuclei reaches a maximum (SATO and INOUÉ, 1964).

Both of these problems, i.e, the structure of the " post-nuclear cap " and nuclear organization, are amenable to study by the fine structural technique known as freeze-etching which has been developed during the past few years. This method provides at least two advantages over conventional chemical fixation studies which can provide fresh insight into the structural problems introduced above. The first of these advantages is that the cells can be examined without chemical fixation of any kind. The only step necessary in their preparation consists of freezing to low temperatures. Techniques have been developed which assure that many species of spermatozoa can not only be well preserved by freezing, but can be revived after thawing to demonstrate motility and fertilizing capacity (PARKES, 1960). The second advantage is related to the replication technique employed in making freeze-etching preparations. This type of specimen reveals extended surface views of internal as well as external cellular structures including membranes and membrane associated material. It is this property which makes the freeze-etching method particularly valuable in the study of the structure and distribution of the " post-nuclear cap ". Also, the factors which obscure or alter nuclear detail in chemically fixed sperm might be expected to play little or no role in cells prepared by the physical process or freezing. This paper will extend freeze-etching studies initially undertaken with bovine spermatozoa (KOEHLER, 1966 a, b) to several other vertebrate species.

MATERIALS AND METHODS

Spermatozoa of the rainbow trout (*Salmo gardeneri*), rabbits, and humans were the primary specimens utilized in this study. Trout sperm were obtained by stripping mature fish of milt, rabbit sperm were collected by artificial vagina and human sperm from normal students by masturbation. The trout sperm were diluted with fish Ringer containing glycerol to give a final concentration of 10%. Rabbit and human sperm were treated in the same manner as bovine sperm studied earlier (KOEHLER, 1966 a) using a milk-glycerol diluent and incubated at 4° C several hours before freezing. Small droplets of concentrated (centrifuged) spermatozoa were frozen either slowly or ultra-rapidly and stored in liquid nitrogen until needed for the freeze-etching preparation. Instrumentation and the methods used for freeze-etching are the same as described earlier (KOEHLER, 1966 a).

Aliquots of the freshly ejaculated spermatozoa were also taken for chemical fixation in each case. No glycerolation or ether pretreatment was utilized prior to chemical fixation. One percent osmic acid in 0.10 M phosphate buffer was used either as primary fixative or subsequent to glutaraldehyde fixation (2.4% in 0.10 M phosphate buffer). Fish Ringer appeared to be a more effective vehicle for the fixative in the case of trout sperm. These cells were exceptionally difficult to fix well. Extensive membrane damage was the rule rather than the exception with all fixatives tried, including permanganate. Chemically fixed spermatozoa were embedded in Epon 812, sectioned with a Porter Blum II ultramicrotome, and examined in an RCA EMU-3 G electron microscope after staining with uranyl acetate and lead citrate.

RESULTS

Fig. 1 illustrates a freeze-etching image a rabbit spermatozoon head. Consideration of the shadow direction (arrow, top left) and the shape of the sperm head lead to the conclusion that this is a view of the *outer* aspect. Features of the portion covering the acrosomal region include clusters of small, closely packed particles (*P*) interrupted by circular areas (*C*) which are completely free of particles. The boundary between acrosomal and post-nuclear regions (*B*) bears a remarkable " picket fence "-like array of uniform triangular structures. Analysis reveals that the " pickets " with points toward the acrosome lie in the plane of the rest of the material seen in association with the post-nuclear region, and that the complimentary triangles (pointing toward the tail) lie beneath this layer. The rest of the post-nuclear region bears small elongated depressions (*D*) except near the implantation fossa where " stria " (*S*) of material coursing at various angles can be observed.

Occasionally, images are seen which can be interpreted as revealing the mirror image impression of this membrane complex. Fig. 2 illustrates such a view. Notice that the so-called complimentary pickets (with points facing the tail) now appear to be elevations rather than recessed structures. Similarly, the former depressions (Fig. 1) dispersed throughout the post-nuclear region are now seen as elevations and conversely, the stria surrounding the implantation fossa appear recessed rather than elevated. In the region covering the acrosome, the smooth circular domains and surrounding particle laden areas are much less distinct. Fig. 3 shows a view of a rabbit sperm head from chemically fixed and embedded material in the approximate plane of the flattened aspect. Included in the section are portions of nuclear material (*N*), the acrosome (*A*), and post-nuclear cap complex. Notice that in the equatorial region one can detect several profiles of triangular structures (circle) which are undoubtedly equivalent to the freeze-etching " pickets ". The electron dense material of the post-nuclear region can be seen to be continuous with the pickets. The sectioned equivalents of the small depressions (*D*, Fig. 1) are seen as electron transparent specks in the homogeneous matrix of post-nuclear cap material.

A freeze-etching image of a human spermatozoon is seen in Fig. 4. The acrosome-post-nuclear cap junction is not nearly so regularly constructed as that of the rabbit spermatozoon but is nevertheless quite obvious in freeze-etching images. The anterior, or acrosomal region of the head (*A*) is covered by a rather uniform granular textured membrane, whereas the posterior is more coarsely ornamented with ridges and cords of material. The unique scalloped " belt " (*T*) toward the base of the head is a distinctive feature of human spermatozoa.

Spermatozoa of lower vertebrates appear not to display many of the features described above in mammalian species. Fig. 5 illustrates several rainbow trout sperm head surfaces as prepared by freeze-etching. Nothing in the way of unusual or distinctive landmarks can be detected on such surfaces. The unsual, randomly distributed small particles often associated with cellular membranes are present but no highly differentiated regions similar to those seen on mammalian spermatozoa can be visualized.

Surface aspects of sperm head structure are, of course, not the only relationships that can be studied in freeze-etch preparations. Quite often the sperm are fractured in a way which reveals internal organization including that of the nucleus. Fig. 6 shows a rabbit sperm head which has been cross fractured perpendicular to its flattened dimension. The acrosomal material (*A*) is finely granular and quite homogeneous in appearance. The nucleus is characterized by the occurrence of well organized stacks of lamellae extending the entire length of the nucleus. The number of layers appear to be fairly constant among various rabbit sperm nuclei and usually lie between ten and twelve. Extended surface views of such lamellae have also been seen suggesting that these structures are not filamentous, but plate-like in construction. Although the lamellar organization has been observed in a number of mammalian sperm nuclei (as discussed below), this structural pattern is by no means universal among vertebrates. Cross fractures of trout sperm nuclei (Fig. 7) reveal only rounded clumps of closely packed material exhibiting no obvious periodic order.

Spermatozoa were also examined in a polarizing microscope to determine if birefringence could be detected and if it depended on sperm orientation. Sperm heads having a flattened dimension (rabbit, human) showed birefringence only when the cells were oriented with their flattened surface parallel to the optic axis. The ellipsoidal trout sperm exhibited birefringence which did not depend in any obvious way on cell orientation.

Conclusion

It was shown in earlier freeze-etching studies on bovine spermatozoa (Koehler, 1966 a, b) that the area of the post-nuclear cap is occupied by a morphologically recognizable complex consisting of several components. Among these are a compact cytoplasmic layer having close contact with both nuclear and plasma membranes and a system of " basal stria " composed of oriented cords of material surrounding the implantation fossa. Although a finely filamentous or granular material can be detected in the post-nuclear region in thin sections of many mammalian spermatozoa, the stria are either sufficiently dispersed and irregular to remain undetected by the sectioning approach or are altered by chemical fixation.

A similar system has now been described in the case of rabbit spermatozoa. The basal stria are not as extensive in number or regular in orientation as seen in the bovine spermatozoa. Preliminary observations on human sperm show even less organizational detail in the post-nuclear area and studies with trout sperm indicate a complete lack of structural differentiation in this region. Since the size of the sperm heads in this series progressively decreases from almost 10 microns (bull) to less than 2 microns (trout), it is not unreasonable to suggest that the basal stria and post-nuclear cap complex act as a reinforcement to maintain the integrity of the basal membrane system and head-neck attachment. Mechanical stability of the membranes in this region has been noted in chemically fixed material and this kind of function for the post-nuclear cap has been suggested before (see Fawcett, 1965); however, the freeze-etching observations may make such a speculation more convincing. The basal striations do indeed give the appearance of a " basket-weave "–like reinforcing structure around the implantation fossa.

The organization of the acrosome-post-nuclear cap junction appears to be a definite characteristic of the species. In the bull (Koehler, 1966 a), this junction is rather irregular with some small excursions between the two layers. In the case of the rabbit, however, this region is characterized by a precise array of triangular contours as if cut by pinking shears. The transition in human spermatozoa is less precise than in the rabbit, and somewhat similar to that of the bull. Penetration of the zona pellucida as well as the egg itself in many mammals seems to involve a lateral aspect of the sperm head (see review by Austin, 1968). Pikó and Tyler (1967) have suggested that sperm penetration in the rat initially involves the post-nuclear cap area, and Barros and Franklin (1968) have convincingly shown that sperm penetration in the hamster involves membrane apposition in the region of the equatorial segment. It is tempting to speculate that this acrosomal-post-nuclear cap junction region may play an important role in sperm-egg recognition, attachment or other interaction.

In the Salmonid sperm an acrosome is apparently lacking (GINSBERG, 1963) and little, if any, post-nuclear cap exists, so that the appearance of a relatively smooth surface covering the head in freeze-etch preparations, free of junctions, stria, or other ornamentations should not be surprising.

Very few would quarrel with the contention that the term post-nuclear cap does not convey an accurate description of this sometimes delicate and vague structure, particularly as seen in sectioned material. If, however, we discard the term as FAWCETT (1965) suggests, we are faced with finding a new nomenclature to more adequately describe this structure while at the same time coexisting with the extensive post-nuclear cap terminology already well entrenched in the literature. The " intermembranous dense lamina " which FAWCETT suggests is an appropriately descriptive term, however, it does not immediately relate the uninitiated to the fact that this is the equivalent of the classical post-nuclear cap. An alternative might be to let the admittedly inadequate term stand while at the same time defining precisely the morphological features which we would assign to this region. The offending " cap " might alternatively be replaced by " lamina " or " sheath ". The freeze-etching work in particular has shown that the post-nuclear cap in some species consists of a rather elaborate and complex arrangement of membrane associated, cytoplasmic material. The densely staining region which early workers identified as a uniform structure is most likely composed of several descrete but interlinked components as visualized by fine structural methods. Thus, in terms of semantics, the post-nuclear cap takes up a position somewhat anlogous to the light microscopical basement membrane which has been shown to consist of several components (basal lamina, collagen, etc.) and indeed is not a membrane at all. The term basement membrane, however, remains a useful term despite its limitations and so probably will the post-nuclear cap at least until the precise role of this region can be determined and a more functionally oriented nomenclature established.

The nuclear lamellae seen in the rabbit spermatozoa provide an identical image to that seen in the bovine sperm even to the numbers of such lamellae present (10 to 12). The lamellae are observed in spermatozoa which are either cooled quite slowly (best for viability) or in those quenched ultra-rapidly and are, therefore, probably not a result of crystallization phenomena during preparation. The lamellae represent one of the few instances where freeze-etching preparations have demonstrated a structure not observable with conventional fixation and sectioning methods. The freeze-etching result is, however, compatible with results of polarization microscope observations made in our laboratory and elsewhere. RANDALL and FRIEDLANDER (1950) showed that strong birefringence is exhibited by flattened mammalian spermatozoa (ram) only when the head was tipped on its side. Sperm with similarly shaped heads (bull, rabbit) were observed in our laboratory to exhibit similar birefringence behavior. The ellipsoidal trout sperm, on the other hand, appear to lack the directional dependence on birefringence and also the nuclear lamellations. The elegant work of INOUÉ and SATO (1966) has shown that the arrangement of DNA in spermatozoa of certain insects can be described as a " coiled coil " giving rise to helical patterns of birefringence. The nuclear lamellae described here cannot be easily explained on the same terms, but the concept of a continuous DNA superstructure including confluence of chromosome segments is consistent with the lamellar arrangement particularly since there appear to be interconnections between lamellae.

These preliminary observations can form the basis of a great deal of subsequent experimentation including the freeze-etching analysis of changes which take place in nuclear structure during chemical fixation.

Acknowledgement. — The author was fortunate in having the cooperation of Dr. DONALD SMITH, Department of Obstetrics and Gynecology who supplied the rabbit spermatozoa and Dr. LAUREN R. DONALDSON, School of Fisheries who provided trout spermatozoa. Mrs. J. KRIVACÉK assisted in many phases of the work.

REFERENCES

AUSTIN C. R. (1968) – *Ultrastructure of Fertilization*, Chapter 2, page 51. Holt, Rinehart and Winston, New York.

BARROS C. and FRANKLIN L. E. (1968) – *Behavior of the gamete membranes during sperm entry into the mammalian egg.* « J. Cell Biol. », 37, c13-c18.

DASS C. M. S. and RIS H. (1958) – *Submicroscopic organization of the nucleus during spermiogenesis in the grasshopper.* « J. Biophys. Biochem. Cytol. », 4, 129–132.

FAWCETT D. W. (1965) – *The anatomy of the mammalian spermatozoa with particular reference to the guinea pig.* « Z. für Zellforsch. », 67, 279–296.

FAWCETT D. W. and ITO S. (1965) – *The fine structure of bat spermatozoa.* – « Am. J. Anat. », 116, 567–610.

GATENBY J. B. and WIGODER S. B. (1929) – *The post-nuclear body in the spermatogenesisis of* Cavia cobaya *and other animals.* « Proc. Roy. Soc. », B, 104, 471–480.

GIBBONS I. R. and BRADFIELD J. R. G. (1956) – *The fixation of cell nuclei by osmium tetroxide.* – Biochem. Biophys. Acta, 22, 506–513.

GINSBERG A. S. (1963) – *Sperm-egg association and its relationship to the activation of the egg in Salmonid fishes.* « J. Embryol. and Exptl. Morph. », 2, 13–33.

INOUÉ S. and SATO H. (1966) – *Deoxyribonucleic acid arrangement in living sperm. Molecular Architecture in Cell Physiology.* Hayashi and Szent-Gyorgyi (eds.). Prentice Hall Inc., New Jersey.

KOEHLER J. K. (1966 a) – *Fine structure observations in frozen-etched bovine spermatozoa.* « J. Ultrastructures Res. », 16, 359–375.

KOEHLER J. K. (1966 b) – *Electron microscope observations on the post-nuclear region of bovine spermatozoa. Correlation between frozen-etched and chemically fixed material.* « Anat. Rec. », 154, 370 (Abstract).

NATH V. (1965) – *Animal Gametes (Male).* Chapter 1, page 10. – Asia Publishing House, New York.

PARKES A. S. (1960) – *Marshall's Physiology of Reproduction.* A. S. Parkes (ed.), Chapter 9 – Longmans Green and Co., London.

PIKÓ L. and TYLER A. (1964) – *Fine structural studies of sperm penetration in the bat.* Proceedings of Fifth International Congress of Animal Reproduction, Trento. Vol. II, 372–377.

RANDALL J. J. and FRIEDLANDER M. A. G. (1950) – *The microstructure of ram spermatozoa.* « Exptl. Cell Res. », 1, 1–32.

SATO H. and INOUÉ S. (1964) – *Condensation of the sperm nucleus and alignment of DNA molecules during spermiogenesis in* Loligo pealii. « Biol. Bull. », 127, 357.

EXPLANATION OF FIGURES

Fig. 1. – Rabbit sperm head as seen from external view. The plasma membrane over the acrosomal region is characterized by patches of small particles (*P*) and circular " smoth " areas (*C*). The acrosome-" post-nuclear cap " boundary (*B*) is the site of a sharply serrated band. Small depressions (*D*) are uniformly scattered over the post-nuclear cap and cord-like stria (*S*) occur around the implantation fossa. ×18,500.

Fig. 2. – Rabbit sperm head membrane complex as seen in impression view. The pattern of relief of the various components is reversed to that shown in Fig. 1. ×22,000.

Fig. 3. – Chemically fixed rabbit sperm sectioned tangentially along the flattened surface of the head. Nuclear (*N*) and acrosomal (*A*) material appears in the plane of section along with a portion of surface structure (circle) clearly showing the serrated pattern visualized in the freeze-etchings. ×11,500.

Fig. 4. – Human spermatozoan head exhibiting a uniform particle studded acrosomal region (*A*) and a characteristic scalloped belt (*T*). ×28,000.

Fig. 5. – Several rainbow trout sperm heads are seen in this freeze-etch preparation. No regional, surface differences can be detected. ×18,000.

Fig. 6. – Rabbit spermatozoon cross fractured to expose internal nuclear structure. The lamellar arrangement of the nucleoplasm is clearly illustrated. Acrosomal material (*A*). ×27,000.

Fig. 7. – When trout sperm are seen in cross fractured views such as this, one can detect no lamellar ordering. Small closely packed clumps of material appear to fill the nucleus. ×21,000.

Discussion

NICANDER. – 1) BEDFORD has recently demonstrated that the first area of the sperm head in rabbits to make contact with the egg plasma membrane does include the equatorial region of the acrosome.

2) Could the columns you see at the base of the head correspond to the chromatin threads seen in this area in conventional electron microscopy?

KOEHLER. – 1) Thank you. I am happy to hear about this confirmation.

2) I am not certain that I understand what you mean by « chromatin threads » at the base of the head. In any case, the columns (cords) seen in freeze–etchings appear to be surface structures not concerned with intranuclear material.

FAWCETT. – Do you believe that the basal belt which you describe might not be the same as the basal plate which has also been described as having periodic substructure?

KOEHLER. – I feel that the basal belt is a surface or near-surface structure which could not be identical to the basal plate which is deeply recessed in the insertion fossa.

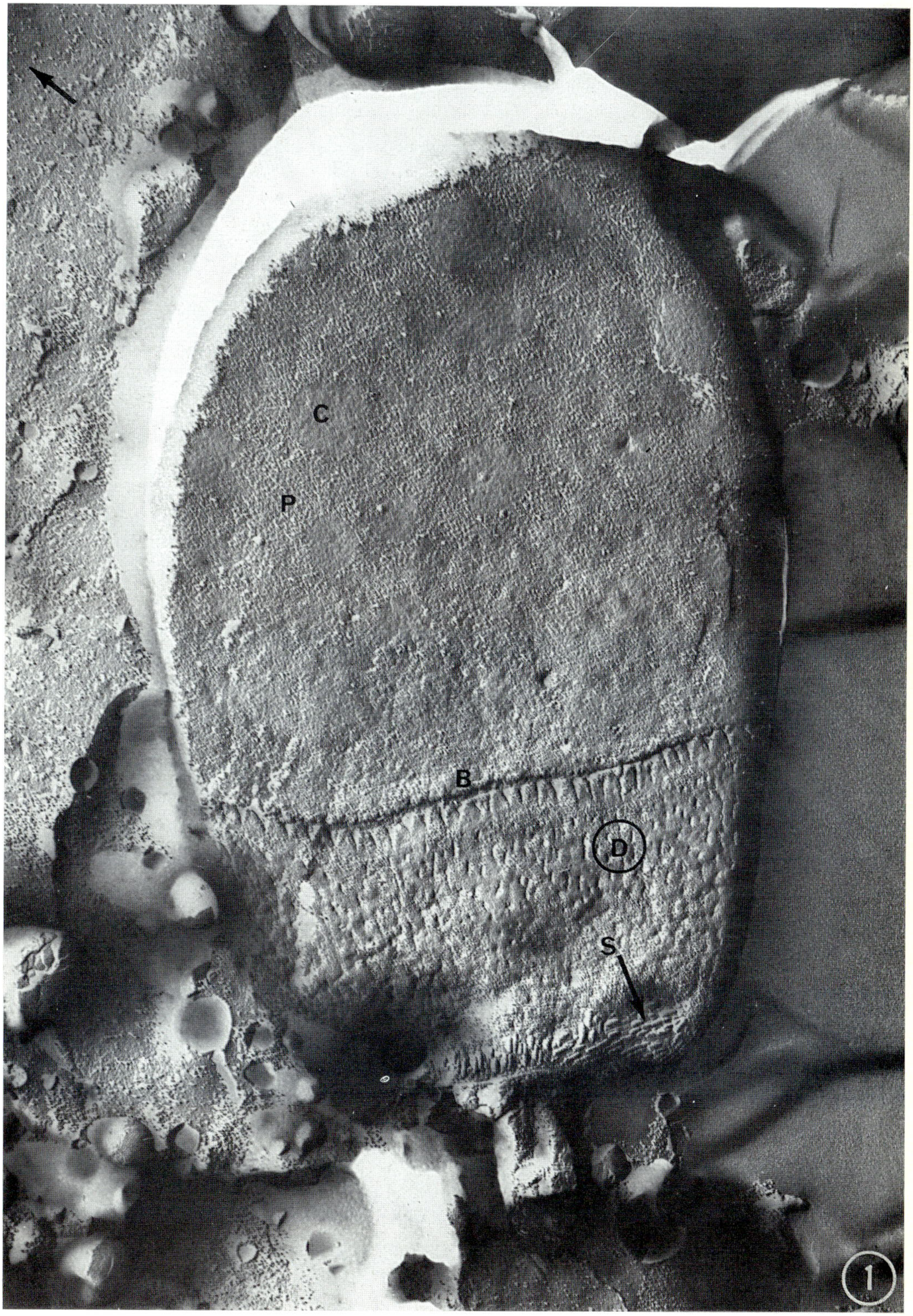
C
P
B
D
S
1

JAMES K. KOEHLER – *Freeze-etching studies on spermatozoa with particular reference to nuclear and post-nuclear cap structure.*

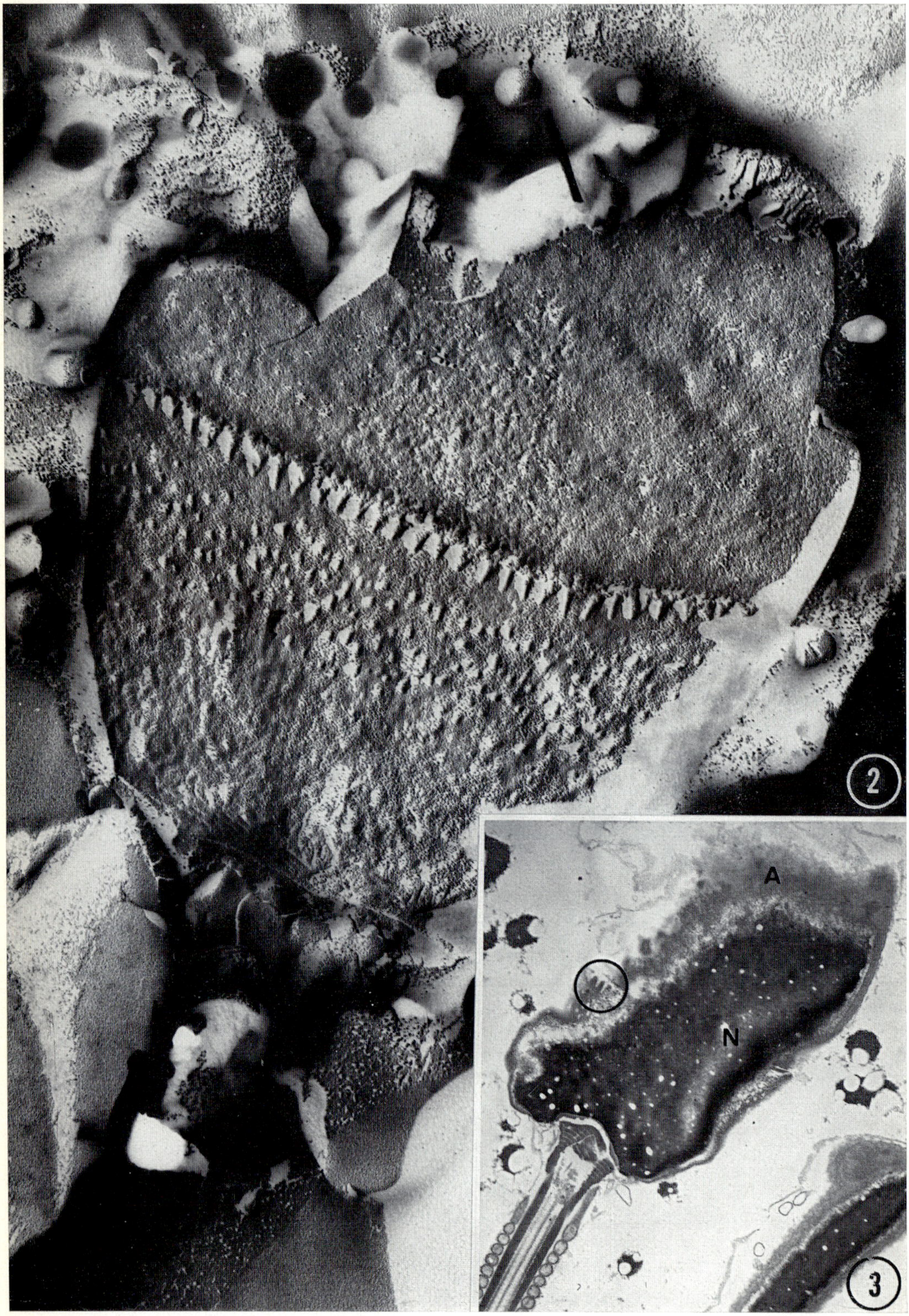

JAMES K. KOEHLER – *Freeze-etching studies on spermatozoa with particular reference to nuclear and post-nuclear cap structure.*

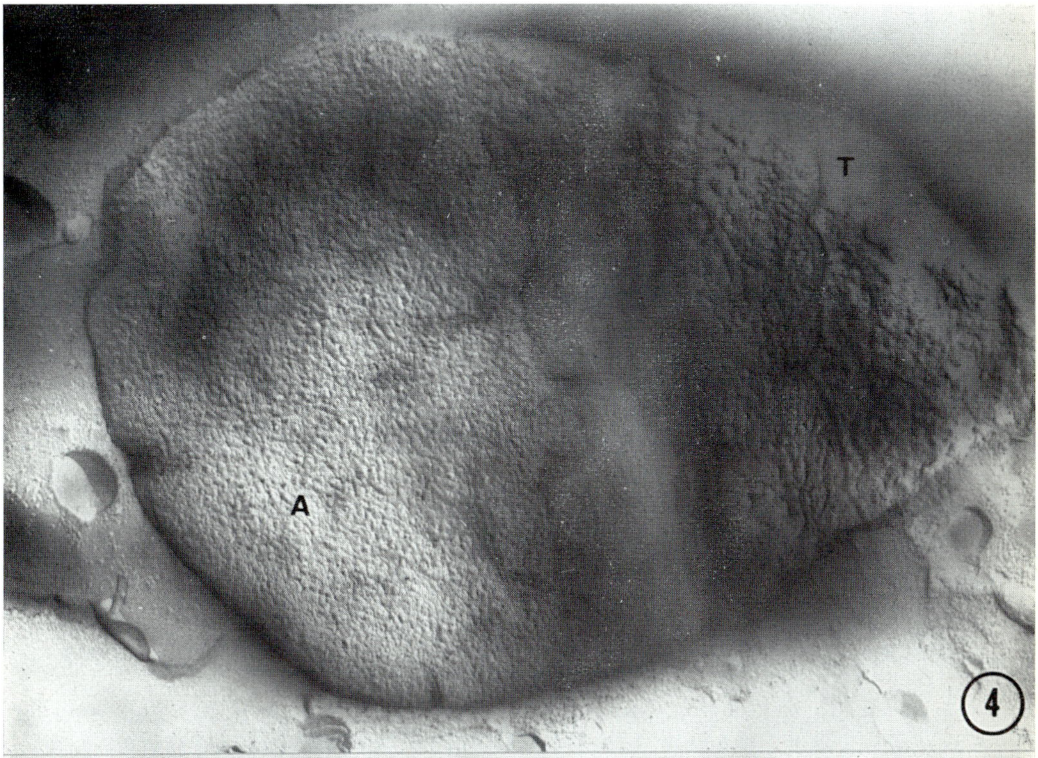

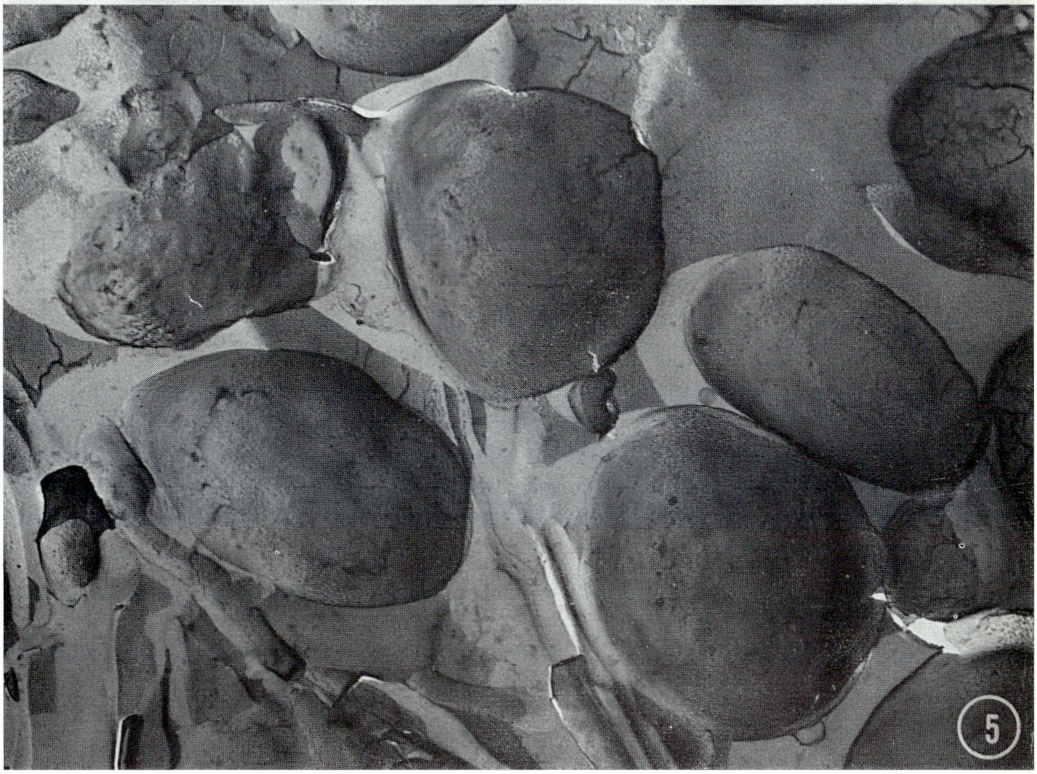

James K. Koehler – *Freeze-etching studies on spermatozoa with particular reference to nuclear and post-nuclear cap structure.*

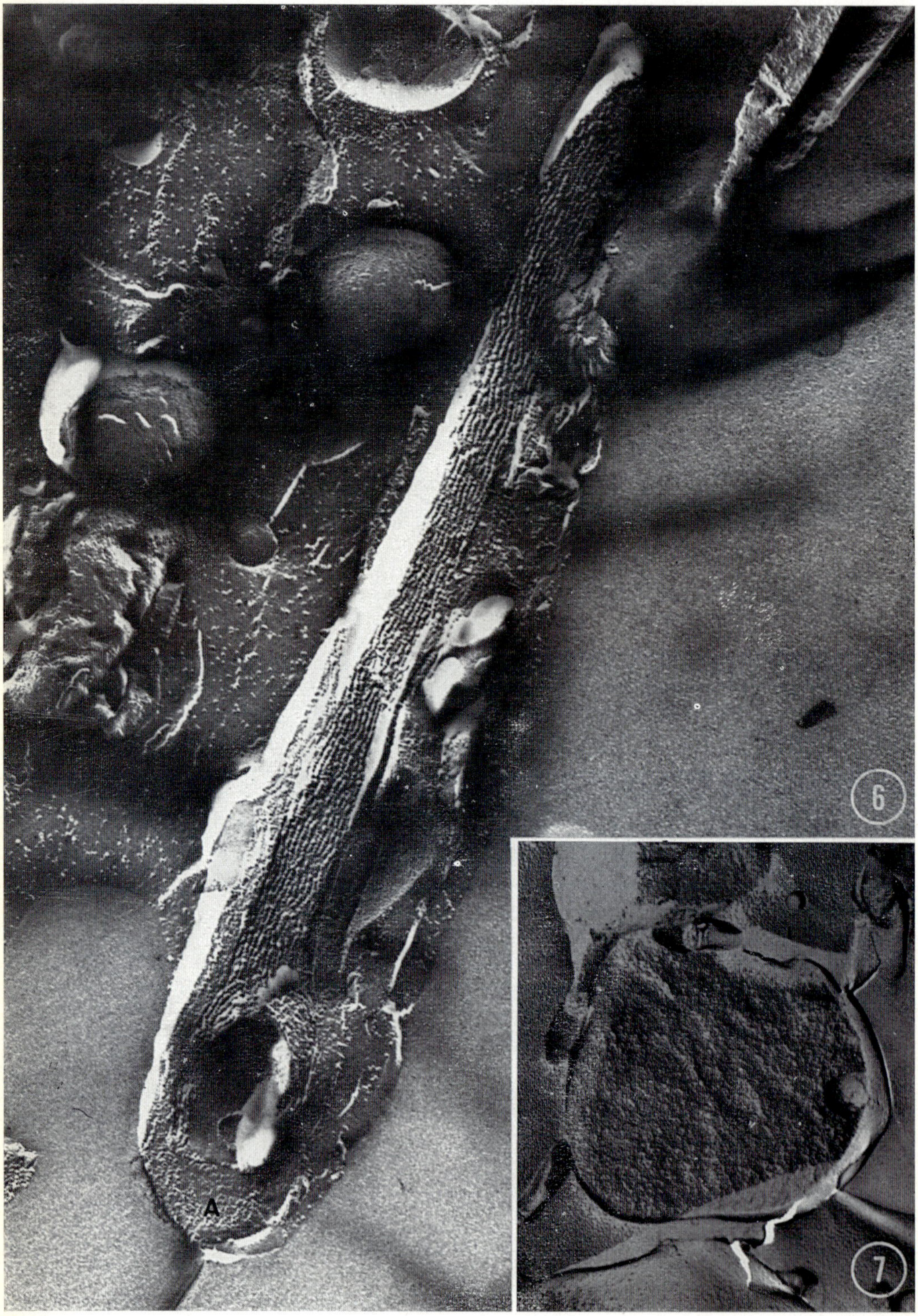

M. ELISA PEROTTI (*)

THE NECK REGION IN MATURE SPERM OF *DROSOPHILA MELANOGASTER* (**)

SUMMARY. — The neck region in mature sperm of *Drosophila melanogaster* contains a short centriole derivative encased within a deep nuclear "implantation fossa". The centriole derivative is conical in shape with an apical tapering end, it is accompanied for most of its length by the principal mitochondrial derivative, whereas the second mitochondrial derivative appears near its distal end. Finely granular electronopaque material is present in large amount within the nucleus indentation and closely surrounds the centriole derivative, the mitochondrial derivatives and the nucleus caudal part. The centriole derivative consists of 9 peripheral triplets and a central pairs of fibres. The triplet arrangement differs from that of triplets of a typical centriole and a rather unusual system of connections is present among them. All the fibres of the centriole derivative are continuous with the fibres of the tail axial filament: namely, the central fibres with the tail central pair, the triplet C-fibres with the outer fibres, the triplet A–and B–fibres with the A–and B–subfibres of the peripheral doublets.

RIASSUNTO. — La zona del « collo » dello spermatozoo maturo di *Drosophila melanogaster* contiene un derivato centriolare molto corto incastrato entro una profonda incavatura del nucleo (« fossa d'impianto »). Tale derivato ha forma conica con estremità appuntita diretta cefalicamente ed è accompagnato per quasi tutta la sua lunghezza dal derivato mitocondriale principale, mentre il secondo derivato mitocondriale compare soltanto all'estremità caudale del derivato centriolare. Nell'incavatura del nucleo è presente materiale elettropaco finemente granulare che circonda il derivato centriolare, i due derivati mitocondriali e l'estremità caudale del nucleo. Il derivato centriolare è costituito da nove triplette periferiche e da due fibre centrali; le triplette differiscono per la loro organizzazione dalle tipiche triplette centriolari e sono connesse tra di loro da un insolito sistema di legami. Tutte le fibre del derivato centriolare si continuano con le fibre del filamento assiale del flagello: le fibre centrali con la coppia centrale, le fibre C delle triplette con le fibre esterne, le fibre A e B delle triplette rispettivamente con le subfibre A e B delle coppie periferiche.

At the submicroscopic level, the neck region has been extensively studied in different vertebrates, especially in mammals. In different species the axial filament complex is derived from the distal centriole, the centriole pair migrating to a juxtanuclear position early during morphogenesis of germ cells. In mature sperm, the proximal centriole, when present, retains its typical configuration and does not exhibit any relationship with the flagellum. The distal centriole is oriented in the axis of the flagellum and constitutes

(*) Institute of Human Anatomy University of Milano. – Italy.

(**) Research supported by the grant No. 115–1150–1080 from C.N.R.

its basal body. It usually undergoes so deep modification during sperm maturation that in most of the mature sperms so far studied it is no longer identifiable. The loss of a typical basal body is generally associated with the presence within the neck of structures like homogeneous or segmented " columns ", " neck cylinder ", " côtes ", etc., so that the connecting piece is regarded as a modified centriole only because it is usually accepted that a basal-body structure is essential for movement of cilia and flagella.

Only scarce attention has been paid so far to this region in mature sperm of Insects. Therefore, we have carried out investigations on the completely mature sperm of *Drosophila melanogaster*.

Fig. 1 shows an early spermatid before nucleus elongation. The flagellar centriole is already inserted against the nucleus. In a later stage (Fig. 2), when the nucleus begins to elongate and before the chromatin condensation, an electron-opaque structure is associated with the flagellar centriole, consisting of electron-opaque grains closely packed. Some vacuoles are present within it, which, as the cell differentiates, reduce in number up to two. The occurrence of a similar pattern seems to be widespread among most of the insects so far studied and observed in *Drosophila* itself (ANDERSON, 1967; SHOUP, 1967), and called " juxtanuclear body " or, more recently, " centriole adjunct ". At this stage of maturation, ANDERSON (1967) observed in *Drosophila* spermatid a second centriole arranged perpendicular to the distal end of the flagellar centriole. It seems therefore that the terminology usually employed for vertebrate sperm centriole should be reversed here, since it is the flagellar centriole (corresponding to the distal centriole in other sperms) which is juxtapposed to nucleus whereas the second centriole, not connected with flagellum, lies in a distal position with respect to the nucleus.

As far as the mature sperm is concerned, only serial sectioning allowed to elucidate the fate of the two centrioles and the organization of the neck region in *Drosophila*.

Figs. 3 to 8 are serial sections from proximal to distal. Near its caudal end, the nucleus displays a little indentation where some electron-opaque material, highly condensed, is present. In more distal sections the indentation becomes deeper and the electron-opaque material more abundant and extending with thin laminar expansions adherent to the nucleus (Fig. 4). This substance is very compact and without vacuoles when compared to the spermatid centriole adjunct to which it corresponds in localization. In a more caudal position (Fig. 5), the nucleus size abruptly decreases and within the dense material an oval structure appears. It displays a dense core and a wall consisting of numerous microtubules cross-sectioned. They are so closely apposed that it is difficult to count them exactly. Between them, some triplets of fibres, reminiscent the centriolar ones, can be identified. One of the triplets microtubules, (the C microtubule of the centriole terminology) appears less developed than the others (A and B). More distally (Fig. 6), the structure of this complex changes as follows: (1) it becomes roundish, within it 9 triplets of fibres are present and spaced enough to identify easily the centriole blade; (2) the C fibres are here as developed as the A and B fibres; (3) in the centre of the centriole a pair of tubules is present similar in size and shape to the triplet members. The angle formed by the triplet plane with the centriole radius is much greater than in the former section, thus determining an increase of the centriole diameter. Between the centriole and the nucleus a new structure appears on a side of the centriole (Fig. 6), which the serial sections allowed to identify as the principal mitochondrial derivative. Also the total cross diameter of the sperm is increasing, so that in the next section (Fig. 7) it attains the value of 0.4 μ which will be retained for most of the sperm length. At this level, the mitochondrial derivative size is larger, the nucleus is reduced to a very thin crescent-shaped portion

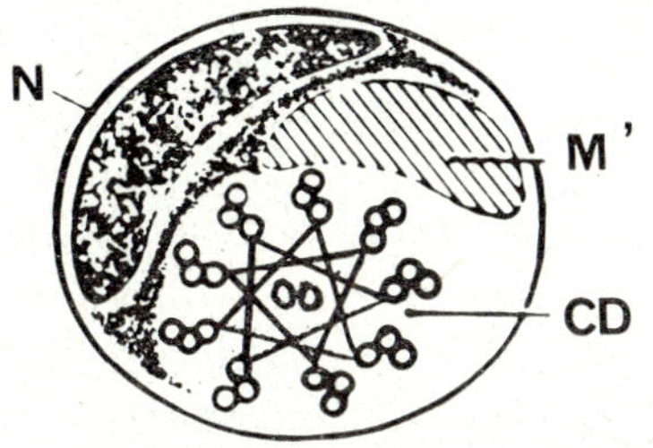

Diag. 1. – Diagram illustrating the system of connections present among the centriole triplets and forming a 9–pointed star pattern.

N = nucleus *M'* = principal mitochondrial derivative *CD* = centriole derivative.

eccentrically placed with respect to the sperm central axis. The centriole organization is changing also, as the C fibres are no more aligned with A and B but are laterally displaced and connected with a dense granule (Fig. 7). Meanwhile, the A and B fibres are tilted to an orientation tangential to the centriole wall. The secondary fibres are present nearby the A fibres. The granular material is still present between nucleus, mitochondrial derivative and forms a partial sheath around the centriole apparatus.

Eventually, at the most caudal level (Fig. 8), the nucleus has disappeared, the principal mitochondrial derivative already shows a paracrystalline structure and also the second mitochondrial derivative is present. The displacement of the triplets members is completed so that the fibres arrangement typical for the tail axial filament is recognizable, except for the lack of radial links between central and peripheral fibres.

Some electronopaque material is still present between the principal and the second mitochondrial derivative. From the triplets of fibres two electronopaque lines, 80 Å wide, diverge at a constant angle of 60 degrees (Fig. 8) and connect a triplet with two others. Presumably, a complex system of links is present forming a 9–pointed star connecting the triplets three by three (Diag. 1). Probably, the connecting system of every group of triplets lies in its own plane, since in a section only the links related to a triade of triplets is present.

The flagellar basal body is on the whole long 0.1–0.15 μ and its three-dimensional feature is conical with the tapering pointed end facing the nucleus. The " implantation fossa " present at the caudal end of the nucleus appears in *Drosophila* sperm particularly deep so that the relationship between nucleus, apical basis of the tail and the mitochondrial derivative is particularly intimate. Recent observations (FAWCETT and ITO, 1965; ANDERSON and PERSONNE, 1967) pointed out that mitochondria can occur also in the neck region. In the *Drosophila* sperm the mitochondrial derivative extend very cephalad up to the nucleus so that it bears very close and extensive relations to the flagellar basal body. The fact that in practice there is nearly no area in the neck region free of mitochondrial derivative and that the principal mitochondrial derivative is here so closely applied to the basal body as in the tail to the axial filament, strongly supports the idea that, like mitochondria in the neck region of bat and *Helix*, it is essential for the functions of this region, probably providing energy for the role of initiation of the wave movement ascribed to the basal bodies.

The results of this research demonstrated that only one centriole derivative, whose typical centriole structure has undergone modification, is present within the neck. Its centriolar origin can be deduced only from the presence of triplets of fibres, which, on the other hand, for the most of their extent do not display the arrangement typical for the centriole triplets. Serial sectioning showed that the tail fibres are continuous with the fibres of the centriole derivative. In particular, it seems noteworthy the fact that the axial filament outer fibres are continuous with the C fibres, the central fibres with the central pair of the basal body. This is of particular interest as far as the outer fibres are concerned. In fact, the presence in the axial filament of a row of fibres outer to the peripheral doublets appears to be widespread among most of the Insects so far studied. These fibres (BAIRATI and PEROTTI, this Symposium) have been demonstrated to have a microtubular ultrastructure similar to that of the other axial filament fibres. The origin of the outer row of fibres has been so far still unsettled in all cases of which we are aware, as well as, on the other hand, the fate of the C–fibre of basal bodies.

CAMERON (1965) stated that in *Tenebrio* sperm each outer fibre originates from the B–subfibre of the corresponding doublet. This interpretation now should be reinvestigated in view of our observations about the continuity between C–fibres and outer fibres existing in mature sperm, and it would be interesting to elucidate the behaviour of the outer fibres in other insects to establish the possibility of homologies between the different species endowed with this additional set of fibres, with particular reference to those in which these fibres apparently do not show a tubular structure. Since it is generally accepted that the tubular components of cilia and flagella are contractile elements, it derives that all the members of the connecting piece play in *Drosophila* a tensile role. This is of interest for comparative remarks, as it is still under discussion the role of structures such as the dense " columns " present within the neck of vertebrates and mollusca sperms. They are supposed to be contractile, with particular reference to those exhibiting a cross striated structure (FAWCETT and ITO, 1965; ANDERSON and PERSONNE,

1967), and probably to contribute with the connecting piece to bend an elaborate mid-piece.

The presence for the largest extension of the centriole derivative of two central fibres and of the links between the triplets testifies for the profound changes that have occurred in this structure as compared to a typical centriole. Actually, the presence of a central pair of fibres is not typical of a true centriole. A central pair of fibres is present in the centriole of snake sperm (HAMILTON and FAWCETT, 1968), but detailed information about their extent is not provided.

While in all the other instances so far studied the central fibres appear to end before the beginning of the typical centriole, we have seen the central pair run the length of the basal body from the flagellar shaft to a point very close to its proximal end, namely, to the electrondense centre of the most apical portion of centriole.

As to the links organization, the functional significance of the star-shaped pattern can only be a matter of speculation. These links appear when the triplet members displacement has begun, but the radial spokes characteristic of the axial filament are not yet present. They might therefore substitute the radial spokes for the functions generally ascribed to them in localizing the effects of the fibres contraction to the particular region of the flagellum in which they are taking place. Links are commonly present in basal body of cilia, although, unlike this case, they usually connect adjacent triplets. Anyway, this system of links does not correspond in morphology to the cart-wheel, with hub and spokes, characteristic of basal bodies of cilia from different organism. A pattern of connections similar to that observed in the centriole of *Drosophila* sperm has been found in the flagellum basal body of *Clamydomonas* (LANG, 1963). Corresponding comparative remarks on the flagellar basal bodies of other sperms cannot be made as extensive investigations on this subject have not been so far carried out.

As to the second centriole observed by ANDERSON (1967) in spermatid, it is impossible to state whether it is completely lost during sperm maturation or, deeply modified, takes part in some way in the formation of the neck in mature sperm.

Some comments are appropriate relative to the compact electron-opaque material present in the neck between nucleus, centriole and mit. derivative. It corresponds in localization to the juxtanuclear body or centriolar adjunct observed in spermatid. Since it is still present in large amount in mature sperm, it can be excluded that it represents precursor substances for the formation of microtubules (either of the " manchette " or of the flagellar shaft) as suggested for the pericentriolar densities observed in crayfish spermatid (ANDERSON and ELLIS, 1967). On the contrary, as it is more abundant in mature sperm than in spermatid, it is possible that the material originating from disintegration of the " manchette " microtubules, which present in spermatid are completely absent from mature sperm, contributes to the increase in density and amount of this substance. The principal function of the centriole adjunct in insects is still conjectural. Recently (BACCETTI *et al.*, 1969) it has been stated that it consists of ribonucleoproteins. In default of histochemical data on this region in *Drosophila* sperm, it can only be conjectured that this material, which closely sheathes the neck components encasing them in a coherent structure, might act as a device for maintaining cohesion among the neck components and the nucleus during flagellar bending. Similar distribution of electron-opaque material has been observed in the neck of Lampetra (STANLEY, 1967). On the other hand, this material differs in distribution and extent from the so-called "basal plate" present in mammals and snake sperm, whose origin from the proximal centriole has been recently pointed out (HAMILTON and FAWCETT, 1968).

REFERENCES

ANDERSON W. A. (1967) – *Cytodifferentiation of spermatozoa of* Drosophila melanogaster: *the effect of elevated temperature on spermiogenesis.* «Mol. Gen. Genetics», 99, 257–273.

ANDERSON W. A. and ELLIS R. A. (1967) – *Cytodifferentiation of the crayfish spermatozoa: acrosome formation, trans formation of mitochondria and development of microtubules.* «Z. Zellforsch. Mikroskop. Anat.», 77, 80–94.

ANDERSON W. A. and PERSONNE P. (1967) – *The fine structure of the neck region of spermatozoa of* Helix aspersa. «J. Microscopie», 6, 1033–1042.

BACCETTI B., DALLAI R. and ROSATI F. (1969) – *The spermatozoon of Arthropoda.* III. *The lowest holometabolic insects.* «J. Microscopie.», 8, 233–248.

CAMERON M. L. (1965) – *Some details of ultrastructure in the development of flagellar fibres of* Tenebrio *sperm.* «Can. J. Zool.», 43, 1005–1010.

FAWCETT D. W. and ITO S. (1965) – *The fine structure of bat spermatozoa.* «Am. J. Anat.», 116, 567–610.

HAMILTON D. W. and FAWCETT D. W. (1968) – *Unusual features of the neck and middle piece of snake spermatozoa.* «J. Ultrastruct. Res.», 23, 81–97.

LANG N. G. (1963) – *An additional ultrastructural component of flagella.* «J. Cell. Biol.», 19, 631–634.

SHOUP J. R. (1967) – *Spermiogenesis in wild type and a male mutant of* Drosophila melanogaster. «J. Cell. Biol.», 32, 663–675.

STANLEY H. P. (1967) – *The fine structure of spermatozoa in the lamprey* Lampetra planeri «J. Ultrastruct. Res.», 19, 84–99.

EXPLANATION OF FIGURES

Fig. 1. – Longitudinal section of an early spermatid examined before the nucleus elongation. The flagellar centriole is already inserted against the nucleus. ×18,750.

FC = flagellar centriole. *M* = mitochondrial derivatives. *N* = nucleus.

Fig. 2. – Stage of spermatid differentiation later than in Fig. 1: the nucleus elongation is in progress but the chromatin is still uncondensed. Granular material (*G*) forming the so-called «centriole adjunct» is visible surrounding the flagellar centriole and within it two vacuoles are present. ×20,000.

N = nucleus. *F* = flagellum.

Figs. 3–8. – Serial sections from proximal to distal of the neck region of mature sperm, showing the relationship between nucleus, centriole derivative and mitochondrial derivatives. The different features the centriole derivative displays from its cephalic to caudal end are illustrated in Figs. 5 to 8. The electronopaque material present in the nuclear indentation (Fig. 4) closely surrounds the mitochondrial derivatives and the centriole derivative (Figs. 5–8). ×120,000.

N = nucleus *M'* = principal mitochondrial derivative *M''* = second mitochondrial derivative *C* = C fibre of the centriole triplets *SF* = secondary fibres.

Discussion

FAWCETT. – I would draw your attention to certain other examples of the extension of the central pair of tubules into the interior of the centriole Several years ago ROTH described such a relationship in the basal bodies of a ciliate protozoan. In our own work on development of mammalian spermatozoan, we found that the central pair of microtubules secondarily extend into the distal centriole during differentiation of the striated columns of the connecting-piece.

AFZELIUS. – Have you considered the similarity between your triangular cross-links and the stellate pattern described by MANTON?

MANTON. – The so-called " stellate-pattern " present in the transition region of the green algae other derivatives (i.e. *archegoniate*) involves connections between alternate doublets and not, as suggested here, connections between every third doublet.

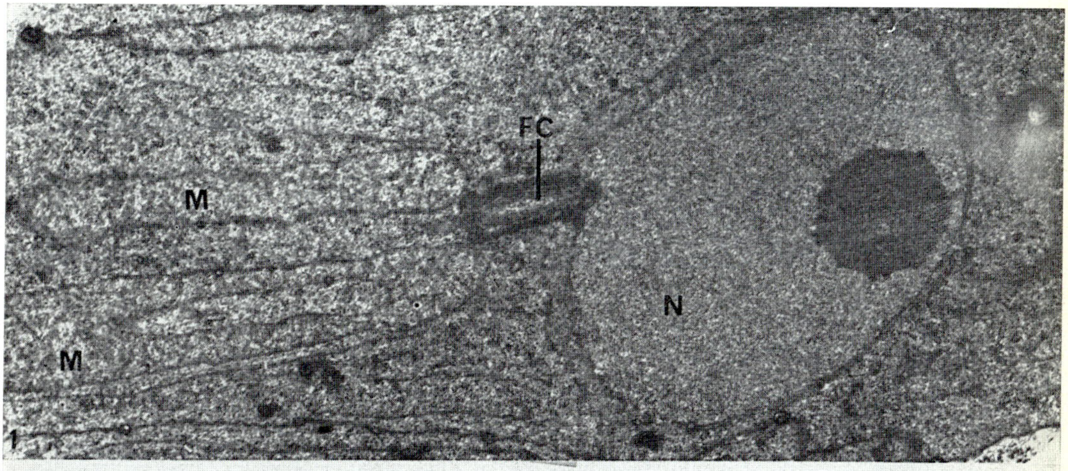
FC
M
M
N
1

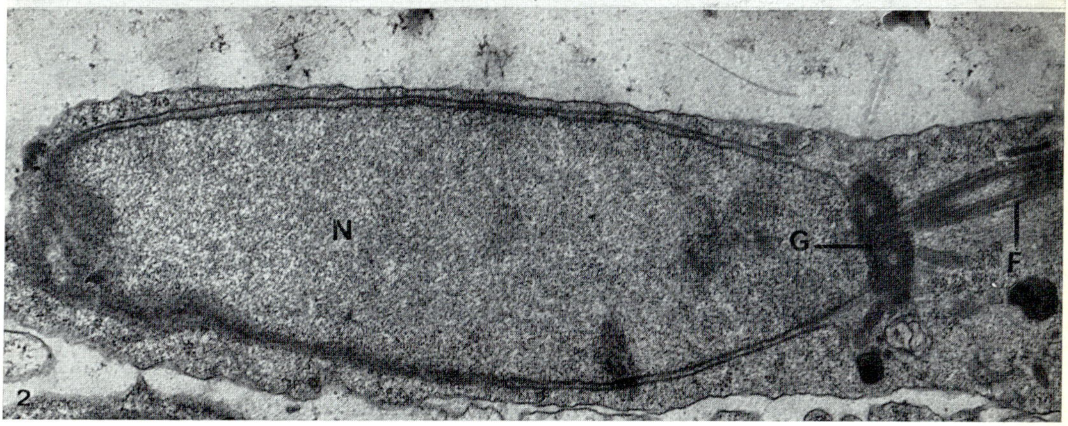
N
G
F
2

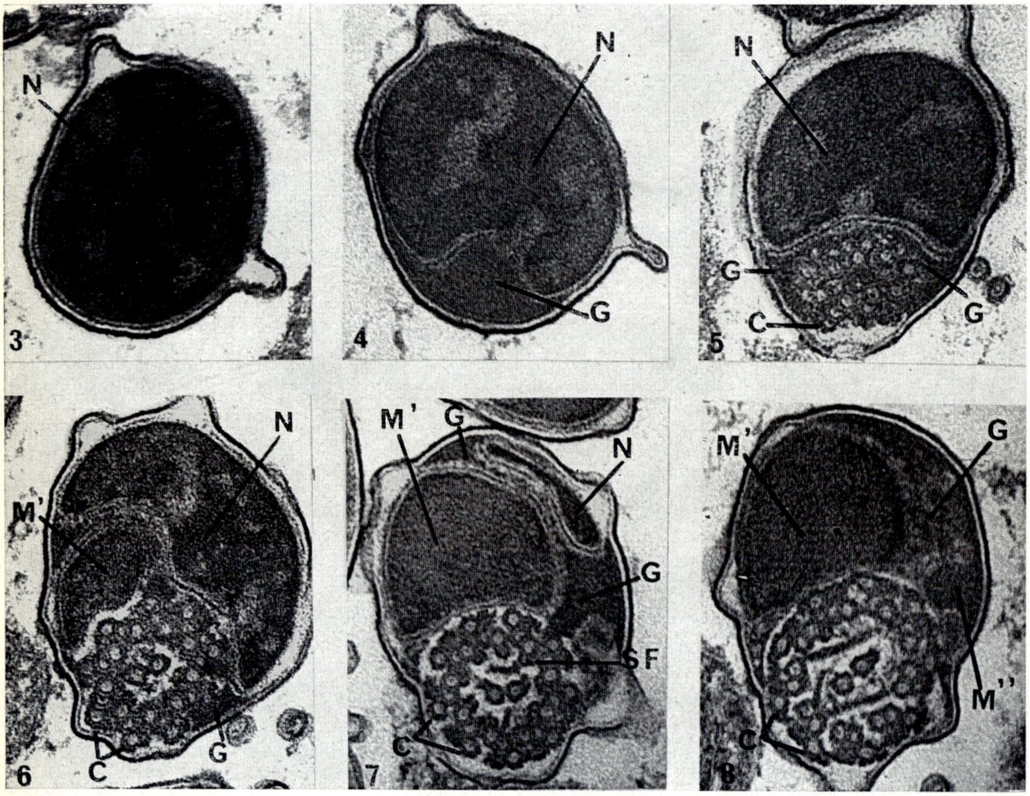
N
3
N
G
4
N
G
C
G
5
N
M'
G
C
6
M'
G
N
G
SF
C
7
M'
G
M''
C
8

RICHARD G. KESSEL (*)

SPERMIOGENESIS IN THE DRAGONFLY WITH SPECIAL REFERENCE TO A CONSIDERATION OF THE MECHANISMS INVOLVED IN THE DEVELOPMENT OF CELLULAR ASYMMETRY (**).

SUMMARY. — The present communication is concerned with a detailed description of the nuclear and cytoplasmic changes which occur during spermiogenesis in the dragonfly as observed with the electron microscope. Particular attention is directed toward a system of microtubules which display a special relationship to the nucleus and mid-piece structures during the development of asymmetry. The observed relationships and changes are discussed in terms of possible functional significance.

RIASSUNTO. — Vengono descritti i cambiamenti nucleari e citoplasmatici osservati al microscopio elettronico durante la spermiogenesi della libellula. Con particolare attenzione viene osservato un sistema di microtubuli che è in relazione con il nucleo e con le strutture della regione intermedia durante lo sviluppo dell'asimmetria. Tali relazioni e cambiamenti sono discussi in termini di possibile significato funzionale.

INTRODUCTION

During the past few years, one of the more exciting aspects to the study of differentiation in male germ cells has involved an appreciation of the extent to which microtubules are utilized or involved in the morphogenetic processes during maturation of these cells as well as the extent to which these structures are utilized in the permanent cytoarchitecture and or motility of the mature cells. On the basis of what must now be considered a very extensive bibliography on the subject, it is clearly apparent that microtubules constitute a ubiquitous and abundant organelle not only in developing spermatozoa (e.g. BAWA, 1964; YASUZUMI and ŌURA, 1965), but in all eucaryotic cells. Probably, in part, because microtubules vary considerably in their number, disposition and relationships to other structures in the male germ cell, a variety of functions have been proposed for them. In some species, either a straight or spiraling system of microtubules is thought to constitute a device for support (SILVEIRA and PORTER, 1964; LUMSDEN, 1965; BURTON, 1966b).

(*) Department of Zoology, The University of Iowa, Iowa City, Iowa, U.S.A.

(**) The investigations on which this presentation is based were supported by the United States Public Health Service and the National Science Foundation. It is a pleasure to acknowledge the skillful technical assistance of Mrs. Robert Decker.

Furthermore, microtubules appear to function in the development of motility as, for example, in certain non-flagellate, but motile sperm (CHRISTIANSEN, 1961; MOSES and COLEMAN, 1964; ROBISON, 1966). Moreover, in a number of different species, an extensive system of microtubules closely invests the nucleus of the spermatid during the remarkable elongation which it undergoes during spermiogenesis to result in a highly attentuated structure. In some cases, the microtubules are initially arranged in a spiral or helix of variable pitch around the elongating spermatid nucleus and then subsequently unwind during the process (TANDLER and MORIBER, 1966; MCINTOSH and PORTER, 1967; CLARK, 1967). In other species, the microtubules associated with the elongating spermatid nucleus appear to remain remarkably straight and rigid in appearance during the process (BURGOS and FAWCETT, 1955; BRADKE, 1963; SCHIN, 1965; PORTER, 1965; KESSEL, 1966; FAIN-MAUREL, 1966; ANDERSON, *et al.*, 1967).

Microtubules which are associated with elongating spermatid nuclei may, in some species, disappear after spermiogenesis is complete (NAGANO, 1962; KESSEL, 1966, 1967; WERNER, 1966; REGER, 1967; ANDERSON, *et al.*, 1967; HOAGE and KESSEL, 1968). In other species microtubules are present in both elongating spermatids and mature spermatozoa as, for example in cestodes (SILVEIRA and PORTER, 1964; BONSDORFF and TELKKA, 1965; ROSARIO, 1964), ticks (REGER, 1963), and the fungus gnat (MAKIELSKI, 1966, PHILLIPS, 1966 a, b).

From these studies, there are suggestions that the microtubules may play a causative role in the development of nuclear and cellular asymmetry associated with spermiogenesis (KESSEL, 1966; CLARK, 1967; MCINTOSH and PORTER, 1967). Conversely, PORTER (1965) has suggested that the caudal sheath of microtubules associated with the nuclei of mouse spermatids may serve a cytoskeletal function and that the microtubules may act as a framework to guide the elongation of the nucleus. An essentially similar function has been proposed for the manchette microtubules in earthworm spermatids (ANDERSON, *et al.*, 1967).

While some of the earlier studies were quick to ascribe a functional role for these microtubules in the development and maintenance of the highly asymmetric condition so characteristic of spermiogenesis in many forms, the fact currently remains that little or no direct information is available to support the view that microtubules may be responsible for the asymmetry which develops not only in the spermatid as a cell, but in the various components within the cell. An exception is provided by the brief report by SHOUP (1966) dealing whith the microtubules in spermatids from normal and mutant *Drosophila*. A large bundle of microtubules running parallel to the long axis of the spermatid nucleus is present in normal spermatids. However, in a male sterility mutant, the nucleus fails to elongate and the bundle of microtubules is not observed. These observations strongly suggest that the bundle of microtubules associated with the concave surface of the normal differentiating spermatid nucleus is intimately related to its elongation.

The spermatid of the dragonfly has proven to be a unique and useful system in which problems relating to the functional role of microtubules can be investigated (KESSEL, 1966). Therefore, it is the purpose of this presentation to describe further details in the association of microtubules with other components of the dragonfly spermatid throughout the developmental period required for spermiogenesis and to attempt to relate form and changes in form with function.

MATERIALS AND METHODS

The dragonflies (Odonata, Aeschnidae) examined were collected in the vicinity of Iowa City, Iowa. Testes were dissected in cold fixative which consisted of a 3% solution of glutaraldehyde in 0.1 M phosphate buffer. After fixation for 1–2 hours, pieces of the testes were rinsed in several changes of cold phosphate buffer for a period of 12 hours and then transferred to a cold, 1% solution of phosphate-buffered osmium tetroxide for 2 hours. After dehydration in alcohol, the tissues were embedded in Epon 812 (LUFT, 1961), sectioned on a Sorvall MT-II ultramicrotome, stained with uranyl acetate (WATSON, 1958) and lead citrate (REYNOLDS, 1963), and examined in an RCA EMU-3 G electron microscope.

DESCRIPTION

An extensive system of microtubules becomes associated with the dragonfly spermatid nucleus shortly after the transition from spermatocyte to spermatid. During the course of nuclear elongation which costitutes one of the events associated with spermiogenesis in this and many other species, microtubules display a unique and special relationship with the nuclear surface as well as more posterior structures in the cell. Some of the events and relationships have been characterized previously (KESSEL, 1966), but subsequent studies have resulted in additional morphological details in the process. It is pertinent at this point to be reminded that while the spermatid nucleus initially is approximately spherical, it becomes (when considered overall) oval, then elliptical and eventually conical in shape. In fact, for the greater part of the process of spermiogenesis, it appears that the spermatid nucleus is conical and that the cone is progressively flattened to a point late in the process so that the nucleus might then be considered as a long cylinder with rounded ends. It is also pertinent to point out at this juncture that since the longitudinally oriented microtubules follow the contour of the nucleus and mid-piece structures from the beginning to the end of spermiogenesis, so too will their overall configuration change when considered as a group. Spermatogenesis in the dragonfly at the light microscope level has been studied and described by SESHACHAR and BAGGA (1963).

A longitudinal section of an early spermatid is illustrated in Fig. 1 where it can be demonstrated that a single microtubule extends parallel with and very close to the surface of the nucleus. Because of the small size and disposition of the microtubules, however, transverse sections of early spermatid nuclei demonstrate more favorably some aspects of the close relationship between the nucleus and microtubules. Transverse sections of early spermatid nuclei just prior to or during initial stages of chromatin clumping reveal a gentle scalloping in the nuclear surface (Fig. 2). As a result the nuclear surface is arranged in alternate furrows and ridges. Initially, the depressions in the nuclear surface are extremely shallow so that there is only sufficient space for one or two microtubules in each. In the particular section illustrated in Fig. 2, those microtubules associated with the right side of the nucleus are sectioned transversely while those associated with the left side of the nucleus appear somewhat obliquely sectioned. Those portions of the nuclear envelope adjacent to the microtubules already appear extremely electron-opaque. The full compliment of microtubules associated whith this early spermatid nucleus is not yet established (Fig. 2). A slightly later stage of nuclear elongation is displayed by transversely sectioned spermatids in Figs. 3–5. In these nuclei, initiation of chromatin condensation has clearly begun. The microtubules surrounding the nuclei appear to be more numerous and the scalloping of the nuclear surface is more apparent. In Fig. 3, some of the microtubules are sectioned transversely while others are somewhat obliquely sectioned; a feature which could suggest that the microtubules are not oriented precisely longitudinal with respect to the nuclear grooves. In Fig. 5 as well, not all of the microtubules surrounding the nucleus appear to be sectioned in exactly the same plane. In other cases such as illustrated in Figs. 5 and 22, all the microtubules associated with the transverse sections of these nuclei appear to be sectioned in approximately the same plane.

Longitudinal sections of early spermatids provide some additional details to the relationships between the microtubules and the changing shape of the nucleus (Figs. 6–11). The region of the ridges and grooves in the nuclear surface can be identified in such sections; the latter by the electron-opaque nuclear envelope (Figs. 7–11). When the nuclear grooves are sectioned so as to include a considerable portion of their length, it is apparent that the adjacent microtubules can also be traced in the section for a considerable distance. From these relationships it is clear that the microtubules are not arranged in a low pitch around the nucleus as has been demonstrated in certain other species (McIntosh and Porter, 1967; Clark, 1967). The microtubules do, however, closely follow the changing contour of the nucleus (Fig. 10). It is also apparent from such sections that the posterior portion of the elongationg nucleus is truncated and abuts upon a fairly extensive region of the cytoplasm which consists of a heterogeneous and granular substance which tapers as it extends into the elongating mid-piece (Figs. 6, 7, 11). The proximal centriole is located in the center of this granular material and touches the posterior aspect of the nucleus. Many of the microtubules surrounding the nucleus extend posteriorly so as to also invest the post-nuclear granular accumulation. In this region as well, the microtubules closely follow the contour of the mid piece structures (Figs. 6, 7).

An early spermatid nucleus, approximately 1.4 microns in diameter, is illustrated in Fig. 22. At this stage, the alternate furrows and ridges in the nuclear surface are apparent, but not extensive. It is clear that a single row of microtubules is positioned in each of the shallow furrows and, further, that the center-to-center spacing of the microtubules in the furrows is remarkably constant. A total of 87 microtubules, nearly all of which are sectioned transversely, closely invests this spermatid nucleus. It is also apparent, however, that the number of microtubules in each of the furrows associated with the spermatid nucleus in Fig. 22 is not constant, but is related to the furrow length. The number of tubules in the furrows ranges from 2 to at least 12 (Fig. 22). The nuclear envelope in this early spermatid nucleus is extremely dense in the furrow area; as a result, an inner and outer layer of the nuclear envelope is apparent only in the ridge areas (Fig. 22). A narrow, discontinuous band of condensed chromatin is located just inside the nuclear envelope with small masses of chromatin dispersed rather uniformly throughout the remainder of the nucleus at this stage (Fig. 22).

During the course of the development of nuclear asymmetry; that is, as the nucleus elongates and as its cross-sectional diameter decreases, the furrows associated with the surface of the nucleus and the nuclear envelope progressively deepen (Figs. 13–15). Probably as a result, the ridges in the nuclear surface bounded by nuclear envelope in this area become more extensive and apparent. Associated with these changes, a number of interesting features become more apparent. First, that portion of the nuclear envelope contained within the nuclear furrows remains remarkably dense and it is obvious that this density is due to the presence of a substance within the perinuclear cistern in this particular region (Figs. 15, 18). However, the dense product is not present within the perinuclear cistern in that portion of the nuclear envelope comprising the nuclear ridges (Fig. 15). Rather, the inner and outer layers of the nuclear envelope, the perinuclear cistern, as well as the nuclear pores are all clearly evident in the ridges of the nucleus formed by the scalloping of the nuclear envelope (Figs. 15, 34). The density of the substance within the perinuclear cistern of the furrow region is as dense or denser than that displayed by the condensing chromatin (Figs. 13–15).

Another point of interest here is that the layer of investing microtubules are only positioned against the nucleus in the region of the furrows; that is, adjacent to the dense substance which obliterates the perinuclear cistern in these regions (Figs. 13–18). In the furrows, the microtubules are separated from the nuclear surface by a distance of approximately 90–100 Å (Figs. 15–18). The diameter of the tubules ranges from 240–300 Å and the center-to-center spacing of the tubules ranges from 350–400 Å.

From the initiation of nuclear elongation to its completion, those microtubules located in the furrows of the nucleus are attached to each other as well as to the surface of the nucleus (Figs. 16–18). These connections are achieved by exceedingly thin filaments 50–100 Å thick. The filamentous connections between the adjacent microtubules and between the microtubules and nuclear surface are illustrated in Figs. 16–18. Those filaments extending between the tubules and nuclear surface appear to become continuous with the matrix material obliterating the former perinuclear cistern (Figs. 16–18). Thus, all of the microtubules in a furrow are « anchored » or stabilized by both intertubular attachments and tubular-nuclear attachments.

Due to the changes in overall shape of the spermatid nucleus during the elongation process, it is to be expected that a single nucleus early in the process would have a maximum cross-sectional diameter either at the middle or posterior region of the nucleus and that its diameter would be less toward the anterior end. It would then become of interest to determine what relationships exist between the microtubules and the nuclear surface in these regions. In Figs. 19–22, there are ilustrated four transverse sections through different regions of spermatid nuclei all of which are at an approximately similar stage of elongation as determined from the nature of the condensing chromatin. The anterior-most section is illustrated in Fig. 19. In this region, seven shallow furrows and ridges are present in the nuclear surface. A total of 41 microtubules surrounds the nucleus at this level. The minimum number of tubules in a furrow is 4 while the maximum number of tubules in a furrow is 8. Note that the plasma membrane is closely applied to the microtubules in this anterior section (Fig. 19). In a somewhat posterior section (Fig. 20), there are eight furrows and ridges in the nuclear surface. The total number of tubules associated with the nucleus in this region is 62. The minimum number of tubules in a furrow is 5 while the maximum number of tubules in a furrow is 12. Still further posteriorly in the nucleus (Fig. 21), there are 13 furrows and ridges associated with the nuclear surface with a total of 67 microtubules. The minimum number of microtubules is 2 while the maximum number is 9. Finally, more posteriorly in the spermatid nucleus (Fig. 22), there are approximately two dozen furrows and ridges associated with the nuclear surface with a total of 83 microtubules. The number of tubules per furrow ranges from 1 to 7.

The progression of nuclear elongation and the resulting reduction in nuclear cross-sectional diameter result in further morphological changes. The furrows in the nucleus deepen and the ridges become larger. As a result the ridges eventually become extensive loops in the nuclear envelope (Figs. 29–34). During this process also, the nuclear chromatin has continued the condensation process so that it is now extremely dense with little internal detail. The process appears to be initiated in the central most portion of the nucleus with coarse chromatin particles extending more peripherally in the nucleus (Fig. 15). These dense chromatin particles which initially may occur in the ridges and loops formed by the nuclear envelope (Fig. 15) by some means are attracted to or migrate toward the nuclear center since they are never observed in the more extensive loops evident later in spermiogenesis (Figs. 29–34).

Again, it is of interest to compare the number of furrows and ridges in the nuclear surface as well as the number of microtubules occurring within the furrows after considerable elongation of the nucleus has occurred.

The sections illustrated in Figs. 23–26 depict various regions sectioned transversely along the axis of a spermatid nucleus approximately midway through the elongation process as established by the maximum cross–sectional diameter of the nucleus, the degree of condensation of the chromatin, and by the extent of nuclear loop development. In Fig. 23, which represents a transverse section through the anterior portion of the nucleus near its tip, no loops or furrows are evident, but a lamella of endoplasmic reticulum partially encircles the microtubules and the nucleus. In a slightly more posterior section, 5 loops and furrows are evident (Fig. 24). Some 22 microtubules surround the nucleus at this level. In a section posterior to that just described, a total of 6 loops and furrows are associated with the spermatid nucleus (Fig. 25). The total number of microtubules present is 38 and the number per furrow ranges from 4 to 8. Still more posteriorly (Fig. 26), 8 furrows and ridges in the nuclear surface are apparent. A total of 50 microtubules are present in this particular section and the number per furrow varies from 4 to 9.

Thus, it can be established that the number of furrows and loops associated with the spermatid nucleus as well as the total number of microtubules associated with the nucleus varies within a single spermatid depending upon the cross-sectional diameter of the nucleus. Clearly the number of loops, furrows and microtubules is related to the width of the nucleus as reflected in its cross-sectional diameter from furrow to furrow. It appears that as elongation of the nucleus proceeds, the number of furrows and ridges in the nuclear surface decreases if point to point comparisons are made between nuclei at different stages in spermiogenesis. Thus, the number of ridges in the nuclear envelope of an early spermatid at its maximum width may approach two dozen, but in sections through the maximum width of a spermatid nucleus well along with the elongation process, only 7 or 8 ridges or loops are evident. Such a condition is apparent by a comparison of Figs. 22 and 31. Since the number of furrows tend to decrease toward the end of spermiogenesis, it follows also that the total number of microtubules associated with the nucleus also decreases since the effective nuclear surface available for microtubules has decreased. Thus, the maximum number of microtubules associated with an early spermatid nucleus may approach 90 (Fig. 22) while only some 50–60 microtubules are associated with a spermatid nucleus in which maximum development of nuclear loops has been achieved (Fig. 31).

Clearly, some of the microtubules surrounding the dragonfly spermatid may not reach the anterior tip of the spermatid. Thus, there are never as many microtubules surrounding the anterior tip of the nucleus or acrosome as there are associated with the widest portion of the nucleus at similar periods of development. Thus, it is conceivable that only some of the microtubules in each of the nuclear furrows (as seen in transverse sections) reach the anteriormost tip of the spermatid.

It is reasonable to suspect that if the number of microtubules associated with the nucleus gradually decreases during its elongation, images in what might be interpreted as the breakdown of microtubular integrity should be encountered. Indeed at all stages of spermiogenesis examples are found in which the microtubules have lost their integrity in the sense that they are no longer tubular. In many cases (Figs. 4, 15, 33), « C », « S », and « 6 »-shaped structures are observed. Such images may well represent instances in the breakdown of microtubular structure. Generally, it is those tubules which are most peripherally placed in the furrows which lose their integrity (Fig. 33).

As the final elongation of the nucleus is achieved, the remaining loops in the nuclear envelope become completely constricted proximally (Figs. 30, 32). By this time, the condensation of chromatin is largely complete and the nucleoplasm within the loops is devoid of chromatin (Figs. 29–34). At this point in nuclear elongation the dense furrows in the nuclear envelope appear to be compressed against the entire surface of condensed chromatin (Fig. 29–34).

It is apparent that the loss of loops in the nuclear envelope proceeds throughout spermiogenesis, but it is especially noticeable toward the end of the process since it is at this time that the loops are the most extensive and they are at this point also probably detaching within a comparatively short period of time. It is thus a favorable period in which to determine the mechanisms by which this activity occurs. In some cases, (Fig. 34) single annulated membranes are present in the perinuclear cytoplasm, and it is not difficult to envision such a configuration resulting from a detachment of a loop in the nuclear envelope and its subsequently assuming a lamellar configuration. In some cases also, loops of the nuclear envelope toward the end of nuclear elongation assume a configuration reminiscent of a « myelin figure » and such an image might be interpreted as a step in the degeneration or breakdown in the loop structure (Fig. 32).

After all remaining loops have detached from the nucleus, transverse sections reveal the nucleus to be circular in shape, much reduced in cross-sectional diameter, and surrounded by a complete investment of 30–40 longitudinally oriented microtubules (Figs. 35, 36). A single row of microtubules then completely encircles the nucleus and they remain uniformly spaced. They also retain their close relationship with the surface of the nucleus (Fig. 37). At this point in development, the plasma membrane and a loop of endoplasmic reticulum are closely applied to the outer surface of the microtubules (Figs. 35, 37). Transverse sections through « fields » of nuclei at a stage just described illustrate remarkable uniformity in cross-sectional diameter compared to earlier stages in nuclear elongation (Fig. 35). However, slight variations in nuclear cross-sectional diameter are still noted. Those sections illustrating nuclei of smaller cross-sectional diameter probably represent the anterior, narrowed tip of the sperm (Fig. 27). Oblique sections of these nearly mature sperm, demonstrate that the microtubules are disposed in a straight configuration (i.e., parallel with the longitudinal axis of the nucleus) over considerable distances (Fig. 36).

The content of the late spermatid nucleus in many cases appears uniformly dense with no apparent internal structural detail (Figs. 35-37).

Occasionally, however, one or more small areas of low electron density is apparent within the late spermatid or mature sperm nucleus (Fig. 35). The completely condensed chromatin of the late spermatid nucleus is surrounded by a thin electron lucent layer and an outer thicker layer which exhibits similar electron density as that of the chromatin (Fig. 37). This outermost layer represents the product deposited within the perinuclear cistern of early spermatid nuclei and, as such, represents a unique specialization of the nuclear envelope (Fig. 37).

One of the final steps in the nuclear elongation process involves the complete loss of investing microtubules. In the completely mature sperm, no microtubules are associated with the nucleus (Fig. 38). That the microtubules disappear after nuclear elongation is finished suggests that they are no longer functionally necessary for the cell.. The microtubules appear to breakdown and disappear at approximately the same time since only on occasion are nearly mature nuclei observed with only a few microtubules surrounding them (Fig. 46).

The anterior region of the dragonfly sperm is provided with an elongated acrosome. Longitudinal and transverse sections of this structure are illustrated in Figs. 39–44. The plasma membrane is closely applied to the acrosome and anterior-most portion of the nucleus in this region and the layer of microtubules associated with the nucleus terminate at the level of the acrosome where they are closely applied to its surface (Figs. 40–43). Thus, the anterior termination of the microtubules is in a narrow wedge of cytoplasm between the plasma membrane and acrosome. In some instances, a loop of endoplasmic reticulum is positioned between the microtubules and plasma membrane in this region (Figs. 42–43).

It was previously noted that an accumulation of granular material is associated with the posterior region of the spermatid nucleus. The paired mitochondrial derivatives and flagellum extend posteriorly from the granular material. During the extension of the spermatid, there is also some lengthening of the post-nuclear granular material as well as the mitochondrial derivatives. In addition, the flagellum grows to accomodate itself to the elongation of the cytoplasm. It is of interest that microtubules are also intimately associated with the mid-piece structures during spermiogenesis and, further, that at least some of the microtubules encircling the nucleus also extend into the mid-piece where they form an investing sheath around the components in this region (Figs. 47-51). It is apparent from Fig. 47 that the previously truncated posteror aspect of the spermatid nucleus tappers to a point which is partially surrounded by the granular material (Fig. 47).

Aggregations of granular and electron-opaque material have been described in association with the centrioles of a number of spermatid species. Because the nucleus-associated or manchette microtubules are closely associated with this material early in their formation (KESSEL, 1967) or appear to insert in this material (CLARK, 1967), it has been suggested that this aggregation of granular material, termed centriolar satellite or satellite derivative by CLARK (1967), may participate in the formation of caudal sheath microtubules (KOEHLER and BIRKY, 1966; CLARK, 1967). No information relating to this particular problem was obtained in the study of the dragonfly spermatid.

The posterior tip of the nucleus as well as the granular material associated with it are invested by a single, but closely packed layer of microtubules (Fig. 47). All of the aforementioned structures are in turn surrounded by a complete or discontinuous membranous lamella (Fig. 47) which appears to represent a differentiation of the smooth endoplasmic reticulum. Fine filamentous interconnections between adjacent microtubules as well as between the microtubules and the mid-piece structure are still evident in this region of the spermatid (Figs. 48, 53). Discontinuity in the wall of some of the microtubules is also observed in this region (Fig. 47). In a slightly more posterior section (Fig. 48) which includes only the centriole and granular aggregation of material the microtubules still exhibit their close association with the surface of the mid-piece structures. Again, a single loop of endoplasmic reticulum partially or completely surrounds the microtubules. At a still more posterior section level, including in this case the paired mitochondrial derivatives and flagellum, it is apparent that the mid-piece structures are still invested by a layer of microtubules which in turn are surrounded by a membranous lamella similar to those previsiously described (Fig. 49). Even at more posterior levels of the mid-piece, the same relationships hold; namely, that the mid-piece structures are surrounded by microtubules which in turn are enveloped by a membranous lamella of endoplasmic reticulum (Figs. 50, 51). The point to be emphasized is that the membranous differentiations of the endoplasmic reticulum display a consistent and close relationship to the microtubules which surround the elongating mid-piece structures as well as with the anterior portion of the spermatid nucleus (Fig. 39). From this special association, it would appear that this membranous differentiation is functionally important in the morphogenesis and differentiation of the spermatid.

As the dragonfly sperm reaches maturity, those microtubules associated with the mid-piece structures disappear. Stages in the partial to complete loss of the microtubules in this region of the sperm are illustrated in Figs. 45 and 46. From the variations noted in tubular structure during this time, it apperas that a break in the wall of the microtubule is an initial stage in its complete breakdown with the result that a variety of configurations formed by « open » microtubules are evident (Figs. 45, 46). As the microtubules are lost in the mid-piece of the sperm, so too is there a disappearance of the lamellae of endoplasmic reticulum which formerly surrounded the microtubules (Figs. 45, 46).

The flagellum of an early spermatid is illustrated in Fig. 52. Subfiber A of the peripheral doublets contains an electron-opaque material which is also present in later stages of spermiogenesis (Fig. 53). Prominent hooks extend from subfiber B of the doublet and in some cases they establish connections with straight arms extending from subfiber A (Fig. 52). At this period of development, patches of increased density can be noted just peripheral to each of the flagellar doublets. In late spermatids, an accessory microtubular system has formed (peripheral singlets) and is closely associated with the flagellum. As illustrated in Fig. 53, nine microtubules are placed peripheral to and between the flagellar doublets. The position in which the microtubules form is essentially in that region occupied by the prominent hooks from subfiber B earlier in development. From the morphological variations noted, it appears that the large hooks extending from subfiber B may represent a stage in the formation of the accessory microtubular system (*c.f.* BEHNKE and FORER, 1967). After the microtubules have been formed, it can can be noted that both the microtubules and subfiber B eastablish continuity by means of small filaments or arms extending from each of the structures (Fig. 53). The arms extending from subfiber A of the doublets, however, rarely establish contact with the peripheral and singlet microtubules (Fig. 53). The accessory microtubules associated with the flagellum persist in mature sperm and PHILLIPS (1969) has noted that these peripheral singlets are in a position analogous to that of the nine outer dense fibers of mammalian spermatozoa (FAWCETT, 1965; FAWCETT and ITO, 1965) and may have similar functions. In late spermatids also, a double-layered membrane forms an envelope around the flagellum and the peripheral singlet microtubules (Fig. 53). In two opposing regions of this membranous sheath, the membranes are curved and the cytoplasm associated with the inner membrane is more electrone-opaque (Fig. 53). This particular membranous differentiation in association with the flagellum persists in the mature spermatozoan (Fig. 45).

CONCLUSIONS

Since a system of microtubules (1) closely invests the spermatid nucleus and mid-piece structures prior to their elongation, (2) persists throughout the process of nuclear and mid-piece elongation and (3) subsequently disappears after nuclear and mid-piece elongation are completed, there is strong evidence for the premise that the microtubules play an important role in this process. Unfortunately morphological observations alone do not provide conclusive evidence that the microtubules play a *causative* role in the development of nuclear and mid-piece asymmetry so characteristic of spermiogenesis in many forms. Thus, whether the microtubules actually provide the motive force or simply give direction to the translocation of protoplasm caused by forces generated elsewhere is not known. What seens to occupy a position of special significance in the case of the dragonfly spermatid is the fact that compression occurs symmetrically around the nucleus *only* in the region of the furrows. Furthermore, it is only in these specific areas that microtubules are found.

An alternative function that might be proposed for the perinuclear system of microtubules involves the suggestion that they may act as or provide cytoskeletal support for the elongation of the nucleus and that the forces necessary for the generation of this asymmetry are derived from other sources. What sources might be involved are unknown, but it seems worthwhile to speculate about certain unusual features which are apparent during nuclear elongation in the dragonfly. One such unusual feature is the deposition of a dense material within selected areas of the perinuclear cistern very early in spermiogenesis; as a result this portion of the nuclear envelope appears as a thick, dense line. It is of interest that those areas containing the dense product which obliterates the perinuclear cistern in a number of regions are also those areas which comprise the furrows in the elongating spermatid nucleus. The furrows, in turn, represent those regions in which a reduction of nuclear cross-sectional diameter is most intense. Such areas alternate with loops of the nuclear envelope which progressively become longer and extend into more peripheral areas of the cytoplasm. On the basis of these relationships, it might be suggested that the product which is deposited early within selected sites of the perinuclear cistern might also play a significant and, perhaps, causative role in the elongation process. The fact that microtubules are located against the spermatid nucleus only in a position adjacent to that area of the nuclear envelope containing the dense product and, further, on the basis of the continuity between the microtubules and this region of the nucleus by means of the thin filaments, it is reasonable to suggest that the two are interrelated in their role of nuclear elongation. Both the microtubules as well as the product within the selected regions of the perinuclear cistern are present very early in spermiogenesis, but it has been impossible to determine if one precedes the other or whether the two develop at approximately similar times. It does appear, however, that the product is present in the perinuclear cistern before *all* of the microtubules are formed. At the end of spermiogenesis, moreover, it obvious that the microtubules disappear but the product within the perinuclear cistern not only persists but completely envelops the nucleus. The morphological observations, in fact, do not negate the possibility that the product in the perinuclear cistern plays a role in the assembly of microtubules.

If it can tentatively be accepted that the microtubules in the dragonfly do play an active role in nuclear elongation, it becomes appropriate to consider those aspects concerning the disposition of the microtubules which might relate to such an activity. One question raised in such a consideration concerns whether or not the tubules are disposed in some sort of helical arrangment. It was previously pointed out that in some transverse sections of early spermatids (*i.e.*, in those spermatids in which the microtubular investment of the nucleus had been nearly or completely established), all of the tubules surrounding the nucleus appear in cross-section as clearly defined circles; a feature which tends to support a view that the microtubules are longitudinally oriented along the nucleus. In a few spermatids of similar stage, however, sections cut so that the tubules on one side of the nucleus appear in cross-section as clearly defined circles reveal tubules on the opposite side of the nucleus to appear somewhat blurred; a feature which suggests that the tubules are obliquely inclined with respect to the section plane and perhaps, spirally arranged about the nucleus. The latter condition, since it is not uniformly observed, conceivably could also result from localized variations involving deformations of nuclear shape even if the microtubules were longitudinally oriented. On the other hand, transverse sections of nuclei in which all microtubules appear to be disposed in the same plane with respect to the section might occur even if the microtubules were arranged in a spiral provided this involved an extremely shallow pitch. If this were the case, it is difficult to envision how an uncoiling of such a shallow pitch might effectively contribute a force for the elongation of the nucleus. In studies describing the helical arrangement of microtubules around spermatid nuclei of other species (McINTOSH and PORTER, 1967; CLARK, 1967), the pitch of the microtubules is quite steep. In chicken spermatids, McINTOSH and PORTER (1967) have described a tightly coiled system of microtubules around the nucleus. They suggested that fine cross-bridges (Maxwellian demons) between the microtubules might expand the helix and serve to straighten the tubules and thereby lengthen and compress the nucleus. Indeed, a tightly coiled system of microtubules capable of contraction around a nucleus constitutes an intriquing operational mechanism for nuclear elongation especially in view of recent studies which have demonstrated that the protein extracted from microtubules has several similar biochemical properties to that of muscle actin (STEPHENS, 1968 a, b). Thus, the amino acid composition and molecular weight of the protein isolated from microtubules closely resembles that of muscle actin as does its capacity to bind one mole of nucleotide per 60,000 gm of protein (review by TILNEY, 1968). On the basis of the aforementioned considerations, however, it must be concluded that in the dragonfly, the microtubules are eiter longitudinally oriented with respect to the long axis of the elongating nucleus or are arranged initially in such a shallow pitch so as to be difficult to demonstrate in thin sections. Clearly, during later stages of spermiogenesis, the microtubules are longitudinally oriented with respect to the nucleus and mid-piece structures.

It was previously pointed out that during its elongation, the dragonfly spermatid nucleus undergoes a series of transitions in geometry. However, regardless of section level or shape of the nucleus, the microtubules remain positioned at a constant distance from the surface of the nucleus. Such a condition, if visualized in three dimensions, indicates that the microtubules surrounding the nucleus follow the curvature of the nucleus which progressively changes during the elongation process. Thus, the microtubules have an orientation with respect to the nucleus and mid-piece structures much like that for the staves in a barrel. As the final elongation of the nucleus is achieved, and the nucleus is relatively constant in cross-sectional diameter regardles of the section level, the microtubules approach a condition of maximum straightness.

The anterior termination of the microtubules is at a point adjacent to the acrosome near the anterior tip of the cell. In this region, the microtubules are closely positioned to the surface of the acrosome on the one hand and are in turn closely invested by differentiations of the endoplasmic reticulum or by the plasma membrane depending upon the particular section level. The posterior extent of the system of microtubules is near the terminus of the mid-piece. In all regions of the elongating cell the microtubules are closely positioned with respect to the surface of the nucleus or to the structures contained within the mid-piece. In the anterior and posterior portions of the cell, the specialization of the endoplasmic reticulum described, when considered in three–dimensions, forms an investing sheath around the microtubules. In these areas, the diposition of the endoplasmic reticulum is such as to suggest that it may play a role in preventing the lateral displacement of the system of microtubules.

If one entertains the notion that the microtubules surrounding the dragonfly spermatid nucleus exert compressional forces on the nucleus and thereby assist with the elongation process, then it would appear that the following sequence of events is compatable with the morphological observations: (1) The microtubules at the anterior tip of the spermatid extend slightly beyond the nucleus and « insert » in a narrow wedge or band of cytoplasm between the plasma membrane in this area and the wall of acrosome. The tubules in this region may be « attached » to the surface of the acrosome. The microtubules are also attached to each other and the surface of the nucleus throughout their length. In this region also, « loops » of endoplasmic reticulum surround the microtubules and nucleus. Assuming that the plasma membrane in this region and the wall of the acrosome were relatively inflexible, then the microtubules could be thought of as wedged within this narrowed anterior tip of the spermatid much like the point of insertion of a lever. (2) The microtubules are arranged longitudinally (or possibly a very shallow helix) along the elongating spermatid nucleus. Thus, the microtubules when considered in three dimensions along their total course are « bowed ». This condition may develop as a result of or reflect the original shape of the spermatid nucleus (spherical) which subsequently changes to an extremely attenuated form. (3) Some of the microtubules which surround the spermatid nucleus extend into the elongating mid-piece where they form an investing layer around the structures contained in this area (*e.g.*, mitocondrial nebenkern or derivative). Furthermore, these tubules appear to be maintaned in their position in this region not only by cross-bridges between themselves and the mid-piece structures, but by enveloping cisternal differentiation of the endoplasmic reticulum. Thus, it could be envisioned that this differentiation of the endoplasmic reticulum might act as a posterior « lasso » which assists with the maintenance of the « bowed » condition of the microtubules around the nucleus. Furthermore, there is evidence to suggest that there is a tendency for microtubules to become straight rather than remain in an « unnaturally bowed » configuration; a condition which would cause the microtubules to exert a continuous pressure on the spermatid nucleus at its maximum width. The trasmission of this pressure would then tend to gradually and continuously compress the nucleus into more elongate form; *i.e.*, to reduce its cross-sectional diameter especially in the tubule-associated furrow region. Thus, the microtubules would continue to exert a force on the nucleus until it achieved a nearly uniform cross-sectional diameter throughout its length; at this time then, the microtubules would be « freed » of their original and unatural « bowed » condition (and any helical arrangement would be obliterated). It has previously been noted that microtubules in general are relatively rigid and elastic and possess a tendency to assume a straight form when they are distorted (PORTER, 1966). Further, PEASE (1963) has noted that microtubules tend to break rather than bend sharply.

The small filaments which connect adjacent microtubules and which also serve to connect the microtubules with the surface of the nucleus and the mid-piece structures throughout the cell possibly serve to (1) prevent the displacement of microtubules from their close and constant position with respect to these structures and (2) to interconnect the entire microtubular system so that all the individual microtubules might function more nearly as a unit. The presence of specific types of connecting links between microtubular subunits in *Actinosphaerium* has been suggested as related to the determination and maintenance of the overall pattern of microtubules in this cell (TILNEY, 1968). The presence of connections between microtubules in other cell types as well (BURTON, 1966 a, b) has generated the notion that they may, at least in part, be involved in the formation and maintenance of patterned assemblages of microtubules.

During the nuclear elongation process, it was described that the chromatin condensation generally occurred in the center of the nucleus and that smaller pieces of chromatin were dispersed more peripherally and even extended into the loops of the nucleus. It was also indicated that the ultimate fate of these loops is to constrict proximally and to subsequently detach from the nucleus. This activity serves to decrease the amount of nuclear envelope as well as the volume of the nuclear contents and is probably related to the overall decrease in volume of the nucleus during elongation. It is clear, that as a result of the process, considerable amounts of nucleoplasm are removed from the nucleus. The nature of the materials removed from the nucleus in this manner is unknown, but in mature sperm of some species no basic proteins are present in the nucleus (VAUGHN, 1968). The fact that chromatin is never observed within those loops which appear in section to be completely closed off from the remainder of the nucleus or in the process of detaching from it, implies that some rather specific mechanism exists for the segregation of the chromatin to insure that none of this material escapes from nucleus. Perhaps attraction forces or differential charges exist between the main mass of condensing chromatin in the center of the nucleus and the smaller units of chromatin more peripherally placed. Further, the dense substance in the perinuclear cistern which is positioned in such a manner as to constitute a « gate » into the nuclear loops, may contribute to what appears to be a very effective system against loss of chromatin during the nuclear elongation process. Further, the role of physical furces such as osmotic phenomena should not be overlooked.

It was earlier noted that as the dragonfly spermatid nucleus decreased in cross-sectional diameter, the number of nuclear loops and furrows as well as the number of microtubules associated with the nucleus decreased. A reduction in number of both furrows and ridges might be accomplished by a compression of a loop by the microtubules in adjacent furrows. This condition implies that small ridges (loops) in the nuclear surface may be « pinched off » or released into the cytoplasm (or alternatively, compressed inward) throughout the elongation process. By the time, however, that most of the compression in the nuclear furrow region has been achieved, seven or eight large loops in the nuclear envelope remain which must then detach within a relatively short time. The spermatid nucleus of many forms undergoes a considerable reduction in volume during spermiogenesis and redundant portions of the nuclear envelope containing nucleoplasm have been described on numerous occasions especially in mammalian species (*cfr.*, FRANKLIN, 1968). These portions of the nuclear envelope form a loop from the base of the nucleus back into the neck region of the spermatozoan and it has been suggested that redundant portions of the nuclear envelope seen in spermatozoa may represent accommodation of the nuclear envelope to reduction in nuclear volume which occurs during spermiogenesis (FAWCETT, 1965).

Because the microtubules are arranged in only a single layer around the dragonfly spermatid nucleus and because of the rather constant center-to-center spacing of the microtubules, it is apparent that the number of microtubules must progressively decrease in order to conform to a reduction in nuclear surface. Throughout nuclear elongation, microtubules are encountered which appeared to have lost their integrity and may thus represent those tubules in the process of disappearing in an accommodation to the decreasing nuclear (furrow) surface. Generally, these microtubules are peripherally placed in the furrows. Incomplete or C-shaped microtubules have been described previously (KESSEL, 1966; BEHNKE, 1967) as respresenting a breakdown or depolymerization of microtubules. It has since been demostrated that such C-shaped microtubules are also formed during reassembly of microtubules (BEHNKE, 1967; TILNEY, 1968) so that caution must be exercised in the interpretation of such profiles.

CLARK (1967) in considering the manchette associated with elongating nuclei of lizard spermatids has commented that if microtubules were arranged around an elongating spermatid nucleus much like the staves of a barrel, then at the end of elongation there would be perhaps a 5 fold excess of microtubules. CLARK (1967) further notes that such as excess might be avoided either by (1) arranging the microtubules in a helix of sufficiently steep pitch so that they would be longitudinally oriented only after nuclear elongation was completed, or (2) providing for a selective deletion of microtubules during the elongation process and addition to the ends of those remaining microtubules. From the observations described in the dragonfly, it appears that the latter condition is employed.

Only a single layer of closely packed microtubules completely engirdles the mature and highly attenuated spermatid nucleus. These tubules do not, however, persist for a very long time since they are no longer found in mature sperm. The factors causing the complete breakdown of nuclear tubules at this particular period constitute one of several interesting, but unanswered questions in the dragonfly spermatid. It was also demonstrated that almost the entire system of microtubules originally present in the mid-piece of the spermatid also breaks down since it is no longer present in mature sperm. The fact that the microtubules associated with the nucleus and mid-piece disappear after spermiogenesis in the dragonfly suggests that these structures are not needed for the *maintenance* of the high degree of asymmetry shown by this spermatozoan. Based on the morphological evidence it is, however, likely that they helped to produce it.

Those microtubules located in the mid-piece region of developing dragonfly spermatid vary considerably in their diameter. Even adjacent microtubules often exhibit such variations so that it is unlikely that fixation or embedding procedures could have produced the condition. The size differences noted may then be due to differences in the size and/or arrangement of the subinits comprising the microtubules.

References

ANDERSON W. A. WEISSMAN A. and ELLIS R. A. (1966) – *A comparative study of microtubules in some vertebrate and invertebrate cells.* « Zeit. Zellforsch. », 71, 1–13.

BAWA S. R. (1964) – *Electron microscope study of spermiogenesis in a fire-brat insect,* Thermobia domestica. I. *Mature spermatozoan.* « J. Cell Biol. », 23, 431–446.

BEHNKE O. and FORER A. (1967) – *Evidence for four classes of microtubules in individual cells.* « J. Cell Sci. », 2, 169–192.

BONSDORFF C. H. v. and TELKKA A. (1965) – *The spermatozoon flagella in* Diphyllobothrium latum (*Fish tapeworm*). « Zeit. Zellforsch. », 66, 643–648.

BRADKE D. L. (1963) – *Special features of spermatogenesis in* Lumbricus terrestris. « Anat. Rec. », 145, 360.

BURGOS M. H. and FAWCETT D. W. (1955) – *Studies on the fine structure of the mammalian testis.* I. *Differentiation of the spermatids in the cat* (Felis domesticus). « J. Biophys. Biochem. Cytol. », 1, 287–300.

BURTON P. R. (1966 a) – *Substructure of certain cytoplasmic microtubules: An electron microscopic study.* « Science », 154, 903–805.

BURTON P. R. (1966 b) – *A comparative electron microscopic study of cytoplasmic microtubules and axial unit tubules in a spermatozoon and a protozoan.* « J. Morph. », 120, 397–424.

CHRISTENSEN A. K. (1961) – *Fine structure in an unusual spermatozoan in the flatworm* Plagiostomum. « Bio. Bull. », 121, 416.

CLARK A. (1967) – *Some aspects of spermiogenesis in a lizard.* « Am. J. Anat. », 121, 369–400.

FAIN–MAUREL M. (1966) – *Contribution a l'histologie et a 'a caryologie de quelques Isopods. Spermiogenese et infrastructure du spermatozoide des Oniscides et des Cymothoides.* « Ann. Sci. Nat. Zool. », 8, 1–188.

FAWCETT D. W. (1965) – *The anatomy of the mammalian spermatozoon with particular reference to the guinea pig.* « Zeit. Zellforsch. », 67, 279–296.

FAWCETT D. W. and ITO S. (1965) – *The fine structure of bat spermatozoa.* « Am. J. Anat. », 116, 567–610.

FRANKLIN L. E. (1968) – *Formation of the redundant nuclear envelope in monkey spermatids.* « Anat. Rec. », 161, 149–162.

HOAGE T. R. and KESSEL R. G. (1968) – *An electron microscope study of the process of differentiation during spermatogenesis in the drone honey bee* (Alpis mellifera *L*) *with special reference to centriole replication and elimination.* « J. Ultrastruct. Res. », 24, 6–32.

KESSEL R. G. (1966) – *The association between microtubules and nuclei during spermiogenesis in the dragonfly.* « J. Ultrastruct. Res. », 16, 293–304.

KESSEL R. G. (1967) – *An electron microscope study of spermiogenesis in the grasshopper with particular reference to the development of microtubular systems during differentiation.* « J. Ultrastruct. Res. », 18, 677–694.

KOEHLER J. K. and BIRKY C. W. (1966) – *An electron microscope study of the dimorphic spermatozoa of* Asplanchna (*Rotifera*). « Zeit. Zellforsch. », 70, 303–321.

LUFT J. (1961) – *Improvements in epoxy resin embedding methods.* « J. Biophys. Biochem. Cytol. », 9, 409–414.

LUMSDEN R. D. (1965) – *Microtubules in the peripheral cytoplasm of cestode spermatozoa.* « J. Parasit. », 51, 929–931.

MAKIELSKI S. K. (1966) – *The structure and maturation of the spermatozoa of* Sciara coprophila. « J. Morph. », 118, 11–42.

MCINTOSH J. R. and PORTER K. R. (1967) – *Microtubules in the spermatids of the domestic fowl.* « J. Cell Biol. », 35, 153–173.

MOSES M. J. and COLEMAN J. R. (1964) – *Structural patterns and the functional organization of chromosomes.* – In: *The Role of Chromosomes in Development,* M. Locke, Ed., Academic Press, New York, pp. 11–49.

NAGANO T. (1962) – *Observations on the fine structure of the developing spermatid in the domestic chicken.* « J. Cell Biol. », 14, 193–205.

PEASE D. C. (1963) – *The ultrastructure of flagellar fibrils.* « J. Cell Biol. », 18, 313–326.

PHILLIPS D. M. (1966 a) – *Fine structure of* Sciara coprophila *sperm.* « J. Cell Biol. », 30, 249–259.

PHILLIPS D. M. (1969) – *Exceptions to the prevailing pattern of tubules* (9+9+2) *in the sperm flagella of certain insect species.* « J. Cell Biol. », 40, 28–43.

PORTER K. R. (1965) – *Illustrations of cell fine structure.* – In: « *Ideas in Modern Biology* ». J. A. Moore, Ed., The Natural History Press, Garden City, New York, pp. 95–124.

PORTER K. R. (1966) – *Cytoplasmic microtubules and their functions.* In: *Ciba Foundation Symposium, Principles of Biomolecular Organization.* G. E. W. Wolstenholme and M. O' Connor, Eds., J & A Churchill, Ltd. London, pp. 308–346.

REGER J. F. (1963) – *Spermiogenesis in the tick,* Amblyomma dissimili, *as revealed by electron microscopy.* « J. Ultrastruct. Res. », 8, 607–621.

REGER J. M. (1967) – *A study on the fine structure of developing spermatozoa from the oligochaete,* Enchytraeus albidus. « Zeit. Zellforsch. », 82, 257–269.

REYNOLDS E. S. (1963) – *Use of lead citrate at high pH as an electronopaque stain in electron microscopy.* « J. Cell. Biol. », 17, 208–212.

ROBISON W. G. (1966) – *Microtubules in relation to the motility of a sperm syncytium in an armored scale insect.* « J. Cell Biol. », 29, 251–265.

ROSARIO B. J. (1964) – *An electron microscope study on spermatogenesis in cestodes.* « J. Ultrastruct. Res. », 11, 412–427.

SCHIN K. S. (1965) – *Meiotische Prophase und Spermatidenreifung bei* Gryllus domesticus *mit besonderer Berucksichtigung der Chromosomenstruktur.* « Zeit. Zellforsch. », 65, 418–513.

SESHACHAR B. R. and BAGGA S. (1963) – *Cytology and cytochemistry of spermiogenesis in two dragonflies* Ictinogomphys rapot (*Rambur*) *and* Pantala flovescens (*Fabricius*). « J. Morph. », 113, 267–274.

SHOUP J. R. (1966) – *Spermiogenesis, with special reference to nuclear differentiation in wild type and in a male sterility mutant of* Drosophila melanogaster. « J. Cell Biol. », 31, 107 A.

SILVEIRA M. and PORTER K. R. (1964) – *The spermatozoids of flatworms and their microtubular systems.* « Protoplasma (Wien) », 59, 240–265.

STEPHENS R. E. (1968 a) – *On the structural protein of flagellar outer fibers.* « J. Mol. Biol. », 32, 277–283.

STEPHENS R. E. (1968 b) – *Reassociation of microtubule protein.* « J. Mol. Biol. », 33. 517–519.

TANDLER B. and MORIBER L. G. (1966) – *Microtubular structures associated with the acrosome during spermiogenesis in the water-strider,* Geris remigis (*Say*). « J. Ultrastruct. Res. », 14, 391–404.

TILNEY L. G. (1968) – *The assembly of microtubules and their role in the development of cell form.* – In: *The Emergence of Order in Developing Systems.* M. Locke, Ed., Academic Press, New York. Dev. Biol., Suppl. 2, 63–102.

VAUGHN J. C. (1968) – *Changing nuclear histone patterns during development.* I. *Fertilization and early cleavage in the crab.* Emerita analoga. « J. Histochem. Cytochem. », 16, 473–479.

WATSON M. L. (1958) – *Staining of tissue sections for electron microscopy with heavy metals.* « J. Biophys. Biochem. Cytol. », 4, 475–485.

WERNER G. (1966) – *Untersuchungen über Spermiogenese bei einen Laufkäfer,* Carabus catenulatus *Scop., und der Skorpion-Wasserwanze,* Nepa rubra *L.* « Zeit. Zellforsch. », 73, 576–599.

YASUZUMI G. and ŌURA C. (1965) – *Spermatogenesis in animals as revealed by electron microscopy.* XV. *The fine structure of the middle piece in the developing spermatids of the silkworm.* Bombyx mori. « Zeit. Zellforsch. », 67, 502–520.

EXPLANATION OF FIGURES

Fig. 1. – Longitudinal section of early spermatid. Nucleus (*N*), nebenkern (*NK*), flagellum (*FL*), granular accumulation (*G*), Golgi complex (*GC*), endoplasmic reticulum (*ER*). Note single microtubule (arrows) extending close to and parallel with the surface of the nucleus. ×22,000.

Fig. 2. – Transverse section of early spermatid nucleus (*N*). Microtubules (arrows) surround the nucleus, but at this stage are not yet maximally developed. Only one or two microtubules are associated with each of the small, shallow furrows in the nuclear surface. Note that the microtubules surrounding left side of nucleus are sectioned somewhat obliquely while those microtubules associated with the right side of the nucleus are sectioned transversely. ×25,000.

Fig. 3. – Transverse sections at different levels of two early spermatid nuclei (*N*). Note that some of the microtubules associated with the nucleus are obliquely sectioned (single arrows) while the remainder are transversely sectioned (double arrows). ×37,500.

Figs. 4 and 5.– T ransverse section of early spermatid nuclei (*N*) illustrate initial clumping of chromatin. The alternate furrows (*F*) and ridges (*R*) in the nuclear surface are clearly demonstrated. A dense substance (*PC*) occupies the perinuclear cistern of the nuclear envelope in furrow region only. Note that the microtubules are present only in the furrows of the nuclear surface and that all microtubules in Fig. 4 appear to be sectioned transversely. A few obliquely sectioned microtubules (arrows) occur in Fig. 5. Incomplete microtubules indicated at arrows in Fig. 4. Fig. 4, ×25,000; Fig. 5, ×50,000.

Figs. 6–9. – All figures illustrate longitudinal or oblique sections of spermatids at a stage (based on degree of chromatin (*CH*) clumping) similar to that in Fig. 5. Portions of the furrows (*F*) and loops (*L*) in the nucleus are identified in Fig. 9. Dense substance in perinuclear cistern of furrow (Fig. 8, PC). The heterogenous, granular accumulation of material at the posterior end of the nucleus is illustrated in Figs. 6, 7, and 9 at (*G*). Microtubules (MT and arrows). Note that many of the microtubules extend for considerable distances in these longitudinal sections in Figs. 7 and 8. Some of the microtubules adjacent to the nucleus extend posteriorly into the mid-piece in which case they follow the curvature of the associated structures (Fig. 6, arrows). Endoplasmic reticulum (*ER*). Fig. 6, ×25,500; Fig. 7, ×37,500; Fig. 8, ×25,500; Fig. 9, ×25,500.

Fig. 10. – Longitudinal section of spermatid. A furrow (*F*) region on each side of the nucleus is sectioned so as to include a considerable distance. The adjacent microtubules in each case (*MT*) can also be traced over a similar distance where they are positioned adjacent to the nuclear surface and closely follow its contour. ×25,200.

Fig. 11. – Posterior region of nucleus and associated granular product (*G*). Furrows (*F*) and ridges or loops (*L*) in nucleus identified. Microtubules (*MT*). Endoplasmic reticulum (*ER*). ×43,700.

Fig. 12. – Mid-piece of spermatid illustrates the paired mitochondrial nebenkern (*NK*). A microtubule (*MT*) extends parallel with and closely applied to the surface of the nebenkern. Endoplasmic reticulum (*ER*). ×43,700.

Fig. 13. – Transverse section of spermatid nucleus to illustrate arrangement of alternate furrows (*F*) and ridges (*R*) in the nuclear surface. Microtubules are restricted to the furrow region of the nucleus adjacent to the dense substance in the perinuclear cistern of nuclear envelope (*PC*) in this region. All microtubules appear to be sectioned approximately at right angles to their long axis. ×43,750.

Fig. 14. – Transverse section through spermatid nucleus in which greater clumping of chromatin (*CH*) is apparent. Alternate furrows (*F*) with microtubules and ridges (*R*) in nuclear surface. ×37,500.

Fig. 15. – In this transverse section of spermatid, chromatin (*CH*) is condensed into a large central mass with smaller aggregations more peripherally placed. Inner and outer membranes of the nuclear envelope are apparent in ridges (*R*) or loops of the nuclear envelope. Microtubules (*MT*). Dense substance in perinuclear cistern of nuclear envelope in furrows (*PC*). ×87,500.

Figs. 16–18. – Details of relationships between microtubules and nuclear surface. Fine filaments (arrows) or cross-bridges interconnect some of the adjacent microtubules and they extend between the microtubules and nuclear surface as well (arrows). The dense substance (*PC*) obliterating the perinuclear cistern of the nuclear envelope is favorably illustrated in Fig. 18. Fig. 16, ×118,800; Fig. 17, ×140,000; Fig. 18, ×274,500.

Figs. 19–22. – Sections extending progressively through anterior to middle portion of spermatid nuclei at approximately similar stages of nuclear elongation to illustrate differences in number of furrows and ridges associated with the nuclear surface in the different regions. Note also variation in number of microtubules in each of the furrows at the different section levels. All microtubules in Figs. 21 and 22 are sectioned transversely. Figs. 19–21, ×37,500; Fig. 22, ×45,300.

Figs. 23–26. – Transverse sections extending progressively from anetrior to posterior in spermatids at approximately similar stage of elongation and chromatin condensation but at a later stage of spermiogenesis than that illustrated in Figs. 19–22.

Again, note variation in number of ridges and furrows in nuclear surface at the different levels along the elongating nuclei. Condensing chromatin (*CH*). Figs. 23–25, ×46,800; Fig. 26, ×50,000.

Fig. 27. – Transverse sections of late spermatids to illustrate variation in cross-sectional diameter of nuclei (*N*). ×37,500.

Fig. 28. – Transverse section of mature sperm to illustrate variation in cross-sectional diameter of nucleus (*N*). Microtubules (arrow). ×37,500.

Figs. 29–34. – Transverse sections of late spermatid nuclei. In all cases, the chromatin has condensed and only on occasion are electron-lucent areas present within the nuclear chromatin. The loops (*L*) of the nuclear envelope are now extensive and number 6–8. In some cases there is a continuity between the nucleoplasm within the loops formed by the nuclear envelope and the chromatin (Figs. 29, 31), while in other cases the proximal constriction of the loops appears to have effectively segregated the two components of the nucleus (Fig. 32). The dense substance within selected areas of the perinuclear cisternae of the nuclear envelopes is still prominent and microtubules, sectioned transversely, still reside in the furrows adjacent to the intracisternal product. The loops of the nuclear envelope in some cases (Fig. 32, L) appear to lose their integrity. In other instances single profiles of annulate membranes are present in the perinuclear cytoplasm (Fig. 34, A). Note that some of the microtubules in peripheral areas of the furrows are incomplete (Fig. 33, arrows). Considerable variation in size is noted in those microtubules adjacent to the mitochondrial derivative of the mid-piece (Fig. 31, MT). Figs. 29, 34, ×37,500; Fig. 30, ×50,000; Figs. 31, 33, 54,300; Fig. 32, ×42,500.

Fig. 35. – Transverse sections of spermatid nuclei from which the loops in the nuclear envelope and their contents have separated. A single, but closely packed layer of microtubules (*MT*) now completely surrounds the nucleus. The layer of microtubules in this particular area is, in turn, completely surrounded by a double-layered membrane representing a differentiation of the endoplasmic reticulum (*ER*). ×31,500.

Fig. 36. – Oblique section of spermatid nucleus similar to those illustrated in Fig. 35. Microtubules (*MT*). ×63,300.

Fig. 37. – Enlargement of late spermatid nuclei. The dense product (*PC*) within the perinuclear cisterna of the nuclear envelope now forms a complete outer covering for the chromatin both of which have similar densities. The two are separated from each other by a thin electron-lucent layer. Microtubules (*MT*). Incomplete microtubule at arrow. ×85,400.

Fig. 38. – Transverse section through nuclei of completely mature sperm. Microtubules have now completely disappeared and the chromatin is surrounded by the plasma membrane. ×34,000.

Fig. 39. – Longitudinal section of anterior portion of nearly mature spermatid. Nucleus (*N*). Acrosome (*AC*). Microtubule (*MT*) oriented parallel with the nucleus. Differentiations of the endoplasmic reticulum (*ER*). ×37,500.

Figs. 40–43. – Transverse sections through different levels of the acrosome during spermiogenesis. Acrosome (*AC*), Microtubules (arrows), lamellae of endoplasmic reticulum (*ER*). Fig. 40, ×54,300; Fig. 41, ×73,200; Fig. 42, ×37,500; Fig. 43, ×48,800.

Fig. 44. – Longitudinal section through acrosome (*AC*) of mature sperm. ×37,500.

Figs. 45 and 46. – The figures illustrate transverse sections of the mid-piece region of nearly mature sperm. In some cases, the mid-piece structures are surrounded by a loop of endoplasmic reticulum (*ER*). Numerous incomplete microtubules (*IM*) are located in some of the mid-oieces, while only a few intact microtubules (*MT*) are present. In some of the mid-pieces, the microtubules and loops of endoplasmic reticulum have completely disappeared (*MM*) leaving only the flagellum with its specialized membranous envelope and the mitochondrial derivatives. ×19,000.

Fig. 47. – Transverse sections of spermatid illustrating posterior tip of the nucleus (*N*) which is partially surrounded by a homogeneous, granular accumulation (*G*). Microtubules (*MT*) form a complete, but single layer around the aforementioned structures. The microtubules are surrounded by a loop of endoplasmic reticulum (ER). ×50,000.

Figs. 48–51. – Transverse sections at various levels through the mid-piece of spermatids to illustrate relationships between the granular material (*G*) and the mitochondrial derivatives (*MD*), flagellum (*FL*), microtubules (*MT*), and the loops of endoplasmic reticulum (*ER*). Note also that the flagellum is surrounded by a double-layred envelope (*FE*). Centriole, (*C*) in Fig. 48. Figs. 48–51, ×50,000.

Fig. 52. – Flagellum of early spermatid. Note presence of hooks or filaments emanating from subfiber B of the doublet which in some cases appears to be continuous with a projection from subfiber A of an adjacent doublet (arrow). Irregular, amorphous masses are positioned peripherally to each of the flagellar doublets. ×184,300.

Fig. 53. – Mid-piece region of late spermatid. Mitochondrial derivative (*MD*), Post-nuclear granular product (*G*). Microtubules (*MT*), endoplasmic reticulum (*ER*). Note thin connections between microtubules and mid-piece structures (arrows). Those microtubules surrounding the flagellum possess hooks which connect with similar structures originating from subfiber B of the flagellum (B, arrow). Projections from subfiber A of the flagellum (A, arrow) less frequently make a connection with the peripheral microtubules. Note specialized membrane (*FM*) surrounding flagellum. ×184,300.

RICHARD G. KESSEL – *Spermiogenesis in the dragonfly with special reference to a consideration of the mechanisms involved in the development of cellular asymmetry.*

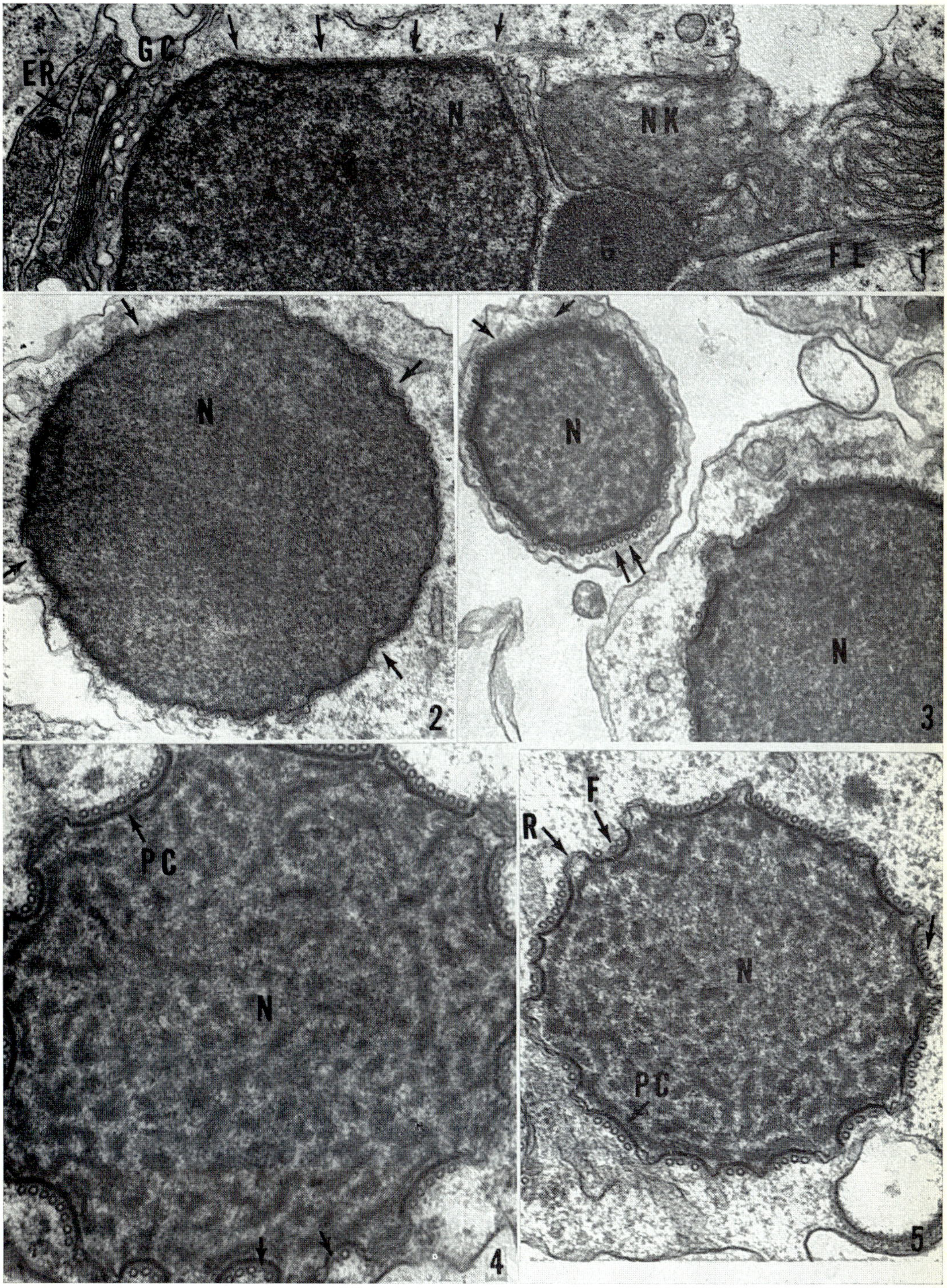

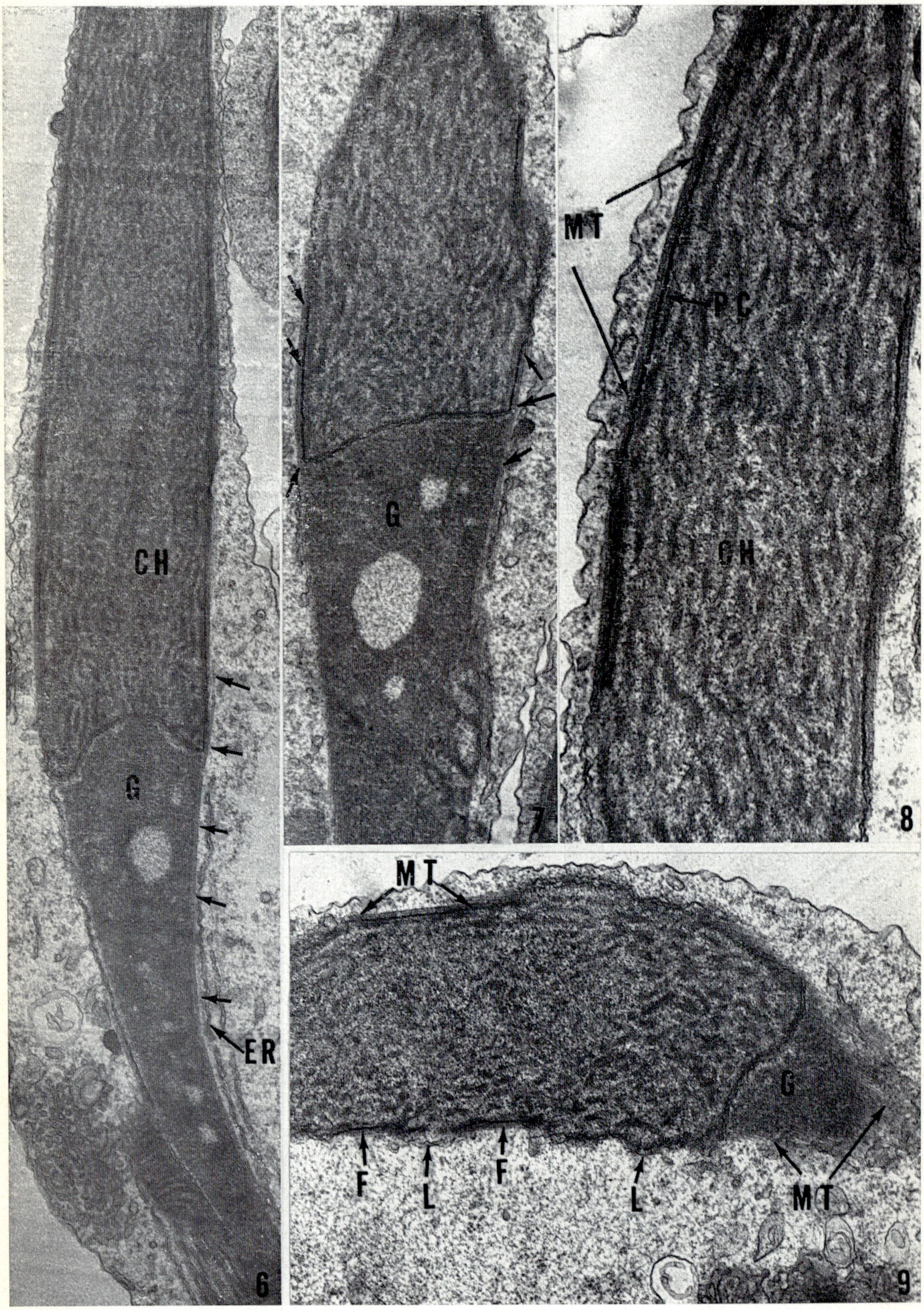
CH
G
ER
6
G
7
MT
PC
CH
8
MT
G
F
L
F
L
MT
9

RICHARD G. KESSEL – *Spermiogenesis in the dragonfly with special reference to a consideration of the mechanisms involved in the development of cellular asymmetry.*

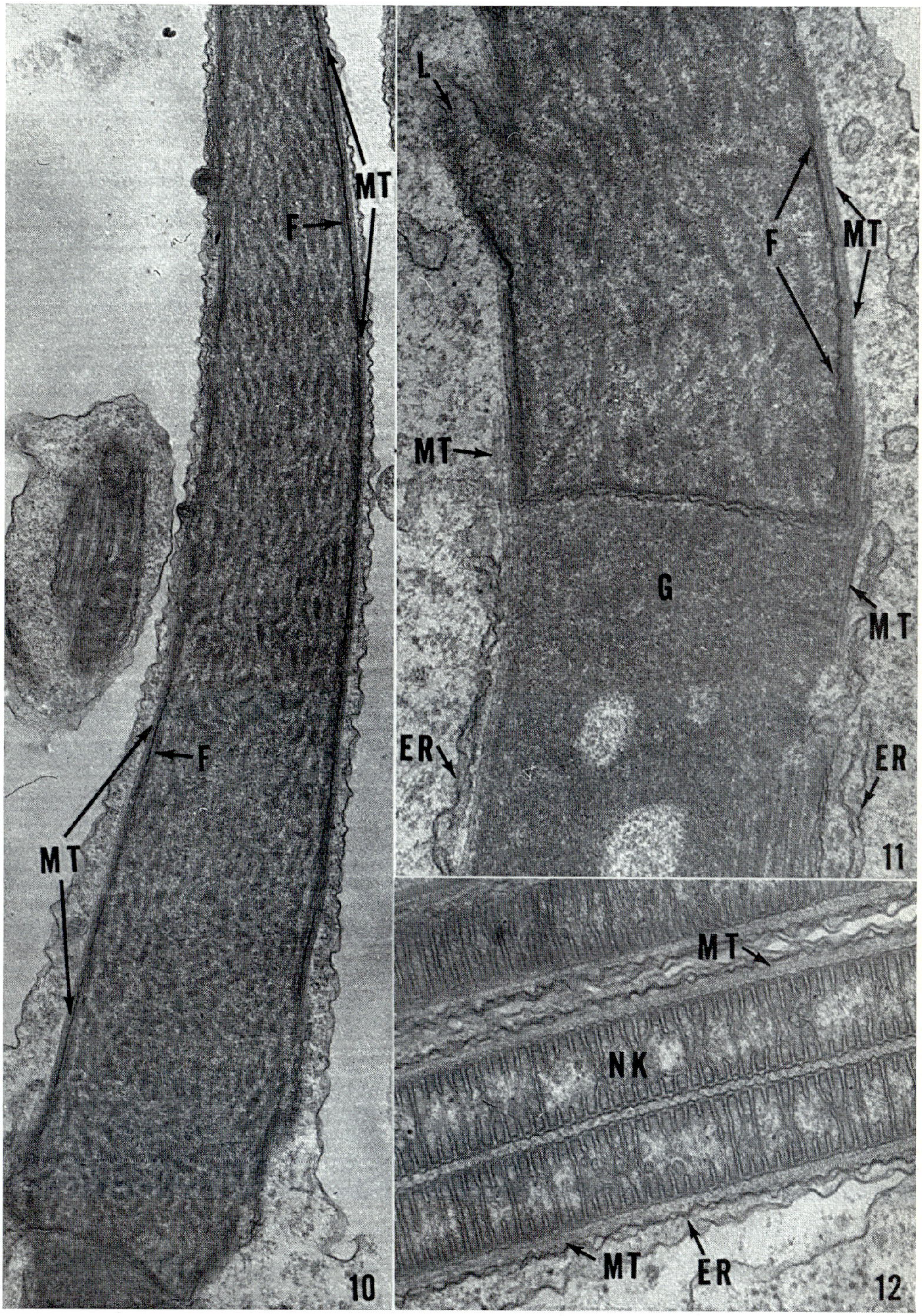

RICHARD G. KESSEL – *Spermiogenesis in the dragonfly with special reference to a consideration of the mechanisms involved in the development of cellular asymmetry.*

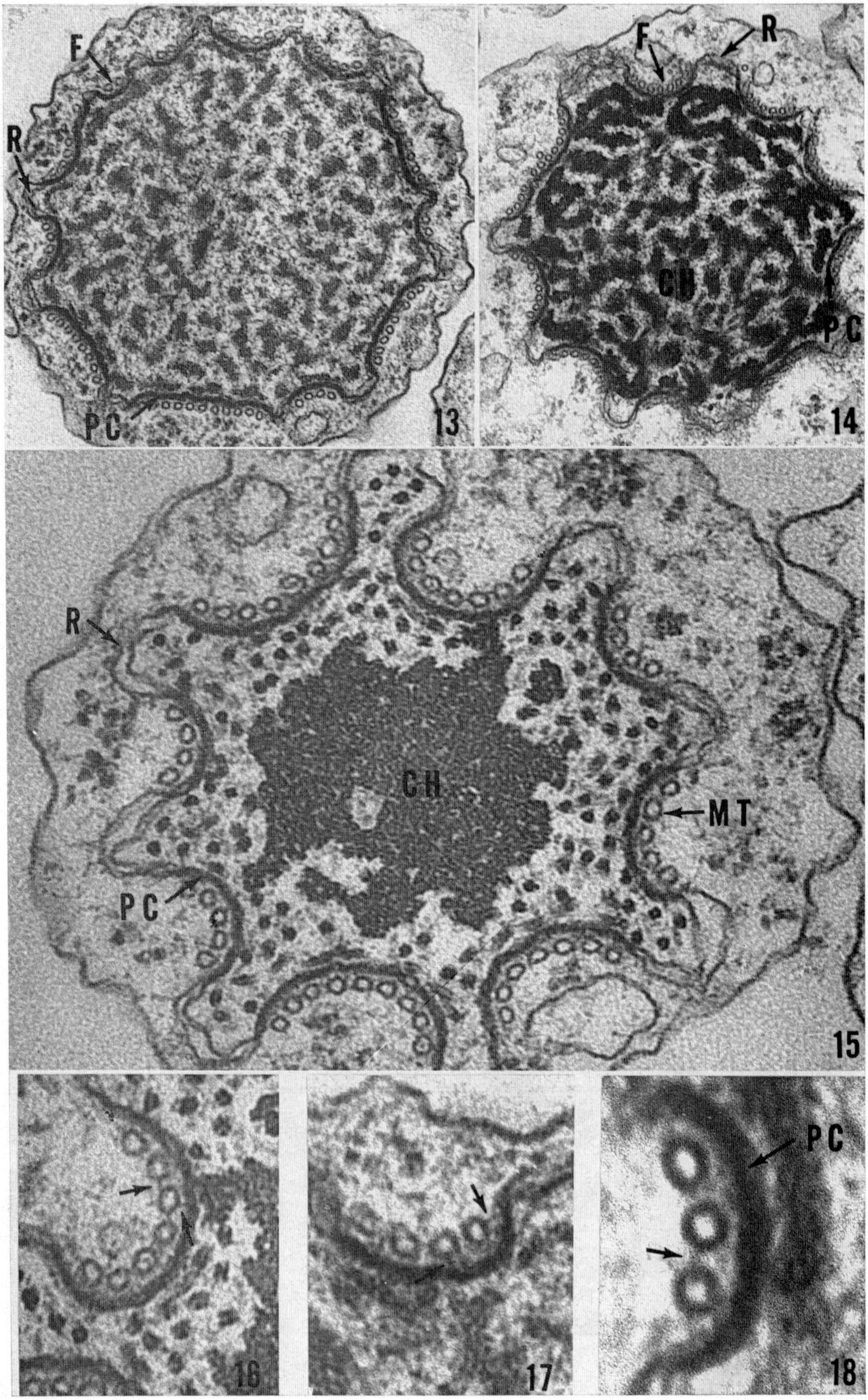

RICHARD G. KESSEL – *Spermiogenesis in the dragonfly with special reference to a consideration of the mechanisms involved in the development of cellular asymmetry.*

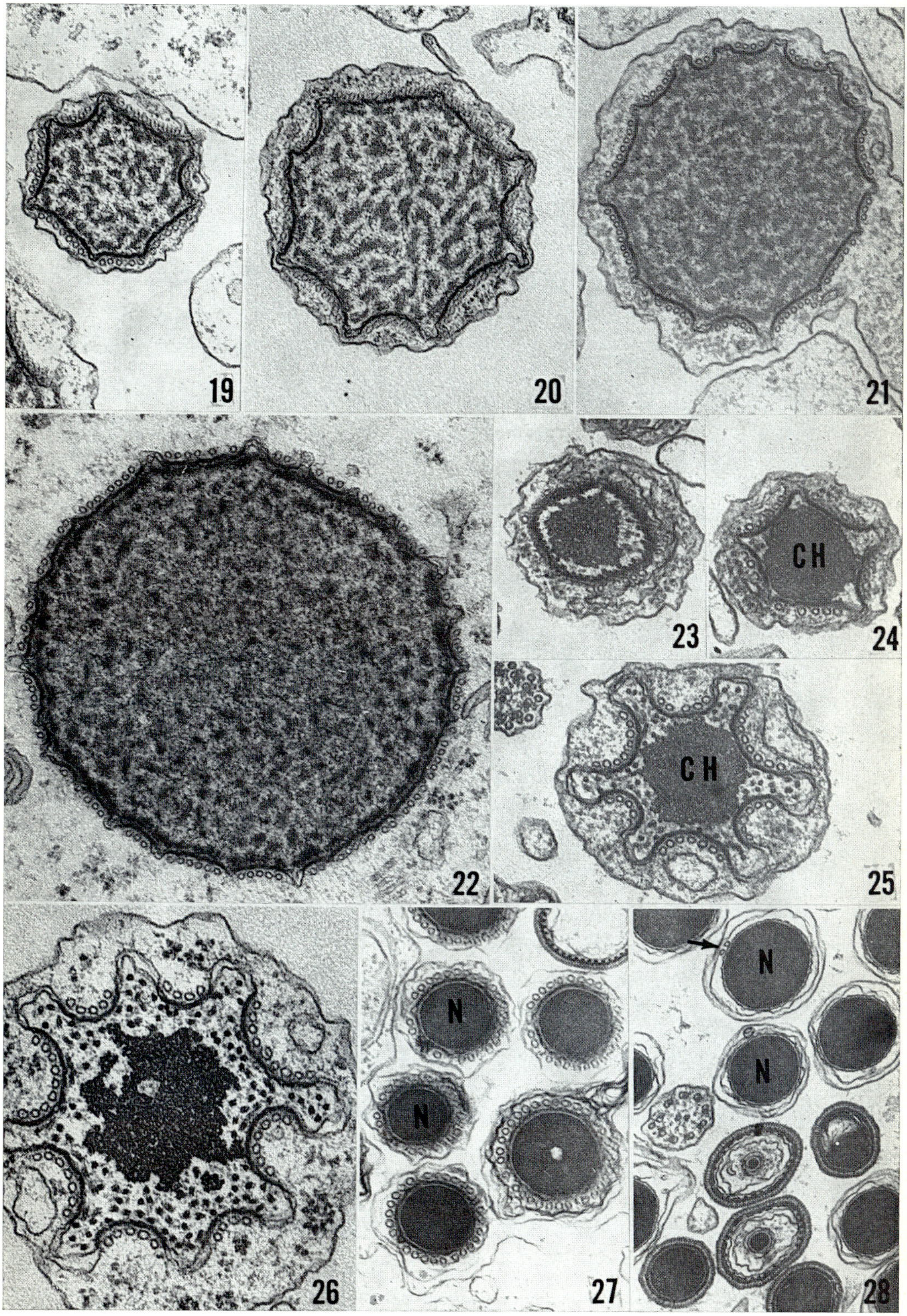

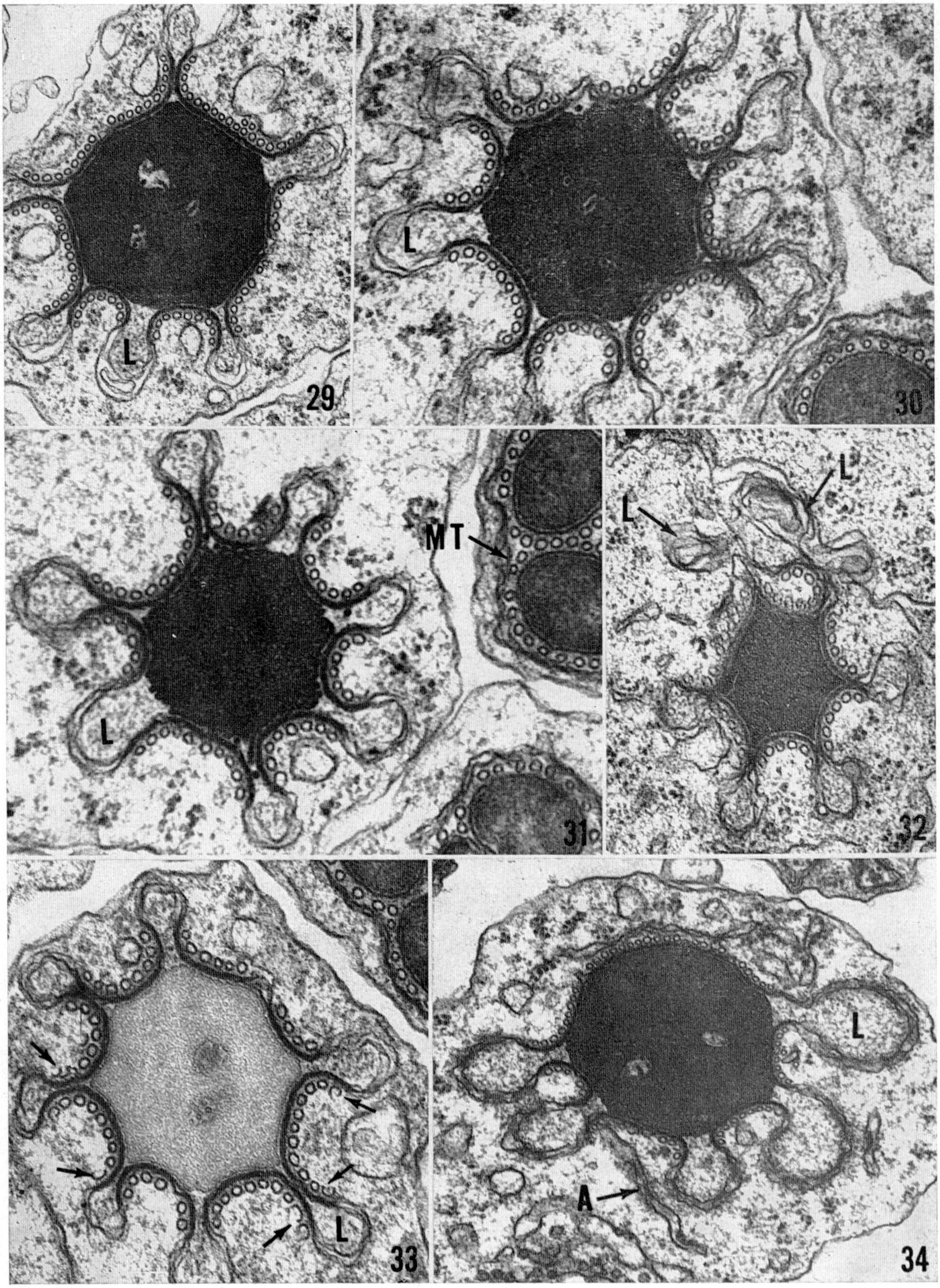
29
L
30
L
31
L
MT
32
L
L
33
L
34
L
A

RICHARD G. KESSEL – *Spermiogenesis in the dragonfly with special reference to a consideration of the mechanisms involved in the development of cellular asymmetry.*

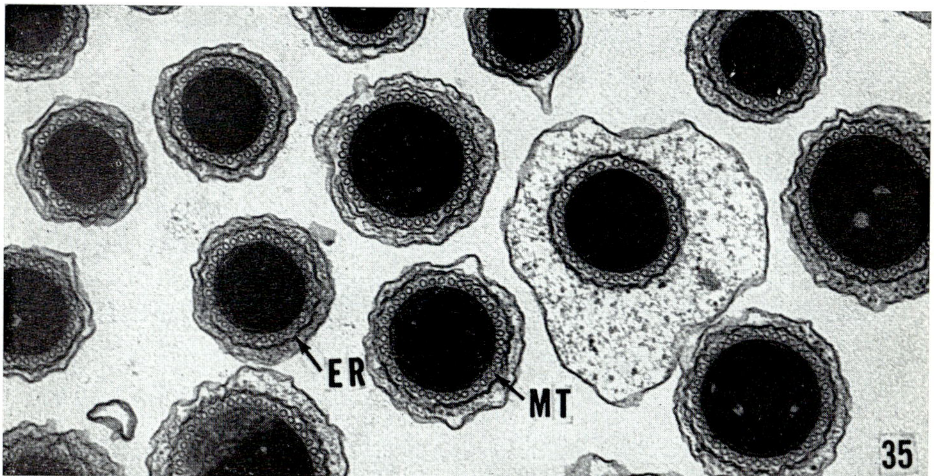

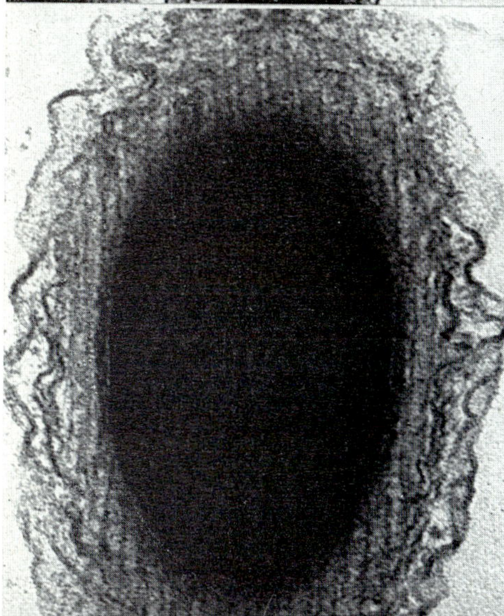

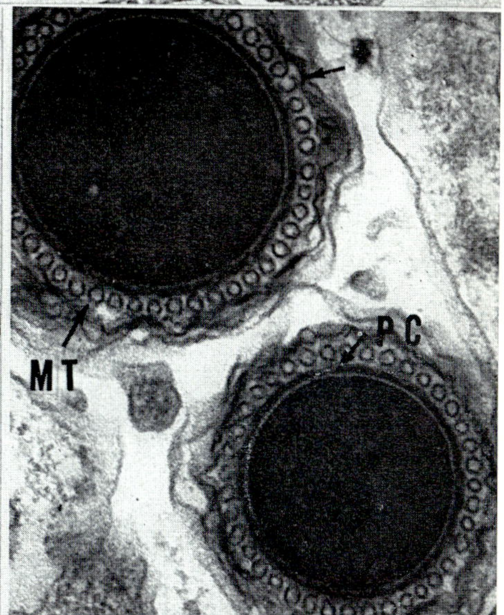

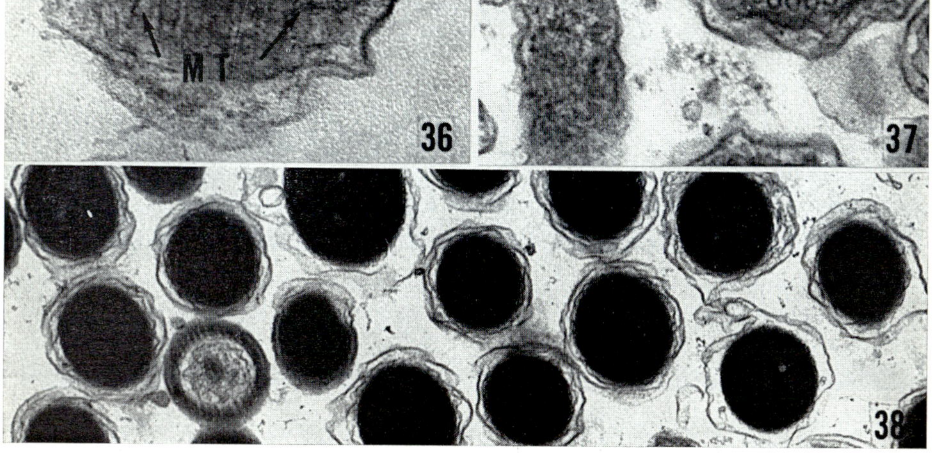

RICHARD G. KESSEL – *Spermiogenesis in the dragonfly with special reference to a consideration of the mechanisms involved in the development of cellular asymmetry.*

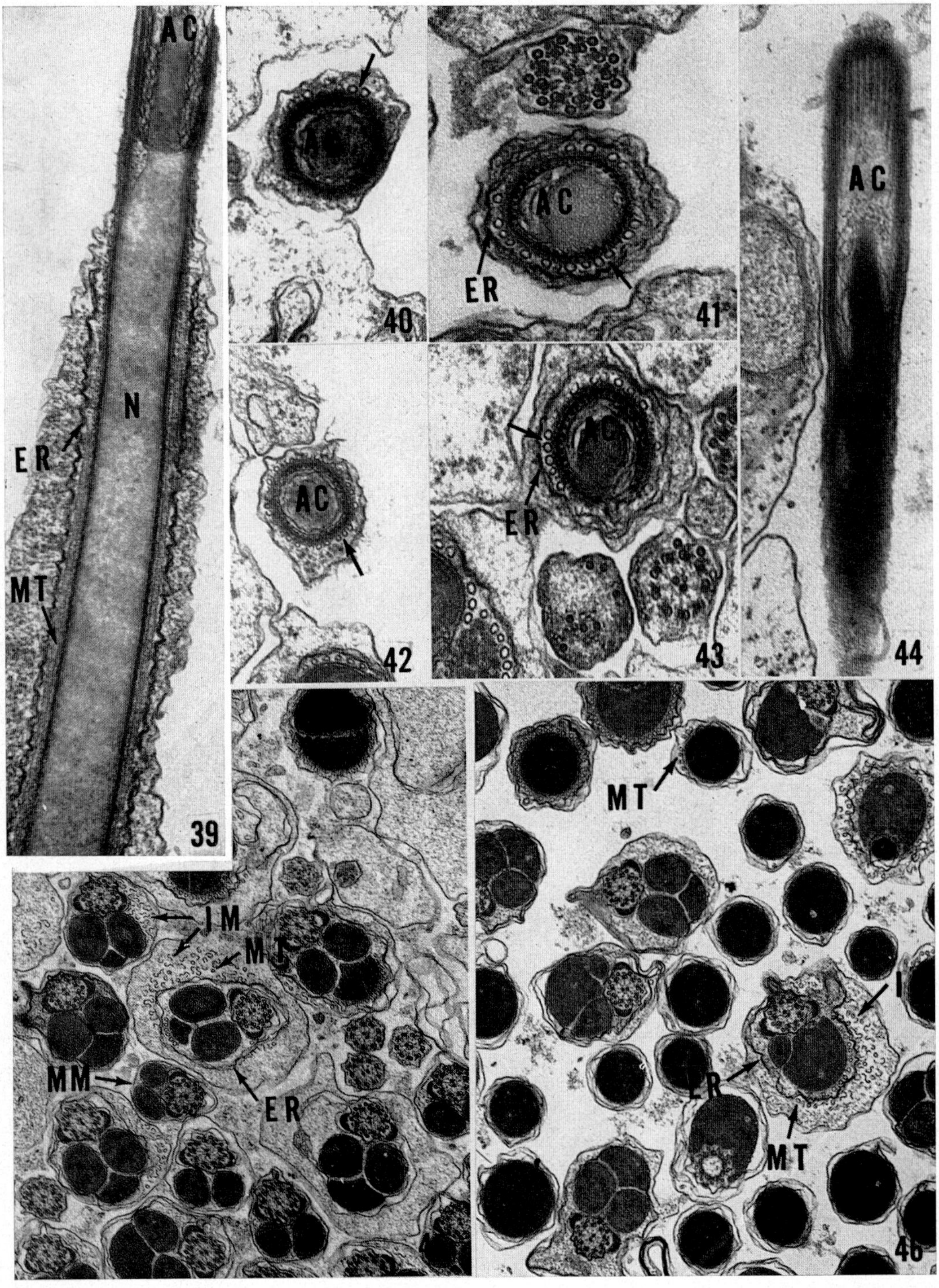

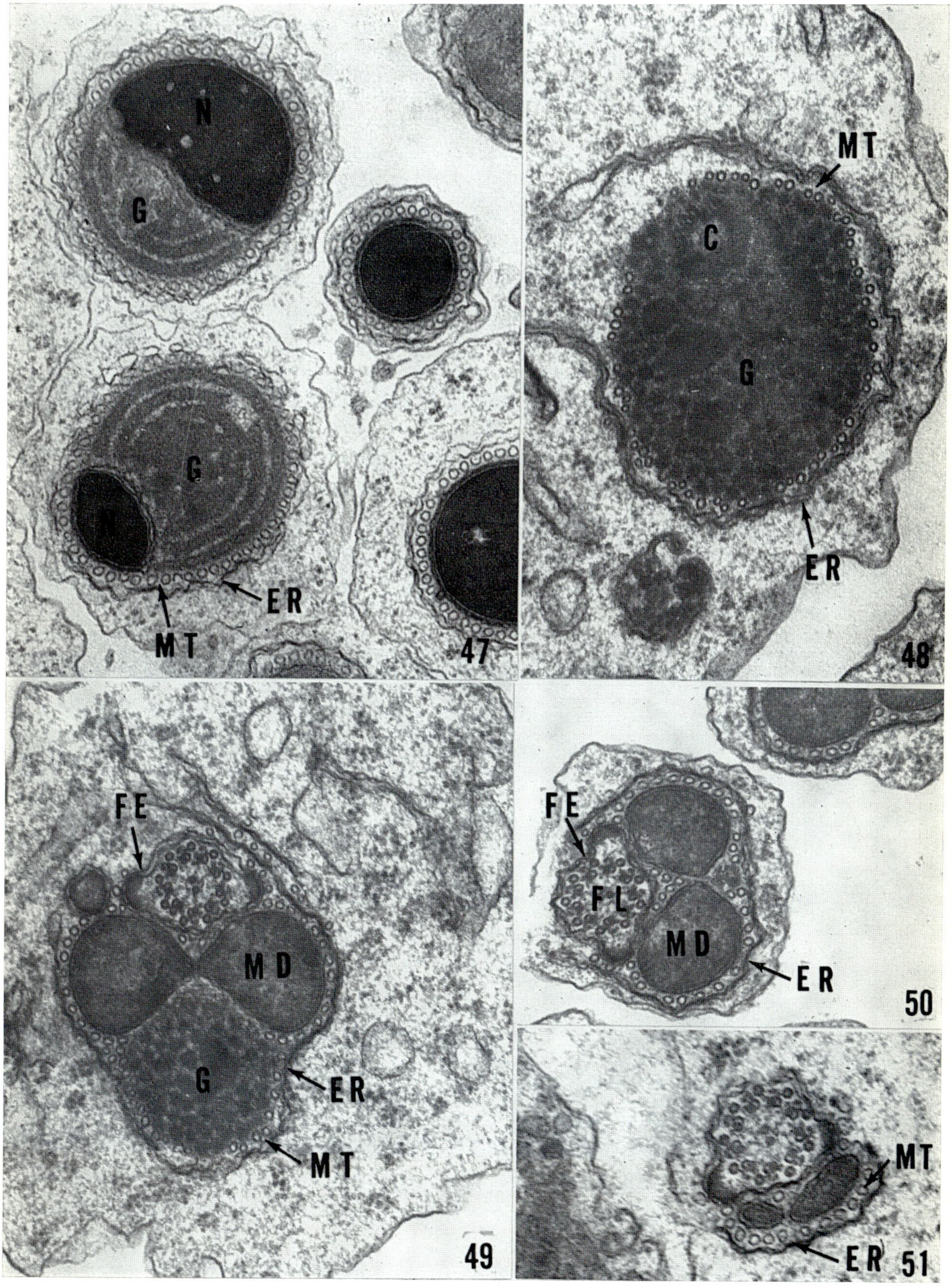
N
G
G
N
ER
MT
47
MT
C
G
ER
48
FE
MD
G
ER
MT
49
FE
FL
MD
ER
50
MT
ER
51

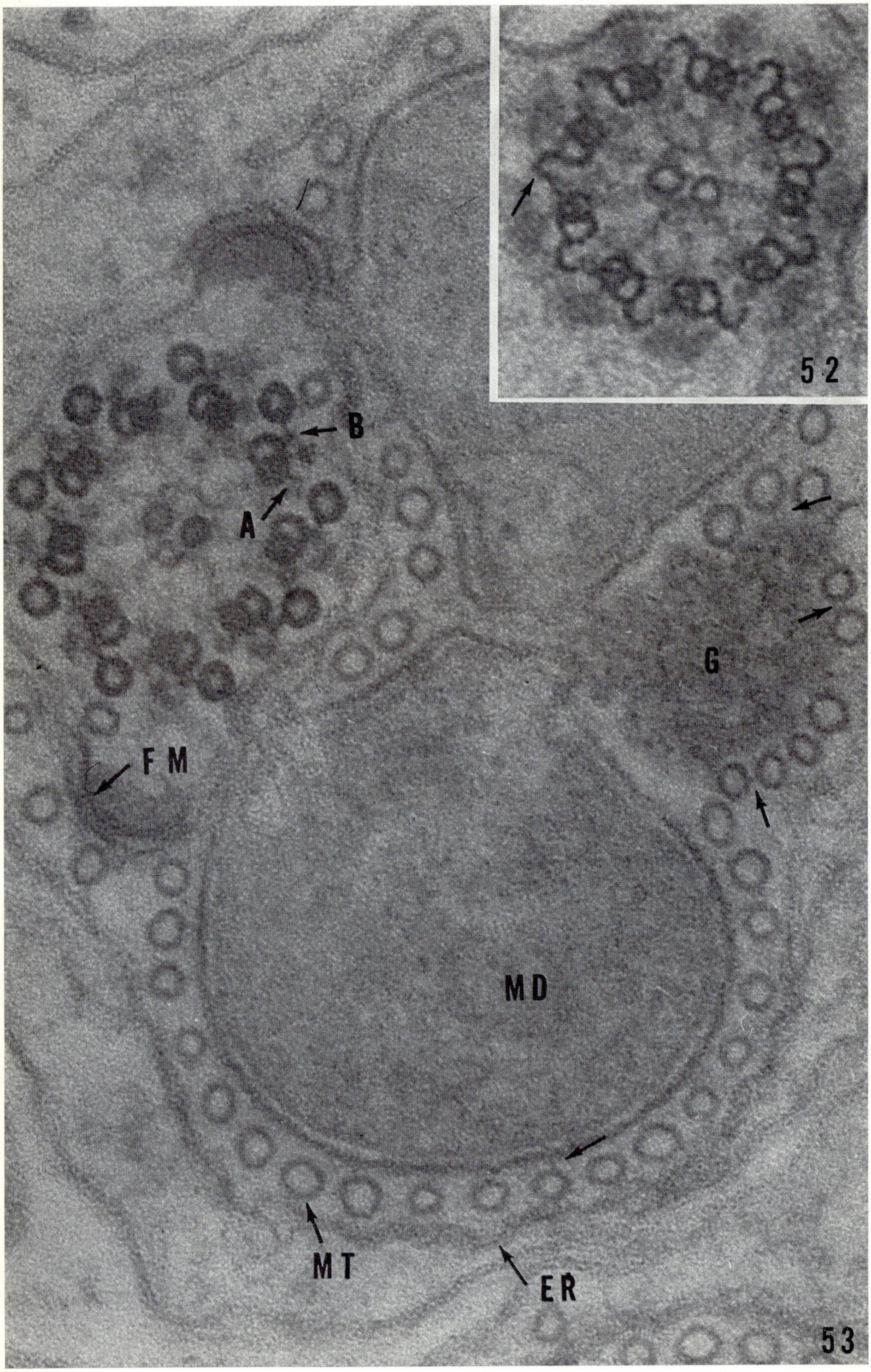
52
B
A
G
FM
MD
MT
ER
53

ANNE-MARIE CANTACUZÈNE (*)

L'ANNEXE CENTRIOLAIRE DU SPERMATOZOÏDE DES INSECTES

SUMMARY. — There is a centriolar adjunct in the spermatozoa of nearly all Insects. The structure is described as " typical centriolar adjunct " in the majority of Insects but other pericentriolar structures are described as well. The different hypotheses upon the origin of centriolar adjunct material are presented and discussed. Personal studies are made of these organelles in *Locusta migratoria* (*Orthoptera*), particularly on the question of its chemical nature which has been proved to be proteic.

The fields proposed for investigation in the future are:

1) the precise determination of chemical nature of the organelle.
2) the origin of its material.

RIASSUNTO. — Negli spermatozoi di quasi tutti gli insetti vi è un aggiunto centriolare. Nella maggioranza degli insetti questa struttura è descritta come « tipico aggiunto centriolare » ma sono descritte anche altre strutture pericentriolari. Vengono presentate e discusse le differenti ipotesi sull'origine del materiale costituente l'aggiunto centriolare. Sono stati fatti studi personali su questi organuli in *Locusta migratoria* (Ortotteri), particolarmente riguardo alla loro natura chimica che è stata trovata essere proteica.

Le vie proposte per l'indagine futura sono:

1) la precisa determinazione della natura chimica dell'organulo;
2) l'origine di questo materiale.

L'apparition, dans la spermatide jeune, d'un matériel dense péricentriolaire et son expansion rapide le long du flagelle constituent des caractères assez constants de la spermiogenèse des Insectes.

Dès 1929, des structures différenciées associées au centriole furent observées au microscope photonique par GATENBY et WIGODER. La morphologie de ces organites ne put cependant être connue que grâce à la microscopie électronique. Dès les premières observations effectuées à l'échelle ultrastructurale, GATENBY et TAHMISIAN (1959) constatèrent que les organites péricentriolaires des spermatozoïdes d'Insecte et de certains autres Invertébrés différaient des structures post-nucléaires des spermatozoïdes de Vertébrés et ils proposèrent de réserver le terme «centriole adjunct» à ces formations péricentriolaires.

L'état actuel de nos connaissances sur « l'annexe centriolaire » sera présenté ici dans la seule classe des Insectes.

(*) Laboratoire de Biologie Animale C, Faculté des Sciences, Paris, France. (Laboratoire de Microscopie electronique appliquée à la Biologie. CNRS).

TABLEAU.

					Annexe centriol.
APTERYGOTES		Thysanoures	*Lepisma saccharina*	WERNER, 1964	+
			Thermobia domestica	BAWA, 1964	?
		Collemboles	*Anurida maritima*	DALLAI, com. pers.	+
PTERYGOTES	Paléoptères.	Odonates	*Argia sp.*	BRELAND *et al.* 1966	+
	Néoptères Hétéro-métaboles.	Orthoptères	*Gelastorrhinus bicoler*	YASUZUMI *et al.*, 1957	+
			Laplatacris dispar	DE ROBERTIS *et al.*, 1957	+
			Chortophaga viridifasciata	DASS *et al.*, 1958	+
			Melanoplus differentialis	GATENBY *et al.* 1959	+
				KESSEL, 1967	+
			Locusta migratoria	CANTACUZÈNE	+
			Nemobius sp.	GATENBY *et al.*, 1959	+
			Acheta domestica	KAYE, 1962	+
				SCHIN, 1965	+
			Pachyrhamma fasifer	BERTAUD *et al.*, 1961	+
			Ceutophilus secretus	SHAY *et al.*, 1968	+
		Psocoptères	*Atropos pulsatorium*	BACCETTI *et al.*, 1969	+
		Mallophages	*Menopon gallinae*	BACCETTI *et al.*, 1969	+
		Thysanoptères	*Chriptothrips latus*	BACCETTI *et al.*, 1969	+
		Hétéroptères	*Gerris remigis*	TANDLER *et al.*, 1966	+
			Oncopeltus fasciatus	BARKER *et al.*, 1966	+
			Gelastocoris oculatus	PAYNE, 1966	+
			Nepa rubra	WERNER, 1966	*spc*
			Euchistus sp.	PHILLIPS, 1969 Sienne	+
		Homoptères	*divers Auchénorhynches*	FOLLIOT, 1969 Sienne	+
			Peregrinus maidis	HEROLD *et al.*, 1967	?
			Parlatoria oleae	ROBISON, 1966	?
			Pseudococus obscurus	ROSS *et al.*, 1969	?
	Néoptères holométabo-les.	Plannipennes	*Hesperoleon, Corydalis*	BRELAND, 1966	+
			Chrysopa, Eumicromus	BACCETTI *et al.*, 1969	+
		Coléoptères	*Cicindela campestris*	WERNER, 1965	*spc*
			Carabus sp.	WERNER, 1966	+
		Mécoptères	*Panorpa nuptialis*	BRELAND, 1966	+
			Panorpa annexa	BACCETTI, 1969	+
		Lépidoptères	*Pieris brasicae*	ZYLBERBERG, 1968	+
		Diptères	*Culex pipiens*	NUÑEZ, 1963	+
			Culex molestus	BRELAND *et al.*, 1966	+
			Anopheles punctipennis	BRELAND *et al.*, 1966	+
			Culiseta inornata	BRELAND *et al.*, 1966	+
			Aedes aegypti	BRELAND *et al.*, 1966	+
			Drosophila melanogaster	BRELAND *et al.*, 1966	+
			Drosophila viridis	BRELAND *et al.*; 1966	+
			Drosophila melanogaster	PEROTTI, 1969 Sienne	+
			Sciara coprophila	PHILLIPS, 1966	+
		Hyménoptères	*Apis melifera*	HOAGE *et al.*, 1968	+

+ : annexe centriolaire granulaire dans la spermatide.
? : aucune mention de cet organite.
spc : autre type des structures péri ou juxta-centriolaire.

Depuis le travail de GATENBY et TAHMISIAN, une annexe centriolaire a été décrite dans la plupart des ordres d'Insectes. On trouvera ci-dessous la liste des espèces pour lesquelles il existe quelque information sur la région centriolaire (ces informations étant parfois réduites à une seule micrographie). La morphologie de l'organite, ses rapports avec les autres organites du spermatozoïde, sa nature chimique et son rôle seront ensuite successivement envisagés.

MORPHOLOGIE

La très grande majorité des Insectes possède une annexe centriolaire pouvant être qualifiée de « typique » et qui est indiquée dans le tableau par le signe +.

– Dans quelques espèces, des structures péricentriolaires quelque peu différentes ont été décrites: spc.

– Dans l'ordre des Homoptères Sternorhynches, la morphologie du spermatozoïde est très modifiée et aucune structure ne peut, semble–t–il, être assimilée à l'annexe centriolaire.

Structure typique.

Dans la plupart des cas, l'annexe centriolaire de la spermatide jeune est hémisphérique. Elle coiffe la partie postérieure du noyau et englobe le centriole flagellaire (Figs. 1–4). Sa structure est granulaire; la taille des granules ne parait pas dépendre des fixateurs utilisés (OsO_4 ou fixation double) mais varie selon les espèces: 160 Å chez *Laplatacris* (Orthoptère), 200 à 300 Å chez *Atropos* (Psocoptère), 300 Å chez *Locusta* (Orthoptère), 320 Å chez *Chrysopa* (Planipenne). Chez certains Diptères, Lépidoptères et Hyménoptères, les grains sont, à l'examen des clichés, du même ordre de grandeur.

Par contre, dans le cas d'*Acheta* (Orthoptère), de *Carabus* et de *Cicindela* (Coléoptère), la substance péricentriolaire est plus finement granuleuse. Barker et Riess comparent ces granules à des ribosomes dans le cas d'*Oncopeltus* (Hétéroptère).

Dans l'annexe centriolaire « jeune » on note la présence constante au sein de la masse granulaire d'une ou deux zones claires dont la signification n'a jamais été envisagée.

– La morphologie de l'annexe centriolaire est la même dans les spermatozoïdes atypiques des Thysanoures où le centriole flagellaire est en position très antérieure. Chez *Lepisma*, il semble bien que le matériel péricentriolaire soit non pas un acrosome, mais unc annexe centriolaire qui donne, après allongement, le corps post–nucléaire.

Autres structures péricentriolaires.

Chez *Cicindela* (Coléoptère), la substance granulaire est organisée en couches concentriques autour du centriole et une sorte de gouttière arquée très opaque est associée de manière constante au matériel péricentriolaire. L'origine de cette structure est inconnue mais sa taille est proche de celle d'un centriole. Les deux éléments s'étendent vers l'arrière le long du flagelle en restant en contact.

Chez *Nepa* (Hétéroptère), le matériel qui se condense près de la membrane nucléaire, et à proximité du centriole, forme une double lame opaque ne présentant aucune ressemblance morphologique avec une annexe centriolaire typique.

Dans le cas général où le spermatozoïde possède une annexe centriolaire typique celle–ci s'accroît et se transforme en un organite compact qui persiste dans le spermatozoïde mûr. Cette transformation a été peu étudiée, elle sera illustrée ici par l'exemple de *Locusta* (Orthoptère). (Figs. 5–8).

Pendant l'allongement de la spermatide, la masse granulaire s'étend le long du flagelle de façon dissymétrique, une pointe médiane très nettement marquée s'engageant entre les deux dérivés mitochondriaux. Dans le même temps, elle enveloppe vers l'avant la base du noyau. Pendant cet allongement, les granules fusionnent de manière irrégulière (Fig. 5). Dans une spermatide d'âge moyen (chromatine en réseau), l'annexe centriolaire est devenue une masse relativement dense avec des zones claires irrégulièrement distribuées (Fig. 6). Ces zones confluent pendant la phase terminale de l'allongement et forment des lames courbes partageant l'annexe centriolaire en plusieurs éléments longitudinaux (Fig. 7). A ce stade, la structure primitive granulaire est encore visible mais elle devient ensuite tout à fait compacte. Au cours de cette évolution, l'organite a acquis une symétrie bilatérale; son plan de symétrie contient les deux fibres centrales du filament axial (Fig. 8). On ne constate pas cette même symétrie quand le spermatozoïde ne contient qu'un seul dérivé mitochondrial comme chez *Panorpa* (Mécoptère).

Rapports anatomiques entre l'annexe centriolaire et les autres organites du spermatozoïde

Noyau.

Dans la spermatide jeune, les grains de l'annexe centriolaire sont disposés régulièrement à une certaine distance de la membrane nucléaire (250 Å chez *Locusta*) (Fig. 3). Cette zone du noyau est caractérisée par un épaississement de ses deux membranes et est entourée par une aire différenciée où les pores nucléaires sont nombreux et rapprochés. Dans certains cas (*Cicindela*, (Coléoptère), la substance s'accumule plus précisément en face d'une zone nucléaire différenciée particulièrement « poreuse ». En ce qui concerne la chromatine, elle se condense préférentiellement dans la zone juxta–centriolaire (Fig. 2). Le cas de la spermatide de *Gryllus* (Orthoptère) où la chromatine est répartie sur le pourtour du noyau sauf dans la zone juxta–centriolaire est exceptionnel à cet égard (Kaye, 1962; Schin, 1965). Condensations chromatiniennes, abondance de pores nucléaires et aspect granulaire de l'annexe centriolaire sont autant d'éléments qui ont suggéré une origine nucléaire du matériel péricentriolaire (BARKER et RIESS pour *Oncopeltus*; WERNER pour *Cicindela*). Des extrusions parfois très abondantes de matériel nucléaire ont en effet été décrites dans les cellules sexuelles mâles (MAILLET et GOURANTON, 1965). On observe chez *Locusta* des figures semblables, et souvent dans les régions voisines de l'annexe centriolaire mais le matériel accumulé dans le cytoplasme et en relation topographique avec les pores nucléaires, n'a pas la structure granulaire de l'annexe centriolaire. L'existence de telles figures ne suffit pas à prouver l'origine nucléaire du matériel péricentriolaire mais justifierait semble-t-il de nouvelles recherches conduites avec l'aide de traceurs radioactifs.

Centriole.

Contrairement à de nombreux groupes animaux, la plupart des Insectes ont un spermatozoïde à un seul centriole: le centriole flagellaire (SOTELO et TRUJILLO-CENOZ, 1958; BRELAND *et al.*, 1968). Le dépôt du matériel granulaire ne commence qu'à partir du moment où ce centriole est en contact avec le noyau. La croissance de l'annexe centriolaire est alors très brusque et ceci explique l'absence d'observation sur les premiers stades de sa formation. Seuls GATENBY et TAHMISIAN ont noté la coalescence de granules encore peu nombreux et dispersés. Le rôle inducteur du centriole sur l'organisation de ces granules est très net. On le constate directement lorsqu'il y a organisation de la substance en couches concentriques (*Cicindela*). On l'observe également à l'occasion d'anomalies de la spermiogenèse. Chez les Orthoptères, une irradiation par les rayons X (TAHMISIAN et DEVINE, 1961) ou un déséquilibre endocrinien (CANTACUZÈNE, 1969) peut empêcher le formation de l'annexe centriolaire. Inversement, une multiplication aberrante des centrioles s'accompagne d'une multiplication des annexes correspondantes. (Figs. 10, 11). Chaque centriole joue alors manifestement le rôle d'un centre organisateur. Dans le cas très particulier de *Sciara coprophila* (Diptère) dont le centriole est géant, la production d'un matériel dense est également observée au contact des fibres périphériques (PHILLIPS, 1966), mais le manchon péricentriolaire disparait dans la suite de la spermiogenèse. Dans tous les cas, la substance granulaire est au contact direct des fibres centriolaires externes.

Réticulum endoplasmique et Polysomes.

Des citernes du réticulum endoplasmique ont été signalées à proximité de l'annexe centriolaire (DE ROBERTIS et RAFFO, 1957); on en remarque sur un cliché de SOTELO et TRUJILLO-CENOZ, et ANDERSON en a observé également chez *Carausius* (com. pers.). Chez *Locusta*, il existe parfois autour de l'annexe centriolaire un véritable anneau constitué par des citernes de réticulum à contenu relativement opaque aux électrons. Cette situation est peut-être temporaire car on l'observe rarement, mais par contre des éléments isolés de réticulum endoplasmique sont toujours assez nombreux dans cette région (Fig. 3).

Malgré des relations topographiques parfois étroites, aucune figure ne suggère qu'il y ait passage de matériel depuis ces citernes du réticulum vers l'annexe centriolaire.

Les nombreux polysomes qui se trouvent dans le cytoplasme de la spermatide jeune pourraient mieux, peut-être, jouer un rôle dans l'élaboration des protéines de l'annexe centriolaire ces protéines étant ensuite polymérisées au contact du centriole. Il s'agirait, dans ce cas d'un processus très semblable à celui qui intervient dans la formation des fuseaux de division.

Microtubules.

C'est autour de l'annexe centriolaire qu'aparaissent les premières concentrations de microtubules dans la spermatide chez *Melanoplus* (KESSEL, 1967). Chez *Locusta*, dans les cas d'anomalies cités plus haut, et du fait d'un blocage probable, de nombreuses spermatides contiennent des ilots de substance granulaire entourés par une couronne de microtubules (Fig. 9). Dans la spermiogenèse normale, ce stade est de courte durée et aucune hypothèse n'a été avancée sur les relations existant entre ces deux structures cellulaires.

L'origine des matériaux qui constituent l'annexe centriolaire n'est donc pas élucidée à l'heure actuelle et nous verrons que leur nature chimique est également encore mal connue.

NATURE CHIMIQUE DU MATERIEL DE L'ANNEXE CENTRIOLAIRE

Dans le spermatozoïde de *Chrysopa* (BACCETTI, DALLAI et ROSATI, 1969) le matériel de l'annexe centriolaire est digéré par la trypsine à forte concentration, par la RNASE et par la diestérase extraite du venin de Crotale, mais non par la pepsine ou la papaïne. Les auteurs concluent à la nature ribonucléoprotéique de ce matériel.

Dans le cas de *Locusta*, le groupement des spermatozoïdes en spermatodesmes permet l'étude cytochimique en microscopie photonique d'organites dont la taille est inférieure au pouvoir de résolution du microscope. (CANTACUZENE, 1968). En effet, les spermatozoïdes sont disposés en grand nombre et parallèlement les uns aux autres. Dans ces conditions, une région chromophile bien visible correspond à l'ensemble des annexes centriolaires alignées. Cette zone n'est pas pyroninophile, elle n'est colorée ni par l'A.P.S. (polysaccharides), ni par les colorants des lipides. Elle donne par contre une réaction positive à de nombreux tests des protéines, y compris ceux qui caractérisent les protéines basiques. Par la méthode d'ALFERT et GESHWIND (1953) au Fast green à *p*H 8,2, on colore entièrement la tête du spermatozoïde si on fait précéder la coloration d'une extraction par l'acide trichloracétique, et, électivement la zone centriolaire, si on ne procède pas à cette extraction.

Les affinités tinctoriales de cette zone dans les colorations topographiques utilisant les seuls colorants « acides » (azorubine, par exemple), suggèrent également la présence de protéines basiques. Le fait demande a être confirmé mais il s'accorderait à ce que l'on sait actuellement de l'existence de protéines basiques extranucléaires. Celles–ci ont été mises en évidence dans la capsule des spermatozoïdes de Crustacés Décapodes (CHEVAILLIER, 1967) ou dans l'acrosome de divers spermatozoïdes (DAS *et al.*, 1967).

A l'échelle ultrastructurale, la nature protéique de l'annexe centriolaire du spermatozoïde est mise en évidence par des digestions enzymatiques (Figs. 12–13). Celles–ci sont conduites selon le protocole indiqué par MONNERON et BERNHARD (1966), puis par ANDERSON et ANDRÉ (1968), pour des tissus inclus dans le mélange Araldite–Epon. Les résultats les plus nets sont obtenus sur des coupes relativement épaisses: les deux fibres internes et les neufs fibres accessoires périphériques du filament axial sont partiellement digérées, l'annexe centriolaire est totalement détruite. La pepsine et la pronase sont également actives à la concentration de 0,2 %, alors que la trypsine donne des résultats inconstants. Les résultats obtenus sur les spermatides jeunes sont tout différents. Dans les coupes soumises à la digestion enzymatique (pepsine, pronase et trypsine à 0,2 et 0,5 %), l'opacité du matériel granulaire n'est pas diminuée par rapport à celle de coupes témoins flottées sur l'eau pendant le même temps et à la même température. Deux hypothèses peuvent être avancées pour expliquer ces résultats:

L'attaque enzymatique d'une structure compacte (annexe centriolaire du spermatozoïde) pourrait être plus aisée que celle d'une structure diffuse inclue dans une masse relativement importante de résine (annexe centriolaire de la spermatide).

Des remaniements chimiques pourraient accompagner les transformations morphologiques de l'annexe centriolaire: un matériel protéique venant s'ajouter au matériel granulaire préexistant.

Il conviendrait donc, malgré l'absence de pyroninophilie, de rechercher la présence de ribonucléoprotéines dans l'annexe centriolaire. Quoiqu'il en soit, nos résultats indiquent, dès à présent, que dans la spermatozoïde de *Locusta*, cette structure est riche en matériel protéique.

ROLE

Pour GATENBY (1959, 1961), la localisation anatomique du « centriole adjunct » des spermatozoïdes d'Insectes indique clairement son rôle mécanique. De manière générale, il constitue effectivement une structure de jonction efficace entre la tête rigide et le flagelle mobile, mais on peut se demander si c'est là son seul rôle. La présence de protéines basiques dans l'annexe centriolaire soulève notamment un problème. On sait qu'au cours de la spermiogenèse, les protéines basiques du noyau (histones somatiques) sont remplacées par des histones riches en Arginine. (LECHENAULT, 1968). Le moment où s'effectue cette « transition des histones » est facilement repéré par une incorporation massive d'Arginine tritiée dans les noyaux. Chez *Locusta*, une heure après une injection intra-abdominale (20 μC de L–Arg H 3) (1), les noyaux des spermatides jeunes sont fortement radioactifs. Or, l'annexe centriolaire se forme à ce stade de la spermiogenèse ou un peu antérieurement. Ne pourrait–on envisager dès lors une relation entre sa formation et le rejet des histones somatiques?

Pour mieux comprendre les fonctions de l'annexe centriolaire du spermatozoïde des Insectes, il serait très utile de pouvoir comparer cet organite aux diverses structures occupant une situation analogue dans d'autres types de spermatozoïdes. La morphologie de la région centriolaire diffère profondément selon les groupes zoologiques mais la présence de substances plus ou moins granulaire autour du centriole ou du flagelle est néanmoins fréquente. Aucune comparaison valable ne semble cependant possible à l'heure actuelle puisqu'on ignore à la fois l'origine et la nature chimique précise de ces composés. Les réponses apportées à ces deux questions conduiront peut–être à ré–envisager le rôle de l'annexe centriolaire dans la physiologie du spermatozoïde.

Bibliographie

Alfert M. et Geschwind I. I. (1953) – *A selective staining method for the basic protein of cell nuclei.* « Proc. Nat. Acad. Sc. U. S. », 39, 991–999.

Anderson W. A. et Andre J. (1968) – *The extraction of some cell components with pronase and pepsine from thin sections of tissues embedded in an Epon–Araldite mixture.* « J. Microscopie », 7, 343–354.

Baccetti B., Dallai R. et Rosati F. (1969) – *The spermatozoon of Arthropoda.* III. *The lowest insects.* « J. Microscopie », 8, 233–248.

Baccetti B., Dallai R. et Rosati F. (1969) – *The spermatozoon of Arthropoda.* IV. *Corrodentia, Mallophaga, Thysanoptera.* « J. Microscopie », 8, 249–262.

Barker K. et Riess R. W. (1966) – *An electron microscope study of spermateleosis in the Hemipteran:* Oncopeltus fasciatus. « La Cellule », 66, 41–54.

Bawa S. R. (1964) – *Electron microscope study of spermiogenesis in a firebrat insect: Thermobia domestica.* I. *Mature spermatozoon.* « J. Cell. Biol. », 23, 431–446.

Bertaud W. et Gatenby J. (1961) – *The mitochondrial nebenkern and centriole complex in* Pachyrhamma fasifer. *An electron microscope study.* « La Cellule », 61, 153–170.

Breland O. P., Cummings R. B., Gassner III G. et Biesele J. J. (1965) – *Phase and electron microscopy studies of the centriole adjunct in Insects.* « Amer. Zool. », 5, 245–246.

Breland O. P., Gassner G., Riess R. et Biesele J. J. (1966) – *Certain aspects of the centriole adjunct, Spermiogenesis and the mature sperm of Insects.* « Canad. J. Genet. Cytol. », 8, 759–773.

Breland O. P., Barker K. R., Eddleman C. D. et Biesele J. J. (1968) – *Centriole in the spermatids of insects.* « Ann. Entomol. Soc. Amer. », 61 (4), 1037–9.

Breland O. P., Eddleman C. D. et Biesele J. J. (1968) – *Studies of Insect spermatozoa.* « Entomol. News. U.S.A. », 79, n°8, 197–216.

(1) « Act. spec. », 18 C/mM, C.E.A.

CANTACUZÈNE A. M. (1968) – *Recherches morphologiques et physiologiques sur les glandes annexes ♂ des Orthoptères.* III. *Modes d'association des spermatozoïdes d'Orthoptères.* « Z. Zellforsch. », 90, 113–126.

CANTACUZÈNE A. M. (1969) – *Données ultrastructurales sur la spermiogènese de* Locusta migratoria *après implantation de corps allates.* « Bull. Soc. Fr. Zool. » 94, 290.

CHEVAILLIER PH. (1967) – *Mise en évidence et étude cytochimique d'une protéine basique extranucléaire dans les spermatozoïdes de crustacés décapodes.* « J. Cell. Biol. », 32 (3), 547–556.

DALLAI R. (1967) – *Lo Spermatozoo degli Artropodi.* I. Anurida maritima *ed* Orchesella villosa (Insecta, Collembola). « Atti. Accad. Fisiocritici Siena », 16, 468–476.

DAS N. K., MICOU–EASTWOOD J. et ALFERT M. (1967) – *Cytochemical and biochemical properties of basic proteins of* urechis *acrosome* (*ver echiuride*). « J. Cell Biol. », 2, 455–458.

DASS C. M. et RIS H. (1958) – *Submicroscopic organization of the Nucleus during Spermiogenesis in the grasshoper.* « J. Biophys. Biochem. Cytol. », 4, 129–132.

DE ROBERTIS E. et FRANCO RAFFO H. (1957) – *Submicroscopic organization of the mitochondrial body and other cytoplasmic structures of insect testis.* « Exp. Cell. Res. », 12, (1), 66–79.

FOLLIOT R. (1969) – *Fine structure of spermiogenesis and spermatozoa of different Insects in the Order* Homoptera. Symp. on comparative Spermatology, Siena.

GATENBY J. B. et TAHMISIAN T. N. (1959) – *Centriole adjunct, Centrioles, Mitochondria and Ergastoplasm in Orthopteran spermatogenesis.* « La Cellule », 60, 105–134.

GATENBY J. B. et WIGODER S. (1929) – *The effect of X radiation on the Spermatogenesis of the guinea pig.* « Proc. Roy. Soc. B. », 104–351.

GATENBY J. B. (1961) – *The electron microscopy of centriole, flagellum and cilium.* « J. Roy. Micr. Soc. », 79, 299–317.

HEROLD F. et MUNZ K. (1967) – *Ultrastructure of Spermatozoa of* Peregrinus maïdis, Homoptera (Delphacidae). « Z. Zellforsch. », 83, 364–374.

HOAGE T. R. et KESSEL R. G. (1968) – *An electron microscope study of the process of differentiation during spermatogenesis in the Drone Honeg bee* (Apis mellifera) *with special reference to centriole replication and elimination.* « J. Ultrastructure Res. », 24, 6–32.

KAYE J. S. (1962) – *Acrosome formation in the House cricket.* « J. Cell. Biol. », 12, 411–431.

KAYE J. S. et MASTER–KAYE (1966) – *The fine structure and chemical composition of nuclei during spermiogenesis in the house Cricket.* I. *Initial stages of differentiation and the loss of non histone protein.* « J. Cell. Biol. », 31, 159–179.

KESSEL R. G. (1967) – *An electron microscopic study of spermiogenesis in the grasshopper with particular reference to the development of microtubular systems during differentiation.* « J. Ultrastructure Res. », 18, 677–694.

LECHENAULT H. (1968) – *Les protéines basiques nucléaires et cytoplasmiques au cours de la gamétogenèse animale.* « Ann. Univers. et A.R.E.R.S. », 6, 37–43.

MAILLET P. L. et GOURANTON J. (1965) – *Sur l'expulsion de l'acide ribonucleoprotéique nucléaire par les spermatides de* Philaenus spumarus (Homoptera, Cercopidae). « C. R. Acad. Sc. », 261, 1417–1419.

MONNERON A. et BERNHARD W. (1966) – *Action de certaines enzymes sur des tissus inclus en Epon.* « J. Microscopie », 5, 697–714.

NUÑEZ J. A. (1963) – *Über den Feinbau der Spermienschwanzes von* Culex pipiens. « Biol. Zentrb. », 82, 1–7.

PAYNE F. (1966) – *Some observations on spermatogenesis of* Gelastocoris oculatus (Hemiptera) *with the aid of the electron microscope.* « J. Morph. », 119, 357–382.

PEROTTI M. E. (1969) – *The neck region in mature sperm of* Drosophila melanogaster. Symp. on Comparative Spermatology. Siena.

PHILLIPS D. M. (1966) – *Observations on spermiogenesis in the Fungus gnat* Sciara coprophila. « J. Cell. Biol. », 30, 477–497.

ROBISON G. W. (1966) – *Microtubules in relation to the mobility of a sperm syncytium in an armored scale insect* Parlatoria oleae (Homoptera, Coccoïdea). « J. Cell. Biol. », 29, 251–265.

SCHIN KI SAU (1965) – *Meiotische prophase und spermatidezelfung bei* Gryllus domesticus *mit besonderer berücksichtung der Chromosomen strucktur.* « Z. Zellforsch. », 65, 481–513.

SHAY J. W. et BIESELE J. J. (1968) – *Ultrastructural observations on spermiogenesis in the Cave cricket,* Ceutophilus secretus. « La Cellule », 67, 269–282.

SOTELO J. R. et TRUJILLO-CENOZ O. (1958) – *Electron-microscope study of the kinetic apparatus in animal sperm cells.* « Z. Zellforsch. », 48, 565–601.

TAHMISIAN T. N. et DEVINE R. L. (1961) – *The influence of X-rays on organelle induction and differentiation in grasshopper spermatogenesis.* « J. Biophys. Biochem. Cytol. », 9, 20–45.

TANDLER B. et MORIBER L. G. (1966) – *Microtubular structures associated with the acrosome during spermiogenesis in* Gerris remigis. « J. Ultrastructure Res. », 14, 391–404.

WERNER G. (1964) – *Untersuchungen ueber die spermiogenese beim Silber fischchen* Lepisma saccharina. « Z. Zellforsch. », 63, 880–912.

WERNER G. (1965) – *Untersuchungen ueber die Spermiogenese beim Sandlaüfer* Cicindela campestris. « Z. Zellforsch. », 66, 255–275.

WERNER G. (1966) – *Untersuchungen ueber die Spermiogenese beim einem laüf käfer,* Carabus catenulatus *und der Skorpion–Wasserwanze,* Nepa rubra. « Z. Zellforsch. », 73, 576–599.

YASUZUMI G. et ISHIDA H. (1957) – *Spermatogenesis in animals as revealed by electron microscopy.* IV. *Fine structure of spermatid nuclei in early stage of maturation.* « J. Electr. Microsc. », 5, 38–42.

ZYLBERBERG L. (1968) – *Contribution à l'étude de la double spermatogenèse chez un Lépidoptère* (Pieris brasicae, Pierideae). Thèse, Paris.

LÉGENDES DES FIGURES

Locusta migratoria.	Fixation:	Glutaraldéhyde–OsO4
	Inclusion:	Araldite–Epon ou metacrylate (fig. 3)
	Coloration:	Acétate d'uranyle–Plomb.

Fig. 1. – Coupe longitudinale de la Spermatide jeune.

A.C. annexe centriolaire
C fl centriole flagellaire
Fl flagelle
R E réticulum endoplasmique

Fig. 2. – Coupe oblique de la spermatide jeune: Noter l'abondance des pores nucléaires PN au voisinage immédiat de l'annexe centriolaire A C.

Nk nebenkern

Sur les deux clichés, la flèche indique les zones claire de l'annexe centriolaire.

Fig. 3. – Spermatide jeune. Les pores nucléaires sont indiqués par la flèche. Noter la concentration du matériel chromatinien dans la zone juxta-centriolaire. Dans le cytoplasme qui entoure l'annexe centriolaire, citernes de réticulum à contenu dense *RE* et microtubules *Mt.*

Fig. 4. – Spermatide en cours d'allongement: la chromatine est organisée en une lame dense postérieure *Ch* et en fibres longitudinales. Un ou deux corps denses granulaires *CD* se trouvent de manière constante à proximité de l'annexe centriolaire *AC.* Celle–ci est séparée des membranes nucléaires par un espace de 250 Å.

Fig. 5. – Début de l'allongement de l'annexe centriolaire. La flèche indique le niveau à partir duquel une pointe médiane s'engage entre les dérivés mitochondriaux.

Fig. 6. – Spermatide d'âge moyen. La chromatine du noyau *N* est organisée en réseau. L'annexe centriolaire *AC* est devenue compacte et vacuolisée.

Fig. 7. – Coupe longitudinale d'une spermatide en fin d'allongement. L'annexe centriolaire est divisée en plusieurs éléments longitudinaux par les lames cytoplasmiques claires. (flèches blanches).

Fig. 8. – Coupe transversale dans le flagelle d'une spermatide d'âge avancé. L'annexe centriolaire, découpée en 4 éléments, est localisée entre les deux dérivés mitochondriaux. L'abondance des microtubules indique que l'allongement de la spermatide n'est pas achevé.

Figs. 9–11. – Anomalies de la spermiogenèse consécutives à une implantation de corps allates durant la vie larvaire. Substance granulaire de l'annexe centriolaire en forme d'ilôt entouré de microtubules (Fig. 9); la multiplication des centrioles s'accompagne d'une multiplication des annexes centriolaires (Figs. 10 et 11).

Fig. 12. – Sections transversales de spermatozoïdes dans la vésicule séminale. Digestion de l'annexe centriolaire par la pronase.

Fig. 13. – Sections obliques. Digestion par la Pepsine.

A C emplacement de l'annexe centriolaire
N noyau
C Fl centriole flagellaire.

Les digestions sont conduites selon le protocole de MONNERON et BERNHARD (1966) après oxydation par l'acide périodique à 10%.

Discussion

ANDRÉ. – Did you try the Thiéry technique for polysaccharides, and, if so, what are the results?

CANTACUZÈNE. – The results of the Thiéry technique are entirely negative on the centriolar adjunct. The control of the reaction is given by the outer fibers of flagella which contains glycogen and stains strongly.

ANDRÉ. – What results did you obtain for –SH groups and acid proteins?

CANTACUZÈNE. – For SH groups, in light microscopy, I obtained positive results with the DDD method which gives good contrast and has a good specificity. No special test has been done for acid proteins: In all general methods, the region of centriole adjunct stains with acid dyes.

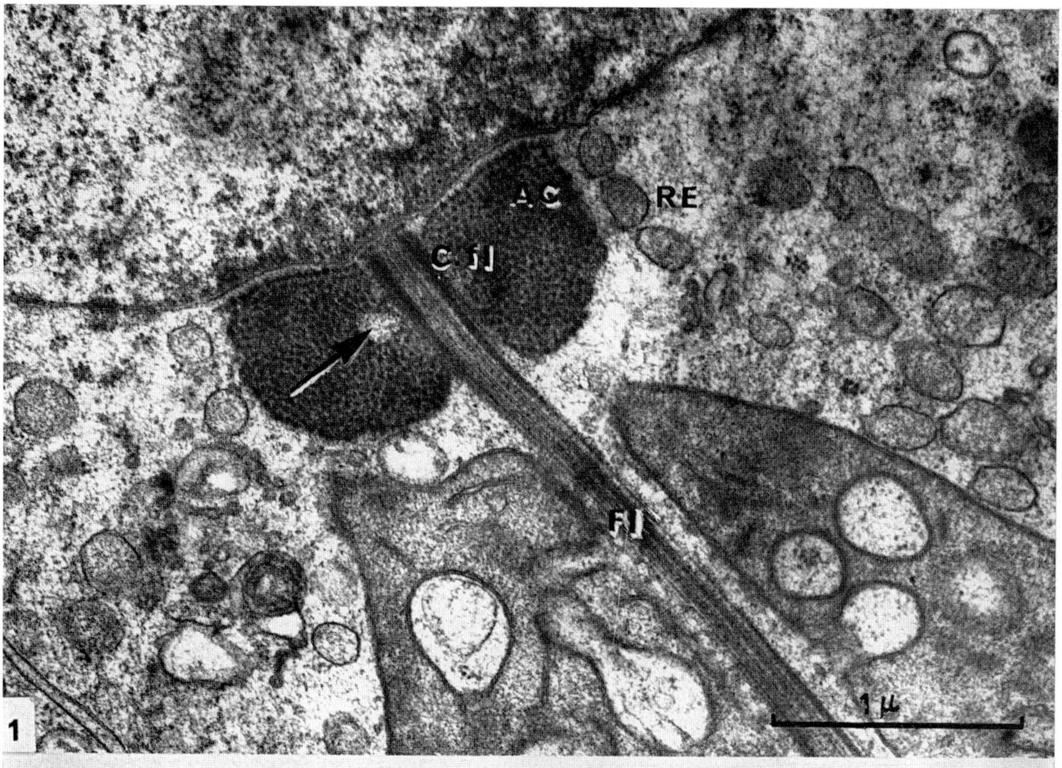
AC
RE
C fl
Fl
1 μ
1

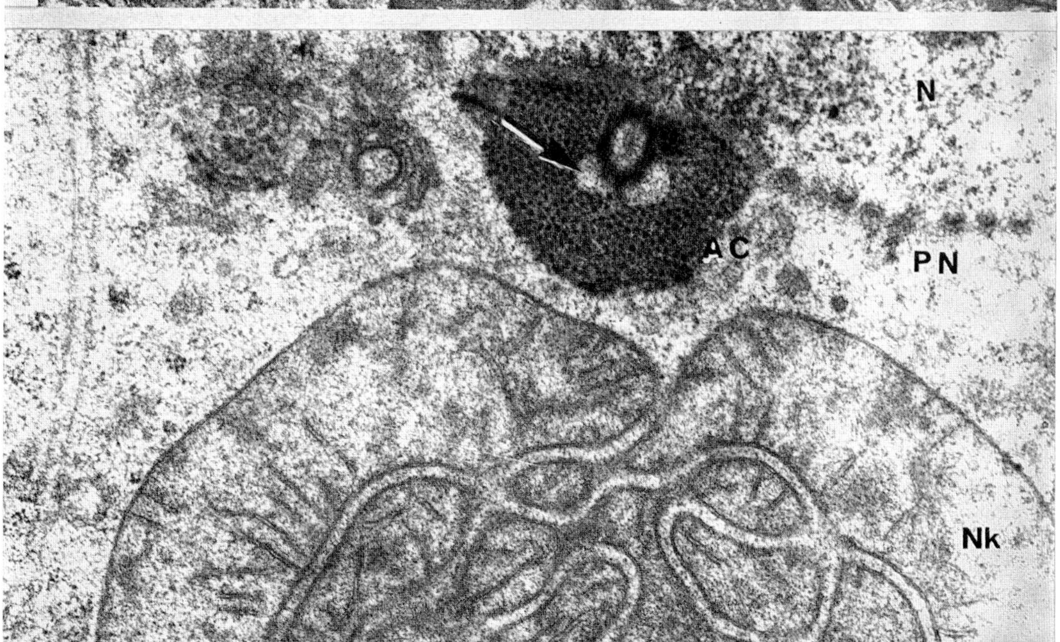
N
AC
PN
Nk
1μ

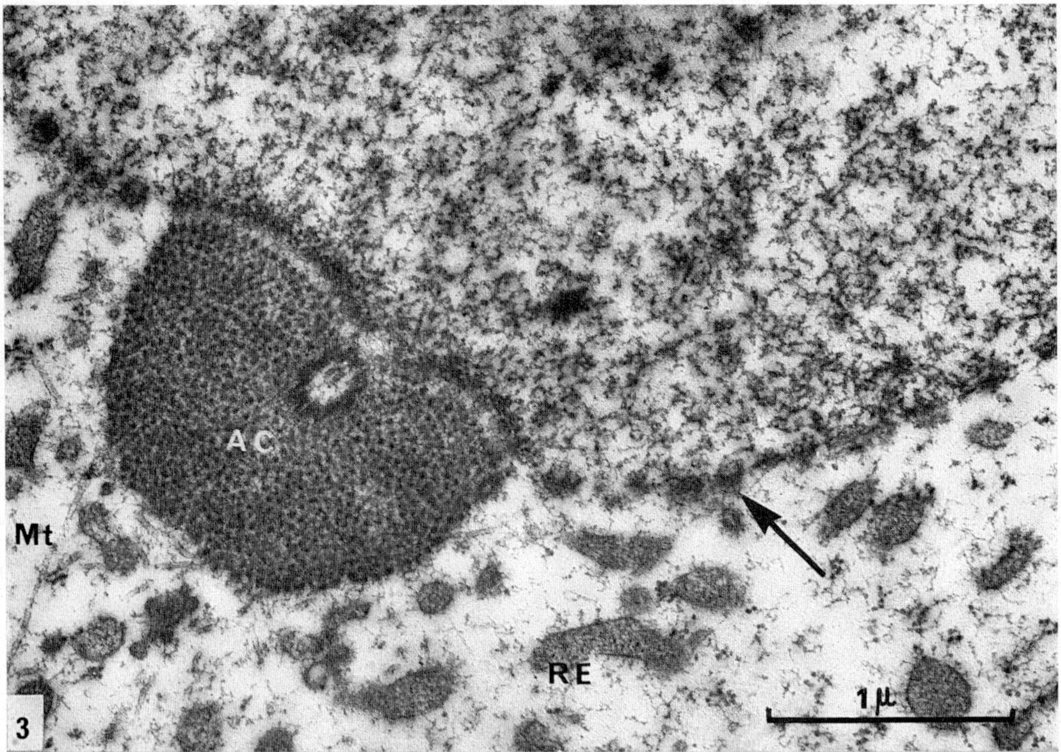
AC
Mt
RE
1µ
3

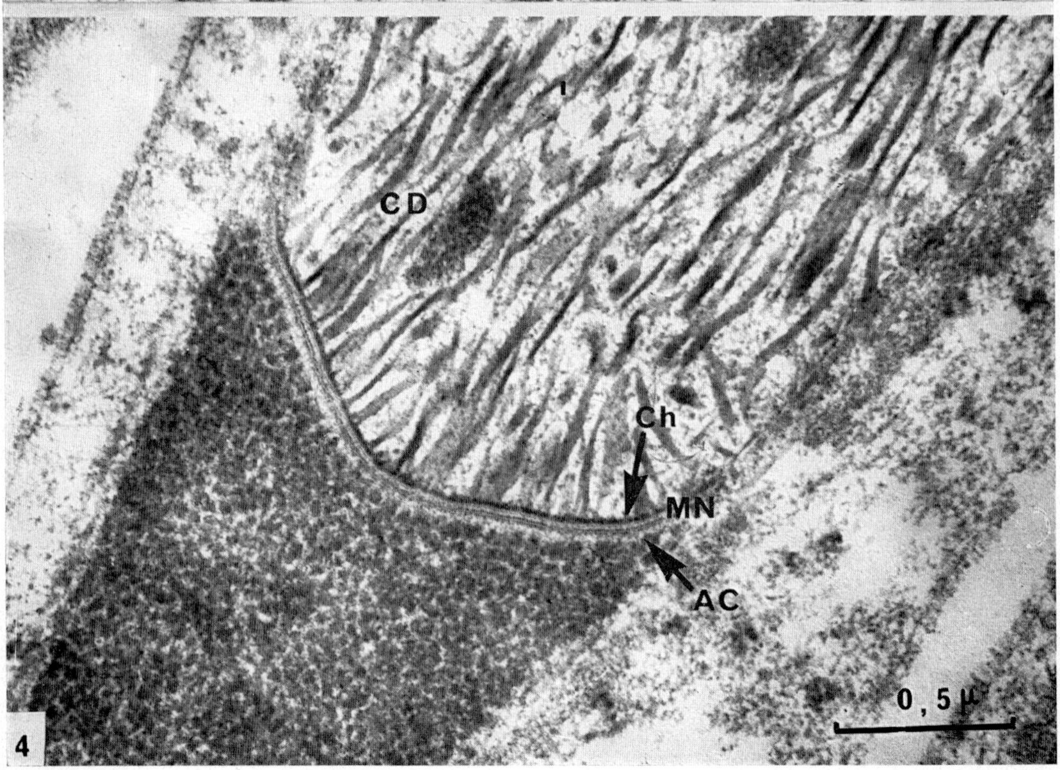
CD
Ch
MN
AC
0,5µ
4

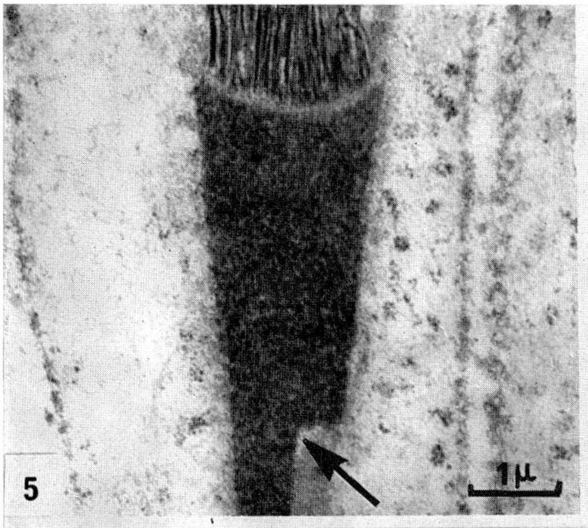
5
1μ

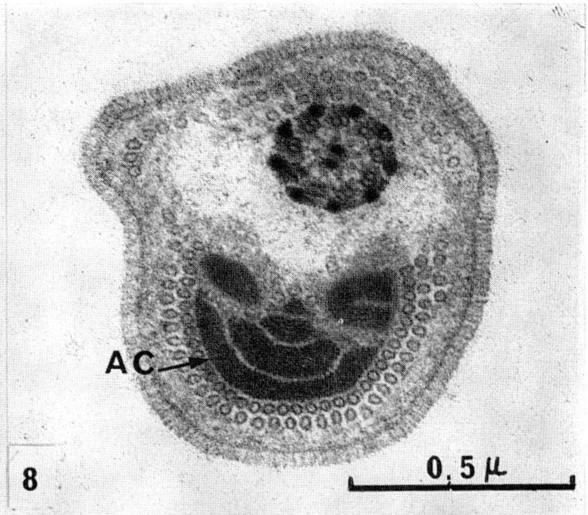
8
AC
0,5 μ

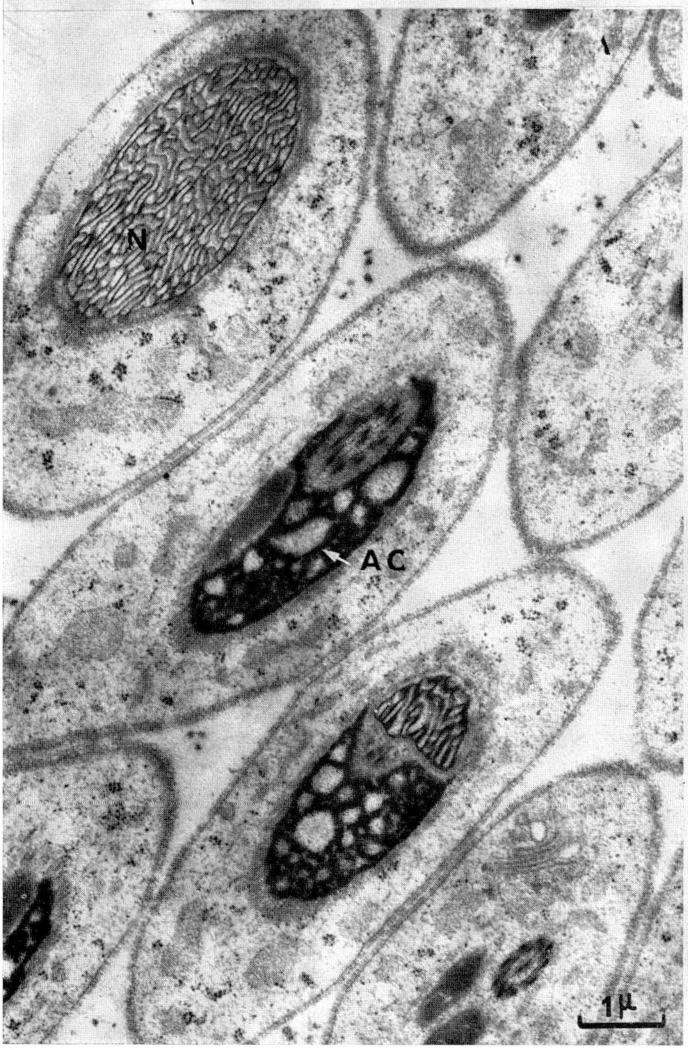
N
AC
1μ

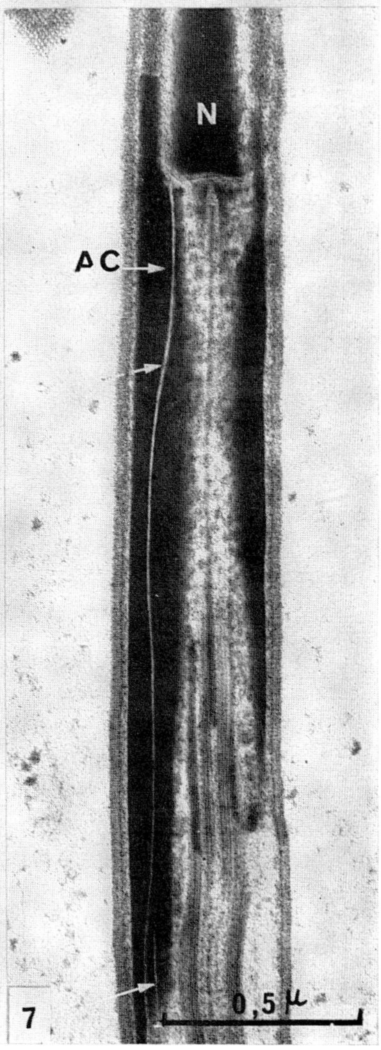
N
AC
7
0,5 μ

B. A. AFZELIUS (*)

THOUGHTS ON COMPARATIVE SPERMATOLOGY

SUMMARY. — In order to recognize the constituents of the spermatozoon it is necessary to analyse their derivation during spermiogenesis. Such a study may not however reveal the physiological role. It is essential to make a clear distinction between the function of an organelle and its derivation. Examples illustrating this point are given. The article also lists some problems in spermatology which seem promising for future investigations.

RIASSUNTO. — Per conoscere i costituenti dello spermatozoo è necessario analizzare la loro derivazione durante la spermiogenesi. Un tale studio non può tuttavia rivelare il loro ruolo fisiologico. È essenziale fare una chiara distinzione tra la funzione di un organello e la sua derivazione. Sono dati esempi che illustrano questo punto. Vengono enunciati anche alcuni problemi di spermatologia che sembrano interessanti per indagini future.

" The sperm seems never to transgress the few rules which govern the production of its fundamental parts, but in the arrangement of these parts every sperm (flagellate or non-flagellate) seems to be a law unto itself ".

The above quotation is from a paper by ROBERT BOWEN dealing with the homologies of different sperm types. BOWEN pointed out that a tapering part of the sperm must not necessarily be the tail and a round portion at the front of the sperm not necessarily the head. He expressed his notion like this: " It is the nucleus which makes the head, not the head which makes the nucleus ". BOWEN's recipe for recognizing the constituents of the spermatozoon was to analyse their derivation during spermiogenesis. This concept certainly is a fruitful one. HENDELBERG employed it, as presented at this symposium, and was able to convince us that he had indeed been able to make " head and tail " of the polyclad spermatozoon.

Activation versus hereditary transfer.

The question may be raised: which are the necessary sperm constituents? The question becomes easier to answer if the following question is first considered: which are the functions of the spermatozoon?

The traditional answer to the second question goes like this: the spermatozoon has a dual function; to activate the egg and to transmit paternal hereditary factors to the egg.

This answer is certainly quite correct although usually incomplete. Other functions will be listed below. Activation and hereditary transfer are normally

(*) Wenner-Gren Institute, University of Stockholm, Sweden.

coupled. The same spermatozoon brings about the two phenomena. There are however known cases of a distinction between egg activation and the transmission of hereditary factors. The best example is provided by the peculiar case of the Amazon black molly, *Molliensia formosa* or *Poecilia formosa*, as clarified by CARL HUBBS and his co-workers (1932 and 1955). (See also SCHULTZ and KALLMAN, 1968).

The little fish has females only, no males have ever been found. The female has to be mated in order to get an offspring. The male to mate with her may be the related fish species *M. latipenna* or *M. sphenops*. Evidently the egg becomes activated by the " fertilizing " spermatozoon, but the spermatozoon either does not enter the egg or it enters but has no influence on the egg (other than by activating it). The spermatozoon triggers off the cellular events leading to cell division and eventually to the formation of a new individual – again a female. This unusual example of activation without transfer of hereditary material can be regarded as one of Nature's experiments on living organisms. Similar cases of parthogenetic development initiated by sperms have been suspected to occur among some strains of salamanders (MC GREGOR and UZZEL, 1964), earthworms (MULDAL, 1952 and CHRISTENSEN and O'CONNOR, 1958) and a beetle (MOORE *et al.*, 1956, and SANDERSON 1960). There are several examples of laboratory experiments where activation and hereditary transfer can be experimentally separated (LILLIE, 1912).

HIRAMOTO has been able to inject a sea urchin sperm into the egg from the same species (1962). The sperm remains inside the egg and nothing happens. The paternal hereditary material of the spermatozoon undoubtedly has been transferred to the egg, but the activation step has been omitted.

When the phenomenon of egg activation becomes better understood, it is possible that the activating capacity of the spermatozoon can be subdivided into several components.

Given the two functions of the sperm, the activating one and the transfer of hereditary factors, one may put the question: which is the minimum number of sperm constituents to fulfill these two roles? Perhaps the answer is " A nucleus ", perhaps " A nucleus plus a membrane ". Closest to this minimum is the sperm of the coccid insect as described by HUGHES-SCHRADER (1946, and 1948), NEBEL (1957) and ROBISON (1966 and this symposium). It is composed almost entirely of nuclear material and microtubules. It lacks flagella, centrioles, mitochondria and problably also an acrosome, perhaps also nuclear membrane or cell membrane.

The case of the coccid sperm is interesting as a group of spermatozoa are clumped together into a functional unit of a higher organizational order, the sperm bundle. The sperm bundle has a complex structure reminiscent of a typical insect spermatozoon. It thus has an enveloping membrane, a corkscrew-shaped anterior end resembling an acrosome and a tapering taillike end. What is lacking in the single spermatozoon seems to be present in the sperm bundle.

Functions of the spermatozoon.

This case hence leads back to the question of the necessary functions of the spermatozoon. The spermatozoon usually has to be mobile. Motility is perhaps of importance as a means to announce to the egg that a healthy spermatozoon is approaching (BROKAW, personal communication). Motility will also aid in bringing the spermatozoon close to the egg. A flagellum may give the spermatozoon the power to swim in a fluid medium, and a set of microtubules may furnish it with the capacity to wriggle through a more viscous medium, such as the body tissue of the female. The motile spermatozoon can be expected to consume some fuel during its swimming which usually would necessitate the presence both of mitochondria and a source of fuel, which may be intrinsic (a stored nutrient) or extrinsic.

As the egg may be protected by follicle cells, jelly coat, vitelline membrane, and perhaps other protective envelopes, it can be regarded as a treasure hidden by many seals, locked by many locks. The spermatozoon has to perform the unlocking. It must possess the proper keys, and these may be immunological, enzymatic, or mechanical. Perhaps the sperm may also provide the egg with a necessary component, for instance a missing division center.

Other roles of the spermatozoon can be conceived of. It may be of importance to the sperm to have the proper size and form to fit into the female ducts. The narrowness of the oviduct may be useful for aiding the spermatozoon towards the eggs (REINIUS 1969). Barbs such as can be seen on the grasshopper spermatozoon (RETZIUS, 1909) may act just as barbs do. There may also be other types of handles on the spermatozoon for letting the female tract grip the sperm and carry it forward. In cases where the sperm equals the egg in size, one may wonder whether the sperm too may contain nutritive substances to be used by the new individual. The same may also be the case in functionally polyspermic species.

If these are the demands of the functioning spermatozoon then the following sperm components can be expected:

1) A *nucleus* containing the paternal hereditary material *plus* possibly other structures containing geneting information, such as plastids, mitochondria, and perhaps a centriole.

2) A *flagellum* providing the sperm with motility *or* some other device for locomotion.

3) A *mitochondrion* furnishing the locomotor apparatus with ATP *or* some other type of biochemical machinery with this role.

4) *Glycogen or* some other substrate for the mitochondrial (or equivalent) oxidations.

5) An *acrosome* to unlock some of the barriers around the egg cytoplasm and for making gamete fusion possible *or* some other structure with these roles.

6) A *cell membrane* having several functions, one of which may be to carry specificity factors, *or* this particular functions may have been taken over by an extra-cellular layer, a glycocalix.

7) A *centriole* which may or may not control the flagellar movements and which may or may not provide the egg with a missing division center.

8) Et cetera.

This list is based on functions rather than homologies. A particular component may have a different function than that expected from its derivation in spermiogenesis. The following two examples illustrate this point. The Füsschen of the gnathostomulid sperm (GRAEBNER, this symposium) may be partly derived from the Golgi apparatus and hence homologous to the acrosome. They seem however to be motile and are then the functional equivalent to the tail. The opposite situation may exist in some algae where the tip of the flagellum has taken over the roles of the acrosome (MANTON, this symposium). It is hence necessary to make a distinction between the physiological role of a structure and its derivation. Tracing the homologies of the sperm components is not sufficient for a proper understanding of the spermatozoon. Even DNA itself may have new functions in the sperm (YASUZUMI, this symposium).

Unsolved problems in sperm morphology.

In spite of the great efforts to solve the problems in comparative spermatology we find ourselves confronted with more questions than answers. New riddles have appeared whenever we think a riddle has been solved. It may be appropriate to list here some topics which seem promising for a future attack.

Acrosome. G. G. BROWN has remarked in this symposium that the role at fertilization of each sperm component has to be studied. This is particularly true when it comes to the acrosome region.

The complex sequence leading to the formation of an acrosome filament in some invertebrate spermatozoa certainly is an interesting event. A detailed comparison has to be made between two species with preformed acrosome filaments, the horseshoe crab, *Limulus polyphemus*, and the lamprey, *Lampetra fluviatilis*. In both cases the newly ejected filament seems to be surrounded by a membrane. Is this a case of the cell membrane stretching, as seems likely from the data presented by NICANDER (this symposium)? Or how else can the very rapid membrane formation be accounted for?

The notable diversity in shape of the mammalian acrosome, as shown to us by FAWCETT (this symposium), is perplexing. As asked by him: why do the acrosomes have complicated forms if they are just made to get dissolved? The acrosomes have a structural and presumably also a chemical heterogeneity which has to be investigated.

Cell surface. Most cells are surrounded by a polysaccharide–containing layer, a glycocalyx according to BENNETT (1963). So is the sea urchin spermatozoon (ANDERSON, 1968). Its role in fertilization remains obscure. ANDRÉ (1963) has suggested that a polysaccharid layer provides the cell surface with a negative charge which facilitates the separation between sperm cell ad sertoli cell.

Centriole. The time–honored hypothesis of the sperm centriole as missing division center (BOVERI, 1889, 1895) needs a reinvestigation. It is believed that the egg cannot start its cell divisions unless it receives a centriole at fertilization, but is this nice old story true? See also LILLIE and JUST (1924).

What is the function of the centriolar adjunct in vertebrate spermatozoa or elsewhere?

Mitochondria. SUSAN PRATT has demonstrated to us the remarkable sequences of mitochondrial twisting and untwisting in the insect sperm Nebenkern. What could possibly be the meaning of this complicated process and which are the forces behind it? The events are reminescent of the chromosomal crossing-over process, but an interpretation along such a line would hardly seem meaningful.

It has certainly been fascinating to find that the sperm mitochondria have DNA–fibers (NASS *et al.*, 1965). The full significance of this finding has yet to be explored. Geneticists may some day have to take these cytoplasmic factors into account. A start has been taken by MCDANIEL and SARKISSIAN (1966).

Giant mitochondrial derivatives such as shown in the *Notonecta glauca* spermatozoon (Fig. 1) also give rise to questions. Are they beautifully powerful mitochondra as believe ANDRÉ and FAVARD (this symposium) or are they simple, degenerated structures, as I am more inclined to believe.

In his thesis ANDRÉ (1962) described how the mitochondria at a certain stage seemed to be cemented together by a material which evidently came from the nucleus. This mitochondrial cement has not been mentioned during the symposium, although many reports on such material have lately been published. There are several diverging ideas about its role in the morphogenetic events of mitochondria and even of the Golgi bodies (WARD and WARD, 1969).

The dense matrix granules may also have a role in mitochondrial growth (BARNARD and LINDBERG, 1969), but they seem to have been nearly totally neglected by the spermatologists.

Nucleus. With respect to the nucleus there are likewise many unsolved problems. The chromatine condensation occuring during spermiogenesis in most animals and some plants is a perplexing phenomenon. So are the regular patterns seen before the final condensation stage has been reached: arrays of fibers, concentric lamellae, or honey combs.

The sperm nucleus of the myzostomid worm *Myzostomum cirriferum* consists of a string of beads, described by RETZIUS (1910) and JÄGERSTEN (1934) and depictured in Figure 2. Are they balls made up of the separate chromosomes and if so, do the chromosome occupy well determined positions along the length of the nucleus? Evidence for fixed positions of the separate chromosomes and chromosome segments have come from the work by HUGHES-SCHRADER (1946, 1948) and more recently from MEYER (1963).

Sperm tail. Insect spermatozoa may have 0, 1 or 2 flagella (BACCETTI, ROBISON, PHILLIPS, this symposium). Fish spermatozoa may have 0, 1 or 2 flagella (MATTEI, this symposium and 1967, BOISSON *et al.*, 1967 and STANLEY, 1965). Annelid spermatozoa may have 0, 1 or 2 flagella (FRANZÉN, this symposium and 1958). Flatworm spermatozoa may have 0, 1 or 2 flagella (HENDELBERG, this symposium, and GRESSON, 1962). The insect sperm flagellum may have an axonemal pattern (excepting the coarse filaments) of 9 + 0, 9 + 1, 9 + 2, 9 + 3, 9 + 7 or something else (PHILLIPS, this symposium). The fish sperm 9 + 0 or 9 + 2 (BOISSON *et al.*, 1967 b). The annelid sperm 9 + 0 or 9 + 2 (AFZELIUS, 1962). The flatworm sperm 9 + 0, 9 + a big 1, or 9 + 2 (BEDINI, HENDELBERG, this symposium, and COSTELLO *et al.*, 1969).

In animal groups other that insects, fish, annelids, and flatworms the variation does not seem to be as great. Does this fact mean that these four animal groups are better studied than others? Do we need BACCETTIS and PHILLIPSES to examine other animal phyla? Or do these four groups show " evolutionary explosions " with regard to their sperm tails?

The phylogenetic significance of the various sperm tail patterns will have to be further investigated.

The 9 coarse fibers and their satellite fibers have been characterized morphologically by FAWCETT (this symposium) and biochemically by NELSON (this symposium). Do they perform mechanical work and if so, how?

What is the significance of the striations in the tail matrix described by PEDERSEN (this symposium)? Do they fit with the glycogen described by ANDERSON (this symposium).

Morphology of spermatozoon. One of the most striking features of the spermatozoa is their remarkably precise form and the high degree of their internal organization. This poses some questions: which forces shape the spermatozoon? How much information is needed as building instructions for the spermatozoon? Where is it stored and how is it used?

GÜNTHER MEYER has shown us the direct method for examining some of these questions (this symposium). By changing the chromosomal complement it has been possible to interfere with the morphogenesis of the spermatozoon and to get spermatozoa of novel shapes. This approach seems very rewarding.

Some sperm shapes pose a problem of their own. There are the two peculiar enantiomorphic forms of the spermatozoa of the hemipteran *Dahlbomian*, that is right hand twisted and left hand twisted forms (Lee and WILKES, 1965). There are further the twin spermatozoa described from some animals, which may be a related case: those of the marsupial mammal *Didelphys virginiana* (HOLSTEIN, 1965), the apterygot insect *Thermobia domestica* (BAWA, 1964), the coleopteran insect *Dytiscus* (Retzius, 1909), and the gastropod mollusc *Turritella terebra* (RETZIUS, 1910). There are finally the often remarked situation that some spermatozoa seem to have a bilateral cross–section (see for example PHILLIPS, this symposium).

Since spermatozoa are built of molecules which cannot have bilateral symmetry, this type of symmetry cannot exist at the molecular level of organization. Bilateral symmetry implies that one part looks like the mirror image of the other part and a perfect bilateral symmetry (also called mirror or inversion symmetry) cannot exist in cells. It is hence a safe prediction that the apparent bilateral symmetry of the spermatozoon will turn out to be false when a higher degree of resolution is reached. The 9 + 2 pattern was once regarded as an example of bilateral symmetry but is now seen to be an asymmetric structure. The 9 + 0 and 0 + 1 patterns have cyclic symmetries.

The above list of unsolved problems could have been made much longer. Still, it suffices to indicate that the next symposium of this kind will contain many new and stimulating facts and findings.

Acknowledgement. Parts of the study has been supported by the Swedish Natural Science Resarch Council. The *Myzostomum* material has been obtained from the Kristineberg Zoological Station, Fiskebäckskil, Sweden, and the *Notonecta* from the neighborhood of Stockholm. My thanks are due to Dr. B. SWEDMARK and Mr. N. GONNERT respectively for help in obtaining this material. Technical assistance by Mrs EVA FJELLSTEDT is gratefully acknowledged.

REFERENCES

AFZELIUS B. A. (1962) – *The contractile apparatus in some invertebrate muscles and spermatozoa.* « Proc. 5th Internat. Congr. Electron Microscopy, Philadelphia », M 1.

ANDERSON W. A. (1968) – *Cytochemistry of the sea urchin gametes II. Ruthenium red staining of gamete membranes of sea urchins.* « J. Ultrastruct. Res. », 24, 322–333.

ANDRÉ J. (1962) – *Contribution à la connaissance du chondriome: Etude de ses modifications ultrastructurales pendent la spermiogenèse.* « J. Ultrastruct. Res. », Suppl. 3, 1–185.

ANDRÉ J. (1963) – *Some aspects of specialization in sperm.* in *General Physiology of Cell specialization* (D. Mazia and A. Tyler, editors) McGraw Hill Inc., N. Y., 91–115.

ANDRÉ J. (1965) – *A propos d'une leçon sur la Limule.* « Ann. Fac. Sci », 26, 27–38.

BARNARD T. and LINDBERG O. (1969) – *Ultrastructural changes in the chondriome during perinatal development in brown adipose tissue of rats.* « J. Ultrastruct. Research », 29, 293–310.

BAWA S. R. (1964) – *Electron microscope study of spermiogenes in a fire–brat insect, Thermobia domestica Peck,* I. *Mature spermatozoa.* « J. Cell Biol. », 23, 431–446.

BENNETT H. S. (1963) – *Morphological aspects of extracellular polysaccharides.* « J. Histochem. Cytochem. », 11, 14–23.

BOISSON C., MATTEI C. and MATTEI X. (1967) – *Troisième note sur la spermiogenèse de Protepterus annectens* (*Dipneuste*) *du Senegal.* « Bull. Inst. Fondam. Afrique Noir », 29, 1097–1121.

BOISSON C., MATTEI X. and MATTEI C. (1967) – *Le flagelle de type* 9 + 0 *et la remarquable extension du centriole proximal dans les spermatides de Lycodontis afer* (*Bloch 1795*) (*Poisson Muraenidae*). « Compt. rend. Acad. Sci. (Paris) », 264, 2909–2912.

BOVERI T. (1887) – *Ueber den Antheil des Spermatozoon an der Theilung des Eies.* « Sitzungsber. Gesellsch. Morphol. Physiol. München », 3, 151–164.

BOVERI T. (1888) – *Ueber partielle Befruchtung.* « Sitzungsber. Gesellsch. Morphol. Physiol. München », 4, 64–72.

BOVERI T. (1895) – *Ueber das Verhalten der Centrosomen bei der Befruchtung des Seeigeleies nebst allgemeinen Bemerkungen über Centrosomen und Verwandtes.* « Verh. Physiol. Med. Gesellsch. », Würzburg, 29, 1–75.

BOWEN R. H. (1925) – *Further notes on the acrosome of animal sperm. The homologies of non-flagellate sperms.* « Anat. Record », 31, 201–231.

CHRISTENSON B. and O'CONNOR F. G. (1958) – *Pseudofertilization in the genus Lumbricillus (Enchytraeidae).* « Nature » 181, 1085–1086.

COSTELLO D. P., HENLEY C. and AULT C. R. (1969) – *Microtubules in spermatozoa of Childia (Turbellaria, Acoela) revealed by negative staining.* « Science », 163, 678–679.

FRANZÉN Å. (1958) – *On sperm morphology and acrosome filament formation in some annelida, echiuroidea and tunicata.* « Zool. Bidrag Uppsala », 33, 1–28.

HIRAMOTO Y. (1962) – *Microinjection of the live spermatozoa into Sea urchin eggs.* « Exp. Cell. Res. », 27, 416–426.

HOLSTEIN A. – F. (1965) – *Elektronenmikroskopische Untersuchungen am Spermatozoon des Opossum (Didelphys virginiana Kerr).* « Z. Zellforsch. », 65, 905–914.

HUBBS C. L. (1955) – *Hybridization between fish species in nature.* « System. Zool. », 4, 1–20.

HUBBS C. L. and HUBBS L. C. (1932) – *Apparent parthenogenesis in nature, in a form of fish of hybrid origin.* « Science », 76, 628–630.

HUGHES-SCHRADER S. (1946) – *A new type of spermiogenesis in iceryine coccids – with linear alignment of chromosomes in the sperm.* « J. Morphol. », 78, 43–83.

HUGHES-SCHRADER S. (1948) – *Cytology of Coccids (Coccoidea–Homoptera).* « Adv. Genetics », 2, 127–203.

JÄGERSTEN G. (1934) – *Studien über den histologischen Bau der männlichen Geschlechtsorgane und die Ausbildung des Spermiums bei Mysostomum.* « Zool. Bidrag, Uppsala », 15, 1–22.

LEE P. E. and WILKES A. (1965) – *Polymorphic spermatozoa in the hymenopterus wasp Dahlbominus.* « Science », 147, 1445–1446.

LILLIE P. E. and JUST E. E. (1924) – Cap. *Fertilization* in *General Cytology* (Cowdry, editor) Univ. of Chicago Press, 451–536.

MC DANIEL R. G. and SARKISSIAN I. V. (1966) – *Heterosis: Complementation by mitochondria.* « Science », 1526, 1640–1642.

MCGREGOR H. C. and UZZELL JR. T. M. (1964) – *Gynogenesis in salamanders related to Ambystoma jeffersonianum.* « Science », 143, 1043–1045.

MATTEI X., BOISSON C., MATTEI C. and REIZER C. (1967) – *Spermatozoïdes aflagelles chez un poisson: Gymnarchus niloticus (Teleostéen, Gymnarchidae).* « Compt. rend. Acad. Sci. » (Paris), Ser. D, 265, 2010–2012.

MEYER G. F. (1963) – *Die Funktionsstrukturen der Y-Chromosoms in den Spermatozytenkerne von Drosophila hydei, D. neohydei, D. repleta und einigen anderen Drosophila-arten.* « Chromosoma », 14, 207–255.

MOORE B. P., WOODROFFE G. E. and SANDERSON A. R. (1956) – *Polymorphism and parthenogenesis in a ptinid beetle.* « Nature » 177, 847–848.

MULDAL S. (1952) – *The chromosomes of the earthworms. I. The evolution of polyploidy.* « Heredity » 6, 55–76.

NASS M. M. K., NASS S. and AFZELIUS B. A. (1965) – *The general occurence of mitochondrial DNA.* « Exp. Cell Res. », 37, 516–539.

NEBEL B. R. (1957) – *Chromosomal and cytoplasmic microfibrillae in sperm of an iceryne coccid.* « J. Heredity », 48, 51–56.

PANTEL J. and de SINÉTY R. (1906) – *Les Cellules de la lignée mâle chez le Notonecta glauca L avec des details plus étendus sur la periode d'accroissement et sur celle de transformation.* « Cellule », 23, 87–303.

REINIUS S. (1969) – *Morphology of oviduct, gametes and zygotes as a basis of oviductal function in the mouse.* Thesis, Uppsala and « Intern. J. Fertility » 1970 in press.

RETZIUS G. (1909) – *Zur Kenntnis der Spermien der Insekten.* « Biologische Untersuchungen, N. F. », 14, 55–56.

RETZIUS G. (1909) – *Die Spermie von Didelphys.* « Biologische Untersuchungen, N. F. », 14, 123–126.

RETZIUS G. (1910) – *Weitere Beiträge zur Kenntnis der Spermien mit besonderer Berücksinchtung der Kernsubstanz.* « Biologische Untersuchungen N. F. », 15, 63–82.

ROBISON JR. W. G. (1966) – *Microtubules in relation to the motility of a sperm syncytium in an armored scale insect.* « J. Cell Biol. », 29, 251–265.

ROSARIO B. (1964) – *An electron microscope study of spermatogenesis in cestodes.* « J. Ultrastruct. Res. », 11, 412–427.

SANDERSON A. R. (1960) – *The cytology of a diploid bisexual spider beetle, Ptinus clavipes Panzer and its triploid gynogenetic form mobilis.* « Proc. Roy. Soc. Edinburgh », 67, 333–350.

SCHULZ R. J. and KALLMAN K. D. (1968) – *Triploid hybrids betwen the all-female teleost Poecilia formosa and Poecilia sphenops.* « Nature », 219, 280–282.

STANLEY H. P. (1965) – *Electron microscopic observations on the biflagellate spermatids of the teleost fish Porichtys notatus.* « Anat. Record », 151, 477.

WARD R. T. and WARD E. (1968) – *The multiplication of Golgi bodies in the oocytes of Rana pipiens.* « J. Microscopie », 7, 1007–1020.

EXPLANATION OF FIGURES

Fig. 1. – Cross-section through the tail region of some *Notonecta* spermatozoa. These spermatozoa belong to the longest known. Note the presence of six pseudocrystalline regions in each tail (arrows). Magnification. ×70,000.

Fig. 2. – Section along part of the head of some spermatozoa of *Myzostomum*. There is a row of dense bodies in each nucleus. Magnification. ×53,000

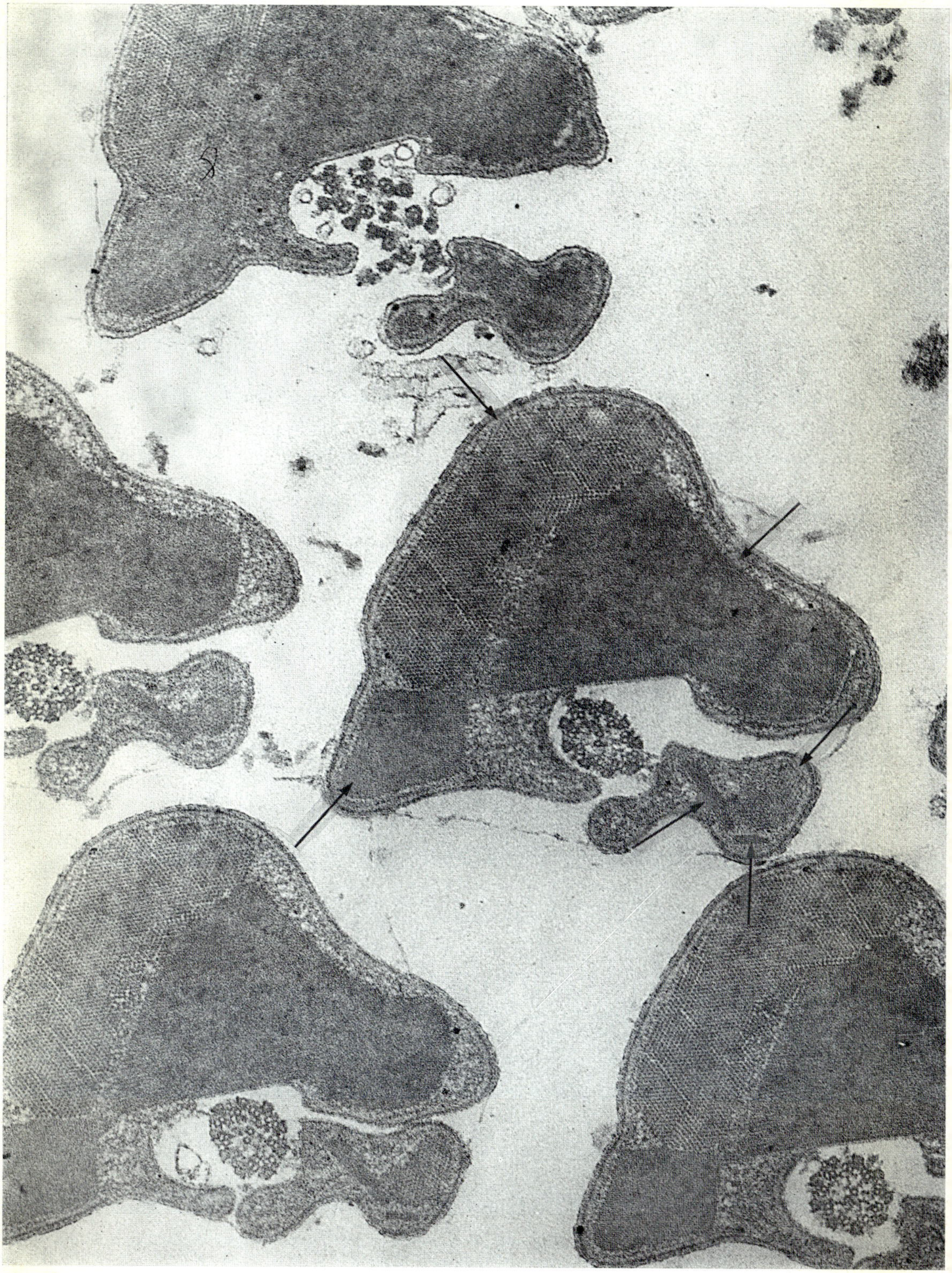

Fig. 1.

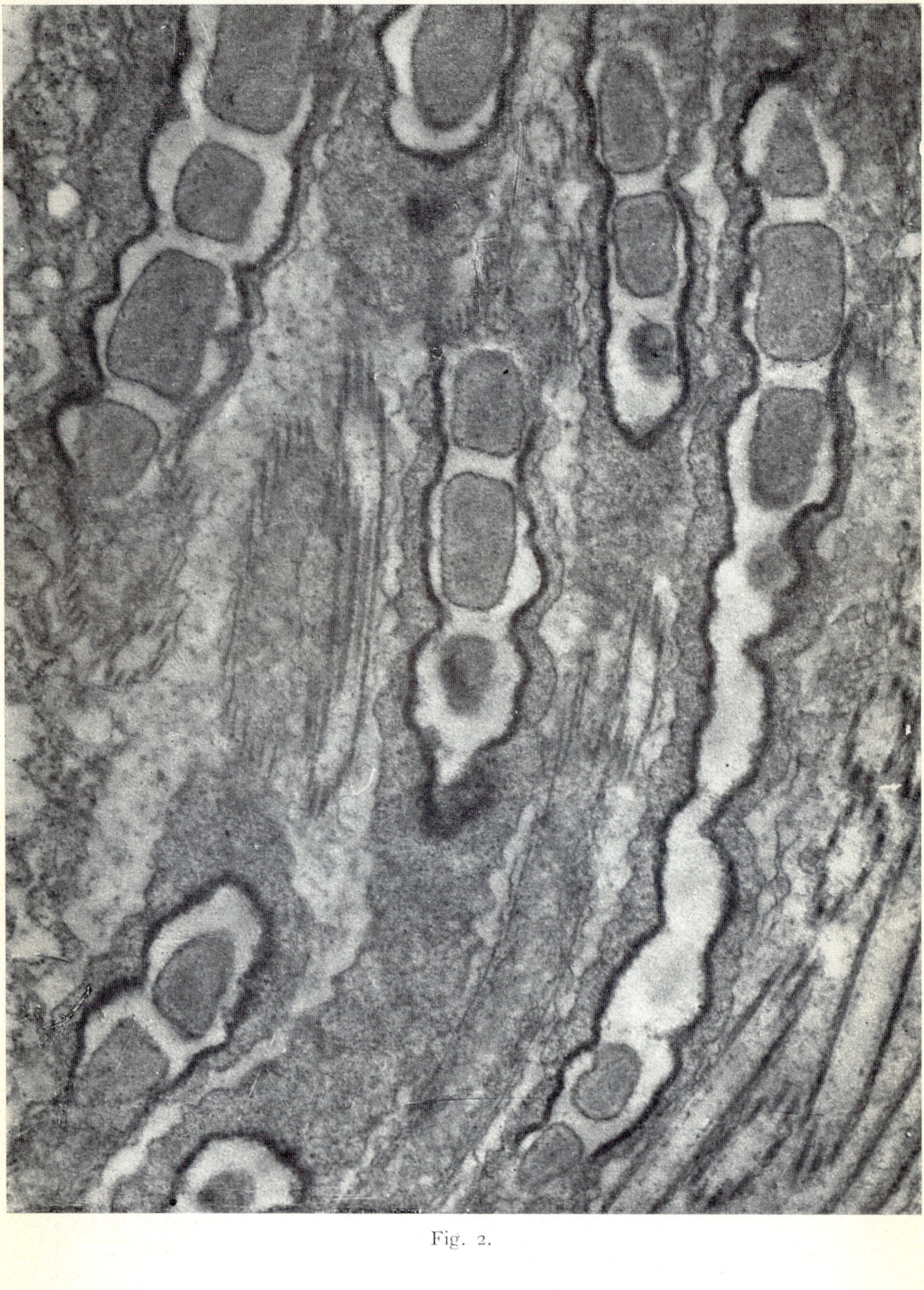

Fig. 2.